Nursing *for* Wellness in Older Adults
Theory and Practice

Nursing *for* Wellness in Older Adults

Theory and Practice

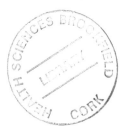

FOURTH EDITION

Carol A. Miller, MSN, RN,C

Gerontological Clinical Nurse Specialist and Certified Nurse Case Manager
Care & Counseling, Miller/Wetzler Associates
Cleveland, Ohio

Clinical Faculty
Frances Payne Bolton School of Nursing
Case Western Reserve University
Cleveland, Ohio

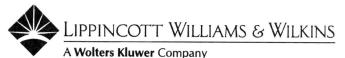

LIPPINCOTT WILLIAMS & WILKINS
A **Wolters Kluwer** Company
Philadelphia • Baltimore • New York • London
Buenos Aires • Hong Kong • Sydney • Tokyo

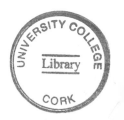

Senior Acquisitions Editor: Quincy McDonald
Developmental Editors: Melanie Cann and Michael Porter
Editorial Assistants: Sharon Nowak and Marie Rim
Senior Production Editor: Rosanne Hallowell
Senior Production Manager: Helen Ewan
Managing Editor / Production: Erika Kors
Art Directors: Brett MacNaughton and Carolyn O'Brien
Interior Designer: Melissa Olson
Senior Manufacturing Coordinator: Michael Carcel
Manufacturing Manager: William Alberti
Indexer: Angie Wiley Indexing Services
Compositor: TechBooks
Printer: Quebecor-World/Versailles

Fourth Edition

Cover image: Franz Kupka, *Disks of Newton, Study of Fugue in Two Colors.* Philadelphia Museum of Art: The Louise and Walter Arensberg Collection, 1950. Copyright 2003, Artists Rights Society (ARS), New York/ADAGP, Paris.

9 8 7 6 5 4 3 2 1

Library of Congress Cataloging-in-Publication Data
Miller, Carol A.
    Nursing for wellness in older adults : theory and practice / Carol A. Miller.— 4th ed.
        p. cm.
    Previous editions have title: Nursing care of older adults : theory and practice.
    Includes bibliographical references and index.
    ISBN 0-7817-3808-3 (alk. paper)
        1. Geriatric nursing.   I. Miller, Carol A. Nursing care of older adults.   II. Title.

    RC954.M55   2003
    618.97'0231—dc22

                                        2003058816

Care has been taken to confirm the accuracy of the information presented and to describe generally accepted practices. However, the author, editors, and publisher are not responsible for errors or omissions or for any consequences from application of the information in this book and make no warranty, express or implied, with respect to the content of the publication.

The author, editors, and publisher have exerted every effort to ensure that drug selection and dosage set forth in this text are in accordance with the current recommendations and practice at the time of publication. However, in view of ongoing research, changes in government regulations, and the constant flow of information relating to drug therapy and drug reactions, the reader is urged to check the package insert for each drug for any change in indications and dosage and for added warnings and precautions. This is particularly important when the recommended agent is a new or infrequently employed drug.

Some drugs and medical devices presented in this publication have Food and Drug Administration (FDA) clearance for limited use in restricted research settings. It is the responsibility of the health care provider to ascertain the FDA status of each drug or device planned for use in his or her clinical practice.

I lovingly dedicate this book to my parents, Margaret and Bob Miller,
who have always given me boundless support, encouragement, and inspiration.
My mother continues to be a shining example of living life to its fullest.

I also dedicate this work to the many older adults and their families who have taught me
countless lessons about successfully navigating the challenges of older adulthood.

Reviewers

Katherine Ash, RN, BA, BSN, MN
Associate Professor
University of Saskatchewan
Saskatoon, Saskatchewan

Valerie J. Benedix, RN, BSN
Nursing Instructor
Clovis Community College
Clovis, New Mexico

Mary Bliesmer , DNSc, RN
Professor, School of Nursing
Minnesota State University, Mankato
Mankato, Minnesota

Margaret R. Colyar, DSN, APRN, C-FNP/C-PNP
Assistant Professor
University of Utah, College of Nursing
Salt Lake City, Utah

Linda Cornell, RN, BSN, MEd
University-College Professor
Malaspina University-College
Nanaimo, British Columbia

Joan Anne Leach, BSN, MSN, MEd
Professor of Nursing
Capital Community College
Hartford, Connecticut

Margie Maddox, EdD, CRNP, CS
Associate Professor of Nursing
University of Scranton
Scranton, Pennsylvania

Elizabeth Jean Mistretta, PhD, RN
Chair and Associate Professor
Department of Nursing
Georgia Perimeter College
Clarkston, Georgia

Janice Z. Peterson, RN, PhD
Assistant Professor
University of Central Florida
Orlando, Florida

Billie Rhea Phillips, PhD, RN, CDFS
Assistant Professor
Tennessee Wesleyan College
Knoxville, Tennessee

Patsy Ruppert Rider, RN, BSN, MSN, CS
Clinical Instructor in Nursing
The University of Texas at Austin
  School of Nursing
Austin, Texas

Ellen Shannon, MSN, RN
Assistant Professor
East Stroudsburg University of Pennsylvania
East Stroudsburg, Pennsylvania

Kathleen Zajic, RN, MSN
Associate Professor of Nursing
College of Saint Mary
Omaha, Nebraska

Foreword

Leaders in health care are acutely aware of the urgent need to address the unique needs of older adults, who comprise the fastest growing part of our population. The population group designated as "older adults" has a broad range of health care needs, which is widening as "baby boomers" are beginning to join the ranks of the "young-old," and the number of people categorized as "old-old," including centenarians, is rapidly increasing. In addition, the population of older adults in the United States is growing in cultural diversity, as the life expectancy of racial and ethnic groups is increasing and more immigrants of all ages come here. Despite the diverse makeup of this segment of the population, however, one theme permeates the approach taken when caring for older adults: helping the older adult to remain healthy and functional, and to maintain the best quality of life. To that end, nurses must address a broad continuum of health care needs of older adults, ranging from primary and secondary prevention interventions to issues related to end-of-life care.

In addition to recognizing the need to address the wide range of health care needs of older adults, health care leaders are expressing grave concerns about the serious shortage of nurses and the impact of this shortage on older adults. Because of the growing number of older adults and the concurrent decreasing number of nurses, a priority in nursing education today is ensuring that new graduates are adequately prepared to care for older adults, the segment of the population that consumes the greatest amount of health care services in hospitals, home care agencies, and long-term care settings. Thus, efforts are being directed toward "gerontologizing" the curriculum so all nurses are prepared to address the unique needs of this diverse population.

Nursing for Wellness in Older Adults: Theory and Practice, which is a product of more than 3 decades of Carol A. Miller's work with older adults, meets the need for a gerontological nursing text that focuses on the unique and diverse health care needs of older adults. The functional consequences theory of gerontological nursing provides a framework for this text and distinctively blends a theoretical base with a practical application of knowledge to address the unique health care needs of older adults in a variety of settings. Using this framework, Miller examines age-related changes and risk factors that interfere with optimal health and functioning in older adults. In addition, she identifies practical strategies for assessing and improving health and functioning, with emphasis on health promotion interventions. Throughout this text, pertinent information about cultural diversity is incorporated, as is information about up-to-date research on issues related to the nursing care of older adults.

A book that spans the nursing curriculum, *Nursing for Wellness in Older Adults: Theory and Practice* provides practical, research-based information that will assist nurses in all settings to help older adults improve their level of functioning and achieve wellness. As such, it addresses the current need to prepare nurses to address the unique health care needs of this highly diverse and rapidly growing population. Moreover, its life-affirming and positive approach will stimulate enthusiasm for the challenge of providing nursing care that promotes wellness in older adults.

May L. Wykle, PhD, RN, FAAN, FGSA
*Dean and Florence Cellar Professor of
Gerontological Nursing
Frances Payne Bolton School of Nursing
Director, University Center on Aging and Health
Case Western Reserve University
Cleveland, Ohio*

Preface

With the exception of nurses who work in subspecialties with younger populations, most nurses spend at least half their time providing care to people categorized chronologically as "old." As nurses address the complex health care needs of this diverse population, they recognize that care of older adults is not simply a variation of care of adults in general. They seek answers to questions such as, *What is unique about the health care needs of older adults?* and *How can nurses effectively care for older adults?* Nurses and nursing students can find answers to these questions in the theories and practical approaches that form the foundation of gerontological nursing. Thus, there is a great need to teach about theory-based practices for nursing care of older adults throughout the nursing curriculum and in a variety of health care settings.

Since the publication of the first edition of this text in 1990, knowledge about aging, older adults, and gerontological nursing has grown rapidly, but this information is not widely integrated into nursing curricula. The intent of this fourth edition, now titled *Nursing for Wellness in Older Adults: Theory and Practice*, is to provide a theory-based framework for nursing students and practicing nurses that will enable them to address the unique health care needs of older adults. A primary focus is on the role of nurses in assisting older adults to achieve improved levels of health and functioning at any point along the continuum of health. Accordingly, this text can be used to integrate concepts pertinent to nursing care of older adults in any setting throughout the nursing curriculum.

Nursing for Wellness in Older Adults: Theory and Practice has been extensively updated to incorporate recent research findings pertinent to gerontological nursing. As in previous editions, this text covers all aspects of physiologic and psychosocial function that distinguish gerontological nursing from other types of nursing. The *functional consequences theory of gerontological nursing* is used in this text to identify age-related changes and risk factors that affect the level of function and quality of life of older adults. Assessment guidelines identify risk factors and functional consequences that nurses can address, and interventions focus on health promotion. As in the first three editions, a major focus is on healthy aging, but this edition places an even stronger emphasis on nursing interventions to reduce risks, prevent disease, and promote health in older adults. For example, wherever applicable, interventions incorporate the recommendations of organizations such as the United States Preventive Services Task Force and the goals and objectives of *Healthy People 2010*. Thus, the title of this edition has been changed to more accurately reflect this focus on wellness.

Organization

Nursing for Wellness in Older Adults: Theory and Practice has 26 chapters, organized into 6 parts. Chapters in Parts 1 and 2 introduce topics relevant to aging, older adults, and gerontological nursing. Chapters in Parts 3 through 6 are organized around the functional consequences theory of gerontological nursing, so each facet of physiologic or psychosocial function is presented according to age-related changes, risk factors, functional consequences, nursing assessment, nursing diagnosis, outcomes, nursing interventions, and evaluation of nursing care.

- Part 1 (Chapters 1 through 3), *Older Adults: An Introduction,* begins with a discussion of the continuum of older adulthood and the diversity and characteristics of older adults. In addition, it reviews theories to explain aging and explicates the functional consequences theory of gerontological nursing.
- Part 2 (Chapters 4 through 6), *Gerontological Nursing,* introduces gerontological nursing as a subspecialty within nursing and addresses the unique challenges of caring for older adults, with an extensive discussion of health promotion in relation to older adults. Roles for gerontological nurses are described in relation to settings that comprise the continuum of health care services for older adults. This section also covers financial, legal, and ethical issues that are pertinent to gerontological nursing.
- Part 3 (Chapters 7 through 10), *Psychosocial Aspects of Function,* extensively reviews cognitive

and psychosocial function and provides guidelines for a comprehensive nursing assessment of psychosocial function, with emphasis on healthy older adults. In addition, this part covers communication techniques and aspects of transcultural nursing applicable to older adults.

- Part 4 (Chapters 11 through 22), *Physiologic Aspects of Function*, begins with a chapter on functional assessment and includes chapters that address each of the following specific aspects of functioning in older adults: hearing, vision, digestion and nutrition, urinary function, cardiovascular function, respiratory function, mobility and safety, skin, sleep and rest, thermoregulation, and sexual function. Although the emphasis of this book is on wellness, coverage of selected common chronic pathologic conditions is included when these conditions affect a particular aspect of functioning in older adults.
- Part 5 (Chapter 23), *Medication Management,* reviews age-related changes, risk factors, functional consequences, assessment, and interventions related to medication use by older adults.
- Part 6 (Chapters 24 through 26), *Impaired Psychosocial Function in Older Adults,* is the one part of this text in which pathological conditions common in older adults are comprehensively covered. The topics of delirium, dementia, and depression are discussed from the perspective of the functional consequences framework because they are conditions that nurses commonly address when caring for older adults in all settings. In addition, the topic of elder abuse and neglect is covered because nurses have important obligations to identify and address this most challenging aspect of caring for older adults.

New and Special Features

Several special features from past editions have been retained in this edition, and several new features have been added.

Pedagogical Features

- **Chapter Outlines** and **Learning Objectives** give the reader an overview of the chapter content and focus his or her reading.
- *NEW!* **Icons** identify the five major components of the functional consequences theory:

  Age-related changes

  Risk factors

  Functional consequences

  Nursing assessment

  Nursing interventions

- **Chapter Summaries** facilitate review of the material.
- **Critical Thinking Exercises**, at the end of each chapter, and **Thinking Points**, interspersed throughout the chapter, help readers gain insight and develop problem-solving skills through purposeful, goal-directed thinking.
- *NEW!* **Progressive Case Studies** provide real-life examples of the effects of age-related changes and risk factors, beginning in young-old adulthood and continuing through all the stages of later adulthood. Thinking Points after each segment of the case assist the student in applying the content of the chapter to the case example.
- **References** give readers additional information about the most up-to-date research that supports evidence-based practice.

Practice-Oriented Features

- **Culture Boxes** help the reader to appreciate cultural differences that may influence his or her approach to a patient, resident, or client.
- *NEW!* **Diversity Notes** give brief information about differences among specific groups (e.g., men and women, whites and African Americans).

- **Assessment displays** provide the reader with specific approaches for nursing assessment. Commonly used assessment tools are described (and in many cases, illustrated).

- **Interventions displays** provide succinct guides for nursing interventions, with a strong focus on health promotion. Guidelines for "best practices" in nursing interventions are given. Many of the Interventions displays can be used as tools for teaching older adults and their

caregivers about how to improve functional abilities. Printable PDF files of Interventions displays that double as teaching tools can be downloaded from the Connection site that accompanies this book, http://connection.lww.com/go/miller.
- **Educational Resources** direct the reader to sources of additional information and patient education materials. Complete contact information (including Internet addresses) is given. Key resources for Canadian readers are noted as well.
- *NEW!* **Future Directions for Healthier Aging boxes,** at the end of many chapters, highlight the current research and foreseeable developments pertinent to a particular aspect of function.

Ancillaries

- *NEW!* **Connection site.** Resources for the gerontological nursing community are housed on the Internet site that accompanies this text, http://connection.lww.com/go/miller. Visit the Connection site for printable PDF files of the Interventions displays that double as patient teaching tools, links to other Internet sites of interest, and abstracts of recently published journal articles. Check the Gerontological Nursing News Alert section for updates of information in the text, such as changes to evidence-based practice recommendations.

- **Instructor's Resource CD.** The Instructor's Resource CD contains the following items:
  - A thoroughly revised and updated **Instructor's Manual,** by Ana Valadez, RN, EdD, CNAA, FAAN, and Tracey A. Woodward, RN, MSN, of the Texas Tech University Health Sciences Center, featuring information about how to integrate gerontology into the curriculum
  - A thoroughly revised and augmented **Test Generator** by Karen Johnson Karner, EdD, RN, CS, containing more than 300 multiple-choice, NCLEX-style questions in Microsoft Word™ format
  - An **Image Bank,** containing illustrations from the book in formats suitable for printing and incorporating into Power Point presentations and Internet sites

Summary

Gerontological nursing provides an opportunity to care for people who are striving to meet the challenges of remaining healthy and functional as they cope with age-related changes and risk factors that affect their functioning and quality of life. The goal of *Nursing for Wellness in Older Adults: Theory and Practice* is to provide nurses and nursing students with a practical approach to assisting older adults in meeting the many challenges of older adulthood in a positive and creative way.

Carol A. Miller, MSN, RN,C

Acknowledgments

I am deeply grateful to my family, friends, and colleagues who have supported me on my journey as this book has grown from a dream to a reality and now into its fourth edition. Pat Rehm, in particular, has constantly supported and encouraged me on my journey as a nurse and author. My family has always encouraged me to believe in my dreams, and my sister, Kathleen Unetic, and sister-in-law, Rosie Miller, enjoy with me the rewards of our nursing profession. Many older adults and their families have taught me valuable lessons that have become part of this text. These experiences, which cannot be learned in books, have taught me to care deeply about, and to care sensitively for, older adults. I thank these older adults and their families and I appreciate their contributions to my life and my writings.

I appreciate and acknowledge the many people who assisted and guided me through all phases of my text-writing journey. Georgia Anetzberger co-authored the chapter on Elder Abuse and Neglect in all four editions; Margaret Andrews, Katharine Kolcaba, and Betsy Todd contributed to earlier editions. The thoughtful comments and suggestions offered by the reviewers were also most helpful.

I want to extend my deepest appreciation to the staff at Lippincott Williams & Wilkins who assisted with all phases of development and production. I am grateful for the enthusiasm and encouragement of Quincy McDonald, Senior Acquisitions Editor, Lippincott Williams & Wilkins. Melanie Cann and Michael Porter, the Developmental Editors, deserve a special word of appreciation for their unending support, guidance, attention to detail, and lessons about editing, as does Claudia Vaughn, Ancillary Editor. I also thank and acknowledge the hard-working production staff: Carolyn O'Brien and Brett MacNaughton, who were responsible for the art and design of the book, and Rosanne Hallowell, who managed the copyediting and coordinated the production process.

I thank all these people, and many unnamed people, for the advice, guidance, support, assistance, and encouragement on my journey through all four editions of *Nursing for Wellness in Older Adults: Theory and Practice.*

Carol A. Miller, MSN, RN,C

Contents

Detailed Contents

CHAPTER 17

Respiratory Function, 363

CHAPTER 18

Mobility and Safety, 381

CHAPTER 19

Skin, 415

CHAPTER 20

Sleep and Rest, 437

CHAPTER 21

Thermoregulation, 457

CHAPTER 22

Sexual Function, 473

PART 5

MEDICATION MANAGEMENT

CHAPTER 23

Medications and the Older Adult, 503

PART 6

IMPAIRED PSYCHOSOCIAL FUNCTION IN OLDER ADULTS

CHAPTER 24

Impaired Cognitive Function: Delirium and Dementia, 541

CHAPTER 25

Impaired Affective Function: Depression, 581

Assessment and Interventions Displays

1

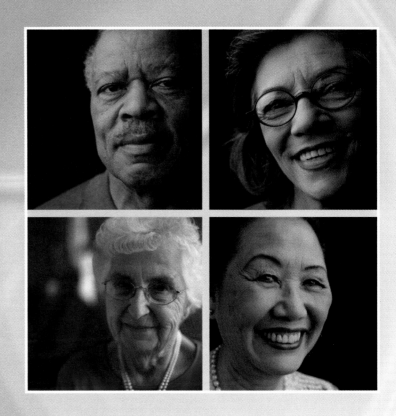

OLDER ADULTS:
AN INTRODUCTION

The Continuum of Older Adulthood

LEARNING OBJECTIVES

1. Describe older adulthood as a continuum.
2. Examine definitions of aging.
3. Recognize attitudes, myths, and sociocultural factors that influence perspectives on aging and older adulthood.
4. Discuss the consequences of ageism.
5. Describe the health and socioeconomic characteristics of older adults.

OLDER ADULTHOOD AS A CONTINUUM

Because this text is entirely about nursing care of older adults, the first question to be addressed is *Who are older adults?* For decades, gerontologists, sociologists, and health care practitioners have been seeking and developing answers to this question. Although the answers to this question are highly diverse, two themes are consistent in most descriptors of older adults. First, older adulthood is part of a life course continuum, and its beginning is not clearly demarcated at any one specific point in time. Second, because there is a great deal of individual variation among people who are placed in the category of "older adults," identifying those characteristics that apply to all older adults is extremely difficult. The best answer to the question of *Who are older adults?* is that they are a diverse group of people moving along the life course continuum and increasing in their diversity as they progress along the continuum. One does not become an "older adult" at any one chronologic point, but some common characteristics accumulate with increasing age so that a person recognizes that he or she has entered the period of life that is viewed as later adulthood.

The peak of physical maturity is reached during younger adulthood, but the peak of psychosocial maturity, with regard to aspects such as wisdom, creativity, spirituality, and emotional growth, is likely to be reached in older adulthood. Thus, from a holistic perspective, older adulthood is a time of increasing opportunities for continued development in many ways. Similarly, the peak of physical health usually occurs in younger adulthood, and illnesses tend to accumulate with increasing age; however, older adulthood is a time of life filled with opportunities for finding ways of improving health and functioning despite the age-related changes and pathologic conditions. Thus, from a *holistic* perspective, nurses have countless opportunities for implementing interventions that are directed toward improving and maintaining health and functioning in older adults and facilitating healthy responses to illnesses and compromised abilities.

This chapter discusses characteristics that best describe older adults and the unique challenges and opportunities of the life course of older adulthood. Chapter 2 addresses questions about where older adults are in families, communities, and the world, and Chapter 3 addresses questions about why people age. Part II addresses issues related to older adults in health care systems. A major focus of this text is on the role of nurses in helping older adults to achieve the highest level of wellness and functioning that is possible. This "highest level of wellness and functioning" for each person is on a continuum and is determined to a small degree by age-related changes, and to a more significant degree by pathologic conditions, risk factors, and other factors that affect one's wellness and functioning. Thus, some older adults will be extremely healthy and maintain a high level of independent functioning throughout old age until their death, whereas other older adults will have significant degrees of physical, mental, or psychosocial impairment for brief or long periods during older adulthood. This text focuses on the factors that influence wellness and functioning of older adults so that nurses can plan interventions to improve health and functioning. When functioning cannot be improved, nurses can plan interventions that help older adults adapt to or compensate for their limitations.

DEFINITIONS OF AGING

Aging is defined objectively, subjectively, and functionally, as well as in a number of other ways, by gerontologists and lay people alike. Objectively, aging is viewed as a universal process that begins at birth; in this context, it applies equally to young and old people. Subjectively, however, aging is associated with being "old" or reaching "older adulthood," and people define aging in terms of personal meaning and experience. Children usually do not view themselves as aging, but they do delight in announcing how old they are. They view birthdays as positive experiences that will permit them to enjoy additional opportunities and responsibilities. Adolescents, likewise, perceive aging as the mechanism that allows them to participate legally in coveted activities, such as driving. In adulthood, however, aging is negatively associated with being "old," and "old age" is often arbitrarily defined as an age that is several years or a decade beyond a person's current age. This perspective is evident in the fact that many people whose chronologic age is 70 years, 75 years, or older refer to "old people" as if they were a group distinct from themselves.

Gerontologists define *age identity* from various perspectives, and all of the following terms have been applied to this concept: *feel-age, subjective age, cognitive age, stereotype age, comparative age,* and *perceived* or *self-perceived age.* Since the 1980s, gerontologists have viewed age identity on a continuum of subjective wellness. This perspective is rooted in the assumption that old age is accompanied by a decline in health. Consequently, people who feel good will feel younger, and people who feel poorly will feel older (Kaufman & Elder, 2002).

Because age identity is significantly influenced by cultural views of aging, people in societies that place a high social value on youth are likely to adopt age identifications that are younger than their chronologic age. That is, beginning at about the fourth decade, people are likely to report their age as younger than their chronologic age. This may be changing, however, as indicated by the results of two almost identical national probability surveys conducted in 1974 and 2000 to identify public and personal perceptions of aging. The researchers found that Americans now date the beginning of older adulthood to later chronologic ages than they did several decades ago. Moreover, Americans do not necessarily view chronologic age as a factor in defining people as "old" (Bradley & Longino, 2001). In addition to societal factors influencing one's age identification, poor health and lower socioeconomic status have been associated with having an older age identification.

Objectively, people define age as the length of time that has passed since one's birth. North American culture is particularly fascinated by numbers, quantities, and relative values that can be measured. Among the questions frequently asked and answered are *How much? How far? How often?* and *How old?* Our fascination with age is particularly evident in newspaper articles, which invariably state the age of the subjects, regardless of the relevance of age to the topic. In addition to being easily measured, another advantage of chronologic age is that it serves as an objective basis for social organization. For example, societies establish chronologic age criteria for certain activities, such as education, driving, marriage, employment, alcohol consumption, military service, and the collection of retirement benefits. To participate legally in these activities, people must provide documentation of a certain chronologic age.

With the passage of the 1935 Social Security Act and the 1965 amendment that created Medicare, the age of 65 years was established as the standard age criterion for eligibility for retirement and health care benefits in the United States. At least part of the basis for this age-based determination for retirement was associated with the socioeconomic condition of the United States following the Depression. Retirement of older workers was seen as a solution to providing much needed jobs for younger workers, and the establishment of Social Security was seen as a solution to the social burden caused by increasing numbers of older people (Hirshbein, 2001). Thus, in America, 65 years of age has been accepted as the designated age for becoming a "senior citizen" and enjoying the benefits of the so-called Golden Age. Even this government-established chronologic age criterion, however, is subject to cross-cultural variation when it is applied to some government-sponsored programs, such as the Older Americans Act (OAA). For example, the qualifying age for American Indians' and Native Americans' participation in OAA-funded programs is 45 years in Montana, but it is 55 years in all other states.

In the early decades of gerontology, gerontologists also viewed 65 years of age as an acceptable chronologic criterion for aging processes. In recent decades, however, gerontologists agree that aging is too complex to be defined only by one's birth date. Consequently, older adulthood is commonly divided into subgroups, such as young-old, middle-old, old-old, and oldest-old. As one of the first gerontologists to challenge the original criterion stated:

We have used sixty-five as the economic marker, then as the social and psychological marker, of old age. A set of stereotypes has grown up that older persons are sick, poor, enfeebled, isolated, and desolated. While these stereotypes have been greatly overdrawn even for the old-old, they have become uncritically attached to the whole group over sixty-five. (Neugarten, 1978, pp. 47–48)

The trend in gerontology to divide old age into chronologic subcategories is an improvement over the categorization of all people older than 65 years of age as one homogeneous group, but it has the disadvantage of creating additional stereotypes and age biases. For example, if a chronologically old-old person needs a complicated or expensive medical treatment to maintain or potentially improve his or her health status, such treatment may be denied or withheld because of the person's advanced age.

Although chronologic age has the advantages of being easily measured, widely accepted, and readily understood, it has many disadvantages, especially in gerontology. From both scientific and humanistic perspectives, a person's age is relatively insignificant. From the perspective of biogerontology, chronologic age has little or no value because no biologic measurement applies to everyone at a specific age; from this perspective, therefore, there is no way of measuring age objectively (International Longevity Center, 2001).

For gerontological practitioners, as well as for most older adults, the important indicators of age are physiologic health, psychological well-being, socioeconomic factors, and the ability to function and socialize to the extent that one desires. Based on this understanding of the meaning of aging, the concept of functional age has been used for several decades by gerontologists as an alternative to chronologic age. This concept is associated with a shift in emphasis from chronologic factors to factors such as whether individuals can contribute to society and benefit others and themselves. Functional age is a concept that is used worldwide, but its definition varies according to the specific cultural context. For example, industrialized societies may associate functional age with self-sufficiency and physiologic function, whereas other cultures might associate it more closely with social or psychological function than with physiologic function.

One advantage of functional definitions of age over chronologic definitions is that the former are associated with higher levels of well-being and with more positive attitudes about aging. Because nursing addresses the response of people to actual or potential health problems, the concept of functional age provides a more rational basis for care than the measurement of how many years have passed since the person was born. Thus, the question *How functional?* becomes more relevant than *How old?* For gerontological nurses, the concept of chronologic age is of minimal importance. More important questions include *How well do you feel?* and *Is there anything that you would like to do that you cannot do?* In this text, "older adults" are defined in relation to the cumulative effects of age-related changes and risk factors that affect their health and functioning. This concept is discussed in detail in Chapter 3.

DIVERSITY OF OLDER ADULTS

Any discussion of the definitions of aging and the characteristics of older adults must first underscore the great degree of variation that exists in how individuals age. Gerontologists agree that aging includes a number of processes that are highly variable and individualized. Most also agree that it is difficult to identify those characteristics that are common in the majority of individuals who are divided chronologically according to age groups. These concepts are in stark contrast to the common perception held during the early decades of gerontology that all people aged 65 years or older could be grouped together as the population of old people. In the past several decades, gerontologists have recognized the need to identify the characteristics of subgroups. For example, articles about the characteristics of nonagenarians or centenarians are commonly found in current gerontological literature.

Another gerontological trend is to differentiate older adults according to their functional abilities, distinguishing between "frail elderly" and those who can be classified as "able elderly," or those experiencing "robust aging" or "successful aging." The frail elderly tend to belong to the oldest-old group, whereas able elderly persons usually belong to the young-old or middle-old groups. Frail elderly is a term applied to older adults who are medically ill or incapacitated most of the time and who, therefore, have the greatest health care needs. This subgroup is the opposite extreme of the majority of older adults who are able to function in the community with little assistance. The medically frail older person typically is 85 years of age or older, is functionally disabled, takes several medications, and has few social supports. What is of concern to health care planners and providers is that the group of people older than 85 years of age has become the fastest growing population group. Because not all people aged 85 years or older are frail and dependent, however, gerontologists are trying to identify characteristics that determine robust aging and successful aging.

Descriptions of healthy aging invariably address not only physical health and functioning but also many aspects of psychosocial health and functioning. Results of a large-scale longitudinal study identified three components of successful aging as an active engagement with life, high cognitive and physical function, and low probability of disease and disability (Rowe & Kahn, 1997). Other studies have confirmed the importance of active engagement with life as an important component of successful and healthy aging (Everard et al., 2000). One study found that psychosocial factors exert an influence on functioning, particularly in older adults with chronic conditions such as diabetes and high blood pressure (Seeman & Chen, 2002). Gerontologists agree that both lifestyle factors and social factors, such as meaningful relationships, have an important bearing on successful aging.

Another aspect of diversity among older adults is the tremendous social and cultural diversity and the increasing numbers of culturally diverse older adults in the United States. This topic is addressed in detail in Chapter 2.

ATTITUDES, AGEISM, AND MYTHS OF AGING

Attitudes Toward Aging in the United States

Although old age has not always been viewed as something to look forward to, until recently it was at least viewed as something to be respected. Fischer (1977) has analyzed trends in attitudes toward old people in the United States from the early 1600s through the 1970s. Data from this analysis indicate that the first period—extending from 1607 to 1820—was characterized by gerontocratic attitudes (veneration of old people). Fischer has emphasized that the median age in 1790 was barely 16 years old, and that respect for age was at least partly attributable to its relative rarity. In early America, then, old age was sometimes hated and feared, but more often, it was honored and obeyed. Fischer cites evidence of a subsequent revolution in attitudes, originating between 1770 and 1820, which sparked a long period of gerontophobia characterized by an idealization of youth. According to Fischer, the "cult of youth . . . became most extreme in the 1960s, when mature men and women followed fashions in books, music, and clothing which were set by their adolescent children. . . . But always, old was out and youth was in" (pp. 132–133). At the same time that youth was being idealized, old age was being identified as a medical problem and labeled as a social problem. Although Fischer did not use the term "ageism" in his book, he discussed the importance of efforts "to oppose the age prejudice which has grown so strong in America" (p. 195).

Another analysis of views of old age in America between 1900 and 1950 concluded that a shift in perception of aging began in the 1930s when "national enthusiasm about extending life and avoiding old age was waning" (Hirshbein, 2001, p. 1558). During this time, American society began to see older adults as a group of people with economic needs. Professional organizations became interested in aging and old age, and by the 1950s, "old age was seen as an economic, social, and medical problem that demanded management by a variety of professional groups" (Hirshbein, 2001, p. 1558). Similarly, an analysis of articles published in health-related journals from 1900 through 1999 identified trends in perceptions of aging and old age (Holkup, 2001). This analysis concluded that awareness of aging-related issues began to emerge in the mid-1940s when increasing life expectancy was acknowledged as a trend in the United States. Initially, gerontologists and health care professionals addressed age-related concerns as problems to be solved, but the focus slowly shifted to concern about how to best manage one's own increased life expectancy (Holkup, 2001). In recent decades, growing older has been gradually shedding its negative aura, and the focus is now on increased vitality and productivity in older adulthood (Holkup, 2001).

Ageism

The term ageism was coined by Robert Butler in 1968 and was first used in a publication, *The Gerontologist,* the next year (Butler, 1969). With the publication of Butler's Pulitzer Prize-winning book *Why Survive? Being Old in America* (1975), ageism became an accepted new word in the English language. Butler defines ageism as "the prejudices and stereotypes that are applied to older people sheerly on the basis of their age. . . . Ageism, like racism and sexism, is a way of pigeonholing people and not allowing them to be individuals with unique ways of living their lives" (Butler et al., 1991, p. 243). Devaluing the contributions of older adults and viewing the pathologies of later life as normal aging processes are common forms of ageism today (Cummings et al., 2000).

Some historians and gerontologists view ageism as an outcome of modernization. It is likely that the increased emphasis on the negative and debilitative aspects of old age correlates with the change in perception of the usefulness of older people brought about by urbanization and industrialization (Covey, 1988). However, Cohen (1988) has proposed that, rather than affecting all old people, ageism affects only those who are disabled. This gerontologist further suggests that discrimination against older disabled people arises from the societal perception of them as "biologically inferior and hence incapable of levels of self-fulfillment and self-realization comparable to those of the dominant reference group" (p. 25). Cohen asserts that older disabled people who are the target of ageism share similarities with other groups who have fought against prejudices. Multiple jeopardy, a similar concept, describes the situation of older adults who are likely to experience added discrimination because of their race or gender. Older women of color, for example, encounter "triple jeopardy," or discrimination based on ageism, sexism, and racism (Cummings et al., 2000).

Ageism continues to be a frequent topic in current gerontological literature, with some emphasis on identifying and addressing its causes. Cohen (2001, p. 576) suggested that "gerontologists and social activists can and should probe more deeply into the nature and sources of ageism." A 20-item survey has been developed to answer questions about types and prevalence of ageism and which subgroups of older people report more ageism (Figure 1-1). When this survey was administered to a test group of older adults, results indicated that the experience of ageism continues to be widespread and frequent in the United States (Palmore, 2001). In an effort to combat ageism, gerontological leaders urge professionals to avoid any ageist terminology in conversations and writing and to substitute neutral or non-ageist terms

---

The Ageism Survey

Please put a number in the blank that shows how often you have experienced that event: Never = 0; Once = 1; More than once =2.
("Age" means older age.)

_____ 1. I was told a joke that pokes fun at old people.

_____ 2. I was sent a birthday card that pokes fun at old people.

_____ 3. I was ignored or not taken seriously because of my age.

_____ 4. I was called an insulting name related to my age.

_____ 5. I was partronized or "talked down to" because of my age.

_____ 6. I was refused rental housing because of my age.

_____ 7. I had difficulty getting a loan because of my age.

_____ 8. I was denied a position of leadership because of my age.

_____ 9. I was rejected as unattractive because of my age.

_____ 10. I was treated with less dignity and respect because of my age.

_____ 11. A waiter or waitress ignored me because of my age.

_____ 12. A doctor or nurse assumed my ailments were caused by my age.

_____ 13. I was denied medical treatment because of my age.

_____ 14. I was denied employment because of my age.

_____ 15. I was denied promotion because of my age.

_____ 16. Someone assumed I could not hear well because of my age.

_____ 17. Someone assumed I could not understand because of my age.

_____ 18. Someone told me,"You're too old for that."

_____ 19. My house was vandalized because of my age.

_____ 20. I was victimized by a criminal because of my age.

Please write in your age: _____

Please check: Male _____ Female _____

What is the highest grade in school that you completed? _____

FIGURE 1-1 The Ageism Survey is being used to measure the prevalence and identify types of ageism. (From Palmore, E. [2000]. *The ageism survey*. Durham, NC: Duke Center for the study of Aging. Used with permission.)

for terms that reinforce negative perceptions of older people (Hogstel, 2001; Levy & Palmore, 2001; Palmore, 2000). A recent article on myths of aging noted that "updating our image of aging and discarding ageist myths require dedication of the same order given racism and sexism" (Thornton, 2002).

Gerontologists also are recognizing and raising questions about the serious and detrimental effects of "implicit ageism." This is defined as "the thoughts, feelings, and behaviors toward elderly people that exist and operate without conscious awareness or control, with the assumption that it forms the basis of most interactions with older individuals" (Levy, 2001, p. 578). Implicit ageism is detrimental in several ways. First, because individuals are not aware that a person's older age has automatically triggered their negative stereotypes of aging, they may attribute their own response to other factors. For example, an employer will attribute the preferential hiring of a younger person to training or experience rather than to age discrimination. Second, Levy points out that older people themselves may accept false explanations for ageist behavior because they do not want to admit that they are members of a stigmatized group (Levy, 2001). Implicit ageism and other forms of ageism can have serious implications for gerontological nurses, as discussed later in this chapter.

Although the concept of ageism is most often used in reference to discrimination against older people, ageism can also apply to other stages of life. For example, older people may hold prejudices against young people, and old people may feel anger and ambivalence toward middle-aged people. Similarly, middle-aged people may experience anger toward both younger and older age groups (Butler, 2001). One study found that older adults often hold negative attitudes about themselves as well as about young people (McGowan, 1996).

Cultural Perspectives on Aging and Ageism

Although ageism is not unique to the United States, it does not exist in all cultures. In the United States, ageism has developed and grown as a result of dominant cultural beliefs and trends, such as the glorification of youth, the ideal of socioeconomic competition, the perception of the individual as autonomous, and the equating of human worth with economic worth. "These values create a cultural environment in which the drawbacks of aging are emphasized, the benefits of aging are ignored, and individual elders are blamed for problems they have not created" (McGowan, 1996, p. 71). A potentially positive outcome of the increasing cultural diversity in the United States is that the dominant cultural values that foster ageism may be challenged by cultural values of other groups. For example,

a study of the self-perceptions of older Anglo-Americans, Chinese Americans, and Chinese in Taiwan found that all three groups held positive views of aging, and that the group that represented the highest degree of industrialization and modernization held the most positive view of aging (Tien-Hyatt, 1986–1987). Culture Box 1-1 summarizes various cultural perspectives on aging, elders, and ageism.

CULTURE BOX 1-1	Cultural Perspectives on Aging, Elders, and Ageism

African Americans, Asian Americans, and Many Other Groups
- Elders are respected and honored and are viewed as a source of wisdom
- Elders often assume responsibility for the care of younger generations in the immediate and extended family.

Native Americans
- Elder status is determined not by age but by the assumption of new social roles, such as teaching, counseling, or grandparenting.
- Expectations of elders include self-control, self-discipline, and positive attitude toward living.

Gypsies
- Elders are highly respected for their ability to survive hardship and their superior knowledge of Gypsy culture and history.
- Elders are feared for their power within the group.

Mexican Americans
- Elders are treated with respect and reverance and in a formal manner.
- Elders are involved in the care and education of children.

Puerto Ricans
- *La abuela(o)* (elders or grandparents) are figures of respect, wisdom, and admiration.

South Asians
- The presence of an elder in a family is considered a blessing; elders are very highly respected.
- Elders usually live with their children; they provide child care and teach religion and cultural values to their grandchildren.

White Americans (Dominant Culture in the United States)
- Aging is viewed as a socioeconomic problem. Stereotypes of older people continue to include images of declining health, social isolation, diminished capabilities, and financial problems (AARP, 1995).
- Ageism is fostered by values that emphasize individualism, economic competition, glorification of youth, and reduction of human worth to economic use (McGowan, 1996).

(From Lipson, J. G., Dibble, L. & Minarik, P. A. (1996). *Culture and nursing care: A pocket guide.* San Francisco: UCSF Nursing Press.)

As the so-called baby-boom generation, one of the most diverse generations in American history, reaches older adulthood, some of the long-held American values that have promoted ageism may be challenged and perhaps even replaced with different values that do not foster ageism. The questions that follow are among those that need to be addressed by gerontologists and others in the United States as planning for the aging baby-boom cohorts proceeds.

Should society automatically marginalize one-fifth of its population because of a chronological age? . . . What roles and responsibilities ought older people to have as individuals to families and to society? . . . Should society care about the quality of life of older persons? . . . Ought society to be concerned if significant numbers of older people are economically poor and/or experience significant health problems? . . . How might we best support the efforts of family members to provide care to persons with significant functional disabilities? (Cornman & Kingston, 1996, p. 24)

Effects of Ageism

As a consequence of ageism, many negative stereotypes about older adults are perpetuated. Although the concepts of "old" and "aging" are not themselves inherently positive or negative, they are generally associated with undesirable characteristics when they are used in reference to people. Because of ageism, older people "are categorized as senile, rigid in thought and manner, and old-fashioned in morality and skills. In medicine, terms like 'crock' and 'vegetable' have been commonly used" (Butler, 2001, p. 26). Other common stereotypes of older adults include perceptions of older people as poor, unproductive, socially isolated, and lacking any interest in or capacity for sexuality. Stereotypes also associate old age with poor health, impaired functioning, and inevitable declines in health and functioning. Although negative stereotypes may have some basis in reality, they usually lead to myths and misunderstandings. Some of the myths about aging that are commonly accepted as truths are listed in Table 1-1. The related realities about each aspect of health and functioning also are identified, along with a reference to the chapter in this text that provides accurate information to dispel the myths.

The effects of negative stereotypes are hard to measure, but attempts have been made to identify some of the effects on both younger and older adults. For the younger generation, ageism may perpetuate the perception that older people are different from themselves; thus, they do not identify with their elders as human beings (Butler, 2001). Negative stereotypes are likely to have a detrimental effect on the self-esteem of older people, and long-term exposure to negative stereotypes may result in internalized ageism and self-hatred (Butler, 1975; Butler, 2001; Levy, 2001). Thus, the consequences of ageism can be quite serious for those older people who believe in the stereotype because it can become a self-fulfilling prophecy. Ryan and colleagues (2002) explored the potential effects of "age excuses," which is the tendency to attribute problems such as forgetfulness to old age rather than to pathologic and potentially treatable conditions. These researchers concluded that age excuses could undermine the self-perceptions of older people and threaten self-esteem if the older person believed the excuse.

Gerontologists have attempted to measure some specific effects of negative stereotypes on various responses of older adults, and some researchers have looked at the effects of subliminal messages conveying either positive or negative age stereotypes. Levy and colleagues found that exposure to negative age stereotypes can result in worse handwriting, lower self-efficacy, diminished memory performance, and even a decreased will to live (Levy, 1996; Levy, 2000; Levy et al., 1999–2000). These gerontologists also demonstrated that self-stereotypes about aging can influence an older adult's physiologic functioning, specifically with regard to cardiovascular response to stress (Levy et al., 2000). In this study, negative aging stereotypes acted as direct stressors, and positive aging stereotypes reduced cardiovascular stress as evidenced by measures of heart rate and systolic and diastolic blood pressures. Levy and colleagues suggest that negative aging stereotypes can have adverse health effects, even when the older person is not aware that he or she is succumbing to the stereotype, and that positive aging stereotypes can serve as interventions to reduce cardiovascular stress.

Some attention has been paid to the association between age stereotypes and health-related behaviors. For example, a negative age stereotype may influence an older adult to perceive health problems as normal aging. Sarkisian and colleagues (2001) found that 13.5% of older women falsely attributed new disability to old age. These researchers concluded that "despite great advances in geriatric medicine, old age is still perceived as a causal agent in functional decline, especially among our oldest patients" (p. 134). When older adults or health care professionals falsely attribute pathologic conditions to normal aging, they are likely to overlook treatable conditions, and significant harm can result from this negligence. An important responsibility of gerontological nurses is to be knowledgeable about the differences between age-related changes and pathologic conditions, so that appropriate nursing interventions

TABLE 1-1 ● Myths and Realities of Aging

Myth	Reality
People consider themselves to be old at the age of 65 years.	People usually feel old based on their health and function, rather than on their chronologic age. *(Chapter 1)*
Gerontologists have discovered that, by the age of 75 years, people are quite homogeneous as a group.	The more gerontologists learn about aging, the more they realize that, with increased age, people become more diverse, and individuals become less like their age-peers. *(Chapter 1)*
Ageism is endemic in all societies.	Ageism is much more common in industrialized societies and is highly influenced by stereotypes and cultural values. *(Chapter 1)*
Gerontologists have recently discovered a theory that explains biologic aging.	Theories about biologic aging continue to evolve, and there is little agreement on any one theory. *(Chapter 3)*
In today's society, families no longer care for older people.	In the U.S. 80% of the care of older adults is provided by their families. *(Chapter 2)*
As people grow older, it is natural for them to want to withdraw from society.	Because older people are unique individuals, each of them responds differently to society. *(Charter 3)*
By the age of 70 years, an individual's psychological growth is complete.	People never lose their capacity for psychological growth. *(Chapter 3)*
Increased disability in older people is attributable to age-related changes alone.	Although age-related changes increase one's vulnerability to functional impairments, the disabilities are attributable to risk factors, such as diseases and adverse medication effects. *(Chapter 3)*
Widowhood and other specific life events have been found to have a consistently negative impact on older people.	No one life event affects all old people negatively. The most important consideration governing the impact of an event is its unique meaning for the individual. *(Chapter 8)*
In old age, there is an inevitable decline in all intellectual abilities.	A few areas of cognitive ability decline in older adulthood, but other areas show improvement. *(Chapter 7)*
Older adults cannot learn complex new skills.	Older adults are capable of learning new things, but the speed with which they process information slows with age. *(Chapter 7)*
Constipation develops primarily because of age-related changes.	Constipation is attributable primarily to risk factors, such as restricted activity and poor dietary habits. *(Chapter 14)*
Urinary incontinence is best managed by using an indwelling catheter or incontinence products.	In most cases, urinary incontinence can be alleviated by addressing its cause. *(Chapter 15)*
Skin wrinkles can be prevented by using oils and lotions.	The best way to prevent skin wrinkles is to avoid exposure to ultraviolet light. *(Chapter 19)*
Older people decrease the level of their sexual activity because they are less able to perform sexually.	If sexual activity in older people declines, it is because of social reasons (e.g., loss of partner) or risk factors, such as diseases and adverse medication effects. *(Chapter 22)*
Older people experience the same adverse medication effects as younger people.	Older people are more likely to experience mental changes as an adverse medication effect. *(Chapter 23)*
Some degree of "senility" is normal in very old people.	"Senility" is an inaccurate term used to refer to dementing conditions, which are always caused by pathologic changes. *(Chapter 24)*
Most old people are depressed and should be allowed to withdraw from society.	About one third of older people exhibit depressive symptoms; however, depression is a very treatable condition at any age. *(Chapter 25)*

can be initiated. An essential first step in planning interventions, especially health promotion interventions, is to identify those factors that are not inherent consequences of aging. Throughout this text, emphasis is placed on differentiating between age-related changes, which cannot be modified, and those factors that can be addressed through interventions.

Negative attitudes about aging are likely to be held by health care workers, who are influenced not only by ageism in society but also by their own experiences in health care, which often are with those older adults

who are most impaired and in need of interventions. It is important, therefore, that all health care workers who care for older adults understand that most older adults are healthy and functional and strive toward improved levels of wellness and functioning. The next sections provide an overview of older adults, with emphasis on characteristics that are most pertinent to understanding their health and functioning.

Attitudes are changed through education, but changing them requires first recognizing their existence. Because ageism is subtle but pervasive in American society, nurses first need to become aware of the attitudes they hold toward older adults. The first critical thinking exercise at the end of this chapter suggests ways of becoming aware of one's own attitudes about older adults.

Because many attitudes about aging are based on myths and misperceptions rather than on realities, providing accurate information about aging has been found to be an effective intervention for reducing negative stereotypes and improving attitudes about aging (Harris & Dollinger, 2001; Lynch, 2000; McGowan, 1996). Reinforcing this information with discussion and practical application is likely to maintain improved attitudes toward aging (Ragan & Bowen, 2001). Table 1-1 can be used as a guide for identifying some of the myths and misperceptions about older adults that are commonly held by older adults as well as health care professionals. Another way of addressing attitudes of nurses and other health care workers toward older adults is through experiential educational activities. For example, *Into Aging* is a simulation game that has been developed by nurses to challenge the myths of aging (see the Educational Resources section toward the end of this chapter). This game has been used successfully in a variety of settings to improve attitudes toward aging and to change staff behaviors (e.g., Samter & Voss, 1992).

Aging Anxiety and Anti-Aging

Gerontophobia, a narrower concept than ageism, refers to an "unreasonable fear and/or irrational hatred of older people" (Palmore, 1972). Although gerontophobia has received less attention than ageism, gerontologists have focused some attention on the similar concept of "aging anxiety." Aging anxiety is defined as "the combination of people's concerns or fears about getting older" (Lynch, 2000, p. 533) Indicators of aging anxiety include worries about social losses, cognitive ability, financial well-being, changes in physical appearance, and declines in health and physical functioning (Lynch, 2000). Aging anxiety is related to negative stereotypes of older adults and the perceptions of younger adults that these problems are likely to occur in their own later life. People with greater knowledge about the aging process are less likely to experience anxiety and worries about later life (Cummings et al., 2000). Gerontologists have found that aging anxiety is lower in people with better health, and higher in women and nonwhites (Cummings et al., 2000; Lynch, 2000). The study by Cummings and colleagues suggests that exposure to serious consequences of aging and the experience of caring for older family

members are two factors that may increase a younger adult's insecurity and fears about growing older.

In the 1990s, anti-aging interventions emerged as popular approaches to staving off the negative consequences of aging. One example of the anti-aging movement is the American Academy of Anti-Aging Medicine, founded in 1993 and publicized as a "healthcare model promoting innovative science and research to prolong the healthy lifespan in humans" (Klatz, 2001–2002, p. 59). A group of more than 50 prominent geriatricians and gerontologists recently published position statements summarizing current scientific evidence about anti-aging interventions and denouncing the pseudoscientific anti-aging industry (Butler et al., 2002; Olshansky et al., 2002). Anti-aging medicine is viewed as ageist because it "puts a profoundly negative connotation on the natural and inevitable occurrence of growing old, emphasizing its negative and depleting aspects. The concept denies all that is enriching and positive about aging in the psychosocial sphere and also goes against the past fifty years of work in gerontology, which has been devoted to differentiating normative and natural aging processes from diseases like arteriosclerosis" (p. 64). Another commentary on the debate about anti-aging medicine suggests that the term "anti-aging" attempts to separate us from our bodies and presumes "that we can choose whether we are 'for' or 'against' our very existence as biologic and temporal beings" (Cole & Thompson, 2001–2002, p. 7). Cole and Thompson see anti-aging as a "broad cultural impulse" that has come about because aging has gone out of style and is currently associated with negative images of decay and decline. Butler (2001–2002) proposes that the term "longevity medicine" be used to convey a more positive approach to extending healthy life.

CHARACTERISTICS OF OLDER ADULTS IN THE UNITED STATES

Two major demographic trends that affect gerontological nursing and the health care system are the rapid growth of the old-old subgroup of older adults and the increasing diversity, including increasing cultural diversity, of the older adult population. The chief implication of the rapid growth of the old-old population is that this group is most likely to have significant functional impairments and, therefore, is most likely to need gerontological nursing care. An implication of the increasing diversity of the older adult population is that the nursing care must be based on an assessment of the unique needs of each individual receiving care. Often, these needs are based on a cultural background that differs from that of the nurse and other health care providers. Because each older adult brings a long and diverse personal history to the health care situation, it is important that gerontological nurses be able to identify those factors that are likely to affect each patient's or resident's personal history.

Information in these next sections and in Chapter 2 is intended to provide a base for identifying the characteristics of older adults that are likely to be most pertinent to the provision of culturally sensitive gerontological nursing care. Keep in mind that older adults are a highly diverse group of individuals and that these characteristics are generalizations that may not apply to a specific older adult. As one well-known gerontologist who was describing the psychosocial profile of older adults noted:

One feature of late life that promises to endure is that of diversity. In ethnic origin, language, health, family relations, intelligence, life style, educational background, and socioeconomic status, it is difficult to pinpoint an average older person. The profile of today's and tomorrow's older people can only be reduced to a series of prototypes drawn with the broadest of strokes that touch on some common denominators. With every broad stroke that is made, it must be assumed there are many exceptions to the rule. (Silverstone, 1996, p. 27.)

Demographic Characteristics

Discussions of current demographic trends in the Untied States inevitably contain the phrase "baby boomers" in reference to the significant influence exerted by the large group of people born between 1946 and 1964. Baby boomers are viewed as the cohort of people who are responsible for the "graying of America." The following statistics from the 2000 census reflect the influence of baby boomers and other recent and current population trends:

- Thirty-five million people are 65 years of age or older and account for 12.4 % of the population.
- The median age of 35.3 years is the highest it has ever been.
- In the year 2000, 5,574 people reached their 65th birthday each day.
- The number of people 65 years of age and older increased by 12 % since 1990; for the first time in the history of the census, the increase in percentage of older people was less than the increase in the total population, which was 13.2 %.
- The number of people aged 45 to 64 years increased by 34 % since 1990—these are the people who will reach 65 years of age during the next two decades.

- Sixteen percent of people 65 years of age and older are members of minority groups; this will increase to at least 25 % in the next 25 years.
- The male-to-female ratio by age groups is 82:100 for ages 65 to 74 years, 65:100 for ages 75 to 84 years, and 41:100 for ages 85 years and older.
- The older adult population can be divided by age groups as follows: 53 % aged 65 to 74 years, 35 % aged 74 to 84 years, and 12 % aged 85 years and older.
- Increases by age groups are highest for those aged 85 years and older and lowest for those aged 65 to 74 years; this trend is expected to reverse starting in 2011, when the largest increase will be in the group of people aged 65 to 74 years.
- The number of centenarians increased by 35 %, from 37,306 to 50,454, between 1990 and 2000.

Socioeconomic Characteristics

Socioeconomic characteristics such as income, education, marital status, and living arrangements vary significantly among young-old and old-old groups. Tremendous differences also exist between men and women and among various racial groups. Perhaps the most obvious disparities are in marital status for men and women, and these disparities increase with increasing age. For example, in 1998, of people age 65 to 74 years, 79 % of men and 55 % of women were married. For people aged 85 years and older, 50 % of men and 13 % of women were married. Percentages of men and women aged 85 years and older who were widowed were 42 % and 77 %, respectively. This variation is attributed to factors such as longer life expectancy for women, the tendency for women to marry men who are slightly older, and higher remarriage rates for older widowed men (Federal Interagency Forum on Aging-Related Statistics, 2000). Figure 1-2 illustrates the marital status of people aged 65 years and older by age groups and sex.

Living arrangements also vary by gender and race, with more older men than women living with their spouses and older women more likely to live alone (Figure 1-3). In 1998, percentages of older women living alone (by racial groups) were as follows: 41 % of African American, 41 % of white, 27 % of Hispanic, and 21 % of Asian and Pacific Islander women. Although 15 % of older white women lived with other relatives, one third of each of the other groups (African American, Hispanic, and Asian and Pacific Islander) lived with other relatives (Federal Interagency Forum on Aging-Related Statistics, 2000).

Educational levels exert a significant influence on quality of life for older adults because higher educational levels are associated with higher incomes, better

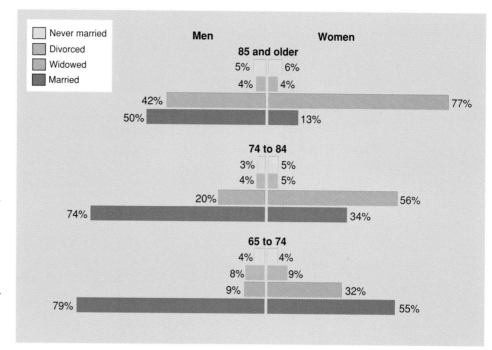

FIGURE 1-2 Marital status of older adults, by sex and age groups, 1998. These data refer to the civilian noninstitutional population. (From Federal Interagency Forum on Aging-Related Statistics. [2000]. *Older Americans 2000: Key indicators of well-being.* Washington, DC: U.S. Government Printing Office.)

health, less disability, and longer life expectancy. Educational levels for older adults are gradually increasing, as indicated by the fact that the number of people aged 65 years and older who had completed high school increased from 18% in 1950, to 28% in 1970, and to 70% in 2000. There are no significant gender differences in the number of older adults who have completed high school, but the rates of older men and women holding a bachelor's degree were 20% and 11%, respectively, in 1998 (Federal Interagency Forum on Aging-Related Statistics, 2000). As with many other socioeconomic indicators, there is tremendous variation among racial and ethnic groups (Figure 1-4).

The number of older people living below the poverty line has diminished from almost 30% in 1967 to 10.2% in 2000, but this does not mean that all older people are economically better off today than they were 40 years ago. Gerontologists and sociologists emphasize that statistics about poverty should be interpreted in relation to a broader perspective on the economic conditions of older adults in the United States. One important consideration is that the official "poverty line" varies for the over-65 and under-65 populations. A person younger than 65 years of age living alone is below the poverty line if his or her income is less than $8,959; however, someone older than 65 years of age is considered poor only when his or her income is less than $8,259. For couples, the levels are $11,531 and $10,409 for people under and over 65 years of age, respectively. By these criteria, income must be 8% lower for individuals and 10% lower for couples for older people to be considered

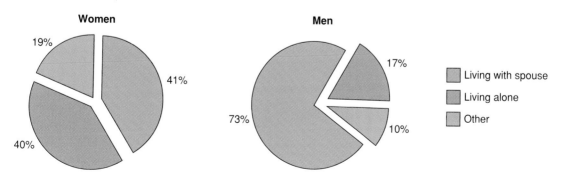

FIGURE 1-3 Living arrangements of people age 65 and older, 2000. (Data from the United States Bureau of the Census. [2001]. *America's families and living arrangements; population characteristics: June, 2001.* Current Population Reports, P20–537; and *The 65 years and over population: 2000,* Census 2000 Brief, October, 2001. Washington, DC: Author.)

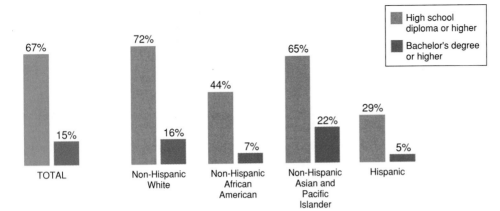

FIGURE 1-4 Educational levels of older adults, by race and Hispanic origin, 1998. Hispanics may be of any race. (From Federal Interagency Forum on Aging-Related Statistics. [2000]. *Older Americans 2000: Key indicators of well-being.* Washington, DC: U.S. Government Printing Office.)

poor (Butler, 2001). Another important consideration is that if the number of people who live within 125% of the poverty line are included as poor (i.e., an annual income of $10,324 for a single person and $13,011 for couples), then almost 17% of older people are living in poverty. A much higher proportion of older people live just above the poverty line in comparison with the overall population (Butler, 2001).

Another major consideration with regard to economic conditions of older adults is the tremendous range in financial status, which varies according to race, gender, and living arrangements. Figure 1-5 illustrates some of the differences in rates of poverty over the past two decades among groups of older adults classified by race and Hispanic origin. Factors that increase the likelihood of an older adult living in poverty are female gender, living alone, advanced old age, having poor health, and not completing high school. Studies suggest that much of the economic disparity for women and minorities can be attributed to occupational segregation and pay differentials during working years (Crown, 2001).

Determination of economic status is based on both income, defined as economic resources available for purchasing power, and net worth, defined as the value of all assets minus outstanding debts. On average, older adults have lower incomes than younger adults, and people aged 85 years and older have the lowest median income. Adults between the ages 65 and 74 years have the highest net worth, but people aged 75 years and older have less net worth than people aged 55 to 64 or 65 to 74 years. It is important to remember that most net worth for older adults is in their homes. Thus, an older adult may live in a house that has substantially appreciated in value over the years, but he or she may not be able to maintain it or cover the expenses of living in it. As with other economic characteristics of older adults, there is a wider range of extremes in both income and assets. For example, the median income of all individuals over 65 years of age was $13,739, but for whites, it was $14,198, and for Hispanics, it was $8,877 (Butler, 2001). Major disparities also exist in net worth: in 1999, net worth for an older African American household was estimated at $13,000, whereas that for an older white household was $181,000 (Federal Interagency Forum on Aging-Related Statistics, 2000). Gender differences also are evident in the 2000 census data that showed

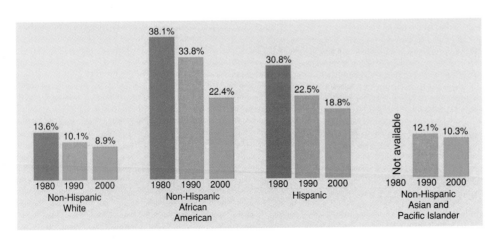

FIGURE 1-5 Percentages of Americans, age 65 years and older, living below the poverty level over the past two decades, by race and Hispanic origin. Hispanics may be of any race. (U.S. Census Bureau. [2000]. Table 3: Poverty status of people by age, race, and Hispanic origin, 1959–2000. In *Current population survey.* Washington, DC: Author.)

median income for older men and women as $19,168 and $10,899, respectively.

In summary, indicators for economic and educational levels are improving for many or most older adults, but disparities are becoming more and more evident, and there is great diversity among various subgroups of older adults. Women are more likely than men to be poor and to live alone. In contrast to whites in the United States, members of minority groups are more likely to be poor and less educated but are more likely to be living with other relatives. Considerations regarding gender differences and different cultural groups of older adults are discussed in greater detail in Chapter 2.

Health Characteristics

Because much of the focus of health care for older adults is on preventing disabilities and maintaining and improving function, gerontologists and health care providers are particularly interested in statistics about chronic conditions and impaired function in daily life. Economists and health care planners also are interested in health characteristics of older adults because the chronic conditions most common among older adults require more care, are more disabling, and are more difficult and costly to treat than the conditions that are common among younger adults (National Academy on an Aging Society, 1999). An example of the significance of chronic illness for older adults can be seen in mortality figures. Of the six leading causes of death in older adults, only pneumonia/influenza, the fifth leading cause, is an acute illness. The other five leading causes of death in older adults—heart disease, cancer, stroke, chronic obstructive pulmonary disease (COPD), and diabetes—are conditions that are likely to be associated with prolonged periods of illness and disability rather

than with rapid mortality. Thus, much of this discussion of health characteristics focuses on chronic conditions and impaired function.

The following facts and statistics present a brief overview of significant health characteristics of older adults in the United States:

- Eighty percent of older adults have at least one chronic condition.
- The most prevalent chronic conditions of older adults are arthritis, hypertension, heart disease, cancer, diabetes, stroke, cataracts, hearing impairments, sinusitis, and orthopedic impairments.
- The percentages of older adults who rated their health as fair or poor in 1996 were 26% of whites, 35.1% of Hispanics, and 41.6% of African Americans.
- Disabilities and limitations on activities as a result of chronic conditions increase gradually with increased age (Figure 1-6).
- There is a strong relationship between having a severe disability and rating one's health as fair or poor.
- Presence of severe disability is associated with lower income levels and educational attainment.

In recent decades, gerontologists have been attempting to estimate trends in disability among older populations. This emphasis came about because of the dramatic increases in life expectancy during the 20th century and the related concern about extending quality of life by preventing disability and delaying the onset of chronic conditions. Several longitudinal studies currently point to a trend toward better health and less disability in recent decades (Fries, 2002; Waidmann & Liu, 2000). An analysis of data from 1982 to 1996 found that disability rates are declining steadily, but the rates varied during that period and no improvements

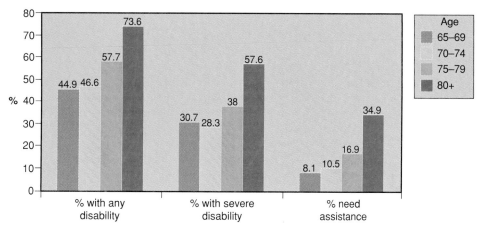

FIGURE 1-6 Percentage of older adults with disabilities, by age group. (Data from Federal Interagency Forum on Aging-Related Statistics. [2000]. *Older Americans 2000: Key indicators of well-being.* Washington, DC: U.S. Government Printing Office.)

were made between 1986 and 1992 (Schoeni et al., 2001). Schoeni and colleagues (2001) found that improvements were widespread and did not vary significantly by race, gender, age group, or marital status. Within educational groups, however, improvements were concentrated among those with the most education. Gerontologists have identified the following factors as underlying reasons for the improved health and functioning of older adults (Fries, 2002; Lan et al., 2002):

- Attitude changes
- Healthier lifestyles
- Environmental changes
- Higher educational levels
- Greater use of assistive devices
- Avoidance of health-risk behaviors
- Improved diagnostic and therapeutic techniques
- Decreased prevalence of chronic conditions

Gerontologists are addressing differences in health and functioning among various subgroups of older adults, such as chronologic subgroups (i.e., young-old, middle-old, old-old, and oldest-old populations) and ethnic populations (e.g., African American and Hispanic older adults). Studies suggest that cultural as well as socioeconomic factors have a significant impact on health and functioning, with strong evidence that older ethnic minority groups have more chronic illnesses, lower functional levels, and poorer self-health ratings than white Americans.

Rural and nonmetropolitan elderly people are other subgroups that have been the subject of gerontological studies in the 1990s. This attention is warranted by the fact that about 25 % of elderly people in the United States live in nonmetropolitan areas. People aged 65 years and older constitute 15 % of the population in nonmetropolitan areas, and this percentage is increasing because of the in-migration of retired persons and the out-migration of younger adults. In contrast to urban older adults, rural older adults are characterized by poorer housing, less formal education, higher poverty rates, less healthy lifestyles, less access to social services, more chronic illnesses and functional disabilities, and more limited access to preventive care and other health services (Rosswurm, 2001).

Implications for Gerontological Nursing

Health characteristics of older adults are of importance to gerontological nurses for several reasons. First, the subgroup of older adults is the population in the United States that receives the most health care services. Although older people constitute 12.4 % of the population, they occupy about half of the available adult hospital beds. Moreover, older adults spent four times as many days in hospitals as younger adults in 1999 (1.6 versus 0.4 days), and they averaged about twice the number of contacts with doctors than did people of all other ages combined (6.8 versus 3.5 contacts). Therefore, with the exception of those nurses who work exclusively with pediatric or young adult populations, nurses focus more of their care on older adults than on any other age group. Second, the health care system is attempting to address the escalating costs of care, and services to older adults are being targeted for cost-cutting measures. Much of this cost cutting has been focused on the high cost of caring for people with chronic illnesses and impaired function. Because of this emphasis, increased attention has been directed toward preventive care and improved function, and there are increasing opportunities for nurses to assist in the development and implementation of health promotion programs for older adults. Identifying the health characteristics of older adults provides a basis for planning these programs. Finally, because the emphasis of gerontological nursing is on improving the health and functioning of older adults, the patterns of functional impairment of this population must be identified. This is especially important in light of the growing recognition that much of the health care that is provided to older people involves chronic care related to functional impairments. This contrasts with the emphasis of health care services in younger populations, which tends to be acute rather than chronic in nature.

In summary, older adults are most likely to have an accumulation of chronic illnesses, and some of these chronic conditions will cause functional impairments in daily activities. These chronic illnesses and functional impairments will increase the vulnerability of the older person to further impairment when an acute illness is superimposed. Because the focus of nursing is on assisting people to respond to actual or potential illness, the goal of gerontological nursing is to assist older adults to attain and maintain the highest level of health and functioning. This theme is discussed at length in the discussion of the functional consequences theory of gerontological nursing in Chapter 3. The chapters in Parts 3, 4, 5, and 6 of this text address specific aspects of health and functioning with emphasis on nursing interventions that are directed toward this goal.

CHAPTER SUMMARY

The older adult population in the United States is characterized by increasing numbers and proportions of old-old people and by a marked growth in diversity. This chapter reviews the health and social characteristics of older adults in the United States, with emphasis on the diversity and cultural aspects of these characteristics. Because attitudes and stereotypes can influence the way a society views and treats its members as well as the way individuals perceive and care for themselves, it is important to recognize and address ageist attitudes and stereotypes as they relate to the care of older adults. Nurses can challenge ageist attitudes by questioning some of the dominant values in American society that foster ageism and by debunking the myths and reinforcing the realities of aging as they care for older adults. Because people become more heterogeneous as they age, the care of older adults is very complex and must be provided with cultural sensitivity and with recognition of the unique history of each older person.

 CRITICAL THINKING EXERCISES

1. In the next few weeks, do the following exercises to increase your awareness of attitudes toward aging and older adults:
   - During the next 2 weeks, as you go about your usual activities, keep a small notebook or note cards handy and jot down examples of images of older adults that you see or hear in the following media: newspapers, magazines, Internet, television, greeting cards, social conversations. Note whether the images convey a neutral, positive, or negative image.
   - During the next 2 weeks, pay attention to your own communication about older adults and identify the terms you use and the images you hold.
   - Re-phrase each of the 20 questions in the Ageism Survey (see Figure 1-1) and ask yourself how often you have done any of those activities in the past few months (e.g., "How often did I tell a joke that pokes fun at old people?"
   - Ask a relative, friend, or acquaintance to fill out the Ageism Survey and discuss his or her experiences.
2. Define old age and aging from each of the following perspectives: chronologic aging, subjective aging, and functional aging.
3. You are asked to staff a booth at a career-day exposition for first-year college students. What information would you give with regard to the following questions?
   - Why is there an increasing need for people to be educated in areas of gerontology?
   - What trends in the United States today will make it interesting and challenging to provide health care to older people in the coming years?
   - What additional areas of study would you recommend (i.e., elective courses) for a nursing student

who wants to specialize in the care of older adults?
- What activities would you suggest a student pursue if he or she is considering a career in gerontological nursing?

EDUCATIONAL RESOURCES

Canadian Institute of Aging
410 Laurier Avenue West, 9th floor
Postal Locator 4209A, Ottawa, ON K1A OW9
http://www.cihr-irse.gc.ca

Into Aging—Understanding Issues Affecting the Later Stages of Life
Boxed Simulation Game
SLACK Inc., 6900 Grove Road, Thorofare, NJ 08086
(800) 257-8290
http://www.slackbooks.com

National Aging Information Center, U.S. Administration on Aging
330 Independence Avenue, SW, Washington, DC 20201
(202) 619-0724
http://www.aoa.gov/naic

National Institute on Aging Information Center
P.O. Box 8057, Gaithersburg, MD 20898
(800) 222-2225
http://nih.gov/nia

United States Census Bureau
Washington, DC 20233
(301) 763-2378
http://www.census.gov

REFERENCES

Bradley, D. E., & Longino, C. F. (2001). How older people think about images of aging in advertising and the media. *Generations (Fall)*, 17–21.

Butler, R. N. (1969). Ageism: Another form of bigotry. *The Gerontologist, 9*, 243–246.

Butler, R. N. (1975). *Why survive? Being old in America.* New York: Harper & Row.

Butler, R. N. (2001). Ageism. In M. D. Mezey (Ed.), *The Encyclopedia of Elder Care* (pp. 26–27). New York: Springer.

Butler, R. N. (2001–2002). Is there an 'anti-aging' medicine? *Generations (Winter)*, 63–64.

Butler, R. N., Fossel, M., Harman, S., Heward, C. B., Olshansky, S. J., Perls, T. T., Rothman, D. J., Warner, H. R., West M. D., & Wright, W. E. (2002). Is there an antiaging medicine? *Journal of Gerontology: Biological Sciences, 57,* B333–B338.

Butler, R. N., Lewis, M. I., & Sunderland, T. (1991). *Aging and mental health* (4th ed.). New York: Merrill/Macmillan.

Cohen, E. S. (1988). The elderly mystique: Constraints on the autonomy of the elderly with disabilities. *The Gerontologist, 28*(Suppl.), 2431.

Cohen, E. S. (2001). The complex nature of ageism: What is it? Who does it? Who perceives it? *The Gerontologist, 41,* 576–577.

Cole, T. R., & Thompson, B. (2001–2002). Introduction: Antiaging: Are you for it or against it? *Generations (Winter)*, 6–8.

Cornman, J. M., & Kingston, E. R. (1996). Trends, issues, perspectives, and values for the aging of the baby boom cohorts. *The Gerontologist, 36,* 15–26.

Covey, H. C. (1988). Historical terminology used to represent older people. *The Gerontologist, 28,* 291–297.

Crown, W. (2001). Economic status of the elderly. In R. H. Binstock & L. K. George (Eds.), *Handbook of aging and the social sciences* (5th ed., pp. 352–368). San Diego: Academic Press.

Cummings, S. M., Kropf, N. P., & DeWeaver, K.L. (2000). Knowledge of and attitudes toward aging among non-elders: Gender and race differences. *Journal of Women & Aging, 12*(1/2), 77–91.

Everard, K. M., Lach, H. W., Fisher, E. B., & Baum, M. C. (2000). Relationship of activity and social support to the functional health of older adults. *Journal of Gerontology: Social Sciences, 55,* S208–S212.

Federal Interagency Forum on Aging-Related Statistics. (2000). *Older Americans 2000: Key indicators of well-being.* Washington, DC: U.S. Government Printing Office.

Fischer, D. H. (1977). *Growing old in America.* New York: Oxford University Press.

Fries, J.F. (2002). Successful aging: An emerging paradigm of gerontology. *Clinics in Geriatric Medicine, 18,* 371–382.

Harris, L. A., & Dollinger, S. (2001). Participation in a course on aging: Knowledge, attitudes and anxiety about aging in oneself and others. *Educational Gerontology, 27,* 657–667.

Hirshbein, L. D. (2001). Popular views of old age in America, 1900–1950. *Journal of the American Geriatrics Society, 49,* 1555–1560.

Hogstel, M. O. (2001). Letter to the editor. *Geriatric Nursing, 22,* 7.

Holkup, P. A. (2001). The 20th century: Looking back at the ambiance of aging from the perspective of age-specific journals and periodicals. *Journal of Gerontological Nursing, 27*(6), 38–46.

International Longevity Center—USA. (2001). *Biomarkers of aging: From primitive organisms to man.* New York: International Longevity Center.

Kaufman, G. & Elder, G.H. (2002). Revisiting age identity: A research note. *Journal of Aging Studies, 16,* 169–176.

Klatz, R. (2001–2002). Anti-aging medicine: Resounding, independent support for expansion of an innovative medical specialty. *Generations (Winter),* 59–62.

Lan, T-Y, Melzer, D., Tom, B. D. M., & Guralnik, J. M. (2002). Performance tests and disability: Developing an objective index of mobility-related limitation in older populations. *Journal of Gerontology: Medical Sciences, 57,* M294–M301.

Levy, B. (1996). Improving memory in old age by implicit self-stereotyping. *Journal of Personality and Social Psychology, 71,* 1092–1107.

Levy, B. (2000). Handwriting as a reflection of aging self-stereotypes. *Journal of Geriatric Psychiatry, 33,* 81–94.

Levy, B. R. (2001). Eradication of ageism requires addressing the enemy within. *The Gerontologist, 41,* 578–579.

Levy, B. R., Ashman, O., & Dror, I. (1999-2000). To be or not to be: The effects of aging self-stereotypes on the will-to-live. *Omega, 40,* 409–420.

Levy, B. R., Hausdorff, J., Hencke, R., & Wei, J. Y. (2000). Reducing cardiovascular stress with positive self-stereotypes of aging. *Journal of Gerontology: Psychological Sciences, 55,* P205–P213.

Levy, B. R., & Palmore, E. (2001). Letters to the editor: Response to "ageism in gerontological language." *The Gerontologist, 41,* 287.

Lynch, S. M. (2000). Measurement and prediction of aging anxiety. *Research on Aging, 22,* 533–558.

McGowan, T. G. (1996). Ageism and discrimination: In J. E. Birren (Ed.), *Encyclopedia of gerontology: Age, aging, and the aged* (Vol. 1, pp. 71–80). San Diego: Academic Press.

National Academy on an Aging Society. (1999). *Chronic conditions: A challenge for the 21st century.* Washington, DC: National Academy on an Aging Society.

Neugarten, B. L. (1978). The rise of the young-old. In R. Gross, B. Gross, & S. Seidman (Eds.), *The new old: Struggling for decent aging* (pp. 47–49). Garden City, NY: Anchor Press/Doubleday.

Olshansky, S. J., Hayflick, L., & Carnes, B. A. (2002). Position statement on human aging. *Journal of Gerontology: Biological Sciences, 57,* B292–B297.

Palmore, E. (1972). Gerontophobia versus ageism. *The Gerontologist, 12,* 213.

Palmore, E. B. (1986). Trends in the health of the aged. *The Gerontologist, 26,* 298–302.

Palmore, E. (2000). Guest editorial: Ageism in gerontological language. *The Gerontologist, 40,* 645.

Palmore, E. (2001). The ageism survey: First findings. *The Gerontologist, 41,* 572–575.

Ragan, A. M., & Bowen, A. M. (2001). Improving attitudes regarding the elderly population: The effects of information and reinforcement for change. *The Gerontologist, 41,* 511–515.

Rosswurm, M. A. (2001). Rural elders. In M. D. Mezey (Ed.), *The Encyclopedia of elder care* (pp. 580–582). New York: Springer.

Rowe, J. W., & Kahn, R. L. (1997). Successful aging. *The Gerontologist, 37,* 433–440.

Ryan, E. B., Bieman-Copland, S., See, S. T. K., Ellis, C. H., & Anas, A. P. (2002). Age excuses: Conversational management of memory failures in older adults. *Journal of Gerontology: Psychological Sciences, 57,* P256–P267.

Samter, J., & Voss, J. B. (1992). Challenging the myths of aging. *Geriatric Nursing, 13,* 17–21.

Sarkisian, C. A., Liu, H., Ensrud, K. E., Stone, K. L., & Mangione, C. M. (2001). Correlates of attributing new disability to old age. *Journal of the American Geriatrics Society, 49,* 134–141.

Schoeni, R. F., Freedman, V. A., & Wallace, R. B. (2001). Persistent, consistent, widespread, and robust? Another look at recent trends in old-age disability. *Journal of Gerontology: Social Sciences, 56,* S206–S218.

Seeman, T., & Chen, X. (2002). Risk and protective factors for physical functioning in older adults with and without chronic conditions: MacArthur studies of successful aging. *Journal of Gerontology: Social Sciences, 57,* S135–S144.

Silverstone, B. (1996). Older people of tomorrow: A psychosocial profile. *The Gerontologist, 36,* 27–32.

Thornton, J. E. (2002). Myths of aging or ageist stereotypes. *Educational Gerontology, 28,* 301–312.

Tien-Hyatt, J. L. (1986-1987). Self-perceptions of aging across cultures: Myth or reality? *International Journal of Aging and Human Development, 24*(2), 129–148.

Van Nostrand, J. F. (Ed.). (1993). *Common beliefs about the rural elderly: What do national data tell us?* Vital and health statistics (Series 3, No.28), Hyattsville, MD: U.S. Department of Health and Human Services.

Waidmann, T. A., & Liu, K. (2000). Disability trends among elderly persons and implications for the future. *Journal of Gerontology: Social Sciences, 55,* S298–S307.

Older Adults in Families, Communities, and the World

LEARNING OBJECTIVES

1. Identify population trends that affect relationships of older adults and their families.

2. Describe characteristics of older adults in the following cultural groups in the United States: African Americans, Hispanics, Asians, and American Indians.

3. Describe characteristics of rural and homeless older adults.

4. Delineate the range of services and housing options for older adults.

5. Discuss trends in world population aging and implications related to health.

OLDER ADULTS IN FAMILIES

Increasing numbers of multigenerational families and other demographic trends in the United States have brought about major changes in family relationships in recent decades. Just as a major defining characteristic of older adults as a group is their increasing diversity, so, too, is increasing diversity a major characteristic of the family relationships of older adults. The phrase "sandwich generation" was coined during the 1990s in reference to the increasing numbers of middle-aged women who must simultaneously juggle the demands of caring for older and younger generations. Another recently coined phrase—"skipped generation households"—reflects the increasing numbers of households in which grandparents have assumed primary responsibility for grandchildren without the presence of a parent of the grandchildren. The following sections explore some of the myths and realities of older adults in families in the United States in the early 2000s.

One of the most significant recent population trends in the United States is the increased number of multigenerational families, a phenomenon that is a direct result of the increasing number of people living into advanced old age. In the early 1900s, great-grandparenthood was something reserved for the minority of people who lived beyond the age of 70 years; in the early 2000s, about half of older adults are great-grandparents, and even great-great-grandparenthood is a common life stage. One-fourth of people aged 58 to 59 years have at least one living parent, and 10% of older people have at least one offspring who is also older than 65 years of age. These statistics represent a dramatic change in the ratio of old-old parents to old children. The *parent support ratio* is the number of people aged 85 years and older per 100 people aged 50 to 64 years. The parent support ratio tripled from 1950 to 1993, and it is expected to triple again by the year 2050 (U.S. Bureau of the

Census, 1996). Demographics such as these have influenced patterns of family caregiving, particularly for women. The mid-1980s, for example, marked the beginning of an era in which the average woman in the United States spent more time caring for her parents than for her children.

Another phenomenon that has emerged from recent social and demographic trends is the dramatic 76% increase over the past 30 years in the number of children younger than 18 years of age living in households maintained by a grandparent. Researchers have estimated that three generations lived together in about two thirds of these households, and that neither parent was present in the remaining third of these households (Fuller-Thomson & Minkler, 2001). Social factors that contribute to this trend include increases in AIDS, unemployment, teen pregnancy, family violence, child maltreatment, maternal substance abuse, and the incarceration of women. Recent changes in child welfare policy favoring placement of children in homes of relatives, rather than in foster care or institutional settings, have also been a significant influence. Articles are appearing more and more frequently in nursing and gerontological journals about health-related and other issues involving older adults who assume long-term caregiving responsibilities for grandchildren (e.g., Davidhizar et al., 2000; Dowdell & Sherwen, 1998).

"Downward extension of households" is being used to describe households in which grandchildren or adult children live with and are in some way dependent on grandparents and older parents. This family configuration contrasts with the more customary upward extension of intergenerational households in the United States in which older adults reside with adult children or grandchildren to receive care. The importance of diversity must be emphasized, however, because the stereotype of dependent older people is being replaced by multiple scenarios in which older adults assume roles as caregivers as well as care receivers, and are involved in complex relationships with peers and with younger and older generations (Silverstone, 1996). The current trend is toward a continuing prevalence of upwardly extended households among whites and downwardly extended households among African Americans (Szinovacz, 1998). One study indicates that caregiving by grandparents is becoming more common in general, but especially among single women, African Americans, and low-income people (Fuller-Thomson et al., 1997).

Although there have been significant increases in multigenerational families and in the numbers of grandparents raising grandchildren, these demographic trends reflect the diversity of family relationships rather than the norm for older adults in relation to their families. Since the preindustrial period, nuclear family living arrangements have always been predominant in Western Europe and the United States. Typically, younger family members establish separate households following marriage, and older family members attempt to maintain independent households for as long as possible. These normative family relationships have been described as "intimacy from a distance," with younger generations residing close to older generations, but not in the same household (Hareven, 2001). For much of American history, the "ideal" relationship between older and younger generations in families has been to be far enough away to preserve independent lifestyles but close enough for social support and emotional connectedness. Moreover, this kind of family relationship provided for meeting occasional caregiving needs of family members while allowing for the maintenance of differing lifestyles for both younger and older generations. Family relationships have been based on the principle of reciprocity across generations, characterized by mutual assistance and extensive exchanges among kin (Hareven, 2001). The current trend in the United States is that caregiving needs are met primarily by spouses and secondarily by adult children, especially daughters and unmarried children.

In recent years, increased rates of divorce and remarriage among younger generations have resulted in the proliferation of varieties of blended families across several generations. In addition, increased rates of remarriage among older adults who are widowed or divorced have led to increasing numbers of later-life blended families. One consequence of these trends is that family dynamics can become quite complicated, particularly when adult "stepchildren" assume new roles as caregivers or decision makers for dependent older adults. For example, it is not uncommon for adult children to share caregiving and decision-making responsibilities regarding their impaired parent with a parent's spouse whom they hardly know. Similarly, adult children may be in positions to assist their parent with caregiving or decision making about a "stepparent" whom they hardly know. Relationships among blended families usually are complicated further by concerns regarding financial resources and questions about inheritance.

Another trend that affects relationships between older adults and their families is differing expectations with regard to attitudes and caregiving practices. In the 1900s, for example, the tradition of deep involvement in generational assistance, reinforced by strong family and ethnic values, was dominant in American culture. After World War II, however, a tradition of individualistic values and lifestyles emerged, and relying on institutions and public agencies to provide care for dependent elderly became acceptable (Hareven, 2001). Current generations of middle-aged daughters also have been influenced by the trend toward having a career and discovering a sense of self-worth that is independent of their roles in families. These trends often cause significant conflict between the expectations of the younger generation of adult children, especially daughters, and older family members who need care.

Despite the complex and evolving social and demographic trends in the United States, some aspects of the relationship between older adults and their families have remained unchanged for many decades. For example, older adults have never been "abandoned" by their children. Studies consistently show that older adults are satisfied with their family relationships and maintain close emotional ties and frequent contact with children and grandchildren. One longitudinal study found that contact with children remained steady for people aged 75 to 84 years and for those aged 85 years and older. Moreover, both old-old and oldest-old participants expressed satisfaction with family relationships and did not feel abandoned by their children (Field & Gueldner, 2001). Another consistent relationship between older adults and their families is that the vast majority of care for dependent older adults is provided by family members and other "informal" sources. Studies indicate that, on average, family members provide as much as 80% of care to dependent older adults. Spousal and filial responsibility are long-standing traditions that have directed family caregiving in the United States for centuries, and this does not seem to be changing. Studies indicate that, in comparison with white families, ethnic minority families provide more informal support and use less formal services for dependent family members. Another difference is that these services are provided by a broader range of immediate and extended family members (Dilworth-Anderson et al., 2002). In recent years, gerontologists have explored non-kin caregiving relationships and are finding that about 10% of community-living dependent older adults receive significant amounts of care from unpaid sources such as friends and neighbors (Barker, 2002).

TRANSCULTURAL PERSPECTIVES OF AGING IN THE UNITED STATES

The study of aging in the United States has primarily been a study of white Americans, but gerontologists have broadened their focus in recent years and paid more attention to the unique characteristics of different cultural groups of older adults. Gerontologists are recognizing the increasing diversity and heterogeneity of older adults in the United States and the importance of identifying the interrelationships among race, ethnicity, aging, and health. Gerontological research regarding cultural aspects of aging began in the 1960s with a focus on African Americans, extended to Hispanic Americans in the 1970s, and then to other groups in the 1980s. Although much progress has been made in research related to diverse groups of older adults, many subgroups continue to be lumped together, and the need to identify within-group differences is great. Within-group differences that need to be addressed in studies include gender difference, differences between immigrants and non-immigrants, and differences between subsequent American-born generations. For example, studies across all racial and ethnic groups in the United States show that immigrants have better health than next generations born in the United States and that this trend is not related to socioeconomic factors. Studies of Hispanic and Asian populations suggest that one explanation for this phenomenon is that greater acculturation leads to detrimental changes in diet and increased use of alcohol, cigarettes, and illicit drugs (Williams & Wilson, 2001). Further research on these kinds of interrelationships may lead to important implications for health care of older adults, particularly with regard to health promotion interventions.

The concept of cultural diversity generally is used in reference to groups of people who share a common heritage. The 2000 census used the following categories for data collection: white, African American, Hispanic origin (of any race), Asian or Pacific Islander, and American Indian or Native Alaskan. Racial and ethnic composition of the United States was discussed in Chapter 1 and is illustrated in Figure 2-1. Between 1995 and 2050, the percentage increase in people aged 65 years and older, grouped by categories, is as follows: white, 114%; African American, 217%; other (Aleuts, Asians, Eskimos, Pacific Islanders, and American Indians), 657%; and Hispanic origin, 815% (National Aging Information Center, 1997). Projections for the year 2050 indicate that the greatest increases in the minority elderly population will be among Hispanics, who will outnumber African Americans as the largest ethnic minority group of older adults. The disproportionate increase in these minority groups is partly attributable to their past and future immigration patterns.

When looking at any data about racial and ethnic groups, it is important to recognize that little or no information about various subgroups was available until the late 1990s. Also, terminology used in reference to subgroups is inconsistent, and there is tremendous variation in definitions of specific

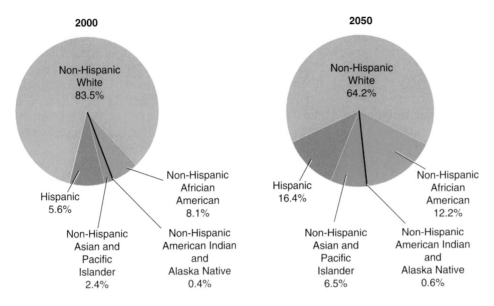

2000

Non-Hispanic
White
83.5%

Hispanic
5.6%

Non-Hispanic
Asian and
Pacific
Islander
2.4%

Non-Hispanic
American Indian
and
Alaska Native
0.4%

Non-Hispanic
African
American
8.1%

2050

Non-Hispanic
White
64.2%

Hispanic
16.4%

Non-Hispanic
Asian and
Pacific
Islander
6.5%

Non-Hispanic
American Indian
and
Alaska Native
0.6%

Non-Hispanic
African
American
12.2%

FIGURE 2-1 Actual and projected distribution of people age 65 and older, by race and Hispanic origin, 2000 and 2050. Data are middle-series projections of the population. Hispanics may be of any race. These data refer to the resident population. (From United States Census Bureau, Population Projections.) (U.S. Census Bureau. [January 2000]. *Population projections of the United States by age, sex, race, Hispanic origin, and nativity: 1999 to 2100.* Washington, DC: Author. http://www.census.gov/population/www/projections/natproj.html.)

groups. To add to the confusion, even the U.S. government defines groups differently. For example, Native Hawaiians are categorized as Asian American or Pacific Islanders in the United States Census, but as Native Americans in the Older Americans Act and in other contexts. Some of the commonly used cultural groupings and subgroupings are as follows:

- Black or African American: African, West Indian, Caribbean Islander
- Hispanic or Latino: Cuban, Spaniard, Mexican, Puerto Rican, and Central or South American
- Asian: Chinese, Japanese, Korean, Filipino, Asian Indians, and Vietnamese
- Native Hawaiian and other Pacific Islander: Native Hawaiian, Samoan, Fijian, and Guamanian
- Native American and Native Alaskan (a.k.a. American Indian and Alaska Native): Aleut, Eskimo, and more than 500 tribes of American Indian

An important aspect of nursing is providing care that is culturally appropriate; for gerontological nurses, this is of particular importance because older adults from racially and ethnically diverse backgrounds bring a long history of cultural influences that affect their health and functioning. Moreover, these factors can significantly affect their relationships with health care providers and their receptivity to interventions. Culturally specific information that is pertinent to nursing assessment of, and interventions for, older adults is incorporated whenever possible in this text and may be found in Culture Boxes and brief Diversity Notes. Nurses are encouraged to supplement this information by reading journals and other references and by obtaining information from the Internet and other sources listed in the Educational Resources section of

this chapter. Many of the organizations listed in the Educational Resources sections at the end of each chapter provide educational materials written and illustrated in other languages. These materials can be important resources for health promotion interventions and are usually available at little or no cost. Additionally, all health care professionals are encouraged to obtain culturally specific information about groups that reside in their locale; such information is often available from local organizations. Information about some specific culturally diverse groups of older adults is discussed in the following sections. Culture Box 2-1 summarizes some of the family caregiving expectations that are associated with selected cultural groups in the United States.

African Americans

Africans were brought to America and bonded into slavery beginning in 1619; by the end of the 19th century, more than 10 million Africans had been sold as slaves. Slavery, therefore, became the way of life that formed the roots of African American culture in a white society. Inherent effects of slavery included poverty, discrimination, and social and psychological obstacles.

Racism continues to affect African Americans today. For example, great disparity exists between the health status of African Americans and whites in the United States as well as in their access to health care. Stroke, cancer, arthritis, diabetes, glaucoma, hypertension, alcoholism, heart disease, and cerebrovascular disease are some of the conditions that have an excess prevalence in African Americans. Life expectancy for African Americans born in 1999 was 6 years lower than that for white Americans. Studies

Family Caregiving Expectations of Some Cultural Groups in the United States

African Americans
- Strong family and kinship networks usually exist, with elder care provided in extended family homes.

American Indians
- Children and grandchildren may provide care for elders.

Chinese Americans
- Elder care is provided by the family with the expectation that the wife becomes part of the husband's family.

Filipinos
- Female family members are expected to provide care at home, and admission of an older person to a nursing home may be viewed as disrespectful.

Japanese Americans
- The family is expected to care for dependent elders.

Koreans
- Elders often live in multigenerational families, with the expectation that the oldest son provides elder care in return for the family inheritance.

Mexican Americans
- Women are expected to care for elders.

Puerto Ricans
- Men and women share responsibilities for elder care in the family.

South Asians
- Elders usually live with a married son and grandchildren; female family members are expected to give care at home.

Source: J. G. Lipson, S. L. Dibble, and P. A. Minarik, (1996), *Culture and nursing care: A pocket guide* (San Francisco: UCSF Nursing Press).

with her grown daughter, and being retired from an unskilled job (Wykle & Kaskel, 1994). Female-headed households are a common family structure, and African American older adults are likely to have a broad base of extended family and social support. Geographically, African Americans live in all states, but their largest populations are in large metropolitan areas and the states of New York, California, Texas, Florida, Georgia, and Illinois. There is a high concentration of African Americans in the South (54%), with 19% living in the Midwest, 18% living in the Northeast, and 10% living in the West. African Americans generally speak standard English, but many also speak black English (Ebonics) or another dialect. Black English is more common in urban areas, whereas Creole dialect is more common in the rural South. In comparison with white older adults, African Americans are more likely to live with their children, grandchildren, or extended family and are less likely to live alone or in a nursing home. African Americans associate good health with harmony in life, and they may view illness as a punishment for sin.

> Mrs. A. is an 81-year-old African American who lives with her daughter, Mildred, and teenaged great-grandson in a two-bedroom apartment in a large metropolitan area of Ohio. Mildred works as a nursing assistant in a nearby nursing home and often works double shifts. Mrs. A. was born in Alabama and lived there until 20 years ago, when her husband died and she moved in with her daughter (who lived alone at the time). Seven years later, Mildred took on responsibility for raising her infant grandson, who is now 13 years old. Mrs. A. has glaucoma, arthritis, and hypertension, and she had a stroke several years ago. She admits to having "a little problem with my memory," but Mildred says "she remembers what she wants to remember." She takes an over-the-counter analgesic as needed for her arthritis and has two prescription medications for hypertension. She also uses prescription eye drops twice daily. Mrs. A. has her blood pressure checked by the parish nurse about once monthly; she sees a doctor and nurse practitioner at a neighborhood clinic for checkups about twice yearly. The parish nurse often tells her that her blood pressure is "a little on the high side" and encourages her to see her doctor, but Mrs. A. has difficulty getting to appointments because she depends on Mildred to take her there. Mrs. A. is about 30 pounds overweight, and she walks very slowly. When she is out of the house, Mildred provides a supportive hand to assist her with steadiness and mobility. Mildred shops for groceries, but Mrs. A. prepares most meals for the family.

suggest that racial differences significantly affect the kind and quality of medical care received, even under the Medicare system. Considerable evidence indicates that systemic discrimination is the most likely explanation for racial disparities in the provision of health care services for older African Americans (Williams & Wilson, 2001). African American older adults are more likely than whites to be impaired in daily activities, and functional declines occur at earlier ages for African Americans than they do for whites. African Americans also have worse self-perceptions of health than do whites. One positive aspect of health differences is that African Americans have a lower rate of osteoporosis than whites.

The "typical" African American elder in the United States can be characterized as poor, female, widowed, separated from her spouse, sharing a home

💭 THINKING POINTS

➤ How might her living arrangements influence Mrs. A.'s health and functioning, both positively and negatively?

➤ What factors are likely to influence the kind of health care Mrs. A. receives?

➤ If you were the parish nurse, what concerns would you have about Mrs. A.'s health?

Hispanics or Latinos

Because the federal government counts race and Hispanic origin as two separate categories, the 2000 census categorizes people by race and by whether or not they are Hispanic or Latino. According to this census data, 12.5% of the total United States population is Hispanic or Latino. A Hispanic or Latino person is a person whose origin is Cuban, Mexican, Puerto Rican, South or Central American, or of other Spanish cultures, regardless of race. Thus, the category of Hispanic includes many heterogeneous groups that immigrated from these countries. Although they have some characteristics in common, they actually represent culturally diverse groups that are categorized together for reasons such as census and research.

Hispanic older adults are divided as follows: 49% Mexican Americans, 15% Cuban, 12% Puerto Rican, and 24% mainly from Central and South American countries (Markides & Miranda, 1997). In the general United States population, although Mexican Americans represent the largest proportion of Hispanics (61%), there are almost three times as many Puerto Ricans (13%) as Cubans (5%). The differences in proportions of younger and older groups of Hispanics can be explained by the immigration patterns of each group.

The initial wave of Mexicans immigrating to America came to what was then the southwest territory during colonial times to build railroads. During the *bracero* period (1940s to 1960s), Mexicans came as agricultural laborers. (*Braceros* were experienced farm laborers who worked in cotton, sugar beet, and other agricultural fields.) The people who came during the bracero period currently comprise the population of older Mexican Americans. Recent Mexican immigrants are younger people, including many who are undocumented immigrants. This group will contribute to the significant increase in older Hispanics that is expected to occur over the next decades (see Figure 2-1).

Cubans initially immigrated to the United States in the late 1800s to work in the tobacco industry, and a second influx occurred between 1940 and 1950 when Cubans came to help with the war industry. The largest number of Cuban immigrants came to the United States between 1959 and 1979 when many middle- and upper-class citizens fled Cuba for political reasons. This accounts for the higher number of older Cubans in relation to younger Cubans.

Puerto Ricans first came to United States in the 1830s and began settling in New York City, but they did not come in great numbers until after World War II. By the 1970s, more than 1 million Puerto Ricans had immigrated to more than 20 cities, motivated primarily by economics, employment, social mobility, and family relationships. Puerto Ricans were granted citizenship status in 1917.

Most Hispanics in the United States are concentrated in major cities in Arizona, California, Florida, New Jersey, New Mexico, New York, and Texas. Despite the significant diversity among these groups, information about them is generally lumped together under the classification of "Hispanics." Health conditions that disproportionately affect Hispanics include diabetes, obesity, malnutrition, and tuberculosis. The rate of heart disease in Mexican Americans is lower than it is in non-Hispanic whites. Like African Americans, Hispanics have lower rates of osteoporosis but higher rates of functional impairments compared with whites. Hispanics have high regard for people by virtue of their age, service, or experience (*respeto*), and this carries over to a strong respect for older people. Hispanic groups have a strong sense of family, and they tend to place the needs of the group or family over those of the individual. Hispanics, like African Americans, are more likely than whites to be living with family or extended family and less likely to be living in a nursing home. Hispanic older Americans, especially those who are Puerto Rican, have higher poverty rates as compared with whites. The educational level of older Hispanics is lower than that of whites or African Americans. Most Hispanics in the United States speak both Spanish and English.

➤ Both Mr. and Mrs. H. are 64-year-old Mexican Americans who came to an urban area of Texas to live with their son, Jose, and daughter-in-law, Maria, about 10 years ago. Mr. and Mrs. H. provide child care for their four grandchildren, while Jose works as a farm laborer and Maria does domestic work. Mr. and Mrs. H. prefer to speak and read in Spanish, and all family members speak Spanish in the home, but they can speak English well enough to communicate when necessary. Jose and Mr. H. each smoke a couple of packs of cigarettes a day. None of the family has health insurance, but this is not of concern to Mr. and Mrs. H. because they have relied on folk healers for many years, and this has been effective for them. In their *curandismo* (traditional healing) system, Mrs. H. is the first person consulted, and she applies the remedies that have been passed on to her from her mother and grandmother. Her remedies are directed toward restoring balance between hot and cold, and she also encourages prayers and lighting of candles at church. In the rare instances when a family member has not gotten better within a couple of days, Mrs. H. takes him or her to a *yerbero* (herbalist) for herbs and other remedies. Once, when Maria had a more serious "female" problem, Mrs. H. took her to a *curandero* (folk healer), who was able to cure the problem.

You are a community health nurse in the county where Mr. and Mrs. H. reside, and you are told to develop a planning committee for a health fair, which is being held at and co-sponsored by the Catholic church attended by many of the community's Mexican Americans. The county health department received a grant from the National Institutes of Health to identify people most at risk for cancer, diabetes, and hypertension as part of the *Healthy People 2010* initiative. At least part of the motivation for receiving this grant was to cut the cost of providing care for people who are not diagnosed until these diseases are advanced. Statistics verify that Hispanics in your county have unusually high rates of diabetes, hypertension, and lung and breast cancer. Statistics also confirm that the cost of treating these conditions is disproportionately high because of complications from untreated and undiagnosed cases. The goal of this health fair, which is part of a larger initiative, is to screen for diabetes and to motivate people to return to future fairs for additional preventive measures. Your target population for this health fair is Hispanic people 45 years of age and older.

 THINKING POINTS

➤ What factors will significantly affect participation in this health fair, both positively and negatively?

➤ What plans would you suggest for overcoming barriers to participation?

➤ Who would you want to be on your committee?

➤ What additional information would you want to have so that you could proceed with planning a successful health fair, and how would you go about finding this information?

Asians and Pacific Islanders

The category of "Asian and Pacific Islanders," like the category of "Hispanics," refers to numerous diverse subgroups of people in the United States who are clustered together for purposes of simplifying data. The 2000 census data distinguish between the Asian population and the Native Hawaiian and Other Pacific Islander population, but previous census data, and much of the available information about subgroups in the United States, lumps together at least 30 subgroups in the one category of "Asian/Pacific Islanders." In the 2000 census, "Asian" refers to people having origins in any of the original peoples of the Far East, Southeast Asia, or the Indian subcontinent (including China, India, Japan, Korea, Thailand, Vietnam, Pakistan, Cambodia, Malaysia, and the Philippine Islands). The largest Asian subgroup in the United States is the Chinese, who account for 30% of the Asian elderly. The next largest groups are the Japanese and Filipinos, each accounting for 24% of the Asian elderly (Williams & Wilson, 2001). Older Chinese and Japanese Americans are the two groups that are represented by both recent immigrants and American-born generations of earlier immigrants. Older Koreans, Vietnamese, Cambodians, and Asian Indians are likely to be recent immigrants to the United States.

The Chinese first migrated as laborers between 1840 and 1882, after which time immigration of Chinese people to America was suspended until 1924 when annual quotas were established. Many of these immigrants came for political or socioeconomic reasons and had little or no education. In 1965, the Quota Act was abolished, and many professional and highly educated Chinese came to the United States. Many Chinese live in metropolitan areas; the states with the largest Chinese populations are California, Hawaii, New York, Illinois, and Texas.

Japanese people began immigrating to America in 1885, and immigration peaked in the early 1900s. In 1924, they were barred from entering the United States, and in 1942, all Japanese people living in the United States were relocated to internment camps. Immigration resumed in the 1950s and increased after 1965 when immigration restrictions were eased. Japanese Americans are the only immigrant group whose members identify themselves according to their generation of birth in the United States. Generation groupings are: *issei*, first-generation immigrants; *nisei*, first American-born generation; *sansei*, third generation; *yonsei*, fourth generation; and *gosei* and *rokusei*, fifth and sixth generations.

Filipinos came to the United States in three waves, beginning in the early 1700s when the "pioneer" group came to New Orleans. This first wave continued through the early 1900s and included agricultural workers in Hawaii and the western states. Beginning in 1934, Filipino immigrants were limited to an annual quota of 50. The second wave of Filipino immigration took place between 1946 and 1965 when the annual quota was raised to 100. During this period, many became United States citizens by joining the armed services or coming as students, professionals, or war brides. The third wave began after quotas were expanded and includes a large proportion of families and young professionals.

Koreans began immigrating to the United States in the 1900s, particularly to Hawaii, where they sought plantation work. Between 1950 and 1965, a second major wave of Koreans came, including many war brides of American servicemen. After 1965, many middle-class and college-educated Koreans, including many health care professionals, came to the United States.

The Vietnamese, who compose the most recent Asian immigrant group, began arriving in the mid-1970s seeking political refuge because of the Vietnam War. Second and third waves of Vietnamese, Cambodians, and Laotians have come to the United States as refugees, including many older adults and other extended family members.

Despite the great diversity among Asian and Pacific Islander groups, some general characteristics may be summarized. Asian and Pacific Islanders cultures are very family oriented and place a strong value on care of older family members. Asian older adults are less likely to live alone than the older population in general in the United States. Most American-born Asians speak English, but some immigrants speak only their native language or are bilingual. In Asian cultures, health is viewed as a state of spiritual and physical harmony, and illness occurs when the yin and yang are out of balance. Yin refers to female energy and is associated with wet, cold, and dark; yang refers to male energy and is associated with dry, hot, and light. Asian and Pacific Islanders have an excess prevalence of diabetes, hypertension, certain cancers, thalassemias (anemia), hepatitis B and other liver diseases, and tuberculosis (including multidrug-resistant strains). They have a lower rate of osteoporosis than whites.

➤ Mrs. C. is a 76-year-old Chinese American widow who lives in an apartment in the Chinatown section of San Francisco. She has lived within the same 1-mile radius since her parents brought her to the United States from Mainland China when she was 9 years old. All three of her children are married; two live about an hour away, and the other one lives on the East Coast. Although she can speak and read English, she prefers to use her native Chinese dialect, and all of her reading materials are in Chinese. She completed a high school education in Chinatown and married a Chinese immigrant when she was 19 years old. She served as her husband's primary caregiver after he developed lung cancer several years ago until his death last year.

Mrs. C. is enrolled in the On Lok Senior Health Program, a health maintenance organization that provides a wide range of health and social services. She attends a daily meal program and sees the nurse at the center for blood pressure checks every month. She has hypertension, arthritis, and coronary artery disease. Mrs. C. sees a local herbalist every few weeks to obtain the herbal medicines that will keep her yin and yang energies in balance, and she chooses foods according to their yin and yang characteristic to keep her energies balanced. She periodically has acupuncture treatments when her arthritis bothers her. Although Mrs. C. believes she can control her heart problem and high blood pressure with herbs and diet, she takes her two medications as prescribed because the nurse at the On Lok clinic has emphasized that these pills are essential for keeping her energy in balance.

Mrs. C. recently had a stroke and received medical treatment and rehabilitation services. She is being discharged to her apartment with a referral to the On Lok home care services for skilled nursing and speech, physical, and occupational therapies. Discharge orders also include the need to instruct Mrs. C. in a low-sodium diet. In addition to having some aphasia and left-sided paralysis, Mrs. C. has some residual memory impairment from the stroke. Before discharge from the rehabilitation program, she said she would not need any home health aide assistance because she expected that her daughter and daughter-in-law would take turns coming over every day and that they would take care of her. You are the nurse assigned to do the initial assessment, and your visit is scheduled for the day after discharge when the daughter-in-law will be there. Although you have been a visiting nurse for several years, you have recently moved to San Francisco, and you began working for On Lok 2 weeks ago.

 THINKING POINTS

➤ What cultural factors might influence Mrs. C.'s acceptance of you, as the skilled care nurse, and of home care services in general?

➤ What would you do to prepare yourself to work with Mrs. C. and other patients in the On Lok health care program?

➤ What strategies would you use to develop an effective and acceptable care plan?

American Indians and Alaska Natives

In the 2000 United States census, the phrase "American Indian and Alaska Native" was used in reference to people having origins in any of the original peoples of North and South America (including Central America) and who maintain a tribal affiliation or community attachment. Native Hawaiians are sometimes categorized as Native Americans, but this is not done consistently, and the 2000 census designates

Native Hawaiians and Other Pacific Islanders as a distinct group. In the United States, there are more than 500 federally recognized American Indian and Native Alaskan tribes and an additional 100 to 200 native societies (unrecognized tribes). American Indians are the only minority group indigenous to the United States. Census 2000 reports that of all the American Indian respondents, 43% lived in the West, 31% in the South, 17% in the Midwest, and 9% in the Northeast. Twenty-five percent of the American Indian population lives in California and Oklahoma, and another 37% lives in Arizona, Texas, New Mexico, New York, Washington, North Carolina, Michigan, Alaska, and Florida.

The typical American Indian elder is poor, has less than a high school education, and lives in a rural area with family or alone. Younger American Indians are likely to speak English, but older American Indians may speak little or no English and are likely instead to speak one of the more than 150 indigenous languages that continue to be spoken. American Indians have the highest prevalence of diabetes and the lowest cancer survival rate of any group. Diabetes is a significant health problem among American Indians, as manifested by high rates of complications such as blindness, lower extremity amputations, and end-stage renal disease. In some American Indian communities, as many as half of all adults have diabetes; the overall rate of diabetes in American Indians aged 65 years and older is almost 21%. Other diseases that are more prevalent among American Indians include cancer, obesity, arthritis, cataracts, alcoholism, tuberculosis, kidney disease, rheumatoid arthritis, and liver and gallbladder disease. American Indians also have a higher-than-average risk for dying from accidents such as falls, fires, and motor vehicle accidents. Compared with whites, they are more likely to have functional impairments and require assistance with daily activities.

> Mrs. I. is a 72-year-old Navajo who lives with her daughter and son-in-law. Like other Navajos, Mrs. I. believes that health is closely linked with being in harmony with the environment, family members, and supernatural forces. She regularly attends native healing ceremonies and protects her family and herself from sickness through songs, stories, rituals, prayers, and sand paintings. Mrs. I.'s mother kept a medicine bundle, called a *jish,* containing stones, feathers, arrowheads, and corn pollen and used this for healing and blessings. Mrs. I.'s older sister now uses the jish that was passed on from their mother. Mrs. I. has had diabetes and hypertension for several years and is about 30 pounds over her ideal weight. She receives medical care at the Indian Health Service, where you are the nurse. During a recent visit, you find that Mrs. I.'s blood pressure was 164/98 mm Hg and that her random blood sugar as measured on the glucometer was 196 mg/dL. You know from previous visits that Mrs. I. does not want to take any prescription medications because she thinks they are not in harmony with spiritual forces. When you explain that both her blood sugar and blood pressure are high, she promises you that she will ask her older sister to use the jish for healing. You know from your experience with the Indian Health Service that nurses have been successful in persuading Navajos to perform physical exercise if it is viewed in a larger cultural context. For example, American Indians at a community health center were receptive to incorporating mild aerobic exercise into their daily routines in the form of traditional dance movements, when the nurse consulted a tribal leader in developing the program.

 THINKING POINTS

> What cultural factors are likely to influence Mrs. I.'s understanding of diabetes and hypertension?

> How might you explain diabetes and hypertension to Mrs. I.?

> What questions would you ask Mrs. I. in order to identify teaching strategies and other interventions that might be successful with regard to her diabetes and hypertension?

> What strategies are likely to be successful in implementing dietary and lifestyle interventions for Mrs. I.?

> What steps would you take to improve your cultural competence in working with Mrs. I.?

OLDER ADULTS IN OTHER DIVERSE COMMUNITIES

In addition to exploring the unique needs of older adults of various ethnic backgrounds, recent gerontological literature also examines the needs of other diverse groups, such as those living in rural areas and homeless older adults. Although most gerontological nurses do not provide care for rural or homeless older adults, they should recognize the numerous, highly diverse subculture groups of older adults who have unique health care needs.

Older Adults in Rural Areas

"Rural" is generally used in reference to people who live outside areas designated as "urban" or "metropolitan" and is determined by population density. Estimates of the percentage of older adults living in rural areas range from one fourth to one third, with only a small minority of these living in farming regions. In many rural areas, older adults constitute more than 20% of the population, in contrast to 12.4% of the population in the entire United States. Although significant local differences exist among rural areas and generalizing about rural elders is difficult, some common characteristics and needs have been identified. Rural elders are usually socioeconomically disadvantaged and have poor housing, higher poverty rates, and less formal education. They are likely to have disabilities associated with arthritis, diabetes, and heart and respiratory diseases. Rural older adults are self-reliant and politically conservative; they are likely to have strong bonds with family, church, and community (Rosswurm, 2001). Because of their geographic remoteness, access to health care is often a problem for rural older adults, and they are more likely to have difficulty getting to the few health care services that are available. A 10-year series of ethnographic studies of a rural subculture of elders, their families, and their health care providers in Colorado identified major cultural themes applicable to health care services for rural older adults. These themes included: (1) availability of significant circles of formal and informal care; (2) a strong integration of faith, spirituality, and family with health status; (3) crisis-oriented decision making during health care transitions; and (4) use of nursing homes as a housing option because of few alternatives (Congdon & Magilvy, 2001).

Appalachia is a specific federally defined rural nonfarming region of the United States that was established by an Act of Congress in 1965. The region spans more than 1000 miles across 13 states, including Ohio, Georgia, Virginia, Alabama, Mississippi, Pennsylvania, New York, and South Carolina. Much of the designated area lies in mountainous territory, causing geographic isolation and lack of access to health care. Appalachian people have been characterized as white, of British or Scotch-Irish descent, and predominantly fundamentalist Protestant religion. Appalachia has a higher poverty rate and lower levels of formal education than the general population. Appalachian families maintain strong bonds, and older family members are honored for their role in transmitting their culture to younger generations. Older family members are likely to live with or very close to their children.

Appalachian people may be reluctant to seek medical care, particularly in a hospital, because they view the hospital as a place to go to die. Similarly, they may be reluctant to use rehabilitative services because they tend to view illness as the will of God and disability as an inevitable consequence of aging. Appalachians are likely to believe that members of the community are called as servants to minister to

people who are disabled and their families (Horton, 1984). These beliefs can present challenges for gerontological nurses and other health care professionals who are attempting to address preventive, rehabilitative, or health promotion needs. One study found that 85% of Appalachian clinic patients were lacking in at least one of six preventive measures; these patients identified cost and lack of knowledge as the primary reasons for omitting the measures. An additional finding from this study is that 72% of those who lacked at least one preventive measure indicated they would obtain the measure if barriers were removed (Elnicki et al., 1995).

Homeless Older Adults

The category of "older homeless" typically extends downward to the age of 50 years because some researchers have observed that homeless people look and behave as if they were 10 to 20 years older than their actual ages and have significant health problems (Brush, 2001). Increased homelessness among older adults is associated with increased poverty rates among certain segments and declining availability of affordable housing. Homeless people aged 65 years and older are entitled to Medicare and Social Security benefits, but homeless people between the ages of 50 and 64 years usually do not qualify for these benefits unless they have been disabled for 2 years. Health characteristics of the homeless elderly include significantly higher mortality rates, higher levels of disability, and higher overall rates of chronic illnesses and mental illness than younger homeless adults or older adults who are not homeless (Brush, 2001). Since the mid-1980s, social service and health care providers have recognized the need to provide rehabilitative services to address health, social, and behavioral problems of homeless elders, in addition to addressing their basic needs for food and shelter. Services that have been developed in recent years specifically for older homeless people include resettlement and rehabilitation programs, drop-in and day care centers, and a variety of long-term housing options (Warnes & Crane, 2000).

CONTINUUM OF LIVING ARRANGEMENTS FOR OLDER ADULTS

Living arrangements for older adults are significantly influenced by such factors as health, family relationships, and socioeconomic conditions. Health is likely to be the most significant variable, particularly in relation to functional levels and abilities to meet one's daily needs. Older people who are able to meet their basic needs with little or no help are likely to live alone or with a spouse. For people who are dependent on others for their daily needs, the willingness and availability of a caregiver is the factor that most strongly determines whether they remain at home or move to a nursing facility. About 90% of the older adult population in the United States lives in houses or apartments, with the remaining 10% about equally divided between nursing facilities and facilities that provide some assistance with daily needs. Data from the 2000 census reveals, for the first time in several decades, a decline in the percentage of people 65 years and over living in nursing homes (from 5.1% in 1990 to 4.5% in 2000). This decline occurred in all age subgroups but was most marked for the group aged 85 years and older, in which the number of people in nursing homes declined from 24.5% in 1990 to 18.2% in 2000. Similarly, the percentage of women aged 75 years and older who live alone increased during the past several decades from 37% in 1970 to 53% in 1998; for men aged 75 years and older during this same period, the percentage increased from 19% to 22%.

Reasons for these changing trends in living arrangements include improved health and functioning, especially for people aged 75 years and older, as well as a broader range of community-based services to provide assistance to people who need help with daily activities but wish to remain in their own homes. Community-based services have been provided through public and private agencies for many decades, and the range of these services is continually broadening. For example, home-delivered meals programs have been available in most metropolitan areas for decades, and in recent years, a variety of home-delivered groceries and prepared meals have become available for delivery within 24 hours through Internet sites or toll-free phone numbers. Although community-based services are widely available, only about one fifth of older adults take advantage of these programs (Anetzberger, 2002). Older adults and their caregivers often are not aware of the great variety of services available to meet the health needs of older adults in their own homes. Even when they are aware of the availability of such services, they may not know the eligibility criteria for publicly funded services to which they are entitled. Also, if community-based services are not culturally relevant, older adults or their families may not use them, even when they are aware of their existence. Because the use of these resources may improve the health, functioning, and quality of life of the older adult, nurses need to address any lack of information about these services. Also, nurses need to assess barriers to the use of community services, as discussed in Chapter 10. Nurses in all settings have many opportunities to suggest the use of the community-based services that are described in Display 2-1.

DISPLAY 2-1
Community Resources for Older Adults

National Eldercare Locator (800-677-1116). This program provides free information about state or local resources in any part of the United States according to the zip code of the location where services are desired. This is a collaborative project of the U.S. Administration on Aging, the National Association of Area Agencies on Aging, and the National Association of State Units on Aging.

Senior Information and Referral Service. This service is often listed in the front of telephone directories under the heading "Community Services" and is sometimes referred to as "Infoline." Callers are given the names of agencies that might address their needs.

Area Agency on Aging. Funded through state, county, and local resources, these agencies provide a range of services. Some area agencies on aging employ social workers and registered nurses to make assessments and provide supportive services (e.g., referrals, case management, assistance with daily living needs). Eligibility for these services is based on economic need and the ability to address the safety and quality-of-life needs of older people living in their home environment.

Senior Centers. Sometimes the sites for hot meals, these community centers provide social, educational, and recreational programs for older adults.

Home-Delivered Meals. This program provides daily home delivery of hot meals to homebound people. Fees generally are based on a sliding scale. Special dietary needs can sometimes be addressed.

Companions and Friendly Visitors. Volunteers visit homebound older adults in their homes. Some also do errands or provide escort service to community activities.

Telephone Reassurance. Volunteers make scheduled, usually daily (sometimes more frequent) telephone calls to older people to provide support and reality orientation.

Personal Emergency Response Systems. This type of program is a home emergency response system that initiates a phone call to designated people when it is activated by a remote-control device. Public funding is available in some areas to assist low-income older adults in acquiring such a system.

Energy Assistance Programs. State and local programs offer financial assistance for utility bills for qualifying people. Older adults should check with local utility companies or the local office on aging.

Home Weatherization and Home Repair Service. Home repairs and maintenance (e.g., insulation, window caulking, and installation) are provided for low-income people by contractors paid by government agencies.

In addition to the growth of community-based services for people who live in their own homes, a wide range of housing options has evolved in recent decades to address the needs of the growing number of older adults who require assistance with their daily needs but do not need full-time care. For example, life-care and continuing-care retirement communities provide a wide range of integrated and comprehensive services addressing health and social needs. Older adults typically enter this type of residential setting when they are relatively healthy and independent, but the arrangement guarantees that their health needs will be met at the most appropriate level until their death. Residents initially reside in an apartment or single home and move to assisted living, skilled nursing, or other areas within the large complex as their needs change. Cost of care is covered primarily through a combination of the entrance fee, a monthly service fee, and long-term care insurance. Some aspects of care may require fee-for-service payment, and some nursing care services may be covered by Medicare and Medicaid. The continuing-care retirement community model provides the most comprehensive type of care, but there are significant financial and other barriers to their use.

Assisted-living facilities have become very popular in recent years and are available in most areas of the country. Although the services provided by these facilities vary widely, basic services generally include a single residential unit, at least one daily meal, and 24-hour availability of assistance. People who live in assisted-living facilities usually need help with three or more daily activities, and some facilities are designed specifically for people who have cognitive impairments. Residence in an assisted-living facility generally costs less than nursing home care or extensive home care services, but it is usually not covered by Medicaid. In recent years, assisted-living facilities have come to be seen as cost-effective ways of providing care to people who otherwise would need care in nursing facilities. Because there is no consistent licensure or regulation of these facilities, however, states have been reluctant to provide Medicaid funds for assisted-living care. Consequently, most people who live in these facilities pay out-of-pocket and move to a nursing facility when their funds are exhausted. This is likely to change in the near future because there is growing recognition of the need for public financial support of this type of facility. Most states are currently considering implementing regulations and licensing for assisted-living facilities, and the Joint Commission for the Accreditation of Healthcare Organizations (JCAHO) began accreditation for assisted-living facilities in 2001.

Because the range of housing options as well as community-based services is rapidly increasing, decisions about staying in one's own home or moving to another type of living facility are becoming more complex. Older adults and their families are likely to seek information and guidance from health care professionals, and nurses need to be aware of these options so that they can educate older adults and their families about their choices. Display 2-2 describes various housing options for older adults that are available in most parts of the United States. It is important to keep in mind that this is one of the most rapidly evolving areas of program development for older adults. Nurses can keep up to date on developments by consulting the Educational Resources listed at the end of this chapter. It is also important to recognize that the continuum of care for older adults includes not just housing options, but, even more importantly, a wide variety of health care services. These services are discussed at length in the chapters in Part 2, which focus on older adults in health care settings.

> Mr. and Mrs. W. are 72 and 74 years old, respectively, and have lived in the same home for 43 years in the same geographic area where you currently live. Their house has three bedrooms and one bathroom on the second floor, and a laundry room and storage area in the basement. The first floor consists of a living room, a large dining room, and a small kitchen with an eat-in dining area. Mr. W. recently had a stroke and is now hemiplegic. He was discharged from a rehabilitation setting several months ago and has been using a hospital bed in the dining room. He gets sponge baths and uses a urinal and bedside commode. Despite months of therapy, he has been unable to regain the ability to go up and down stairs. He has not been out of the house since his stroke, but his son says that he can build a ramp from the back door so that his father can get out in his wheelchair. You have been their visiting nurse and will be discharging Mr. W. because he no longer needs any skilled services. As part of your discharge plan, you need to discuss community resources and housing options to address Mr. and Mrs. W.'s needs. You know they have about $29,000 in savings, they own their home, and their monthly income is about $2,000.

 THINKING POINTS

> Which of the types of services in Display 2-1 would be most appropriate for Mr. and Mrs. W.?

> What additional services might be appropriate for Mr. and Mrs. W. if they wish to stay in their own home?

> What local phone numbers would you give to Mr. and Mrs. W. so that they can obtain further information about community-based services in your geographic area?

> ### DISPLAY 2-2
> *Housing Options for Older Adults*

Family Residence or Apartment. The older person may own, rent, or live with a family member who owns or rents. He or she lives alone, with a spouse or significant other, or with other, often younger, family members. If assistance is needed, the family provides it, or services are provided by outsiders.

Homecare Suite. A fully accessible, modular apartment is installed in the attached garage of a caregiver's home. The unit is fully insulated and contains its own water, heating, and air conditioning systems. It can be purchased, rented, or leased for whatever length of time it is needed.

Foster Care or Board-and-Care Home. The older person lives with unrelated people in a private home. Each resident has a private or shared bedroom and shared use of common space, such as a living room and dining room. The foster family or board-and-care operator usually provides meals, housekeeping, and supervision of, or assistance with, basic and instrumental activities of daily living.

Shared Housing. The older person shares a house or apartment with one or more unrelated people. Each occupant has a private or semiprivate bedroom and shares the rest of the dwelling, expenses, and chores. Offices on aging may coordinate these programs and provide some services.

Congregate Housing. Older people occupy individual apartments within a specially designed, multiunit dwelling.

Supportive services, such as meals, housekeeping, transportation, and social and recreational activities, are provided.

Retirement Community. Self-sufficient older people live in a specially designed residential development with owned or rented units. Recreational programs and support services (e.g., transportation, laundry, and housekeeping) are usually available.

Life-Care or Continuing-Care Retirement Community. Older adults reside in a residential complex that has been designed to provide a full range of services and accommodations to meet each resident's needs as they change. The development includes independent housing, congregate housing, assisted living, and nursing home care. Each resident usually pays a significant fee and enters into a contract with the organization. This legal agreement guarantees lodging, nursing services, and other health-related services for a specified term or for the remainder of the resident's life. Strict admission criteria may apply.

Assisted-Living Facility. Older adults live in their own apartment (usually one or two rooms and a bathroom), and they share common areas for meals and social activities. One to three meals a day are provided. Assistance with laundry, housekeeping, transportation, personal care, and medication administration usually is available, as is some degree of protective supervision and 24-hour emergency services. Fees vary depending on the number of services used, and service agreements may be adjusted as the needs of the resident change.

> ➤ If Mr. and Mrs. W. asked you for information about different housing options, how would you use information in Display 2-2 to discuss the advantages and disadvantages of different living arrangements?
>
> ➤ What local phone numbers would you give to Mr. and Mrs. W. so that they can obtain further information about housing options that are within an hour of where they live?

OLDER ADULTS IN THE WORLD

Because of the recent and continuing expansion of communication technology, people in the United States have extraordinary access to information about the entire world. This unprecedented access to information has resulted in international cooperation and a growing interest in sharing knowledge about issues that affect people in different societies. Major international initiatives have been developed with the goals of sharing information and developing plans to meet identified needs of older adults throughout the world. The first major initiative took place in 1982, when the first

World Assembly on Ageing developed and promulgated an *International Plan of Action on Ageing*, which included 62 recommendations about issues affecting aging of individuals and aging of the global population (United Nations, 1982). The United Nations designated 1999 as "The Year of the Older Person" in recognition of the global population aging. The most recent major initiative was the Second World Assembly on Ageing, which took place in March 2002. This assembly reaffirmed the principles and recommendations of the 1982 action plan and adopted an *International Plan of Action on Ageing 2002,* with the intent of responding to the opportunities and challenges of population aging in the 21st century and promoting the development of a society for all ages (Display 2-3). The Plan of Action on Ageing 2002 addresses 62 recommendations to achieve the objectives; one major priority area of this plan is advancing health and well-being into old age (United Nations, 2002).

Profile of World Population Aging

The attribute that best describes older adults in the United States is their great degree of diversity. Although this applies even more so to older adults in

> **DISPLAY 2-3**
> *Selected Health-Related Objectives and Recommendations from the International Plan of Action on Ageing, 2002*
>
> **Objective 1: Reduce the cumulative effects of factors that increase the risk for disease and potential dependency in older age**
>
> - Give priority to poverty eradication policies to improve the health status of poor and marginalized older people.
> - Set gender-specific targets to improve the health status of older persons and reduce disability and mortality.
> - Identify and address environmental and socioeconomic factors that contribute to disease and disability in later life.
> - Focus health promotion, health education, and prevention policies and information campaigns on major known risk factors associated with unhealthy diet, physical inactivity, and other unhealthy behaviors.
> - Take comprehensive action to prevent the abuse of alcohol and to reduce tobacco use and the involuntary exposure to tobacco smoke.
> - Promote safe use of all medications
>
> **Objective 2: Develop policies to prevent ill-health among older persons**
>
> - Design early interventions to prevent or delay the onset of disease and disability.
> - Ensure that gender-specific primary prevention and screening programs are available and affordable to older persons.
> - Provide training and incentives for health care professionals to teach older persons about self-care and healthy lifestyles.
> - Prevent falls and other unintentional injuries by developing a better understanding of their causes and by implementing prevention programs.
> - Encourage older people to maintain or adopt an active and healthy lifestyle, including physical activity and sport.
>
> **Objective 3: Ensure access to food and adequate nutrition for all older persons**
>
> - Ensure a safe and nutritionally adequate food supply at both national and international levels.
> - Promote lifelong healthy and adequate nutrition, with particular attention to ensuring that specific nutritional needs of men and women throughout the life course are met.
> - Pay particular attention to nutritional deficiency and associated diseases in the design and implementation of health promotion and prevention programs for older people.
> - Educate older persons about specific nutritional needs, including adequate intakes of water, calories, protein, vitamins, and minerals.
> - Promote affordable dental services to prevent and treat disorders that can impede eating and cause malnutrition.
> - Ensure appropriate and adequate provision of accessible nutrition and food for older persons in hospital and other care settings.
>
> *Source:* United Nations. (2002). *International plan of action on ageing 2002.* New York: United Nations.

the global community, some trends and commonalities have been identified in recent years. Most discussions of global aging describe countries and regions as either "developing" or "developed," or as "more developed" or "less developed." Developed regions include Japan, Europe, Australia, North America, and New Zealand; developing regions include all the countries of Africa, Melanesia, Micronesia, Polynesia, Latin America and the Caribbean, and Asia (excluding Japan) (Hayward & Zhang, 2001). It is now widely recognized that the aging of the population that has taken place in recent decades in developed countries also is occurring in developing countries, but at different rates and proportions. It is also widely agreed that the continuing trend in all countries is toward increasing aging of the population.

For many decades, Europe has had the highest proportion of older people, and this is not likely to change. In 1995, about 20% of Western and Southern Europe's populations were 60 years of age or older, with Sweden and Italy having the highest percentages. Worldwide, Greece had the highest percentage (22.1%), whereas less developed regions had the lowest percentage (about 7%). Projections for 2050 indicate that the percentage of the world population aged 60 years or older will be about 21%, similar to that of Europe today (Hayward & Zhang, 2001). Figure 2-2 is a graphical representation of the percentages of people 65 years and older worldwide.

Gerontologists are particularly interested in variations in life expectancy by country because this information contains clues about many of the factors that influence longevity. The highest level of life expectancy is 80 years in Japan; Sweden, Canada, Australia, and Switzerland are some of the countries with an average life expectancy of 79 years. Some developing nations (e.g., Israel, Singapore, and Costa Rica) have life expectancy rates that match or exceed those of many developed countries, but most developing countries have a life expectancy of less than 45 years. The average gap in life expectancy between

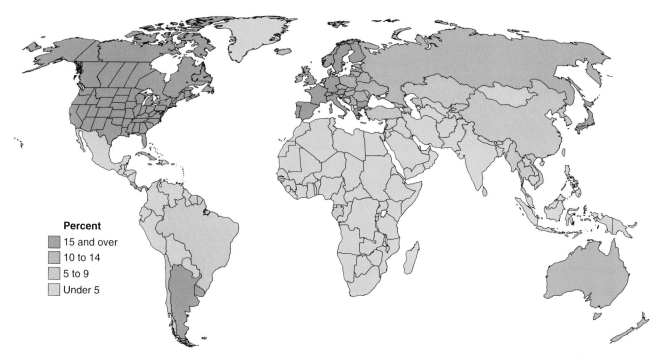

FIGURE 2-2 Percentage of population age 65 years and older: 2000. (From United States Census Bureau, International Data Base; Census 2000 Summary File 1.)

developed and developing nations is 13 years (Kinsella, 2000).

Discussions of global aging usually describe population trends in relation to both fertility (birth) rates and mortality (death) rates. High fertility and low mortality rates result in populations that are younger in age and increasing in number, whereas low fertility and low mortality rates give rise to populations that are older in age and stable or slow-growing in number. An analysis of population age structures around the world since 1950 and projected to 2050 indicates that there have been wide gaps in both fertility and mortality rates between developed and developing nations. Fertility and mortality rates have been declining worldwide, but the declines are greatest in developing countries; thus, these gaps are gradually narrowing. For example, fertility rates for the most and least developed regions in 1950 were 2.8 and 6.5; in 1950, these rates were 1.7 and 5.5; and by 2050, fertility rates for all regions are projected to be 2.1. Similarly, life expectancy—an indicator of mortality rates-has been increasing in all regions, but the magnitude has been greatest in the least developed regions. The end result of these expected demographic trends is that the same demographic revolution that has caused the aging of populations in developed countries will cause the aging of populations in developing countries. One difference, however, is that the trends toward population aging are even more dramatic in developing countries than they have been in developed countries; consequently, by 2050, there

will be little or no international differences in fertility and mortality (Hayward & Zhang, 2001). Another consequence of current demographic trends is that by mid-century, the worldwide proportion of people aged 60 years and older will be about equal to the number of children.

Life expectancy at birth varies significantly by gender, and these differences are largest in the more developed countries. The gap has been widening in European and North American countries since the 1900s; the widest gender gap is in the former Soviet Union, where female life expectancy is 13 years longer than that of men. In developed countries, the gender gap is about 7 years, and in developing countries, it ranges between 3 and 6 years. In a few South Asian and Middle Eastern societies, the gender difference in life expectancy is higher for men than women; this is thought to be associated with cultural factors such as low female status and a preference for male offspring (Kinsella, 2000). Figure 2-3 illustrates differences in life expectancy for men and women in developed and developing regions in 1950, in 1995, and projected for 2050. It is clear from looking at this graph that gaps are narrowing because life expectancies are increasing at different rates. A related trend is that the proportions of older men to older women differ, with greater differences in more developed countries. Current sex ratios, in developing and developed countries, respectively, are 88 and 71 men per 100 women. Projections for 2050 suggest that the gap between developing and developed

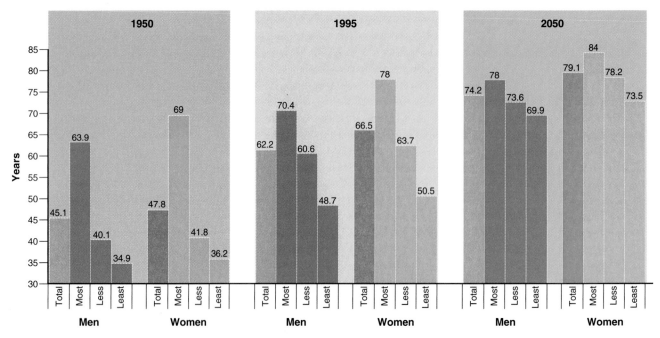

FIGURE 2-3 Actual and projected life expectancies in the most, less, and least developed regions. (From United Nations. [1996]. *World population prospects: The 1996 revision.* New York: Department for Economic and Social Information and Policy Analysis, Population Division.)

countries will narrow and the ratios will be 87 and 78 (United Nations, 2002).

In recent years, much attention has focused on questions about active (healthy) life expectancy, the number of years a person lives in good health. In 1998, 49 nations had estimates of active life expectancy, and long-term data were available for many developed nations. Studies clearly indicate a trend toward diminished disability and improved functioning in older adults, with no developed countries experiencing declines in active life expectancy (Hayward & Zhang, 2001; Kinsella, 2000). Similar data are not currently available for developing countries.

Another demographic trend that has implications for global aging is the differences in living arrangements of older people in developing and developed countries. The overwhelming majority of older persons in developed countries live in urban areas, but the majority of older people in developing countries live in rural areas. Projections suggest that the proportion of older people living in rural areas in developing countries is likely to increase (United Nations, 2002). Another significant difference in living arrangements is that in developing countries, a large proportion of older people live in multigenerational households. A recent study of living arrangements of older adults in 43 developing countries found that most older adults in these countries live in large households and are likely to be living with an adult child, who is more likely to be male than female

(Bongaarts & Zimmer, 2002). Bongaarts and Zimmer also found a strong association between higher levels of education and the likelihood of living alone or in smaller households.

In summary, the following statistics from the United Nations (2002) provide a brief profile of world aging in the early 2000s:

- The number of people in the world aged 60 years and older will increase from about 600,000,000 in 2000 to almost 2,000,000,000 by 2050.
- The fastest growing group of the older population is the group of people aged 80 years and older.
- The proportion of older adults is projected to increase globally from 10% in 1998 to 15% by 2025.
- In Europe, the proportion of older adults will increase from 20% in 1998 to 28% in 2025.
- Increases in the numbers of older adults will occur more dramatically in developing countries, where the older population is expected to quadruple in the next 50 years.
- By mid-century, the old and young will represent equal proportions of the world population.

World Aging and Health Issues

Health issues affecting world populations are similar to those affecting people in the United States. Throughout the world, health care providers are focusing on assuring quality of life to accompany the extended quantity of life that is taking place in all population groups. There is increasing recognition of the need to focus on the chronic conditions that affect functioning as well as on those conditions that cause death. In 1982, the United Nations recognized the importance of health promotion measures directed toward combating the detrimental effects of premature aging (United Nations, 1982). Specific recommendations of the *International Plan of Action on Ageing* addressing health concerns stated:

> *The care of elderly persons should involve their total well-being, taking into account the interdependence of the physical, mental, social, spiritual and environmental factors. Health care should therefore involve the health and social sectors and the family in improving the quality of life of older persons. . . . The promotion of health, the prevention of disease and the maintaining of functional capacities among elderly persons should be actively pursued. . . . A very important question concerns the possibilities of preventing or at least postponing the negative functional consequences of ageing. Many life-style factors may have their most pronounced effects during old age when the reserve capacity usually is lower. (*United Nations, 1982, Recommendations 2, 11, 14)*

Twenty years later, the United Nations reaffirmed the principles and recommendations of the 1982 *International Plan* and expanded the recommendations. The political declaration of the Second World Assembly made a commitment to "provide older persons with universal and equal access to healthcare and services including physical and mental health services and we recognize that the growing needs of an ageing population require additional policies, in particular care and treatment, the promotion of healthy lifestyles and supportive environments" (United Nations, 2002, Article 12). The detailed discussion of health issues emphasized that health promotion and disease prevention activities throughout life need to focus on maintaining independence, preventing and delaying the onset of disease and disability, and improving the quality of life of older persons who already have disabilities. Discussion further emphasized that the leading causes of disease, disability, and mortality in older persons can be alleviated through health promotion and disease prevention measures that focus on nutrition, physical activity, and smoking cessation (United Nations, 2002). All of the recommendations promulgated in the *International Plan on Ageing 2002* are applicable to people in all countries and regions of the world.

CHAPTER SUMMARY

Population trends that most significantly affect older adults in the United States today include increasing numbers of multigenerational families, increasing numbers of older adults who are assuming responsibility for raising their grandchildren, and greater-than-ever diversity of family constellations. In addition, the growing cultural diversity in the United States significantly influences the provision of health care and other services to older adults. Other aspects of diversity among older adults include the unique needs of rural and homeless elders. Nurses and other health care providers need to become knowledgeable about numerous diverse groups of older adults in order to provide culturally appropriate health care. The range of community-based services and housing options is rapidly growing to meet the varied and multiple needs of older adults, as summarized in Displays 2-1 and 2-2. World population trends are of increasing interest to health care providers because communication technology has nearly eliminated boundaries between peoples of the world. Wide gaps have existed between the most and least developed countries in health indicators such as life expectancy, but these gaps are narrowing. The United Nations' *International Plan of Action on Ageing 2002* provides valuable guidelines for addressing health-related issues of older adults; these are just as applicable in the United States as they are in other countries (see Display 2-3.)

 CRITICAL THINKING EXERCISES

1. Identify the culturally diverse groups of older adults that you are likely to work with if you practice gerontological nursing in your current geographic area. Contact the agencies and organizations that serve these groups and find out what services they offer; ask about unique health care issues affecting these particular groups.
2. Go to the Internet site of one of the culturally specific organizations and find information that you might use if you were presenting a health education program to a group of older adults who are of a particular cultural background (e.g., Chinese, African American).

EDUCATIONAL RESOURCES

Association of Asian Pacific Community Organizations
439 23rd Street, Oakland, CA 94612
(510) 272-9536
http://www.aapcho.org

Culture and Nursing Care: A Pocket Guide
UCSF Nursing Press
Box 0608, San Francisco, CA 94143
(415) 476-4992
http://www.ucsf.edu

National Alliance for Hispanic Health
1501 Sixteenth Street NW, Washington, DC, 20036
(202) 387-5000
http://www.hispanichealth.org

National Asian Pacific Center on Aging
P.O. Box 21668, Seattle, WA 98101
(206) 624-1221
http://www.napca.org

National Caucus and Center on Black Aged, Inc.
1401 New York Avenue NW, Suite 1100, Washington,
   DC 20005
(202) 638-6222
http://www.ncba-aged.org

National Hispanic Council on Aging
2713 Ontario Road NW, Washington, DC 20009
(202) 265-1288
http://www.nhcoa.org

National Indian Council on Aging
10501 Montgomery Boulevard NE, Suite 210, Albuquerque,
   NM 87111
(505) 292-2001
http://www.nicoa.org

National Resource Center on Native American Aging
P.O. Box 9037, Grand Forks, ND 58202-9037
(701) 777-3437
http://www.medical.nodak.edu/crh/nrcnaa

National Rural Health Association
One West Armour Boulevard, Suite 203, Kansas City,
   MO 64111
(816) 756-3140
http://www.nrharural.org

Native Elder Health Care Resource Center
University of Colorado Health Sciences Center
P.O. Box 6508, Mailstop F800, Aurora, CO 80045
http://www.uchsc.edu/ai/nehcrc/

Office of Minority Health Resource Center
P.O. Box 37337, Washington, DC 20013
(800) 444-6472
http://www.omhrc.gov

Organization of Chinese Americans
1001 Connecticut Avenue NW, #601, Washington, DC 20036
(202) 223-5500
http://www.ocanatl.org

Statistics Canada
R. H. Coats Building, Holland Avenue, Ottawa,
   ON K1A OT6
(800) 263-1136
http://www.statcan.ca

United Nations Programme on Ageing
Department of Economic and Social Affairs, United Nations,
   New York, NY 10017
http://www.un.org/esa/socdev/

REFERENCES

Anetzberger, G. A. (2002). Community resources to promote successful aging. *Clinics in Geriatric Medicine, 18,* 611–626.

Barker, J. C. (2002). Neighbors, friends, and other nonkin caregivers of community-living dependent elders. *Journal of Gerontology: Social Sciences, 57,* S158–S167.

Bongaarts, J., & Zimmer, Z. (2002). Living arrangements of older adults in the developing world: An analysis of demographic and health survey household surveys. *Journal of Gerontology: Social Sciences, 57,* SS145–S157.

Brush, B. (2001). Homelessness. In M. D. Mezey (Ed.), *The encyclopedia of elder care* (pp. 354–355). New York: Springer.

Congdon, J. G., & Magilvy, J. K. (2001). Themes of rural health and aging from a program of research. *Geriatric Nursing, 22,* 234–238.

Davidhizar, R., Bechtel, G. A., & Woodring, B. C. (2000). The changing role of grandparenthood. *Journal of Gerontological Nursing, 26*(1), 24–29.

Dilworth-Anderson, P., Williams, I. C., & Gibson, B. E. (2002). Issues of race, ethnicity, and culture in caregiving research: A 20-year review (1980-2000). *Gerontologist, 42,* 237–272.

Dowdell, E. B., & Sherwen, L. N. (1998). Grandmothers who raise grandchildren: A cross-generational challenge to caregivers. *Journal of Gerontological Nursing, 24*(5), 8–13.

Elnicki, D. M., Douglas, K., Morris, M., & Shockcor, W. (1995). Patient-perceived barriers to preventive health care among indigent, rural Appalachian patients. *Archives of Internal Medicine, 155,* 421–424.

Field, D., & Gueldner, S. H. (2001). Oldest-old versus old-old. *Journal of Gerontological Nursing, 27*(8), 20–27.

Fuller-Thomson, E., & Minkler, M. (2001). American grandparents providing extensive child care to their grandchildren: Prevalence and profile. *Gerontologist, 41,* 201–209.

Fuller-Thomson, E., Minkler, M., & Driver, D. (1997). A profile of grandparents raising grandchildren in the United States. *Gerontologist, 37,* 406–411.

Hareven, T. K. (2001). Historical perspectives on aging and family relations. In R. H. Binstock & L. K. George (Eds.), *Handbook of aging and the social sciences* (5th ed., pp. 141–159). San Diego: Academic Press.

Hayward, M. D., & Zhang, A. (2001). Demography of aging: A century of global change, 1950–2050. In R. H. Binstock & L. K. George (Eds.), *Handbook of aging and the social sciences* (5th ed., pp. 69–85). San Diego: Academic Press.

Horton, C. F. (1984). Women have headaches, men have backaches: Patterns of illness in an Appalachian community. *Social Science and Medicine, 19,* 647–654.

Kinsella, K. (2000). Demographic dimensions of global aging. *Journal of Family Issues, 21,* 541–558.

Markides, K. S., & Miranda, M. R. (Eds.) (1997). *Minorities, aging and health.* Thousand Oaks, CA: Sage Publications.

National Aging Information Center. (1997). *Aging into the 21st century.* Washington, DC: Administration on Aging.

Rosswurm, M. A. (2001). Rural elders. In M. D. Mezey (Ed.), *The encyclopedia of elder care* (pp. 580–582). New York: Springer.

Silverstone, B. (1996). Older people of tomorrow: A psychosocial profile. *Gerontologist, 36,* 27–32.

Szinovacz, M. E. (1998). Grandparents today: A demographic profile. *Gerontologist, 38,* 37–52.

United Nations. (1982). *International plan of action on ageing.* New York: United Nations.

United Nations. (2002). *International plan of action on ageing 2002.* New York: United Nations.

U.S. Bureau of the Census. (1996). *Sixty-five plus in the United States: Current population reports, special studies* (Series P23–190). Washington, DC: U. S. Government Printing Office.

Warnes, A. M., & Crane, M. A. (2000). The achievements of a multiservice project for older homeless people. *Gerontologist, 40,* 618–626.

Williams, D. R., & Wilson, C. M. (2001). Race, ethnicity, and aging. In R. H. Binstock & L. K. George (Eds.), *Handbook of aging and the social sciences* (5th ed., pp. 160–178). San Diego: Academic Press.

Wykle, M., & Kaskel, B. (1994). Increasing the longevity of minority older adults through improved health status. In J. S. Jackson (Ed.), *Minority elders: Five goals toward building a public policy base* (pp. 32–39). Washington, DC: The Gerontological Society of America.

The Phenomenon of Aging

LEARNING OBJECTIVES

1. Explain the role of theory in understanding aging.
2. Discuss biologic theories of aging and their relevance to gerontological nursing.
3. Discuss sociologic theories of aging and their relevance to gerontological nursing.
4. Discuss psychological theories of aging and their relevance to gerontological nursing.
5. Explain the role of theory in the nursing care of older adults.
6. Explicate the functional consequences theory of gerontological nursing.

Three of the most universally asked queries about aging are *How long can we live? Why do we age?* and *How can we prevent the deleterious effects of aging?* Since the time of the ancient Greeks, scientists and philosophers have been attempting to find answers to these questions by developing theories about aging. Gerontological health care practitioners are particularly interested in finding ways of preventing the deleterious effects of aging and look to theories about aging to provide the foundation for answers to this question.

In the early 1990s, "anti-aging medicine" was popularized as a branch of medicine aimed at finding ways of preventing aging. Hayflick (2001–2002) views the concept of anti-aging as an oxymoron because aging is a universal phenomenon; furthermore, the belief that it is possible or desirable to overcome the natural aging process reinforces fears about aging (see Chapter 1). Moreover, it denies all the positive and enriching aspects of aging from the psychosocial perspective (International Longevity Center, 2001). In recent years, the term "longevity medicine" has been promoted as a more positive approach to finding "all means that would extend healthy life, including health promotion, disease prevention . . . and new discoveries as a result of basic research" (International Longevity Center, 2001, p. 12). Although the "fountain of youth" formula has not yet been found, much progress is being made in identifying methods of delaying the onset of disabilities and chronic illnesses. Progress also is being made in identifying health promotion interventions that will prevent dependency and promote the highest level of functioning.

LIFE EXPECTANCY, MORBIDITY, AND MORTALITY

Questions about how long we can live are best answered in terms of life expectancy, morbidity, and mortality. *Life expectancy* is defined as the predictable length of time that one is expected to live from a specific point in time, such as birth. Life expectancy differs from *life span*, which is defined as the maximum survival potential for a particular species. Life span for humans—between 110 and 122 years—has stayed somewhat stable for the last 100,000 years. Most researchers and gerontologists agree that the human life span is relatively fixed, with barely perceptible extensions occurring in the broad evolutionary time scale. In contrast, tremendous changes are taking place in life expectancy. Hayflick (2001–2002) uses the analogy of a 24-hour clock to illustrate the timeframe for the evolution of human life expectancy. If

the total time in which the human species has existed were imagined on a 24-hour time scale, the changes in life expectancy that most people today experience would occur only a few seconds before midnight, and the life expectancy of humans until this time would have been 25 years or less.

Life expectancy in developed countries has increased from 49 years in 1900 to 74.1 years (for men) and 79.5 years (for women) in 2000—an increase that is equivalent to the entire increase in life expectancy that took place in the previous 2000 years (Hayflick, 2001–2002) (Figure 3-1). Similarly, in 1900, people reaching the age of 65 years could expect to live another 12 years, in the year 2000, men reaching the age of 65 years could expect to live an average of 16.3 years longer and women could expect to live another 19.2 years. Life expectancy for people reaching 85 years in 2000 is 6.7 years for women and 5.6 years for men. Another way of looking at this is to consider that, in 1940, about 7% of people who reached the age of 65 years could expect to survive to 90 years. In 2000, that percentage was 26%, and by 2050, that percentage is expected to increase to 42%. Projections for 2050 estimate that life expectancy will be 82 years and that people aged 65 years and older will represent about 20% of the population.

In addition to gender variation, significant racial variation exists in life expectancy rates. In 2000, life expectancy for whites and African Americans, respectively, was 77.3 and 71.4 years at birth and 17.9 and 16.2 years at age 65 years. By the age of 85 years, life expectancy for African Americans and whites is the

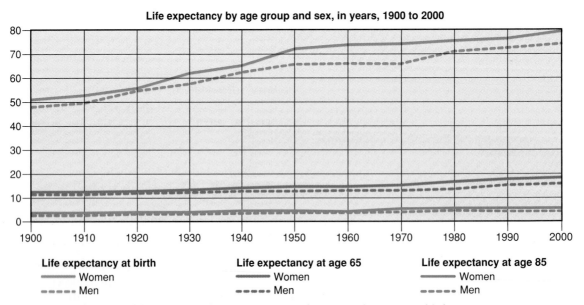

Life expectancy by age group and sex, in years, 1900 to 2000

Life expectancy at birth	Life expectancy at age 65	Life expectancy at age 85
———— Women	———— Women	———— Women
----- Men	----- Men	----- Men

FIGURE 3-1 Changes in life expectancy from 1900 to 2000 for men and women, at birth, age 65, and age 85. (From National Vital Statistics System.)

same, at 6.3 years. The life expectancy of Asians and Pacific Islanders is higher than that of any other group in the United States.

Mortality rates can be graphically represented in a survivorship curve, which illustrates the changes occurring in death rates over different periods of time (Figure 3-2). The vertical axis designates the percentage of survivors, whereas the horizontal axis represents the age of survivorship. As is evident from this graph, the curves are becoming increasingly elongated—nearly rectangular, in fact—owing to changes caused by various significant factors occurring at different points in time. The first major change in survival resulted from improved housing and sanitation practices, and the second major change was brought about by the advent of immunization programs and other advances in public health practices. The third major change, occurring between 1960 and 1980, is attributable to biomedical breakthroughs, such as organ transplantations, heart–lung machines, and increasingly effective cancer treatments. During the

later part of the 20th century and early part of the 21st century, the rate of increase in average longevity has continued to rise, but the pace of increase has decelerated because the causes of mortality have shifted to chronic diseases of middle and later adulthood. This change in pace has resulted in the squaring, or rectangularization, of the human survival curve, meaning that for people who reach the age of 75 or 80 years, longevity is not increased, and life expectancy is not prolonged significantly.

The concept of the rectangularization of the curve has been traced back to the 1920s, and it was first applied to gerontology in the 1960s. In the early 1980s, interest in this concept was stimulated by a growing awareness of the increasing number of older people. In 1980, James Fries, a physician, stirred much controversy with the publication of an article about the compression of morbidity in the *New England Journal of Medicine* (Fries, 1980). Fries argued that the onset of significant illness could be postponed but that one's life span could not be extended

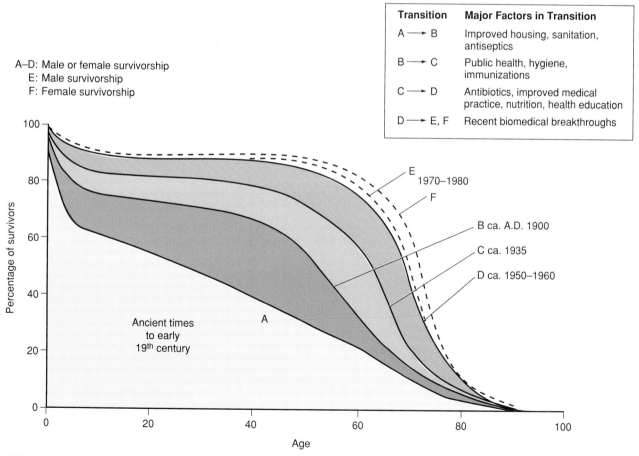

FIGURE 3-2 Human survivorship curve. (Adapted from Strehler, B. L. [1975]. Implications of aging research for society. *Proceedings of the Federation of American Societies for Experimental Biology, 34*, 6. Used with permission.)

to the same extent. Consequently, disease, disability, and functional decline would be "compressed" into a period averaging 3 to 5 years before death. Fries and a colleague emphasized that efforts must be directed toward postponing the onset of chronic illnesses through preventive approaches (Fries & Crapo, 1981). In the past two decades, data on average longevity, health care utilization, and functional and socioeconomic status have provided support for Fries' theory (Hazzard, 2001).

Projections for the mid-21st century are that average life expectancy will level off at the age of 85 years, barring unforeseen breakthroughs in biotechnology (Hazzard, 2001). This is because the inherent teleology of human beings indicates that we seem to be programmed genetically to live for about 100 years, even under the best of circumstances. People today are surviving illnesses that led to early deaths in previous decades, but they still tend to suffer from chronic illnesses that do not lead to death. As a consequence, people today spend a relatively greater proportion of their lives in a state of some level of dependency. This has prompted geriatricians and gerontologists to begin to address the concept of active life expectancy as an indicator of quality of life during older adulthood. This concept is based on the number of years spent at a high functional level. Function may be evaluated on a continuum of four states, ranging from inability to perform activities of daily living to full ability to perform activities and instrumental activities of daily living (Crimmins et al., 1996). The United States Department of Health and Human Services recently addressed this issue of active life expectancy and stated that "one of the overarching goals of *Healthy People 2010* is to increase the quality and years of healthy life"(Wagener et al., 2001, p.1).

Although many researchers have found support for the compression of morbidity theory, some recent evidence suggests that morbidity is expanding rather than contracting because life expectancy is increasing faster than the number of years of active (healthy) life (Laditka & Laditka, 2000). Despite the questions about the compression or expansion of morbidity, gerontologists agree on the following: (1) even in the absence of disease, death will occur as a result of declining organ reserves; (2) the rate of mortality increases exponentially after age 30 years; (3) projections about aging can be dramatically altered in the future by unpredictable events such as warfare, new diseases, or medical breakthroughs; (4) chronic diseases have replaced acute illness as the major threats to life and health; (5) the overriding concern about longevity should focus on quality of life rather than length of life (Laditka & Laditka, 2000).

Successful aging is the ultimate task of older adulthood. As one gerontologist stated, "to age successfully is to live a life of highest quality, maximal longevity, and minimal disease and disability" (Hazzard, 2001). This chapter will review current theories that attempt to answer the questions of how long we can live, why we age, and how the deleterious effects of aging can be avoided or delayed. It also will address the role of theory in nursing and explicate a theory for the practice of gerontological nursing.

THE ROLE OF THEORY IN UNDERSTANDING AGING

Theories make sense of phenomena; they provide order and a perspective from which to view facts. Since early times, scientists have theorized about the universal human phenomenon of aging, with most of the early theories being limited to biologic aging. For example, Aristotle, Hippocrates, Galen, and other early philosopher-scientists associated aging with a decrease in body heat and fluid. As scientists expanded their knowledge, improved their research methods, and discovered more about aging, it became clear that aging is, in fact, an extremely complex and variable process. During the 20th century, biologists, sociologists, and psychologists developed theories to explain the phenomenon of aging from their three different perspectives, leading to the suggestion that aging could be defined in the following ways: (1) biologic age, encompassing measures of functional capacities of vital or life-limiting organ systems; (2) sociologic age, involving the roles and age-graded behaviors of people in response to the society of which they are a part; and (3) psychological age, referring to the behavioral capacities of people to adapt to changing environmental demands.

As discussed throughout this chapter, contemporary gerontologists are particularly interested in trying to determine how we can improve the quality of life as well as extend the quantity of life. Gerontologists also are recognizing the importance and value of expanding the traditional Western perspective and incorporating non-Western views into theories about aging. As a result, aging is now viewed as a highly complex phenomenon that must be addressed from a multicultural, as well as a multidisciplinary, perspective.

Health care practitioners in disciplines that include subspecialties in gerontology, such as geriatric medicine and gerontological nursing, are now focusing much attention on maintenance of health and independent functioning and proposing theories about phenomena related to the unique aspects of care of older adults. In the next sections, some of the biologic, sociologic, and psychological theories of aging are reviewed, and their relevance to gerontological nursing is discussed. Because of the inherent multidisciplinary nature of gerontology, knowledge of these theories is helpful to gerontological nurses in their care of older adults. For example, if a problem, such as discrimination against older people, exists in a larger societal framework, solutions may be found in sociology.

Phenomena related to aging, older adults, and older adulthood are highly complex, and the answers to questions about these phenomena are rooted in several disciplines. Improved function in older adults, for instance, usually depends on a number of interacting influences, including physiologic, psychosocial, and environmental factors. Gerontological nurses and other gerontological practitioners, therefore, must draw on many perspectives to synthesize particular theories on which to base the care of older adults. Furthermore, because nursing views the health of the whole person in relation to his or her environment, theories from other disciplines contribute to an understanding of the inherent complexity of the older adults for whom nurses care. Increasingly, nurses are recognizing the value and necessity of aging theories that are holistic, multidisciplinary, and based on a life span focus (Haight et al., 2002). As several nurse-researchers stated, "A good gerontological theory integrates knowledge, tells how and why phenomena are related, leads to prediction, and provides process and understanding. In addition, a good theory must be holistic and take into account all that impacts on a person throughout a lifetime of aging" (Haight et al., 2002, p. 14).

All gerontological practitioners draw from many of the same theories, but each discipline has a unique approach to assessing situations, planning care, and solving problems. For example, geriatric medicine relies on biologic theories to explain how age-related changes affect the physiologic function of the human body. Likewise, disciplines such as nursing, psychiatry, and sociology have integrated theories of aging with the unique perspective of their own profession. Nurses focus on individuals who have nursing problems, psychiatrists try to identify and cure psychopathologic conditions, and sociologists inquire about cohorts of people with common characteristics. Each profession has a prescribed realm of practice, but each is enriched by drawing on theories from the others. Although theories based in other disciplines are relevant to nurses, they cannot explain the unique relationship between the nurse and the older person. Thus, in the last section of this chapter, a theory for gerontological nursing is proposed.

BIOLOGIC THEORIES OF AGING

Biologic theories of aging address questions about the basic aging processes that affect all living organisms. These theories answer questions such as *How do cells age?* and *What triggers the process of aging?* In addition, biologic aging theories attempt to identify those physiologic processes that occur independently of external or pathologic influences. Leonard Hayflick, one of the first gerontologists to propose a theory of biologic aging, emphasized that a theory of aging or longevity must explain several types of age-related changes, including changes that are: (1) *deleterious,* resulting in reduced function; (2) *progressive,* occurring gradually; (3) *intrinsic,* not attributable to modifiable environmental agents; and (4) *universal,* affecting all members of a species if given the opportunity by virtue of age (Hayflick, 1988). Two additional criteria that have been widely accepted for several decades are that age-related changes are *irreversible* and *genetically programmed* (Blumenthal, 1999). Although for many decades gerontologists have accepted these criteria as the decisive factors for differentiating inherent age-related changes from disease-related processes, recent findings suggest that this theoretical distinction is blurring. For example, recent findings of deposits of amyloid in the heart, brain, and other body organs suggests that this phenomenon—typically viewed as a disease-related process—may, in fact, meet at least one criterion (universality) for inherent aging (Blumenthal, 2001). As researchers discover more and more information about biologic processes in humans, more questions will be raised about biologic theories of aging.

The process of biologic aging is multidimensional, and ongoing debate about biologic mechanisms of aging is important for the growth of theory development. Because of the great deal of variability among people, no single theory will suffice to explain the complex phenomenon of aging that involves many processes and mechanisms. All biologic theories attempt to explain the characteristics of age-related changes, and each theory attempts to explain a particular aspect of aging from a particular perspective. Major biologic theories are considered in this chapter, but these are only a sampling of the various perspectives that have been proposed and that continue to evolve.

Genetic Theories

Genetic theories, which emphasize the role of genes in the development of age-related changes, are one of the most complex types of biologic theories. They are also among the most intensely studied and rapidly evolving types of theories in the 21st century. One of the earliest of the genetic theories is the program theory of aging, proposed by Hayflick in the 1960s. This theory states that the life span of animals is predetermined by a genetic program, or a so-called biologic clock (Hayflick, 1965). In humans, for instance, the program allows for a maximum of about 110 years. Hayflick (1974) estimates that normal human cells divide 50 times in this number of years and argues that cells are genetically programmed to stop dividing after achieving 50 cell divisions, at which time they begin to deteriorate. The number of times cell division takes place is different for each species of animal, and the longer a species' life expectancy, the more cell divisions that animal has in its genetic program. Abnormal cells, however, are not subject to this predictable program and can proliferate an indefinite number of times. Some genetic theories, called *mutation theories,* suggest that aging is the result of mutations of somatic cells or alterations in DNA repair mechanisms.

Genetic theories of aging are supported by studies that indicate that life expectancy is genetically preprogrammed within a species-specific range. Many studies of life expectancies of twins, siblings, and several generations of family members have confirmed a genetic component to aging and to extreme longevity. Recent studies also suggest that genetic variables include longevity-enabling genes as well as disease-resistance genes (Perls et al., 2002). In recent years, genetic research has been focusing on the presence and absence of specific apolipoprotein alleles and their roles in both risk for, and protective effects against, disease.

Currently, one area of focus for research leading to genetic theories of aging is on the relative effects of genetic and environmental influences on aging. Estimates of the degree of genetic influence on longevity and healthy aging range from 20% to 33%, with the remaining influences being attributable to environment and health-related behaviors (Frisoni et al., 2001; Perls et al., 2002). Researchers are also studying how genes can be manipulated to influence specific manifestations of aging. For example, scientists have found a way to "switch off" the genes that regulate a protein responsible for manifestations of skin aging, so that the life of skin cells can be doubled (Moody, 2002). The year 2000 saw many advances in genetic research as scientists involved with the Human Genome Project successfully identified the location of each human gene, facilitating the identification of specific genes that influence both biologic aging and age-related diseases. Ongoing developments of the Human Genome Project are likely to contribute significantly to emerging biologic theories

of aging, particularly with regard to the complex interactions between aging and disease processes.

Wear-and-Tear Theories

The first wear-and-tear theory was based on a 19th-century theory that attempted to explain the difference between immortal "germ plasm" cells—those that are capable of reproducing—and mortal "somatic" cells—those that die. In the late 1880s, August Weismann theorized that normal somatic cells were limited in their ability to replicate and function. He further postulated that death occurred because worn-out tissues could not forever renew themselves and living organisms surrendered to the "wear and tear" of life. According to the wear-and-tear theory, the body can be likened to a machine that is expected to function well during the period of its warranty but that will wear out at a fairly predictable time. Parts can be fixed or replaced, but eventually, the machine no longer functions because of the extensive accumulation of wear and tear. Like the machine, the longevity of the human body will be affected by the care it receives as well as by its genetic components. Unlike the machine, however, the human body can repair many of its own parts well into old age.

Harmful stress factors, such as smoking, poor diet, alcohol abuse, or muscular strain, can exacerbate the wearing-out process. The wear-and-tear theory of aging is supported by microscopic signs of wear and tear in all nerve and striated muscle cells. Osteoarthritis, a degenerative joint condition, is an age-related process that can be explained by this theory.

Immunity Theories

Immunity theories are based on the knowledge that immune system components—particularly the thymus and immunocompetent cells in the bone marrow—are affected by the aging process. Because of this age-related diminished function of the immune system, called *immunosenescence* or immunodeficiency, the older person has fewer defenses against foreign organisms. Consequently, older people are more susceptible to cancer, infections, and autoimmune diseases, such as lupus or rheumatoid arthritis. Immunosenescence may also explain the significant increase in incidence and severity of diarrhea and other gastrointestinal infectious diseases because the gastrointestinal tract represents more than half of the human immune system (Effros, 2001). Immunity theories also attempt to explain a relationship between diminished immune functioning and an increase in the body's autoimmune responses. When autoimmunity occurs, the body reacts against itself and produces antibodies in response to its own constituents. Autoimmunity theory could explain the fact that older adults often manifest allergies to food and environmental conditions that they previously never experienced.

Current research on immunity theories is focusing on links between immune function and age-associated diseases such as Alzheimer's disease and cardiovascular disease (Effros, 2001).

Cross-Linkage Theory

The cross-linkage theory proposes that molecular structures that are normally separated may be bound together through chemical reactions. According to this theory, a cross-linking agent attaches itself to a single strand of a DNA molecule and damages that strand. Natural defense mechanisms usually repair the damage, but increasing age weakens these defense mechanisms, allowing the cross-linkage process to continue until irreparable damage occurs. The end result is an accumulation of cross-linking compounds that causes mutations in the cell and renders the cell unable to eliminate wastes and transport ions. This irreversible damage to the cells that form collagen-type substances eventually leads to tissue and organ failure because the protein system becomes inelastic and ineffective. This theory would explain arteriosclerosis and age-related skin changes.

Lipofuscin and Free Radical Theories

The free radical theory, first proposed in the mid-1950s (Harman, 1956), continues to provide the basis for much of the current research on aging. One discussion of biologic theories of aging suggested that "the free radical theory of aging is the only aging theory to have stood the test of time" (Grune & Davies, 2001, p. 41). Free radicals are highly unstable and reactive molecules (particularly oxygen molecules) that are formed when an electron pair is separated. Free radicals can be produced by normal metabolism, reactions to irradiation, chain reactions with other free radicals, and oxidation of certain environmental pollutants, such as ozone, pesticides, and air pollutants.

Free radicals and their conjugated compounds are capable of attacking other molecules because they possess an extra electric charge, or free electron. Because they are so highly reactive, free radicals rapidly interact with and damage cellular components such as lipids, proteins, and nucleic acids. Fortunately, the human body has protective mechanisms that can interfere with oxidation activity and remove and repair damaged cells. Antioxidants, including beta-carotene and vitamins C and E, are one of the major

defense mechanisms against oxidative damage from free radicals. Despite these natural mechanisms that guard against free radicals, however, a low level of oxidation occurs continuously.

The free radical theory postulates that protective mechanisms decrease, or free radical formation increases, with advancing age. When free radicals attack molecules, they damage the cell membranes; aging is thought to occur because of cumulative cell damage that eventually interferes with function. Early support for the free radical theory came from the discovery of lipofuscin, a pigmented waste material that is rich in lipids and proteins. This discovery led to research on lipid peroxidation, with many studies showing an age-related increase in oxidation of lipids following stress (Grune & Davies, 2001).

Research currently is focusing on developing interventions to modify or prevent the age-related accumulation of free radicals. One approach is through supplementation with natural or synthetic antioxidants, such as melatonin, L-carnitine, and vitamins C and E. Of the substances studied to date, vitamin E is one agent that has been shown to have beneficial antioxidant actions in humans (Grune & Davies, 2001). Studies also are addressing interventions that diminish the formation of free radicals through restricted intake of calories, proteins, or certain types of fats.

Neuroendocrine Theories

Neuroendocrine and neurochemical theories are the focus of intense interest, but they are still in the early stage of development. These theories postulate that changes in the brain and endocrine glands cause aging. One such theory—the neurotransmitter theory—proposes that an imbalance of thought-transmitting chemicals in the brain interferes with cell division throughout the body. Neuroendocrine theories are based on the understanding that the neuroendocrine system integrates body functions and facilitates adaptation to changes in both internal and external environments. These theories suggest that the numerous alterations of the endocrine system may actually represent the mechanisms of age-related changes in organ function (Bartke & Lane, 2001).

Apoptosis Theory

In recent years, gerontologists have expressed much interest in exploring the relationship between apoptosis and aging, and new biologic theories of aging are emerging based on this concept. Apoptosis is a mechanism of cell death, first described in the 1970s, that is distinct from necrosis (Kerr et al., 1972). Although necrosis is an inflammatory response to trauma and is characterized by an uncontrolled breakdown of cellular and organelle structure, apoptosis is a noninflammatory, gene-driven process. Necrosis is characterized by cell swelling and loss of membrane integrity, whereas apoptosis is characterized by cell shrinkage and maintenance of membrane integrity (Kerr et al., 1972). Apoptosis is considered a normal developmental process that occurs continuously throughout life. When apoptosis is properly regulated, it is beneficial to the organ because a balance is maintained between cells that should be retained and those that should be eliminated. Apoptosis can be described as a gene-directed biologic program that has evolved to remove extra cells during development, in order to optimize the pattern and shape of each organ (Wang et al., 2001). This is analogous to the process involved in writing a research paper. Researchers collect large amounts of data, then select the information that actually will be incorporated into the text and discard the information that is not germane.

Recent research suggests that this process is regulated by an interplay between two opposing families of genes. Members of one gene family promote elimination of cells, and members of the opposing gene family promote survival of cells. Theories are currently trying to answer questions about "why, during aging, the apoptotic program is dysregulated and how this dysregulation precipitates the disability and degeneration associated with the aging process" (Wang et al., 2001, p. 260). Some studies suggest that one cause of this dysregulation is age-related changes in the levels of proteins and other factors that control apoptosis (Joaquin & Gollapudi, 2001). The apoptosis theory might explain the increased incidence of cancer, autoimmune disease, and cardiovascular and neurodegenerative disorders in older adults. Studies are currently addressing potential effects of medications in regulating apoptosis, either beneficially or detrimentally. These studies may have significant clinical implications, particularly with regard to cardiovascular disease (Joaquin & Gollapudi, 2001).

Longevity and Senescence Theories

Longevity and senescence theories focus on why people live as long as they do. As discussed earlier, this question is particularly important to gerontological practitioners because of the increasing focus on adding quality, not just quantity, to life. Although many studies of centenarians have found that people who live to age 100 years and older are relatively healthy and functional, other studies have found a high prevalence of chronic illness among centenarians. Authors of one study concluded that "reaching the age of 100 years today is not reserved for people free from potentially mortal disease" (Andersen-Ranberg et al., 2001, p. 906). In the United States and other industrialized countries, 85% of centenarians are women, but their physical and cognitive functioning is not as good as that of men who are centenarians (Perls, 2001). By studying long-lived people who are healthy and functional, we may find answers to the most important question of all: *How can we live a life that is not only long but also functional, productive, and satisfying?*

Alexander Leaf observed three groups of people who were both healthy and long-lived (1973a, 1973b, 1973c). Although his observations are not entirely scientific, they do provide some information about factors that contribute to healthy aging. A summary of findings regarding long-lived healthy people identified the following significant influences: (1) genetic factors; (2) physical environment; (3) physical activity throughout life; (4) consumption of moderate amounts of alcohol; (5) sexual activity persisting into advanced years; (6) dietary factors, such as low animal fat intake; and (7) factors relating to social environment, such as an acquired status of wisdom and dignity (Pelletier, 1986).

Kohn (1982) proposed the senescence theory, which is based on postmortem studies of 200 people who died at the age of 85 years or older. Death certificates of at least 26% of that group listed no pathologic process that experienced pathologists would accept as a cause of death. Kohn determined this by comparing findings from extensive postmortem examinations with the listed cause of death. When decisions about the accuracy of the cause of death were questionable, the evaluations were weighted in favor of the listed cause. Based on the results of these autopsies, Kohn concluded that, had the same degree of disease occurred in middle-aged people, the condition would not have been fatal. Thus, aging itself was thought to be the actual cause of death in a large fraction of the aged population (Kohn, 1982). Kohn further suggested that, when death in older people cannot be ascribed to a disease process that would cause death in middle-aged people, the cause of death should be listed on the death certificate as senescence. According to Kohn, the relationship between aging and disease is very clear: "The aging syndrome should be viewed as a universal, progressive, and ultimately fatal disease" (1982, p. 2797).

A variation of the senescence theory has been proposed to explain the relationships among aging, health beliefs, and health behaviors (Newquist, 1987). According to Newquist, there are three models for viewing these relationships. In the *siege model*, illness is viewed as a necessary concomitant of being old. The attitude of people with this perspective is "Get ready to be sick, you're old." In the *senescence model*, illness and aging represent the same entity. Illnesses are viewed as age-induced changes ("just old age") and are not seen as pathologic conditions. In the *vanquished model,* sickness is viewed as pathologic, but it is seen as something to be accepted if one is old. According to this model, not only does sickness invariably accompany old age, it is untreatable because of old age (Newquist, 1987). This model illustrates an approach that is in stark contrast to that taken currently by gerontological health care practitioners.

Current theories attempt to identify the determinants of longevity so that interventions can be devised to delay the onset of senescence and associated chronic diseases (Kirkland, 2002). These theories address both genetic and environmental factors that significantly influence the ability to live to advanced old age. One specific focus is on distinguishing between the genetics of aging and the genetics of exceptional longevity, as occurs in healthy centenarians (Perls et al., 2002).

> Imagine that you are 72 years old and your parents are still living. Your mother is 96 and your father is 95. You have a brother who died last year at the age of 70 and you have a sister who is 69 years old. You have two children, three grandchildren, and two great-grandchildren. Using your imagination and what you learned about biologic theories of aging in this chapter, answer the following questions.

 THINKING POINTS

> Using the concepts of the rectangularization of the curve and the compression of mortality, what would you expect the health, functioning, and life expectancy to be for each of the five generations in your family?

> Pick the biologic theory of aging that you think is most applicable to your family and use it to explain to your great-grandchildren why their great-great grandparents are still living.

Active Life Expectancy and Functional Health Theories

Spurred partly by the compression of morbidity theory, gerontologists have been trying to predict the probable active life expectancy for older people. This issue is of particular interest to health planners and policy makers because the cost of medical care is significantly related to the degree of an individual's disability. Health care providers are also interested in this issue because quality of life depends significantly on the level of function. Using life table methods and the activities of daily living index as a measure of health,

Katz and coworkers (1983) analyzed data for noninstitutionalized older people in an attempt to predict active (healthy) life expectancy. The results showed that people entering the age category of 65 to 69 years had 10 years of functional well-being remaining, whereas those in older groups had progressively fewer years. For people 85 years of age or older, the active life expectancy was 2.5 years. More recently, the U.S. Department of Health and Human Services calculated and published life expectancy and active life expectancy data for white females in the United States (Figure 3-3).

An article that appeared in 1983 in the *Journal of the American Medical Association* (Kennie, 1983) was viewed as an early attempt to articulate the functional approach to geriatric medical care. The Scottish geriatrician who wrote it stated that "the most important and distinguishing aspect of good health care for the elderly is the switch in emphasis away from dealing strictly with pathology and organ-specific disease [and] toward restoring the patient's resultant loss of function" (Kennie, 1983, p. 770). During the following

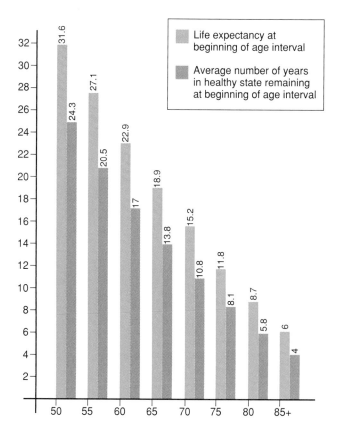

FIGURE 3-3 Graphic illustration of life expectancy and active (healthy) life expectancy for white females in the United States, 1995. (Data from Molla, M. T., Wagener, D. K., & Madans, J. H. [2001]. *Summary measures of population health: Methods for calculating healthy life expectancy.* Washington, D.C.: U.S. Department of Health and Human Services.)

year, an article appearing in the *Journal of the American Geriatrics Society* proposed a conceptual framework for a functional approach to the care of the elderly (Becker & Cohen, 1984). It emphasized the complex relationships between the social, biologic, and psychological variables that influence a person's functional abilities and well-being. Moreover, it emphasized that age-related, as well as disease-related, changes can interfere with functional status. Accordingly, the ultimate goal of the clinician is to orchestrate compensatory responses in an effort to restore, maximize, and maintain a person's functional status and independence for as long as possible (Becker & Cohen, 1984, p. 928). In the late 1980s, the American College of Physicians and the American Geriatrics Society cited the importance of incorporating a functional assessment into routine clinical geriatrics as a major component of quality of life and as a critical component of appropriate health care. Additional concepts pertinent to functional assessment are discussed in Chapter 11, and a nursing model for functional assessment is presented, along with guidelines for its use. The current and dominant emphasis of gerontological health care practitioners on finding ways of improving quality of life for older adults also is strongly associated with the functional health theories.

Medical Theories

Geriatric medical theories try to explain how biologic changes associated with the aging process affect the physiologic function of the human body. Biogerontology is a recent subspecialization, the aim of which is to determine the connections between specific diseases and aging processes (Miller, 1997). These theories address specific questions, such as how aging and disease processes are related and distinguished, and what is different about the medical care of older people. In recent years, many questions have been raised about conclusions drawn from cross-sectional studies, which shed light on age differences rather than age-related changes. As more sophisticated research methods have been used and more data have been collected from healthy subjects in longitudinal studies, some of the conclusions drawn from these cross-sectional studies have been challenged. For example, the common belief that renal function declines with increased age has been called into question by data derived from the Baltimore Longitudinal Study of Aging (Williams, 1987). Increasing emphasis is also being placed on individual variability.

Throughout this text, theoretical explanations of specific functional aspects of aging are discussed in the sections on age-related changes; sometimes opposing conclusions and controversial findings are cited as explanations for age-related or disease-related changes. Whenever possible, theories and conclusions that have generated the greatest concordance are summarized. In all cases, an attempt is made to reflect accurately the current theoretical base. It is important to keep in mind, however, that all theories of aging are in a state of intense flux and growth. As knowledge of this population continues to expand at a rapid pace, current theories may be challenged or supplanted by other theories.

As knowledge about aging and disease increases, more questions are being raised about the relationship between these processes. For example, if aging and disease are interdependent processes, then longitudinal studies must attempt to describe the natural history of diseases and their underlying processes as part of the overall aging process (Fozard et al., 1990). One discussion of theories about biologic theories of aging concluded that aging and disease are not synonymous and that aging proceeds even in the absence of disease, but "aging clearly includes increased *vulnerability* to disease" (Austad, 2001). The noted gerontologist Leonard Hayflick described the complex relationship between aging and disease as analogous to the "weak links" in automobiles. According to his analogy, both humans and particular makes and models of cars are characterized by weak links that increase the probability of component failure. For cheap cars, the "mean time to failure" is 4 or 5 years; for Americans born today, it is about 76 years. The weakest links for people in developed countries are the vascular system and the cells in which cancer commonly occurs. "The aging process increases vulnerability to the pathologies that become the leading causes of death" (Hayflick, 2001–2002, p. 21).

Although the early medical theories of aging were limited in scope to questions about the relationship between disease and aging, more recent medical theories of aging focus on assessing and improving the functional health of older people. Beginning in the 1990s, the focus of geriatric research and practice shifted from an emphasis on disease processes per se to an emphasis on the functional losses that are of key importance to older people. Evolving theories about active life expectancy and functional health are particularly important because they help explain the current emphasis on health promotion interventions and provide goals for healthy aging.

Relevance of Biologic Theories of Aging to Gerontological Nursing

Increasing interest in the compression-of-morbidity perspective has led to a growing emphasis on the role of lifestyle, environment, and other factors as determinants of aging. *Healthy People 2010* emphasized that the effect of changes in life expectancy in the United States has lead to a shift in focus from longevity to improving functioning and preventing disability (Molla et al., 2001). This trend is likely to continue as gerontologists and older adults themselves increasingly view quality of life issues as equal to or even more important than the simple extension of life.

Closely related to this trend, gerontologists have attempted to distinguish between "primary" and "secondary" aging. Primary aging is viewed as the process that occurs late in life and leads to "natural death" at the age genetically programmed for the individual. This process involves "parallel, irreducible declines in physiological efficiency in all systems proceeding from aging per se" (Hazzard, 2001, p. 447). In contrast, secondary aging involves "disease processes that may accelerate and, hence, mimic the phenotype of primary aging, but are at least potentially amenable to being retarded through environmental, biomedical, or behavioral interventions" (Hazzard, 2001, p. 447). Differentiating between aging and disease is important, especially in light of how often people ascribe changes in their own abilities, or in those of a family member or patient, to age ("What do you expect? I'm/he's/she's old!"). Studies suggest that "many older people still have not been hearing (or do not agree with) the messages that the geriatric and gerontological community have been advocating for years, namely that *old age itself is not a disease* and as such should not cause health problems such as disability" (Sarkisian et al., 2001, p. 139).

Recognizing the distinction between aging and disease will facilitate the identification of interventions that can be directed toward delaying the onset of secondary aging processes. Ideally, "preventive gerontology" practices would be implemented throughout life, beginning at conception, and people would have a life of maximal quality and quantity. Preventive gerontology strategies include a range of health promotion interventions that enhance vitality in social, physical, and psychological domains (Hazzard, 2001). Although these health promotion interventions are most effective when they are initiated early in life, it is important to recognize that people of any age move along a health–illness continuum. Many factors determine where a person is on his or her health–illness continuum at any point in time, and some of these factors can be controlled by the individual, for example, through lifestyle modifications. A primary role of gerontological nurses is to help older adults identify the modifiable factors that are associated with secondary aging and to plan interventions to address these factors. The functional consequences theory, discussed later in this chapter, provides a framework for identifying those factors

that are modifiable in older adults. Throughout this book, each aspect of functioning is addressed from this perspective, with emphasis on those factors that are associated with secondary aging and can be addressed through health promotion interventions.

The relevant question for gerontological nursing that is addressed in biologic theories of aging is how aging affects physiologic function. The answers to this question provide a basis for identifying ways to use the nursing process to improve the health and functioning of older adults, which is the focus of this gerontological nursing text. Conclusions that can be drawn from biologic theories of aging include the following:

1. Biologic aging affects all living organisms.
2. Biologic aging is natural, inevitable, irreversible, and progressive with time.
3. The course of aging varies from individual to individual.
4. The rate of aging for different organs and tissues varies within individuals.
5. Biologic aging is influenced by nonbiologic factors.
6. Biologic aging processes are different from pathologic processes.
7. Biologic aging increases one's vulnerability to disease.

With this knowledge of the aging process, gerontological nurses can begin to understand the differences between age-related changes and the risk factors that affect the functional status of older adults. For example, it is important to distinguish between biologic aging changes and pathologic processes that commonly affect older adults. This knowledge can be used in teaching older adults that certain conditions are not inevitable just because a person has reached a certain age.

Concepts from specific theories are also useful to gerontological nurses. For example, the knowledge that the immune system is affected by aging may explain the altered response to infections among older adults. Applying this knowledge, gerontological nurses can be increasingly vigilant about preventing infections and observing for subtle signs of infections in older adults. Concepts gleaned from wear-and-tear theories provide a rationale for gerontological nurses to plan interventions aimed at reducing the effects of psychological and physiologic stress.

In contrast to the studies that treat aging as strictly a biologic phenomenon, the studies of healthy and long-lived people offer a more holistic perspective on older people. Gerontological nurses must be as concerned about improving the quality of life in later adulthood as they are about extending the quantity of life. Because so many of the factors that contribute to a long and healthy life are within the realm of health behaviors, health promotion interventions can significantly increase both longevity and healthy life expectancy. For example, nurses can educate all adults about the importance of physical exercise, emphasizing its role in improving function in later adulthood. Psychosocial interventions, such as those directed toward increasing the quality of social supports, are also important for older adults. Gerontological nurses often work with older adults and their caregivers in addressing many quality-of-life issues. Theories about longevity can be used, along with sociologic and psychological theories, to provide a framework for addressing challenging questions about choices involving quality of life or prolongation of life. By identifying factors that contribute to longevity as well as to quality of life, older adults and their caregivers can make informed choices about lifestyles, health practices, and medical interventions.

Like nurses, primary care providers are asking questions that address the uniqueness of caring for older people as well as questions pertaining to how the functional abilities of older adults can be improved. Unlike nurses, however, primary care providers focus primarily on disease processes. When function is diminished in an older person, these practitioners attempt to identify a pathologic cause of the problem and then initiate appropriate medical interventions. Theories about disease and aging, therefore, provide a basis for addressing the disease-related factors that influence functional abilities. As is emphasized throughout this text, gerontological nursing considers not only the pathologic factors involved but also the many additional risk factors that may significantly influence the functional status of older adults.

Although functional assessment theories provide the most rational approach to the medical care of older people, many primary care providers base their practice on different theoretical perspectives. It is helpful, therefore, for nurses to be familiar with some of the other medical approaches. If medical care is based on the "what do you expect—you're old" perspective, for example, primary care providers might ignore treatable disease conditions. Similarly, if primary care providers ascribe to the theory that aging is an ultimately fatal disease, their attitude may reflect a hopelessness that pervades their approach to caring for older patients. In these situations, nurses may have to focus their assessments specifically on the identification of treatable, disease-related factors. However, in any situation, gerontological nurses can apply a holistic perspective to their own approach to care of older adults.

Because nurses generally spend more time with patients than do primary care providers, nurses are a vital communication link between older adults and their care providers. In this role, nurses have many opportunities to inform older adults of the alternative, more rational, functional approach to health care when other, more disease-focused, approaches are being applied. In this role, too, gerontological nurses can act as advocates for older adults whose care might be based on outdated or narrow approaches. Using the functional consequences theory of gerontological nursing, which is explained later in this chapter, nurses can encourage all health care providers to apply the functional approach to their care of older adults.

Although biologic theories highlight the need for good health care to minimize the damage that can be caused by disease, if these were the only theories of aging, there would be reason to be pessimistic or even fatalistic about the aging process. After all, these theories point to unalterable and detrimental physiologic changes that eventually lead to death. If these theories were the only ones applied, there would be a tendency to adhere to ageist attitudes. Biologic theories do not take into consideration the significant influence of nursing, medical, and psychosocial interventions that can improve a person's functioning and life expectancy. From a broader perspective, aging is more than an unrelenting progression of cellular deterioration. Survival to old age is an accomplishment that denotes strong will and the ability to adapt. As emphasized throughout this text, older adulthood is a dynamic part of the life span continuum and has the potential to be a most rewarding part of the life cycle, during which one experiences personal growth and self-understanding, fulfillment of potential, and the ability to establish clear priorities. These aspects of aging are addressed in the following sections, which describe sociologic and psychological theories of aging.

➤ Imagine, again, that you are 72 years old and your parents live in an assisted living apartment. Your mother is moderately obese and has osteoarthritis, hypertension, glaucoma, and type II diabetes. Functionally, she uses a walker, needs help with getting in and out of the bathtub, and has some trouble reading but can still see well enough to watch television and get around familiar environments. Your father has hypertension, osteoarthritis, and a recent diagnosis of prostate cancer. Functionally, he is independent in his basic activities of daily living but is quite hearing impaired. Both of your parents have some memory impairment, but the support services at the facility where they live address their needs for meals, medication administration, and reminders about getting to activities.

THINKING POINTS

➤ Pick a medical theory or a theory about active life expectancy and functional health and use it to respond to your mother's statement, "I'm 95 years old—what does it matter if I follow a diabetic diet? If the sugar hasn't killed me so far, then eating two donuts this morning isn't going to kill me. It's old age that will take me, not my diet."

➤ Pick a medical theory or a theory about active life expectancy and functional health and use it to respond to your father's declaration that "Of course I have prostate cancer! I'm 96 years old!"

➤ What theoretic approach would you want your father's primary care provider to use in addressing your father's prostate cancer?

SOCIOLOGIC THEORIES OF AGING

Sociologic theories of aging attempt to explain how a society influences its old people and how old people influence their society. Early sociologic theories of aging, developed during the 1960s, focused on adjustments of old people to losses within the context of roles and reference groups. Disengagement, activity, subculture, and continuity theories are some of the theories based on this theme. Early sociologic theories were narrow and tended to address older adults as a problem in society. Beginning in the 1970s, social gerontologists broadened their perspective to focus on larger societal and structural factors that influence aging, but they still tended to view older adults in the context of societal problems. Sociologists are now focusing on theories that challenge this traditional perspective that aging members of society are a societal problem, and have begun to explore the complex interrelationship between old people and their physical, political, and socioeconomic environments.

Sociologic theories of aging currently address issues related to the tremendous diversity of older adults in industrialized as well as developing societies. For example, one focus of social gerontologists is the application of feminist perspectives to sociologic theories of aging. These perspectives critique the dominant male-centered view of aging based on the experiences of white, middle-class men (Lynott & Lynott, 1996). Similarly, emerging sociologic theories are addressing inequality in aging societies by attempting to explain how and why group differences emerge. These theories attempt to explain power hierarchies and address questions about how and why different groups are oppressed (McMullin, 2000).

Some sociologic theories focus on aging as a part of the life course; these theories are discussed in detail in the section on Psychological Theories of Aging. The principles of the life-course perspective that social gerontologists agree on include: (1) aging is a lifelong process, (2) aging influences and is influenced by social processes, and (3) the age structure changes over time and is experienced differently by different cohorts (Marshall, 1996). The following sections present a sampling of the more well-developed sociologic theories of aging.

Disengagement Theory

In 1961, Cumming and Henry published the first sociologic theory of aging in their book, *Growing Old: The Process of Disengagement* (Cumming & Henry, 1961). According to this theory, the maintenance of social equilibrium is achieved by a mutually beneficial process of reciprocal withdrawal between society and older people. This process occurs systematically and inevitably and is governed by society's needs, which override individual needs. Their theory further states that older people desire this withdrawal and are happy when disengagement occurs. As the number, nature, and diversity of the older peoples' social contacts diminish, disengagement becomes a circular process that further limits opportunities for interaction. The original theory was later amended so that it was more reflective of the complexity and diversity of older people.

The usefulness of this theory lies in the controversies it has inspired by challenging traditional beliefs about the relationship between a person and society. For instance, considerable controversy has arisen regarding whether the disengagement process is, in fact, universal, inevitable, and beneficial to the person. Controversy also has focused on the fact that this theory ignores the unique responses of individuals to aging and society. Although the disengagement theory is now viewed as flawed and is no longer widely accepted, it still influences some aspects of aging. For example, the disengagement theory has been used to explain the widespread withdrawal of older adults from productive activities such as work and volunteering (Uhlenberg, 2000).

Activity Theory

The widely held belief that the best way to age successfully is to keep active was first proposed in the early days of social gerontology. Havighurst and Albrecht (1953) are credited with the first explicit statement about the importance of social role participation in positive adjustment to old age. During the next two decades, the term *activity theory* was coined to reflect this point of view, and the theory was formalized. The activity theory is based on the supposition that older people remain psychologically and socially fit if they remain active. This theory reflects the belief that one's self-concept is affirmed through activities associated with various roles and that the loss of roles in old age negatively affects life satisfaction. Lemon and colleagues (1972) tested this theory and found a significant relationship between informal activity and life satisfaction. They concluded that the quality or type of interaction was more important than the quantity of activity. A replication of this study revealed that informal activities promoted well-being, whereas formal, structured activities led to lowered life satisfaction, and solitary activities had little or no effect on life satisfaction (Longino & Kart, 1982). Busywork, for example, did not promote self-esteem, but meaningful interaction with one or more people did.

Continuity Theory

The continuity theory was first advanced by Neugarten and colleagues (1968) because neither the activity theory nor the disengagement theory adequately explained successful aging. These social gerontologists believed that what was missing in these theories was the relationship of personality to successful aging. Thus, they proposed a personality-continuity, or developmental, theory of aging (Neugarten et al., 1968). According to this theory, a person's characteristic coping strategies are in place long before old age, even though personality features are also dynamic and continually evolving. According to this theory, the best way to predict how a person will adjust to being old is to examine how that person has adjusted to changes throughout life. Some longitudinal studies confirm that stability of personality is the rule rather than the exception and suggest that some of the personality traits that are sometimes attributed to age-related changes may instead reflect generational trends that are the result of early socialization of cohorts.

Subculture Theory

The subculture theory, first proposed by Rose in the early 1960s, states that old people, as a group, have their own norms, expectations, beliefs, and habits; therefore, they have their own subculture (Rose, 1965). The theory also maintains that older people are less well integrated into the larger society and interact more among themselves, as compared with people from other age groups. Moreover, the theory

holds that the formation of an aged subculture is primarily a response to the loss of status resulting from old age, which is so negatively defined in the United States that people do not want to be viewed as old. In the aged subculture, individual status is based on health and mobility, rather than on the occupational, educational, or economic achievements that were previously important. Rose envisioned that one outcome of the aged subculture would be the development of an aging group consciousness that would serve to improve the self-image of older people and change the negative cultural definition of aging (Rose, 1965).

Because the aged subculture has millions of members in this country, it constitutes a minority group that can organize and make public demands. The growth of groups such as the American Association of Retired Persons (AARP), whose membership exceeds 34 million people, is evidence of the social importance of the aged subgroup. When considered along with the activity theory, the subculture theory supports the social gerontological view that there is a strong relationship between peer group participation and the adjustment process of aging.

Age Stratification and Age Integration Theories

The age stratification theory, first proposed by Riley and colleagues (1972), addresses the interdependencies between age as an element of the social structure and the aging of people and cohorts as a social process. This theory emphasizes the following concepts: (1) people pass through society in cohorts that are aging socially, biologically, and psychologically; (2) new cohorts are continually being born, and each experiences a unique sense of history; (3) a society can be divided into various strata according to age and roles; (4) society itself is continually changing, as are the people and their roles in each age strata; and (5) a dynamic interplay exists between individual aging and social change. Thus, aging people and the larger society are constantly influencing each other and changing both the cohorts and the society. In recent years, the age stratification theory has evolved into the Aging and Society Paradigm, which seeks to explain the processes underlying the movement of age cohorts through time and age-related social structures (McMullin, 2000).

Social gerontologists in recent years are addressing concepts related to age segregation, the study of relationships among members of different age groups outside the family (Hagestad & Dannefer, 2001). This issue is being addressed particularly in relation to age-segregated residential settings for older adults. Age segregation is being challenged because of an increasing recognition of the importance of age integration.

An age-integrated part of society is one in which chronologic age is not used as a criterion for entrance, exit, or participation. The two related components of age integration are the absence of age barriers and the presence of cross-age interactions (Uhlenberg, 2000). One recent viewpoint suggests that age integration is part of a continuum. That is, some societies may be more age integrated than others, and the degree of age integration in any society changes over time. Similarly, some social structures may be more age integrated than others, and some people may experience more age integration than others (Uhlenberg, 2000). Age integration is seen as an important factor in combating ageism and improving quality of life, not only for older adults, but also for younger generations.

Person–Environment Fit Theory

The person–environment fit theory considers the interrelationships between personal competence and the environment (Lawton, 1982). According to this theory, personal competence involves the following factors, which collectively contribute to a person's functional ability: ego strength, motor skills, biologic health, cognitive capacity, and sensory-perceptual capacity. The environment is viewed in terms of its potential for eliciting a behavioral response from the person. Lawton asserts that, for each person's level of competence, there is a level of environmental demand, or environmental press, that is most advantageous to that person's function. People who function at relatively lower levels of competence can tolerate only low levels of environmental press, whereas people who function at higher levels of competence can tolerate increased environmental demands. An often-quoted correlate is that the more impaired the person, the greater the impact of the environment. This theory is often used in planning appropriate environments for older adults with disabilities.

The person–environment fit theory has stimulated further research and theory development in the field of environmental gerontology, as evidenced by the development of six major models to explain relationships between aging and environmental influences. Person–environment theories currently are addressing questions about aging in private homes and institutional settings as well as questions about relocation and decisions about place of residence (Wahl, 2001).

Relevance of Sociologic Theories of Aging to Gerontological Nursing

Sociologic theories of aging help nurses view older adults as people who function in relation to their environments and who are influenced by the society in which they live. Some of the influences that are addressed in theories of social gerontology are culture, family, education, community, ascribed roles, cohort effects, home and living setting, and personal and political economics. Although there are patterns of similar responses among cohorts in specific cultures, the theories remind health care workers that, within those larger patterns, each person is unique. Some may achieve their identity in an elderly subculture, others may define successful aging in relation to their activities, and still others may find new roles in society. Sociologic theories of aging can shed light on the unique ways that older people cope with stress, respond to illness, and achieve healthy aging.

Gerontological nurses can apply concepts from the continuity theory, particularly when they assess coping mechanisms and plan interventions to facilitate healthy adjustments. For example, it is helpful to understand that the way in which people respond to changes in older adulthood is probably an extension of the way they learned to cope throughout their lifetimes. By identifying usual activity patterns and coping mechanisms from the past, nurses can help older adults find new activities that will contribute to self-fulfillment and effective coping. Onega and Tripp-Reimer (1997) discuss the application of the continuity theory to gerontological nursing practice and provide an excellent case example.

Emerging theories about age integration are stimulating interest in broadening the environments of institutional settings to include pets and intergenerational activities. Theories addressing questions of diversity encourage nurses to consider the cultural needs of individual older adults. Similarly, theories addressing power hierarchies and inequalities encourage nurses to be more aware of opportunities to empower older adults. For example, many of the health promotion interventions discussed throughout this text emphasize the importance of educating older adults about choices they can make that influence their health and functioning. Another implication of theories addressing inequalities is the increased recognition of residents' rights (in institutional settings) as well as increased recognition of the importance of respecting autonomy for all older adults.

Using concepts from the person–environment fit theory, gerontological nurses can appreciate the importance of environmental adaptations as interventions to improve functional status, especially when working with dependent older adults. In addition, these theories emphasize the importance of assessing both environmental and psychosocial factors that influence the functioning of an older person. Lawton's theory also suggests that when an older person has impaired functioning, coping interventions can be directed toward improving personal competency, decreasing environmental demands, or both. Some of the risk factors discussed throughout this text identify environmental factors that interfere with the health and functioning of older adults. Similarly, many of the nursing interventions discussed in this text identify ways of modifying the environment to improve the functioning of older adults.

➤ Imagine that you are 87 years old and have been retired for 10 years. Create an image of yourself at that age, making sure that you incorporate some changes that are likely to occur as you grow older. Describe the people who are an active part of your relationships during a typical month. Describe the activities you would engage in during a typical week for each of the following aspects of your life: leisure activity, physical activity, intellectual stimulation, emotional growth, social interaction, spiritual nurturing. Would you be active in any volunteer organizations? What would your health and functioning be, and where would you be living? Based on the image of yourself at 87 years old that you just created, answer the following questions:

 THINKING POINTS

➤ How could you apply either the activity theory or the disengagement theory to the life you describe at age 87 as it compares with your life at your present age?

➤ What aspects of your lifestyle at 87 years old could be explained by the continuity theory?

➤ Would any of the concepts in the subculture, age stratification, or age integration theories explain your activities and relationships?

➤ How would the person–environment fit theory explain the relationship between you and your environment?

PSYCHOLOGICAL THEORIES OF AGING

Psychological theories of aging address questions about the behavioral and developmental aspects of later adulthood: *How is behavior affected by aging? Do patterns of behavior change over time in any identifiable way?* and *What is the relationship between older adults and the broader universe?* These theories are broad in their scope because psychological aging is influenced by biologic and social factors and involves the use of adaptive capacities for exercising behavioral control or self-regulation. These adaptive capacities include learning, memory, feelings, intelligence, and motivation. A recent

discussion of the development of psychological theories of aging emphasized that the history of geropsychology clearly points to the conclusion "that age itself doesn't cause anything. Age is a convenient index to group phenomena, but it does not reflect the dynamic processes that bring about the changes associated with age" (Birren & Schroots, 2001, p. 25). Some of the major psychological theories of aging are reviewed in the following sections. Because nursing addresses psychosocial, as well as physiologic, aspects of function, these theories are especially relevant to gerontological nurses. In addition to the theories discussed in this chapter, theories about cognitive function, stress and coping, and depression—also among the psychological theories of aging—are discussed in Chapters 7, 8, and 25 because of their specific relevance to those chapters.

Human Needs Theory

Many psychological theories address the concepts of motivation and human needs. Maslow's hierarchy of needs is one such theory that has been used by gerontologists. According to Maslow's theory (1954), the five categories of basic human needs, ordered from lowest to highest, are: physiologic needs, safety and security needs, love and belongingness, self-esteem, and self-actualization. The attainment of lower-level needs takes priority over higher-level needs; self-actualization can occur only when lower-level needs are met to some degree. People continually move between the levels but always strive toward higher levels. This theory is particularly applicable to older adults because Maslow describes self-actualized people as fully mature humans who possess such desirable traits as autonomy, creativity, independence, and positive interpersonal relationships.

Life-Course and Personality Development Theories

Some psychological theories of aging, referred to as personality development theories, identify personality types as predictive forces for successful or unsuccessful aging. Other theories, referred to as life-course theories (also called life span theories), attempt to address old age within the context of the timeframe of the person's life span or life cycle. According to these theories, one's life course is divided into stages, and one moves through these stages in certain patterns. Like Maslow's human needs theory, life-course theories describe some progression through various stages and suggest that successful progression is related in some way to successful accomplishments in prior stages. A central theme of life span models is that successful aging is accomplished when older adults can engage in life tasks that they consider important despite a reduction in their energy (Birren & Schroots, 2001). There is a great deal of overlap between some of the concepts in personality development theories and those in life-course theories; indeed, these terms are often used interchangeably by different authors to refer to the same theories.

Personality development theories, like the theory of continuity discussed previously in this chapter, address the question of whether the personality changes or remains the same throughout the life course. Although researchers agree that personality in later life is characterized by both change and stability, many questions remain unanswered about the extent of change or stability and about variations in change and stability across the life span (Ryff et al., 2001). Sociologic as well as psychological theories of aging are attempting to address such questions.

Based on their belief that neither the activity nor the disengagement theory adequately explained personality differences, Neugarten and colleagues (1968) conducted a study of personality types and identified four basic personality patterns in older adults: integrated, armored-defended, passive-dependent, and unintegrated. Most of their older subjects had made positive adjustments to aging and were assigned to the mature, or integrated, personality group. They further divided this group of high-functioning older subjects into three categories based on their level of role activity: (1) reorganizers, who were engaged in a wide variety of activities; (2) focused people, who had become selective in their activities; and (3) disengaged people, who had voluntarily moved away from role commitments. People in the armored-defended group either held on to patterns of middle age as long as possible or closed themselves off from the world. Those with passive-dependent personalities were found to have strong dependency needs or to be apathetic "rocking-chair" people. Those in the unintegrated personality group formed the smallest group and were the least well adjusted. This group included those with psychological problems, those who exhibited irrational behavior, and those who failed to cope with activities of daily living (Neugarten et al., 1968).

Most theories of adult personality development are based on the theories of Carl Jung or Erik Erikson. Jung's theory (1960) categorizes personalities as either extroverted and oriented toward the external world or introverted and oriented toward subjective experiences. A balance between the two orientations, both of which are present to some degree in all people, is essential for mental health. Jung further theorized that people tend to be more extroverted in their younger years because of the nature of the demands and responsibilities associated with family and social roles. As these demands change and diminish, beginning at about the age of 40 years, people become more introverted. Jung (1954) describes later adulthood as a period of taking stock, a time during which a person looks backward rather than forward and is responsible for devoting serious attention to self. Successful aging, according to Jung's theory, is dependent on accepting one's diminishing capacity and increasing number of losses.

Jung's theory set the stage for later revisions in the disengagement theory of Cumming and Henry (1961) and for Neugarten's (1968) theory of interiority. Based on studies of middle-aged and older adults, Neugarten suggested replacing the term "disengagement" with the phrase "increased interiority of the personality" (1968). Neugarten's definition of interiority was similar to Jung's definition of introversion, but she identified the middle years as beginning at 50, rather than 40, years of age. Neugarten described the middle years of life as the time when "introspection seems to increase noticeably, and contemplation and reflection and self-evaluation become characteristic forms of mental life" (Neugarten, 1968, p. 140). Like Jung, she proposed that, with increasing age, ego functions are increasingly turned toward the self and away from the outer world.

Erik Erikson's original theory (1963) about the eight stages of life has been used widely in relation to older adulthood. Erikson defines the stages of life as trust versus mistrust, autonomy versus shame and doubt, initiative versus guilt, industry versus inferiority, identity versus identity diffusion, intimacy versus self-absorption, generativity versus stagnation, and ego integrity versus despair. Each of these stages presents the person with certain conflicting tendencies that must be balanced before he or she can move successfully from that stage. As in other life-course theories, how one stage is mastered lays the groundwork for successful or unsuccessful mastery of the next stage. In works published between 1950 and 1966, Erikson emphasized the life course from childhood to young adulthood; in later publications, however, he reconsidered the meaning of these stages. In 1982, when he was 80 years old, Erikson described the task of old age as balancing the search for integrity and wholeness with a sense of despair. He believed that the successful accomplishment of this task, achieved primarily through life review activities, would result in wisdom.

Peck (1968) expanded Erikson's original theory and divided the eighth stage—ego integrity versus despair—into additional stages occurring during middle age and old age. The stages described by Peck as specific to old age are ego differentiation versus work-role preoccupation, body transcendence versus body preoccupation, and ego transcendence versus ego pre-occupation. Recent psychological theories on aging continue to use Erikson's construct of generativity in addressing questions about how generativity is linked to other aspects of personality and about how the life course shifts into and out of midlife generativity (Ryff et al., 2001).

Departing from theories that begin with infancy or childhood, some of the more recently developed life-course theories concentrate on middle or later adulthood. For example, Havighurst (1972) defines the tasks of late life as (1) adjusting to decreasing physical strength and health; (2) adjusting to retirement and reduced income; (3) adjusting to the death of a spouse; (4) establishing an explicit association with one's age group; (5) adapting to social roles in a flexible way; and (6) establishing satisfactory physical living arrangements. Another life-course theory defines the tasks of later maturity as (1) coping with physical changes of aging; (2) redirecting energy to new roles and activities, such as retirement, widowhood, and grandparenting; (3) accepting one's own life; and (4) developing a point of view about death (Newman & Newman, 1984).

Psychological Theories About Gender and Aging

In recent decades, a number of psychological theories of aging, particularly those that center on life span perspectives, have focused on relationships between gender and aging. Some of these studies have addressed diverse populations, such as lesbians, gay men, and transgendered persons. Three purposes of gender-related psychological theories of aging studies have been: (1) to compare and contrast male and female performance data, (2) to examine the nature of change in gender roles, and (3) to study the relationship between gender role differences and social roles and social power (Sinnott & Shifren, 2001). Gender-specific aspects of psychology and aging that have been studied include intelligence, personality, caregiving, self-efficacy, body attitudes, verbal ability, social ties, self-reported health, sense of control, and medical decision-making processes (Sinnott & Shifren, 2001). Results of some of these studies are reported in chapters of this text related to these topics (e.g., health characteristics in Chapter 1, caregiver characteristics in Chapter 2, and cognitive functioning in Chapter 7).

Gender role development across the life span is one specific topic addressed by psychological theories of aging. Many researchers believe that gender roles evolve from being narrowly defined in adolescence and younger adulthood to becoming more amorphous in later adulthood. Although many questions about adult role development remain unanswered, an analysis of research on this subject concluded that "gender role development in old age appears to involve transforming and even transcending such roles, at least as they are conceptualized in earlier life, to continue the construction of identity, meaning, and community for the aging person" (Sinnott & Shifren, 2001, pp. 470–471). This same analysis suggested that rather than focusing on whether there are gender differences as we age, the psychological theories of aging should focus on the question of *Why is there a gender difference as we age?* (Sinnott & Shifren, 2001). Throughout this text, some studies that have addressed gender differences in various aspects of health and functioning of older adults are designated in the Diversity Notes. Gender differences relevant to health and aging also are discussed in detail in Chapter 4. It is important to keep in mind, however, that this is a newly evolving area of research and that findings are likely to develop rapidly and may even change during the early part of the 21st century.

Recent and Evolving Theories

Behavioral genetic research, which encompasses both genetic and environmental factors as well as how these factors influence aging, attempts to answer questions such as *Why do people age so differently?* Studies are usually longitudinal and include twins, adoptees, and families of origin. They address issues related to longevity, personality, life events, social support, cognitive functioning, family environment, and health and disease (Bergeman & Plomin, 1996). Evidence from behavioral genetic studies supports the concept of increasing heterogeneity among older adults and debunks the myth that decline is an inevitable part of aging (Pedersen, 1996). Both these conclusions are particularly relevant to gerontological nurses. Some theories, called developmental behavioral genetic theories, merge developmental psychology with behavioral genetics, exploring both the origins of change and the continuity in development.

The branching theory is an evolving psychological theory of aging that is based on the principle of gerodynamics, which draws on chaos theory and general systems theory. The basic theme of this theory is the bifurcation or branching behavior of a person at the social, biologic, or psychological level of function. Simply stated, each person passes critical points (i.e., bifurcation or branching points) and can branch off into higher-order and lower-order processes in relation to mortality, morbidity, and quality of life. For example, traumatic life events may result in lower-order structures that result in an increased probability of dying, whereas a healthy lifestyle may result in higher-order structures that lead to a decreased probability of dying (Schroots, 1996). According to this theory, aging is defined as a series of transformations toward increasing disorder and order in form, pattern, or structure (Schroots, 1988).

Gerotranscendence is another emerging theory that was proposed in the early 1990s by Lars Tornstam (1994) and has become widely recognized in Sweden and other Scandinavian countries. This theory proposes that human aging is a process of shifting from a rational and materialistic metaperspective to a more cosmic and transcendent vision. This shift includes the following aspects: decreased self-centeredness; decreased fear of death; increased time spent in meditation; decreased interest in material things; decreased interest in superfluous social interaction; increased feelings of cosmic union with the universe; increased feelings of affinity with past and coming generations; and a redefinition of one's perception of time, space, and objects (Ruth, 1996). One review of this theory suggests that gerotranscendence theory is an extension of disengagement theory that attempts to "re-enchant aging" by replacing performance-oriented characteristics of people in midlife with alternative qualities such as play, rest, wisdom, creativity, and relaxation (Jonson & Magnusson, 2001). Emerging psychological theories of aging also are addressing questions about the complex relationships between aging and health behaviors and about the origins of later life changes in behavior. Questions also are being addressed about the inner experience of aging and being old (Birren & Schroots, 2001). Some of the theories that address questions about wisdom, creativity, and spiritual outlook are briefly discussed in other chapters of this text (e.g., Chapters 7 and 8).

Relevance of Psychological Theories of Aging to Gerontological Nursing

In caring for older adults, gerontological nurses can use psychological theories of aging as a framework for addressing certain issues, such as response to losses and continued emotional development. Maslow's framework is useful for conceptualizing the nature of interventions in institutional or home settings. For instance, if older adults are unable to purchase food, they are unlikely to feel secure. Likewise, if older adults feel insecure about being able to meet their shelter needs, they are unlikely to have a sense of trust. Older adults who have already met their lower-level needs, however, can be encouraged to focus on higher-level achievements such as self-actualization.

In addition, psychological theories imply that older adults should devote some time and energy to life review and self-understanding. Nurses can facilitate this process by asking sensitive questions and by listening attentively to older adults as they share information about their past. Reminiscence is a positive experience that is essential for continued psychological development, and it can be promoted by nurses either on an individual or group basis.

Finally, both the sociologic and psychological theories of aging can be valuable in dispelling some of the commonly held myths about old age. An understanding of the continued potential for psychological development might help older adults and their caregivers appreciate the positive attributes of growing older, such as the wisdom and creativity that can be derived from life experiences.

Life-course models can help nurses identify those areas of personality that are likely to change and those that are more likely to remain stable. Gerontological nurses can apply the principles of the branching theory to provide insights into the behaviors of older adults as attempts at bringing order out of disorder (Porter, 1995). Based on this theory, Porter suggests that gerontological nurses should (1) identify the unique ways in which older adults bring order out of disorder, (2) describe these processes in relation to each person's uniqueness, and (3) use this knowledge to develop creative nursing interventions.

Nurses have used life span theories to develop a multidisciplinary Theory of Thriving (Haight et al., 2002). This model proposes that thriving is achieved when there is concordance between the person and the human and nonhuman environment; that is, when these three elements are mutually engaged, supportive, and harmonious. In contrast, failure to thrive is the result of discordance among these three elements, causing a failure of engagement and mutual support, and disharmony (Haight et al., 2002). In addition to these implications for gerontological nurses, implications regarding specific aspects, such as intellectual function and coping responses, are discussed in Chapters 7 and 8 of this text and should be considered in the context of psychological theories of aging.

➤ Imagine, again, that you are 87 years old, and add the following information to the description of yourself that you created for the discussion of sociologic theories. Describe your personality, including, but not limited to, the following characteristics: emotional stability, adjustments to losses, contentedness with life, optimism versus pessimism, engagement in activities versus withdrawal from activities, and feelings of self-efficacy versus feelings of powerlessness. Describe your beliefs about your gender-specific roles (i.e., those aspects of roles that are defined by you being a woman, or a man). Based on this image of yourself at 87 years old, answer the following questions:

 THINKING POINTS

➤ Where do you think you would be in Maslow's or Erikson's stages, and how would you have moved between the levels in the past decades?

➤ How would any concepts in the personality development theories apply to you?

➤ Based on your own experiences, how has your perception of your role as a woman (or man) changed over time?

A THEORY FOR GERONTOLOGICAL NURSING: THE FUNCTIONAL CONSEQUENCES THEORY

Gerontological nurses derive theories from existing nursing knowledge and from relevant theories about aging, such as those discussed in this book. Nursing theories are distinctive because they are conceptualizations of some aspect of reality, viewed from the perspective of nursing, used to describe, explain, predict, or prescribe nursing care (Meleis, 1997). Theories about aging can explain various aspects of older adulthood, but only a theory of gerontological nursing can answer the question posed by one gerontological nurse scholar: "What is there about being aged that requires a difference in nursing care?" (Wells, 1987, p. 22). A gerontological nursing theory, therefore, explains the care needs that are unique to older people and provides a basis for addressing those needs from a nursing perspective.

One approach to nursing theory development is to look for observable data and trends and generate theories to explain them. The functional consequences theory of gerontological nursing presented in this text has evolved from this approach. Because this theory underpins all other material presented in this text, it is the theory of gerontological nursing that will be fully explicated. Before the functional consequences theory is discussed, however, an overview of nursing theory will be presented to offer a broader perspective.

Gerontological Nursing Theory in Perspective

Despite the fact that Florence Nightingale is often referred to as the first nurse-theorist, formal articulation of nursing theories did not begin until the mid-1950s. Early nursing theories were built on theories borrowed from other disciplines. Like other nurses, gerontological nurses used theories from other disciplines to underpin their beliefs and practice. By the 1980s, nurses were developing their own theories about phenomena unique to nursing, and nursing subspecialties were identifying the need for theories to explain their particular areas. During the 1990s, nurses developed mid-range theories and situation-specific theories to explain nursing phenomena that were limited in scope (Meleis, 1997).

In 1987, an issue of the *Journal of Gerontological Nursing* addressed the need for theory development in gerontological nursing (Whall, 1987). One article emphasized that this need was "based less on any perceived inadequacies in current models but rather on a call for extension of [the] current theoretical thinking that encompasses gerontological nursing" (Cowling, 1987, p. 12). Moreover, Cowling emphasized the need for theories that shed light on both the "general and unique perspectives that encompass the world of gerontological nursing practice" (1987, p. 12). The recency of interest in gerontological nursing theory is also evident in the American Nurses Association (ANA) Standards of Gerontological Nursing Practice. The 1976 standards contain no reference to theory, but the 1987 revision calls for nurses to participate in the generation and testing of theory. In recent years, nurses have continued to recognize the need for mid-range theory as a step toward knowledge development and a way of supporting nursing practice (McEwen & Wills, 2002).

Theory Development in Nursing

Since the time of Florence Nightingale, nurses have tried to define the domain of nursing and to distinguish nursing knowledge from medical knowledge. Despite this long history, however, only recently have nurses agreed on the concepts that constitute the unique domain of nursing: nursing, health, person, and environment. The purpose of nursing theories is to link these concepts and explain their interrelationships. Frameworks for nursing theories are developed along distinct research traditions, or paradigms, and each paradigm provides a different philosophical approach to theory development and research. The following research traditions or paradigms have been dominant in nursing:

1. The *empiricist* paradigm stresses objectivity, inductive reasoning, measurable variables, and value-free assumptions (Meleis, 1997). Research follows the classic scientific method and removes, as much as possible, variations in findings that

could be caused by the uniqueness of people and their situations.

2. The *historicist* paradigm emphasizes that human phenomena necessarily exist within a sociocultural context. All truths are relative, there are always multiple truths, and the context must be taken into account when compiling findings (Meleis, 1987).

3. The *phenomenological* paradigm seeks to examine the significance of meaning in understanding human behavior, meanings for both the person and the environment that result from transactions between the two. In this paradigm, the nurse is considered to be part of the client's environment, and the meaning of the interaction between the person and the environment is examined. Phenomenologists also look for patterns that incorporate variables related to the phenomenon (Meleis, 1987).

4. The *feminist,* or *gender-sensitive,* perspective is the most recently developed paradigm. The goal of this perspective is understanding, rather than simply knowing, and it can be used to develop an understanding of all nursing clients, without regard for race, gender, or culture (Meleis, 1997). Feminist methodology aims to raise the consciousness of researchers about feminist and other views of nursing phenomena, which are equal in importance to masculine and other dominant views.

A recent analysis of current approaches to theory development in nursing stated that nurses are not in agreement about whether nursing theory should emphasize a holistic and humanistic perspective or an objective and scientifically derived perspective. This analysis concludes that what is needed is an open philosophy that ties empirical concepts that can be validated through the senses with theoretical concepts of meaning and value" (McEwen & Wills, 2002). Although these paradigms may seem irrelevant to nurses caring for older adults, they are reviewed here to provide a philosophical framework for understanding and evaluating the functional consequences theory of gerontological nursing.

The functional consequences theory is based on the historicist perspective. The following three characteristics describe the context from which the functional consequences theory has evolved. First, from a historicist perspective, the relevant element in evaluating a theory is its problem-solving effectiveness. Accordingly, a theory's progress is defined by the degree to which it solves more scientific problems than its rivals (Silva & Rothbart, 1984, p. 6). Second, data for nursing theory development include the day-to-day experiences of

nurses, the common beliefs of the community of nurses, the social and psychological factors affecting the profession of nursing, and the reasoning patterns of individual nurse-theorists (Silva & Rothbart, 1984). Third, concepts pertinent to a discipline at any one time are those problems encountered by the practitioners; thus, as problems change and grow, so do the concepts that explain and inform the discipline (Ramos, 1987).

Finally, before explicating the functional consequences theory, the issue of theory testing through research must be addressed. The functional consequences theory was formulated over a period of almost two decades of gerontological nursing practice. As such, its approach is "from the ground up" rather than "from the grand down" (Wells, 1987, p. 21). It is a response to the challenge posed in the *Journal of Gerontological Nursing*: "examine existing knowledge and, through a process of synthesis, derive models that provide directions for practice" (Wells, 1987, p. 22). As a mid-range theory, it can be tested through nursing research, and it can provide a basis for nursing care of older adults.

The Functional Consequences Theory

The functional consequences theory postulates that older adults experience functional consequences because of age-related changes and additional risk factors. Without interventions, many functional consequences are negative; with them, however, functional consequences can be positive. The role of the gerontological nurse is to identify the factors that cause negative functional consequences and to initiate interventions that will result in positive ones. The ultimate goal of these interventions is to enable older people to function at their highest level despite the presence of age-related changes and risk factors.

This theory, diagrammed in Figure 3-4, can be illustrated by the following example. One negative functional consequence of age-related changes affecting the eye is an increased sensitivity to glare. Thus, older people are less able to see clearly when they face bright lights or when lights reflect off shiny surfaces. They have increased difficulty, for instance, driving into the sunlight or reading shopping mall maps that are enclosed in glass cases. In addition to this age-related change, an older adult might have a disease-related risk factor that causes similar negative functional consequences. Cataracts, for instance, may cause blurred vision and increase an individual's sensitivity to glare. Environmental factors may also pose risk factors: white paint, bright lights, and highly polished floors intensify glare. The combination of these age-related changes and risk factors can interfere with

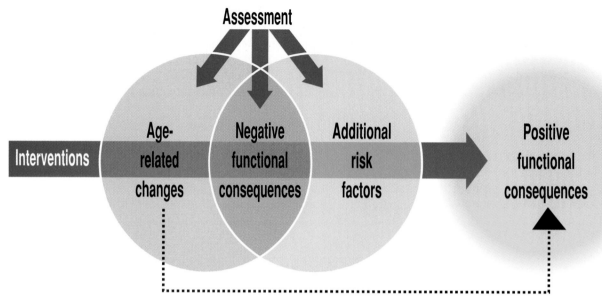

FIGURE 3-4 The functional consequences model of gerontological nursing. Age-related changes and additional risk factors combine to cause negative functional consequences. The shading symbolizes that age-related changes have less impact than risk factors, but together these factors have a cumulative effect. Nurses assess the age-related changes, risk factors, and negative functional consequences, and initiate interventions to counteract or minimize their effects. The outcome of these interventions are positive functional consequences.

the functional capacity of an older adult to the extent that the person stops performing certain activities or performs them in an unsafe manner.

To counteract these negative functional consequences, interventions can be initiated by the older person or suggested by a gerontological nurse. Interventions directed toward the age-related change include wearing sunglasses and using other glare-reducing devices. Interventions directed toward the risk factors include cataract surgery and environmental modifications, such as the use of nonglare glass. The result of these interventions is the positive functional consequence of improved and safer function of the older adult. In addition, the person's quality of life might be enhanced because of positive functional consequences.

CONCEPTS UNDERLYING THE FUNCTIONAL CONSEQUENCES THEORY

The functional consequences theory draws from nursing theories and from nonnursing disciplines to delineate the unique aspects of aging and older adults that distinguish gerontological nursing from nursing in general. The domain concepts of person, environment, health, and nursing are linked together in the functional consequences theory, specifically in relation to older adults. Before discussing these domain concepts,

however, the concepts of functional consequences, age-related changes, and risk factors are examined. Display 3-1 summarizes the key concepts in the functional consequences theory of gerontological nursing.

Functional Consequences

Functional consequences, which may be positive or negative, are the observable effects of actions, risk factors, and age-related changes that influence the quality of life or day-to-day activities of older adults. Actions include, but are not limited to, purposeful interventions initiated either by the older person or by nurses and other caregivers. Risk factors can originate in the environment or arise from physiologic and psychosocial influences. Functional consequences are positive when they facilitate the highest level of performance and the least amount of dependency. Conversely, they are negative when they interfere with a person's level of function or quality of life or increase a person's dependency.

Negative functional consequences typically occur because of a combination of age-related changes and risk factors, as illustrated in the previous example of impaired visual performance. They also may be caused by interventions, in which case the interventions become risk factors. For example, constipation resulting from the use of an antidepressant medication is an example of a negative functional consequence caused

---

DISPLAY 3-1

Concepts in the Functional Consequences Theory of Gerontological Nursing

Functional Consequences. The observable effects of actions, risk factors, and age-related changes that influence the quality of life or day-to-day activities of older adults.

Negative Functional Consequences. Those that interfere with the person's level of functioning or quality of life.

Positive Functional Consequences. Those that facilitate the highest level of performance and the least amount of dependency.

Age-Related Changes. Inevitable, progressive, and irreversible changes that occur during later adulthood and are independent of extrinsic or pathologic conditions.

Risk Factors. Conditions that increase the vulnerability of older people to negative functional consequences. Common risk factors are diseases, environment, lifestyle, support systems, psychosocial circumstances, adverse medication effects, and attitudes based on lack of knowledge.

Person (Older Adults). People whose functional abilities are affected by the acquisition of age-related changes and risk factors. When older adults are affected by age-related changes and risk factors to the extent that they are dependent on others for daily needs, their caregivers are considered an integral focus of gerontological nursing.

Nursing. The goals of gerontological nursing are to minimize the negative effects of age-related changes and risk factors and to promote positive functional consequences. Goals are achieved through the nursing process, with particular emphasis on interacting with older adults and caregivers of dependent older adults to eliminate risk factors or minimize their effects.

Health. The ability of older adults to function at their highest capacity, despite the presence of age-related changes and risk factors. This state includes quality of life and encompasses psychosocial as well as physiologic function.

Environment. External conditions, including caregivers, that influence the function of older adults. These conditions are risk factors when they interfere with function and are interventions when they enhance function.

---

by an intervention. In this case, the medication is both an intervention for the depression and a risk factor for impaired bowel function.

Positive functional consequences are usually brought about by automatic actions or purposeful interventions. Often, older adults bring about positive functional consequences when they compensate for age-related changes without conscious intent. For example, an older person might increase the amount of light for reading or begin using sunglasses without realizing that these actions are compensating for age-related changes. At other times, interventions are initiated in response to a recognized need. In the impaired visual performance example cited earlier, improved function would likely result from purposeful interventions, such as cataract surgery or environmental modifications. In a few instances, positive functional consequences are caused directly by age-related changes. For example, a woman may view the postmenopausal inability to become pregnant as a positive effect of aging. As a consequence, her enjoyment of sexual activities may be enhanced in later adulthood. Similarly, positive functional consequences, such as increased wisdom and maturity, can result from psychological growth in older adulthood.

The concept of functional consequences draws on nursing and nonnursing theories regarding functional assessment. Nonnursing theories are derived primarily from geriatric and rehabilitative medicine (discussed in the earlier section on Medical Theories and in Chapter 11). Many gerontological nursing texts now focus on functional assessment, and nurses commonly address functional health patterns. The gerontological literature discusses functional assessment as a framework for research and as a method for planning health services for dependent people. From a clinical perspective, health care practitioners view the multidimensional functional assessment as an important component in the care of older people. None of the literature, however, suggests an assessment of functional consequences. To date, this aspect has not been developed, and it is unique to the functional consequences theory of gerontological nursing.

The functional consequences theory draws on concepts regarding functional assessment but extends far beyond an assessment of function. The functional consequences theory significantly differs from functional assessment in the following ways: (1) it defines functional consequences and differentiates between positive and negative consequences; (2) it emphasizes the identification of age-related changes and risk factors that affect a person's function, rather than simply identifying a person's functional level; (3) it attempts to distinguish between age-related changes that increase a person's vulnerability and risk factors that interfere with a person's function; and (4) it addresses from a functional perspective, not only assessment, but also interventions.

Age-Related Changes and Risk Factors

Age-related changes and risk factors are concepts crucial to the functional consequences theory because they distinguish the care of older adults from the care of other people. Differentiating between age-related changes and risk factors is essential because the interventions for age-related changes differ from those for risk factors. Age-related changes cannot be reversed or altered, but it is possible to compensate for their effects and to intervene so that positive functional consequences occur. By contrast, risk factors often can be modified or even eliminated, and their effects may be reversed or compensated for through interventions.

The nonnursing theories that underpin the concept of age-related changes have been addressed in earlier sections of this chapter. Biologic theories of aging, for example, are useful in understanding the concept of age-related changes. Our knowledge regarding age-related changes, however, is rapidly evolving. A noted geriatrician underscored this point: "I find I must learn and relearn all the time, namely, to accept no symptom or loss of function in older persons as being simply 'old age.' Rather, professionals should search for explanations, which will almost always be found in one or more diseases that are present, or in life style (such as incremental disuse), or in the environment" (Williams, 1986, p. 347). Although the functional consequences theory challenges the "what-do-you-expect-you're-old" syndrome, it also recognizes that there are not always clear distinctions between age-related and disease-related processes. Even if apparent distinctions are identified, they may be questioned at a later time as new theories evolve. The functional consequences theory views age-related changes, not as the sole cause of negative functional consequences, but rather as factors that increase the vulnerability of older people to the negative impact of risk factors.

Nursing theories have not yet encompassed age-related changes, but at least one gerontological nurse scholar has suggested that nursing research should address this question (Wells, 1987). Nursing theories have, however, addressed risk factors in relation to health. Rose and Killien (1983) analyzed the concepts of risk and vulnerability and identified their distinguishing features in an article that is particularly applicable to the functional consequences theory. Their model was developed from the perspective of pediatric nurses, but it provides a basis for understanding the differences, as well as the relationship, between age-related changes and risk factors in older adults. Rose and Killien conceptualize risks as potentially stressful factors in the person's environment, which includes the immediate surroundings as well as direct and indirect influences of the broader physical and sociocultural environment. Applying this to the functional consequences theory, examples of risk factors would be poor lighting, barriers to mobility, lack of social supports, and myths and misunderstandings about aging. Rose and Killien conceptualize vulnerability as a dynamic continuum that is affected by both constitutional and acquired factors. Constitutional factors are reflected in a person's internal environment and neurophysiology, whereas acquired factors are those resulting from experiences and life events. Applying this to the functional consequences theory, constitutional factors would be the age-related changes that interfere with a person's ability to respond to stresses. Acquired factors would be disease-related conditions and adverse psychosocial influences, such as multiple losses in a short period. According to the functional consequences theory, however, only the constitutional factors (i.e., age-related changes) would be viewed as vulnerability characteristics, whereas the acquired factors (e.g., chronic illnesses) would be considered risk factors.

One of the implications of this model, according to Rose and Killien (1983), is that interventions to improve a person's state of health can be directed toward either reducing risk or changing the person's level of vulnerability. According to these authors, it is often more feasible to modify the environment than it is to change a person's level of vulnerability, particularly if that vulnerability is primarily due to genetic or constitutional factors (Rose & Killien, 1983, p. 68). Although their theory focuses on modification of risk factors, they also emphasize that levels of vulnerability are not static. This viewpoint is consistent with that of the functional consequences approach to gerontological nursing.

Person

The functional consequences theory's conceptualization of person as the focus of nursing care can be linked to the nursing theory of Imogene King (1981). In King's framework, people are social beings who are rational and sentient and who use language to communicate thoughts, actions, customs, and beliefs. They are further characterized by the ability to feel, think, perceive, set goals, make decisions, choose between alternative courses of action, and select the means to achieve goals. Because they possess these characteristics, they are reacting beings. This emphasis on the ability of responsible people to establish and achieve goals is relevant to the functional consequences theory, in which older adults are viewed as being capable of achieving positive functional consequences, despite the presence of age-related changes and risk factors. Furthermore, older adults are viewed as unique individuals who achieve positive functional consequences through interactions with their environment and with people in their environment. The interactions between nurses and older adults are especially important in achieving positive functional consequences.

The functional consequences theory of gerontological nursing is based on a holistic nursing approach that views the older adult as a complex and unique person whose functioning is influenced by the relationships between many internal and external factors. Because this theory is specific to gerontological nursing, *person* is defined in relation to the age category called *older adults*. Using the nonnursing theories discussed in this text, older adult is defined, not just by chronologic age, but also by the acquisition of physiologic and psychosocial characteristics that are associated with maturity. On the positive side, these characteristics include increased wisdom and creativity and advanced levels of personal growth based on experience. On the negative side, these characteristics include a slowing down of physiologic processes, increased vulnerability to chronic illnesses, and a diminished ability to respond to physiologic stress.

Because aging is a complex and gradual process, a person does not discover that he or she has suddenly become an older adult at a particular chronologic age. Rather, people who live long enough recognize at some point that they have reached a stage of life that society categorizes as older adulthood. Although this concept has the distinct disadvantage of being difficult to measure, it has the advantage of accurately reflecting the realities of older adulthood being a part of the life-course continuum. Because people increase in heterogeneity rather than homogeneity as they age, any definition of the older adult must, by its nature, be broad. According to the functional consequences theory, a person is considered to be an older adult when he or she manifests several or many functional consequences attributable to age-related changes alone or to age-related changes in combination with risk factors. Stated simply, the accumulation of age-related functional consequences defines someone as an older adult.

The older adult is further conceptualized in the context of his or her relationships with others because a person is not an isolated entity, but rather a dynamic being who continually influences and is influenced by the environment and other people. This context is particularly important for older adults because the more functionally impaired a person is, the more important are his or her support resources. When negative functional consequences accumulate to the extent that the older adult is very dependent on others for daily needs, the primary focus of gerontological nursing shifts from the older adult to his or her caregivers. Even for older people with few functional impairments, this context is important because older

people have a long history of interpersonal relationships that influence their health behaviors.

Nursing

The conceptualization of nursing in the functional consequences theory draws on many nursing theorists, beginning with Florence Nightingale, who viewed nursing as the provision of an environment conducive to healing and health promotion (Nightingale, 1954 [1859]). In recent decades, nursing has been viewed as a profession that "has a social mandate to provide health care for clients at different points in the health-illness continuum" (McEwen & Wills, 2002, p. 4). The ANA statement on the scope of gerontological nursing, discussed in Chapter 4, also is applicable to the definition of nursing as outlined by the functional consequences theory. Bahr's definition is also applicable to this theory: "The goal of gerontological nursing care is to help elderly clients function as fully as possible by realizing their highest potential" (Bahr, 1981, p. 24). Finally, King's theory of nursing is particularly relevant to the concept of nursing presented in the functional consequences theory.

The crux of nursing in King's theory is the nurse–client transaction, which is defined as a purposeful interaction that leads to goal attainment. Nursing itself is defined as "a process of action, reaction, and interaction whereby nurse and client share information about their perceptions in the nursing situation. Through purposeful communication they identify specific goals, problems, or concerns. They explore means to achieve a goal and agree to means to the goal" (King, 1981, p. 2). Outcomes of these transactions include satisfaction in performing activities of daily living, success in performing activities in one's usual roles, and achievement of immediate and long-range goals. One example of this kind of nursing activity is community nurses who perform health assessments of older adults and "engage in mutual goal setting to help older individuals function in their usual roles" (King, 1981, p. 3).

According to the functional consequences theory, the goals of gerontological nursing are to minimize the effects of negative functional consequences and to promote positive functional consequences in older adults. Through the nursing process, age-related changes and risk factors are assessed, interventions are planned and implemented, and functional outcomes are evaluated. Most often, the goals are achieved through educating older adults and the caregivers of dependent older adults about interventions that will eliminate risk factors or minimize their effects. The educational aspects are particularly important when myths and misunderstandings contribute to negative functional consequences. For example, the gerontological nurse can provide information about age-related changes and risk factors to an older person who believes that functional impairments are a necessary consequence of old age and identify ways of minimizing the effects of the risk factors and compensating for the effects of age-related changes.

The focus and goals of gerontological nursing vary according to the setting. In acute care settings, the focus is on pathologic conditions that create serious risks and that are expected to respond to short-term interventions. Goals of gerontological nurses in these settings include helping vulnerable older adults to maintain their level of functioning and to facilitate recovery from illness. In long-term care settings, the focus is on multiple risk factors that are not immediately responsive to short-term interventions and that interfere with functional abilities to the extent that the older adult is dependent on others in several functional areas. Goals include improving levels of functioning and quality-of-life issues. In home and community settings, the focus is on short-term and long-term interventions aimed at age-related changes and risk factors. As in long-term care facilities, goals include improving or at least preventing declines in functioning and addressing quality-of-life concerns. Goals in community-based settings often address health promotion interventions that are wellness oriented rather than illness oriented.

Health

Health is defined in King's theory as the "dynamic life experiences of a human being, which implies continuous adjustment to stressors in the internal and external environment through optimal use of one's resources to achieve maximum potential for daily living" (1981, p. 5). Health involves performance of the activities of daily living, but the ultimate purpose of doing so is maintaining quality of life. Furthermore, this performance is significantly influenced by one's environment. The functional consequences theory defines health as the ability of older adults to function at their highest capacity, despite the presence of age-related changes and risk factors. It encompasses psychosocial as well as physiologic function, and also considers the quality of life of the person. According to this theory, therefore, health is individually determined, based on the functional capacities that are perceived as important by that person. For example, one person might define the desired level of function as a capacity for intimate relationships, whereas another might define it as being able to perform aerobic exercise for half an hour daily.

Theories of health have been proposed by many nonnursing sources, and several are particularly relevant to the functional consequences theory of gerontological nursing. First, in 1959, the World Health Organization (WHO) defined health in older adults: "Health in the elderly is best measured in terms of function . . . degree of fitness rather than extent of pathology may be used as a measure of the amount of services the aged will require from the community" (WHO, 1959). For more than four decades, this definition has been accepted worldwide, and it underscores the idea that with increasing age, diagnostic labels become less important, and the person's level of functioning and well-being increases in importance.

Second, the perspective of older people themselves has been incorporated into the functional consequences theory. For older adults, there is a very strong relationship between health and functioning, and the relationship is not limited to physical aspects of functioning but also includes many aspects of psychosocial functioning. Older adults typically define health in terms of functional levels that are desirable (e.g., being active, sociable, productive, and helpful to others). Conversely, they typically define illness in terms of an inability to perform certain tasks (e.g., eating, sleeping, or walking).

Third, gerontologists and gerontological health care practitioners have recognized the close relationship between the concepts of health and functioning. One nursing study of the meaning of health for women aged 55 to 104 years identified the following five themes: humor, flexibility, self-acceptance, being other-centered, and interacting with a being greater than themselves (Maddox, 1999). Another nursing study found that perceptions of health for people aged 65 to 79 years was associated with self-esteem and a sense of coherence; for people aged 80 years and older, a sense of mastery was strongly associated with perceived health (Forbes, 2001). Gerontological nurses must identify an older person's beliefs about health, functioning, and the relationship between health and aging because these beliefs can significantly influence his or her approach to health care. The functional consequences theory provides a perspective from which these concepts can be linked and is particularly pertinent to health promotion interventions, as discussed in the next chapter.

Environment

The concept of environment as it is defined in the functional consequences theory of gerontological nursing is similar to King's definition. The *internal environment* transforms energy to enable human beings to adjust to continual external environmental changes. The *external environment* is defined as "an organized boundary system of social roles, behaviors, and practices developed to maintain values and the mechanisms to regulate the practices and rules" (King, 1981, p. 115). The nurse, of course, is part of the environment as well.

In the functional consequences theory, the concept of environment has several meanings, some of which might even seem contradictory. For example, environment can be both a risk factor for negative functional consequences and a source of interventions for positive functional consequences. The environment includes the setting where the care is provided; for dependent older adults, the environment also includes their caregivers. These conceptualizations are consistent with King's theory, in which a transaction is defined as observable behavior of human beings interacting with their environment. The purpose of transactions is to attain goals, which focus on improved function in activities of daily living. In turn, the hoped-for outcome is a "relatively useful, satisfying, productive, and happy life" (King, 1981, p. 4).

A nonnursing theory that sheds light on the concept of environment in the functional consequences theory is Lawton's person—environment fit theory (discussed in the Sociologic Theories section of this chapter). Gerontologists have used this theory, along with the person–environment congruence model of Kahana (1975), to examine the specific attributes of the environment that are important in the interactions between older people and their environments (Windley & Scheidt, 1980). Considerations identified by these gerontologists that are applicable to the functional consequences theory include the following:

1. Is the environment comfortable?
2. How does the spatial organization influence orientation and direction finding?
3. Can the type and amount of visual and auditory stimuli be controlled?
4. How does the environment compensate for sensory deficits?
5. Does the environment allow for choices in the degree of privacy and personal use of space?
6. How does the environment affect activities of daily living?

These attributes are central components of the environment, according to the functional consequences theory, because they represent specific environmental factors that directly influence the functional status of older people. In summary, environmental characteristics can cause negative functional consequences, but with interventions, they can also be the best sources of positive functional consequences.

To recap the functional consequences theory, this mid-range nursing theory explains the unique relationships among the concepts of person, health, nursing, and environment from the perspective of gerontological nursing. It proposes that combinations of age-related changes and risk factors increase the vulnerability of older people to negative functional consequences, which interfere with the person's level of functioning or quality of life. Gerontological nurses assess the age-related changes, risk factors, and negative functional consequences, with particular emphasis on identifying the risk factors that can be addressed through nursing interventions. The ultimate goal is to enable older people to function at their highest level despite the presence of age-related changes and risk factors.

CHAPTER SUMMARY

Theories of aging attempt to develop answers to questions about how and why we age. From a holistic perspective, the most important question is *How can we live a life that is both long and healthy?* Each gerontological health care practitioner addresses this question from her or his particular perspective. However, because care of older adults is provided in a multidisciplinary context, each profession draws on theories from other disciplines. Gerontological nurses, for example, address this question from a holistic nursing perspective that focuses on interventions that facilitate the older adult's optimal level of healthy functioning. Biologic theories of aging help gerontological nurses understand how aging affects physiologic function, and sociologic theories of aging help nurses understand the relationships between older adults and their social environments. Psychological theories of aging provide a framework for addressing certain psychosocial issues that are common among older adults (e.g., responses to losses and continued emotional development). Although theories of aging developed by other disciplines provide a base for caring for older adults from a broad and holistic perspective, they do not provide a framework to guide nursing care of older adults. The functional consequences theory of gerontological nursing is a mid-range nursing theory that offers a specific, practical, and theory-based approach to nursing care of older adults. It answers two crucial questions: *What is unique about the care needs of older adults?* and *How can gerontological nurses effectively care for older adults?*

CRITICAL THINKING EXERCISES

You are doing an admission assessment on an 87-year-old woman who is being admitted to the hospital with congestive heart failure for the third time in the past 2 years. She does not have any cognitive impairment, and she lives alone in her own home. When you ask her why she came to the hospital, she states, "I'm 87 years old, you know, isn't that a good enough reason to be sick? Don't you think you'll be in the hospital when you're my age?"

1. How do you respond to her?
2. What additional assessment information would you want?
3. What health teaching would you think about incorporating into your care plan?

EDUCATIONAL RESOURCES

American Federation for Aging Research
70 West 40th Street, New York, NY 10018
(212) 703-9977
http://www.afar.org and http://www.infoaging.org

Canadian Association on Gerontology
100-824 Meath Street, Ottawa, ON K1Z 6E8
(613) 728-9347
http://www.cagacg.ca

International Longevity Center—USA
60 East 86th Street, New York, NY, 10028
(212) 288-1468
http://www.ilcusa.org

National Institute on Aging Information Center
P.O. Box 8057, Gaithersburg, MD 20898
(800) 222-2225
http://www.nih.gov/nia

REFERENCES

Andersen-Ranberg, K., Schroll, M., & Jeune, B. (2001). Healthy centenarians do not exist, but autonomous centenarians do: A population-based study of morbidity among Danish centenarians. *Journal of the American Geriatrics Society, 49,* 900–908.

Austad, S. N. (2001). Concepts and theories of aging. In E. J. Masoro & S. N. Austad (Eds.), *Handbook of the biology of aging* (5th ed., pp. 3–22). San Diego: Academic Press.

Bahr, S. R. T. (1981). Overview of gerontological nursing. In M.O. Hogstel (Ed.), *Nursing care of the older adult* (pp. 3–29). New York: John Wiley & Sons.

Bartke, A., & Lane, M. (2001). Endocrine and neuroendocrine regulatory functions. In E. J. Masoro & S. N. Austad (Eds.), *Handbook of the biology of aging* (5th ed., pp. 297–323). San Diego: Academic Press.

Becker, P. M., & Cohen, H. J. (1984). The functional approach to the care of the elderly: A conceptual framework. *Journal of the American Geriatrics Society, 32,* 923–929.

Bergeman, C. S., & Plomin, R. (1996). Behavioral genetics. In J. E. Birren (Ed.), *Encyclopedia of gerontology: Age, aging, and the aged* (Vol.1, pp. 163–172). San Diego: Academic Press.

Birren, J. E., & Schroots, J. J. F. (2001). The history of geropsychology. In J. E. Birren and K. W. Schaie (Eds.), *Handbook of the psychology of aging* (5th ed., pp. 3–28). San Diego: Academic Press.

Blumenthal, H. T. (1999). A view of the aging–disease relationship from age 85. *Journal of Gerontology: Biological Sciences, 54,* B255–B259.

Blumenthal, H. T. (2001). Milestone or genomania? The relevance of the human genome project to biological aging and the age-related diseases. *Journal of Gerontology: Medical Science, 56A,* M529–M537.

Cowling, R. W. (1987). Metatheoretical issues: Development of new theory. *Journal of Gerontological Nursing, 13*(9), 10–13.

Crimmins, E. M., Hayward, M. D., & Saito, Y. (1996). Differentials in active life expectancy in the older population of the United States. *Journal of Gerontology: Social Sciences, 51,* S111–S120.

Cumming, E., & Henry, W. (1961). *Growing old: The process of disengagement.* New York: Basic Books.

Effros, R. B. (2001). Immune system activity. In E. J. Masoro & S. N. Austad (Eds.), *Handbook of the biology of aging* (5th ed., pp. 324–350). San Diego: Academic Press.

Erikson, E. H. (1963). *Childhood and society* (2nd ed.). New York: W. W. Norton.

Forbes, D. A. (2001). Enhancing master and sense of coherence: Important determinants of health in older adults. *Geriatric Nursing, 22,* 29–32.

Fozard, J. L., Metter, E. J., & Brant, L. J. (1990). Next steps in describing aging and disease in longitudinal studies. *Journal of Gerontology: Psychological Science, 45,* P116-P127.

Fries, J. F. (1980). Aging, natural death, and the compression of morbidity. *New England Journal of Medicine, 303,* 130–135.

Fries, J. F., & Crapo, L. M. (1981). *Vitality and aging: Implications of the rectangularization of the curve.* San Francisco: W. H. Freeman.

Frisoni, G. B., & Louhija, J., Geroldi, C., & Trabucchi, M. (2001). Longevity and the ε2 allele of apolipoprotein E: The Finnish centenarians study. *Journal of Gerontology: Medical Sciences, 56,* M75–M78.

Grune, T., & Davies, K. J. A. (2001). Oxidative processes in aging. In E. J. Masoro & S. N. Austad (Eds.), *Handbook of the biology of aging* (5th ed., pp. 25–58). San Diego: Academic Press.

Hagestad, G. O., & Dannefer, D. (2001). Concepts and theories of aging: Beyond microfication in social sciences approaches. In R. H. Binstock & L. K. George (Eds.), *Handbook of aging and the social sciences* (5th ed., pp. 3–21). San Diego: Academic Press.

Haight, B. K., Barba B. E., Tesh, A. S., & Courts, N. F. (2002). Thriving: A life span theory. *Journal of Gerontological Nursing, 28*(3), 14–22.

Harman, D. (1956). Aging: A theory based on the free radical and radiation chemistry. *Journal of Gerontology, 11,* 298–300.

Havighurst, R. J. (1972). *Developmental tasks and education* (3rd ed.). New York: David McKay.

Havighurst, R. J., & Albrecht, R. (1953). *Older people.* New York: Longmans, Green.

Hayflick, L. (1965). The limited in vitro lifetime of human diploid cell strains. *Experimental Cell Research, 37,* 614–636.

Hayflick, L. (1974). The longevity of cultured human cells. *Journal of American Geriatrics Society, 22,* 1–12.

Hayflick, L. (1988). Aging in cultured human cells. In B. Kent & R. N. Butler (Eds.), *Human aging research: Concepts and techniques.* New York: Raven Press.

Hayflick, L. (2001–2002). Anti-aging medicine hype, hope, and reality. *Generations, 20,* 20–26.

Hazzard, W. R. (2001). Aging, health, longevity, and the promise of medical research: The perspective of a gerontologist and geriatrician. In E. J. Masoro & S. N. Austad (Eds.), *Handbook of the biology of aging* (5th ed., pp. 445–456). San Diego: Academic Press.

International Longevity Center (2001). *ILC Workshop report: Is there an "anti-aging" medicine?* New York: International Longevity Center.

Joaquin, A. M., & Gollapudi, S. (2001). Functional decline in aging and disease: A role for apoptosis. *Journal of the American Geriatrics Society, 49,* 1234–1240.

Jonson, H., & Magnusson, J. A. (2001). A new age of old age? Gerotranscendence and re-enchantment of aging. *Journal of Aging Studies, 15,* 317–331.

Jung, C. G. (1954). Marriage as a psychological relationship. In W. McGuire, H. Reed, M. Fordham, & G. Adler (Eds.) (R. F. C. Hull, trans.), *The collected works of C. G. Jung: Vol. 17. The development of personality.* New York: Pantheon Books.

Jung, C. G. (1960). The stages of life. In W. McGuire, H. Reed, M. Fordham, & G. Adler (Eds.) (R. F. C. Hull, trans.), *The collected works of C. G. Jung: Vol. 8. The structure and dynamics of the psyche* (pp. 387–403). New York: Pantheon Books.

Kahana, E. (1975). A congruence model of person-environment interaction. In P. G. Windley, T. Byerts, & E. G. Ernst (Eds.), *Theoretical developments in environments for aging* (pp. 181–214). Washington, DC: Gerontological Society of America.

Katz, S., Branch, L. G., Branson, M. H., Papsidero, J. A., Beck, J. C., & Greer, D. S. (1983). Active life expectancy. *New England Journal of Medicine, 309,* 1218–1224.

Kennie, D. C. (1983). Good health care for the aged. *Journal of the American Medical Association, 249,* 770–773.

Kerr, J. F., Wyllie, A. H., & Currie, A. R. (1972). Apoptosis: A basic biologic phenomenon with wide-ranging implications in tissue kinetics. *British Journal of Cancer, 26,* 239–257.

King, I. M. (1981). *A theory for nursing.* New York: John Wiley & Sons.

Kirkland, J. L. (2002). The biology of senescence: Potential for prevention of disease. *Clinics in Geriatric Medicine, 18,* 383–462.

Kohn, R. R. (1982). Cause of death in very old people. *Journal of the American Medical Association, 247,* 2793–2797.

Laditka, J. N., & Laditka, S.B. (2000). The morbidity compression debate: Risk, opportunities, and policy options for women. *Journal of Women & Aging, 12*(1/2), 23–38

Lawton, M. P. (1982). Competence, environmental press, and the adaptation of older people. In M. P. Lawton, P. G. Windley, & T. O. Byerts (Eds.), *Aging and the environment: Theoretical approaches* (pp. 33–59). New York: Springer.

Leaf, A. (1973a). Every day is a gift when you are over 100. *National Geographic, 93,* 110–143.

Leaf, A. (1973b). Getting old. *Scientific American, 229,* 45–52.

Leaf, A. (1973c). Unusual longevity: The common denominators. *Hospital Practice, 8*(10), 74–86.

Lemon, B., Bengston, V. L., & Peterson, J. A. (1972). An exploration of the activity theory of aging: Activity types

and life satisfaction among in-movers to retirement community. *Journal of Gerontology 27,* 511–523.

Longino, C. F., & Kart, C. S. (1982). Explicating activity theory: A formal replication. *Journal of Gerontology 37,* 713–722.

Lynott, R. J., & Lynott, P. P. (1996). Tracing the course of theoretical development in the sociology of aging. *Gerontologist, 36,* 749–760.

Maddox, M. (1999). Older women and the meaning of health. *Journal of Gerontological Nursing, 25*(12), 26–33.

Marshall, V. W. (1996). Theories of aging: Social. In J. E. Birren (Ed.), *Encyclopedia of gerontology: Age, aging, and the aged* (Vol. 2, pp. 569–572). San Diego: Academic Press.

Maslow, A. H. (1954). *Motivation and personality.* New York: Harper & Row.

McEwen, M., & Wills, E. M. (2002). *Theoretical basis for nursing.* Philadelphia: Lippincott Williams & Wilkins.

McMullin, J. A. (2000). Diversity and the state of sociological aging theory. *Gerontologist, 40,* 217–530.

Meleis, A. I. (1987). Theoretical nursing: Today's challenges, tomorrow's bridges. *Nursing Papers/Perspectives on Nursing, 19*(1), 45–57.

Meleis, A. I. (1997). *Theoretical nursing: Development and progress* (3rd ed.). Philadelphia: J.B. Lippincott.

Miller, C. A. (1974, August 28). *Healthy aging.* Unpublished notes for a group discussion with residents of Lakeview Towers, Cleveland, OH.

Miller, R. A. (1997). When will the biology of aging become useful? Future landmarks in biomedical gerontology. *Journal of the American Geriatrics Society, 45,* 1258–1267.

Molla, M. T., Wagener, D. K., & Madans, J. H. (2001). *Summary measures of population health: Methods for calculating healthy life expectancy.* Washington, DC: U.S. Department of Health and Human Services.

Moody, H. R. (2002). *Aging: Concepts and controversies.* Thousand Oaks, CA: Sage Publications.

Neugarten, B. L. (1968). Adult personality: Toward a psychology of the life cycle. In B. L. Neugarten (Ed.), *Middle age and aging* (pp. 137–1477). Chicago: University of Chicago Press.

Neugarten, B. L., Havighurst, R. J., & Tobin, S. S. (1968). Personality and patterns of aging In B. L. Neugarten (Ed.), *Middle age and aging* (pp. 173–177). Chicago: University of Chicago Press.

Newman, B. M., & Newman, P. R. (1984). *Development through life: A psychosocial approach* (3rd ed.) Homewood IL: Dorsey Press.

Newquist, D. D. (1987). Voodoo death in the American aged. In J. E. Birren & J. Livingston (Eds.), *Cognition, stress, and aging* (pp. 111–133). Englewood Cliffs, NJ: Prentice-Hall.

Nightingale, F. (1954). Notes on nursing: What it is and what it is not. In L.R. Seymer (Ed.), *Selected writings on Florence Nightingale* (pp. 123–220). New York: Macmillan (original work published 1859).

Onega, L. L., & Tripp-Reimer, T. (1997). Expanding the scope of continuity theory: Application to gerontological nursing. *Journal of Gerontological Nursing, 23*(6), 29–35.

Peck, R. C. (1968). Psychological developments in the second half of life. In B. L. Neugarten (Ed.), *Middle age and aging* (pp. 88–92). Chicago: University of Chicago Press.

Pedersen, N. L. (1996). Gerontological behavior genetic. In J. E. Birren & K.W. Schaie (Eds.), *Handbook of the psychology of aging* (4th ed.). San Diego: Academic Press.

Pelletier, K. R. (1986). Longevity: What can centenarians teach us? In K. Dytchwald (Ed.), *Wellness and health*

Gerontological Nursing and Health Promotion

LEARNING OBJECTIVES

1. Define the scope of gerontology and geriatrics.
2. Discuss the practice of gerontological nursing as a specialty.
3. Describe the factors that contribute to the unique challenge of providing nursing care for older adults.
4. Identify health promotion interventions that are important for older adults.

GERONTOLOGY AND GERIATRICS

What emerges from the information in Part 1 is a picture of older adults as a diverse group of men and women with various sociocultural backgrounds who are more heterogeneous than homogeneous. Stereotypes of older adults are becoming more inaccurate as the population increases in diversity and gerontologists learn more about the unique characteristics of numerous subgroups of older adults. What is becoming clear is that, as people age, they become less and less like others of the same age. Indeed, the most universal characteristic of increasing age is increasing uniqueness and diversity. Thus, as the discussion of characteristics of older adults and theories of aging illustrates, answers to any questions about older adults or aging are multifaceted. Because the provision of health care and other services to this complex and heterogeneous population is so complicated, several branches of science have evolved to address the unique issues related to aging and older adults.

Gerontology is the branch of science that deals with aging and older adults. Gerontology was first recognized as a specialty in the mid-1940s with the establishment of the Gerontological Society of America and the publication of the first issue of the *Journals of Gerontology*. Since its inception, gerontology has addressed problems that "transcend the knowledge and methods of any one discipline or profession" (Frank, 1946, p. 1). Gerontology continues to be multidisciplinary and is a specialized area within various disciplines, such as nursing, psychology, social work, and certain allied health professions. Although gerontology is defined as the study of aging processes, it commonly has been associated with the study of various problems of aging and older adults. In recent years, however, gerontologists have placed less emphasis on the problems of aging and more emphasis on normal and successful aging.

As gerontologists have become more aware of the increasing diversity among older people, health care providers also have become more aware of the increasing complexity of caring for older people. Consequently, the health care specialties of geriatric medicine and gerontological nursing have emerged. Geriatrics is associated with the diseases and disabilities of old people, and geriatric medicine is recognized as a subspecialty of internal medicine or family practice that focuses on the medical problems of older people. In 1942, the American Geriatrics Society was established, and the editorial of its first publication, *Geriatrics*, called for physicians to "alleviate the inevitable deficiencies and limitations inherent in growing old" (Touhy, 1946, p. 17). In 1953, the society changed the name of their journal to the *Journal of the American Geriatrics Society* and broadened their focus to address a variety of issues that affect the health and functioning of older adults. This change reflected the beginnings of a shift in geriatrics from medically oriented care to care that is more preventive—a shift from curing to caring—as the recent use of the phrase *longevity medicine* suggests. Other recent and evolving trends in geriatrics are increasing emphasis on quality-of-life issues, a focus on maintaining optimal levels of functioning, and the importance of health promotion as a means of delaying the onset of disability (Morley, 2003).

GERONTOLOGICAL NURSING

The History of Gerontological Nursing

In the early 1900s, nurses first recognized the need for a specialization to address the unique needs of older adults, but it was not until the 1960s that geriatric nursing evolved as a nursing subspecialty (Figure 4-1). In 1962, the American Nurses Association (ANA) convened a focus group on gerontological nursing practice. Four years later, they formally recognized this specialty area by establishing a Division of Geriatric Nursing Practice and publishing a monograph entitled *Exploring Progress in Geriatric Nursing Practice*. In 1969, the ANA published its first nursing practice standards, *Standards of Practice for Geriatric Nursing*. By the mid-1970s, the ANA was advocating the use of the term *gerontological nursing*, rather than geriatric nursing, because the former more accurately reflected the scope of nursing. Geriatric nursing implies a focus of care primarily on the disease conditions of older people, which, for the most part, are much the same as those that affect all adults. Because nurses focus on the response of individuals both to actual and potential health problems, gerontological nursing is more appropriate. In recognition of this, the ANA Division of Geriatric Nursing Practice

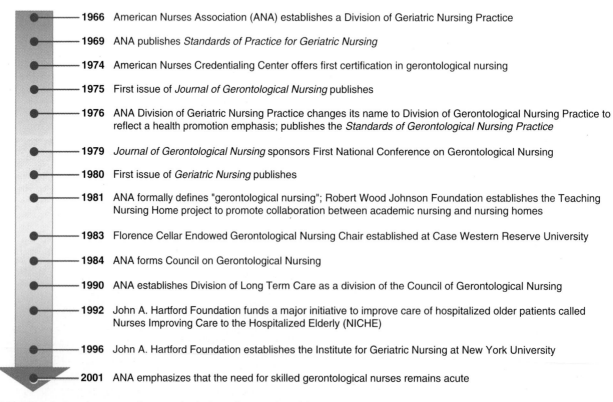

1966 American Nurses Association (ANA) establishes a Division of Geriatric Nursing Practice

1969 ANA publishes *Standards of Practice for Geriatric Nursing*

1974 American Nurses Credentialing Center offers first certification in gerontological nursing

1975 First issue of *Journal of Gerontological Nursing* publishes

1976 ANA Division of Geriatric Nursing Practice changes its name to Division of Gerontological Nursing Practice to reflect a health promotion emphasis; publishes the *Standards of Gerontological Nursing Practice*

1979 *Journal of Gerontological Nursing* sponsors First National Conference on Gerontological Nursing

1980 First issue of *Geriatric Nursing* publishes

1981 ANA formally defines "gerontological nursing"; Robert Wood Johnson Foundation establishes the Teaching Nursing Home project to promote collaboration between academic nursing and nursing homes

1983 Florence Cellar Endowed Gerontological Nursing Chair established at Case Western Reserve University

1984 ANA forms Council on Gerontological Nursing

1990 ANA establishes Division of Long Term Care as a division of the Council of Gerontological Nursing

1992 John A. Hartford Foundation funds a major initiative to improve care of hospitalized older patients called Nurses Improving Care to the Hospitalized Elderly (NICHE)

1996 John A. Hartford Foundation establishes the Institute for Geriatric Nursing at New York University

2001 ANA emphasizes that the need for skilled gerontological nurses remains acute

FIGURE 4-1 Development of gerontological nursing as a specialty.

changed its name to the Division on Gerontological Nursing Practice in 1976 and published the *Standards of Gerontological Nursing Practice*. These standards emphasize the role of gerontological nurses in maximizing independence in daily activities and in promoting, maintaining, and restoring health (ANA, 1976).

In 1981, the ANA formally defined gerontological nursing in *A Statement on the Scope of Gerontological Nursing Practice*. In 1987, the ANA issued the combined *Standards and Scope of Gerontological Nursing Practice*, which was revised in 1995 and 2001. The 2001 revision identified gerontological nursing as "one of the profession's most challenging practice areas" and called for gerontological nurses to "meet the special needs of the increasing numbers of older adults, particularly those over 85 years of age, minorities, and those with decreased financial and social resources" (ANA, 2001, p. 7). The ANA published the 2001 edition jointly with the National Gerontological Nursing Association, the National Conference of Gerontological Nurse Practitioners, and the National Association of Directors of Nursing Administration in Long Term Care. The document summarizes the scope of practice for gerontological nursing and emphasizes that older adults in home, hospital, or various community and long-term care agencies require "comprehensive care that focuses on individualized health promotion and disease prevention, ongoing assessment of functional and cognitive status, rapid identification of acute problems, rehabilitation and restorative care, ongoing education, and appropriate referrals" (ANA, 2001, pp. 7–8). The document also delineates standards of clinical gerontological nursing care and professional gerontological nursing performance (Display 4-1).

The development of professional journals and the establishment of certification provide additional evidence of the growth of gerontological nursing as a specialty. The *Journal of Gerontological Nursing* was first published in 1975, followed by *Geriatric Nursing* in 1980; both journals continue to be published today. The American Nurses Credentialing Center offered the first certification in gerontological nursing in 1974. Today, certification is offered in the following gerontological nursing areas: Gerontological Nurse, Clinical Specialist in Gerontological Nursing, and Gerontological Nurse Practitioner. Home Health Nurse and Nursing Case Manager are additional certification areas that are particularly relevant to gerontological nurses.

Education of Gerontological Nurses

Care of older adults is compromised when the health care practitioner lacks knowledge about the unique manifestations of aging and disease and the relationships between diseases and age-related changes.

DISPLAY 4-1
Standards of Professional Gerontological Nursing Performance

I. **Quality of Care.** The gerontological nurse systematically evaluates the quality of care and effectiveness of nursing practice.

II. **Performance Appraisal.** The gerontological nurse evaluates his or her own nursing practice in relation to professional practice standards and relevant statutes and regulations.

III. **Education.** The gerontological nurse acquires and maintains current knowledge applicable to nursing practice.

IV. **Collegiality.** The gerontological nurse contributes to the professional development of peers, colleagues, and others.

V. **Ethics.** The gerontological nurse's decisions and actions on behalf of older adults are determined in an ethical manner.

VI. **Collaboration.** The gerontological nurse collaborates with the older adult, the older adult's caregivers, and all members of the multidisciplinary team to provide comprehensive care.

VII. **Research.** The gerontological nurse interprets, applies, and evaluates research findings to inform and improve gerontological nursing practice.

VIII. **Resource Utilization.** The gerontological nurse considers factors related to safety, effectiveness, and cost in planning and delivering patient care.

Although this knowledge deficit is diminishing, nurses and other health care practitioners still lack the necessary skills to assess and treat common geriatric conditions accurately and effectively. Recently, two gerontological nursing leaders stated that "Most new graduates and virtually all practicing nurses have had inadequate preparation in geriatrics. Practicing nurses receive little continuing education in geriatrics" (Mezey & Fulmer, 2002). •

In the 1980s, nursing organizations, schools of nursing, and institutions of higher learning began developing undergraduate, graduate, and continuing educational programs to prepare nurses and nursing students for gerontological nursing. Despite these efforts, however, the Bureau of Health Professions of the Health Resources and Service Administration reported a serious shortage of registered nurses that most seriously affected the following groups of older adults: rural elders, older women, minority elders, people in long-term care settings, and older adults with mental health problems (Klein, 1997). The current nursing shortage has important implications for the delivery of health care to all people, but its impact on older adults is likely to be even more serious.

Nationally recognized leaders in gerontology published a document entitled *A National Agenda for*

Geriatric Education (Klein, 1997), which summarized recommendations to address the identified needs. Two recommendations in this document were mandatory continuing education in gerontological nursing and the incorporation of model gerontological nursing curricula at both undergraduate and graduate levels. Some progress has been made in implementing these recommendations, but articles in a variety of nursing and health care journals continue to emphasize the need for educational programs to prepare nurses for gerontological nursing practice. One emphasized "the responsibility of the nursing profession as a whole" to address negative attitudes about and misperceptions of gerontological nursing and to "produce a more accurate and positive representation of gerontology" (Happell & Brooker, 2001).

Since the late 1990s, the nursing profession has recognized that it is imperative to "prepare all practicing nurses with basic geriatric competencies as a way to ensure that older adults experience appropriate nursing care" (Mezey & Fulmer, 2002, p. M439). To accomplish this, the John A. Hartford Foundation established and funded the Hartford Institute for Geriatric Nursing to promote excellence in nursing care and to increase all nurses' understanding of geriatric practice. This mission is accomplished through major initiatives in practice, research, education, and policy and consumer education. Current efforts are directed toward "gerontologicalizing" all practicing nurses and toward developing geriatric competencies and curriculum materials for nursing education programs (Mezey & Fulmer, 2002).

Advanced practice gerontological nurses are registered nurses who hold a master's, nursing doctorate, or higher degree and demonstrate advanced knowledge and clinical expertise in the care of older adults (ANA, 2001). Categories include geriatric nurse practitioners (GNPs) and gerontological clinical nurse specialists (GCNSes). Because state boards of nursing define and regulate the practice of advanced practice nurses, their scope varies to some extent. In general, however, all have some degree of prescriptive authority (as of 1999), and they are viewed as expert practitioners in their specialty area. Roles of advanced practice nurses include educator, researcher, consultant, administrator, expert clinician, independent practitioner, care/case manager, individual/group counselor, and multidisciplinary team member/leader. GNPs are likely to be primary care practitioners; in this role, they manage some acute and many chronic conditions of older adults. GNPs and GCNSes are knowledgeable about normal aging changes as well as common pathologic conditions of older adults.

Their skills include comprehensive assessments of older adults and in-depth prevention and health promotion services.

Research Imperatives for Gerontological Nurses

Standard VII of the *Standards of Professional Gerontological Nursing Performance* states that gerontological nurses "are responsible for improving current nursing practice and the future healthcare for older adults by participating in the generation, testing, utilization, and evaluation of research findings" (ANA, 2001, p. 25). This standard mandates that nurses at the basic level of practice ask questions about the care of older adults, participate in studies to address these questions, and apply research findings to improve clinical care of older adults. At the Advanced Practice Nursing level, the gerontological nurse can fully participate in the generation, testing, utilization, critical evaluation, and dissemination of knowledge related to gerontological health care research (ANA, 2001). For example, in long-term care facilities, a geriatric clinical nurse specialist can improve quality of care by identifying resident care problems and developing solutions that are relevant, clinically correct, and up to date (Popejoy et al., 2000). Major accomplishments of gerontological nursing research in the last two decades include changing the paradigm for the use of physical restraints, improving the assessment and management of pressure ulcers and urinary incontinence, and developing strategies to improve bathing, feeding, and managing difficult and disruptive behaviors (Mezey & Fulmer, 2002).

In 1993, the 7-year-old National Center for Nursing Research was elevated to the status of a national institute within the National Institutes of Health (NIH). The National Institute of Nursing Research (NINR) supports multidisciplinary studies on innovative approaches to promoting health and preventing disease, minimizing the effects of acute and chronic illness and disability, and speeding recovery from disease. In the late 1990s, NINR-funded studies addressed such issues as prevention of pressure sores, decisions about hormonal therapy, the use of hip pads to prevent fractures, and quality of life for Alzheimer's patients and their caregivers. The NINR strategic plan for 2000 to 2004 identifies eight areas of nursing research, all of which are pertinent to gerontological nursing. These areas are symptom management, chronic illness experiences, implications of genetic advances, cultural/ethnic health considerations, telehealth interventions and monitoring, health promotion and disease prevention, end-of-life/palliative care, and quality of life and quality of care (NINR, 1999). Nurses are encouraged to contact the NINR or visit their Internet site (www.nih.gov/ninr) for information about these important areas of nursing research.

A working paper on the state of the art in gerontological nursing identified research priorities of the Hartford Foundation Centers for Geriatric Nursing Excellence in addressing needs of frail elders. Priorities included addressing specific care issues; preventing, delaying, or shortening institutionalization; improving outcomes and decreasing costs of care; facilitating transitions for older adults across the continuum of care; testing effective ways to promote health and improve quality of life; and demonstrating the unique contributions of professional nurses in the care of at-risk and vulnerable older adults and their caregivers (Strumpf, 2000). Another working paper, described as a "think piece" for the John A. Hartford Foundation, proposed the following goal for nursing's research-practice agenda in the third millennium: "May we prevent disease where possible, may we minimize morbidity and maximize quality of life where we cannot prevent disease, and may we have the wisdom to reconcile the two" (McBride, 2000, p. 26).

One of the nation's most recognized gerontological nursing leaders, May L. Wykle, PhD, RN, FAAN, also proposed an agenda for gerontological nursing research addressing the following priorities:

- Developing interdisciplinary research activities
- Addressing diversity issues related to race, gender, and culture
- Promoting health and preventing disease for individuals, families, and communities
- Providing elder care resources that are community focused and home care based
- Testing various gerontological nursing practice models for providing evidence-based practice
- Addressing long-term care issues such as physical care activities, interventions for behavior problems, end-of-life care, and staffing patterns and nursing staff mix
- Attracting students to gerontology and nurses to employment in long-term care (Wykle, 2001)

UNIQUE CHALLENGES OF GERONTOLOGICAL NURSING

Several factors distinguish the care of the older adult population from that of other populations and make the provision of health care for older adults challenging for gerontological nurses. These influencing factors include the unique and complex relationships between aging and disease, the particular manifestations of various disease states in this population, and the functional consequences of these illnesses. Gender differences, which affect people of all ages, also may play a more significant role in older adults. Other influences, such as multiculturalism and complementary and alternative medicine, are increasingly affecting the provision of health care to older adults in the United States.

Geriatricians and other gerontological health professionals have long recognized that not only are the manifestations of illness less predictable in the elderly, but also the causes of illness are more variable and the consequences are more far-reaching. Several factors are responsible for the complexity of illness in older adults.

First, the typical older person in the health care system has a combination of chronic conditions that need to be addressed on a continuing basis and occasional acute episodes that need to be addressed periodically. Chronic conditions, rather than acute conditions, account for most of the health care needs of older adults. Even when acute conditions are the focus of care, the care is likely to be affected by an interplay between chronic conditions and one or more acute conditions. Therefore, older adults are usually moving forward or backward along a health—illness continuum. Goals of gerontological health care providers are to facilitate forward movement toward improved health and functioning whenever that is possible and to prevent backward movement by addressing acute illnesses and preventing complications of chronic illnesses.

- Second, manifestations of illness, even acute illness, tend to be subtler and less predictable in older adults than in other segments of the population. For example, an older adult with an infection is much more likely than his or her younger counterparts to experience mental changes rather than an elevated temperature. Similarly, older adults are likely to experience changes in their level of functioning as manifestations of physiologic disturbances or adverse medication effects. This diversity of signs and symptoms of illness is further complicated by the fact that for any one manifestation of illness in an older adult, there are usually at least three possible explanations. For example, changes in function usually are related to a combination of several of the following conditions: (1) acute illness, (2) psychosocial factors, (3) environmental conditions, (4) age-related changes, (5) a new chronic illness, (6) an existing chronic illness, or (7) an adverse effect of medications or other treatments. Assessment of a physiologic illness becomes even more difficult in older people who are depressed, cognitively impaired, or otherwise psychosocially compromised. For example, cognitive impairment can diminish the ability to describe symptoms accurately, and depression can cause the person either to ignore or exaggerate symptoms of physical illness. In many cases, by the time illness in an older adult is detected and attended to, the underlying physiologic disturbance is in an advanced stage, and additional complications have developed.

Finally, the consequences of illness are likely to have a stronger impact on the older adult, and they may combine with other factors to compromise the person's functional status and quality of life. For example, an older person who has a fractured hip is much more likely than a younger counterpart to become permanently impaired. If the older person had previously lived alone and managed independently, but marginally, any functional impairment secondary to the fracture might result in a permanent move to a setting where dependency needs can be met. In addition to the functional consequences of illness in this population, serious psychosocial consequences also often result. For example, older people who have experienced a fall may develop an exaggerated fear of falling, and they may limit their mobility as a safety precaution. In the United States, fear of being "put away" in a nursing home is a common—although usually unfounded—worry among older people. Because of this anxiety, older people may deny symptoms of illness for fear that the solution will result in a loss of independence. In addition, older adults may avoid the health care system and experience unnecessary anxiety about minor or treatable illnesses.

Because of all of these factors, the assessment of illness in older adults may require a detective-like approach rather than the usual diagnostic process. In a health care system in which patients and providers have become accustomed to quick answers based on readily available diagnostic measures, such a time-consuming, puzzle-solving process often ends up being shortened, to the detriment of the older person. Moreover, our current health care system does not provide compensation for time spent listening to lengthy explanations or exploring multiple causes, so that the complex health care needs of the older person may be disregarded. Accordingly, the gerontological nurse often is the health care practitioner who ensures that the assessment approach addresses the complexity of the older individual's situation.

Gender and Aging

In addition to addressing the complex and unique relationship between aging and disease, gerontological nurses also are challenged by the significant role that gender differences play in providing health care to older adults. A major current trend in health care

as well as gerontology is to identify and address gender-specific health-related issues.

In the late 1980s, women in the United States began raising questions about the predominance of male subjects in the vast majority of health-related studies. Reasons for the exclusion and underrepresentation of women in clinical trials included concern about the effects on fetuses and reproductive functions, the false perception that physiologic function in men and women is similar, and myths about the inferiority of women's bodies and their diminished ability to withstand effects of clinical research. In response to increasing awareness of the importance of including women in various aspects of research, the Office of Research on Women's Health was established as a branch of the NIH in 1990. Much of the research focuses on issues that are relevant to middle-aged and older women, and many of the studies focus on preventive medicine and health promotion.

Several large-scale and longitudinal studies have been funded, but some of the early results of these studies are controversial or have already been questioned by results of other studies. Because many of these first-phase studies are epidemiologic and are not able to identify cause-and-effect relationships, further studies and clinical trials are necessary before accurate and meaningful conclusions can be drawn. For example, epidemiologic studies suggested that the benefits of hormonal therapy outweigh the risks for many women, but in 2002, this conclusion was reversed by findings of the Women's Health Initiative study. Health care professionals must keep up to date on research and pay particular attention to results of long-term clinically controlled trials.

The Women's Health Initiative (WHI), funded in 1991 by the National Heart, Lung, and Blood Institute of the NIH, is a well-known ongoing study with many implications for women's health. This longitudinal and large-scale study of women between the ages of 50 and 79 years focuses on cancer, osteoporosis, and cardiovascular disease. WHI goals include collecting baseline clinical data on women's health, improving diagnostic methods for breast cancer, studying the nutritional requirements for optimal health, examining the psychosocial determinants of health, studying gender-specific effects of drugs, and identifying factors related to the higher rate of mental illness in women (Ransdell, 2001). One major study focus is to examine the risks and benefits of hormonal therapy in healthy menopausal women. Although the study was scheduled to run until 2005, a main component (i.e., the estrogen-progesterone group) was halted prematurely in July 2002 because of statistically significant increases in the risk for stroke, blood clots, heart disease, and breast cancer associated with hormonal therapy. The study found reduced rates of hip fracture and colorectal and endometrial cancers in the hormonal therapy group; however, the overall health risks exceeded benefits (Women's Health Initiative, 2002). At the end of 2002, the estrogen-only arm of the study was continuing, and the NIH was establishing an expert panel to review study results and make recommendations.

The Nurses Health Study (NHS) is another well-known longitudinal study that continues to generate new and controversial findings. The NHS, which was funded by the NIH, began recruiting registered nurses between the ages of 30 and 55 years in 1976 and has since collected interview and laboratory data from more than 120,000 of them at regular intervals. This study focuses on diseases and health-related factors (e.g., diet, smoking, and hormone use) that influence the development of cancer, cardiovascular disease, and other major medical conditions in women. Some of the findings drawn from this study that were not controversial in 2002 are as follows: heavier women have a lower risk for osteoporotic fracture; there is an inverse relationship between intake of calcium, potassium, and magnesium and the risk for ischemic stroke; and there are inverse associations between vitamin A intake and breast cancer risk and between vitamin E intake and heart disease risk (Ransdell, 2001).

The Women's Health Study (WHS), another ongoing study, has focused more narrowly on the association between low-dose aspirin and vitamin E in primary prevention of cancer and cardiovascular disease. The WHS was designed as a randomized, double-blind, placebo-controlled trial that will test whether results are due to a single agent or a synergistic effect (Ransdell, 2001). As with the WHI, conclusive results of the WHS will not be available for several years. Because studies of women's health issues are an emerging topic, nurses are encouraged to keep up to date with findings by visiting the Internet sites listed in the Educational Resources section at the end of this chapter.

As a spin-off of the movement to address women's health issues, men have become increasingly aware of health issues that are unique to them, particularly in middle and later adulthood. It is not unusual to see articles with titles such as "Health Issues Unique to the Aging Man" (Philpot & Morley, 2000) in geriatric journals or to see sections of health care publications designated as "Men's Health." Similarly, terms such as *viropause* and *andropause* are increasingly found in professional and lay literature in relation to the effects of hormonal declines that occur in middle-aged and older men.

The most widely studied men's health issue is the potential effects of declining testosterone and the risks and benefits of testosterone replacement therapy. Hypogonadism, defined as total serum testosterone levels below 250 ng/mL, is the medical term that describes this treatable condition affecting as many as one third of men 50 years of age and older. In 2001, the National Institute on Aging Advisory Panel on Testosterone Replacement in Men published a report addressing questions about testosterone levels and androgen therapy in older men. A major recommendation of this report is that clinical trials be carried out on various aspects of androgen therapy (National Institute on Aging, 2001). Androgen therapy is particularly pertinent to age-related changes in sexual functioning (see Chapter 22), but it is being addressed in relation to other aspects of physiologic function as well. For example, the role of testosterone in both preventing and treating osteoporosis in men is being investigated (see Chapter 18). A recent review of studies concluded that testosterone therapy in healthy older men may have beneficial effects on angina, libido, muscle strength, body composition, bone mineral density, general well-being, low-density lipoprotein cholesterol, exercise-induced cardiac ischemia, and certain aspects of cognitive function (Matsumoto, 2002). As with hormonal therapy for women, however, little is known about the long-term effects and risks of androgen therapy, and men are being cautioned that the potential risks may outweigh any benefits.

Gynecomastia, breast cancer, prostate cancer, and benign prostatic hyperplasia are other aspects of men's health that are receiving increased attention in geriatric research and literature. Questions about shorter life expectancies of men also are being raised as topics for concern and study. Some efforts have been made to promote the establishment of an Office of Men's Health in the NIH, but it is doubtful that this will happen in the very near future. Internet sites that provide up-to-date information on health issues specific to aging men are listed in the Educational Resources section of this chapter.

In summary, although many gender-specific health-related issues have been identified that are relevant to older adults, research on these topics is still in its infancy. Many questions remain about the roles of hormones and the effects of age-related declines in various hormones on numerous aspects of functioning in both men and women. In the next decades, we are likely to find answers to some of the questions about hormonal therapy and androgen therapy, but these answers often generate further questions. Because gender-specific research is a recent and evolving specialty, it may be years before clear conclusions and clinically relevant findings emerge. Throughout this text, information about gender-related differences is incorporated wherever possible, and current research is summarized.

Multiculturalism and Complementary and Alternative Medicine

The increasing cultural diversity of American society and an increasing acceptance and use of complementary and alternative medicine are two trends that need to be addressed in all areas of health care practice, including gerontological nursing. As emphasized in earlier chapters, the number and proportion of older adults in culturally diverse groups is increasing dramatically in the United States, and this trend will continue at an accelerated rate during the next few decades. Pertinent multicultural information about older adults in the United States has only recently become available, but this is a rapidly evolving area of interest in gerontology. Each chapter in this text attempts to include information that is relevant to different cultural groups.

Similarly, information about complementary and alternative medicine is incorporated in this text when pertinent. Nurses are encouraged to use the Internet to gather up-to-date information about alternative health care practices. However, caution must be exercised because groups that stand to benefit from the use of those alternative health care products and practices provide much of the information on the Internet. The National Center for Complementary and Alternative Medicine (NCCAM) which is part of the NIH, is a good resource for reliable and professional information (see the Educational Resources listed at the end of this chapter).

HEALTH PROMOTION

Health Promotion and Aging

Health promotion is a broad term that refers to activities whose goals are to prevent disease and disability and to limit the effects of diseases and disabilities. Health promotion is evolving as a major focus of health care services in the United States, as evidenced by the development of several major national health initiatives since 1979. These initiatives, which apply the concept of healthy aging to adults of all ages, emphasize that everyone can benefit from preventive health care (Infeld & Whitelaw, 2002). Students in nursing and other health care professions are encouraged to study the initiatives that are most relevant to care of older adults, including the *Guide to Clinical Preventive Services* (USDHHS, 1996a), the *Surgeon General's Report on Physical Activity and*

Health (USDHHS, 1996b), and the *Clinician's Handbook of Preventive Services* (USDHHS, 1998) (Haber, 2002). Display 4-2 lists 11 national health initiatives that are applicable to health promotion for older adults. Resources for health promotion materials that are especially useful for gerontological nurses (including Internet sites for many of the national health initiatives) are listed in the Educational Resources section at the end of this chapter.

Healthy People 2010, launched in January 2000 as an extension of the *Healthy People 2000* campaign that was implemented during the 1990s, is a well-known national health initiative with many aspects particularly applicable to older adults. The program—designed as a roadmap for improving the health of all people in the United States—outlines a comprehensive, nationwide agenda for promoting health and preventing illness, disability, and premature death. The two major goals are increasing quality and years of healthy life and eliminating health disparities. For older adults, the first goal is associated with preventing chronic illness as well as exacerbations of illnesses that already exist. The second goal addresses some of the health disparities that disproportionately affect specific older populations. Examples of common health disparities include hypertension in African Americans, diabetes in Hispanic and Native American Indian groups, obesity in Hispanic and African American women, and smoking in American Indians and Alaska Natives (Burggraf & Barry, 2000). Nurses are encouraged to use the Internet site listed in the Educational Resources section of this chapter to find more information and to keep up to date on this national program.

The emergence and expansion of interest in health promotion interventions can be attributed in part to the national initiatives and in large part to the current emphasis on both cost-effectiveness of health care services and quality of life for health care consumers of all ages. Health care planners are increasingly recognizing that health promotion activities can be cost-effective when they prevent or delay the onset of disease or disability. Although Medicare and many managed care systems have traditionally focused on acute and episodic care, the focus is now shifting, and health care systems are addressing and managing risk factors and helping people maintain independence as ways of controlling health care costs (Given & Given, 2001). A discussion of health promotion and disease prevention specifically with regard to older adults concluded that "concepts such as function preservation, disability prevention and postponement, chronic-disease management, and independence enhancement must become central concerns of our health care system" (Given & Given, 2001, p 220). Another

---

DISPLAY 4-2
National Health Initiatives and Resources Important to Older Adults

Medicare. Medicare covers the following preventive services: glaucoma screening, breast examinations, screening mammograms, bone density measurements, influenza and pneumonia immunizations, Pap smears and pelvic examinations, colorectal cancer screening procedures, prostate-specific antigen tests and digital rectal examinations, and diabetes education and self-management benefits.

Healthy People 2010. *Healthy People 2010* focuses on leading health indicators for which measurable baseline and target levels have been established (e.g., mental health, physical activity, and access to quality health services).

Eliminating Racial and Ethnic Disparities in Health. This initiative addresses disparities in health status that are applicable to racial and ethnic older adults (e.g., diabetes, immunizations, cardiovascular disease, and cancer screening and management).

Healthy Aging Project. Part of the Centers for Medicare and Medicaid Service, the Healthy Aging Project reviews available literature on health promotion and disease prevention interventions for older people and publishes evidence-based recommendations (e.g., *Smoking Cessation and Medicare*).

Program of All-Inclusive Care for the Elderly (PACE). PACE provides an integrated, community-based multidisciplinary care model with a strong emphasis on health promotion.

National Institute on Aging. The Institute's goals for 2001 to 2005 include understanding healthy aging processes, reducing health disparities among older people and groups, improving health and quality of life for older people, and enhancing resources to support high-quality research.

Put Prevention in Practice: Staying Healthy at 50+. This educational booklet offers recommendations about living habits, screening tests, and immunizations.

Exercise: A Guide From the National Institute on Aging. This video and booklet focus on a safe and effective exercise program for older adults.

Healthfinder. From the U.S. Department of Health and Human Services, Healthfinder provides reliable information on the Internet about health topics (e.g., prevention, self-care).

National Resource Center on Aging and Injury. The Center provides information about preventing unintentional injuries to older adults. It is a division of the National Center for Injury Prevention of the Centers for Disease Control and Prevention.

National Center for Chronic Disease Prevention and Health Promotion. The Center provides educational materials on healthy aging.

(From Infeld, D. L., & Whitelaw, N. [2002]. Policy initiatives to promote healthy aging. *Clinics in Geriatric Medicine, 18,* 627–642.)

---

article concluded that "the net effect of primary prevention will be to reduce and compress disability into a shorter period toward the end of life, to decrease overall lifetime disability, and consequently, to reduce the associated health care burden" (Hubert et al., 2002, p M347).

A dominant theme of current gerontological health promotion efforts is to add life to years, not just more years to life (Drewnowski & Evans, 2001a; Mehr & Tatum, 2002; Rejeski & Mihalko, 2001). The concept of health-related quality of life—a phrase that is becoming commonplace in gerontological literature—is being promoted as an alternative to morbidity and mortality data as an indicator of health status. Definitions of health-related quality of life include characteristics such as social functioning, emotional well-being, a personal sense of physical and mental health, and overall life satisfaction and happiness (Drewnowski & Evans, 2001a). Health promotion activities, such as exercise, nutrition, and other lifestyle modifications, improve health-related quality of life by improving the ability of older adults to live independently and care for themselves (Chernoff, 2002). Gerontologists emphasize that "there is no single segment of our society that can benefit more from regular exercise and

improved diet than older adults. Maintenance of function permits older adults to care for themselves, maintain their independence, and enjoy improved quality of life" (Drewnowski & Evans, 2001b, p. 5). A recent review of preventive interventions concluded that "perhaps the best antiaging medicine is exercise" (Fisher & Morley, 2002, p. M637). Because older adults are likely to view nurses as important providers of health education and other health promotion interventions, nurses have numerous opportunities for improving the quality of life for older adults through health promotion interventions (Dubbert et al., 2002; Hawranik & Pangman, 2002).

Goals of Health Promotion Interventions for Older Adults

The focus of health promotion activities varies for different age groups. For older adults, health promotion activities focus on (1) prevention and postponement of disease and disability and (2) early identification and effective management of disease conditions. Specific goals for health promotion and disease prevention for older adults include reduced premature mortality, enhanced quality of life, expanded active life expectancy, and maintenance of functional independence for as long as possible (Bloom, 2001). Major emphasis is placed on modifiable lifestyle factors because lifestyle choices account for as much as 10 years of life expectancy, and they strongly influence health, functioning, quality of life, and the onset of disability (Fraser & Shavlik, 2001; Mehr & Tatum, 2002; Hubert et al., 2002).

Despite the proliferation of evidence that health promotion interventions are cost-effective ways of preventing disease and disability and improving functioning and quality of life for older adults, evidence indicates that older adults as a group receive fewer prevention and screening health care services than other populations. Misconceptions that have interfered with the development of health promotion programs for older adults include: (1) normal aging processes diminish the benefits of prevention, (2) prevention is not effective after the onset of chronic illness, and (3) older adults are less responsive to health education and promotion interventions. Researchers have recently debunked all three of these myths (Bhalotra & Mutschler, 2001), providing even more impetus for the development of health promotion programs for older adults.

Many organizations disseminate guidelines for health promotion interventions, and they are not always in agreement, especially with regard to recommendations for older adults. The American Cancer Society, the U.S. Preventive Services Task Force, and the Agency for Healthcare Research and Quality are some of the organizations that play a prominent role in developing and promulgating guidelines for preventive care. Display 4-3 summarizes some of the more widely agreed-on guidelines for older adults, which gerontological nurses can follow when educating older adults about health promotion interventions.

Types of Health Promotion Interventions for Older Adults

Interventions to promote physical and psychosocial well-being include screening programs, risk reduction interventions, environmental modifications, and health education to promote good health practices. In addition to addressing all aspects of physical function, health promotion activities for older adults are likely to address psychosocial aspects of function such as dementia, depression, mental health, substance abuse, and elder abuse and neglect. This is appropriate because gerontologists frequently identify active engagement in life as an important component of successful aging (Anetzberger, 2002). Social supports and social interaction on a regular basis have positive effects on many aspects of mental health and some

aspects of physiologic function, such as cardiovascular health. Religion and spiritual practices are aspects of psychosocial functioning that are increasingly being recognized as factors that significantly affect health and functioning. A multidisciplinary model of health promotion has been developed as an intervention for incorporating spirituality into a successful aging intervention with older adults (Parker et al., 2002).

Screening Programs

Screening programs are particularly important for the early detection of serious and progressive conditions that can readily be detected and treated, such as glaucoma, diabetes, hypertension, hyperlipidemia, osteoporosis, hypothyroidism, and skin cancer. The following criteria have been identified for effectiveness of screening tests: (1) the test must be able to detect the condition or risk factor earlier than without screening and without excessive false-positive or false-negative results, and (2) early intervention must be superior to waiting until signs or symptoms of disease are present (Mehr & Tatum, 2002).

Although the incidence of many types of cancer increases with age, and cancer screening programs have been widely recommended for skin, breast, colon, prostate, and other cancers, cancer screening for older adults, particularly for those older than 75 years of age, has always been somewhat controversial. Recently, controversy about mammography for older women and prostate-specific antigen (PSA) testing for older men has increased because of conflicting study findings, concerns about cost-effectiveness, and questions about the risks and benefits of treatment options. Because geriatric practitioners are focusing more on increasing years of healthy living and less on extending the quantity of life, decisions about screening tests can be based on the person's active life expectancy and health-related quality of life. These decisions also are based on individual values, which are shaped in large part by culture and religion (Mehr & Tatum, 2002). For example, if these principles were applied to the use of the PSA screening test, this test would not be recommended for a man with a life expectancy of less than 10 years, nor would it be offered to a man with dementia because the interventions would not contribute to short-term well-being. However, it would be given to a man older than 70 years of age if he still requested it after a discussion of its advantages and disadvantages (Mehr & Tatum, 2002).

Risk Reduction Interventions

Risk reduction interventions include any activity that is directed toward reducing the chance that a disease condition will develop; these interventions are based on

DISPLAY 4-3

Guidelines for Prevention and Health Promotion Interventions for Older Adults

Immunizations

For All Older Adults

- **Tetanus-diphtheria** primary series every 10 years
- **Influenza** annually at beginning of influenza season
- **Pneumovax** once after age 65 years, then booster after 5 years of age if initial vaccination was before age 65 years or if other risk factors are present

For At-Risk Older Adults

- **Hepatitis A or B**
- **Measles, mumps, rubella** if evidence of lack of immunity and significant risk for exposure
- **Varicella** if evidence of lack of immunity and significant risk for exposure

Screening

For All Older Adults

- **Blood pressure** checks at least annually, more frequently if range is 130–139 mm Hg systolic or 85–90 mm Hg diastolic or if other risk factors are present (e.g., diabetes, African American race)
- **Serum cholesterol** every 5 years, more frequently in people with risk such as personal or family history of cardiovascular disease
- **Fecal occult blood and rectal exam** annually
- **Sigmoidoscopy** every (3 to) 5 years after age 50 years
- **Visual acuity and glaucoma screening** annually
- **Breast exam:** self-exam monthly, annually by primary care practitioner

For Women

- **Pap smear and pelvic exam** annually until three consecutive negative exams, then every 2 to 3 years; discontinue after 65 years of age if three consecutive negative exams
- **Mammogram** annually or biannually between 50 and 69 years, every 1 to 3 years between 70 and 85 years

For Men

- **Digital rectal exam** annually

For At-Risk Older Adults

- **Blood glucose level**
- **Thyroid function**
- **Heart function (electrocardiograph)**
- **Bone density**
- **Mental status assessment**
- **Screening for dementia, depression, substance abuse**
- **Urinary incontinence assessment**
- **Functional assessment**
- **Screening for adverse medication effects and drug interactions**
- **Skin cancer assessment**
- **Fall risk assessment**
- **Pressure ulcer assessment**
- **Elder abuse or neglect assessment**

For Men

- **Prostate-specific antigen (PSA) blood test**

Health Promotion Counseling

For All Older Adults (Unless Contraindicated)

- **Exercise:** at least 30 minutes of moderate-intensity physical activity daily
- **Nutrition:** adequate intake of all vitamins and minerals, especially calcium and antioxidants
- **Dental care** and prophylaxis: every 6 months
- **Protective measures:** seatbelts, sunscreens, smoke detectors, fall risk prevention

For Older Adults if Applicable

- **Smoking cessation**
- **Substance abuse cessation**

an assessment of the degree of risk for developing a particular condition. Some risk reduction interventions (e.g., vaccinations) are applicable to all older adults, and other interventions vary according to the specific risk factors and the level of health or frailty of an older person. Risk assessment tools have been developed for a variety of conditions, including falls, incontinence, heart disease, pressure ulcers, and elder abuse and neglect. These tools often include a rating scale to identify people who are most likely to develop a particular condition so that health care professionals can plan and implement preventive interventions for people at higher risk. These tools also serve as a way of identifying the risk factors that can be addressed through preventive interventions.

Even without assessment tools, health care professionals can usually identify risk factors that can be addressed to prevent disease or disability. Priority usually is given to reducing the risk factors that are most dominant or are likely to have the most serious negative consequences. For example, health promotion interventions for a relatively healthy older adult with a history of hypertension, hypercholesterolemia, and family history of heart attacks would address risk factors for heart disease for that person. Health promotion interventions for a frail older adult who is in a skilled care unit recovering from a fractured hip would focus on fall prevention and safe mobility. For any older adult, risk reduction interventions include lifestyle factors such as exercise, optimal nutrition, physical activity, stress-relieving techniques, and smoking cessation (if applicable). Health promotion activities to reduce risk may also include the use of over-the-counter medications (e.g., low-dose aspirin), nutritional supplements (e.g., vitamins), and complementary and alternative medicine (e.g., yoga). The Health Enhancement Program is one example of a risk reduction program for community-dwelling older adults at risk for functional decline in which a nurse works with each participant to develop a "health action plan" that addresses at least one disability risk factor identified in an initial assessment (Phelan et al., 2002). Positive outcomes of this program after 1 year of participation include improved health status, decreased burden of disability, and no decline in functional status.

Environmental Modifications

Environmental modifications are within the realm of health promotion activities when they are implemented to reduce risks or to improve a person's level of functioning. For example, reduction of fall risks involves numerous environmental modifications (discussed in Chapter 18). Environmental modifications also are effective in improving hearing and vision and in preventing urinary incontinence, as discussed in Chapters 12, 13, and 15. The National Resource Center on Supportive Housing and Home Modifications (listed in the Educational Resources section) is an example of an initiative to promote healthy aging through environments designed to facilitate optimal functioning. This center disseminates information, conducts research, and provides training and education for older adults, caregivers, providers, and policymakers (Infeld & Whitelaw, 2002).

Health Education to Promote Good Health Practices

Health education is a key component of most health promotion interventions, with a focus on teaching people to engage in self-care activities that are preventive in their scope. Health education addresses health practices such as nutrition, dental care, exercise and physical activity, and avoidance of smoking and environmental tobacco smoke. Because health education about nutrition, dental care, and smoking cessation are addressed in Chapters 14 and 17, this chapter will focus on health education related to exercise and physical activity.

Articles about the need for increased physical activity are ubiquitous in lay and professional literature, and physical activity is probably the most widely promulgated health promotion intervention today. Gerontologists emphasize that physical inactivity is an independent risk factor for a wide range of chronic conditions, and older adults are at particular risk for

leading sedentary lifestyles (King, 2001). A summary of research concluded that older adults should be screened for sedentary lifestyle at all major encounters with health care professionals, "given its role as a potent risk factor for all-cause and cardiovascular mortality, obesity, hypertension, insulin resistance, cardiovascular disease, diabetes, stroke, colon cancer, depression, osteoporosis, recurrent falls, and disability, among other conditions" (Singh, 2002, p. M276). Numerous well-designed studies support the recommendation that exercise should be the standard of care for all older adults because "there is no group of individuals who can benefit more from increased levels of physical activity than elderly people" (Evans, 2002, p. M260). Even moderate levels of physical activity—defined as 30 minutes of participation in activities of moderate intensity such as walking or gardening on most days of the week—can have substantial health benefits (DiPietro, 2001).

Despite the wealth of undisputed evidence about the beneficial effects of physical activity for older adults, less than one third of older people in the United States engage in it regularly. Factors associated with lower levels of physical activity are female sex, being a smoker, having poor health or medical concerns, having lower income and less education, and lacking experience with physical activity. Barriers that have been identified in older adults include impaired health, fear of injury, unpleasant sensations associated with exercise, lack of access to appropriate facilities, and lack of knowledge about the benefits of exercise (Resnick, 2002). Motivational factors that are associated with higher levels of physical activity include a desire to improve physical fitness and appearance, fewer perceived barriers to being physically active, positive beliefs about the value of physical activity, and a higher level of confidence about being able to undertake successfully physical activity (King, 2001).

Nurses take many roles in promoting physical activity for older adults. Because many older adults do not perceive the benefits of physical activity and, in fact, may falsely believe that physical activity should be avoided, nurses need to assess the person's beliefs about and understanding of both the beneficial and detrimental effects of physical activity. Nurses also assess for and address other factors that positively or negatively influence an older adult to participate in regular physical activity. Nurse researchers found an association between self-efficacy and motivation to participate in exercise and physical activity (e.g, Allison & Keller, 2000). Health-related barriers that interfere with physical activity in older adults include pain, fatigue, and sensory and mobility impairments (Cooper et al., 2001). Cooper and colleagues (2001) proposed a variety of nursing interventions to help overcome these barriers. For example, pacing the exercise program and taking prescribed antiinflammatory medications before physical activity are interventions that address pain. The WALC model—Walk, Address pain, fear, fatigue; Learn about exercise, Cue by self-modeling—is one example of a nursing intervention that has been used effectively to increase participation of older adults in exercise and can be implemented in a variety of settings (Resnick, 2002). The University of Iowa Gerontological Nursing Interventions Research Center has developed an evidence-based protocol that provides nursing guidelines for teaching older adults about exercise promotion (Titler, 2002). Singh (2002) summarizes current research on exercise and aging and makes comprehensive recommendations for an exercise and physical activity program for health promotion and disease prevention in older adults. Other examples of nursing interventions to promote exercise interventions for older adults are found in nursing journals (e.g., Melillo et al., 2001; Resnick & Spellbring, 2000; Schlicht, 2000). Nurses can use Display 4-4 as a guide to teaching older adults about recommended exercises.

DISPLAY 4-4
Types of Exercise

Physical activity is any skeletal muscle activity that causes energy expenditure.
Exercise refers to structured and repetitive body movements performed with the goal of attaining physical fitness.

	Definition	Benefits	Intensity	Frequency	Examples
Aerobic (dynamic or endurance) activity	Activity that requires the body to use oxygen to produce the energy necessary for the activity	Lowers blood pressure, strengthens heart muscle, decreases triglycerides, increases low-density lipoproteins, diminishes blood glucose, decreases intraabdominal fat, decreases risk for cardiovascular disease, improves self-esteem, relieves symptoms of anxiety and depression	Identify your target heart rate by subtracting your age in years from 220 (this is the maximum heart rate) and multiplying by 0.65	30 minutes, 5 times weekly	Brisk walking, jogging, walking up stairs
Strength training (resistance training, weight-training, muscle-building) activity	Performance of muscle contractions against a resistance that is greater than usual for that muscle; slow and controlled movements of major muscled groups such as arms, back, hips, chest, and shoulders, with exhalation during exertion and inhalation during return to the starting position	Improves balance and diminishes risk for falls, strengthens musculoskeletal system, improves function and independence, decreases risk for osteoporosis, favorably modifies risk factors for cardiovascular disease and type II diabetes	You should be able to repeat the movement 8 consecutive times, but not more than 12 times, before experiencing significant muscle fatigue	8 to 10 different sets of exercises working all major muscle groups, each repeated 8 to 12 times, several days a week	Resistance bands, weight training, strap-on sandbags, bicep curls for the arms, bench presses for the chest, bent-over rows for the upper back
Stretching	Activity that improves body flexibility	Increases flexibility, reduces muscle soreness, improves performance of daily activities	Stretch muscle groups, but not to the point of pain, and hold for 10 to 30 seconds	Repeat each stretch at least 4 times, a minimum of 2 to 4 times weekly	Yoga, stretching of all joints and muscle groups, range-of-motion exercises

Other Interventions

Additional types of health promotion interventions that are relevant for some older adults include addressing their pain and comfort concerns and issues related to the use of multiple medications. Active management of pain is an essential aspect of disability prevention because chronic pain leads to depression and diminished physical activity (Morley & Flaherty, 2002). Interventions for polypharmacy are considered health promotion activities when they are directed toward identifying and preventing medication interactions and other adverse effects of medications. Gerontological nurses have important responsibilities for monitoring therapeutic as well as adverse medication effects and for educating older adults and their caregivers about medication effects. These responsibilities are discussed in Chapter 23.

The Transtheoretical Model of Health Promotion

Many disease prevention and health promotion interventions require a change from detrimental health-related behaviors to those that prevent disease and promote wellness. Once behavior change has been initiated, the new healthier behaviors must be maintained. Initiation and maintenance of these changes involve both motivation and action steps. The more ingrained and rewarding or pleasurable the behaviors that must be changed, the more difficult it is to refrain from these activities. Some unhealthy behaviors, such as cigarette smoking, have a strong addictive component that increases the difficulty of behavior change. Similarly, the more comfortable a person is with the absence of healthy behaviors, such as physical activity, the more difficult it will be to develop healthier behaviors. The role of gerontological health care professionals in health promotion interventions is to lead and support the older person through the stages of change involved in replacing unhealthy behaviors with health-promoting behaviors.

The *Transtheoretical Model* (TTM), developed two decades ago (Prochaska & DiClemente, 1982), has been widely used by health care professionals to explain stages of behavior change. Stress management, sun exposure, smoking cessation, medication compliance, alcohol and drug cessation, diet and weight control, and screening for breast and cervical cancer are health promotion areas in which the TTM has been used successfully (Burkholder & Evers, 2002). One gerontological nursing article described the TTM as "an integrative model of behavior change that is applicable to older adults and can be used easily by nurses in any health care setting. . . . Further, the recommendations from the TTM are well suited to nurses working with

older people and can be used both in individual interactions or group sessions" (Burbank et al., 2000, p. 32). Application of this model specifically in gerontological health care settings is described in detail in *Promoting Exercise and Behavior Change in Older Adults* (Burbank & Riebe, 2002).

The TTM is called the *stages-of-change model* because it describes five specific stages through which a person progresses in accomplishing behavior changes. In the first stage, *Precontemplation*, the person is unaware of the problem, is in denial of the need for change, or is resistant to change. At this stage, the person has no intention of changing his or her behaviors within the next 6 months. Appropriate health promotion interventions for a person in this stage include providing information about the problem behavior and providing unconditional encouragement for thinking about behavior change. When working with an older adult in this stage, gerontological nurses can offer information, discuss their own beliefs, and help the person identify the personal benefits of the health-promoting behaviors. The nurse also can acknowledge the person's perspective and point out the negative consequences of current behaviors.

The second stage, *Contemplation*, is characterized by an intention to change in the foreseeable future, based on some acknowledgement of the negative consequences of current behaviors and positive consequences of different behaviors. The person is likely to ask questions and to seek information about the short- and long-term risks and benefits of various behaviors. He or she is likely to be ambivalent about giving up a rewarding activity or taking on an activity that is viewed as difficult or less enjoyable. During this stage, the gerontological nurse can help the person see that the benefits outweigh the disadvantages, even though the person may not experience the benefits immediately. Appropriate health promotion interventions for this stage include providing additional information about the risks and benefits and exploring with the person how he or she can begin establishing personal goals for a healthier lifestyle. Interventions also include increasing the person's sense of self-efficacy by helping the person to see himself or herself practicing these new behaviors. When working with an older adult in this stage, it is helpful to express confidence in the person's ability to develop health-promoting behaviors.

Stage three, the *Preparation* stage, is characterized by some ambivalence about the unhealthy behavior, but a stronger inclination to change to healthier behaviors. The person acknowledges the need for change, expresses serious intent to adopt the healthier behaviors within the next month, and begins to identify strategies for implementing them. During this stage, people usually benefit from support from family and friends and are likely to state their intentions and seek help from others in accomplishing their goals. Gerontological nurses can support and provide positive reinforcement for the person's intent to change; they also can point out the progress that the person already has made in developing an action plan. An important role for nurses is to assist with developing a plan and identifying the person's goals and small-step strategies to achieve them. Although discussing the barriers to changing behaviors might be necessary, it is important to focus on the benefits of the new behavior. Planning strategies for dealing with anticipated difficulties in implementing the plan is also helpful.

Action, the fourth stage, occurs when the person has already made the behavior change, but the changes have taken place for less than 6 months. At this stage, people usually do not fully experience the benefits of the new behavior and are vulnerable to resuming prior unhealthy behaviors or giving up the new healthy behaviors. At the same time, they are likely to have high levels of self-efficacy and to feel good about the progress they have made. Health promotion interventions during this stage are directed toward reinforcing the progress that has been made as well as toward identifying any barriers to continuing the healthy behaviors. Gerontological nurses can help the older adult identify motivators, establish a reward system, and plan strategies for overcoming the identified obstacles. They also can ask about support from friends and family and help the person identify ways of extending his or her support system if necessary.

Stage five, *Maintenance*, occurs when the person has continued the healthy behaviors for 6 months or longer. By this time, the person is experiencing positive effects of the healthier behavior, and the risk for relapse is less. During this stage, levels of self-efficacy are usually high, and the person is motivated to maintain the healthier lifestyle. Because the person has less need for external support, the role of the gerontological nurse diminishes. Health promotion interventions during this stage include reinforcement of progress and positive feedback about the healthier behaviors. In addition, the nurse can ask about any difficulties in maintaining the progress and help the person identify strategies to overcome any difficulties.

> Mrs. H. is 72 years old and visits the local senior center three times weekly for meals and social activities. Once a month, she comes to see you to have her blood pressure checked. You have recently studied the Transtheoretical Model and are interested in applying it to your clinical work in the Senior Wellness Program. Mrs. H. takes medication for high blood pressure and has expressed concern

about heart disease. When you discuss risk factors for heart disease with Mrs. H., she says that she would like to incorporate more physical activity into her daily life. She agrees to begin meeting with you regularly to develop a plan. Table 4-1 shows how you might apply the Transtheoretical Model to your work with Mrs. H.

THINKING POINTS WITH REGARD TO THE PRECONTEMPLATION STAGE

> From a health promotion perspective, how would you assess Mrs. H.'s understanding of the role of exercise in prevention of heart disease? What misconceptions would you want to address?

> What are the goals of your teaching interventions at this stage?

THINKING POINTS WITH REGARD TO THE CONTEMPLATION STAGE

> How would you assess Mrs. H.'s perception of the advantages and disadvantages of increased levels of exercise?

> What are the goals of your teaching interventions at this stage?

> What additional teaching points would you incorporate in your health promotion interventions at this time?

THINKING POINTS WITH REGARD TO THE PREPARATION STAGE

> What additional assessment questions would you ask Mrs. H.?

> What are the goals of your teaching interventions at this stage?

> What additional teaching points would you incorporate, particularly with regard to Mrs. H.'s concerns about arthritis?

THINKING POINTS WITH REGARD TO THE ACTION STAGE

> What concerns would you have about Mrs. H. during this stage, and what additional questions would you ask?

> What additional teaching points would you make?

TABLE 4-1 • Applying the Transtheoretical Model to Mrs. H.

Stage	Nurse	Mrs. H.
I: Precontemplation		
Assessment	"I know you're concerned about preventing heart disease because you've talked with me about your high blood pressure and you pay attention to avoiding high-fat foods. How do you think you rate on a scale of 1 to 10, with 1 being the lowest level and 10 being the best, in level of physical activity for preventing heart disease?"	"I would rate myself about 10. I take the dog out for a 5-minute walk every morning. My friend says we don't need more than 10 minutes of walking a day after we're 70 years old."
Intervention	"Did you know that there is extremely good evidence that 30 minutes of physical activity every day—even if it's not done all at once—is a good measure for protecting against heart disease? Would you be willing to read this pamphlet from the American Heart Association and let me know what you think when I see you again next week?"	"I've seen that before, but I'll try to read it this week if I have a chance."
II: Contemplation		
Assessment	"Now that you've had a chance to read that brochure, what's your understanding of the role of physical activity in preventing heart problems?"	"I think the Heart Association is on an exercise kick—they must think we all want to participate in marathons! Maybe they have a point about walking more than 15 minutes a day, but don't they realize that those of us who are in our 70s have a lot of problems walking? Most of us have arthritis. I think that brochure was written for people in their 20s, but on the other hand, maybe they do know what they're talking about."
Intervention	"From what I know, the Heart Association focuses on helping people prevent heart disease through healthy habits. They strongly urge everyone to do physical exercise for 30 minutes every day to keep the heart healthy. Many studies of people of all ages support this recommendation. You already walk 5 minutes with your dog every day, so you've gotten a good start on daily exercise. I bet your dog would love to go just a little farther each day and you would be quite capable of increasing your walk by just a little bit."	"Well, the dog is getting pretty fat, and it would probably do her good to get out for another walk in the evening. But it's hard enough for me to get out once a day with the weather as cold as it is right now. With my arthritis, I think I should wait a couple of months until the weather is warmer."
III: Preparation		
Assessment	"Since we met a couple of months ago, what are your current thoughts about increasing your walking?"	"I've been doing a lot of thinking about what we discussed, and now that spring is finally here, I think it's time to increase my walking time by a little bit each day. I just hope my arthritis doesn't get worse if I walk more."
Intervention	"So, have you thought of a plan that might work for you? Can you identify people who might be helpful in supporting your efforts?"	"Well, to begin with, I thought I could walk for 10 minutes every morning instead of 5—my dog sure would like that. I could increase that by 5 minutes every few weeks until I get up to 30 minutes a day. I've told my daughter that I'm trying to do more walking, and she said she might come over and walk with me and the dog on Saturdays. I do worry about my arthritis, though."
IV: Action		
Assessment	"It's so good to hear that you've been increasing your walking time for 3 months now. Congratulations on getting up to 30 minutes a day. How are you feeling about that?"	"My dog sure likes it, but I'm not sure that it's doing any good for me. I guess it feels good to pay attention to my health, but I haven't noticed that I'm feeling any better physically—at least not yet. My daughter came with me for the first few weeks and that was a good chance to see her, but she hasn't been coming for the last 3 weeks."
Intervention	"You deserve a lot of credit for accomplishing your goal—do you give yourself any rewards? It sounds as though you're disappointed that your daughter stopped walking with you—is there anyone else who might walk with you?"	"I guess I do deserve some credit—I did buy myself a new pair of walking shoes last week. A neighbor lady has talked to me about my walking and she said she'd like to get out there and join me, but I didn't encourage that because I thought my daughter would be coming with me. Maybe I'll invite her along—she could use the exercise, too."
V: Maintenance		
Assessment	"Congratulations on walking for 30 minutes every day for 7 months—that's quite an accomplishment and a nice gift for yourself and your health. You also deserve credit for getting your neighbor to join you at least a couple of days a week. Are you concerned about any temptations to cut down on your walking routine?"	"Thanks for the encouragement—my neighbor says she appreciates me inviting her along, and I enjoy the chance to keep up on neighborhood happenings by chatting with her when we walk. I am a little concerned about keeping up with the walking during the winter. I don't even take the dog out when it snows."

(continued)

Stage	Nurse	Mrs. H.
TABLE 4-1 • (Continued)		
Stage	Nurse	Mrs. H.
Intervention	"Have you thought about walking in the mall when the weather is bad? I'm not sure if you can take the dog along, but the mall opens every day an hour before the stores open so that walkers can come. I understand there's quite a group that walks there in the mornings."	"That sounds like a good idea—my neighbor mentioned that we might go there in bad weather. I think I'll try that out—maybe if I went to the mall, I could get my daughter to meet me there on Saturdays."

THINKING POINTS WITH REGARD TO THE MAINTENANCE STAGE

➤ What additional assessment questions would you ask Mrs. H.?

➤ What additional teaching points would you make?

CHAPTER SUMMARY

Geriatrics and gerontology are areas of professional specialization that have evolved since the mid-1940s to study and address the unique needs of older adults. These specialties initially focused on problems associated with aging, but the current focus is on quality-of-life issues and promoting optimal health and functioning. Gerontological nursing was first recognized as a nursing specialty during the 1960s, and major initiatives continue to encourage the development of this much-needed area of expertise. Major initiatives currently endorse geriatric competencies for all nurses and nursing research that focuses on nursing interventions to meet the unique needs of older adults.

Care of older adults is exceptionally challenging for gerontological nurses because of factors such as the unique and complex relationships between aging and disease and the unique and complex manifestations and consequences of illness in older adults. Recent trends that influence the practice of gerontological nursing are a focus on gender-specific health-related issues, the increasing cultural diversity of American society, and the increasing use of complementary and alternative medicine.

Health promotion is evolving as a major focus of health care in the United States, as evidenced by major national initiatives such as *Healthy People 2010*. Gerontological health care practitioners are increasingly recognizing that health promotion interventions are essential if older adults are to achieve and maintain high levels of health and functioning. Goals of health promotion for older adults focus on (1) the prevention and postponement of disease and disability, and (2) early identification and effective management of disease conditions. Types of health promotion interventions that are applicable to older adults include screening programs, risk reduction interventions, environmental modifications, and health education to promote good health practices. Gerontological nurses can apply the Transtheoretical Model of Health Promotion to address the many disease prevention and health promotion interventions that require a change in health-related behaviors.

CRITICAL THINKING EXERCISES

1. Describe the development of gerontological nursing from the 1960s to the present time.

2. You are asked to give a presentation to beginning nursing students to recruit them for an elective class called "Nursing for Wellness in Older Adults." What topics would you expect to be covered in this course and what points would you make to encourage them to enlist in this course?

3. You are discussing with your fellow students the choices you will be making about a practice area after graduation. You tell them that you are planning to specialize in gerontological nursing, and they challenge your decision with statements such as, "You'll be bored to death taking care of old fogies. Why don't you specialize in something exciting like trauma care? Besides, there's not much to do about the conditions of older folks, and what's the challenge in taking care of people who aren't going to get better?" How do you respond to these statements?

4. Identify one health-related behavior that you would like to change in your life (e.g., smoking cessation, increased level of exercise, decreased dietary fat intake) and develop a care plan for your behavior change using the Transtheoretical Model of Health Promotion (as in the case study).

EDUCATIONAL RESOURCES

American Association of Retired Persons (AARP)
601 E Street, NW, Washington, DC 20049
(800) 424-3410
http://www.aarp.org

American Nurses Association (ANA)
600 Maryland Ave, SW, Suite 100 West, Washington, DC 20024
(800) 274-4262
http://www.nursingworld.org

Centers for Medicare & Medicaid Services
Healthy Aging Project
7500 Security Blvd, Baltimore, MD 21244-1850
http://www.cms.hhs.gov

Fifty Plus Fitness Association
Box 20230, Stanford, CA 94309
(650) 323-6160
http://www.50plus.org

National Center for Chronic Disease Prevention and Health Promotion
Centers for Disease Control and Prevention
1600 Clifton Road, Atlanta, GA 30333
(404) 639-3311
http://www.cdc.gov/nccdphp

National Center for Complementary and Alternative Medicine
NCCAM Clearinghouse
P.O. Box 7923
Gaithersburg, MD 20898
(888) 644-6226
http://nccam.nih.gov/

National Gerontological Nursing Association (NGNA)
7794 Grow Drive, Pensacola, FL 32514
(800) 723-0560
http://www.ngna.org

National Institute on Aging
Building 31, Room 5C27
31 Center Drive, MSC 2292, Bethesda,MD 20892
(301) 496-1752
http://www.nia.nih.gov

National Institute of Nursing Research
Building 31, Room 5B13, Bethesda, MD 20892-2178
(301) 496-0207
http://www.nih.gov/ninr

National Resource Center on Aging and Injury
San Diego State University Center on Aging
College of Health and Human Services
5500 Campanile Drive, San Diego, CA 92182-1872
http://www.nrcai.org

National Resource Center on Supportive Housing & Home Modifications
USC Andrus Gerontology Center
3715 McClintock Avenue
Los Angeles, CA 90089-0191
(213) 740-1364
http://www.homemods.org

Office of Disease Prevention and Health Promotion
U.S. Department of Health and Human Services
200 Independence Avenue, SW, Room 738G, Washington, DC 20201
(202) 401-6295
http://www.osophs.dhhs.gov
http://www.health.gov/healthypeople (*Healthy People 2010*)

Office of Minority Health Resource Center
P.O. Box 37337, Washington, DC 20013-7337
(800) 444-6472
http://www.omhrc.gov

Partnership for Prevention
1015 18th Street, NW, Suite 200, Washington, DC 20036
(202) 833-0009
http://www.prevent.org

REFERENCES

Allison, M. J., & Keller, C. (2000). Physical activity maintenance in elders with cardiac problems. *Geriatric Nursing, 21*, 200–203.

American Nurses Association (ANA). (1976). *Standards of gerontological nursing practice.* Kansas City, MO: Author.

American Nurses Association (ANA). (2001). *Scope and standards of gerontological nursing practice* (2nd ed.). Washington, DC: Author.

Anetzberger, G. J. (2002). Community resources to promote successful aging. *Clinics in Geriatric Medicine, 18,* 611–626.

Bhalotra, S. M., & Mutschler, P. H. (2001). Primary prevention for older adults: No longer a paradox. *Journal of Aging and Social Policy, 12*(2), 5–22.

Bloom, H. G. (2001). Preventive medicine: When to screen for disease in older patients. *Geriatrics, 56*(4), 41–45.

Burbank, P. M., Padula, C. A., & Nigg, C. R. (2000). Changing health behaviors of older adults. *Journal of Gerontological Nursing, 26*(3), 26–33.

Burbank, P. M., & Riebe, D. (Eds.) (2002). *Promoting exercise and behavior change in older adults.* New York: Springer.

Burggraf, V., & Barry, R. J. (2000). Healthy people 2010: Protecting the health of older individuals. *Journal of Gerontological Nursing, 26*(12), 16–22.

Burkholder, G. J., & Evers, K. A. (2002). Application of the transtheoretical model to several problem behaviors. In P. M. Burbank & D. Riebe (Eds.), *Promoting exercise and behavior change in older adults* (pp. 85–145). New York: Springer.

Chernoff, R. (2002). Health promotion for older women: Benefits of nutrition and exercise programs. *Topics in Geriatric Rehabilitation, 18,* 59–67.

Cooper, K. M., Bilbrew, D., Dubbert, P. M., Kerr, K., & Kirchner, K. (2001). Health barriers to walking for exercise in elderly primary care. *Geriatric Nursing, 22,* 258–262.

DiPietro, L. (2001). Physical activity in aging: Changes in patterns and their relationship to health and function. *Journal of Gerontology, 56A*(Special Issue II), 13–22.

Drewnowski, A., & Evans, W. J. (2001a). Nutrition, physical activity, and quality of life in older adults: Summary. *Journal of Gerontology, 56A*(Special Issue II), 89–94.

Drewnowski, A., & Evans, W. J. (2001b). Introduction. *Journal of Gerontology, 56A*(Special Issue II), 5.

Dubbert, P. M., Cooper, K. M., Kirchner, K. A., Meydrech, E. F., & Bilbrew, D. (2002). Effects of nurse counseling on walking for exercise in elderly primary care patients. *Journal of Gerontology: Medical Sciences, 57A,* M733–M740.

Evans, W. J. (2002). Guest editorial: Exercise as the standard of care for elderly people. *Journal of Gerontology, 57A,* M260–M261.

Fisher, A., & Morley J. E. (2002). Antiaging medicine: The good, the bad and the ugly. *Journal of Gerontology, 57A,* M636–M639.

Frank, L. K. (1946). Gerontology. *Journal of Gerontology, 1*(1), 1–11.

Fraser, G. E., & Shavlik, D. J. (2001). Ten years of life: Is it a matter of choice? *Archives of Internal Medicine, 161,* 1645–1652.

Given, B. A., & Given, C. W. (2001). Health promotion for older adults in a managed care environment. In E. A. Swanson, T. Tripp-Reimer, & K. Buckwalter (Eds.), *Health promotion and disease prevention in the older adult* (pp. 219–241). New York: Springer.

Haber, D. (2002). Health promotion and aging: Educational and clinical initiatives by the federal government. *Educational Gerontology, 28,* 253–262.

Happell, B., & Brooker, J. (2001). Who will look after my grandmother? Attitudes of student nurses toward the care of older adults. *Journal of Gerontological Nursing, 27,* 12–17.

Hawranik, P., & Pangman, V. (2002). Perceptions of a senior citizens' wellness center: The community's voice. *Journal of Gerontological Nursing, 28*(11), 38–44.

Hubert, H. B., Bloch, D. A., Oehlert, J. W., & Fries, J. F. (2002). Lifestyle habits and compression of morbidity. *Journal of Gerontology: Medical Sciences, 57A,* M347–M351.

Infeld, D. L., & Whitelaw, N. (2002). Policy initiatives to promote healthy aging. *Clinics in Geriatric Medicine, 18*(3), 627–642.

King, A. C. (2001). Interventions to promote physical activity by older adults. *Journal of Gerontology, 56A*(Special Issue II), 36–46.

Klein, S. M. (1997). *A national agenda for geriatric education.* New York: Springer.

Matsumoto, A. M. (2002). Andropause: Clinical implications of the decline in serum testosterone levels with aging in men. *Journal of Gerontology: Medical Sciences, 57A,* M76–M99.

McBride, A. B. (2000). Nursing and gerontology. *Journal of Gerontological Nursing, 26*(7), 18–27.

Mehr, D. R., & Tatum, P. E. (2002). Primary prevention of disease in old age. *Clinics in Geriatric Medicine, 18,* 407–430.

Melillo, K. D., Williamson, E., Houde, S. C., Futrell, M., Read, C. Y., & Campasano, M. (2001). Perceptions of older Latino adults regarding physical fitness, physical activity, and exercise. *Journal of Gerontological Nursing, 27*(9), 38–46.

Mezey, M. D. (2001). Advanced practice nursing. In M. D. Mezey (Ed.), *The encyclopedia of elder care* (pp. 24–26). New York: Springer.

Mezey, M., & Fulmer, T. (2002). The future history of gerontological nursing. *Journal of Gerontology: Medical Sciences, 57A,* M438–M441.

Morley, J. E. (2003). Hot topics in geriatrics [Editorial]. *Journal of Gerontology: Medical Sciences, 53A,* 30–36.

Morley, J. E., & Flaherty, J. H. (2002). It's never too late: Health promotion and illness prevention in older persons. *Journal of Gerontology: Medical Sciences, 57A,* M338–M342.

National Institute on Aging. (2001). Report of the National Institute on Aging Advisory Panel on testosterone replacement in men. *Journal of Clinical Endocrinology and Metabolism, 86,* 4611–4614.

National Institute of Nursing Research (NINR). (1999, November). *Strategic planning for the 21st century.* [On-Line] Available http://www.nih.gov/ninr/strategicplan.htm.

Parker, M. W., Bellis, J. M., Bishop, P., Harper, M., Allman, R. M., Moore, C., & Thompson, P. (2002). A multidisciplinary model of health promotion incorporating spirituality into a successful aging intervention with African American and white elderly groups. *Gerontologist, 42,* 406–415.

Phelan, E. A., Williams, B., Leveille, S., Snyder, S., Wagner, E. H., & LoGerfo, J. P. (2002). Outcomes of a community-based dissemination of the Health Enhancement Project. *Journal of the American Geriatrics Society, 50,* 1519–1524.

Philpot, C. D., & Morley, J. E. (2000). Health issues unique to the aging man. *Geriatric Nursing, 21,* 234–239.

Popejoy, L. L., Rantz, M. J., Conn, V., Wipke-Tevis, D., Grando, V. T., & Porter, R. (2000). Improving quality of care in nursing facilities: Gerontological clinical nurse specialist as Research Nurse Consultant. *Journal of Gerontological Nursing, 26*(4), 6–13.

Prochaska, J. O., & DiClemente, C. C. (1982). Transtheoretical therapy: Toward a more integrative model of change. *Psychotherapy: Theory, Research, and Practice, 19,* 276–288.

Ransdell, L. B. (2001). A chronology of the study of older women's health: Data, discoveries, and future directions. *Journal of Women & Aging, 13,* 39–55.

Rejeski, W. J., & Mihalko, S. L. (2001). Physical activity and quality of life in older adults. *Journals of Gerontology, 56A*(Special Issue II), 23–35.

Resnick, B. (2002). Testing the effect of the WALC intervention on exercise adherence in older adults. *Journal of Gerontological Nursing, 28*(6), 40–49.

Resnick, B., & Spellbring, M. (2000). Understanding what motivates older adults to exercise. *Journal of Gerontological Nursing, 26*(3), 34–42.

Schlicht, J. (2000). Strength training for older adults: Prescription guidelines for nurses in advanced practice. *Journal of Gerontological Nursing, 26*(8), 25–32.

Singh, M. A. F. (2002). Exercise comes of age: Rationale and recommendations for a geriatric exercise prescription. *Journal of Gerontology: Medical Sciences, 57A,* M262–M282.

Strumpf, N. E. (2000). Improving care for the frail elderly: The challenge for nursing. *Journal of Gerontological Nursing, 26*(7), 36–44.

Titler, M. (2002). Evidence-based protocol. *Exercise promotion: Walking in elders.* Iowa City: University of Iowa Gerontological Nursing Interventions Research Center.

Touhy, E. L. (1946). Geriatrics: The general setting. *Geriatrics: Official Journal of the American Geriatrics Society, 1*(1), 17–20.

U.S. Department of Health and Human Services (USDHHS). (1996a). *Guide to clinical prevention services* (2nd ed.). U.S. Preventive Services task force. Baltimore: Williams & Wilkins.

U.S. Department of Health and Human Services (USDHHS). (1996b). *Surgeon General's report on physical activity and health.* Washington, DC: U.S. Government Printing Office.

U.S. Department of Health and Human Services (USDHHS). (1998). *Clinician's handbook of preventive services.* Washington, DC: U.S. Government Printing Office.

Women's Health Initiative Investigators. (2002). Risks and benefits of estrogen plus progestin in healthy postmenopausal women: Principal results from the Women's Health Initiative randomized controlled trial. *Journal of the American Medical Association, 288*(3), 321–333.

Wykle, M. L. (2001). Gerontological nursing research: Challenges for the new millennium. *Journal of Gerontological Nursing, 27*(4), 7–9.

Gerontological Nursing and the Continuum of Care for Older Adults

LEARNING OBJECTIVES

1. Describe the services that are included in a continuum of care for older adults.

2. List the characteristics of specialized acute care for the elderly (ACE) programs.

3. Describe the levels of care in nursing homes and trends in nursing home care.

4. Discuss roles of gerontological nurses in acute care and long-term care settings.

5. Describe the levels of home care services, including sources of payment and types of services.

6. Describe each of the following types of community-based services: adult day centers, respite services, health promotion programs, and geriatric care management programs.

7. Discuss roles of gerontological nurses in home care and community-based services.

8. Describe the role of Medicare, Medicaid, private insurance, and PACE programs in paying for health care services for older adults.

Although nurses have always cared for older adults, it has been only since the late 1960s that health care organizations have recognized and addressed the unique health care needs of older adults by developing new programs. Because of these new programs, a continuum of care for older adults has gradually evolved over the past several decades, and health care services are increasingly addressing specific needs of older adults during different phases of health and illness. Another outcome of these new programs is the emergence of countless new roles for gerontological nurses because nurses provide specific health care services at each point along this continuum. This chapter presents an overview of the continuum of health care services for older adults that began in the late 1960s and continues to evolve today; it also discusses roles of gerontological nurses in these programs.

DEVELOPMENT OF A CONTINUUM OF CARE

The establishment of Medicare in 1965 (discussed later in this chapter) stimulated major changes in the delivery of health care services to older adults, and nurses have taken prominent roles in developing gerontological health care programs. For example, during the early 1970s, home care and community health nurses recognized the central role they play in coordinating services for older adults, and they spearheaded the development of multidisciplinary models of health care in home and community settings. Around this same time, nurses in nursing home settings recognized the vital leadership roles they play in developing models for skilled, rehabilitative, and long-term nursing care of older adults. By the 1980s, health care providers acknowledged that most existing acute care models did not comprehensively address the health and functioning of older adults, and they began developing innovative and cost-effective models for inpatient care. During the 1990s, health care programs began emphasizing health promotion, prevention of disease, improvement in functioning, and enhancement of quality of life. In 1992, an amendment to the Older Americans Act enabled the federal Administration on Aging to expand its support of health promotion and wellness programs nationwide. By the early 2000s, a continuum of innovative health care services had emerged, and programs continue to be developed to meet the complex needs of diverse groups of older adults in numerous settings. Although some of these programs have arisen from an increased concern about health expenditures, many are the result of an increased awareness of the importance of meeting chronic care needs of older adults in a way that addresses both financial concerns and quality-of-life issues.

Long-term care refers to health care services that address the chronic care needs of older adults. Traditionally, this term was associated with care provided in nursing homes because they were the primary resource, and usually the only formal resource, for people who needed more care on a long-term basis than could be provided by family members in home settings. But this narrow perception of long-term care has become outdated. In recent decades, numerous types of services have been developed to address the needs of people of all ages who need long-term care. Currently, long-term care refers to any personal care

and assistance that an individual might need because of a long-term disability or chronic illness—indicated by physical and cognitive impairments—that limits the person's ability to function, as measured by impairments in activities of daily living (ADLs) (Borrayo et al., 2002; Kane, 2001). Many long-term care services are provided in nursing homes, assisted-living facilities, and other institutional settings, but these services are also provided in apartments, private homes, and other community settings.

Aging in place refers to a range of services that allow older adults to remain in one setting and receive different levels of care as their needs change. Aging-in-place programs often are established in institutional settings that are able to provide services ranging from meals and housekeeping for people who are relatively independent to hands-on nursing care for more dependent people. Some models are limited to addressing the needs of a specific group of people. For example, a model called *in-place progression* provides services for people with Alzheimer's disease who remain in the same bedroom and on the same nursing care unit from the middle stages of the disorder until the time of death (Weaverdyck et al., 1998).

Continuum of care (sometimes called *seamless continuum of care*) is evolving to replace the traditional concept of long-term care. Continuum of care programs holistically address the comprehensive needs of older adults in a variety of settings and include all those services designed to provide care for people at different stages of dependence for an extended period. Life-care or continuing-care retirement communities (described in Chapter 2) are examples of continuum of care programs. Continuum of care models usually include all or most of the following services: primary and preventive care, acute care, transitional care, rehabilitation services, extended care, respite care, social services, home health care, adult day centers, and care management services. By nature, these programs provide multidisciplinary and coordinated services, often using a care manager. Some models use a continuing care pathway to assess a person's readiness for transition from one part of the program to another. For example, the Pathway Project uses a care management model to assess, plan, implement, coordinate, monitor, and evaluate services effectively to meet the acute and long-term care needs of frail elders (Tichawa, 2002).

Programs providing a continuum of care covered by health care insurance are not widely available in the United States, but two well-known and relatively long-standing programs are the On Lok Program and the Program of All-inclusive Care for the Elderly (PACE), which is discussed later in this chapter. Even without formal continuum of care models, however, numerous long-term care services are provided in many settings ranging from traditional nursing homes to innovative community-based settings. People with complex needs usually require a combination of services. For example, a person with early dementia who lives with her daughter may attend an adult day center 3 days a week, receive home-delivered meals twice weekly, and have a companion service on weekends. Combinations of services also are needed when two or more people with long-term care needs live together (e.g., siblings, couples, or parents and adult children). When combinations of long-term care services are needed, family members or care managers must coordinate care.

ACUTE CARE

Inpatient hospital stays now are viewed as one part of a continuum of care that necessitates careful preadmission and postdischarge planning and coordination of services. As with other aspects of health care, hospital care of older adults is rapidly changing, with many of these changes being determined in large part by health insurance coverage. For example, because the current Medicare reimbursement policy provides financial incentives for earlier discharge from acute care settings, hospitals have developed *subacute care units* (also called *transitional care units*). These units provide skilled nursing care under Medicare and other insurance programs; hence, reimbursement is lower than that for acute care. In general, subacute care patients are medically complex or need skilled rehabilitation following acute episodes such as a stroke or orthopedic surgery. Examples of typical subacute care services include chemotherapy; intravenous therapy; complex wound care; enteral and parenteral nutrition; speech, physical, and occupational therapies; and management of complex respiratory care (e.g., ventilator, tracheostomy). In recent years, some nursing homes also have developed subacute care units.

Many hospitals are addressing acute care needs of older adults by establishing separate geriatric units—often referred to as *acute care for elders* (ACE) units—staffed by a specially trained multidisciplinary team. The rationale for these units is that older adults have unique needs that can be anticipated and addressed to prevent functional decline during hospitalization (Miller, 2002). Compared with patients who receive usual hospital care, patients who receive care in ACE units have improved functional status, fewer discharges to nursing homes, and a better 1-year survival rate (Thomas, 2002), and there is increasing evidence of the effectiveness of these units (Morley, 2003). The

focus of ACE programs is to assist older adults who have complex problems to remain at their highest level of function. Key elements of ACE units are: (1) a specially adapted environment; (2) a multidisciplinary team approach; (3) patient-centered care, including care plans for rehabilitation and prevention of disability; (4) intensive review of care to minimize the adverse effects of medications and procedures; and (5) discharge planning with the goal of returning the patient to his or her home (Counsell et al., 2000; Siegler et al., 2002). In addition to gerontological nurses, the teams typically include a geriatrician, pharmacist, social worker, various rehabilitation therapists (e.g., speech, physical, or occupational therapists), and mental health professionals (e.g., psychologists or psychiatrists). Some teams also include a geriatric care manager and music, activity, or horticultural therapists.

Other acute care programs focus on specific target conditions, such as delirium, with an emphasis on comprehensive improvement of one aspect of geriatric care in hospital settings (Fulmer et al., 2002). For example, the Hospital Elder Life Program is a hospital-wide program that screens patients on admission for the risk factors of immobility, dehydration, sleep deprivation, vision impairment, hearing impairment, and cognitive impairment (Inouye, 2000). This program uses a multidisciplinary team to implement interventions to prevent cognitive and functional decline in older patients. Another model, called Together We Improve Care of the Elderly (TWICE), has achieved significant improvements in care of hospitalized older adults using nursing protocols, staff development, and geriatric resource staff (Swauger & Tomlin, 2002).

Emergency departments of acute care settings also have developed innovative programs to address the complex needs of frail elders. The Systematic Intervention for Geriatric Network of Evaluation and Treatment (SIGNET) model was developed to improve case finding of at-risk older patients, improve care planning and referral of at-risk older people, and create a coordinated network of existing medical, nursing, and social services (Mion et al., 2001). This program demonstrated the feasibility of implementing an assessment and linkage model to address the needs of frail older adults in emergency departments.

Roles for Gerontological Nurses in Acute Care Settings

As acute care settings have developed programs to address the unique needs of hospitalized older patients, new roles have emerged for gerontological nurses, particularly for advanced practice nurses.

Gerontological nurses are likely to serve as consultants and role models for staff nurses and often take leadership roles in developing and implementing specialized care programs and protocols for hospitalized older adults. The Geriatric Resource Nurse Model has been successful in developing bedside experts in geriatric care through mentoring by advanced practice nurses (Turner et al., 2001). The following positive outcomes have been associated with the use of advanced practice nurses in acute care settings: (1) shorter lengths of stay; (2) reduced morbidity following discharge; (3) fewer readmissions and less use of emergency room after discharge; and (4) significant reductions in morbidity, including preventing or reducing the incidence of delirium and other syndromes that commonly occur in hospitalized older patients (Mezey, 2001).

Since the early 1990s, the Yale Geriatric Care Program has been using a unit-based and nursing-centered model of care to prevent functional decline in hospitalized older adults (Fulmer, 1991; Inouye et al., 1993a, 1993b). Primary nurses, designated as Geriatric Resource Nurses, identify risks for conditions associated with functional decline in older adults and implement preventive measures. Older patients who receive care in a unit staffed with Geriatric Resource Nurses have less functional decline in ADLs than patients on similar units without the specialized care (Turner et al., 2001). This model has been supported by the Nurses Improving Care to the Hospitalized Elderly (NICHE) program of the John A. Hartford Foundation and is now widely used (Fulmer et al., 2002; Guthrie et al., 2002; Lee & Fletcher, 2002; Pfaff, 2002; Salinas et al, 2002). The functional assessment guide used in these programs is described in Chapter 11.

NURSING HOMES

Nursing home care refers to nursing care that is provided in a residential institutional setting. Nursing homes are licensed by a state or federal agency and must be certified as a Medicare and/or Medicaid facility if they receive funds from those programs. Nursing homes are required to have continuous on-site supervision by a registered nurse or licensed practical nurse. Sixty-six percent of all nursing homes are for-profit, whereas 36% are not-for-profit, and 8% are government owned (Mitty, 2001). In addition to medical care and nursing services, nursing homes must provide dental, podiatry, medical specialty consultation services, and rehabilitation therapies (e.g., physical and occupational therapies).

Gerontologists have identified the reasons why older people are admitted for nursing home care.

Factors that increase the likelihood of being admitted to a nursing home include poverty, white race, female gender, living alone, advanced age, hospital admission, confinement to bed, impaired mental status, lack of informal supports, and loss of self-care ability (Mitty, 2001). The most common diagnoses leading to nursing home admission are dementia, heart disease, and hypertension (Mitty, 2001). People with a combination of cognitive impairment and ADL limitations are significantly more at risk for being admitted to a nursing home, and this risk increases with the severity of the cognitive impairment (Borrayo et al., 2002).

Although the basic criterion for admission to a nursing home is that the person be sick enough to require continuous nursing care but not sick enough to require hospital care, not everyone meeting this criterion goes to a nursing home. Many people needing continuous nursing care—as well as less intense levels of nursing care—are cared for in their own homes or in other settings. Since the 1970s, gerontologists have recognized that the chance of being admitted to a nursing home is determined not only by the characteristics of the person who needs the care but also by the availability of capable and willing caregivers. The combination of dependence in performing ADLs and lack of caregiver resources brings older people to nursing homes for long-term care. Thus, many older people move to a nursing home not because their condition has changed, but because there has been a change in the availability or abilities of the caregiver.

Nursing home care is generally categorized as *skilled nursing* or *skilled rehabilitation* (usually short-term) or *intermediate care* (usually long-term). Skilled nursing home care, usually provided for 6 months or less, is associated with posthospital care. Medicare and other health insurance programs cover the cost of skilled nursing or skilled rehabilitation services for up to 100 days if the care is medically necessary and the person is progressing; however, people generally meet these criteria for only 32 days (Mitty, 2001). Long-term or intermediate nursing home care refers to nursing services provided for chronically ill people who need assistance with daily activities. The average length of stay for long-term residents is 2.5 years (Mitty, 2001). Medicare does not cover costs of long-term nursing care, but some long-term care insurance policies provide limited coverage. Sources of payment for long-term nursing home care are as follows: Medicaid (about 50%); private pay, which is also called out-of-pocket (about 33%); and other insurance (Yeaworth, 2002). Seventy-five to 85% of all public long-term care dollars (primarily from Medicaid and Medicare) is spent for care in institutions such as nursing homes rather than for community-based care (Borrayo et al., 2002).

Trends in Nursing Home Care

Recent changes in the health care services for older adults have significantly influenced both long-term and short-term nursing home care. On any given day, between 4% and 5% of people older than 65 years in the United States live in a nursing home. This percentage has declined slightly since the 1970s (Hays et al., 2003). However, about 40% of people older than 65 years of age are likely to spend some time in a nursing home, and this is likely to increase to 46% by the year 2020 (Spillman & Lubitz, 2002). These statistics reflect two major trends in health care services for older adults in the United States. First, the emphasis on shorter lengths of hospital stays has led to more people being admitted to nursing homes for short-term care since the late 1980s. Between 1985 and 1997, the percentage of nursing home residents who returned to community settings increased from 18% to 30% of all nursing home residents (Hays et al, 2003). Second, the rapid growth of assisted-living facilities and community-based long-term care services has led to less demand for long-term nursing home care because many services that used to be provided only in nursing homes are now provided in other settings. For example, assisted-living facilities provide some of the basic nursing home services (e.g., meals and laundry) at a lower cost, and additional services (e.g., dementia care and medication management) can often be purchased as the need arises (Hujer et al., 2000). These *housing-and-service settings* are now widely available and often are viewed as an alternative to long-term nursing home care for people with disabilities (Kane & Kane, 2001).

As a result of these trends, most nursing homes provide a combination of skilled care services for short-term residents and intermediate care services for long-term residents. Because the skilled care provided in nursing homes today is similar to the care that used to be provided to patients in hospitals, residents often are able to stay in the nursing facility during acute illnesses rather than being admitted to a hospital. Another result of these trends is that the percentage of long-term residents who are more dependent in ADLs has gradually increased in recent years because people who are less dependent now receive care in other settings.

A recent development in nursing homes is the establishment of special care units (SCUs), which are separate units designed to address the needs of specific groups of residents who meet explicit admission criteria. Dementia-care units, or Alzheimer's units,

are a common type of SCU; other types are acquired immunodeficiency syndrome (AIDS), subacute care, oncology, ventilator-dependent, pressure ulcer, and traumatic brain injury units. SCU staff members receive specialized training, and care plans address unique needs of the residents. Support and educational programs often are provided for residents and families. About 7% of all nursing home beds are in SCUs; they are more common in larger and not-for-profit nursing homes (Mitty, 2001).

In recent years, health care providers have emphasized quality of care and quality of life in nursing homes. This focus stems in part from consumer pressure that began during the 1970s and in part from legislation passed during the late 1980s (see Chapter 6). Terms such as *resident-centered care* refer to the shift from the traditional nursing home focus on the efficient provision of physical care to frail and impaired individuals to a focus on quality of life for residents. Goals for resident-centered care include supporting opportunities for continued growth, encouraging meaningful connections with family and the community, respecting the individual needs and desires of each resident, and honoring the life patterns and accomplishments of each person in the setting (Calkins, 2002).

Models of Nursing Home Care

Concerns about quality of care and quality of life have prompted a limited but growing effort to bring about a "culture change" in the provision of nursing home care (Kane, 2001). For example, the Pioneer Network in Long-Term Care is a group of providers who strive to implement care in nursing homes that exemplifies values such as putting people before tasks and responding to the needs of the spirit, mind, and body. To this end, nursing homes are making efforts to permit spontaneity, foster neighborhood groupings, include residents in decision making, break down the rigidities of routines, empower both residents and certified nursing assistants, and foster more normal and meaningful relationships between residents and staff (Kane, 2001; McGilton, 2002).

The Eden Alternative is a model developed in the mid-1990s by Dr. William Thomas, with the intent of creating a "human habitat" to combat boredom, loneliness, and lack of meaning in nursing homes (Thomas, 1994). The Eden Alternative is a comprehensive program of transforming the organizational culture as well as the physical, spiritual, psychosocial, and interpersonal environments of a facility. An essential component is the systematic introduction of pets, plants, and children to create a home-like setting and improve the quality of life of residents.

The program incorporates strategies to engage and empower staff in bringing about the environmental change (Thomas, 1994). Many nursing homes are adopting this comprehensive model or implementing some components of it.

Nurses in particular have expressed much interest in incorporating aspects of the Eden Alternative in nursing homes. Nursing research "supports the conclusion that the Eden Alternative or other environmental transformation may be feasibly undertaken by facilities of any sort, large or small, private or public, rural or urban" (Tesh et al., 2002, p. 33). Barba and colleagues (2002) describe the implementation of this model in one nursing home and discuss some of its risks, benefits, and challenges from a nursing perspective. The Eden Alternative web site (www.edenalt.com) provides further information about this program.

Roles for Gerontological Nurses in Nursing Homes and Long-Term Care Settings

Nurses have always assumed strong leadership roles in nursing homes and other long-term care settings, and opportunities for role expansion are skyrocketing because of some of the trends just discussed. The focus on improved quality of care and quality of life encouraged the use of nurses to implement innovative changes in delivery of care in nursing homes and other long-term care settings. Currently, gerontological nurses have almost unlimited opportunities to develop and implement cost-effective programs directed at improving care in nursing homes and other long-term care settings. Some of the most common roles for gerontological nurses in long-term care settings include team leader, restorative nurse, wellness nurse, and director of nursing.

In the late 1990s, numerous opportunities opened up for gerontological nurses in long-term care settings when Medicare and Medicaid began to reimburse for advanced practice nurses. For example, advanced practice nurses in assisted-living facilities may provide staff education, assist with program development, develop plans for clients with dementia, provide for acute and chronic care needs, establish support groups for clients and families, and act as advocates for clients and their families (Bonnel, 2002). The following positive outcomes of the use of advanced practice nurses in nursing homes have been identified: (1) fewer hospitalizations, (2) better resident assessments, (3) decreased use of emergency rooms, (4) better illness prevention and case finding, (5) lower use of physical restraints and psychotropic medications, (6) improved nursing outcomes for health problems such as pressure ulcers, urinary incontinence, and aggressive behaviors, and (7) successful and cost-effective management of an anticoagulation treatment program for residents taking warfarin (Allen et al., 2000; Mezey, 2001; Ryden et al., 2000). Other roles for advanced practice nurses in long-term care include consultation regarding conditions such as dementia and depression. Eisch and colleagues (2000) found that positive behavioral changes occurred in 62% of the residents who had been referred by the nursing home staff for agitation, disruptive behaviors, depressive symptoms, or a decline in ADLs when recommendations of a geriatric nurse practitioner consultant were implemented.

HOME CARE

Older people and other dependent populations have always received much of their health care at home, and visiting nurse services have existed in the United States since the late 1880s. But the delivery of home care services dramatically changed after 1965 when Medicare funds became available for these services. In 1975, the Older Americans Act and Title XX Social Services Act allocated federal funds for home-based services, and the federal Health Services Program funded grants for the establishment, operation, or expansion of programs providing home health services. By the late 1970s, thousands of home care agencies had been established, and their number escalated exponentially over the course of the next two decades.

Although the federal government had envisioned Medicare home health care services as a short-term supplement to acute care services for people who needed skilled care, consumers came to view these services as an extension of long-term care for people with chronic illnesses. By the 1990s, home care had become the fastest growing component of the Medicare program, and costs had increased so drastically that Congress included cost-containment measures in the Balanced Budget Act of 1997. A major goal of the Act was to reduce Medicare payments substantially for home health care services. In practical terms, however, home care agencies reduced their spending through screening, fewer visits, earlier discharges, and reduction or elimination of specialized staffing (Smith et al., 2000). In the 2 years after this legislation went into effect, Medicare spending on home health care decreased 45%, the number of beneficiaries dropped from 3.6 to 3.0 million, and about 3,000 home health agencies closed for financial reasons (Leff & Burton, 2001; Martin, 2001). The new payment system established by the Act "wrought the biggest changes to the home care industry since the inception of the Medicare program 30 years ago" (Marrelli, 2001, p. 217). The impact was larger on people in rural areas where home care was already in short supply (Anetzberger, 2002).

While the federal government was cutting funding for home care, state governments were recognizing the need for increased funding for home- and community-based services. Motivated both by cost-containment and consumer preference, state long-term care policy shifted from a focus on institutional care to a focus on noninstitutional services. As a result, more state funds became available for home care and other community-based long-term care services. Although many state-funded programs are limited to people who would be eligible for Medicaid if they were in a nursing home, many affordable services have become widely available through public, private, and nonprofit agencies. Skilled home care services and long-term home care services are the main types of home care services for older adults in the United States that evolved because of these trends.

Skilled Home Care

Home care services provided under Medicare and some other health insurance programs have always been limited to skilled care and restricted to people who meet all of the following criteria:

- The person must be homebound (i.e., leaving the home requires considerable and taxing effort).
- The services must be ordered by a primary care provider.
- There must be a need for skilled nursing or rehabilitative services.
- The person must require intermittent, but not full-time, care.

People often qualify for skilled home care following a hospitalization or a stay in a skilled nursing or rehabilitation setting for an acute illness. Conditions that are likely to necessitate skilled home care services are strokes, fractures, and congestive heart failure.

Medicare covers the following types of home care services for people who meet the criteria: skilled nursing, physical therapy, occupational therapy, nutrition counseling, speech-language therapy, medical social work, the assistance of a home health aide, and medical supplies and equipment. A licensed professional nurse or therapist provides or directs the services. Types of skilled nursing services covered by Medicare home care benefits include case management, medication management, infusion therapy, intravenous antibiotics, and psychiatric nursing services. Home health aides can provide some of the care (e.g., assistance with bathing, linen changes, range-of-motion exercises, and assistance with transfers and ambulation), and their services are provided

under the directions of a licensed nurse or therapist. Because skilled home care services are meant to be short-term, a major focus is on teaching the older person and caregivers about self-care activities.

Typical skilled care recipients are: (1) people who are homebound but able to manage most of their daily care at some level of independence; and (2) people who, although homebound and dependent in many functional areas, receive help from families, friends, or paid caregivers to supplement the skilled care services. If people reach a level of independence so that they are no longer homebound, they cannot continue receiving skilled care services. Likewise, people no longer qualify for skilled care after they achieve self-care goals. Many people receiving skilled care, however, still need some level of home care services after the skilled services are discontinued.

Long-Term Home Care

A wide spectrum of long-term home care services are available for the large majority of older adults who need home care but do not meet the criteria for skilled care. At one end of the spectrum is nonskilled care provided by companions, homemakers, and home health aides. The most common services are meal preparation, light housekeeping, assistance with personal care, accompaniment to medical appointments, and grocery shopping and other errands. These services are often supplemented by community-based services such as transportation and home-delivered meals (discussed in Chapter 2). Frequency of service ranges from periodic to 24 hours daily, and some agencies and independent caregivers require a minimum number of hours weekly. A licensed nurse may assess the client and supervise the services, and a registered nurse usually assists with medication management, if needed. At the other end of the spectrum is skilled care for people who need this type of care but do not meet Medicare criteria. Virtually any skilled service available under Medicare is available as a self-pay service, but these services are usually quite expensive.

Payment for Home Care Services

Sources of payment for home care services are self-pay, public funds for people who qualify, and some long-term care insurance for the small minority of older adults who have these policies. Self-pay has been the primary source of payment for long-term home care, but public funds through Medicaid waiver programs have been increasing gradually since the early 1990s. In addition, sliding-scale fees for home care and other community-based services are increasingly becoming available through public and nonprofit agencies.

Home care services are available through formal sources (e.g., agencies) or informal sources (e.g., independent caregivers). Agencies usually provide initial assessments, arrange for services, assign workers, provide ongoing supervision, and collect payment for services. They are responsible for hiring, training, directing, scheduling, and firing workers. Some agencies provide a wide range of services, including care management. Other agencies provide only a limited type of service, such as the provision of home health aides. Some so-called agencies, however, are little more than a registry or referral service. When services are obtained from informal sources rather than from agencies, the care recipient or a surrogate decision maker is responsible for performing the organizational tasks that agencies normally perform (e.g., hiring, firing, and supervising the caregiver). In this case, sometimes the aid of a geriatric care management service (discussed later in this chapter) is enlisted to arrange for services and oversee the care. A common way of finding independent caregivers and other home care resources is through a word-of-mouth network, in which names are obtained from friends, families, churches, or local offices on aging.

People who self-pay for home care obtain services from agencies or from informal sources. Traditionally, when home care services are covered by insurance or public funds, they have been provided by agencies under contractual arrangements. This is changing, however, as an increasing number of states are allowing care recipients to choose and direct independent providers (Wiener, 2001). In some situations, Medicaid waiver programs compensate family members for providing home care services.

Roles for Gerontological Nurses in Home Care Settings

Nursing services have always been the foundation of skilled home care services, but the roles of nurses have been limited and determined largely by Medicare policies. Two recent trends in health care—a change in the Medicare reimbursement system and the development of telehealth technology—are creating opportunities for expanded roles for home care nurses. Because of the October 2000 change in the Medicare reimbursement system, home health agencies have more incentives and fewer barriers to using advanced practice nurses (Pierson, 2001). Several models have demonstrated the effectiveness of advanced practice nurses in home care settings for consultation, home visits, comprehensive assessments, and staff education and mentoring (Milone-Nuzzo & Pike, 2001). The transitional care model, which uses advanced practice nurses to promote continuity of care from hospital to home for older

hospitalized patients who were at high risk for readmission, has consistently demonstrated reduced costs, fewer hospital readmissions, and reduced lengths of stay when readmissions were necessary (Bourbonniere & Evans, 2002). Home care roles for gerontological nurses are likely to continue expanding as Medicare and other health insurance programs address cost-effectiveness and quality-of-care issues.

Developments in telecommunication technology also are creating new roles for nurses, particularly in home care settings. *Telehealth* is the use of audio, video, and other electronic information processing technologies in the provision of health services or professional health education at distant sites (Field, 1996). Subsets of telehealth include *telemedicine* (remote health care facilities interact with facilities that provide specialized services), *telenursing* (nurses deliver services through telecommunication devices), *telehomecare* (home health care services are delivered through telecommunication devices), and *telemonitoring* (health data is transmitted from site to site over a telecommunications network (Tran et al., 2002). Nurses are advocating for the use of telehealth technology to improve access and availability of health care services for older adults, particularly those who are homebound or live in rural, remote, or underserved areas (Wakefield et al., 2001). Telehealth technology typically is used to collect information through physiologic monitors connected to a computer in the home. Assessment data are then sent through a telephone connection to a nurse or other health care professional who verbally communicates with the patient to obtain additional information. Some systems use videophones to allow for visual as well as audio communication.

Since the late 1990s, Medicare and a few other health insurance programs have reimbursed providers for telehealth services, and insurance coverage is likely to increase as studies demonstrate the effectiveness and cost benefits of particular telehealth programs. For example, Jenkins and McSweeney (2001) found that telehealth assessments provided information that was comparable to in-home nursing assessments of older adults with congestive heart failure. Assessment parameters included weight, edema, blood pressure, respiratory effort, heart rate and rhythm, lung and heart sounds, and color of the patient's lips, face, and nails. Nurses and older clients expressed satisfaction with the telehealth assessment. Additional benefits of telehealth technology include quicker access of home health nurses to their patients, decreased patient anxiety and stress, and substantial cost and time savings without any loss of quality of care (Jenkins & McSweeney, 2001). Telehealth technology in home care settings also can reduce hospital readmissions for people who have congestive heart failure and for patients who are recovering from cardiac surgery (Frantz et al., 2002). Tran and colleagues (2002) described the effective use of telehealth technology in home care settings to support and educate caregivers of stroke patients.

COMMUNITY-BASED SERVICES

Adult Day Centers

Adult day centers, first developed in the 1970s, have become a major community-based resource for care of dependent older adults. They offer structured, comprehensive programming to functionally impaired older people in a congregate setting for less than 24 hours per day (Anetzberger, 2002). Adult day centers provide meals and structured social and recreational activities in a group setting, and they may also provide transportation services. Some adult day centers provide medication management, assistance with personal care, and other health-related services and therapies. Adult day centers generally provide supervised care on weekdays for 8 hours a day with about 5 hours of formal programming during that time and the other 3 hours being used for social interaction and other unstructured activities. Less commonly, services are available for longer hours and on weekends and holidays.

Participants in adult day centers usually are impaired to the point that they need supervision or assistance in several functional areas. Most participants are cognitively impaired, but depression and physical disabilities also are common conditions among adult day center participants. Participants typically live with a family member, but some live independently or in group settings.

The goals of these programs are to maintain or improve the functional abilities of impaired older people; to delay or prevent the need for institutional care; to provide relief for caregivers of dependent older adults; and to improve the quality of life for impaired older adults and their caregivers. Researchers have evaluated the effects of adult day center care on both dependent older adults and their caregivers. For example, Zank and Schacke (2002) found a significant decline in health in the control group and an improvement or stabilization of subjective well-being and dementia symptoms in a group of adult day center participants.

Costs of adult day center programs vary widely, as does the source of payment. Although families have been the primary source of payment for most costs of adult day center care, public funds are increasingly

becoming available because of the growing recognition of the benefits and cost-effectiveness of this kind of community-based service. Some programs are subsidized by nonprofit organizations, and some have a sliding fee scale. Only a few health insurance policies cover adult day center programs. The PACE model (discussed later in this chapter) is a very successful, but atypical, model that uses adult day centers as a core component of long-term care services. It is projected that adult day centers will become more integral to the community. For example, they are likely to be located in places where caregivers work and may be regarded as an employment benefit in the future (Anetzberger, 2002).

Respite Services

Respite generally refers to any service whose primary goal is periodically to relieve caregivers from the stress of their usual caregiving responsibilities. The term first appeared in the gerontological literature in the late 1970s when gerontologists first recognized that caregivers had substantial risk for developing social isolation, clinical depression, psychological distress, and other problems directly related to the burden of caregiving. As such, respite services are provided for people who are living in a home setting and are being cared for by family members or other unpaid help. Goals of respite services include improved well-being for caregivers and delayed institutionalization of dependent older people. Types of respite services include adult day center care, overnight and short-term nursing home care, and provision of in-home companions or home health aides.

Health Promotion Programs

Because of the growing emphasis on health promotion, many community-based programs address the needs of older adults who are relatively healthy and functional (see Chapter 4 for more details). Periodic health screenings and other health promotion activities are increasingly being offered in senior centers and other places where older adults gather. Among the health promotion activities offered by these programs are blood pressure checks; safe driving courses; smoking cessation classes; health screening (e.g., cancer, vision, hearing); flu shots and other immunizations; medication assessment, management, and education; and various types of exercise, such as walking, aerobics, aquatics, and tai chi. Health education topics include nutrition, stress management, general health care, and seasonal health issues such as hypothermia, heat-related illness, and colds and flu.

Organized group activities, such as senior wellness programs, frequently take place in or are sponsored by community-based senior centers that exist in almost every community. Hospitals and other health care institutions are becoming more involved in providing this kind of program and are employing nurses to address the needs of older adults in the community. Programs are sometimes sponsored jointly by senior centers and health care agencies. For example, senior health fairs, which address the specific health needs of a specific population, provide the opportunity for follow-up and referral of identified medical issues. Thus, they can provide a valuable health promotion service for older adults while increasing the potential patient base for health care providers. Recommended health promotion activities for a senior health fair include the provision of information about interventions for maintaining good health and screenings for diabetes, glaucoma, cholesterol, and blood pressure (Hatchett & Duran, 2001).

Geriatric Care Management Services

Services provided to older adults in their own homes constitute one of the most rapidly growing components of health care services. Although family and other unpaid workers provide 85% of all in-home care, informal and formal paid caregivers provide the remaining 15%. Family caregiving has become more complex and difficult as more and more family members have moved away from their hometowns. In addition, the entry of more women into the paid workforce has significantly diminished the availability of traditional family caregivers. These trends, along with the significant increase in the number of people aged 85 years and older, have led to the need for professional geriatric care management services.

As the range of services for older adults has expanded, identification of appropriate services and coordination of care has become more necessary and more challenging. Although family members sometimes take on these tasks, many family members are not prepared to assume this challenge, and many older adults do not have any family members available. In these situations, the older adult may receive care (or case) management services. A geriatric care manager serves as the primary coordinator who is responsible for implementing a long-term care plan in the absence of family members who have the ability to do so.

Care management involves comprehensive assessment, care planning, implementation, monitoring, and reassessment. Professional geriatric care management services are provided by individual professionals and by not-for-profit and for-profit groups and organizations. These services are often provided by a nurse who assesses the needs for a variety of long-term care services and then plans, coordinates, and oversees the services. Care management has created many opportunities for gerontological nurses in agencies or in private practice settings.

Roles for Gerontological Nurses in the Community

Gerontological nurses play a leading role in developing and implementing health promotion and other community-based health care programs for older adults. For example, gerontological nurses can establish wellness centers to provide well-adult care, including screening, counseling, and skill enhancement programs for older adults. Services can include assessment of nutrition, blood glucose, blood pressure, mood states, and risks for falls (Belza & Baker, 2000). *Parish nursing*, first established in the early 1970s and recognized by the American Nurses Association as a specialty practice since 1998, is a community-based health promotion program that has been called "one of the most significant developments in modern geriatric nursing" (Ebersole, 2000, p. 148). Parish nursing is a holistic approach to addressing the physical, emotional, and spiritual health care needs of members of church-based congregations, with a focus on health promotion activities such as screenings and education. Although parish nurse programs serve people of all ages, a high percentage of care recipients are older adults or people with chronic illnesses. Roles for parish nurses specific to older adults include meeting health needs, providing health education and counseling, training volunteers to assist with visiting people, and acting as referral agent and liaison with other community services (Matteson et al., 2000; Weis & Schank, 2000).

Innovative roles are being increasingly developed for gerontological nurses involved in the care or counseling of older adults living in the community, dependent older adults in various institutional settings, and caregivers of dependent older adults. In addition to the health care needs of older adults, there is growing concern about the needs of the caregivers of dependent older adults; gerontological nurses have many opportunities for expanding their roles to address those needs. Geriatric care management services and caregiver counseling and education are rapidly becoming essential components of gerontological nursing, and gerontological nurses are frequently involved in formally assessing not only the needs of older adults but also the needs of their caregivers, who may or may not be older adults themselves. Interventions are directed as much toward the caregivers of dependent older people as toward the older people themselves. It has become increasingly common for gerontological nurses to work in collegial relationships with other members of a multidisciplinary team, including primary care providers, psychiatrists, social workers, physical therapists, and other health care providers, to address the needs of older adults as well as their caregivers.

Attention in recent years also has focused on the health care needs of culturally diverse older adults and groups such as rural elders. There is a tremendous need for gerontological nurses who can develop and implement health care programs that are designed to meet specific needs of groups such as African Americans, Asian Americans, Native Americans, and Hispanic Americans. Gerontological literature has also focused in recent years on the health care needs of two population groups that exhibit characteristics of old age beginning in their 50s: prisoners and homeless people (e.g., Dubler, 2001). Chow (2002) described the role of a gerontological nurse in organizing and implementing a long-term care nursing service for aging inmates. Clearly, there are no limits to the creativity that nurses can use in developing health care services for older adults.

PAYING FOR GERONTOLOGICAL HEALTH CARE SERVICES

At a minimum, gerontological nurses must be knowledgeable enough about current health care policies relating to older people to understand some of the barriers and challenges of implementing nursing care plans and discharge plans. For example, knowing the Medicare criteria for skilled home care services enables the nurse to make referrals for this type of nursing care when appropriate. In addition, nurses need to keep up to date on recent changes, not only so that they can guide older adults in the many choices of health care delivery systems that are now available but also so that they can identify opportunities for new roles for gerontological nurses. The roles of gerontological nurses are expanding rapidly, and much of this expansion directly relates to changes in health insurance and health care delivery systems. For example, after several decades of anticipation, Medicare reimbursement for advanced practice nurses finally became a reality in the late 1990s.

Medicare

Medicare is a health insurance program that was established by Congress in 1965 as an entitlement program for people who are eligible for Social Security benefits. Medicare covers primarily hospital and physician services, with very limited coverage for some skilled care services in homes and nursing homes. It does not cover dental care, most vision care, most routine or preventive services, or nonskilled long-term care. It also does not cover prescriptions, but this is one of the most hotly debated issues in recent years. Various bills have been introduced in Congress to provide Medicare prescription drug coverage, but none had been approved in 2002. Medicare is divided into Part A, funded through payroll taxes, and Part B, financed through monthly premiums paid by beneficiaries and by general revenues. Medicare, therefore, is part of the national budget and is subject to the same political processes that affect other budget items. For instance, the Balanced Budget Act of 1997 scheduled regular increases in the Part B premium so that it will reach $105 per month by 2007.

Hospital insurance (Part A) covers medical and psychiatric inpatient care in a hospital and in a skilled nursing facility after a hospital stay. It also covers some of the approved costs of durable medical equipment and skilled home care services and hospice care for those patients who qualify. Beneficiaries are responsible for a co-pay amount for hospital services that increases every year and is the equivalent of the average cost of 1 day of hospital care. Reimbursement for hospital and skilled nursing facility care is based on benefit periods. A benefit period begins on the first day of hospital admission and ends 60 days after the person no longer qualifies for care in a hospital or skilled nursing facility. Strict criteria must be met for coverage of services in a skilled nursing facility, and the number of days that are covered is limited. The Medicare home care benefit is intended to provide medically oriented, acute or restorative, skilled nursing care on an intermittent, short-term basis to homebound patients who are under the care of a physician.

Supplemental medical insurance (Part B) covers all or part of the cost of approved physician's services and other outpatient services, such as diagnostic imaging and laboratory services. Additional services covered under Part B include certain ambulance services, durable medical equipment used at home, and the services of certain specially qualified, nonphysician health care practitioners (e.g., nurse practitioners).

A major limitation of traditional Medicare has been its lack of coverage for preventive services. This is changing, however, because of the increasing recognition of the importance of these services in delaying the onset of chronic illnesses and improving the health and function of older adults. In recent years, Medicare began paying for the following preventive services: diabetes education; glaucoma screening; bone density measurements; colorectal cancer screening; mammograms and breast examinations; Pap smears and pelvic examinations; influenza, pneumonia, and hepatitis B vaccinations; and prostate-specific antigen (PSA) tests and digital rectal examinations. Additional preventive and screening coverage that has been proposed for Medicare coverage includes hypertension screening, osteoporosis screening and counseling, and counseling for cessation of tobacco use (Infeld & Whitelaw, 2002).

In the past four decades, Medicare has always achieved its original goal of paying for basic medical services, but program implementation has undergone significant changes. When Medicare was first established, there was a limit on the types of services covered but little regulation of the amount of reimbursement for these services. A fee-for-service system reimbursed providers directly for the cost of services. During the first 10 years of Medicare, health care costs increased an average of 141% per year, compared with an 11.4% increase in the gross national product. Causes of this unprecedented rise in health care costs included the availability of federal funds under Medicare, the high rate of inflation in the general economy, and the even higher rate of inflation in the health care industry. Other contributing factors were malpractice concerns, expensive technology, duplication of equipment and services, lack of less costly alternatives to institutional care, and the legal and ethical constraints that encourage the use of high technology to prolong life.

Because the federal government had not anticipated the dramatic rise in health care costs that began in the late 1960s, they grossly underestimated the projected spending for the 1970s and 1980s. In an attempt to control the rapidly growing costs of this federal program, Congress amended Medicare in 1972 and established Professional Standard Review Organizations to review use of services. Despite the need to control costs, these same amendments expanded Medicare coverage to include adults of any age who had end-stage renal disease or were disabled for 2 years or more as a result of any disease. Although these amendments provided some control over the use of services, the costs of the program continued to escalate far beyond the cost estimates.

In the early 1980s, the federal government took a serious look at health care expenditures and began to deal with the problem of cost containment. Other goals of the federal government during this period included increasing expenditures for defense and diminishing the role of the government in health and social programs. One way of accomplishing these goals was to target for reduction the large part of the federal budget that went toward Medicare, Medicaid, Social Security, and other programs for older people. The three-pronged approach that was adopted to cut health care costs included an increase in the amount paid by individual participants, restriction of the amount of Medicare payment for services, and promotion of voluntary reductions in costs of health care services.

In 1982, the federal government established a system of prospective payment as the basis of fee-for-service payments. This system reimbursed providers on a predetermined rate based on the expected cost of treating a patient with a specific diagnosis, which was classified according to a diagnosis-related group (DRG). Initially, this system was applied only to Medicare patients, but insurance companies now use it almost universally. Thus, hospitals are no longer guaranteed payment for actual services rendered. Rather, they are financially rewarded when the cost of patient care is less than that allowed for the relevant DRG and are penalized when the cost of patient care is more than that allowed for the relevant DRG. This system promotes the early discharge of hospitalized patients, who tend to be relatively sicker at the time of discharge, and shifts the burden of care from hospitals to families, nursing homes, and other community-based care providers. This approach has given rise to the phrase "quicker and sicker," which became the theme of discharge planning in the 1980s. Other results are a dramatic increase in the number of outpatient procedures and the development of postacute and subacute care programs.

In addition to radically changing the Medicare reimbursement system, the 1982 federal legislation allowed Medicare beneficiaries to enroll in approved Medicare managed care organizations. This marked the first time that Medicare payments were based on criteria other than a fee-for-service basis. People in managed care programs pay little or nothing for premiums, deductibles, and co-insurance amounts. For each enrollee in their program, the managed care organization receives capitation payments of 95% of the average amount paid to fee-for-service providers in the same geographic area. The major advantage to participants is that these plans generally cover all or part of the costs of medications, vision care, and some other services not covered under traditional Medicare. In addition, preventive services are covered, and many plans strongly encourage health promotion services. In contrast to the traditional Medicare plan, managed care plans do not require a 3-day hospital stay to qualify for skilled nursing services. The major disadvantage for some participants is that the choice of health care providers is limited, and permission is needed from a primary care provider before services can be obtained from specialists.

Medicare managed care organizations initially evolved very slowly, but the Balanced Budget Act of

1997 promoted the growth of managed care by creating Medicare Plus Choice (M + C) plans (also called Medicare Part C). This legislation provided Medicare funds for a variety of managed care organizations, including preferred provider organizations and provider-sponsored organizations. By the early 2000s, many types of managed care plans were available under Medicare as alternatives to the traditional fee-for-service Medicare plan. The main differences among managed care plans are the amount of choice allowed to participants, the amount of co-payments and other out-of-pocket costs, and the optional services covered (e.g., dental care, eye care, and prescription drugs).

Medicaid

Medicaid legislation was enacted at the same time as Medicare to provide health insurance for poor people. Although Medicare falls entirely under the jurisdiction of the federal government, Medicaid is a state-run program that receives partial funding from federal sources and is subject to certain federal guidelines. To qualify for Medicaid, people must meet medical and financial criteria. Financially, they must have a very low income and limited assets. If income is more than the lower eligibility level and medical expenses account for a high proportion of income, people can qualify by spending down to the eligible income level. Each state determines the specific income and asset limits, and rules differ considerably among the states. State and federal regulations restrict the transfer of assets from one family member to another to qualify for Medicaid, but federal legislation enacted in 1988 protects the income and assets of a married person when his or her spouse is in a nursing facility for at least 30 days. Although a high proportion of nursing home residents qualify for Medicaid, fewer than 10% of noninstitutionalized older adults receive Medicaid (Crystal et al., 2000).

States have some discretion with regard to eligibility criteria for Medicaid, but the federal government mandates that states pay for certain medical services, including skilled and intermediate levels of nursing home care, for all eligible adults. Because the cost of nursing home care is so high—about $50,000 per year in the early 2000s—many older adults with modest incomes meet the eligibility criteria by having limited assets and medical expenses that account for a very high proportion of their income. Thus, Medicaid has become increasingly important as a source of payment for long-term care for older adults, covering about half of nursing home costs. It is less important for noninstitutionalized older adults, however, because it accounts for less than 2% of health care expenditures for this group (Crystal et al., 2000).

Traditionally, Medicaid has been biased toward paying for institutional care rather than community-based long-term care, but this is gradually changing. Since the 1980s, states have been able to apply for Medicaid waivers to provide community-based services to people who otherwise would need nursing home care. Between 1989 and 1999, the proportion of Medicaid funding for long-term care devoted to home-based care doubled from 13% to 26% (Feder et al., 2001). As with other components of Medicaid, the federal government mandates some long-term care services, whereas states have discretion over the provision of other services. Home care services are mandatory, but optional services include personal care, case management, and medically oriented day care (Wiener, 2001).

Private Insurance

Because of the many limitations of Medicare as a health insurance program, about three fourths of older adults purchase additional insurance coverage from private companies. Private health insurance policies include all of the following types: medigap, managed care, hospital indemnity, specific diseases, long-term care, and continuation of employer-provided policies. These supplemental policies attempt to fill the gap between the services covered by Medicare and the services paid for out of pocket. All supplemental policies cover the premiums and co-payments for services covered by Medicare Parts A and B, but additional benefits vary according to each policy.

Employer-sponsored policies usually provide the best supplemental insurance—sometimes covering prescription drugs and limited long-term care services—but they are available only to retired people (or their spouses) who continue coverage under the health insurance policy offered by their employer. Retirees who held higher-paying jobs and attained higher educational levels are more likely to have these policies (Crystal et al., 2000). Because many retirees are required to pay all or part of the premium, it is estimated that 27% of people who are offered employer-sponsored health insurance do not accept the insurance (Crystal et al., 2000). As employers address current major economic concerns, employee-sponsored policies are likely to be less available and more costly for retirees.

Hospital indemnity policies pay cash amounts for each day of inpatient hospital care; they may also include benefits for surgical procedures or days spent in a skilled nursing facility. Specific disease policies are limited to paying for services related to a specific disease and are likely to duplicate benefits covered under Medicare or other primary insurance policies.

Medigap policies are designed to supplement Medicare benefits and are now regulated by federal and state laws. The National Association of Insurance Commissioners has developed 10 standard plans that insurance companies must follow in the provision of medigap policies. Plan A contains basic benefits, such as coverage for co-insurance payments and additional payments for hospital days. Other plans (B through J) cover Part A deductible and additional services, such as preventive medical care, skilled nursing co-insurance, and medical care in foreign countries. The most comprehensive policies cover the cost of medications. Limits are applied to the drug benefit and some of the other benefits. A relatively new type of supplemental policy is the Medicare Select policy, which provides the same coverage as medigap policies, but only when services are provided by a designated preferred provider.

Long-term care insurance is a recent development in the health insurance industry. When these policies were introduced in the late 1980s, they were unregulated, and many of the policies contained large loopholes and significant barriers to receiving benefits. During the 1990s, many states enacted laws mandating standards suggested by the National Association of Insurance Commissioners. Suggested requirements for long-term care insurance policies include inflation protection and caps on rates. A good long-term care policy will provide payment for a range of options, including home care services, assisted-living facilities, and nursing home care. In addition, policies should be open enough that they include services that may be developed in the future but are not available at the time the policy is initiated. For example, the first long-term care policies that were developed were limited to nursing home care because few other options were available at that time. A major drawback of this type of insurance for older people is that the premiums are based on the age of the person when he or she initially signs up for the policy. For most older adults, therefore, the cost of the policy will outweigh the benefits. These policies will likely become increasingly important, particularly for young-old and middle-aged people, because recent proposals promote private long-term care insurance rather than public programs (Wiener, 2001).

Out-of-Pocket Spending

Despite the major contribution of health insurance programs in paying for health care services, older adults currently spend a larger percentage of their income—about 20%—on their health care needs than ever before. Out-of-pocket health care expenses have been increasing steadily in the past four decades, and that burden falls disproportionately on poor people. Crystal and colleagues (2000) found that increases in out-of-pocket expenses were consistent with increases in income, but that the out-of-pocket expenditures account for much larger proportions of income (31.5%) for people in the lowest income quintile than for those in the highest income group (8.5%).

In the early 2000s, this issue emerged as one of the most hotly debated aspects of Medicare reform legislation and stirred great conflict among groups concerned about the increasing costs of both providing and paying for health care services. In particular, many groups are concerned about the significant financial burden associated with prescription drugs and long-term care. Many of the proposals that Congress considered during the early 2000s attempt to limit the rate of Medicare growth. If this goal is accomplished, out-of-pocket expenses will inevitably increase, and the financial burden will fall most heavily on the people who already experience high out-of-pocket expenses: those with lower incomes and chronic illnesses (Crystal et al., 2000).

Comprehensive Models

Consumer demand for noninstitutional long-term care services and persistent increases in health care costs for Medicare and Medicaid programs have stimulated the development of new models of health insurance and health care delivery. Since the 1980s, the federal government has funded innovative models of long-term care for people with chronic conditions that are both comprehensive and cost-effective. These Medicare and Medicaid waiver programs—sometimes called Social Health Maintenance Organizations—provide a wide range of social and medical services on a capitated managed care basis. The prototype of this model is the On Lok Senior Services program, which was developed in the early 1970s in the Chinatown area of San Francisco and still exists today in a greatly expanded form. On Lok—Cantonese for "peaceful happy abode"—successfully addresses the health care system issues that most strongly affect older adults: expense, fragmentation, and lack of creativity in community-based care (Pierce, 2002).

The success of On Lok prompted the development of 10 similar programs, called Programs of All-inclusive Care for the Elderly (PACE), in the late 1980s. Based on data from On Lok, it is estimated that the cost of care for frail elders in PACE programs is 15% less than the cost in traditional fee-for-service programs (Mui, 2002). The Balanced Budget Act of 1997 established PACE models as permanently recognized Medicare and Medicaid providers. By the end of 1998, 17 PACE programs were fully funded under dual Medicare and Medicaid capitation, and 14 programs were in development (Mui, 2002). In 2000, two private foundations—the Robert Wood Johnson Foundation and the John A. Hartford Foundation—supported the expansion of these models of care. By the end of 2002, 25 demonstration sites were eligible for permanent federal funding, and more than 70 organizations in 30 states were developing or implementing PACE models. Clearly, it is possible that this model will revolutionize how long-term care is provided in the future.

The target group for PACE is people who are eligible for both Medicare and Medicaid services, live in the community, and qualify for nursing home care. Distinguishing features of the model are: (1) the provision of comprehensive and community-based long-term care services to nursing home–eligible clients, (2) an emphasis on preventive services, (3) integrated service delivery through adult day health centers, (4) case management through multidisciplinary teams, and (5) full funding on a capitation basis (similar to health maintenance organizations). Core components of PACE programs are nutrition, transportation, home care, acute care, respite care, primary care, social services, restorative therapies, prescription drugs, long-term care, adult day care, medical specialty care, durable medical equipment, and multidisciplinary case management. The hallmarks of PACE programs are an emphasis on interdisciplinary teamwork, a reliance on day care centers as the base of services, and a commitment to keeping enrollees out of institutions (Kane et al., 2002).

CHAPTER SUMMARY

The establishment of Medicare and Medicaid in 1965 provided a major financial stimulus for the development of health care programs for older adults. By the early 1970s, home care agencies and nursing home facilities had emerged as the primary avenue for addressing health care needs of older adults outside of acute care settings. During the 1980s, geriatricians, gerontologists, and health care providers became aware of the need to develop more cost-effective and innovative ways of providing health care services to older adults. This awareness arose in part because of concern about the dramatic increases in federal expenditures for health care and in part because of consumer demand for more choices and improved quality of health care, particularly long-term care, for older adults. By the early 2000s, a wide continuum of health care services was available to address the complex needs of older adults. Gerontological nurses assume many roles in the diverse settings that compose the continuum of care for

older adults. Changes in Medicare reimbursement policy have created opportunities for advanced practice nurses, particularly in acute care settings, nursing homes, and home care agencies.

Older adults who have chronic conditions that affect their level of functioning and quality of life typically need long-term care services. Although long-term care has traditionally been associated with nursing home care, it is currently associated with a continuum of care services that are provided in many institutional and community-based settings. Acute care settings, which are part of the continuum of care, have developed subacute care units and specialized geriatric units for addressing the complex needs of hospitalized older adults. Nursing home care plays an important role in the continuum of health care by providing short-term skilled nursing for people who are recovering from acute conditions and intermediate nursing care for chronically ill people who need assistance with daily activities. Because of federal legislation and consumer demand, nursing homes are currently addressing many issues about quality of care and quality of life for their residents.

Home care services are widely available and are generally classified as skilled and long-term. Skilled home care services, which are covered under Medicare and other health insurance programs, provide short-term skilled nursing or rehabilitative services for homebound people who meet medical criteria. Long-term home care includes a wide spectrum of services ranging from unskilled care, such as meal preparation and grocery shopping, to full-time hands-on nursing care. Medicaid and other government or insurance programs cover the full or partial cost of some long-term home care services for those who meet financial and other criteria, but older adults or their families pay for most of these services out of pocket. Community-based services, which include adult day centers, health promotion programs, and geriatric care management services, play important roles in meeting the long-term needs of older adults.

Medicare is the health insurance program that covers hospital and medical care and some skilled care services. In the 1970s, Congress began making major changes to Medicare because costs were exceeding estimated expenditures, and these changes continue today. By the early 2000s, Medicare benefits to providers had been reduced significantly, and many types of managed care plans were available as alternatives to the traditional fee-for-service Medicare plan. Medicaid was a health insurance program established to provide medical care for poor people, but it has evolved to being the primary source of payment for nonskilled long-term care for older adults. Medicaid has traditionally been slanted toward payment for nursing home care rather than community-based care, but this has been changing in recent years. Private insurance is available from many sources to supplement Medicare coverage, but older adults spend a larger percentage of their income—about 20%—on their health care than ever before. Programs of All-inclusive Care for the Elderly, which are comprehensive models of health care first developed in the late 1980s, are becoming more widely available.

 CRITICAL THINKING EXERCISES

1. You are on a panel of nursing students who are presenting information about opportunities for nurses to work in various settings. Your topic is "Roles for Gerontological Nurses in Home, Institutional, and Community Settings." Describe the content of your 20-minute presentation.
2. Mrs. F. is a resident in the skilled care section of the nursing home where you work. She had been living alone in her own home before being admitted to the hospital with a fractured hip 4 weeks ago. She has regained much of her independence and walks with a walker and one-person assist. She expects to ambulate independently using a walker within 2 weeks, at which time she expects to return to her own home. She asks you what kind of services would be available in her own home. What additional information would you want to know before you answered her questions? What information would you give to her? What suggestions would you make?
3. Your grandmother, who is 64 years old, asks your advice about health insurance choices that she needs to make when she is 65. How would you explain her choices and what suggestions would you make to her?

EDUCATIONAL RESOURCES

Administration on Aging
Washington, DC 20201
Eldercare locator: (800) 677-1116
http://www.aoa.gov

American Association of Retired Persons (AARP)
601 E Street, NW, Washington, DC 20049
(800) 424-3410
http://www.aarp.org

Centers for Medicare & Medicaid Services
7500 Security Boulevard, Baltimore, MD 21244-1850
http://www.cms.hhs.gov

National Association of Professional Geriatric Care Managers
1604 Country Club Road, Tucson, AZ 85716-3102
(520) 881-8008
http://www.caremanager.org

National Institute on Aging
Building 31, Room 5C27
31 Center Drive, MSC 2292, Bethesda, MD 20892
(301) 496-1752
http://www.nia.nih.gov

National PACE Association
801 N. Fairfax Street, Suite 301, Alexandria, VA 22314
http://www.npaonline.org

REFERENCES

Allen, L. A., Mihalovic, S. J., & Narveson, G. G. (2000). Successful protocol-based practitioner management of warfarin anticoagulation in nursing home patients. *Annals of Long-Term Care, 8*, 60–71.

Anetzberger, G. J. (2002). Community resources to promote successful aging. *Clinics in Geriatric Medicine, 18*(3), 611–626.

Barba, B. A., Tesh, A. S., & Courts, A. F. (2002). Promoting thriving in nursing homes. *Journal of Gerontological Nursing, 28*(3), 7–13.

Belza, B., & Baker, M. W. (2000). Maintaining health in well older adults: Initiatives for schools of nursing and the John A. Hartford Foundation for the 21st Century. *Journal of Gerontological Nursing, 26*(7), 8–17.

Bonnel, W. B. (2002). Assisted living: Strategies for initiating an advanced practice nurse clinic. *Journal of Gerontological Nursing, 28*(1), 5–11.

Borrayo, E. A., Salmon, J. R., Polivka, L., & Dunlop, B. D. (2002). Utilization across the continuum of long-term services. *Gerontologist, 42*, 603–612.

Bourbonniere, M., & Evans, L. K. (2002). Advanced practice nursing in the care of frail older adults. *Journal of the American Geriatrics Society, 50*, 2062–2076.

Calkins, M. C. (2002). The nursing home of the future: Are you ready? *Nursing Homes/Long Term Care Management, 51*(6), 42–47.

Chow, R. K. (2002). Initiating a long-term care nursing service for aging inmates. *Geriatric Nursing, 23*, 24–27.

Counsell, S. R., Holder, C. M., Liebenauer, L. L., Palmer, R. M., Fortinsky, R. H., Kresevic, D. M., et al. (2000). Effects of multicomponent intervention on functional outcomes and process of care in hospitalized older patients: A randomized controlled trial of acute care for elders in a community hospital. *Journal of the American Geriatrics Society, 48*, 1572–1581.

Crystal, S., Johnson, R. W., Harman, J., Sambamoorthi, U., & Kumar, R. (2000). Out-of-pocket health care among older Americans. *Journal of Gerontology: Social Sciences, 55*, S51–S62.

Dubler, N. N. (2001). Prison-residing elders. In M. D. Mezey (Ed.), *The encyclopedia of elder care* (pp. 528–531). New York: Springer.

Ebersole, P. (2000). Parish nurse leaders. *Geriatric Nursing, 21*, 148–149.

Eisch, J. S., Brozovic, B., Colling, K., & Wold, K. (2000). Nurse practitioner geropsychiatric consultation services to nursing homes. *Geriatric Nursing, 21*, 150–155.

Feder, J., Komisar, H. L., & Niefeld, M. (2001). The financing and organization of health care. In R. H. Binstock & L. K. George (Eds.), *Handbook of aging and the social sciences* (5th ed., pp. 387–405). San Diego: Academic Press.

Field, M. J. (1996). *Telemedicine: A guide to assessing telecommunications in health care.* Washington, DC: National Academy Press.

Frantz, A. K., Colgan, J., Palmer, K., & Ledgerwood, B. (2002). Lessons learned from telehealth pioneers. *Home Healthcare Nurse, 20*(6) 363–366.

Fulmer, T. T. (1991). The geriatric nurse specialist role: A new model. *Nursing Management, 22,* 91–93.

Fulmer, T., Mezey, M., Bottrell, M., Abraham, I., Sazant, J., Grossman, S., & Grisham, E. (2002). Nurses Improving Care for Healthsystem Elders (NICHE): Using outcomes and benchmarks for evidenced-based practice. *Geriatric Nursing, 23,* 121–123.

Guthrie, P. F., Edinger, G., & Schumacher, S. (2002). A NICHE program at North Memorial Health Care. *Geriatric Nursing, 23,* 133–138.

Hatchett, B. F., & Duran, D. A. (2001). Older adults share opinions: Senior health fairs. *Activities, Adaptation & Aging, 25*(3/4), 59–71.

Hays, J. C., Pieper, C. F., & Purser, J. L. (2003). Competing risk of household expansion or institutionalization in late life. *Journals of Gerontology: Social Sciences, 58B,* S11–S20.

Hujer, M., Mann, A., & Mion, L. C. (2000). Assisted living facilities. In J. J. Fitzpatrick & T. Fulmer (Eds.), *Geriatric nursing research digest.* New York: Springer.

Infield, D. L., & Whitelaw, N. (2002). Policy initiatives to promote healthy aging. *Clinics in Geriatric Medicine, 18,* 627–642.

Inouye, S. K. (2000). The hospital elder life program: A model of care to prevent cognitive and functional decline in older hospitalized patients. *Journal of the American Geriatrics Society, 48,* 1697–1706.

Inouye, S. K., Acampora, D., Miller, R. L., Fulmer, T., Hurst, L. D., & Cooney, L. M. (1993a). The Yale geriatric care program: A model of care to prevent functional decline in hospitalized elderly patients. *Journal of the American Geriatrics Society, 41,* 1345–1352.

Inouye, S. K., Wagner, D. R., Acampora, D., Horwitz, R. I., Cooney, L. M., & Tinetti, M. E. (1993b). A controlled trial of a nursing-centred intervention in hospitalized elderly medical patients: The Yale geriatric care program. *Journal of the American Geriatrics Society, 41,* 1353–1360.

Jenkins, R. L., & McSweeney, M. (2001). Assessing elderly patients with congestive heart failure via in-home interactive telecommunication. *Journal of Gerontological Nursing, 27*(1), 21–27.

Johnson-Mekota, J. L., Maas, M., Buresh, K. A., Gardner, S. E., Frantz, R. A., Specht, J. K. P., et al. (2001). A nursing application of telecommunications: Measurement of satisfaction for patients and providers. *Journal of Gerontological Nursing, 27*(1), 28–33.

Kane, R. A. (2001). Long-term care and a good quality of life: Bringing them closer together. *Gerontologist, 41,* 293–304.

Kane, R. L., Homyak, P., & Bershadsky, B. (2002). Consumer reactions to the Wisconsin partnership program and its parent, the Program for All-inclusive Care of the Elderly (PACE). *Gerontologist, 42,* 314–320.

Kane, R. L., & Kane, R. A. (2001). Emerging issues in chronic care. In R. H. Binstock & L. K. George (Eds.), *Handbook of aging and the social sciences* (5th ed., pp. 406–425). San Diego: Academic Press.

Lee, V. K., & Fletcher, K. R. (2002). Sustaining the geriatric resource nurse model at the University of Virginia. *Geriatric Nursing, 23,* 128–132.

Leff, B., & Burton, J. R. (2001). The future history of home care and physician house calls in the United States. *Journals of Gerontology: Medical Sciences, 56A*(10), M603–M608.

Marrelli, T. M. (2001). Prospective payment in home care: An overview. *Geriatric Nursing, 22,* 217–218.

Martin, K. S. (2001). Home health care. In M. D. Mezey (Ed.), *The encyclopedia of elder care* (pp. 351–353). New York: Springer.

Matteson, M. A., Reilly, M., & Moseley, M. (2000). Needs assessment of homebound elders in a parish church: Implications for parish nursing. *Geriatric Nursing, 21,* 144–146.

McGilton, K. S. (2002). Enhancing relationships between care providers and residents in long-term care: Designing a model of care. *Journal of Gerontological Nursing, 28*(12), 13–21.

Mezey, M. M. (2001). Advanced practice nursing. In M. D. Mezey (Ed.), *The encyclopedia of elder care* (pp. 24–26). New York: Springer.

Miller, S. K. (2002). Acute care of the elderly units: A positive outcomes case study. *AACN Clinical Issues, 13*(1), 34–42.

Milone-Nuzzo, P., & Pike, A. (2001). Advanced practice nurses in home care: Is there a role? *Home Health Care Management & Practice, 13*(5), 349–355.

Mion, L. C., Palmer, R. M., Anetzberger, G. J., & Meldon, S. W. (2001). Establishing a case-finding and referral system for at-risk older individuals in the emergency department setting: The SIGNET model. *Journal of the American Geriatrics Society, 49,* 1379–1386.

Mitty, E. L. (2001). Nursing homes. In M. D. Mezey (Ed.), *The encyclopedia of elder care* (pp. 452–455). New York: Springer.

Morley, J. E. (2003). Hot topics in geriatrics [Editorial]. *Journal of Gerontology: Medical Sciences, 53A,* 30–36.

Mui, A. C. (2002). The program of all-inclusive care for the elderly (PACE): An innovative long-term care model in the United States. *Journal of Aging and Social Policy, 13*(2/3), 53–67.

Pfaff, J. (2002). The geriatric resource nurse model: A culture change. *Geriatric Nursing, 23*(3), 140–144.

Pierce, C. A. (2002). Program of all-inclusive care for the elderly in 2002. *Geriatric Nursing, 23*(3), 173–174.

Pierson, C. (2001). APN elder home care: A successful model. *Home Health Care Management & Practice, 13,* 375–379.

Ryden, M. B., Snyder, M., Gross, C. R., Savik, K., Pearson, V., Kirchbaum, K., & Mueller, C. (2000). Value-added outcomes: The use of advanced practice nurses in long-term care facilities. *Gerontologist, 40,* 654–662.

Salinas, T. K., O'Connor, L. J., Weinstein, M., Lee, S. Y., & Fitzpatrick, J. J. (2002). A family assessment tool for hospitalized elders. *Geriatric Nursing, 23,* 316–319, 335.

Siegler, E. L., Glick, D., & Lee, J. (2002). Optimal staffing for acute care of the elderly (ACE) units. *Geriatric Nursing, 23,* 152–155.

Smith, B. M., Maloy, K. A., & Hawkins, D. J. (2000). An examination of Medicare home health services. *Care Management Journals, 2*(4), 238–247.

Specht, J. P. K., Wakefield, B., & Flanagan, J. (2001). Evaluating the cost of one telehealth application connecting an acute and long-term care setting. *Journal of Gerontological Nursing, 27*(1), 34–39.

Spillman, B. C., & Lubitz, J. (2002). New estimates of lifetime nursing home use: Have patterns changed? *Medical Care, 40,* 965–975.

Swauger, K., & Tomlin, C. (2002). Best care for the elderly at Forsyth Medical Center. *Geriatric Nursing, 23,* 145–150.

Tesh, A. S., McNutt, K., Courts, N. F., & Barba, B. A. (2002). Characteristics of nursing homes: Adopting environmental transformations. *Journal of Gerontological Nursing, 28*(3), 28–34.

Thomas, D. R. (2002). Focus on functional decline in hospitalized older adults. *Journal of Gerontology: Medical Sciences, 57A,* M567–M568.

Thomas, W. (1994). *The Eden alternative: Nature hope and nursing homes.* New York: Eden Alternative Foundation.

Tichawa, U. (2002). Creating a continuum of care for elderly individuals. *Journal of Gerontological Nursing, 28*(1), 46–52.

Tran, B. Q., Buckley, K. M., & Prandoni, C. M. (2002). Selection and use of telehealth technology in support of homebound caregivers of stroke patients. *CARING Magazine, March,* 16–21.

Turner, J. T., Lee, V., Fletcher, K., Hudson, K., & Barton, D. (2001). Measuring quality of care with an inpatient elderly population: The Geriatric Resource Nurse Model. *Journal of Gerontological Nursing, 27*(3), 8–18.

Wakefield, B., Flanagan, J., & Specht, J. K. P. (2001). Telehealth: An opportunity for gerontological nursing practice. *Journal of Gerontological Nursing, 27*(1), 10–14.

Weaverdyck, S. E., Wittle, A., & Delaski-Smith, D. (1998). In-place progression: Lessons learned from the Huron Woods' staff. *Journal of Gerontological Nursing, 24*(1), 31–39.

Weis, D., & Schank, M. J. (2000). Use of a taxonomy to describe parish nurse practice with older adults. *Geriatric Nursing, 21,* 125–130.

Wiener, J. M. (2001). Long-term-care policy. In M. D. Mezey (Ed.), *The encyclopedia of elder care* (pp. 4403–4406). New York: Springer.

Yeaworth, R. C. (2002). Long-term care and insurance. *Journal of Gerontological Nursing, 28*(11), 45–51.

Zank, S., & Schacke, C. (2002). Evaluation of geriatric day care units: Effects on patients and caregivers. *Journal of Gerontology, 57B*(4), P348–P357.

Legal and Ethical Concerns

LEARNING OBJECTIVES

1. Define the following terms: autonomy, competency, and decision-making capacity.

2. Describe the following advance directives: living wills, advance medical directives, and durable power of attorney for health care.

3. Discuss nursing responsibilities in relation to advance directives.

4. Describe at least three ways that the Omnibus Budget Reconciliation Act (OBRA) of 1987 has affected care for nursing home residents.

5. Discuss the role of the nurse in assisting families and older adults with end-of-life decisions.

In the past two decades, various legislative efforts have attempted to address issues related to the rights of older adults and their quality of life. During the early 1980s, for example, state and federal governments began addressing issues related to vulnerable elders and, during the later part of that decade, began focusing on issues related to rights of patients and nursing home residents, end-of-life decisions, and the quality of care provided under Medicaid and Medicare programs. Many of these legislative and policy initiatives have created ethical issues for gerontological health care practitioners. For example, questions often arise about the extent to which an older person is able to make health care decisions about his or her care. Although legislation can provide legal guidelines for these questions, laws do not resolve ethical dilemmas that arise when no advance directive was provided or when conflicts exist about an advance directive's interpretation. The next sections review some of the pertinent legal and ethical issues that are relevant to nursing care of older adults. Additional legal and ethical considerations regarding vulnerable elders are discussed in Chapter 26.

AUTONOMY AND RIGHTS

Autonomy is the personal freedom to direct one's own life as long as it does not impinge on the rights of others. An autonomous person is capable of rational thought and is able to recognize the need for problem solving. The person can identify the problem, search for alternatives, and select a solution that allows their continued personal freedom, as long as it does not cause any harm to another's rights or property. Loss of autonomy and, therefore, loss of independence, is a very real fear among the elderly. Gerontological nurses are likely to encounter ethical dilemmas related to autonomy when questions arise about medical interventions and health care decisions, particularly for people who are cognitively impaired. In these situations, nurses need to be familiar with legal and ethical guidelines related to competency and decision-making capacity. Nurses have a responsibility to assist older people and their families, often as impartial mediators, when issues concerning personal autonomy arise. However, if the safety of the older person becomes jeopardized by risk-taking behaviors arising from impaired decision-making abilities, nurses must refer older people to the appropriate community agencies (e.g., Adult Protective Services) for further evaluation (see Chapter 26).

Competency

Competency is a legal term that refers to the ability to fulfill one's role and handle one's affairs in an adequate manner. All adults are presumed to be competent, and state laws designate the age of competency—usually 18 years—for participating in legally binding decisions. Because competent people are guaranteed all the rights granted by the Constitution and state laws, all adults who have not been declared incompetent by a judge have the right to make their own decisions about medical treatment and health care. However, families or health care providers often raise questions about an older person's ability to make reasonable decisions, particularly when the person is cognitively impaired.

When questions are raised about the person's ability to participate in decisions about medical care, the health care proxy (discussed in the section on Advance Directives) may assume decision-making responsibility. In the absence of a health care proxy or when conflicts exist among the people involved with making and implementing decisions, a petition can be filed with probate court to determine whether the person is competent. Often, these petitions are filed because a health care provider (usually a physician) is concerned that appropriate decisions be made for a person who does not seem able to make reasonable decisions about medical treatments. Usually a family member files the petition, but if no qualified family member is available or if family members are in conflict about the petition, an attorney or other person may file. If the court determines that the person is incompetent (i.e., incapable of making decisions on one's own behalf), the judge assigns either a partial or a full *guardianship* (also called a *conservatorship*). With a partial guardianship, the incompetent person is permitted to make limited decisions; with a full guardianship, the person loses all of his or her rights to make such decisions. Although guardianship can be revoked or reversed, it usually is long-term and terminates only when the incompetent

person dies. Because guardianship is a drastic legal measure that takes away legal rights (even the right to vote) and entails initial court proceedings and ongoing court monitoring, it is viewed as a last resort when other legal interventions, such as durable power of attorney, are not appropriate. The need for guardianship often can be avoided if the person establishes comprehensive and legally binding advance directives, including a durable power of attorney for health care, before any questions arise about his or her mental capacities.

Decision-Making Capacity

Decision-making capacity refers to the ability of a person to consent to or refuse a specific medical treatment or procedure. In contrast to competency—which is determined by a court of law—decision-making capacity is determined by health care practitioners or by an interdisciplinary health care team. Capacity is based on a person's having the following characteristics: (1) appreciation of the right to make a choice, (2) understanding of the risks and benefits of the medical intervention and lack of intervention, (3) ability to communicate about the decision, (4) stability over time, and (5) consistency with the person's usual beliefs and values. Determination of decision-making capacity should not be based on a particular diagnosis, nor should it be influenced by a person's chronologic old age. Rather, it should be based on a careful evaluation of the person's ability to understand the issues involved in a specific decision-making situation and to communicate about these issues. For example, a person with dementia may be able to participate in a decision about a health care proxy but not be able to participate in a complex decision about medical interventions for prostate cancer. In this situation, it might be reasonable for the person to designate his wife or one of his children to make the treatment decision for him.

Determination of decision-making capacity also takes into consideration that cognitive abilities can fluctuate from day to day and hour to hour and may be significantly influenced by factors such as medications, dementia, depression, and many acute and chronic medical conditions. Thus, health care professionals are responsible for identifying and addressing the factors that influence cognitive functioning (e.g., sensory impairments, medication effects), so that the person's decision-making abilities are at their best level. For example, even such a relatively simple measure as ensuring that a hearing-impaired person use his or her hearing aid may improve communication and thereby have a positive effect on decision-making abilities. Similarly, if a person with dementia has better cognitive abilities in the morning or when he or she is rested, then efforts can be made to discuss health care decisions during this time rather than when the person is more confused.

The terms *decisional autonomy* and *executive autonomy* are sometimes used in relation to the concept of decision-making capacity. Decisional autonomy is the ability and freedom to make decisions without external influence, and executional autonomy is the ability to implement the decisions (Collopy, 1988). These concepts call attention to the complexity of decision-making capacity and the importance of evaluating the person's ability not only to make reasonable decisions but also to carry out all of the actions necessary for implementing decisions. Medical ethicists point out that the traditional narrow focus on decisional autonomy is inadequate because it ignores the importance of evaluating a person's capacity to make, adapt, and implement plans (McCullough et al., 2001). This is particularly important in relation to people with impaired executive control functions, which are the cognitive skills involved in successfully planning and carrying out goal-oriented behavior such as self-care tasks. Conditions that are likely to cause impaired executive control functions include dementia, major depression, Parkinson's disease, and traumatic brain injury. These situations are particularly difficult to evaluate because the person may retain the capacity to understand and make decisions (i.e., decisional autonomy) but may not have the capacity to carry them out (executive autonomy). Therefore, assessment of both decisional and executive autonomy is essential (McCullough et al., 2001). Chapter 10 discusses guidelines for nursing assessment of executive control functions.

ADVANCE DIRECTIVES

The Patient Self-Determination Act (PSDA), enacted by Congress in 1990, became effective on December 1, 1991. It has had far-reaching consequences, particularly regarding end-of-life care (discussed later in this chapter). The primary intent of this legislation is to protect health care consumers by requiring that health care providers do all of the following: (1) inform patients of their right to refuse treatments and make health care decisions, (2) provide written information about their state's provisions for implementing advance directives, (3) ask each person whether an advance directive has been completed, (4) include documentation of patients' advance directives in their medical records, and (5) provide education for their staff and the community on advance directives. The PSDA applies to all hospices, hospitals, home health agencies, extended care facilities, and health maintenance organizations that receive

federal funds. Because of this legislation, nurses in all settings routinely inquire about advance directives and facilitate communication about patient's wishes.

Advance directives are legally binding documents that allow competent people to document what medical care they would or would not want to receive if they were not capable of making decisions and communicating their wishes. Advance directives also enable people to appoint a proxy decision maker, who is a person responsible for communicating their wishes if they are incompetent or unable to communicate. Many advocacy groups encourage all adults to establish advance directives and to make known to their families and health care providers their wishes about health care decisions, particularly end-of-life care issues. For example, Aging With Dignity promotes the use of the *Five Wishes* document (available in English or Spanish) for use as an advance directive document (see Educational Resources section). The *Five Wishes* document addresses the following questions: (1) Who do I want to make care decisions for me when I cannot make them for myself? (2) What kind of medical treatment do I want or not want when I am very sick and unable to speak for myself? (3) What would help me feel comfortable while I am dying? (4) How do I want people to treat me? and (5) What do I want my loved ones to know about me and my feelings after I am gone? (Aging With Dignity, 2001).

Advance care directive documents must be drawn up when the person is capable of understanding their intent, and they become effective only when the person lacks the capacity to make a particular health-related decision. This is particularly relevant to people who are in early-stage dementia because, although loss of decisional capacity is a predictable outcome of this progressive condition, most people in early-stage dementia are capable of executing advance directives. For people with dementia, advance directives can provide important guidelines for families and health care providers when decisions about hospitalization, resuscitation, tube feeding, renal dialysis, antibiotic use, and end-of-life treatment issues need to be addressed (Mezey et al., 2000; Michel et al., 2002). Feinberg and Whitlach (2002) found that people with mild to moderate cognitive impairment are able to communicate their wishes about daily care and to choose a surrogate decision maker.

In the absence of written advance directives, oral advance directives are often respected, but they may be challenged legally if family members are not in agreement about the person's wishes. Oral advance directives are more likely to be accepted if the statements were: (1) made known on a serious occasion, (2) repeated and consistent with the person's usual values, (3) made by a mature person who understood the underlying issues, or (4) made shortly before the need for a treatment decision or with some specificity to the actual conditions of the person (Bottrell, 2001).

All states and the District of Columbia have laws defining and addressing advance directives, but only about 20% of people in the United States have advance directive documents. Most states require a periodic update of the advance directives (e.g., every 5 to 7 years). State laws vary regarding the scope and other details (e.g., type of document included, conditions under which it applies) of advance directives, and not all states honor out-of-state advance directives. This is particularly problematic for older adults who travel between or reside in more than one state. Gerontologist and law makers have called for standards and more uniformity among states regarding advance care directives and recommend the use of one document that comprehensively addresses all of the issues related to health care decisions (Gunter-Hunt et al., 2002). Nurses need to have up-to-date information about their own state's legal requirements for advance directives, which is widely available in health care institutions. Common types of advance directives are *living wills* and *durable power of attorney for health care*.

Living Wills and Advance Medical Directives

Living wills are legal documents whose purpose is to allow people to specify what type of medical treatment they would want or not want if they became incapacitated and terminally ill. They evolved as a component of the first right-to-die statute that was enacted in 1976 in California. People must be competent to initiate a living will, and they can revoke or change it at any time. A major goal of living wills is to affirm the right of the person to refuse treatment, but they do not always specify the particular type of treatment that can be refused. In addition to expressing wishes about refusal of treatment, living wills may express the person's preferences about pain management, organ donation, place of death, and specific treatments he or she would want to receive. A limitation of living will directives is that they apply only to situations in which the person is considered terminally ill. Definitions of terminal illness are not always clear, and there may be disagreement about whether the person is terminally ill. In general, someone is considered to be terminally ill when a physician determines that the person's predictable life expectancy is 6 months or less.

Most states and the District of Columbia recognize the validity of living wills, but the scope and details of living wills differ from state to state. For example, some states require that living wills specifically address certain procedures, such as the withholding or withdrawal of artificial sustenance when the person is terminally ill. However, in one third of the states, living wills do not explicitly address the use of artificial sustenance for people who are in a persistent vegetative state (Gunter-Hunt et al., 2002). Advocacy groups and health care professionals are encouraging all adults to draw up living wills and to take steps to ensure that all their health care providers have copies of these documents. For example, the U.S. Living Will Registry (listed in the Educational Resources section) electronically stores living wills and health care proxy documents and provides immediate access to living will documents for a small fee.

Advance medical directives are similar to living wills in specifying wishes for medical treatment, but they apply to a broader range of circumstances. For example, living wills are applicable when people are terminally ill, but advance medical directives can address circumstances (e.g., irreversible brain damage) that do not meet criteria for being a terminal illness. A *Do-Not-Resuscitate (DNR)* order is a very specific type of medical directive that directs health care providers to refrain from cardiopulmonary resuscitation if the person is no longer breathing and has no heart beat. In addition to focusing on the right to refuse treatments, medical directives address the person's desires for medical treatment that should be provided in certain circumstances. These directives can provide instructions about specific interventions, such as antibiotics, food and nutrition, and admissions to the hospital. These documents afford reassurance to people who fear that medical treatments or pain control and comfort measures will not be provided when they are sick and cannot express their own wishes. Although they do guarantee that the person's preferences will be considered, they do not guarantee that a medical intervention will be provided regardless of the circumstances. Because of the inability to predict medical treatments that might become available, and because of the changing health condition of the person executing the document, medical directives should be reviewed and updated periodically. Given the restrictions of living wills and the complexity of medical directives, older people who wish to use them should be encouraged to consult their attorneys and to fill out a durable power of attorney for health care as well. In this way, the person will have legally recognized advance directives that facilitate decision making about end-of-life issues.

Durable Power of Attorney for Health Care

A durable power of attorney for health care is an advance directive that takes effect whenever someone cannot, for any reason, provide informed consent for health care treatment decisions. It allows a surrogate health care decision maker, also called a *health care proxy*, to voice the wishes of the person who is incapacitated. Like other powers of attorney, the durable power of attorney for health care must be initiated when the person is competent, and it takes effect only when the person is incapacitated. The document usually provides the surrogate with written guidelines stating the person's wishes, such as with regard to termination of life support. It is imperative that the health care proxy includes a copy of all advance directives and periodically discusses the person's wishes about medical treatments and end-of-life issues. Because language in advance directive documents can sometimes be vague, it is advisable to encourage older people to discuss their wishes with their primary care provider, other health care workers, and their designated surrogate before a crisis develops.

Role of Nurses

Older adults generally prefer that family members, rather than health care providers, be surrogate decision makers, and they trust that family members will make appropriate choices. Although most older people are willing to discuss their wishes about medical treatments, they usually expect health care professionals to initiate the topic. In light of this, nurses have an obligation to older adults and their surrogate decision makers to assist them in the decision-making process by providing accurate information on rights and statutes, answering questions concerning their care, listening to patient and family needs, and acting as liaisons with primary care providers when necessary. Nurses are encouraged to initiate discussion of advance directives and end-of-life wishes with older adults when they are well, rather than waiting until they are ill (Inman, 2002; Vig et al, 2002). For example, nurses working with people who have early-stage dementia can suggest that the person execute advance directives. Combs and Stahl (2002) developed an excellent protocol for implementation of advance directives in adult day care centers. When an advance directive exists, it is the nurse's responsibility to inform other members of the health care team and to make certain that it is readily accessible in the chart. Each caregiver should read the directive and know what it covers. In addition, nurses should encourage patients to provide copies of advance directives to their family members, their designated surrogate, and anyone who is likely to be involved with decisions about their medical care. When written advance directives do not exist, nurses can initiate discussion of relevant medical care and end-of-life treatment preferences and document any statements made that express a patient's wishes.

In addition to providing information about advance directives, an important role for nurses is to provide information and support to proxy decision makers. When complex decisions must be made, an interdisciplinary team—composed of a social worker, minister, therapists, nurses, and primary care provider—may provide information and support to proxy decision makers. Decision-making assistance from professionals may relieve families and proxy decision makers of some of the guilt they may experience when making and implementing difficult decisions, particularly when difficult end-of-life decisions are being discussed.

NURSING HOMES

As the regulator of Medicare and Medicaid programs, Congress is responsible for ensuring that dollars expended for health care are well spent. In response to cited examples of poor quality of care in nursing homes dating back to the 1960s, Congress mandated an Institute of Medicine study entitled *Improving the Quality of Care in Nursing Homes*, which was published in 1986. Recommendations of the study included the increased use of registered nurses, the use of standardized resident assessments, and the implementation of nurse's aide training and certification. Subsequently, the Nursing Home Reform Act was included as part of the Omnibus Budget Reconciliation Act (OBRA) of 1987. It has had far-reaching consequences since 1990, when it began to be implemented. For example, it established regulations for care of nursing home residents with particular emphasis on residents' rights and quality of life, and it established requirements for institutional staffing, training, and evaluation (Meyers, 2002). The provisions of OBRA that apply to nursing homes were developed through joint efforts of health care professionals, the Health Care Financing Administration, the National Citizens Coalition for Nursing Home Reform, the American Association for Retired Persons, and representatives from the long-term care industry.

OBRA states that each resident in a long-term care facility is to be at his or her highest practicable level of physical, mental, and psychosocial well-being and that the long-term care facility is to accomplish this in an atmosphere that emphasizes residents' rights. To assist facilities in accomplishing this goal, OBRA mandates that all Medicaid- and Medicare-funded facilities use a standardized form, known as the Minimum Data Set (MDS) for Resident Assessment and Care Planning. This form includes a Resident Assessment Instrument (RAI), which is a structured, multidimensional resident assessment and problem identification system (discussed in Chapter 11). OBRA requires that within 14 days of admission and at least annually thereafter, nursing facility staff members perform a comprehensive, interdisciplinary assessment of every resident. Also, a care plan must be developed from that assessment, with the goal of continually evaluating the resident's highest functional level and preventing any deterioration unless it is assessed and clearly documented that the deterioration was unavoidable. A primary responsibility of nurses is to ensure that the comprehensive assessment is done at the appropriate times. Also, the nurse must ensure that the assessment tool is used as a basis for planning care that addresses the changing needs of the resident. By October of 1991, the RAI was being used in all Medicaid- and Medicare-funded nursing homes; in 1995, a second version of the MDS was developed to replace the first version.

In addition to addressing the development and documentation of care plans in nursing homes, OBRA strengthened the government oversight of nursing homes and addressed the many issues related to quality of care in nursing homes, which had been a focus of consumer advocacy groups since the 1970s. Improvements in nursing home care that have been attributed to the enactment of OBRA include decreased use of indwelling catheters, decreased prevalence of dehydration and pressure ulcers, increased presence of geriatricians and nurse practitioners, and reduced use of physical restraints and psychotropic drugs (Kane, 2001; Mitty, 2001; Sirin et al, 2002; Weintraub & Spurlock, 2002).

The focus on quality of care in nursing homes has recently extended to a focus on quality of life for nursing home residents (Calkins, 2002; Kane, 2001). Rosalie Kane, a prominent gerontologist, proposed that "a good quality of life should be elevated to a priority goal for long-term care rather than a pious afterthought to quality of care" (2001, p. 297). Kane identified the following 11 quality-of-life domains for nursing home residents: security, comfort, meaningful activity, relationships, enjoyment, dignity, autonomy, privacy, individuality, spiritual well-being, and functional competence (2001). She further recommended that rules and regulations for long-term care place less emphasis on "the best quality of life as is consistent with health and safety" and place more emphasis on "the best health and safety outcomes possible that are consistent with a meaningful quality of life" (Kane, 2001, p. 296). This recommendation represents a shift in emphasis that sometimes leads to ethical issues related to autonomy. For example, a person with a history of falls may express a desire to walk freely around the nursing home, but nursing home staff may want to limit that person's activity to reduce the risk for falls. This situation may present an ethical dilemma about the value of freedom over the value of safety.

Residents' rights are another major component of OBRA legislation that has had far-reaching consequences for nursing home staff and residents. The Nursing Home Residents' Bill of Rights states that "the resident has a right to a dignified existence, self-determination, and communication with and access to persons and services inside and outside the facility (Code of Federal Regulations, Title 42, Section 483.10). Display 6-1 lists some of the rights explicitly defined by this bill.

Autonomy issues may arise in nursing homes because it is not always easy to balance the individual resident's freedom of choice with the organizational needs of the institution. Examples of autonomy issues that are commonly addressed in nursing homes are: using physical restraints (see Chapter 18); restricting cigarette smoking; allowing residents to refuse treatments, social activities, and food or fluid; and providing more care assistance than necessary because this is more time-efficient for the staff (Mullins & Hartley, 2002). Another autonomy issue that is currently being addressed in nursing home settings is the right to express sexual interests and activities (see Chapter 22).

END-OF-LIFE CARE

Quality End-of-Life Care

Health care providers currently are focusing much attention on developing appropriate approaches to the end-of-life period for older adults, which can stretch over a period of 2 years (Morley, 2003). A major challenge of gerontological nursing is assisting with and implementing decisions about end-of-life care, which often involve ethical questions such as, "Is the length of life the ultimate value, or is the quality of life the ultimate value?" (Matzo & Sherman, 2001). Nurses in long-term care settings inevitably and frequently face this question and address issues about end-of-life care because death is part of the culture of nursing homes, dubbed by one nurse researcher as "heaven's waiting room" (Forbes, 2001). As a result of the PSDA, discussion of decisions affecting end-of-life care have become commonplace, nursing homes have policies addressing end-of-life care issues, and residents and their health care proxies have become more dominant in decision making about end-of-life care (Wurzbach, 2002). Despite the progress made since 1990, however, discussions about end-of-life care continue to be among the most stressful situations for nurses. For example, one major source of stress for gerontological

DISPLAY 6-1
Some Rights of Nursing Home Residents

The Right to Be Fully Informed
- The right to daily communication in their language
- The right to assistance if they have a sensory impairment
- The right to be notified in advance of any plans to change their room or roommate
- The right to be fully informed of all services available and the charge for each service

The Right to Participate in Their Own Care
- The right to receive adequate and appropriate care
- The right to participate in planning their treatment, care, and discharge
- The right to refuse medications, treatments, and physical and chemical restraints
- The right to review their own record

The Right to Make Independent Choices
- The right to make personal choices, such as what to wear and how to spend their time
- The right to reasonable accommodation of their needs and preferences
- The right to participate in activities, both inside and outside the nursing home
- The right to organize and participate in a Resident Council

The Right to Privacy and Confidentiality
- The right to private and unrestricted communication with any person
- The right to privacy in treatment and in personal care activities

- The right to confidentiality regarding their medical, personal, or financial affairs

The Right to Dignity, Respect, and Freedom
- The right to be treated with the fullest measure of consideration, respect, and dignity
- The right to be free from mental and physical abuse
- The right to self-determination

The Right to Security of Possessions
- The right to manage their own financial affairs
- The right to be free from charge for services covered by Medicaid or Medicare

Rights During Transfers and Discharges
- The right to remain in the facility unless a transfer or discharge is necessary, appropriate, or required
- The right to receive a 30-day notice of transfer or discharge

The Right to Complain
- The right to present grievances without fear of reprisal
- The right to prompt efforts by the nursing home to resolve grievances

The Right to Visits
- The right to immediate access by their relatives
- The right to reasonable visits by organizations or individuals providing health, social, legal, or other services

(Adapted from the U. S. Code of Federal Regulations, Title 42, Section 483.10, with permission.)

---

nurses working with older adults who have a progressive chronic condition such as dementia is the difficulty of determining the point at which the person has a terminal illness. In these situations, decisions about end-of-life measures are often avoided or addressed only when a major medical crisis occurs.

Major obstacles to initiating and implementing end-of-life care in nursing homes are lack of communication among decision makers and failure of clinicians to recognize that curative and restorative treatments are futile (Travis et al., 2001). Other barriers to implementing quality end-of-life care in nursing homes include inadequate staffing, the strong emphasis of quality indicators on rehabilitation and improved functioning, staff who are not prepared to address the needs of dying residents, and the task-oriented nature of care that does not adequately address cultural and psychosocial needs (Forbes, 2001;

Kayser-Jones, 2002; Raudonis et al, 2002). Gerontological nurses are actively trying to address these barriers through research and the development of clinical guidelines published in nursing journals (e.g., Baggs & Mick, 2000; Briggs & Colvin, 2002; Burack & Chichin, 2001; Norton & Talerico, 2000; Travis et al., 2002; Valente, 2001).

One approach to providing quality end-of-life care is to apply principles of palliative care. Although palliative care has traditionally been associated with hospice services, it is increasingly being offered to people with dementia, end-stage organ disease, and other degenerative diseases. *Palliative care nursing*, defined as "the art and science of quality end-of-life care," incorporates holistic caring with aggressive management of pain and symptoms associated with advanced diseases (Matzo & Sherman, 2001, p. 288). In recent years, more and more nursing homes are incorporating palliative care principles and using hospice/palliative care services to address end-of-life needs of residents. Rather than focusing interventions on improved functioning, hospice/palliative care nurses focus on ensuring comfort and psychosocial and spiritual well-being. They also provide support for caregivers and manage distressing symptoms (e.g., pain, thirst, nausea, dyspnea, constipation, dry mouth). An important responsibility of gerontological nurses is to recognize the appropriateness of a referral for hospice/palliative care and to initiate discussion of this option with older adults and their families.

Artificial Nutrition and Hydration

Gerontological nurses commonly deal with ethical aspects of decisions about artificial nutrition and hydration in many settings. Questions about initiating, continuing, withholding, or withdrawing artificial nutrition and hydration have been hotly debated since the early 1980s when percutaneous endoscopic gastrostomy (PEG) tubes became commonplace medical treatments. PEG tubes were initially developed for use in children with swallowing difficulties, and they have been found to be useful for people recovering from acute episodes such as stroke (Post, 2001). In recent years, however, it has become commonplace to use PEG tubes for long-term nutrition and hydration in people who have progressive and irreversible conditions such as dementia. Proxy decision makers for people in middle and late stages of dementia almost inevitably face decisions about placement of a PEG tube. These decisions are fraught with legal, ethical, and emotional dilemmas; often, it is the nurse who assumes a dominant role in providing information and support.

There is growing evidence that people with dementia do not benefit from long-term tube feeding (Gillick & Mitchell, 2002). Contrary to common perceptions, there is no published evidence that PEG feeding maintains weight, improves function, prolongs survival, provides palliation, prevents aspiration pneumonia, or reduces risks for pressure sores or infections in patients with advanced dementia (Daly, 2000; Finucane et al., 1999; Post, 2001). Another common perception that is not supported by research is that inadequate fluid and nutrition will cause undue suffering. A detrimental effect is that PEG tubes are associated with increased use of physical restraints (Gillick, 2000). Another detrimental effect for people who are still able to enjoy the sensation of food is the deprivation of that simple pleasure when a PEG tube is used for nutrition and hydration.

Discussions about PEG tubes may be initiated when the person with dementia requires considerable assistance with oral fluid and nutrition. Often, a concern about weight loss precipitates the question. In these situations, a major contributing factor may be the lack of a caregiver who will spend the significant amount of time required for assisted feeding. At least some of the intent of inserting a PEG tube might be to provide a more efficient method of assuring adequate nutrition and fluid. Discussions about PEG tubes also are initiated when the person with dementia is no longer able to swallow and cannot obtain adequate fluid and nutrition intake through assisted oral feedings. This is likely to be viewed as a terminal stage. Much research supports the view that the withholding of artificial hydration and nutrition at this stage is not associated with suffering as long as good oral care and desired sips of water are provided (Daly, 2000; Post, 2001). The consensus is that diminished fluid and nutrition stimulates the release of natural endorphins that provide an analgesic effect and protect the person from discomfort (Critchlow & Bauer-Wu, 2002; Daly, 2000; Post, 2001).

When families face complex decisions about using PEG tubes, nurses are responsible for providing up-to-date information and answering questions about the advantages and disadvantages of artificial fluid and nutrition. They also take a strong role in supporting and facilitating other decisions about end-of-life care (e.g., considering referrals for hospice care, discussing decisions about sending a nursing home resident to a hospital when medical problems arise). Guidelines and recommendations for these decisions are available from nursing organizations such as the National League for Nursing (NLN) and the American Nurses Association (ANA). For example, in 1992, the ANA published a position statement on foregoing nutrition and hydration with specific recommendations about the role of nurses. Many excellent educational resources are available for nurses and consumers to provide information about end-of-life decisions (see Educational Resources section). For example, *Making Choices: Long Term Feeding Tube Placement in Elderly Patients* is a workbook and cassette tape designed to assist families in making a decision about placing a feeding tube in an elderly patient (Mitchell et al., 2000).

CULTURAL ASPECTS OF LEGAL AND ETHICAL ISSUES

Health care providers need to be aware of the strong Anglo-centric bias of certain laws, such as the PSDA. There are many significant cultural differences with regard to patterns of decision making about medical interventions and health care services. For example, some families may believe it is a sign of respect to protect an elder from the burdens of receiving information about their health status and making decisions about medical interventions and long-term care plans. This may present a conflict for health care professionals who believe that all competent adults are entitled to information about their own health. It is imperative that health care providers determine culturally influenced patterns of decision making with such questions as, Whom do you talk to about your health care decisions? or Who will help you decide about where you are going to live? In some situations, it may be appropriate to ask a family member about decision-making patterns. It is especially important to be sensitive to cultural differences when discussing advance directives and end-of-life issues. Culture Box 6-1 summarizes some cultural considerations related to legal and ethical aspects of gerontological nursing care.

CHAPTER SUMMARY

Nurses frequently address ethical concerns and dilemmas with regard to rights, autonomy, and decision-making capacity of older adults. All adults have the right to make health-related decisions, unless they have been declared incompetent by a judge. This legal right can be questioned, however, when the older person's decision-making capacities are impaired. In these

---

CULTURE BOX 6-1   Cultural Considerations Relating to Legal and Ethical Aspects of Care

Autonomy and Decision-Making Patterns

Decision-making patterns in many non-Western cultures are centered on the good of the group rather than the good of the individual and are based on the social framework paradigm rather than the autonomy paradigm. Family and kinship patterns delineate the different roles, status, and power of each member of the group, and the social hierarchy governs decision making. For example, among traditional Japanese, group members are expected to honor and obey the elder male because he is accorded higher status and authority and carries a sense of responsibility for the entire group (Pacquiao, 2003). In these cultures . . .

- Patients may prefer not to be informed about medical conditions or involved with decisions about their care.
- Decisions about medical care may be based on the good of the family, rather than the good of the individual.
- Families may expect that medical information will be given to the designated family authority figure, who then will decide what to do with the information.
- Decisions are likely to be made by a designated authority figure, although opinions of all adult family members are acknowledged.
- As a sign of respect, elders may be protected from the burden and responsibility of making decisions about their own health care.
- The primary health care provider may be seen as the authority figure who should make decisions without discussing options with patients or their families.

Advance Directives

- Cultures with strong family ties may not see the need for advance directives because they expect the family members to make decisions, and advance directives may represent a conflict between individual autonomy and family solidarity (Pacquiao, 2003).
- Cultures that see the cycle of birth, life, and death as natural (e.g., Native Americans) may see no need for advance directives.
- Cultures that believe in fatalism (e.g., Filipino) are likely to resist any discussion about planning for events that are beyond one's control, such as illness or death, because this is viewed as tempting fate and will likely bring the potential event into reality (Pacquiao, 2003).
- African Americans may be suspicious of advance directives and equate these with abandonment by health care practitioners based on the legacy of slavery and past experiences with medical research (e.g., the Tuskegee experiments) (Crawley et al., 2002; Dupree, 2000).
- Filipino and Chinese nurses may be uncomfortable discussing advance directives because they view this as conflicting with their role as caregivers; they may prefer that clergy or pastoral care services discuss advance directives with hospitalized patients (Pacquaio, 2001).

End-of-Life Issues

- In many cultures, it is taboo to discuss impending death or end-of-life issues with the person who is terminally ill because these discussions imply hopelessness, are considered harmful to the person's well-being, and are viewed as increasing the person's suffering and hastening the inevitable outcome (Kramer, 2001).
- Although it might be taboo for Asians to discuss end-of-life treatment issues, it may be acceptable and common to discuss funeral arrangements and preferences for burial (Cheng, 1997).
- Health care providers need to identify any culturally based rituals that are done at the time of death and need to be addressed in a health care setting. For example, in Judaism, the collective presence of family and members of the community at the bedside when someone is dying manifests communal obligations that are part of that culture (Pacquiao, 2003).
- Health care providers need to identify any culture-based beliefs that may influence acceptance of comfort measures and medical interventions at the end-of-life. For example, a Hindu person who is dying may refuse pain medication because this is in direct conflict with the goals of maintaining awareness and experiencing what is to come as an integral part of preparing for a good death (Pacquiao, 2003).

situations, legal documents, such as living wills, advance medical directives, and a durable power of attorney for health care, are used to guide decision makers in identifying and carrying out the person's wishes. The PSDA delineates federal guidelines for advance directives, but advance directives are defined by state laws and can vary significantly. It is imperative that all adults draw up these legal documents and make them available to all people who are likely to be involved with decisions about their medical care. Nurses play important roles in initiating discussions about advance directives, making sure that advance directives are available to health care providers, and documenting conversations about the person's wishes with regard to medical care and end-of-life issues.

Legal and ethical issues have particularly affected staff and residents of nursing homes since the late 1980s. Because of OBRA, nursing homes must meet certain requirements with regard to the care of residents, and they must provide documentation of comprehensive assessments and care plans. Aspects of nursing home care that have improved because of OBRA include decreased use of indwelling catheters, reduced use of physical and chemical restraints, and lower prevalence of dehydration and pressure ulcers. Another outcome of OBRA is increased emphasis on quality of care and quality of life for nursing home residents. The Nursing Home Bill of Rights establishes the rights of nursing home residents to dignity, self-determination, and communication. Nurses in nursing home settings frequently address autonomy issues because it is not always easy to balance the rights of residents with the needs of the organization.

One of the most challenging aspects of gerontological nursing is assisting with and implementing decisions about end-of-life care, and nurses can apply principles of palliative care to their care of terminally ill older adults. Gerontological nurses are likely to be involved with decisions about artificial nutrition and hydration, and this issue is particularly difficult with regard to people with dementia. Because cultural differences can have a significant impact on the way decisions are made regarding health care and end-of-life issues, nurses need to be familiar with cultural considerations relating to legal and ethical aspects of care. Many resources are available to provide guidelines and information about legal and ethical issues encountered by gerontological nurses.

CRITICAL THINKING EXERCISES

1. You have been assigned to work with Mrs. M., an 85-year-old white widowed woman who is in the hospital with congestive heart failure. Her son and daughter tell you they would like to arrange for her to be discharged to a nursing home because they don't think she takes her medications correctly and they are tired of her being admitted to the hospital every couple of months "to get her straightened out." The son and daughter live in another state and visit only when their mother is in the hospital. Mrs. M. has told you that she thinks her son and daughter would like to have her "put away in one of those homes" but she is adamantly opposed to leaving her home. She also has told you that they think she is "senile" and should stop driving her car, but she thinks she is quite capable of living alone, driving her car, and taking care of herself. Your observations are that she needs a lot of direction to take medications and participate in self-care activities, and she seems to be somewhat confused later in the day. What steps would you take to address her competency and decision-making abilities?

2. A Mexican American woman, aged 78 years old, is being admitted to the hospital with hemiplegia following a stroke. There are no advance directives on her chart. What information would you want to know before you approached her about a living will and durable power of attorney for health care? How would you explain these documents to her?

3. Mr. S. is 78 years old and has been admitted for hip surgery following a fall-related fracture. He has had dementia for 5 years, and his family provides care for him in his home. His son is designated as his durable power of attorney for health care, but the son will not make any decisions unless his three sisters agree on the decision. Mr. S. does not have any other advance directives, and the family says he never talked much about what medical care he would want. He always told his family that they could make whatever decisions are best for him. The physician has asked the family to consider placement of a PEG tube because Mr. S.'s food and fluid intake are inadequate to meet his needs and one pressure area is beginning to develop on his buttocks. Mr. S.'s son and one daughter think that their father would have wanted to have everything possible done in such a situation, and they think the PEG tube will improve his comfort and prevent the pressure ulcer. The other two daughters adamantly state that their father would never agree to such an invasive procedure and that they are not sure it will make him any more comfortable. They also worry that he will need to be restrained to keep him from pulling the tube out. You are a member of the multidisciplinary team that is meeting with the family to help them come to a decision about a PEG tube. What points would you want to make during this family conference?

EDUCATIONAL RESOURCES

Aging With Dignity
P.O. Box 1661, Tallahassee, FL 32302-1661
(850) 681-2010
http://www.agingwithdignity.org

American Association of Colleges of Nursing (AACN)
End-of-Life Nursing Education Consortium Project
One Dupont Circle, NW, Suite 530, Washington, DC 20036
(202) 463-6930
http://www.aacn.nche.edu/elnec

American Association of Retired Persons (AARP)
601 E Street, NW, Washington, DC 20049
(800) 424-3410
http://www.aarp.org

American Bar Association Commission on Law and Aging
740 Fifteenth Street, NW, Washington, DC 20005-1019
(202) 662-1000
http://www.abanet.org/aging

American Bar Association, Senior Lawyers Division
750 North Lake Shore Drive, Chicago, IL 60611
(312) 988-5000
http://www.abanet.org/srlawyers/home.html

American Nurses Association (ANA)
Center for Ethics & Human Rights
600 Maryland Avenue, SW, Suite 100 West, Washington, DC 20024
(800) 274-4262
http://www.nursingworld.org/ethics

Midwest Bioethics Center
1021-1025 Jefferson Street, Kansas City, MO 64105
(800) 344-3829
http://www.midbio.org

National Senior Citizens Law Center
1101 14th Street, NW, Suite 400, Washington, DC 20005
(202) 289-6976
http://www.nsclc.org

U.S. Living Will Registry
523 Westfield Ave., P.O. Box 2789, Westfield, NJ 07091-2789
(800) 548-9455
http://www.uslivingwillregistry.com

REFERENCES

Aging With Dignity. (2001). *Five wishes.* Tallahassee, FL: Author.

Baggs, J. G., & Mick, D. J. (2000). Collaboration: A tool addressing ethical issues for elderly patients near the end of life in intensive care units. *Journal of Gerontological Nursing, 26*(9), 41–47.

Bottrell, M. M. (2001). Advance directives. In M.D. Mezey (Ed.), *The encyclopedia of elder care* (pp. 21–24). New York: Springer.

Briggs, L., & Colvin, E. (2002). The nurse's role in end-of-life decision-making for patients and families. *Geriatric Nursing, 23,* 302–310.

Burack, O. R., & Chichin, E. R. (2001). A support group for nursing assistants: Caring for nursing home residents the end of life. *Geriatric Nursing, 22,* 299–306.

Calkins, M. C. (2002). The nursing home of the future: Are you ready? *Nursing Homes/Long Term Care Management, 51*(6), 42–47.

Cheng, B. K. (1997). Cultural clash between providers of majority culture and patients of Chinese culture. *Journal of Long-Term Home Health Care, 16*(2), 39–43.

Collopy, B. J. (1988). Autonomy in long term care: Some crucial distinctions. *Gerontologist, 28*(Suppl.), 10–17.

Combs, P. L., & Stahl, L. D. (2002). Implementing a do-not-resuscitate order in an adult day care center. *Geriatric Nursing, 23,* 312–315.

Crawley, L. M., Marshall, P. A., Lo, B., & Koenig, B. A. (2002). Strategies for culturally effective end-of-life care. *Annals of Internal Medicine, 136,* 673–678.

Critchlow, J., & Bauer-Wu, S. M. (2002). Nurses' perceptions of dehydration. *Journal of Gerontological Nursing, 28*(12), 31–39.

Daly, B. J. (2000). Special challenges of withholding artificial nutrition and hydration. *Journal of Gerontological Nursing, 26*(9), 25–31.

Dupree, C. Y. (2000). The attitudes of Black Americans toward advance directives. *Journal of Transcultural Nursing, 11*(1), 12–18.

Feinberg, L. F., & Whitlach, C. J. (2002). Decision-making for persons with cognitive impairment and their family caregivers. *American Journal of Alzheimer's Disease and Other Dementias, 17,* 237–244.

Finucane, T. E., Christmas, C. & Travis, K. (1999). Tube feeding in patients with advanced dementia: A review of the evidence. *Journal of the American Medical Association, 282,* 1365–1370.

Forbes, S. (2001). This is heavens waiting room: End of life in one nursing home. *Journal of Gerontological Nursing, 27*(11), 37–45.

Gillick, M. R. (2000). Rethinking the role of tube feeding in patients with advanced dementia. *New England Journal of Medicine, 342,* 206–210.

Gillick, M. R., & Mitchell, S. L. (2002). Facing eating difficulties in end-stage dementia. *Alzheimer's Care Quarterly, 3,* 227–232.

Gunter-Hunt, G., Mahoney, J. E., & Sieger, C. E. (2002). A comparison of state advance directive documents. *Gerontologist, 42*(1), 51–60.

Inman, L. (2002). Advance directives. Journal of *Gerontological Nursing, 28*(9), 40–46.

Kane, R. A. (2001). Long-term care and a good quality of life bringing them closer together. *Gerontologist, 41*(3), 293–304.

Kayser-Jones, J. (2002). The experience of dying: An ethnographic nursing home study. *Gerontologist, 42*(Special Issue III), 11–19.

Kramer, B. J. (2001). Cultural assessment. In M. D. Mezey (Ed.), *The encyclopedia of elder care* (pp. 176–179). New York: Springer.

Matzo, M. L., & Sherman, D. W. (2001). Palliative care nursing: Ensuring competent care at the end of life. *Geriatric Nursing, 22,* 288–293.

McCullough, L.B., Molinari, V., & Workman, R. H. (2001). Implications of impaired executive control functions for patient autonomy and surrogate decision making. *Journal of Clinical Ethics, 12,* 397–405.

Meyers, E. M. (2002). Physical restraints in nursing homes: An analysis of quality of care and legal liability. *Elder Law Journal, 10*(1), 217–262.

Mezey, M. D., Mitty, E. L., Bottrell, M. M., Ramsey, G. C., & Fisher, T. (2000). Death and dying: Advance directives—older adults with dementia. *Clinics in Geriatric Medicine, 16*(2), 255–268.

Michel, J. P., Pautex, S., Zekry, D., Zulian, G., & Gold G. (2002). End-of-life care of persons with dementia. *Journal of Gerontology, 57A,* M640–M644.

Mitchell, S., O'Connor, A., & Tetroe, J. (2000). *Making choices: Long-term feeding tube placement in elderly patients: A book and audiotape for substitute decision makers.* Ottawa, ON: Ottawa Health Research Institute. Available at www.ohri.ca/programs/clinical_epidemiology/OHDEC/decision_aids.asp.

Mitty, E. L. (2001). Nursing homes. In M. D. Mezey (Ed.), *The encyclopedia of elder care* (pp. 452–455). New York: Springer.

Morley, J. E. (2003). Editorial: Hot topics in geriatrics. *Journal of Gerontology, 53A,* 30–36.

Mullins, L. C., & Hartley, T. M. (2002). Residents' autonomy nursing home personnel's perceptions. *Journal of Gerontological Nursing, 28*(2), 35–44.

Norton, S. A., & Talerico, K. A. (2000). Decision-making strategies for communicating and assessing. *Journal of Gerontological Nursing, 26*(9), 6–13.

Pacquiao, D. F. (2001). Addressing cultural incongruities of advance directives. *Bioethics Forum, 17*(1), 27–31.

Pacquiao, D. F. (2003). Cultural competence in ethical decision-making. In M. M. Andrews & J. S. Boyle. *Transcultural concepts in nursing care* (4th ed., pp. 503–532). Philadelphia: Lippincott Williams & Wilkins.

Post, S. G. (2001). Tube feeding and advanced progressive dementia. *Hastings Center Report, 31*(1), 36–42.

Raudonis, B. M., Kyba, F. C. N., & Kinsey, T. A. (2002). Long-term care nurses' knowledge of end-of-life care. *Geriatric Nursing, 23,* 296–299.

Sirin, S. R., Castle, N. G., & Smyer, M. (2002). Risk factors for physical restraint use in nursing homes: The impact of the Nursing Home Reform Act. *Research on Aging, 24,* 513–527.

Travis, S. S., Conway, J., Daly, M., & Larsen, L. (2001). Terminal restlessness in the nursing facility: Assessment, palliation, and symptom management. *Geriatric Nursing, 22,* 308–312.

Travis, S. S., Bernard, M., Dixion, S., McAuley, W. J., Loving, G., & McClanahan, L. (2002). Obstacles to palliation and end of life care in long-term care facility. *Gerontologist, 42,* 342–349.

Valente, S. M. (2001). End of life issues. *Geriatric Nursing, 22,* 294–298.

Vig, E. K., Davenport, N. A., & Pearlman, R. A. (2002). Good deaths, bad deaths, and preferences for the end of life: A qualitative study of geriatric outpatients. *Journal of the American Geriatrics Society, 50,* 1541–1548.

Weintraub, D., & Spurlock, M. (2002). Change in the rate of restraint use and falls on psychogeriatric inpatient unit: Impact of the health care financing administration's new restraint and seclusions standards for hospitals. *Journal of Geriatric Psychiatry and Neurology, 15,* 91–94.

Wurzbach, M. E. (2002). End-of-life treatment decisions in long-term care. *Journal of Gerontological Nursing, 28*(6), 14–21.

3

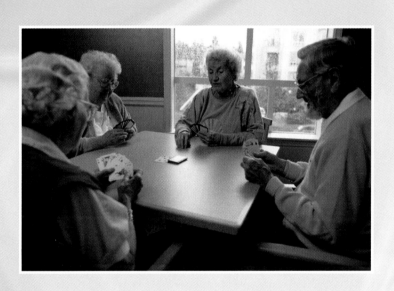

PSYCHOSOCIAL ASPECTS OF FUNCTION

Cognitive Function

LEARNING OBJECTIVES

1. Describe theories about adult intellectual development and age-related cognitive changes, including memory changes.
2. List risk factors that influence cognitive function in older adults.
3. Discuss the functional consequences that affect cognition in older adults.
4. Identify strategies that older adults can use to maintain or improve intellectual performance.

Cognitive function in old age is one of the most controversial areas of psychology, and the debate is becoming more heated as newer theories of cognitive aging are developed. In the late 1970s, psychologists thought that a decline in cognitive abilities was a normal part of the aging process, but by the mid-1980s, this conclusion was widely challenged, particularly because it was based on cross-sectional rather than longitudinal studies of intelligence. Currently, researchers in the field of cognitive aging are looking not only at measures of cognitive ability but also at measures of an older adult's capacity to maintain intellectual skills despite the age-related changes and risk factors that are likely to interfere with cognitive function. Some of the questions that researchers are attempting to answer are, Why do some people show intellectual decrement in early adulthood, whereas others maintain or increase their intellectual skills well into old age? Can interventions prevent, retard, or reverse intellectual decline? And, perhaps most important, How can we enhance cognitive abilities, even in those people who are intellectually intact?

AGE-RELATED CHANGES THAT AFFECT COGNITIVE FUNCTION

The identification of age-related changes that affect cognitive function is clouded by inconsistent definitions and measures of intelligence and by the wide variety of terms that are applied to memory and other aspects of cognitive function. As with many other aspects of function in older adults, researchers are trying to distinguish between age-related and pathologic changes, with much attention on identifying the cognitive changes that occur in healthy older adults and those that occur in older adults with pathologic processes such as dementia (discussed in Chapter 24). Age-related changes of the central nervous system provide a base of information about cognitive function, whereas theories about aging and cognition attempt to explain the complex effects of age-related changes on various aspects of cognitive function.

Central Nervous System Changes

Recent major technological advances in neuroimaging techniques (e.g., functional magnetic resonance imaging) have significantly broadened the base of information on age-related changes in brain structure and function. Additional sources of information about brain aging include clinical, neuropsychological, neuropathologic, and neurochemical investigations (Vinters, 2001). Research on brain aging no longer relies primarily on autopsy studies, and researchers have come much closer to being able to distinguish between pathologic and normal aging changes that commonly occur in older brains. Thus, recent findings sometimes differ from earlier studies. For example, studies continue to provide considerable evidence for age-related decline in some aspects of cognition, but recently there "has been a major revision in our understanding of the type of changes that occur in the brain with advancing age. There is increasing evidence that widespread neuronal loss does not take place and produce ever increasing amounts of cognitive decline over time" (Albert & Killiany, 2001, p. 178). Some of the age-related changes in the brain that may cause cognitive changes in healthy older adults are as follows (Backman et al., 2001; Simensky & Abeles, 2002; Vinters, 2001):

- A gradual reduction in brain weight of 2 to 3 g per year (from an average of 1400 g in adult men and 1250 g in adult women) beginning at about the age of 60 years, due primarily to loss of white matter, particularly in the frontal lobes
- Diminished ratio of brain to skull volume, from 95% at about the age of 60 years to 80% in nonagenarians
- Enlarged ventricles, with average ventricle volume increasing from 15 mL in teens to 55 mL in people older than 60 years of age
- Widening of the sulci
- Shrinkage of larger neurons and possibly some neuronal loss, particularly in frontal and temporal lobes
- Loss of one or more neurotransmitters or their binding sites
- A gradual decrease in dopaminergic function of 6% to 10% per decade from early to later adulthood
- Diminished cerebral blood flow, particularly in the prefrontal cortex
- Accumulation of lipofuscin in nerve cell bodies

Diminished reaction time is widely recognized as an age-related change of the central nervous system that can affect cognitive function, particularly with regard to tasks that are dependent on speed and timing of performance. Diminished sensory abilities, particularly vision and hearing, are other central nervous system changes that can interfere with cognitive function in older adults.

THEORIES ABOUT AGING AND COGNITION

A literature review of aging and cognition identified four distinct phases in the use of psychometric tests to measure adult intelligence (Woodruff, 1983). During phase I, adult intelligence was measured with tests designed to predict school performance in children. In cross-sectional studies using these tests, younger adults consistently scored higher than older adults. Based on these results, it was concluded that intelligence begins to decline in early adulthood. Phase II studies began in the mid-1950s, when questions were raised about the validity of cross-sectional studies. Phase II longitudinal studies, developed to identify patterns of adult intellectual development, consistently showed that intellectual function remained the same or improved up to the age of 50 or 60 years, after which time it gradually declined. A landmark 21-year study that included both longitudinal and cross-sectional data confirmed the findings of the previous studies. That is, the cross-sectional studies showed that adult intelligence peaks at about 35 years of age and then sharply declines, whereas the longitudinal studies indicate that adult intelligence peaks at about 60 years of age and then declines slightly until the ages of 74 to 81 years (Schaie & Willis, 1986).

Phase III studies, begun in the 1970s, were designed to address the question of whether life experiences account for some of the age differences reflected in intelligence scores. Studies were developed that modified adult cognition to test the effects of experience and environment. This approach had the practical benefit of identifying ways to improve cognitive abilities (Woodruff, 1983). According to Botwinick (1984), this approach used modification studies to explore individual plasticity, or the person's possible range of tested behavior. Typically, this testing method involved administration of an initial test, followed by a period of training, and then by a retest using a different type of test. Although this kind of study is still being evaluated and refined, Botwinick concluded, "these studies have shown that the old, like the young, have more potential than is typically measured by the tests" (1984, p. 271).

Phase IV studies, first developed in the 1980s, are based on the discovery that performance on intelligence tests could be improved through interventions. In this phase, researchers have tried to identify cognitive skills that develop over the adult life span, such as those based on wisdom and experience (Woodruff, 1983). Phase IV studies also address new questions about the complex relationship between cognition and other factors, such as speed of response. For example, the results of these studies suggest that older people respond more quickly with practice, and, in fact, improve more than do younger people (Botwinick, 1984, p. 246).

Current research focuses on identifying those people who are at risk for developing cognitive impairment, so that intervention strategies can be implemented to help maintain high levels of intellectual function in later adulthood. Another question that has been posed recently concerns the possible confounding influence of "preclinical dementia," which is the occurrence of subtle but abnormal cognitive changes that develop into dementia within several years. For example, studies of older adults that include subjects who have undetected preclinical dementia may inaccurately attribute cognitive changes to aging rather than to pathologic conditions (Schaie & Hofer, 2001).

Theory of Fluid and Crystallized Intelligence

Cattell and Horn's theory of fluid and crystallized intelligence, first proposed in the late 1960s, is one of the first theories that attempted to explain age-related changes in some cognitive abilities. *Crystallized intelligence* refers to those cognitive skills that are acquired through culture, education, informal learning, and other life experiences. Crystallized intelligence is strongly associated with wisdom, judgment, and life experiences. By contrast, fluid intelligence depends primarily on a person's inherent abilities, such as memory, pattern recognition, and the central nervous system. Fluid intelligence is associated with an ability to identify complex relationships and to draw conclusions from these relationships.

According to this theory, fluid and crystallized intelligence develop concurrently during infancy and childhood and, in fact, are indistinguishable as the central nervous system is maturing. During early adulthood, fluid intelligence begins to decline because of the progressive age-related deterioration of neural structures, which interferes with one's ability to maintain spontaneous alertness, focused intensive concentration, and an awareness of possible organization for otherwise disorganized information (Horn, 1982). By contrast, crystallized intelligence continues to develop throughout adulthood because

of accumulated experiences and learning. Crystallized intelligence, except for those processes that depend on speed of response, does not change with age, and it may even increase because of adult educational experiences. In later adulthood, increased crystallized intelligence can help explain the growth in wisdom that enables older adults to place present issues in a broader context than younger people who have less life experience (Thomson, 2001).

In applying this theory to cognitive aging, specific aspects of fluid and crystallized intelligence can be compared with aspects of traditional tests of intellectual function. For example, components of fluid intelligence, such as reasoning and abstraction, coincide roughly with the Wechsler Adult Intelligence Scale (WAIS) Performance Scale measures and are thought to decline in older adulthood. Similarly, the components of crystallized intelligence, such as information and comprehension, correspond roughly with the WAIS Verbal Scale measures, which do not exhibit a decline with advancing years. Based on this theory, cognitive aging is caused by a disintegration of higher-order functions that normally facilitate the transfer and integration of information. Findings from both cross-sectional and longitudinal studies support this theory, but some questions remain about the age at which declines are initially observed and the extent of the declines (Schaie & Hofer, 2001).

Theories of Adult Cognitive Development

Schaie (1977–1978), expanding on Piaget's theory of intellectual development in childhood and adolescence, proposed a theory of stages relating to adult cognitive development. Schaie reasoned that, if the focus of childhood and adolescence is the acquisition of knowledge, then the focus of adulthood is the application of knowledge. The *achieving stage* of adult cognitive development, which marks the onset of adult cognitive maturity, is characterized by a striving to apply one's newly acquired knowledge to demands and commitments, such as career and family. In this stage, young adults use their intellectual abilities to establish their independence and develop goal-oriented behaviors. The second stage of adult cognitive development, called the *responsible stage*, extends in age from the late 30s to the early 60s. During this stage, people focus on integrating their long-range goals and attending to the needs of their family and society. Some people in this stage have high levels of social responsibilities; these individuals are categorized as being in the *executive stage*. The tasks of the last stage, called the *reintegrate stage*, are to simplify life and to select only those responsibilities that have meaning and purpose. During this stage, rather than asking, What should I know?, the older adult asks, Why should I know?

The theory of cognitive aging and psychological growth postulates that the thinking of older adults becomes increasingly complex and shows progressive reorganization of intellectual skills (Labouvie-Vief & Blanchard-Fields, 1982). Because these skills differ from those of younger adults, they cannot be measured with traditional intelligence tests. Labouvie-Vief and Blanchard-Fields cite numerous examples of studies in which conclusions about cognitive decline are based on standards of youth-oriented cognitive patterns. They suggest that if these studies were interpreted in relation to the advanced psychological development that occurs with mature aging, the conclusions would be different. This, and other theories about the interaction between emotion and cognition, support the increasing recognition that emotional complexity is enhanced with age, although it peaks during the middle years (Magai, 2001). A current focus of research on cognitive aging and psychological growth is the development of wisdom and creativity during later adulthood (Sternberg & Lubart, 2001).

Theories About Memory

A widely held perspective is that memory is a computer-like information-processing system in which information is first perceived, then stored in the primary or secondary memory, and finally, retrieved when needed or wanted. Primary memory has a short duration, a very small capacity, and serves as a holding tank for events of the immediate past few seconds, rather than as a true memory storage system. Information in the primary memory either can be recalled for a brief time or can be transmitted to long-term storage. Secondary memory is longer term and therefore is more important in terms of the retrieval, as well as storage, of information. Retrieval of information from storage is variously referred to as *remote, tertiary,* or *very long-term memory processing,* and skills involved are classified as *recall memory* and *recognition memory.* A popular belief is that older people remember events of long ago better than events of the immediate past, but this has not consistently been supported in studies, which indicate that both types of memory decline equally in older adulthood (Botwinick, 1984). The effect of age-related changes on memory has been succinctly summarized as: "TM [tertiary memory] may or may not hold with age, but even if not, the old have a large store of information, as large as that of younger people. This store is largely of occurrences of long ago" (Botwinick, 1984, p. 333).

In recent years, the information-processing model has been viewed as too simplistic because it ignores the milieu in which the memory operates. Newer theories, called *contextual theories,* have expanded the information-processing model, addressing some of the variables that may affect memory. Some of the factors that may influence memory function, regardless of age, are motivation, expectations, experiences, education, personality, task demands, learning habits, intellectual skills, sociocultural background, physical and mental health, and style of processing information. Because the contextual factor that most consistently affects memory skills in older adults is general processing speed, older adults will have better memory skills when they have more time to process information.

A different theoretical approach is to disregard the storage and retrieval aspects of memory and emphasize the encoding and analyzing aspects. Memory is viewed as a continuum of processing, ranging from shallow to deep levels, and the duration of a particular memory depends on the depth of the processing. According to this theory, the deeper the level at which information is stored, the longer the memory will last. Duration of storage can be influenced by any of the following: (1) the processing techniques, ranging from the shallowest levels used for sensory information to the deepest levels used for highly abstract information; (2) the elaboration, or quality, of processing carried out at any depth level; (3) the distinctiveness of the information, which depends partially on how well it is learned; and (4) the depth and elaboration of retrieval processes (Botwinick, 1984). Several studies based on this framework have concluded that the memory function of older adults is decreased because of faulty processing mechanisms (Botwinick, 1984). This theory provides a framework for current research on the effects of age-related changes in frontal lobe functioning that may affect memory by interfering with organization of material (Simensky & Abeles, 2002).

Another theoretical perspective that views memory as a continuum is the automatic and effortful processing theory (Hasher & Zacks, 1979). At the one end is automatic processing, or those tasks that do not require attention or awareness and do not improve with practice. At the other end is effortful processing, or those tasks that demand high levels of attention and cognitive energy. With practice, effortful tasks require less attention and become more automatic. According to this theory, automatic memory would not be affected by age because these tasks require little or no cognitive energy. Effortful memory, however, would decline with age because only a limited amount of cognitive resources are available for memory functions, and these resources gradually decline, beginning in early adulthood. Studies of automatic processing activities in older adults support the theory of little or no decline in automatic processing and some deficits in effortful encoding tasks (Botwinick, 1984; Rohling & Scogin, 1993). Researchers currently are applying this theoretical base to study the effects of age-related changes in frontal lobe functioning that may affect memory by interfering with attention (Persad et al., 2002).

Metamemory is an evolving concept that refers to self-knowledge about memory or cognitive functions. It includes all of one's knowledge and perceptions about the function and development of memory. Interest in metamemory is based on the belief that metacognitive processes enable a person to influence and regulate the memory processes consciously and to use memory compensation strategies (DeFries et al., 2003). Metamemory is important in everyday activities because if people know what they can remember and how much effort they will need to remember certain things, they can plan efficient and effective strategies for remembering. Older adults tend to perceive themselves as less competent in some cognitive skills than they actually are, and as less competent than younger adults in many cognitive tasks. These false perceptions may lead to anxiety, depression, decreased effort and motivation, and increased dependency on others. Researchers are studying the predictive value of metamemory as an indicator of future cognitive decline and subsequent diagnosis of dementia (Johansson et al., 1997).

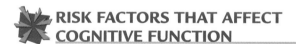 **RISK FACTORS THAT AFFECT COGNITIVE FUNCTION**

Personal Characteristics and Lifestyle Factors

Numerous personal characteristics and lifestyle factors affect cognitive abilities in people of any age, and researchers have tried to identify those that most significantly affect older adults. Years of formal education is the factor that most consistently is associated with cognitive performance in older adults, and this association is independent of race, gender, cultural, geographic, or other variables. There is strong support for the idea that the educational process itself is the underlying factor for maintenance of cognitive health in older adults, but other probable contributing mechanisms include an active lifestyle, past and current socioeconomic status, the content of the educational material, mental stimulation in the workplace, or a combination of these factors (Cagney & Lauderdale,

2002; Turrell et al., 2002). Level of activity is a major lifestyle factor that significantly affects cognitive function, with a strong positive relationship between engagement in social, cognitive, and physical activities and better memory performance in older adults (Backman et al., 2001; Colcombe et al., 2003; Naylor et al., 2000; Rebok & Plude, 2001; Yaffe et al., 2001).

Self-perceptions and expectations also significantly affect cognitive skills and performance on intelligence tests. Low self-efficacy (i.e., the belief in one's ability to perform at a given level) is associated with persistent emotional stress and poor cognitive performance (Ball & Birge, 2002). Low self-esteem also contributes to poor cognitive function. Thus, ageism and diminished expectations of older adults in modern societies can negatively affect cognitive function (Hess et al., 2003).

Sensory Function and Physical and Mental Health Factors

Because the acquisition of information is highly dependent on sensory input, cognitive processes are affected when the quantity and quality of information from the environment is limited because of hearing and vision impairments (discussed in Chapters 12 and 13, respectively). There is a strong correlation between visual acuity, hearing abilities, and cognitive abilities for adults of all ages, and the correlation becomes stronger with increasing age (Fozard & Gordon-Salant, 2001; Park, 2000). Likewise, there is a strong correlation between many aspects of physical health, especially many chronic conditions, and cognitive abilities. Some of the physical conditions associated with impaired cognitive function are the following (Backman et al., 2001):

- Thyroid disorders
- Diabetes and impaired glucose tolerance
- Dementia (e.g., Alzheimer's disease, vascular dementia)
- Circulatory disorders (e.g., stroke, hypertension, transient ischemic attacks)

Anxiety can interfere with cognitive abilities by causing excessive worry and self-centeredness, and this mental health factor is consistently identified as a risk for poor cognitive function. Depression, and even subclinical variations in depressive symptoms, is strongly associated with impaired cognitive function (especially memory), as discussed in Chapter 25 (Backman et al., 2001). Depression contributes to negative self-expectations and interferes with attention and concentration, which are two cognitive skills that significantly affect memory.

Nutritional Factors

Nutritional status has been singled out as a physical health variable that influences cognitive function, particularly memory performance, regardless of a person's age. For example, beta-carotene, B vitamins, and vitamin C can affect cognitive function. Even subclinical deficiencies of B vitamins can have a detrimental effect on memory (Backman et al., 2001; Calvaresi & Bryan, 2001). Recent studies have found that higher intake of vitamin E, in food or supplements, is associated with improved cognitive function in older adults (Morris, 2002; Ortega, 2002). Interest in the role of choline and lecithin stems from the theory that cognitive and memory deficits may be caused by a disruption of normal acetylcholine transmission in the brain. Although the consumption of foods rich in choline or lecithin can increase plasma choline levels, the effectiveness of these interventions on cognitive function has not been determined.

Much of the research on the relationship between alcohol consumption and cognitive function is not age specific, but conclusions can be applied to older adults as well as younger adults. For example, moderate consumption of alcohol is likely to interfere with short-term memory, but not with immediate or long-term memory, and long-term consumption of alcohol in excessive amounts is likely to interfere with memory performance, even during periods of abstention from alcohol.

Medication Effects

Prescription and over-the-counter medications can interfere with memory and other cognitive functions in a variety of ways. For example, anticholinergic ingredients, contained in numerous prescription and over-the-counter medications, significantly affect memory and other cognitive functions and are a common cause of changes in mental status in older adults. Older adults are particularly susceptible to developing adverse cognitive effects from the anticholinergic medications that cross the blood–brain barrier (e.g., atropine, benztropine, dicyclomine, flavoxate, and trihexyphenidyl). Because many medications have direct anticholinergic effects or increase the effects of anticholinergic medications, researchers and geriatric clinicians have paid particular attention in recent years to drug interactions and the cumulative effects of these medications on acetylcholine (a neurotransmitter that directly affects cognitive function) (Tune, 2001). Older adults with dementia are more likely than healthy older adults to develop medication-induced cognitive impairment from anticholinergic medications. Mechanisms of medication action that can interfere with cognitive function are described in detail in Chapter 23.

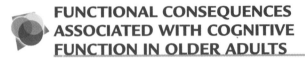

FUNCTIONAL CONSEQUENCES ASSOCIATED WITH COGNITIVE FUNCTION IN OLDER ADULTS

It is widely agreed that some cognitive decline occurs in later adulthood, with subtle, but noticeable, effects occurring after the age of 60 or 70 years. However, there is a great deal of individual variation in the rate and onset of decline, with some older adults showing no decline and a small percentage even showing improvement in cognitive abilities (Aartsen et al., 2002; Field & Gueldner, 2001). In healthy, active, and mentally stimulated older adults, the deficits are generally minimal and do not interfere with daily functioning. In older adults with risk factors, however, the cognitive declines are likely to progress and interfere with daily functioning. A research review concluded that a wealth of evidence suggests that older adults perform well when carrying out routine tasks in familiar environments and that the impact of any cognitive deficits is most pronounced when older adults are in unfamiliar environments or performing new tasks (Park & Hall Gutchess, 2000). The terms *benign senescent forgetfulness* and *age-associated memory impairment* refer to memory deficits that are thought to occur in older adults, even in the absence of any risk factors. These deficits are minor and nonprogressive, and they are most noticeable in association with stressful conditions. In actuality, they are not much different from the kind of forgetfulness that all people experience at times. The major difference is that, when they occur in older people, they may cause more anxiety or be viewed as evidence of so-called senility.

Display 7-1 summarizes some of the conclusions drawn from studies of cognitive aging that have generated the greatest accord and provides information about factors that influence learning in older adults. These factors are important considerations in determining appropriate health education interventions. It is important to keep in mind that conclusions about cognitive aging do not address cultural factors and therefore are limited by the factors cited in Culture Box 7-1. Figure 7-1 summarizes the age-related changes, risk factors, and functional consequences that may affect cognitive function.

DISPLAY 7-1
Functional Consequences Affecting Cognition in Older Adults

Intellectual Abilities

- Healthy older adults show no decline, and perhaps improve, in some cognitive skills, such as wisdom, judgment, creativity, common sense, coordination of facts and ideas, and breadth of knowledge and experience.
- Most older adults show a slight and gradual decline in some cognitive skills, such as abstraction, calculation, word fluency, verbal comprehension, spatial orientation, and inductive reasoning.
- Age-related cognitive declines are thought to begin at about 60 years of age.

Memory

- Short-term memory shows a modest decline in older adulthood.
- Remote memory may or may not be better than recent memory in older adults, but regardless of whether it changes, older adults have a larger store of information about the past than do younger adults.

- The following factors influence cognitive function: motivation, expectations, personality, task demands, learning habits, intellectual skills, educational level, sociocultural background, style of processing information, and actual and self-reported health status.
- Risk factors that interfere with cognitive function include anxiety, depression, sensory function, physical conditions, nutritional status, and level of physical activity and mental stimulation.

Learning Abilities of Older Adults

- Older adults are as capable of learning new things as younger people, but the speed with which they process information is slower.
- Older adults are more cautious in their responses and make more errors of omission.
- Potential barriers to learning in older adults include sensory deficits, lack of relevance, teacher–learner age differences, and values that are incongruent with new knowledge.

NURSING ASSESSMENT OF COGNITIVE FUNCTION

Formal assessment of intellectual performance is accomplished by administering psychometric tests, but nurses can use a functional approach to assess informally memory and cognitive skills. In addition to assessing the intellectual performance of older adults, nurses can assess for risk factors that might contribute to cognitive deficits. For example, a nursing study of the relationships among loneliness, social support, and decline in cognitive function in hospitalized elderly people emphasized the need to assess thoroughly their cognitive status as well as

social support to identify risk factors for negative consequences of hospitalization (Ryan, 1998). Because nursing assessment of cognition is an integral part of the psychosocial assessment, it is addressed comprehensively in Chapter 10, rather than in this chapter.

NURSING DIAGNOSIS

Because age-related changes in cognitive function in healthy older adults do not significantly affect activities of daily living, the only nursing diagnosis that might be applicable is Health-Seeking Behaviors. This is defined as "the state in which an individual in stable health actively seeks ways to alter personal health habits and/or the environment in order to move toward a higher level of wellness" (Carpenito, 2002, p. 466). This diagnosis could be applied to older adults who are aware of some decline in their intellectual abilities and who wish to preserve specific cognitive abilities, such as memory. Nurses working in community settings may have opportunities to address this health-related concern of older adults, perhaps through group health education. The case example and nursing care plan at the end of this chapter illustrate interventions related to cognitive function in older adulthood that might be used for individual or group health education.

CULTURE BOX 7-1	Cultural Factors and Cognitive Function

- It is important to recognize that the standards of intellectual performance used in the United States have been developed for English-speaking white Americans.
- It is important to recognize that cognitive abilities are highly influenced by health, education, and socioeconomic status and that these factors and cultural factors are interrelated.
- Cultural and language factors may influence an older adult's perception and description of memory problems.

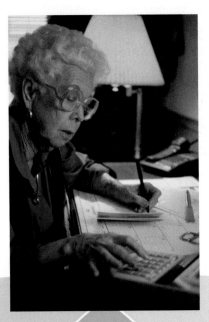

Age-related changes
- Older adults may show decline in some intellectual skills, but they are capable of cognitive growth and intellectual development throughout adulthood

Negative functional consequences
- Slight decline in short-term memory
- No decline in crystalized intelligence (e.g., wisdom, creativity, common sense, breadth of knowledge)
- Slight, gradual decline in fluid intelligence (e.g., abstraction, calculation, spatial orientation, inductive reasoning)
- Slower processing of information

Risk factors
- Impaired sensory function
- Alcohol consumption
- Medications (e.g., anticholinergics)
- Physiologic disorders (e.g., malnutrition)
- Psychosocial influences (e.g., anxiety, depression)
- Environmental distractions
- Lack of motivation
- Lack of stimulation

FIGURE 7-1. Age-related changes and risk factors intersect to negatively affect cognitive function in older adults.

OUTCOMES

An outcome criterion for older adults with Health-Seeking Behaviors related to cognitive function would be that the person takes responsibility for maintaining or compensating for age-related cognitive changes. An indicator of achievement would be that the person participates in activities that address risk factors (e.g., participation in physically and mentally stimulating activities) or compensates for age-related changes (e.g., use of memory-enhancing techniques).

NURSING INTERVENTIONS TO PROMOTE HEALTHY COGNITIVE FUNCTION

Studies have consistently found that good nutrition, stress reduction, lifelong learning, continued social engagement, mental and physical exercise, and primary and secondary prevention of cardiovascular disease and other pathologic conditions are effective health promotion activities for cognitive health in older adults (Fillit, 2002). Thus, many of the health promotion interventions discussed throughout this text are also effective in promoting optimal cognitive function. Also, because vision and hearing impairments can interfere with cognitive abilities, any interventions directed toward improving sensory function (discussed in Chapters 12 and 13) may be effective in improving cognitive function.

During the 1980s, geropsychologists focused on identifying techniques that older adults can use to maintain or increase their cognitive abilities. The Penn State Adult Development and Enrichment Project (ADEPT) was devised to address this issue, and initial findings emphasized that, at any age, there is room for intellectual performance enhancement (Baltes & Willis, 1982).

Willis (1987) described the following types of interventions for older adults with age-related cognitive changes:

- Remediation-in-kind interventions, which directly improve a cognitive skill (e.g., practicing to improve perceptual speed skills)
- Remediation-with-compensation interventions, which involve the improvement of one skill to compensate for a decline in another (e.g., increasing one's level of caution to compensate for a slower speed of performance)
- Compensation interventions, which compensate for irreversible declines (e.g., the use of external devices as reminder systems)

During the 1990s, researchers identified the following strategies that are effective for cognitive performance enhancement in older adults (i.e., a method for performing a particular cognitive task): organization, associations, imagery or visualization, and verbal memory training (Willis, 2001). Recent large-scale studies have confirmed the effectiveness of cognitive training interventions in improving everyday functioning and preventing cognitive decline in older adults (Ball et al., 2002).

Promoting Further Education

In addition to using the interventions discussed here, nurses can encourage older adults to take advantage of the many educational programs that are geared specifically for them. For example, some universities and colleges (particularly community colleges) offer reduced-rate or no-fee courses for students age 60 years and older. Some programs also offer associate degrees, certification programs, or a General Equivalency Diploma (GED) for older adults.

Elderhostel is a national organization that provides numerous opportunities for individuals aged 55 years and older to become involved in educational and social action groups in the United States and world-wide. These educational activities involve short-term residential programs that usually last 4 to 5 days in the United States and 2 to 4 weeks in other countries. The Institutes for Learning in Retirement (ILR) is a network of community-based organizations for retirement-aged learners that develop and implement educational programs in affiliation with a college or university. These sessions typically involve homework and usually are held for a couple of hours weekly for several months (see the Educational Resources section for information about Elderhostel and ILR). Less formal education programs often are available through local senior centers and adult education programs affiliated with local school districts.

Nurses also can actively promote the use of computers by older adults for mental stimulation and practical benefits, such as increased communication with others and the acquisition of information that is relevant to their health and daily functioning. Hendrix and Sakauye (2001) have developed an excellent nursing model for teaching older adults about using computers.

Teaching About Memory and Cognition

The concept of metacognition suggests that an understanding of one's own cognitive processes can influence performance. For example, someone who wants to remember a list of names needs both the intent to remember and knowledge about techniques for remembering. In addition, knowledge about which techniques are most effective would improve his or her performance. The following interventions, therefore, are essential for optimal cognitive function: (1) correction of misinformation and negative expectations; (2) provision of accurate information about age-related changes; and (3) provision of information about techniques to enhance cognitive abilities. Thus, just as health education about techniques for improving physical health is an important nursing intervention, so too is health education about techniques for improving cognitive health.

In community and long-term care settings, group sessions can be effective and efficient ways of addressing many psychosocial aspects of aging, including cognitive function. For example, the Healthy Aging Class (described in detail in Chapter 8) can be used as a model for health education about age-related cognitive changes. A model developed by Turner Geriatric Services at the University of Michigan can be used for either a single- or multiple-session program for older adults. A training manual provides information about developing memory-training programs, and it includes lesson plans and handouts for group leaders (Fogler & Stern, 1994). Display 7-2, which outlines a

DISPLAY 7-2
Memory Training for Older Adults

Introduction

- Forgetting is a normal part of life for all people, but memory skills can be learned. The purposes of this program are to look at some reasons people forget things and to discuss ways of improving memory skills.
- When older adults are forgetful, they may blame it on old age, rather than seeing it as something that happens to everyone, regardless of age.
- Memory problems can be viewed as a challenge. Anyone can improve his or her memory, but as with any other skill, an effort must be made.

Stages of Memory

- *Sensory memory* lasts only a few seconds. It involves the awareness of information obtained through vision, hearing, smell, taste, and touch.
- *Short-term memory* is your working memory, or what's in your conscious thoughts. This, too, is very brief and contains small amounts of information. For example, this type of memory allows you to recall a telephone number as you dial it.
- *Long-term memory* is the memory bank, or what you depend on whenever you need to retrieve information. This memory bank is almost limitless and contains information you just learned, as well as information from long ago.

Memory Changes and Aging

- Aging is blamed for a lot of memory problems, but very few changes occur solely because of aging.
- In older adulthood, the processes of learning new information and recalling old information slow down a little. The overall ability to learn and remember, however, is not significantly affected in healthy older people.

Factors That Interfere with Memory

As people grow older, an increasing number of factors may interfere with their ability to remember, including the following:

- Not being attentive to the situation. This might be attributable, for example, to the fact that the situation is not relevant to you.
- Being distracted by a lot of things that interfere with your ability to concentrate. For example, this might be the result of worry or anxiety.
- Feeling stressed
- Having a physical illness or being tired
- Having vision, hearing, or other functional impairments that interfere with the ability to obtain information
- Feeling sad or depressed, or coping with loss or grief
- Not being intellectually stimulated (principle of "use it or lose it!")
- Not having cues to help you remember
- Not organizing information for easy retention; not being organized in daily life
- Taking medications or alcohol that interfere with mental abilities

- Not being physically fit (e.g., as a result of poor nutrition or lack of exercise)

Ways of Improving Memory Skills

- Write things down (e.g., use lists, calendars, and notebooks).
- Use auditory cues (e.g., timers, alarm clocks) in conjunction with written cues.
- Use environmental cues. (For instance, you might remove something from its usual place, then return it to its normal location after it has served its purpose as a reminder.)
- Assign specific places for specific items and keep the items in their proper place (e.g., keep keys on a hook near the door).
- Put reminders in appropriate places (e.g., place shoes that need to be repaired near the door).
- Use visual images. ("A picture is worth a thousand words.") Create a picture in your mind when you want to remember something; the more bizarre the picture, the more likely it is that you will remember.
- Use active observation: pay attention to details of what's going on around you and be alert to the environment.
- Make associations, or mental connections. (For example, the phrase "spring ahead, fall back" can be recalled to ensure accuracy in changing clocks for seasonal time changes [from daylight savings time to standard time and vice versa].)
- Make associations between names and mental images (e.g., Carol and Christmas carol).
- Rehearse items you want to remember by repeating them aloud or writing the information on paper.
- Use self-instruction; say things aloud (e.g., "I'm putting my keys on the counter so I remember to turn off the stove before I leave").
- Divide information into small parts that can be remembered easily. (For instance, to remember an address or a zip code, divide it into groups [seven hundred sixty, fifty-five].)
- Organize information into logical categories (e.g., shampoo and hair spray, toothpaste and mouthwash, soap and deodorant).
- Use rhyming cues (e.g., "In 1492, Columbus sailed the ocean blue.").
- Use first-letter cues and make associations. (For example, to remember to buy carrots, apples, radishes, pickles, eggs, and tea bags, remember the word CARPET.)
- Make word associations. (For instance, to remember the letters of your license plate, make a word, such as camel, out of the letters CML.)
- Search the alphabet while focusing on what you're trying to remember. (For example, to remember that someone's name is Martin, start with names that begin with A and continue naming names through the alphabet until your memory is jogged for the correct one.)
- Make up a story to connect things you want to remember. (For instance, if you have to go to the cleaners and the post office, create a story about mailing a pair of pants.)

DISPLAY 7-2
Memory Training for Older Adults (Continued)

Conclusion

- Don't try to remember all of these techniques—you'll need another method just to remember them all!
- Select a few techniques that you like, and use these whenever appropriate or needed.
- Minimize any distractions; pay attention to one thing at a time.
- Give yourself time to remember; forgetfulness is most likely to occur when you are in a hurry. Try to prepare in advance, when you have time to concentrate.

- Maintain some sense of organization in your daily life, and devise systems to organize routine tasks, like taking medications.
- Carry a note pad or calendar, and use written records so you don't have to rely entirely on mental cues.
- Relax and maintain a sense of humor. If you become anxious about your memory and are convinced you can't remember, then you will create a self-fulfilling prophecy.

(Adapted, with permission, from Fogler, J., & Stern, L. [1994]. *Improvinig your memory: How to remember what you're starting to forget*. Baltimore: Johns Hopkins University Press.)

sample presentation for older adults based on the material from the Turner Geriatric Clinic, can be used to educate older adults about techniques for memory enhancement. Examples of additional models for group educational programs to enhance cognitive abilities in older adults can be found in gerontological journals (e.g., Rapp et al., 2002; Weinstein & Sachs, 2000; Werner, 2000).

Teaching About Concentration and Attention Enhancement Techniques

When one's ability to attend to the environment and concentrate on visual and auditory cues is limited, the ability to learn and remember is also impaired. Thus, techniques such as relaxation and imagery, which enhance attention and concentration, may also improve memory and learning. Likewise, any method that reduces environmental distractions may also improve one's cognitive abilities. Many of the popular self-help books describe methods of relaxation as a way of opening the mind to new learning. The relaxation technique outlined in Chapter 20 (Display 20-3) can be taught to older adults for a variety of uses, including the enhancement of mental skills. Nurses can encourage older adults to use these techniques as mental health practices that can improve cognitive abilities.

Adapting Health Education Materials for Older Adults

Much of the research on cognitive aging has centered on factors that affect learning in older adulthood. For example, some researchers have found that visual, rather than auditory, presentation of educational materials results in better recall, learning, and retrieval of

information (Constantinidou, 2002). Because many nursing interventions include patient teaching or health education, principles regarding cognitive aging can be used to adapt educational methods and materials to older adults. The suggestions presented in this text for communicating with older adults and compensating for hearing and vision deficits can be applied to health education. Display 7-3 summarizes guidelines

DISPLAY 7-3
Guidelines for Health Education for Older Adults

Conditions That Are Most Conducive to Learning

- Contexts that are supportive and rewarding (e.g., praise), in contrast to those that are neutral, challenging, or critical
- An environment that is pleasant, familiar, brightly lit, and has the least number of distractions possible
- Information that relates to prior experiences and is personally relevant, rather than meaningless
- Information that is concrete rather than abstract

Presentation Methods Most Conducive to Learning

- A self-paced, rather than externally paced, rate
- Emphasis on the integration and application of knowledge and experience, rather than on the acquisition of large amounts of new information
- Use of visual methods for material that is meaningful and lends itself to thoughtful analysis
- Use of auditory methods, alone or in combination with visual ones, for information that is factual and straightforward
- Provision of advance organizers, such as outlines, written cues, and introductory overviews
- Reinforcement of the value of organizing aids

that can be applied to educational interventions for older adults. Examples of models of educational materials that have been adapted to meet the unique learning styles of older adults can be found in the nursing and gerontology literature (e.g., Conn et al., 2001; Rankin & Stallings, 2001; Van Wynen, 2001).

EVALUATING EFFECTIVENESS OF NURSING INTERVENTIONS

Nursing care of older adults who want to maintain a high level of cognitive function is evaluated by the degree to which these adults express satisfaction with their cognitive abilities, such as memory skills. Objectively, it is evaluated by the degree to which they use their cognitive abilities to meet their daily needs. For example, an older adult who forgets to keep appointments might learn to use a calendar or other organizational aids to remember the appointments. In this situation, the effectiveness of interventions would be measured by how well the person remembers to keep appointments.

CHAPTER SUMMARY

Age-related changes affecting some intellectual skills are noticed at about 60 years of age, even in healthy adults. These changes are minor and do not interfere significantly with daily function, especially if compensatory interventions are used. Factors that influence cognitive abilities in older adulthood include chemical effects (e.g., medications), personal characteristics (e.g., educational level), and physical and mental health status (e.g., sensory function). Any major decline in cognitive function is caused by disease conditions, such as dementia or other risk factors, as discussed in Chapter 24. Functional consequences affecting cognition include a slight and gradual decline in some intellectual abilities, such as short-term memory.

Nursing assessment of cognition is reviewed in Chapter 10 as part of the comprehensive psychosocial assessment. Health-Seeking Behaviors is a nursing diagnosis that might be used for older adults with age-related changes in cognitive function. A nursing goal is to teach older adults to use techniques aimed at improving or maintaining intellectual performance. This is accomplished through educational interventions, such as memory training. Nursing care is evaluated by the degree to which the older adult successfully uses memory-training skills to improve his or her functional level.

CONCLUDING CASE STUDY AND NURSING CARE PLAN

▶ Mrs. C. is 71 years old and lives alone in her own home. She attends a local Senior Wellness clinic for blood pressure checks, health screenings (e.g., cholesterol levels), and her annual flu shot. During her monthly visit for a blood pressure check, she confides that she is embarrassed about missing a doctor's appointment last week. She says she has been noticing increased difficulties with memory, and one of her friends has told her that she probably has Alzheimer's disease. She asks if there's a place where she can get a test for Alzheimer's.

■ Nursing Assessment

Your nursing assessment indicates that Mrs. C. has missed a couple of health care appointments during the past year. She said she missed a dental appointment 6 months ago when she was very worried about her daughter, who was undergoing diagnostic tests for a lump in her breast. Last week, when she missed her doctor's appointment, she had been busy shopping for presents for her grandson's wedding. When you ask about additional problems with memory, Mrs. C. admits that she has more difficulty remembering people's names than she used to have. You do not identify any risk factors that might affect Mrs. C.'s cognitive abilities (e.g., depression, medication effects, poor nutrition). Mrs. C. has never used calendars, and she says she remembers her doctor's appointments by keeping the appointment cards in her desk drawer along with her bills and her checkbook. She says that she checks her appointment cards every month, but she had not noticed the cards for the two appointments she missed.

■ Nursing Diagnosis

You use the nursing diagnosis of Health-Seeking Behaviors because Mrs. C. is interested in learning about memory-training skills to assist her in remembering appointments. Mrs. C. has a poor understanding of age-related cognitive changes, and she indicates that she is interested in learning about ways to improve her memory.

■ Nursing Care Plan

The nursing care plan you devise for Mrs. C. is shown in Display 7-4.

DISPLAY 7-4 • NURSING CARE PLAN FOR MR. C.

EXPECTED OUTCOME	NURSING INTERVENTIONS	NURSING EVALUATION
Mrs. C. will express an interest in improving her memory skills.	• Use information in Display 7-1 to teach Mrs. C. about age-related changes that affect cognitive abilities. • Discuss the difference between dementia and age-associated memory impairment. • Emphasize that memory skills can be developed through memory training techniques.	Mrs. C. will agree to participate in a discussion of memory training skills.
Mrs. C. will use memory training techniques to improve her functional level.	• Give Mrs. C. a copy of Display 7-2 and review the information. • Assist Mrs. C. in identifying one or two strategies for remembering appointments (e.g., begin using a calendar). • Assist Mrs. C. in identifying one or two strategies for remembering the names of people she meets (e.g., using visual images).	Mrs. C. will report success in using a method for remembering appointments. Mrs. C. will report success in using a method for remembering names of people.

 CRITICAL THINKING EXERCISES

1. Identify the factors in your own life that interfere with cognitive function.
2. What memory aids do you use in your life? Are they effective? Would you like to develop additional memory aids?
3. You are working in a senior center and have suggested that the center sponsor a series of classes on the memory problems of older adults. This suggestion is based on your observation that many of the older adults have asked you questions about memory problems, and some are concerned about Alzheimer's disease. Address each of the following issues:
   • The center director is a firm believer in the adage, "you can't teach an old dog new tricks." How would you convince the director that the classes you wish to offer are worthwhile?
   • How would you structure the sessions (number and length of sessions, number of participants, and so forth)?
   • Describe the content you would cover and the approach you would use for each topic. Include information about normal cognitive aging, risk factors for impaired cognitive function, and techniques for improving memory and other aspects of cognition.
   • What audiovisual aids, including written materials, would you use?
   • How would you adapt your teaching method and materials for the group?
   • How would you evaluate the sessions?

EDUCATIONAL RESOURCES

Elderhostel Institute Network (EIN)
11 Avenue de Lafayette, Boston, MA 02111-1746
(877) 426-8056
http://www.elderhostel.org/ein/intro.asp

Turner Geriatric Clinic
University of Michigan Health Systems
1500 East Medical Center Drive, Ann Arbor, MI 48109
(734) 764-2556
http://www.med.umich.edu
(Publications include *Improving Your Memory: How to Remember What You're Starting to Forget* and *Teaching Memory Improvement to Adults*)

REFERENCES

Aartsen, M. J., Smits, C. H. M., van Tilburg, T., Knipscheer, K. C. P. M., & Deeg, D. J. H. (2002). Activity in older adults: Cause or consequence of cognitive functioning? A longitudinal study on everyday activities and cognitive performance in older adults. *Journals of Gerontology: Psychological Sciences, 57B*, P153–P162.

Albert, M. S., & Killiany, R. J. (2001). Age-related cognitive change and brain-behavior relationships. In J. E. Birren and K. W. Schaie (Eds.), *Handbook of the psychology of aging* (5th ed., pp.161–185). San Diego: Academic Press.

Backman, L., Small, B. J., & Wahlin, A. (2001). Aging and memory: Cognitive and biological perspectives. In J. E. Birren & K. W. Schaie (Eds.), *Handbook of the psychology of aging* (5th ed., pp. 349–377). San Diego: Academic Press.

Ball, K., Berch, D. B., Helmers, K. F., Jobe, J. B., Leveck, M. D., Marsiske, M., et al. (2002). Effects of cognitive training interventions with older adults: A randomized controlled trial. *Journal of the American Medical Association, 288*, 2271–2281.

Ball, L. J., & Birge, S. J. (2002). Prevention of brain aging and dementia. *Clinics in Geriatric Medicine, 18*, 485–504.

Baltes, P. B., & Willis, S. L. (1982). Plasticity and enhancement of intellectual functioning in old age. In F. I. M. Craik & S. Trehab (Eds.), *Advances in the study of communication and affect* (Vol. 8, pp. 353–389). New York: Plenum Press.

Botwinick, J. (1984). *Aging and behavior* (3rd ed.). New York: Springer.

Cagney, K. A., & Lauderdale, D. S. (2002). Education, wealth, and cognitive function in later life. *Journal of Gerontology: Psychological Sciences, 57B*, P163–P172.

Calvaresi, E., & Bryan, J. (2001). B vitamins, cognition, and aging: A review. *Journal of Gerontology: Psychological Sciences, 56B*, P327–P339.

Carpenito, L. J. (2002). *Nursing diagnosis: Application to clinical practice* (9th ed.). Philadelphia: Lippincott Williams & Wilkins.

Colcombe, S. J., Erickson, K. I., Raz, N., Webb, A. G., Cohen, N. J., McAuley, E., & Kramer, A. F. (2003). Aerobic fitness reduces brain tissue loss in aging humans. *Journal of Gerontology: Medical Sciences, 58A*, 176–180.

Conn, V. S., Armer, J. M., & Hayes, K. S. (2001). Knowledge deficit. In M. L. Maas, K. C. Buckwalter, M. D. Hardy, T. Tripp-Reimer, M. G. Titler, & J. P. Specht (Eds.), *Nursing care of older adults: Diagnoses, outcomes, and interventions* (pp. 503–515). St. Louis: Mosby.

Constantinidou, F. (2002). Stimulus modality and verbal learning performance in normal aging. *Brain and Language, 82*, 296–311.

DeFries, C. M., Dixon, R. A., & Backman, L. (2003). Use of memory compensation strategies is related to psychosocial and health indicators. *Journal of Gerontology: Psychological Sciences, 58B*, P12–P22.

Field, D., & Gueldner, S. H. (2001). The oldest-old: How do they differ from the old-old? *Journal of Gerontological Nursing, 27*(8), 20–27.

Fillit, H. M. (2002). Achieving and maintaining cognitive vitality with aging. *Mayo Clinic Proceedings, 77*, 681–696.

Fogler, J., & Stern, L. (1994). *Teaching memory improvement to adults* (rev. ed.). Baltimore: The Johns Hopkins University Press.

Fozard, J. L., & Gordon-Salant, S. (2001). Changes in vision and hearing. In J. E. Birren & K. W. Schaie (Eds.), *Handbook of the psychology of aging* (5th ed., pp. 1241–266). San Diego: Academic Press.

Hasher, L., & Zacks, R. T. (1979). Autonomic and effortful processes in memory. *Journal of Experimental Psychology: General, 108*, 356–388.

Hendrix, C. C., & Sakauye, K. M. (2001). Teaching elderly individuals on computer use. *Journal of Gerontological Nursing, 27*(6), 47–53.

Hess, T. M., Auman, C., Colcombe, S. J., & Rahhal, T. A. (2003). The impact of stereotype threat on age differences in memory performance. *Journal of Gerontology: Psychological Sciences, 58B*, P3–P11.

Horn, J. L. (1982). The theory of fluid and crystallized psychology and aging in adulthood. In F. I. M. Criak & S. Trehab (Eds.), *Advances in the study of communication and affect* (Vol. 8, pp. 237–378). New York: Plenum Press.

Johansson, B., Allan-Burge, R., & Zarit, S. H. (1997). Self-reports on memory functioning in a longitudinal study of the older old: Relation to current, prospective, and retrospective performance. *Journals of Gerontology: Psychological Sciences, 52B*, P139–P146.

Labouvie-Vief, G., & Blanchard-Fields, F. (1982). Cognitive aging and psychological growth. *Ageing and Society, 2*, 183–209.

Magai, C. (2001). Emotions over the life span. In J. E. Birren and K. W. Schaie (Eds.), *Handbook of the psychology of aging* (5th ed., pp. 399–426). San Diego: Academic Press.

Morris, M. C. (2002). Vitamin E and cognitive decline in older persons. *Archives of Neurology, 59*, 1125–1132.

Naylor, E., Penev, P. D., Orbeta, L., Janssen, I., Ortiz, R., Colecchia, E. F., et al. (2000). Daily social and physical activity increase slow-wave sleep and daytime neuropsychological performance in the elderly. *Sleep, 23*(1), 87–95.

Ortega, R. M. (2002). Cognitive function in elderly people is influenced by vitamin E status. *Journal of Nutrition, 132*, 2065–2068.

Park, D. C. (2000). The basic mechanisms accounting for age-related decline in cognitive function. In D. C. Park & N. Schwarz (Eds.). *Cognitive aging: A primer* (pp. 1–21). Philadelphia: Psychology Press.

Park, D. C., & Hall Gutchess. (2000). Cognitive aging and everyday life. In N. Charness, D. C. Park, & B. Sabel (Eds.), *Aging and communication* (pp. 217–232). New York: Springer.

Persad, C. C., Abeles, N., Zacks, R. T., & Denburg, N. L. (2002). Inhibitory changes after 60 and their relationship to measures of attention and memory. *Journal of Gerontology: Psychological Sciences, 57B*, P223–P232.

Rankin S. H., & Stallings, K. D. (2001). *Patient education: Principles and practice* (4th ed). Philadelphia: Lippincott Williams & Wilkins.

Rapp, S., Brenes, G., & Marsh, A. P. (2002). Memory enhancement training for older adults with mild cognitive impairment: A preliminary study. *Aging & Mental Health, 6*(1), 5–11.

Rebok, G. W., & Plude, D. J. (2001). Relation of physical activity to memory functioning in older adults: The memory workout program. *Educational Gerontology, 27*, 241–259.

Roe, C., Anderson, M. J., & Spivak, B. (2002). Use of anticholinergic medications by older adults with dementia. *Journal of the American Geriatrics Society, 50*, 836–842.

Rohling, M. L., & Scogin, F. (1993). Autonomic and effortful memory processes in depressed persons. *Journal of Gerontology: Psychological Sciences, 48*, P87–P95.

Ryan, M. C. (1998). The relationship between loneliness, social support, and decline in cognitive function in the hospitalized elderly. *Journal of Gerontological Nursing, 24*(3), 19–27.

Schaie, K. W. (1977–1978). Toward a stage theory of adult cognitive development. *Journal of Aging and Human Development, 8*, 129–138.

Schaie, K. W., & Hofer, S. C. (2001). Longitudinal studies in aging research. In J. E. Birren & K. W. Schaie (Eds.), *Handbook of the psychology of aging* (5th ed., pp. 53–77). San Diego: Academic Press.

Schaie, K. W., & Willis, S. L. (1986). *Adult development and aging.* Boston: Little, Brown.

Simensky, J. D., & Abeles, N. (2002). Decline in verbal memory performance with advancing age: The role of frontal lobe functioning. *Aging & Mental Health, 6*, 293–303.

Sternberg, R. J., & Lubart, T. I. (2001). Wisdom and creativity. In J. E. Birren and K. W. Schaie (Eds.), *Handbook of the psychology of aging* (5th ed., pp. 500–522). San Diego: Academic Press.

Thomson, D. (2001). The getting and losing wisdom. *Journal of Religious Gerontology, 12* (3/4), 77–88.

Tune, L. E. (2001). Anticholinergic effects of medication in elderly patients. *Journal of Clinical Psychiatry, 62*(Suppl 21), 11–14.

Turrell, G., Lynch, J. W., Kaplan, G. A., Everson, S. A., Helkala, E-L., Kauhanen, J., et al. (2002). Socioeconomic position across the lifecourse and cognitive function in late middle age. *Journals of Gerontology: Social Sciences, 57B*, S43-S51.

Van Wynen, E. A. (2001). A key to successful aging: Learning-style patterns of older adults. *Journal of Gerontological Nursing, 27*(9), 6–15.

Vinters, H. V. (2001). Aging and the human nervous system. In J. E. Birren & K. W. Schaie (Eds.), *Handbook of the psychology of aging* (5th ed., pp. 135–160). San Diego: Academic Press.

Weinstein, C. S., & Sachs, W. (2000). Memory 101: A psychotherapist's guide to understanding and teaching memory strategies to patients and significant others. *Journal of Geriatric Psychiatry: A Multidisciplinary Journal of Mental Health and Aging, 33*(1), 5–26.

Werner, P. (2000). Assessing the effectiveness of a memory club for elderly persons suffering from mild cognitive deterioration. *Clinical Gerontologist, 22*(1), 3–14.

Willis, S. L. (1987). Cognitive training and everyday competence. In K. W. Schaie & C. Eisdorfer (Eds.), *Annual review of gerontology and geriatrics* (pp. 159–188). New York: Springer.

Willis, S. L. (2001). Methodological issues in behavioral intervention research with the elderly. In J. E. Birren & K. W. Schaie (Eds.), *Handbook of the psychology of aging* (5th ed., pp. 78–108). San Diego: Academic Press.

Woodruff, D. S. (1983). A review of aging and cognitive processes. *Research on Aging, 5*(2), 139–153.

Yaffe, K., Barnes, D., Nevitt, M., Lui, L-Y, & Covinsky, K. (2001). A prospective study of physical activity and cognitive decline in elderly women. *Archives of Internal Medicine, 161*, 1703–1708.

Psychosocial Function

Although the physiologic changes and chronic illnesses associated with older adulthood may affect a person's functional abilities, the psychosocial changes are often the most challenging and demanding in terms of coping energy. Of course, some of the psychosocial challenges arise from physical changes, but many are attributable to changes in roles, relationships, and living environments. Because many of the psychosocial changes are inevitable and somewhat predictable, older adults can prepare for and respond to psychosocial changes by developing and using effective coping strategies. Nurses can identify both the age-related psychosocial changes and the risk factors associated with negative functional consequences with regard to psychosocial function for the older adult. Interventions can then be directed toward supporting effective coping mechanisms and assisting in the development of new coping strategies.

AGE-RELATED CHANGES THAT AFFECT PSYCHOSOCIAL FUNCTION: LIFE EVENTS

Certain life events demand an emotional adjustment on the part of the person experiencing the event, and different challenges are likely to occur during different periods in one's life. For example, younger adults are likely to experience the following life events: establishing a career, moving away from the nuclear family, committing to a partner, buying a house, and beginning a family. The major life events of younger adulthood are familiar to us through either personal experiences or the shared experiences of friends. People usually view these events positively and choose them purposefully. By contrast, the life events of older adulthood might be unknown, unexpected, and, in fact, unwanted or even feared. Also, in contrast to the life events of younger adulthood, many life events associated with old age involve losses, rather than gains. In addition, the losses of older adulthood are likely to be losses of significant others and objects that have been part of life for many decades.

The life events most likely to occur in older adulthood have several characteristics that distinguish them from the life events and adjustments associated with younger adulthood. These distinguishing features include the following:

- They usually involve losses, rather than gains.
- They are likely to occur close together, with less time available to adjust to each event.
- They are longer lasting and often become chronic problems.
- They are inevitable, evoking a feeling of powerlessness.

Some examples of common life events requiring psychosocial adjustments in older adulthood are retirement, relocation, chronic illness and functional impairments, decisions about driving a car, widowhood, death of friends and family, and confrontation of ageist attitudes. The longer a person lives, the more likely it is that all of these events will happen.

Figure 8-1 illustrates some of the major life events that are likely to occur in older adulthood, as well as the related consequences. The illustration attempts to show the interrelatedness among the life events of older adulthood.

Retirement

Retirement from a primary career is viewed as a milestone that marks the passage into later stages of adulthood (Kim & Moen, 2002). Societal attitudes can influence one's adjustment to retirement, particularly in societies like that of the United States, where a strong work ethic is held and people are valued based on their contribution to the workforce. Working people have a higher social status than unemployed people. Moreover, among working people, status is based on the kind of job one holds and the salary one earns. Therefore, when people retire, they inevitably cope with a change in social status, and the psychosocial challenge may be the greatest for people whose self-concept is based on job status. Health and wealth are the factors that most significantly influence the decision to retire, but additional influential factors include job conditions, pension availability, family circumstances, opportunities for continued employment, and continued ability to perform job responsibilities (Eckerdt, 2001). For married couples, the spouse, as well as the worker, must adjust to the changes related to retirement; indeed, the adjustment might be even more difficult for the spouse than for the retiree.

> When women retire they have higher initial levels of depressive symptoms and lower levels of morale, personal control, and perceived income adequacy compared with those of men (Kim & Moen, 2002).

Relocation

Another area of psychosocial adjustment for older adults is the decision to move from the family home. As people grow older and their family situations change, relocation from the family home is likely to be a major decision. Older people in urban areas often find they are living in unsafe or isolated conditions because the neighborhood around them has changed gradually. For example, many older people live in urban areas that were originally settled by people of the same ethnic background. Neighbors who were of the same cultural background may have moved away, leaving one or two socially isolated older people. For people in rural areas, the geographic distance and lack of supportive services may lead to serious consequences for older adults who are functionally impaired, especially if they have few social supports. Additional problems arise when the older homeowner is less able physically and financially to maintain the house and pay for utilities.

In addition to the environmental factors that necessitate relocation, changes in health, functioning, support systems, and life circumstances frequently cause older adults to relocate to more supportive housing. Factors that increase the risk for relocation in later adulthood include loss of spouse, lack of available assistive services, lack of a kinship network or caregiver, chronic conditions and declining functional abilities,

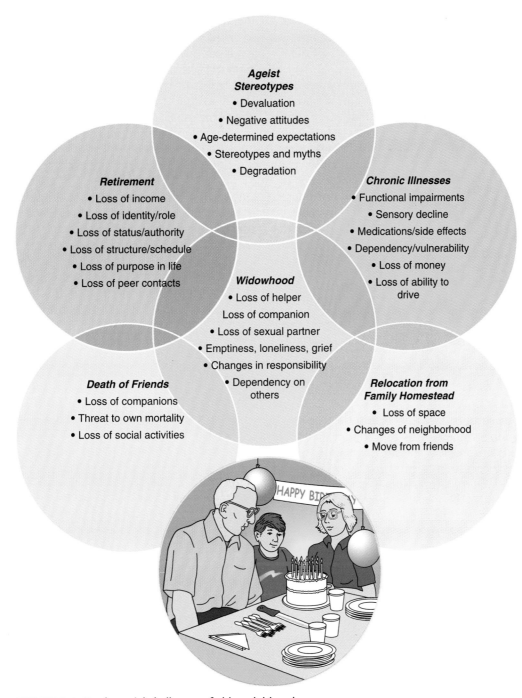

FIGURE 8-1 Psychosocial challenges of older adulthood

and cognitive impairment or psychiatric illness. Relocation occurs more often for women than men, for urban residents than rural residents, and for married couples than widows (Johnson & Tripp-Reimer, 2001).

The three relocations that commonly occur in the last three decades of life are (1) a voluntary move to a desirable geographic location shortly after retirement, (2) a move to be close to family members and medical care, and (3) a move to more supportive housing (e.g., assisted living, senior apartments) when health needs change (Johnson, 2001). Relocation to a nursing home is a significant life event for some older adults. Although only about 5% of people aged 65 years or older in the United States are in a nursing facility at any one time, the chance of being admitted to a nursing facility at some time is about

50% for a person aged 65 years. Because most of these admissions are for short-term stays, nurses caring for older adults in hospitals and nursing homes frequently deal with relocation adjustments of older adults and their families.

In the early 1960s, social gerontologists coined the terms "transfer trauma" and "transplantation shock" in reference to the high mortality rate that was associated with relocation to nursing homes (Aldrich & Mendkoff, 1963). High mortality rates within the first 6 months of being admitted to a nursing facility continue to be the focus of studies. Many variables, including health and social factors, interact to influence adjustment to relocation (Aneshensel et al., 2000). Today, gerontologists do not consider an increased risk for mortality to be an inevitable consequence of relocation per se, and the older adult's degree of willingness to move and level of involvement in decision making are seen as important variables.

> Perceived choice may be of greater importance to older adults of European descent than to those whose cultural background is based on family decision-making values (Johnson & Tripp-Reimer, 2001).

In the American health care system, the decision regarding nursing home care is too often viewed as strictly a medical decision, rather than as a medical–psychosocial decision with serious psychosocial consequences. Medical professionals do not always address the serious financial and emotional significance of decisions regarding long-term care, and it is often the gerontological nurse who deals with these decisions from a holistic perspective. In fact, nurses are the health care professionals who are likely to have the most important role in assisting older adults with this major life event.

Chronic Illness and Functional Impairments

Another major life adjustment for many older adults is coping with chronic illnesses and functional limitations, particularly limitations that curtail their independence. Although chronic illnesses are not an inevitable part of aging, 85% of people older than 65 years of age have one chronic illness, and 50% have two or more. Most older adults are able to function with little or no assistance in daily activities; however, the longer a person lives, the more likely it is that he or she will experience functional limitations.

Most functional limitations necessitate only minor adjustments in daily living, but some functional consequences, such as immobility or sensory impairments, significantly increase a person's dependency on others. Other consequences of chronic illnesses include altered self-concept; changes in lifestyle; trips to primary care providers and hospitals; unpredictability about one's ability to do what one wants; expenditures for assistance, medications, and medical care; and adverse medication effects, which sometimes cause further functional impairments. People who have functional impairments also are more vulnerable to personal crimes and may feel more fearful of crime.

Decisions About Driving a Car

Age-related and disease-related changes in visual abilities, cognitive abilities, musculoskeletal function, and central nervous system function can affect the older adult's ability to drive safely. Factors associated with driving cessation in older adults are female gender, poor memory, advanced age, poor health, depressed mood, visual impairment, and limitations in daily activities (Foley et al., 2002; Marottoli et al., 2000). Gerontologists also have identified factors that are associated with an increased risk for motor vehicle crashes among older adults (e.g., stroke, dementia, visual impairment, and use of certain medications), but increased age and the number of miles driven are the two most consistently identified risk factors (Margolis et al., 2002). When motor vehicle crash rates are adjusted for miles driven, older drivers represent a crash risk equivalent to that of younger drivers (Bedard et al., 2001). Most older drivers gradually change their driving behavior by driving shorter distances, driving more slowly, decreasing or eliminating night and highway driving, and avoiding driving in congested areas or during rush-hour periods (Klavora & Heslegrave, 2002). Decisions about driving a car represent one of the most emotionally charged issues relating to functional impairment that older adults and their families face. Increasingly, these decisions involve gerontological nurses and other health care professionals who are responsible for assessing the person's risk to themselves and society (McGregor, 2002). In the United States, access to an automobile and the possession of a valid driver's license not only provide transportation but also serve as significant indicators of autonomy. In fact, for many older adults, the ability to drive is synonymous with independence, and the possession of a driver's license, even one that goes unused, is a symbol of one's ability to shield oneself from dependence on others.

The loss of an independent means of transportation affects every aspect of an older person's life, from the acquisition of food and medicine to opportunities for social interaction. Because of this global impact, families and older persons may avoid dealing with driving-related issues. Family members may be reluctant to suggest that an older relative give up driving for a number of reasons. For example, family members may not want to assume an authority role, or they may lack acceptable alternatives for transportation. It is not surprising, then, that older adults and their families may avoid or resist the decision to stop driving. Neither is it surprising that when older adults give up or significantly curtail their driving, they face a difficult psychosocial challenge that may be viewed as a major life event.

Widowhood

The example of widowhood as a life event of older adulthood illustrates all of the characteristics listed earlier. For most older couples, widowhood is inevitable, and the chances are greater that the woman will be widowed rather than the man. When widowhood occurs, additional consequences follow. Common additional consequences include loss of one's sexual partner; loss of companionship and intimacy; feelings of grief, loneliness, and emptiness; increased responsibilities and increased dependency on others; loss of income and less efficient financial management; and changes in relationships with children, married friends, and other family members. When a marriage has lasted for many decades, as is common in people who are in their 70s and 80s, the impact of the loss can be tremendous, and the feelings of grief, loneliness, and emptiness may be overwhelming. A study of grief responses of older widows found that being lonely and alone was the most troubling and most frequently cited problem (Hegge & Fischer, 2000).

Another characteristic of widowhood in older adulthood is that the chance of remarriage diminishes with advancing age, especially for women. Thus, there is little potential for resuming the married lifestyle. Last, if the married couple had clearly divided roles, as is common in the cohort of people who are old today, loss of the partner means an adjustment in important day-to-day tasks. For example, older couples often divide tasks so that only one of the two manages money, drives the car, cleans the house, shops for groceries, and does household repairs and maintenance. When the person responsible for a task is no longer able to perform the role, the other person may be unable, unwilling, or unprepared to assume this role.

The presence of a spouse may provide a buffer for older men (but not older women) against declining life satisfaction (Chipperfield & Havens, 2001), and widowhood is more distressing and has a more lasting depressive effect for men than women (Lee et al., 2001).

Death of Friends and Family

Like other life events of older adulthood, the loss of friends and family becomes inevitable with each advancing year. Many people who are in their 80s or 90s have outlived most, if not all, of their friends and many of their relatives. Indeed, people who are in their 90s may not even know anyone who is older than they are. Loneliness and social isolation are two consequences of these losses, particularly for older people with few social supports (van Baarsen, 2002; Wilson, 2001). Moreover, as people are confronted with the death of others who are younger than or similar to them in age, they become increasingly aware of their own mortality. Older people may read obituaries and death notices in the newspaper as a daily activity. Although families may view this activity as a morbid preoccupation, it may, in fact, be an effective way for older people to learn what is happening to their friends.

Ageist Attitudes

A life adjustment that, by its nature, is unique to older adulthood is the acceptance of being old. Because of the ageist attitudes common in modern industrialized societies, many older adults deny that they are old. Frequently, old age in our society is accompanied by feelings of devaluation and degradation. Even if a person has a good self-acceptance of being old, the person may feel that it is socially unacceptable to admit that it is okay to be old.

Because of these societal attitudes, older adults may be confronted with age-determined expectations that dictate appropriate social behaviors. For example, public displays of affection are viewed as socially appropriate for teenagers and younger adults. However, when older adults hold hands or kiss in public, observers are likely to make comments like, "Isn't that cute, look at that old couple holding hands." Having sexual relationships outside of a marriage is another action that is generally overlooked when done by young adults, but that is likely to be criticized when done by older adults.

As an example of age-determined expectations, consider the following scene: A gray-haired man, who was clearly an older adult, was wearing headphones and listening to music on a portable radio. He was briskly moving along in a combination dance–walk tempo on a public sidewalk in an urban area. Observers remarked that the old man looked like he needed psychiatric care, whereas they ignored several teens nearby who were exhibiting the same type of behavior. The only apparent difference between the older adult and the teens was that the younger people were listening to louder music and demonstrated less control in their movements. The primary difference, however, was in the age-determined expectations in the eyes of the beholders!

THEORIES ABOUT AGING AND PSYCHOSOCIAL FUNCTION

Theories about aging and psychosocial function address questions such as, How do emotions develop over the life course? What influences the way older adults respond to life events? Are certain life events more stressful for older adults? How do coping patterns change in older adulthood? In the following sections, a few of the more widely accepted theories about emotional development, stress, and coping are discussed. In addition, some of the recent conclusions about the response of older adults to stressful events are discussed. In keeping with the perspective of this text, these theories are used to explain the age-related changes that can cause positive or negative functional consequences with regard to psychosocial function.

Emotional Development and Aging Theories

For several decades, gerontologists have studied emotional development during later adulthood. Early studies, which focused on institutionalized older adults, suggested that a blunting of emotions and an increase in negative affect occurred in older adulthood, but more recent studies have challenged those assumptions (Magai, 2001). Researchers now emphasize that emotional expression is more complex in older adults, and that they experience events with more poignant, mixed, or bittersweet feelings (Carstensen et al., 2000). Conclusions from a summary of recent studies (Magai, 2001) about emotional development during aging are as follows:

- Affective experience may deepen and become more complex with age, at least up to and through middle age.
- The capacity to regulate emotions improves with age, at least until very old age.
- Older adults are better at avoiding anger and other negative affects (e.g., sadness).

Stress Theories

Hans Selye's stress theory, first proposed in 1956, laid the groundwork for contemporary theories of stress. Selye defined stress as the sum of all the nonspecific effects of factors that act on the body (Selye, 1956). These factors, including normal activities as well as disease states, are called *stressors*, and they are considered to be equally important regardless of whether they are pleasant or unpleasant. According to Selye's theory, people respond to stressors in three stages: alarm, resistance, and exhaustion. A major criticism of Selye's theory is his application of the term *stress* to the external stimuli, the internal consequences, and the actions taken to prevent or neutralize the event. Additional limitations of Selye's theory center on his lack of distinction between pleasant and unpleasant stressors and his failure to address the meaning of events for the person.

In addition to the work of Selye, the work of Holmes and Rahe (1967) is often used as a theoretical basis for investigating stress. According to this framework, stress is viewed as a mediator between a life event and adaptation to that event. Life events are defined as discrete and identifiable changes in life patterns that create stress and that can lead to negative health outcomes. According to this theory, stress causes physical and psychological harm that is in proportion to the intensity of the impact on and duration of a disruption in one's usual life pattern. Holmes and Rahe developed the Social Readjustment Rating Scale (SRRS) as a tool for measuring the duration and intensity of specific life events. The SRRS is a checklist of 43 life events, with relative weights assigned to each according to the usual amount of adaptive effort required by each event.

Because one of the criticisms of the SRRS is its assumption that life events always have a negative impact, researchers have been prompted to consider the meaning of life events for individuals. Variations of the SRRS have taken into account the meaning of life events for the person. Lazarus (1966), for instance, proposed a scale based on his cognitive appraisal approach. According to Lazarus, people initially appraise the significance of an event according to the way it actually or potentially affects their well-being. Secondarily, they appraise the event according to the personal and social resources that are available for coping, as well as the cost of these resources in relation to positive and negative outcomes. Using these concepts, Folkman and Lazarus (1980) proposed the Ways of Coping Checklist to measure individual thoughts, feelings, and actions in response to specific stressful situations. There is much agreement now that the response of different individuals to the same stressful event will show tremendous variability and that life events can have positive as well as negative effects (George, 2001).

In addition to questioning the impact of major life events, researchers also are questioning the impact of daily stresses. Older adults may experience more stress from the ordinary stressors of daily living, called hassles or chronic stress, than from specific life events. Gerontologists now view chronic stressors, defined as those that persist over long periods, as a major component of social stress (George, 2001). Older adults are likely to experience stressful hassles related to their health, income, home maintenance, and long-term caregiving responsibilities.

As life event scales have become more popular, the need for a scale specific to older adults has been identified. Most scales address issues that are pertinent to younger and middle-aged adults, excluding important life events that are relevant to older adults. In 1988, two nurses proposed the Stokes/Gordon Stress Scale (SGSS) for research of and clinical use with older adults (Stokes & Gordon, 1988). The SGSS is a 104-item checklist that can be self-administered and then scored according to a scoring sheet. The end result is a stress score, which can be used as a measure of the level of stress an older person is experiencing at a given time. The items in this checklist were identified through interviews with older adults, a literature review, and consultations with gerontological nurses. Some of the significant stresses, such as decreasing eyesight and hearing, can be addressed through nursing interventions aimed at improving functional abilities. Other significant stresses, such as losses of or changes in relationships, can be addressed through the psychosocial interventions discussed in this chapter. Table 8-1 identifies some of the SGSS items and their corresponding relative weights. The SGSS and a user's guide can be obtained from the Stokes/Gordon Stress Study (listed in the Educational Resources section of this chapter).

Coping Theories

One approach to studying age-related differences in coping has been to examine the internal mechanisms that people use in dealing with stressful situations. These mechanisms include seeking information; maintaining a hopeful outlook; using stress-reduction techniques; denying or minimizing the threat; channeling energy into physical activity; creating fantasies about various outcomes; finding reassurance and emotional support; identifying limited and realistic goals; identifying a positive purpose for the event; getting involved in other activities, such as work and family; and expressing oneself creatively, such as through music, art, or writing.

In the late 1970s, two opposing theories were proposed to explain age-related differences in coping mechanisms. Pfeiffer (1977) theorized that older adults used more primitive defense mechanisms, such

TABLE 8-1 • Stokes/Gordon Stress Scale (SGSS): Selected Items		
Rank	Event or Situation	Weight
1	Death of a son or daughter (unexpected)	100
2	Decreasing eyesight	99
2	Death of a grandchild	99
3	Death of spouse (unexpected)	97
4	Loss of ability to get around	96
4	Death of son or daughter (expected, anticipated)	96
5	Fear of your home being invaded or robbed	93
5	Constant or recurring pain or discomfort	93
6	Illness or injury of close relative	92
7	Death of spouse (expected, anticipated)	90
7	Moving in with children or other family	90
7	Moving to an institution	90
8	Minor or major car accident	89
8	Needing to rely on cane, wheelchair, walker, hearing aid	89
8	Change in ability to do personal care	89
10	Loneliness or aloneness	87
11	Having an unexpected debt	86
11	Your own hospitalization (unplanned)	86
12	Decreasing hearing	85
13	Fear of abuse from others	84
13	Being judged legally incompetent	84
13	Not feeling needed or having a purpose in life	84
14	Decreasing mental abilities	84
15	Giving up long-cherished possessions	82
15	Wishing parts of your life had been different	82
16	Using your savings for living expenses	80
17	Change in behavior of family member	79
18	Taking a relative or friend into your home to live	78
19	Concern about elimination	77
19	Illness in public places	77
20	Feeling of remaining time being short	76
20	Giving up or losing driver's license	76
20	Change in your sleeping habits	76
21	Difficulty using public transportation system	75
23	Uncertainty about the future	73
25	Fear of your own or your spouse's driving	71
27	Concern for completing required forms	69
27	Death of a loved pet	69
29	Reaching a milestone year	67
32	Outstanding personal achievement	64
33	Retirement	63
35	Change in your sexual activity	59

(Adapted, with permission, from Stokes, S. A., & Gordon, S. E. (1988). *User's manual, SGSS*. Pleasautville, NY: Pace University.)

as denial, anxiety, and depression-withdrawal. By contrast, both Haan (1977) and Vaillant (1977) asserted that the use of different coping mechanisms depends on the person's degree of maturity. They maintained that less mature people use mechanisms such as denial and projection, whereas more mature people use mechanisms such as humor and sublimation. In an attempt to address these divergent views, McCrae (1982) studied the response of older and younger adults to stressful life events. McCrae concluded that the difference in the use of coping mechanisms in these populations was not related to the age of the person, but rather to the type of stress with which the person was coping. A study designed to address the complexities of this issue concluded that the types of coping and defense strategies used depend both on the level of ego maturity of the person and the source of stress (Labouvie-Vief et al., 1987).

Some studies of coping styles distinguish between problem-focused and emotion-focused behaviors. Problem-focused coping is directed toward altering the stress-provoking event, whereas emotion-focused coping is directed toward regulating one's emotional response to the event. Within these two categories, specific coping methods include confrontation and cognitive types of problem-focused coping; distancing, self-control, escape-avoidance, accepting responsibility, and positive reappraisal methods of emotion-focused coping; and, for both categories, the seeking of social support (Folkman et al., 1987). The choice of a coping style and method depends, in part, on the way people appraise the situation in terms of its personal significance and their ability to alter the outcomes. For example, when people appraise a situation as high in potential for change (in contrast to having little or no such potential), they tend to use confrontation, positive reappraisal, and planned problem solving and are less likely to use escape-avoidance coping mechanisms (Folkman et al., 1986).

Folkman and colleagues (1987) found "striking and consistent" differences between younger subjects, who were found to use predominantly active and problem-focused forms of coping, and older subjects, who were found to use predominantly passive and emotion-focused coping strategies. Coping mechanisms of older subjects included distancing, positive appraisal, and acceptance of responsibility. The authors suggested that these differences had more to do with the types of stress than with the age differences in the two groups. That is, the coping patterns of older people were consistent with and appropriate for the less changeable types of problems with which they were coping.

A study of coping mechanisms of people aged 85 years and older identified two adaptive techniques that helped sustain a sense of well-being despite experiences of physical and social losses. First, older adults in the study directed their coping strategies toward specific losses (e.g., daily activities were incorporated into a routine to make them more manageable). Second, these older adults developed a sense of control over their lives by redefining their optimal health and functional level and their desired level of social integration (Johnson & Barer, 1993). Another study found that older adults developed new coping strategies to cope with vision loss when their preexisting strategies were ineffective in reducing the perceived threat (Brennan & Cardinali, 2000).

Older men are most likely to use problem-solving coping methods, whereas older women are likely to use positive reappraisal (Dunkle et al., 1992).

Before the 1980s, it was assumed that the impact of major life events associated with older adulthood was negative. Based on this assumption, researchers tried, but failed, to identify specific changes that adversely affect older adults. There is now much agreement that both the strength of the life event (i.e., the meaning of the event to the individual) and the coping resources available to the individual are the factors that determine whether the life event has a negative impact on health (George, 2001; Martin et al., 2001). Thus, researchers have focused on identifying the factors that affect one's ability to cope with life events, with much emphasis on the influence of social resources, such as economic resources and social support, which are particularly powerful resources for offsetting the effects of stress.

It is widely agreed that older adults who are engaged in interaction with supportive social networks have better mental and physical health than older adults who do not maintain meaningful ties with others (Krause, 2001). Social supports are categorized as follows:

- Instrumental support, which provides tangible assistance (e.g., transportation, personal care)
- Informational support, which provides essential information about appropriate resources (e.g., information about community services)
- Emotional support, which provides comfort, self-validation, and companionship from intimate others (George, 2001)

Components of emotional support include information that leads a person to believe that he or she is loved, cared for, esteemed and valued, and belongs to a network of communication and mutual obligations (Krause, 2001).

In addition, health status and psychosocial resources significantly affect the coping abilities of older adults and influence the response of older adults to life events. Gerontologists emphasize the following characteristics that are associated with improved coping abilities in older adults:

- Hardiness
- Self-esteem
- Good social skills
- Good cognitive abilities

- Good physical health and functioning
- Beliefs about self-efficacy
- Greater sense of mastery and personal control
- A sense of person and existential integrity (Blazer, 2002; DiBartolo, 2002; George, 2001; Steverink et al., 2001)

The timing of life events also can affect coping abilities because it is more difficult to cope with cumulative losses or losses that occur close together. Researchers also have explored issues about anticipation of life events and social supports. For example, studies suggest that when older adults can anticipate having social supports they have a "social safety net" that provides a sense of hope (Krause, 2001, p. 274). Studies also have suggested that anticipated and predictable life events are less stressful than unexpected events, but this finding may not apply to death of a spouse for older adults. Carr and colleagues (2001) found that sudden spousal death does not have serious and far-reaching deleterious effects on mental health, and these researchers suggest that the impact of spousal death is affected by much more than the degree of anticipation. Conclusions that can be drawn from studies on stress and coping in older adults are summarized in Display 8-1.

RELIGION, SPIRITUALITY, AND AGING

The topics of religion and spirituality are addressed here because of their importance as both coping resources and as significant aspects of psychosocial function for older adults. Major themes identified in a review of nursing articles related to religion, spirituality, and aging are (1) the need for sensitivity to cultural differences in religious practices and beliefs, (2) the need to encourage support services for caregivers and community-dwelling older adults, and (3) the importance of recognizing and addressing the individual cognitive, emotional, physical, and spiritual needs of older adults (Weaver et al., 2001).

Religion and spirituality are closely related but distinct concepts. Religion and religiosity, which have a strong social component, refer to the beliefs, feelings, and behaviors that are associated with a faith community. Spirituality generally is viewed as a broader concept than religion. For many people, religion is a part of their spirituality; for others, it is not. Florence Nightingale viewed spirituality as intrinsic to human nature and emphasized that it was an individual's deepest and most potent resource for healing. Definitions of spirituality generally include the following concepts: healing; wholeness; social justice; personal growth; interpersonal relationships; a sense of meaning and

---

DISPLAY 8-1
Conclusions About Stress and Coping in Older Adulthood

The Impact of Life Events on Coping
- The unique meaning of a life event must be considered for each person.
- The timing of events can significantly influence a person's ability to cope, with several events in a short period of time having an extremely detrimental effect.
- No one life event has been found to have a consistently negative impact on the older adult.
- The amount of anticipation about an event can influence the ability to cope, with more stress being associated with events that are least anticipated.
- Chronic stressors and daily hassles may demand greater coping energy than major life events.

Coping Resources
- Social supports may be a buffer against stress, particularly through their positive effects on self-esteem and feelings of personal control.
- Financial assets are an important buffer against stressful life events for older adults.
- Religious beliefs are an important coping resource for older adults.
- Although high social status and high feelings of self-efficacy are assets for older adults under normal circumstances, they may be deleterious factors at the time of stressful life events.

Coping Styles
- The choice of coping mechanisms is influenced more by the individual's level of maturity than by chronologic age.
- Passive, emotion-focused coping styles (e.g., distancing, self-control, accepting responsibility) are effective in dealing with situations that have a low potential for change.
- Active, problem-focused coping styles (e.g., confrontation, information-seeking) are effective in dealing with situations that can be changed.

---

purpose to life; a transcendent relationship with a higher being; an association with reverence, mystery, and inspiration; connectedness with nature, other people, and the universe; and feelings of and behaviors arising from love, faith, hope, trust, and forgiveness.

Religious practices are one way of expressing spirituality, and an affiliation with a religious denomination provides a vehicle for formalized religious practices. Other expressions of spirituality include prayer, meditation, centering, forgiveness, creative activities, love and caring, storytelling and reminiscence, finding meaning in life, work in service to others, and rituals and other activities that nourish the spirit.

Gerontologists have looked at various aspects of the role of religion as an aspect of psychosocial function in older adulthood. Some of the research findings are as follows:

- Eighty percent of older Americans belong to a church or synagogue.
- Seventy-three percent of older adults say that religion is very important to them.
- More than 50% of all older people watch religious television programs at least occasionally.
- Fifty-two percent of older adults attend religious services at least once weekly.
- Sixty percent of older adults report that they became more devout as they grew older.
- Older adults are likely to identify religion as their primary way of coping with difficult life events (Weaver et al., 2001).

Researchers also have found the following mental and physical health benefits associated with participation in religious activity:

- Longer life expectancy
- Greater well-being and life satisfaction
- Less anxiety and depression
- Better adaptation to medical illness
- Better immune system function
- Better adaptation to caregiving burden
- Faster recovery from depression
- Fewer hospitalizations and shorter hospital stays
- Higher levels of hope and optimism
- Lower rates of substance abuse
- Lower rates of suicide
- Higher levels of participation in health promotion activities (e.g., increased exercise and smoking cessation (Armer & Conn, 2001; Crowther et al., 2002)

There is strong research support indicating that religion becomes increasingly salient with age and that older adults who are more involved in, and committed to, their faith tend to have better physical and mental health than those who are not as religious (Helm et al., 2000; Krause, 2001). Specifically, religion has been identified as an important coping mechanism for meeting challenges associated with pain, anxiety, depression, suicide, disability, bereavement, alcohol abuse, social isolation, cognitive impairment, and decisions about end-of-life care (Idler et al., 2001). Thus, it is important for gerontological nurses to assess religious affiliation as a social resource and a component of mental health for older adults (as discussed in Chapter 10).

Spirituality, also, becomes increasingly important as an aspect of psychosocial function in later adulthood. Specific dimensions of spirituality that are associated with psychosocial function in older adults identified by Ortiz and Langer (2002) are as follows:

- Interconnectedness between self and others in the community
- A relationship with transcendent forces or powers beyond human associations
- Power for living, which is associated with faith, hope, courage, and determination to face situations that seem beyond human control
- "Meaning making," defined as "making sense of it all" or viewing one's experiences in the context of a larger purpose
- Public or private expression that enables one to stay focused or provide a restorative sense to life

> Hispanics, African Americans, and Native Americans are among the ethnic groups that report high levels of involvement of older adults in both organizational and nonorganizational religious activities.

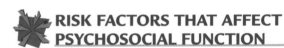

RISK FACTORS THAT AFFECT PSYCHOSOCIAL FUNCTION

Information about risks that can affect psychosocial function can be drawn from the theories of stress and coping and from knowledge about causes of impaired mental health in older adulthood. The following factors have been identified as risks for high levels of stress and poor coping in older adults:

- Poor physical health
- Impaired functional abilities
- Poor social supports
- Lack of economic resources
- An immature developmental level
- The occurrence of unanticipated events
- The occurrence of several daily hassles at the same time
- The occurrence of several major life events in a short period of time
- High social status and high feelings of self-efficacy in situations that cannot be changed

In addition, people who have a rigid set or narrow range of coping skills are more at risk for impaired coping because different types of coping strategies are effective in different situations. People who cannot realistically appraise a situation also may be at increased risk for poor coping because the choice of effective coping behaviors depends partially on the ability to determine the potential for change.

An accurate appraisal is particularly important with regard to health problems, and it depends on the person's knowledge about health changes and potential interventions. For example, older adults who experience urinary incontinence or difficulties with sexual function may consider these changes to be inevitable consequences of age. Based on this appraisal, older adults may use passive, emotion-focused coping mechanisms, trying simply to accept the situation. When older adults view functional decline as an inevitable consequence of aging, they are less likely to seek help for treatable problems (Sarkisian et al., 2002). In addition, they are more likely to experience an unnecessary and unfortunate functional impairment and a diminished quality of life. By contrast, if the situation is appraised more accurately as a potentially treatable condition, more active, problem-focused coping mechanisms are likely to be used. Even if the health problem is accurately appraised as changeable, however, older adults must identify health professionals who understand the problem and who will attempt to find solutions. It is only when both the older adult and the health care professional accurately appraise the situation as changeable that interventions can be initiated to effect positive functional consequences.

A move to an institutional setting is a risk factor for disturbed self-esteem in older adults because adjustment to nursing home settings is associated with loss of rights, wishes, desires, feelings, and initiatives (Groh & Whall, 2001). Older adults who have feelings of high self-efficacy may be particularly susceptible to disturbed self-esteem when they are in situations where they have little control over their environment. Many studies have addressed the relationship between locus of control and psychosocial adjustment, with consistent agreement that lack of perceived control interferes with well-being and increases the risk for feelings of powerlessness (Davidhizar, 2001). Similarly, a sense of mastery or sense of control protects against depression, fosters resilience under stressful situations, and promotes physical and emotional well-being (Jang et al., 2002). Studies also are addressing the effects of involvement or lack of involvement in decision making, particularly on older adults who are cognitively intact. For example, the degree of involvement in everyday decisions, such as routine health care, timing of meals, placement of furniture, and choice of seating in the dining room can significantly affect the well-being of nursing home residents and their adjustment to the institutional setting (Shawler et al., 2001).

The concept of *learned helplessness* has been used to explain the excess dependency that occurs in older adults in hospital or long-term cares settings (Faulkner, 2001). Learned helplessness is the experience of uncontrollable events that leads to expectations that

future events will also be uncontrollable. Thus, actions that increase dependency or disempower older adults (e.g., providing assistance because this is more time efficient rather than allowing the older person to function independently or with only a little assistance) are risk factors for diminished self-esteem and feelings of powerlessness. In addition, learned helplessness may contribute to depression, as discussed in Chapter 25. Similarly, studies suggest that the provision of more assistance than is needed, especially with tasks such as daily activities, results in reduced self-esteem and well-being (Antonnuci, 2001).

 ## FUNCTIONAL CONSEQUENCES ASSOCIATED WITH PSYCHOSOCIAL FUNCTION IN OLDER ADULTS

Since the life events scale of Holmes and Rahe was first proposed in 1967, many studies have been conducted to measure the negative impact of stressful events, with particular emphasis on physical health effects. Although some studies have found an association between a high SRRS rating and the occurrence of certain diseases (e.g., heart attacks), most people who experience life events do not become ill (George, 2001). Because the impact of life events on health is significantly influenced by the strength of the life event and the coping resources and personality characteristics of the individual (George, 2001), a wide range of both negative and positive functional consequences is associated with psychosocial function in older adults.

Negative functional consequences include anxiety, loneliness, depression, and cognitive impairment. About 20% of older adults report clinically relevant symptoms of anxiety, which manifests in older adults as distress, exaggerated fears and concerns about their health, and a heightened awareness of physiologic arousal and discomfort (Frazier et al., 2002). Loneliness—which is associated with increased dependency, lack of intimate relationships, and the losses that commonly occur during later adulthood—is a common functional consequence for older adults, especially those who are widowed or living in institutional settings (Hegge & Fischer, 2000; Hicks, 2000). Stress also may cause negative functional consequences in terms of cognitive impairment (especially memory), as discussed in Chapter 7. Finally, depression (discussed comprehensively in Chapter 25) is another negative functional consequence of stress because it is a common response to the losses that are associated with life events of older adulthood.

Although most studies on psychological aging have focused on anxiety, depression, and other negative emotions, more recent studies are addressing the relationship between positive emotions (e.g., happiness, life satisfaction, emotional well-being) and health in older adults. There is a strong independent relationship between emotional well-being and physical health, and it is commonly believed that a positive attitude toward life leads to better health (Penninx, 2000). Much of the current focus on psychosocial function in older adults is on identifying the factors that affect emotional well-being and thereby improve the health and quality of life of older adults. Gerontologists have identified the following characteristics of older adults that are associated with emotional vitality and improved health:

- Feeling happy
- Enjoying life
- Experiencing autonomy
- Experiencing personal growth
- Having a purpose in life
- Being extroverted and outgoing
- Feeling hopeful about the future
- Having positive relations with others
- Having a sense of self-acceptance
- Having a high sense of personal mastery
- Feeling "just as good" as other people
- Having low measures of anxiety and depression
- Having a sense of religious or spiritual connectedness
- Experiencing a sense of mastery over one's environment

(Koenig, 2000; Ostir et al., 2000; Penninx, 2000)

Using information from these studies, nurses can assess not only the negative but also the positive functional consequences of psychosocial function in older adults (discussed in Chapter 10). Nurses can then identify and facilitate interventions that address the negative functional consequences (e.g., anxiety and depression) and foster positive functional consequences (e.g., enhanced self-esteem, a sense of mastery over one's environment) as discussed in this chapter and in Chapter 25.

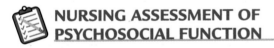

NURSING ASSESSMENT OF PSYCHOSOCIAL FUNCTION

Because psychosocial function encompasses a broad range of social, cognitive, and emotional aspects of functioning that are intertwined, the assessment of psychosocial function is addressed comprehensively in a separate chapter. Readers are directed to Chapter 10 for a thorough review of nursing assessment of psychosocial function.

NURSING DIAGNOSIS

The nursing diagnoses of Self-Esteem Disturbance and Situational Low Self-Esteem are applicable in relation to some of the psychosocial adjustment issues of older adults. Situational Low Self-Esteem is defined as "the state in which an individual who previously had positive self-esteem experiences negative feelings about self in response to an event (loss, change)" (Carpenito, 2002, p. 815). Related factors might be the internalization of ageist attitudes, the loss of roles or financial security, the need for a change to a more supportive living arrangement, and chronic illnesses that affect one's abilities and role identities.

If the nursing assessment identifies threats to the older person's sense of control, an appropriate nursing diagnosis is Powerlessness. This is defined as "the state in which an individual or group perceives a lack of personal control over certain events or situations that affect outlook, goals, and lifestyle" (Carpenito, 2002, p. 687). Common related factors for older adults are forced retirement, loss of the ability to drive a car, lack of involvement in decision making, chronic conditions that cause progressive functional declines (e.g., dementia), and institutional constraints, such as lack of privacy and the need to follow schedules that do not meet the needs of the individual.

Impaired Adjustment is another nursing diagnosis that addresses the psychosocial needs of older adults. This is defined as "the state in which the individual is unwilling to modify his or her lifestyle/behavior in a manner consistent with a change in health status" (Carpenito, 2002, p. 112). For example, this nursing diagnosis would be applicable to an older adult who is driving unsafely because of cognitive or other functional deficits, but who refuses to give up driving. Another nursing diagnosis that might be applied to the psychosocial needs of older adults is Ineffective Individual Coping. Carpenito defines this as a "state in which the individual experiences, or is at risk to experience, an inability to manage internal or environmental stressors adequately due to inadequate resources (physical, psychological, behavioral, and/or cognitive)" (2002, p. 257). She suggests that the diagnosis of Impaired Adjustment might be appropriate during the initial period after a stressful event, whereas the diagnosis of Ineffective Individual Coping would be more applicable to longer-term coping problems.

Social Isolation, which is defined as "the state in which the individual or group experiences or perceives a need or desire for increased involvement with others but is unable to make that contact," is a nursing diagnosis applicable to older adults who have limited or inadequate social supports to address their needs (Carpenito, 2002, p. 892). Because social supports are a major factor that influences the ability of older adults to cope with losses, this important nursing diagnosis is commonly applied to numerous situations in which older adults are adjusting to psychosocial challenges such as life events. A closely related nursing diagnosis is Impaired Social Interaction, defined as "the state in which an individual experiences or is at risk of experiencing negative, insufficient, or unsatisfactory responses from interactions" (Carpenito, 2002, p. 882).

Nurses who are addressing the spiritual needs of older adults might find the diagnosis of Spiritual Distress useful and appropriate if the older person is experiencing conflicts with his or her belief system. Spiritual Distress is defined as "the state in which the individual or group experiences a disturbance in the belief or value system that provides strength, hope, and meaning to life" (Carpenito, 2002, p. 897). If nursing care is directed toward promoting spiritual growth for an older adult, the appropriate nursing diagnosis would be Readiness for Enhanced Spiritual Well-Being.

OUTCOMES

Nursing-sensitive outcomes related to Self-Esteem Disturbance are as follows:

- Verbalization of self-acceptance
- Acceptance of compliments from others
- Diminished levels of anxiety or depression
- Improvements in physical appearance and hygiene
- Increased social interaction and interest in trying new activities (Groh & Whall, 2001)

Nursing-sensitive outcomes for older adults who experience Powerlessness include involvement in decisions and expressions of satisfaction with self-concept, health status, social circumstances, and ability to cope (Davidhizar, 2001). Because a lack of social supports and other important coping resources is a common related factor for older adults with a nursing diagnosis of Ineffective Individual Coping, nursing-sensitive outcomes for this diagnosis include verbalizes need for assistance, uses available social supports, and identifies and uses effective coping strategies (Stolley, 2001). Nursing-sensitive outcomes for Social Isolation include use of resources, evidence of willingness to call on others for help, and reports of having a confidant relationship and receiving assistance when needed (Waterman et al., 2001).

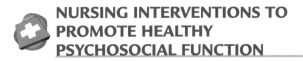

NURSING INTERVENTIONS TO PROMOTE HEALTHY PSYCHOSOCIAL FUNCTION

Nurses have many opportunities to help older adults develop effective coping strategies, with a twofold result: a reduced level of stress and anxiety and an improved quality of life. Nursing interventions are directed toward enhancing self-esteem, promoting a sense of control, fostering social supports, and addressing spiritual needs. Two additional interventions for addressing psychosocial function in older adults are life review and reminiscence processes. Healthy aging classes, described in detail in the interventions section, is a nursing model of a group intervention for assisting older adults to adjust to the challenges typical of older adulthood.

Enhancing Self-Esteem

Self-esteem is an aspect of psychosocial function that has been addressed in the nursing literature for many decades, and it is considered to be an essential component of nursing care, particularly for older adults. Self-esteem is considered an important coping resource and a factor that influences well-being because people with high self-esteem are happier, healthier, less anxious, more independent, more self-confident, and more effective in meeting environmental demands than people with low self-esteem (Groh & Whall, 2001). Thus, an important nursing responsibility is to assist older adults in maintaining or restoring self-esteem.

The following potential threats to self-esteem are likely to occur in older adulthood and can be addressed through nursing interventions: dependence, infantalization, devaluation, depersonalization, functional impairments, and lack of control over one's environment. Many of these actual and potential threats arise from the staff and environments of the institutions where older adults receive their care. Other threats arise from the negative functional consequences that are discussed throughout this text. Thus, to enhance self-esteem in older adults, nursing interventions must address the many threats to self-esteem that are within the scope of nursing care.

Self-esteem depends partially on the perceived appraisal of significant others, which is communicated through verbal as well as nonverbal messages. Nurses must be aware of their ageist attitudes and avoid reflecting these attitudes in verbal statements. For example, even a remark such as "You certainly look good for 85 years old," although said with good intentions, can reinforce ageist attitudes. Hidden messages in this statement may be that it is better to look younger, and that when you are old, you generally do not look good. If ageism is going to be curbed, even subtle messages communicating negative attitudes about old age must be avoided. For instance, a statement such as the following might enhance an older person's self-esteem and challenge ageist attitudes: "At 85 years old, you must have a lot of wisdom. What advice can you give about successful aging?"

Because self-esteem is based partially on the perceived appraisal of significant others, nurses can focus their interventions on increasing the older adult's perception of self-worth. It is important to recognize that nonverbal communication may influence the person's perception of self-worth even more than verbal communication. For example, if a nurse walks past an older person sitting in a hallway without acknowledging his or her presence, the action may be perceived as an indication that the older person is not valued by the nurse. Even though the nurse may have been attending to responsibilities and had no intention of communicating this negative message, this action may negatively affect that older person's self-esteem. In influencing the self-esteem of others, nurses must keep in mind that the perception of their actions is often more important than their actual intent. Therefore, if nurses are aiming to enhance the self-esteem of older adults, they must be aware of any messages that might influence the older person's perceptions. In addition, they must use both verbal and nonverbal messages to communicate feelings of positive regard whenever possible.

Another intervention aimed at challenging ageist attitudes is the redirecting of the negative attributions associated with aging to external factors, such as the environment. Many studies have confirmed the importance of modifying the way people perceive and explain events, shifting attention to factors that can be changed or controlled. In the classic study by Rodin and Langer (1980), whenever a nursing home resident attributed a problem to being old, the staff provided another explanation and identified a causative factor that was amenable to change. For example, when residents attributed feelings of fatigue to being old, they were reminded that they were awakened at 5:30 AM (Rodin & Langer, 1980). Some of the nursing interventions for Powerlessness that can be used to redirect negative attributions associated with aging to external factors are Cognitive Restructuring, Socialization Enhancement, Self-Esteem Enhancement, and Decision-Making Support (Davidhizar, 2001). These and other nursing interventions can assist older adults in developing problem-focused coping mechanisms as an alternative to passive acceptance of the negative functional consequences of aging.

Self-esteem is closely associated with physical health and functional abilities, and it is likely to be diminished at times of illness. Therefore, any intervention directed toward improving functional abilities also can be effective in enhancing self-esteem. Throughout this text, in all the discussions of physiologic function, numerous interventions are discussed for improving functional abilities. An additional intervention that has been found to be effective in improving the physiologic function of older adults, as well as their self-esteem, is participation in physical activity, especially aerobic exercise (McAuley, 2000).

Meaningful roles (e.g., spouse, caregiver, volunteer) are important determinants of feelings of worth, efficacy, and self-esteem. Although role loss is a common occurrence in later adulthood, the development of new roles to compensate for the loss is an effective coping strategy for older adults (Ferraro, 2001). Thus, nurses can discuss current roles with older adults and assist them in identifying new roles. For example, the nurse can ask older persons about their responsibilities as parents, grandparents, or roommates as a strategy for improving their self-perception. In long-term care settings, the nurse can create meaningful roles, such as helper or assistant, for older adults by involving them in tasks that are viewed as productive. When older adults volunteer to assist others, nurses can enhance their self-esteem by acknowledging this contribution with a remark such as, "You certainly help us a lot when you help take Mrs. Smith to the dining room in her wheelchair."

An often overlooked but essential aspect of self-esteem in older adulthood is the acknowledgment of achievements. When people are dependent on others, they often have difficulty feeling a sense of accomplishment, or even a sense of basic usefulness. Therefore, an intervention to increase the self-esteem of people who are physically impaired is to focus attention on nonphysical assets, such as family relationships or a good sense of humor. One way of focusing attention on positive relationships is to acknowledge the receipt of flowers, greeting cards, and other visible signs of concern expressed by others. Asking about a get-well card that someone has received will provide an opportunity for a discussion of positive relationships, and it may also remind the person that others care.

In addition to focusing on present roles and positive relationships, another intervention designed to enhance self-esteem is to focus on past achievements. This may be done within the context of a group exchange or on an individual basis. This intervention may be especially effective for people who have difficulty identifying current accomplishments. On an individual basis, nurses can ask older adults about their past accomplishments in areas such as work and family. Asking questions about family pictures is one way of opening a discussion of successful and positive relationships. Encouraging older people to talk about grandchildren and great-grandchildren is another intervention that may enhance their feelings of accomplishment. Nurses can further enhance self-esteem with comments such as, "You must be proud of your grandchildren" or "You certainly have accomplished a lot." Nursing interventions to promote self-esteem are identified in Display 8-2.

Promoting a Sense of Control

Interventions to improve one's sense of control over the environment and involvement in decision making can be implemented to address Powerlessness in older adults. This is particularly important in settings such as nursing homes and other long-term care institutions where the caregiving environment affects virtually every aspect of daily life for the residents. Any intervention that improves the level of function of an older person (as discussed throughout this text) can be viewed as an intervention for improving the older person's perceived sense of control.

Older people frequently are left out of the decision-making process, even for those decisions that most profoundly affect their lives, such as moving to a nursing home. This lack of involvement occurs for a variety of reasons, related both to the older adult and to the decision makers. Some of the barriers within the older adult are dementia, depression, long-term passivity regarding decisions, and hearing impairments or other communication barriers. Some of the barriers within the decision makers that may thwart the decision-making process include stereotypes of older people as incompetent, perceptions that the older adult is not interested in or capable of making decisions, and an unwillingness to deal with the older person's anticipated resistance to the desired outcome.

Many of the reasons for excluding older adults from the decision-making process are related to the attitudes of the family and of professional caregivers; hence, one nursing intervention is to challenge these attitudes. For example, in acute care settings, nurses can facilitate communication between older patients and their primary care provider to ensure that the older person is included in decisions about medical treatment and discharge plans. In long-term care settings, nurses have numerous opportunities to involve older adults in decisions about their daily care, medical interventions, and discharge plans. In home settings, nurses might work with family members as well as older adults to ensure that the latter are involved in decisions about their care and that their rights are respected. In any setting, nurses may have to remind health professionals, as well as family members and other caregivers, that although people may gain rights by virtue of being a certain age, they do not lose their rights just because they reach a certain age. For a comprehensive discussion of the nurse's role in decisions regarding long-term care for people with dementia, refer to Chapter 24.

Other aspects of decision making that can be addressed in nursing interventions are one's verbal interactions and choice of terminology. With regard to verbal communication, health professionals often talk *about* older adults when in their presence rather than addressing questions *to* them and focusing the conversation *on* them. This commonly occurs when family members or other caregivers are discussing situations with a nurse or other professional and the conversation takes place in the presence of the older person without directly involving him or her. In working with older adults, nurses need to pay particular attention to including older adults in conversations when the topic is directly related to them. When it is not appropriate to include the older adult in the conversation, the nurse can take steps to facilitate the conversation outside the presence of the older person. In these situations, the nurse can ask the older person's permission to discuss his or her situation with family members or caregivers and then report back to the older person, in language that the person can understand, about any discussions that take place or decisions that are made or pending.

With regard to terminology, the word "placement" often is used in reference to an older adult's admission to a nursing home. This term denotes passivity on the part of the older adult; it is closer to the terminology used when objects are placed on a shelf than to words normally used in reference to human beings. Nurses would communicate more positive feelings and a greater sense of control if they referred to an "admission" to a nursing home. The term admission suggests that certain criteria have been met and that an active decision has been made to determine whether the person meets these criteria. Even more important than using the correct terms, nurses must ensure that older adults are, in fact, actively involved in the decision-making process, rather than passively being "placed." Nurses can help older adults and their families with decisions about long-term care by helping them assess their situation and by correcting misinformation and providing accurate information about specific resources and the range of services available (as described in Chapter 5). Nurses frequently assume a primary role in helping older adults and their families assess the need for a move from independent living to supervised settings, and Baldwin and Shaul (2001) describe a nursing framework for this process.

Another area affecting one's perceived control over the environment involves the lack of privacy and loss of individuality that often occur in institutional settings. Nurses can show respect for privacy by knocking on bedroom doors and asking permission before entering, by closing doors when privacy is desired, by asking permission before pulling bed curtains open, and by being careful about moving personal belongings without permission from the older person. Encouraging the person to have personal belongings and to arrange these belongings in whatever fashion is desired also shows concern for individuality.

Fostering Social Supports

Although many of the important social supports that serve as coping resources, such as financial assets, usually are not addressed through nursing interventions, nurses have many opportunities to foster the development of social networks for older adults, and this is an appropriate intervention for addressing social isolation. In some situations, particularly in home and long-term care settings, nurses often become an integral part of the older person's social network. Social isolation is likely to occur because of any of the following factors that commonly occur in older adulthood: hearing impairments and other communication barriers; chronic illnesses that limit activity or energy; lack of opportunities because of caregiving responsibilities; mobility limitations, including an inability to drive a car; mental or psychosocial impairments that interfere with relationships; and loss of spouse, friends, or family through death, illness, or physical distance. Therefore, any intervention directed toward these risk factors also can be an intervention to improve social supports. Because these interventions have been discussed throughout this text, they will not be addressed in this section. However, nurses should appreciate the potential positive effects on social supports that are associated with interventions that improve the functional status of an older person.

In long-term care settings, nurses can create opportunities for social interaction through the use of group activities and the encouragement of conversations at mealtimes. Sometimes, a very simple intervention, such as positioning chairs (including wheelchairs) so that people can interact with each other, can significantly influence social contacts, either positively or negatively. Whenever possible, nurses should arrange room assignments to encourage opportunities for positive social interactions. Reminiscence groups, discussed as an intervention to enhance self-esteem, can also be effective as an intervention for fostering social supports.

In home settings, nurses can identify community resources, such as volunteer friendly visitor and meal

DISPLAY 8-3

Nursing Interventions to Promote Psychosocial Health

Promoting a Sense of Control

- Ask about likes and dislikes and try to address personal preferences.
- Whenever possible, allow the person to choose between two alternatives, even if the options are in a very narrow range (e.g., Would you prefer to wear the yellow sweater or the pink one today?).
- Ensure as much privacy, or perceived privacy, as possible.
- Knock on the door and ask permission before entering a bedroom, even in institutional settings.
- Allow as much expression of individuality as possible in the personal environment (e.g., use personal furniture when possible and display family pictures in full view).
- Make sure that the call light is accessible for people who are confined.
- Do not talk about someone in his or her presence as if he or she does not exist.
- Involve older adults as much as possible in decisions, especially those that affect their care most directly.
- Avoid referring to nursing home placement. Refer instead to an admission, and include the person in the decision-making process.

Facilitating Maximum Independence

- Make sure that the person has access to all necessary assistive devices and personal accessories (e.g., wigs, canes, dentures, walkers, and hearing aids).
- Allow enough time for the person to perform tasks at her or his own pace, and avoid unnecessary dependence that results from an overemphasis on time efficiency.
- Make sure that the environment has been adapted as much as possible to compensate for sensory losses and other functional impairments.

Fostering Social Supports

- Use interventions to deal with hearing impairments and other communication barriers (see Chapter 12).
- Encourage participation in group activities.
- For people in wheelchairs, especially those who cannot move independently, position the chair in a way that promotes social interaction.
- For nursing home residents, plan table and room arrangements in such a way that social relationships are fostered.

---

programs, to decrease social isolation. Support and education groups that primarily focus on coping with a chronic illness (e.g., stroke clubs, or better-breathing groups) also provide excellent opportunities for social contact and the development of friendships with people who are in similar situations. For people who are socially isolated because of caregiving responsibility, caregiver support groups can enhance coping abilities and provide social support. Display 8-3 summarizes the interventions for promoting a sense of control, facilitating maximum independence, and fostering social supports.

Addressing Spiritual Needs of Older Adults

Gerontological nursing literature increasingly is discussing the role of nurses in addressing spiritual needs of older adults (e.g., Hermann, 2000; LeMone, 2001; MacKinlay, 2001; Weaver et al., 2001). Often, the spiritual needs of older adults and their caregivers can be met by intentionally communicating caring and compassion. Many interventions that are an integral part of routine nursing care of older adults also address their spiritual needs. For example, facilitating reminiscence, honoring a person's integrity, providing active and passive listening, making referrals for spiritual care, caring for someone who

feels hopeless, arranging for participation in religious services, and encouraging or facilitating participation in activities such as prayer and meditation are interventions that address spiritual needs. It is imperative that nursing interventions to address the spiritual needs of older adults be individualized and offered only if the person is receptive to the interventions. In addition, it is imperative that nurses not impose their personal beliefs and that they maintain nonjudgmental communication about religion and spirituality. Because cultural factors significantly influence a person's spirituality and religious beliefs, interventions must be culturally sensitive. Andrews and Hanson (2003) provide an excellent overview of specific cultural influences on religion and spirituality, including details about health-related beliefs and practices of selected religious groups in North America.

In addition to addressing spiritual needs as a routine part of psychosocial nursing care, nurses often address spiritual needs during times of spiritual distress. For example, older adults are likely to express spiritual needs when they are coping with the loss of a significant relationship or dealing with news about a serious or terminal illness. Older adults who are caregivers for others, especially a spouse, are likely to express spiritual needs in relation to decisions about the care of the other person. For example, they may

DISPLAY 8-4
Nursing Interventions to Address Spiritual Needs

Therapeutic Communication Interventions

- Use verbal and nonverbal communication to establish trust and convey empathic caring.
- Use active supportive listening.
- Convey nonjudgmental attitudes.
- Communicate respect for individuality.
- Provide a supportive presence.
- Be open to expressions of feelings such as fear, anger, loneliness, and powerlessness.
- Honor a person's integrity.
- Support the person in their feeling of being loved by others and by a higher power (e.g., God, Allah, Jehovah).
- Encourage verbalization of feelings about meaning of illness.
- Provide positive feedback about faith, courage, sense of humor, and other such feelings and experiences.
- Encourage discussion of events and relationships that provide spiritual support.

Actions to Foster Religious and Spiritual Activities

- Facilitate referrals for visits from religious care providers and sources of spiritual care (clergy, rabbis, church members, spiritual directors).

- Facilitate participation in religious services or activities (e.g., tapes, readings, videos, observations of "holy days").
- Assist with obtaining requested religious items (books, music, statues).
- Provide quiet and private time for individual spiritual or religious activities (e.g., prayer, reflection, meditation, guided imagery).
- Provide necessary support for religious rituals (e.g., lighting candles, receiving communion, praying the rosary).
- Encourage participation in relaxing and enjoyable activities (art, music, nature).

Interventions for Specific Circumstances

- Provide support and care during times of suffering.
- Assist in the process of dying.
- Assist a person who is fearful of the future.
- Provide care for the person who feels hopeless.
- Facilitate reconciliation among family members.
- Encourage participation in support groups.

---

experience feelings of guilt about not being able to meet the needs of a dependent loved one, or feelings of "playing God" in regard to decisions about mentally incompetent loved ones. In these circumstances, the provision of support, information, and reassurance from a nurse who has dealt with these decisions in professional experiences may be an effective counseling intervention. At times, information from the primary care provider may be helpful in alleviating spiritual distress associated with end-of-life decisions or decisions about long-term care. In these cases, the nurse may be able to facilitate communication between the primary care provider and the family to alleviate the spiritual distress. Some nursing interventions that address spiritual needs of older adults are listed in Display 8-4.

Encouraging Life Review and Reminiscence

Although the two processes are distinct, reminiscence and life review are often mistakenly viewed as synonymous. Since the 1960s, reminiscence has been promoted as part of a normal life review process for older adults, and it is based on the realization that the end of life is approaching (Butler, 2001). Butler describes life review as a progressive return to consciousness of past

experiences, particularly unresolved conflicts, for reexamination and reintegration. If the reintegration process is successful, reminiscence gives new significance and meaning to life and prepares the person for death by alleviating fear and anxiety (Butler, 2001). Positive effects of life review include accepting one's mortality, righting of old wrongs, taking pride in accomplishments, gaining a sense of serenity, and feeling that one has done one's best (Butler, 2001). Nursing home residents who participated in life review therapy showed significant improvement over a 3-year period on measures of depression, life satisfaction, and self-esteem (Haight, 2000).

In contrast to life review, reminiscence is a less formal and less intense intervention that, nonetheless, is based on the same theoretical framework. An additional difference is that life review addresses both pleasant and unpleasant issues of the past, whereas reminiscence focuses primarily on pleasant and positive experiences. A nursing definition of reminiscence therapy is "using the recall of past events, feelings, and thoughts to facilitate pleasure, quality of life, or adaptation to present circumstances" (Iowa Intervention Project, 2000, p. 554). As a group therapy, the reminiscence group is one of the most widely used interventions for older adults, and it may be particularly effective for older adults who are anxious or depressed (Cully et al., 2001). Although life review interventions require the involvement of a person with advanced mental health skills, reminiscence interventions can be done by an astute and caring person who has some understanding of older adulthood. Nursing literature describes reminiscence groups as a nursing intervention in long-term care settings (e.g., LeMone, 2001; Rantz & Popejoy, 2001).

Promoting Health Through Healthy Aging Classes

When older adults need assistance in coping with specific functional consequences, or when they need education to clarify myths and misunderstandings about age-related changes, individual counseling may be the best intervention. When older adults need counseling about psychosocial adjustments, however, this may be done most effectively through educational groups. Indeed, one model developed to teach resourcefulness skills to older adults found that the group members improved, as measured by adaptive function and life satisfaction, because of their participation in the group. This nurse-led group focused on helping the members develop strategies to enhance self-control, problem-solving skills, and self-efficacy behaviors that would be useful in coping with distress and managing daily activities (Zauszniewski, 1997).

Another example of a nurse-led group intervention that allows for sharing of experiences among peers is the healthy aging class, developed by this author and used successfully during the past two decades in a variety of settings with older adults at various functional levels. This model is based on the belief that older adults who are beginning to recognize age-related physical and psychosocial changes or who are already dealing with such changes can benefit from sharing their experiences with their peers. This model will be described in detail because the healthy aging class is an intervention designed to enhance the coping skills of older adults who are adjusting to any of the challenges of older adulthood.

Goals

The goals for older adults who participate in healthy aging classes are as follows: (1) to recognize the impact of common age-related physical and psychosocial changes; (2) to support and encourage any effective coping mechanisms already being used; (3) to develop coping mechanisms that are not being used but that may prove effective for a particular situation; (4) to obtain information that will facilitate

problem-focused coping mechanisms for stressful situations that are amenable to change; and (5) to provide an opportunity for the sharing of similar experiences with peers.

Setting

Healthy aging classes can be initiated by nurses in any setting, but long-term care institutions are perhaps the most conducive setting for several reasons. First, nurses have many opportunities to establish and lead groups. Second, the residents of long-term care facilities provide a captive audience from which to select group members. Third, residents of long-term care institutions usually are not acutely ill, and they are dealing with psychosocial adjustments that are readily identified. Finally, residents of long-term care settings have in common at least one major life event, which is a temporary or permanent move to a more dependent setting.

Community settings also are conducive to successful healthy aging classes, but nurses may have to be more creative in gathering the group members. Nurses who provide nursing services or health education programs for senior centers or assisted-living facilities might be able to establish ongoing healthy aging classes as part of their nursing responsibilities. In these settings, a healthy aging class may be an efficient, as well as effective, way of providing health education using a format that has the additional advantage of enhancing coping mechanisms.

In acute care settings, nurses usually do not plan and implement group therapies, but in rehabilitative settings, nurses may have the opportunity to initiate healthy aging classes. In psychiatric units, often there are enough older adults among the patients to warrant the implementation of healthy aging classes as a form of group therapy.

Membership Criteria

The primary criteria for group membership are that the person be willing to acknowledge age-related changes and be capable of acquiring insight into his or her adjustment to these changes. This author has led groups ranging from highly functional older adults in community settings to seriously impaired older adults in a hospital-based medical geropsychiatric unit. Group members may be coping with similar psychosocial stresses, but this is not necessarily a criterion for participation. For example, a healthy aging class may be composed of older adults who all have some degree of depression or who are coping with a particular stressful event, such as widowhood. An ideal group includes members who are coping with various life events commonly associated with older adulthood and who are motivated to learn effective coping styles.

The group usually works best if the membership is stable and closed, but this is not always possible. A major disadvantage of an open group is that it is very difficult to develop cohesiveness. If the membership is open and changing, the leader must be more directive, and the group as a whole will not be able to establish ongoing priorities for discussion topics. In addition, with changing membership, the leader has to focus more attention on the exchange of information about group members at the beginning of each session.

Size of Group and Length, Duration, and Frequency of Sessions

Group size can range from 5 to 12 members, with the ideal class numbering about 8 members. Groups can be either ongoing or time limited. When the membership is changing, such as in psychiatric or rehabilitative settings, the group session can be offered as an ongoing mode of therapy. In long-term care or community settings, it is best to schedule group meetings for a predetermined length of time, such as 8 to 10 weeks, and allow for changes in membership at the end of each period. It is recommended that sessions be held at weekly intervals and that the time and place for each meeting be consistent. The length of each session should be about 1 hour. In community settings, the groups might be scheduled to meet in conjunction with a meal program because social relationships usually are formed among participants in these programs. As in institutional settings, a community center offers an audience from which to select the group members, and transportation usually is not a problem. Other potential community-based sites include assisted-living facilities and group settings, such as adult care homes (also called board-and-care homes).

Criteria for and Responsibilities of Group Leaders

One nurse can lead group sessions, but it is often helpful to have a co-leader who has had social service training. An older adult who has made a positive psychosocial adjustment and who can serve as a role model also can be a good co-leader. The nurse must be able to clarify myths and misunderstandings about age-related changes and be skilled in group dynamics. As with the reminiscence group, the healthy aging class is not an intense psychotherapy session; therefore, the group leader is not required to be specially trained in mental health. To lead a healthy aging class, however, a good understanding of both the physiologic and psychosocial aspects of aging is essential.

The primary responsibilities of the group leaders are to facilitate the discussion of psychosocial adjust-

ments of older adulthood and to provide feedback and clarification to the members. As with other groups, the leaders must ensure that all members have an opportunity to participate and that the members attend to the identified topic. The leaders also must ensure that some conclusions are reached before the end of each session so that members leave with a feeling of accomplishment relating to at least one psychosocial challenge of older adulthood.

Format

As in all educational groups, the leader begins with an explanation of the purpose of the group and an introduction of the leaders and members. The leader might also review the details of the sessions, such as their length, the duration of the group, the role of the leader, and the expectations of the members. After the introductory material has been discussed and any questions have been answered, the leader introduces the concepts of life events and adjustments to the challenges of older adulthood. A statement similar to the following can be used: "Throughout life, certain events are likely to occur that affect us emotionally. These events may involve our health, our personal relationships, the place where we live, our job or career responsibilities and opportunities, or other events that require an adjustment on our part. These are sometimes referred to as major life events, and they often occur at certain points of life. To begin our discussion today, let's look at some of the major life events that are likely to occur in younger adulthood, around the age of 20 to 30 years." The group then identifies various life events, such as finding a job, moving from the family home, finding a partner, and starting a family. The members then are asked to identify life adjustments that are likely to occur between 30 and 50 years of age.

After the members have identified these life events, the leader emphasizes that one purpose of the healthy aging class is to identify the life events of older adulthood so as to adjust successfully to the challenges they present. The term *challenges* is used to communicate an active mode of addressing issues. The leader may want to discuss the phrase "challenges of older adulthood" and allow the group members to comment on what they see as challenges in their lives. As the members identify the life events of older adulthood, the leader writes the events on a board or paper so that all the members can see the list. The leader can then ask about events that the members have experienced, as well as those events that the members think they are likely to experience in the next few years. As events are identified, the members also are asked to identify the consequences of the events that require an adjustment.

TABLE 8-2 • Coping Strategies for the Psychosocial Challenges of Older Adulthood

Psychosocial Adjustment	Coping Strategy
Ageist stereotypes	Develop a firm self-identity, challenge the myths, question any behaviors that are based on age-determined expectations.
Retirement	Develop new skills, use time for hobbies and personal pursuits, become involved with meaningful volunteer activities.
Reduced income	Take advantage of discounts for seniors.
Declining physical health	Maintain good health practices (nutrition, exercise, rest).
Functional limitations	Adapt the environment to ensure safety and optimal functional status, take advantage of assistive devices and equipment, accept help when necessary.
Changes in cognitive skills	Take advantage of educational opportunities, enroll in classes, keep mentally stimulated, join a discussion group, use the library, avoid dwelling on the things you cannot do and focus on your abilities, take advantage of increased potential for wisdom and creativity.
Death of spouse, friends, and family members	Allow yourself to grieve appropriately, take advantage of opportunities for group or individual counseling and support, establish new relationships, renew old friendships, cherish the happy memories of the past, realize new freedoms.
Relocation from family home	Look into the broad range of options for housing, appreciate the relief from the responsibilities of home ownership, take advantage of new services and opportunities for socialization.
Other challenges to mental health	Maintain a sense of humor, use stress-reduction techniques, learn assertiveness skills, participate in support groups.

Examples of these life events and consequences were discussed earlier in this chapter, and they are summarized in Figure 8-1. If group members do not identify all the life events, the leader may ask about a certain event, such as coping with one's own or a spouse's retirement. This discussion should continue until all the events and consequences in Figure 8-1 have been identified.

If the group is a closed one with a stable membership, the leader may devote the majority of the first meeting to this discussion. The leader should emphasize that the rest of the meetings will be devoted to discussions of the identified issues, and that the first meeting will set the stage for future sessions. If the group is open and has a changing membership, the leader may need to be more directive during this first phase in order to limit the time spent on this topic. With changing membership, this initial identification of issues would be limited to the first 20 to 30 minutes. The discussion of problem-focused coping mechanisms for one specific issue can then be slated for the latter half of the meeting.

After the issues are identified, the leader summarizes the discussion, referring to the list of challenges written for the members to see. The members are then asked to share ideas about coping strategies that they have found to be helpful in adjusting to these changes. The leader may begin this part with a statement such as: "Now that we've identified the challenges of older adulthood, let's look at what things are helpful in responding to these challenges. I'd like each of you to share with the group one thing you do to help yourself face difficult challenges." After

members have identified general coping mechanisms, the leader can suggest that the group choose one specific life event of older adulthood and discuss specific coping mechanisms that might be used to address this challenge. Examples of coping strategies that might be discussed in relation to specific life events are summarized in Table 8-2. As these coping strategies are identified, they should be written on a board, and members should be encouraged to relate their personal experiences.

As the cohesiveness and trust level among members increase, particularly in closed groups, the sharing of experiences may become very open and revealing. The task of the leader, then, is to keep the discussion focused on appropriate coping mechanisms. In cohesive groups with highly functional members, the leader might have an opportunity to discuss the difference between emotion-focused and problem-focused mechanisms. The depth of discussion will depend on the degree of group cohesiveness and trust, the functional level of the members, and the comfort level and willingness of the leader to deal with the identified issues.

During the last 10 minutes of each session, the leader should attempt to bring the discussion to some closure on at least one issue. This may be accomplished by summarizing the issues and coping mechanisms that were identified. In open groups, the leader would end by encouraging those members who do not return to the group to look at coping mechanisms for their own specific issues, either by themselves or with a friend or confidant. For ongoing groups, the leader would end the session by coming to some agreement on the issues that will be discussed during the next session. The leader also can encourage group members to think about the identified issues in the interim.

EVALUATING EFFECTIVENESS OF NURSING INTERVENTIONS

The effectiveness of nursing interventions for older adults with Self-Concept Disturbance is evaluated by determining the extent to which older adults express positive views of themselves. Another measure of effective nursing care of older adults with such a diagnosis is that they no longer verbalize ageist attitudes. Nursing care of older adults who express a sense of Powerlessness is evaluated by the extent to which they become involved in decisions that affect them and the degree to which they express feelings of control over their lives. Nursing care for older adults with Ineffective Individual Coping would be evaluated by observing behaviors that reflect the use of a variety of coping strategies. For example, an older adult might learn to use problem-focused coping strategies for a situation that he or she previously viewed as hopeless and unchangeable.

CHAPTER SUMMARY

Older adults face many psychosocial challenges that are associated with the life events of later adulthood (e.g., functional limitations and loss of significant relationships). Factors that influence the response of older adults to stressful events include the meaning of the event, the timing of the event, and the degree of anticipation of the event. Social resources and long-term coping styles also influence the response of an older individual to stress. Religion and spirituality become increasingly important as coping resources in later adulthood. Factors that increase the risk for poor coping responses include feelings of powerlessness, lack of social resources, and the occurrence of several major life events within a short period of time. Functional consequences of high levels of stress and poor coping include depression and mental changes.

Nursing diagnoses that might be applicable to psychosocial adjustment issues include Self-Esteem Disturbance, Powerlessness, Impaired Adjustment, Ineffective Individual Coping, Social Isolation, and Spiritual Distress. Nursing interventions are directed toward enhancing self-esteem, promoting a sense of control, fostering social supports, and assisting the older adult with the use of effective coping mechanisms. Nursing interventions include individual and group therapy and education. Communication techniques are other

interventions that are directed toward enhancing self-esteem and challenging ageist attitudes. Effectiveness of nursing interventions is determined by observations that the older adult uses effective coping mechanisms, expresses positive self-esteem, and experiences some degree of control over his or her life.

■ CONCLUDING CASE STUDY AND NURSING CARE PLAN

➤ Mr. P. is 86 years old and has recently been admitted to a nursing facility for long-term care. His medical diagnoses are diabetes, glaucoma, retinopathy, and dementia of the Alzheimer's type. Mr. P. lived with his wife until 6 months ago when she died after a brief illness. After her death, he needed help with all his activities of daily living, and his daughter arranged home care assistance for 6 hours a day. About 1 month ago, he started getting up and wandering outside at night. Once, he wandered off at 3:00 AM, and the police had to take him home. After this episode, he was afraid to be alone, and he agreed to go to a nursing facility because he could not afford to pay for 24-hour assistance at home.

During the first week in the nursing facility, Mr. P. was cooperative with the staff and sociable with the other residents. He was resistant to the morning schedule of getting up at 6:00 AM and eating breakfast in the dining room at 7:30 AM, but he passively complied when the staff firmly directed him. His daughter visited him daily and accompanied him to social and recreational activities with other residents. Mr. P. has been in the nursing facility for 10 days, and he is becoming very resistant to staff efforts to get him dressed for breakfast. When he attends group activities, he is disruptive, yelling about being a hostage in a monastery. Mr. P. tells other residents that he was tricked into coming to this place, and that the only reason he has to stay is because his daughter has taken over his house and is living there with her family. He frequently paces up and down the corridors and says he has to find his daughter to take him home because his wife is sick and she needs him to take care of her. You walk with him in the hallway, and he says, "I don't know why they keep me locked up here. I can't do anything like I used to do at home. It's like a monastery where you have to get up in the middle of the night, and they make you get cleaned up and eat breakfast when it's still dark out."

■ Nursing Assessment

Your nursing assessment shows that Mr. P. needs supervision in all activities of daily living because of poor vision and memory impairment. He needs some assistance with personal care, but he can dress himself if staff set his clothes out for him. When Mr. P. was admitted to the nursing facility, he was assigned

DISPLAY 8-5 • NURSING CARE PLAN FOR MR. P.

EXPECTED OUTCOME	NURSING INTERVENTIONS	NURSING EVALUATION
Mr. P. will feel he has greater control over his morning schedule.	• Take Mr. P. off the "night-shift wakers" list and allow him to sleep until 8 AM. • Allow Mr. P. to wear his pajamas and robe to breakfast and to shower, bathe, and dress after breakfast.	• Mr. P. will no longer verbalize feelings of being locked up in a monastery or a prison.
Mr. P. will function as independently as possible.	• The staff will set out Mr. P.'s clothing and allow him to dress himself. • The staff will give Mr. P. positive feedback for dressing himself.	• Mr. P. will dress himself with minimal supervision. • Mr. P. will carry out his personal care activities at a pace that is comfortable for him.
Mr. P. will engage in a familiar activity that gives him a meaningful role.	• Ask Jane to send a set of bill stubs, old bank statements, and the inactive checkbook so that Mr. P. can do his "work." • Encourage Mr. P. to "work with his papers" in the activity room, where he can interact with other residents. • Give Mr. P. positive feedback when he interacts with other residents. • Compliment Mr. P. about doing his paperwork.	• Mr. P. will resume his former routine of working with his papers and will interact with other residents.

to the "night-shift wakers" group, which means that the night shift is responsible for waking him and getting him ready for breakfast by 7:30 AM. The night-shift nursing assistants help him with showering, shaving, and dressing.

During the admission interview, Mr. P.'s daughter, Jane, said that his typical morning routine at home was to get up at about 8:30 AM and get dressed independently, using the clothes that were set out for him by the home health aide. He ate breakfast at about 9:30 AM and then spent the day "working on his papers." Jane, who lives out of town, would call her father four times a week. When Jane talked with him on the phone, he always told her how busy he was working on his papers. Although Jane was paying all his bills from a joint bank account, Mr. P. would spend hours and hours with bill stubs, old bank statements, and an inactive checking account, thinking he was paying his bills.

Jane was staying at her father's house for the 2 weeks before his admission and for 1 week after admission to the nursing facility. She plans to return to town for a couple of days every other month and will visit her father at those times. The only nearby relative is a sister-in-law who comes to visit Mr. P. every 2 weeks.

■ Nursing Diagnosis

You use the nursing diagnosis of Powerlessness related to relocation to a nursing facility and lack of control over activities of daily living. You select this diagnosis, rather than Impaired Adjustment or Ineffective Individual Coping, because Mr. P. focuses on a theme of loss of control. Your assessment identifies several factors that contribute to his powerlessness, and you address these factors in your nursing care plan.

■ Nursing Care Plan

The care plan you develop for Mr. P. is shown in Display 8-5.

 CRITICAL THINKING EXERCISES

1. Take a sheet of paper and draw two vertical lines to make three equal columns. Think of someone you know in your personal life or professional practice who is 80 years old or older. In the left column, list three or more life events that this person has experienced in later adulthood. In the center column, describe the impact of the life event on the

person's daily life. In the right column, list the coping mechanisms the person has used to deal with the life event. You can guess at the information, as needed, to complete the information in the center and right columns.

2. Think of a recent life event in your own life and answer the following questions: How close in time was the life event to other stressful events in your life? What impact did the life event have, and what were the manifestations of stress in your life (e.g., in your work, your health, your personal life, your relationships with other people)? What coping mechanisms did you use? Were the coping mechanisms effective? What coping mechanisms would you like to develop to prepare yourself for older adulthood?

3. You are asked to lead a 1-hour discussion entitled "Mental Health and Aging" for a group of 10 people at a senior citizen center. Describe your approach to this topic. What would your goals for the class be? How would you involve the participants? What visual aids would you use?

EDUCATIONAL RESOURCES

National Senior Service Corps
1201 New York Avenue, NW, Washington, DC 20525
(800) 424-8867
http://www.seniorcorps.org

Stokes/Gordon Stress Scale
Pace University, Lienhard School of Nursing
861 Bedford Road, Pleasantville, NY 10570
(914) 773-3200
http://www.pace.edu

REFERENCES

Aldrich, C., & Mendkoff, E. (1963). Relocation of the aged and disabled: A mortality study. *Journal of the American Geriatrics Society, 11*(3), 185–194.

Andrews, M. M., & Hanson, P. A. (2003). Religion, culture, and nursing. In M. M. Andrews & J. S. Boyle (Eds.), *Transcultural concepts in nursing care*. Philadelphia: Lippincott Williams & Wilkins.

Aneshensel, C., Pearlin, L. I., Levy-Storms, L., & Schuler, R. H. (2000). The transition from home to nursing home: Mortality among people with dementia. *Journal of Gerontology: Social Sciences, 55B*, S152–S162.

Antonucci, T. C. (2001). Social relations: An examination of social networks, social support, and sense of control. In J. E. Birren & K. W. Schaie (Eds.), *Handbook of the psychology of aging* (5th ed., pp. 427–453). San Diego: Academic Press.

Armer, J. M., & Conn, V. S. (2001). Exploration of spirituality and health among diverse rural elderly individuals. *Journal of Gerontological Nursing, 27*(6), 28–37.

Baldwin, K., & Shaul, M. (2001). When your patient can no longer live independently: A guide to supporting the patient and family. *Journal of Gerontological Nursing, 27*(11), 10–18.

Bedard, M., Stones, M. J., Guyatt, G. H., & Hirdes, J. P. (2001). Traffic related fatalities among older driver and passengers: Past and future trends. *Gerontologist, 41*, 751–756.

Blazer, D. G. (2002). Self-efficacy and depression in late life: A primary prevention proposal. *Aging & Mental Health, 6*, 315–324.

Brennan, M., & Cardinali, G. (2000). The use of preexisting and novel coping strategies in adapting to age-related vision loss. *Gerontologist, 40*(3), 327–334.

Butler, R. N. (2001). Life review. In M. D. Mezey (Ed.), *The encyclopedia of elder care* (pp. 401–402). New York: Springer.

Carpenito, L. J. (2002). *Nursing diagnosis: Application to clinical practice* (9th ed.). Philadelphia: Lippincott Williams & Wilkins.

Carr, D., House, J. S., Wortman, C., Nesse, R., & Kessler, R. C. (2001). Psychological adjustment to sudden and anticipated spousal loss among older widowed persons. *Journal of Gerontology: Social Sciences, 56B*, S237–S248.

Carstensen, L. L., Pasupathi, M., & Mayr, U. (2000). Emotional experience in everyday life across the adult life span. *Journal of Personality and Social Psychology, 79*, 644–655.

Chipperfield, J. G., & Havens, B. (2001). Gender differences in the relationship between marital status transitions and life satisfaction in later life. *Journal of Gerontology: Psychological Sciences, 56B*, P176–P186.

Crowther, M. R., Parker, M. W., Achenbaum, W. A., Larimore, W. L., & Koenig, H. G. (2002). Rowe and Kahn's model of successful aging revisited: Positive spirituality—the forgotten factor. *Gerontologist, 42*(5), 613–620.

Cully, J. A., Lavoie, D., & Gfeller, J. D. (2001). Reminiscence, personality, and psychological functioning in older adults. *Gerontologist, 41*, 89–95.

Davidhizar, R. E. (2001). Powerlessness. In M. L. Maas, K. C. Buckwalter, M. D. Hardy, T. Tripp-Reimer, M. G. Titler, & J. P. Specht (Eds.), *Nursing care of older adults: Diagnoses, outcomes, & interventions* (pp. 562–570). St. Louis: Mosby.

DiBartolo, M. C. (2002). Exploring self-efficacy and hardiness in spousal caregivers of individuals with dementia. *Journal of Gerontological Nursing, 28*(4), 24–33.

Dunkle, R. E., Roberts, B., Haug, M., & Raphelson, M. (1992). An examination of coping resources of very old men and women: Their association to the relationship between stress, hassles, and function. *Journal of Women & Aging, 43*(3), 79–104.

Echerdt, D. J. (2001). Retirement. In M. D. Mezey (Ed.), *The encyclopedia of elder care* (pp. 569–574). New York: Springer.

Faulkner, M. (2001). The onset and alleviation of learned helplessness in older hospitalized people. *Aging & Mental Health, 5*, 379–386.

Ferraro, K. F. (2001). Aging and role transitions. In R. H. Binstock & L. K. George (Eds.), *Handbook of aging and the social sciences* (5th ed., pp. 313–330). San Diego: Academic Press.

Foley, D. J., Heimovitz, H. K., Guralnik, J. M., & Brock, D. B. (2002). Driving life expectancy of persons aged 70 years and older in the United States. *American Journal of Public Health, 92*(8), 1284–1289.

Folkman, S., & Lazarus, R. S. (1980). An analysis of coping in a middle-aged community sample. *Journal of Health and Social Behavior, 21*, 219–239.

Folkman, S., Lazarus, R. S., Pimley, S., & Novacek, J. (1986). The dynamics of a stressful encounter: Cognitive appraisal, coping and encounter outcomes. *Journal of Personality and Social Psychology, 50,* 992–1003.

Folkman, S., Lazarus, R. S., Pimley, S., & Novacek, J. (1987). Age differences in stress and coping processes. *Psychology and Aging, 2,* 171–184.

Frazier, L. D., Waid, L. D., & Fincke, C. (2002). Coping with anxiety in later life. *Journal of Gerontological Nursing, 28*(12), 40–47.

George, L. K. (2001). Life events. In M. D. Mezey (Ed.), *The encyclopedia of elder care* (pp. 396–399). New York: Springer.

Groh, C. J., & Whall, A. L. (2001). Self-esteem disturbance. In M. L. Maas, K. C. Buckwalter, M. D. Hardy, T. Tripp-Reimer, M. G. Titler, & J. P. Specht (Eds.), *Nursing care of older adults: Diagnoses, outcomes, & interventions* (pp. 593–600). St Louis: Mosby.

Haan, N. (1977). *Coping and defending: Processes of self-environment organization.* New York: Academic Press.

Haight, B. K. (2000). The extended effects of life review in nursing home residents. *International Journal of Aging and Human Development, 50,* 151–168.

Hegge, M., & Fischer, C. (2000). Grief responses of seniors and elders: Practice implications. *Journal of Gerontological Nursing, 26*(2), 35–43.

Helm, H. M., Hays, J. C., Flint, E. P., Koenig, H. G., & Blazer, D. G. (2000). Does private religious activity prolong survival? A six-year follow up study of study of 3,851 older adults. *Journal of Gerontology: Medical Sciences, 55A,* M400–M405.

Hermann, C. (2000). A guide to the spiritual needs of elderly cancer patients. *Geriatric Nursing, 21,* 324–325.

Hicks, T. J. (2000). What is your life now? Loneliness and elderly individuals residing in nursing homes. *Journal of Gerontological Nursing, 26*(8), 15–19.

Holmes, T. H., & Rahe, R. H. (1967). The social readjustment rating scale. *Journal of Psychosomatic Research, 11,* 213–218.

Idler, E. L., Kasl, S. V., & Hays, J. C. (2001). Patterns of religious practice and belief in the last year of life. *Journal of Gerontology: Social Sciences, 56B,* S326–S334.

Iowa Intervention Project. (2000). M. Johnson, M. Maas, & S. Moorhead (Eds.), *Nursing interventions classification* (NIC) (3rd ed.). St. Louis: Mosby.

Jang, Y., Haley, W. E., Small, B. J., & Mortimer, J. A. (2002). The role of mastery and social resources in the associations between disability and depression in later life. *Gerontologist, 42,* 807–813.

Johnson, C. L., & Barer, B. M. (1993). Coping and a sense of control among the oldest old: An exploratory analysis. *Journal of Aging Studies, 7*(1), 67–80.

Johnson, R. A. (2001). Relocation stress. In M. D. Mezey (Ed.), *The encyclopedia of elder care* (pp. 563–565). New York: Springer.

Johnson, R. A., & Tripp-Reimer, T. (2001). Relocation among ethnic elders. *Journal of Gerontological Nursing, 27*(6), 22–27.

Kim, J. E., & Moen, P. (2002). Retirement transitions, gender, and psychological well-being: A life course, ecological model. *Journal of Gerontology: Psychological Sciences, 57B,* P212–P222.

Klavora, P., & Heslegrave, R. J. (2002). Senior drivers: An overview of problems and intervention strategies. *Journal of Aging and Physical Activity, 10,* 322–335.

Koenig, H. G. (2000). Positive emotions, physical disability, and mortality in older adults. *Journal of the American Geriatrics Society, 48*(11), 1525–1526.

Krause, N. (2001). Social support. In R. H. Binstock & L. K. George (Eds.), *Handbook of aging and the social sciences* (5th ed., pp. 272–294). San Diego: Academic Press.

Labouvie-Vief, G., Hakim-Larson, J., & Hobart, C. J. (1987). Age, ego level and the life-span development of coping and defense processes. *Psychology and Aging, 2,* 286–293.

Lazarus, R. S. (1966). *Psychological stress and the coping process.* New York: McGraw Hill.

Lee, G. R., DeMaris, A., Bavin, S., & Sullivan, R. (2001). Gender differences in the depressive effect of widowhood in later life. *Journal of Gerontology: Social Sciences, 56B,* S56–S61.

LeMone, P. (2001). Spiritual distress. In M. L. Maas, K. C. Buckwalter, M. D. Hardy, T. Tripp-Reimer, M. G. Titler, & J. P. Specht (Eds.), *Nursing care of older adults: Diagnoses, outcomes, and interventions* (pp. 782–793). St. Louis: Mosby.

MacKinlay, E. (2001). Understanding the *ageing* process: A developmental perspective of the psychosocial and spiritual dimensions. *Journal of Religious Gerontology, 12*(3/4), 111–122.

Magai, C. (2001). Emotions over the life span. In J. E. Birren & K. W. Schaie (Eds.), *Handbook of the psychology of aging* (5th ed., pp. 399–426). San Diego: Academic Press.

Margolis, K. L., Kerani, R. P., McGrovern, P., Songer, T., Cauley, J. A., & Ensrud, K. E. (2002). Risk factors for motor vehicle crashes in older women. *Journal of Gerontology: Medical Sciences, 57A,* M186–M191.

Marottoli, R. A., De Leon, M., Williams, C. S., Cooney, L. M., & Berkman, L. F. (2000). Consequences of driving cessation: Decreased out of home activity levels. *Journal of Gerontology: Social Sciences, 55B,* S334–S3340.

Martin, M., Grunendahl, M., & Martin, P. (2001). Age differences in stress, social resources, and well being in middle and older age. *Journals of Gerontology: Psychological Sciences, 56B,* P214–P222.

McAuley, E. (2000)). Physical activity, self-esteem, and self-efficacy relationships in older adults: A randomized controlled trial. *Annals of Behavioral Medicine, 22*(2), 131–139.

McCrae, R. M. (1982). Age differences in the use of coping mechanisms. *Journal of Gerontology, 37,* 454–460.

McGregor, D. (2002). Driving over 65: Proceed with caution. *Journal of Gerontological Nursing, 28*(8), 22–26.

Ortiz, L. P. A., & Langer, N. (2002). Assessment of spirituality and religion in later life: Acknowledging clients' needs and personal resources. *Journal of Gerontological Social Work, 37*(2), 5–21.

Ostir, G. V., Markides, K. S., Black, S. A., & Goodwin, J. S. (2000). Emotional well-being predicts subsequent functional independence and survival. *Journal of the American Geriatrics Society, 48*(5), 473–478.

Penninx, B. W. (2000). A happy person, a healthy person? *Journal of the American Geriatrics Society, 48*(5), 590–592.

Penninx, B W. J. H., Guralnik, J. M., Bandeen-Roch, K., Kasper, J. D., Simonsick, E. M., Ferrucci, L., & Fried, L. P. (2000). The protective effect of emotional vitality on adverse health outcomes in disabled older women. *Journal of the American Geriatrics Society, 48*(11), 1359–1366.

Pfeiffer, E. (1977). Psychopathology and social pathology. In J. E. Birren & K. W. Schaie (Eds.), *Handbook of the psychology of aging* (pp. 650–671). New York: Van Nostrand Reinhold.

Rantz, M. J., & Popejoy, L. (2001). Diversional activity deficit. In M. L. Maas, K. C. Buckwalter, M. D. Hardy, T. Tripp-Reimer, M. G. Titler, & J. P. Specht (Eds.),

Nursing care of older adults: Diagnoses, outcomes, and interventions (pp. 385–396). St Louis: Mosby.

Rodin, J., & Langer, E. (1980). Aging labels: The decline of control and the fall of self-esteem. *Journal of Social Issues, 36*(2), 12–29.

Sarkisian, C. A., Hays, R. D., & Mangione, C. M. (2002). Do older adults expect to age successfully? The association between expectations regarding aging and beliefs regarding healthcare seeking among older adults. *Journal of the American Geriatrics Society, 50,* 1837–1843.

Selye, H. (1956). *The stress of life.* New York: McGraw-Hill.

Shawler, C., Rowles, G. D., & High, D. M. (2001). Analysis of key decision making incidents in the life of a nursing home resident. *Gerontologist, 5,* 612–622.

Steverink, N., Westerhof, G. J., Bode, C., & Dittmann-Kohli, F. (2001). The personal experience of aging, individual resources, and subjective well-being. *Journal of Gerontology: Psychological Sciences, 56B,* P364–P373.

Stokes, S. A., & Gordon, S. E. (1988). Development of an instrument to measure stress in the older adult. *Nursing Research, 37,* 16–19.

Stolley, J. M. (2001). Ineffective individual coping. In M. L. Maas, K. C. Buckwalter, M. D. Hardy, T. Tripp-Reimer, M. G. Titler, & J. P. Specht (Eds.), *Nursing care of older*

adults: Diagnoses, outcomes, and interventions (pp. 766–777). St. Louis: Mosby.

Vaillant, G. E. (1977). *Adaptation to life.* Boston: Little Brown.

van Baarsen, B. (2002). Theories on coping with loss: The impact of social support and self-esteem on adjustment to emotional and social loneliness following a partner's death in later life. *The Journal of Gerontology, Series B, Psychological Sciences and Social Sciences, 57,* S33–S42.

Waterman, J. D., Blegen, M., Clinton, P., & Specht, J. P. (2001). Social isolation. In M. L. Maas, K. C. Buckwalter, M. D. Hardy, T. Tripp-Reimer, M. G. Titler, & J. P. Specht (Eds.), *Nursing care of older adults: Diagnoses, outcomes, and interventions* (pp. 651–663). St Louis: Mosby.

Weaver, A. J., Flannelly, L. T., & Flannelly, K. J. (2001). A review of research on religious and spiritual variables in two primary gerontological nursing journals. *Journal of Gerontological Nursing, 27*(9), 47–54.

Wilson, N. L. (2001). Social isolation. In M. D. Mezey (Ed.), *The encyclopedia of elder care* (pp. 598–600). New York: Springer.

Zausniewski, J. A. (1997). Teaching resourcefulness skills to older adults. *Journal of Gerontological Nursing, 23*(2), 14–20.

Communication and Transcultural Nursing Care

LEARNING OBJECTIVES

1. Examine barriers to communication.

2. Identify cultural influences on communication.

3. Identify verbal and nonverbal strategies that may be used to enhance communication with older adults.

4. Describe the effective use of communication techniques for assessing psychosocial function in older adults.

5. State at least six steps nurses can take to develop cultural competency.

6. Describe the appropriate use of interpreters.

As discussed in Chapters 1 and 2, increasing diversity is a hallmark of the aging society in which we live, and this increasing diversity affects almost every facet of nursing care for older adults because cultural background significantly affects communication, values, the expression of feelings, health beliefs and health-related behaviors, and many other aspects of functioning. This chapter addresses communication and culture as interrelated concepts that significantly affect nursing care of older adults and are particularly important in addressing psychosocial aspects of function.

COMMUNICATING WITH OLDER ADULTS

Because skillful communication techniques are crucial not only for accurate assessments but also for effective interventions, communication techniques are considered in relation to nursing care of older adults as both an assessment tool and a nursing intervention. Much of the information in this chapter is discussed in relation to the psychosocial assessment because communication techniques are especially important in addressing all aspects of psychosocial function. Just as a stethoscope and other tools are essential for assessing physical aspects of function, the communication tools discussed in this chapter are essential for assessing psychosocial function, which is discussed comprehensively in Chapter 10. Similarly, therapeutic communication skills are essential for implementing interventions to improve cognitive and psychosocial function, such as many of those discussed in Chapters 7 and 8.

Unique Aspects of Communication With Older Adults

Communication involves the following components: a sender, a message, verbal and nonverbal methods of sending the message, a receiver, and feedback

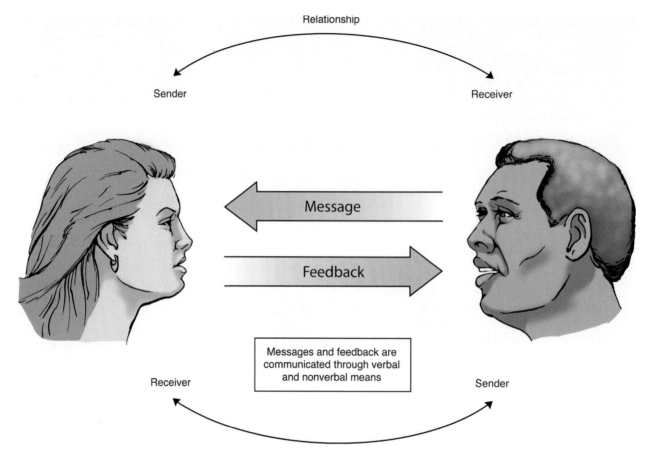

FIGURE 9-1 Communication is an interactive process involving two people and verbal and nonverbal messages.

(Figure 9-1). In terms of the psychosocial assessment, the sender of the message is the nurse, and the message is that information about the person's psychosocial function that is important in planning care for that person. Verbal methods for sending the message include the posing of many open-ended questions. Nonverbal communication methods include the following: touch, clothing, grooming, gestures, physical distance, body language, eye contact, facial expressions, and the tone, rate, and volume of one's voice. A significant source of nonverbal messages is the environment, which can either facilitate or hinder communication. To be effective, verbal and nonverbal messages must convey a nonjudgmental attitude, and the environment must be conducive to good communication. The receiver is the older adult or a caregiver, either of whom may be unfamiliar with psychosocial assessment and thus may be uncomfortable discussing pertinent information. Feedback is important, not only in determining whether the person understood the question, but also in determining the person's receptivity to further questions. Because feedback

includes many subtle and nonverbal messages, excellent listening and observational skills are essential for the gerontological nurse.

Barriers to Communication With Older Adults

Gerontological nurses often encounter communication barriers that can be particularly challenging when discussing personal information such as psychosocial function. It is much easier to communicate effectively when the topic is familiar, such as daily care routines and physical comfort needs. However, usual communication techniques often seem inadequate when the conversation is about sensitive issues or when older adults have a combination of vision and hearing impairments. For example, nurses use nonverbal communication techniques to reinforce verbal messages, but people with visual impairments may not perceive many of the nonverbal messages. Similarly, both the nurse and the older adult may feel uncomfortable speaking loudly about sensitive topics such as the person's feelings about being a widow or adjusting to a move from home.

Sensory overload is another barrier that may interfere with communication, particularly for older adults who are cognitively impaired. Sensory overload can be caused by certain circumstances, such as being asked to receive and process too much information at one time (e.g., responding to questions about social background, cognitive abilities, and emotional function during a single interview), or it may result from too many people trying to communicate at one time (e.g., family members, caregivers, or more than one professional). Sensory overload may also result from environmental noises. These may be particularly bothersome to older adults who use hearing aids because these devices usually magnify background noises. Nurses often become accustomed to background noise in their work environment, learning to tune out stimuli, like alarms and call systems that do not pertain to them. People who are not used to such an environment, however, may be distracted by the noises. In these situations, a simple measure like closing a door or drawing a bed curtain may reduce the sensory input, thereby improving communication.

Internal distractions arise from any physical discomfort that interferes with a person's ability to focus on a conversation. Pain, thirst, hunger, fatigue, bladder fullness, or uncomfortable temperatures all can interfere with a person's attention to psychosocial issues. It is important to assess the older adult for internal distractions so that interventions can be implemented to enhance communication. For example, interventions to alleviate thirst or hunger are often quite simple to implement and can be effective in improving the person's comfort and ability to focus on the conversation. These considerations are especially important when caring for older adults who depend on the nursing staff to meet their basic needs because simply offering water, food, or assistance with toileting may markedly improve the person's ability to attend to the conversation. These simple interventions also may help to establish a trusting relationship because the older adult may then perceive the nurse as someone who understands his or her essential needs.

In an effort to be reassuring, nursing staff and caregivers sometimes offer such remarks as "Why cry over spilled milk?" or "Everything's going to be okay." Although such remarks might be well intentioned and effective in some circumstances, they create barriers to communication in most situations. For example, people who are seriously depressed or coping with an untreatable illness might consider these remarks insensitive. In addition to trite responses and false reassurances, other verbal barriers include

changing the subject, avoiding sensitive issues, jumping to conclusions, giving unwanted advice, and minimizing the person's feelings.

The way the nurse addresses the older person also can be a barrier to communication. For example, many caregivers of older adults consider names like "dear," "honey," or "grandma" to be complimentary, and they habitually use them to address the older adults in their care. However, it is best to avoid these names because they may be perceived as offensive or condescending. Nurses must be aware of any tendency to nickname because even if these terms are not objectionable, they usually do not enhance communication and they do not affirm the older person's individuality. Nurses must also be cautious about addressing people by their first names because many older people interpret that as disrespectful.

Other verbal barriers include inarticulate speech or obstructive mannerisms, such as covering one's mouth or turning one's head away while talking. In institutional settings, much verbal communication takes place while nurses are walking down the hall, pushing a wheelchair, assisting with personal care, or performing other activities. During these activities, nurses can listen and engage in social conversation, but these are not the best times for asking personal questions or giving important information. Not only are the activities a distraction, but also they interfere with the face-to-face positioning that enhances communication and might even be essential for communication with people who are hearing impaired.

Cultural differences can create communication barriers that are difficult, and sometimes impossible, to overcome. For example, if either the older adult or the nurse holds stereotypes or prejudices about the other person, it will be difficult to establish a trusting relationship. Foreign-born people who have a condition that drains their energy or affects their cognitive function may revert to their native language, even if they previously spoke English well. In these situations, family members may be able to facilitate communication, or it may be appropriate to use interpreters, as discussed in the section on Linguistic Competence in Care of Older Adults in this chapter.

Communication barriers can also arise from pathologic disorders and adverse medication effects. For example, neurologic conditions (e.g., aphasia from strokes) often affect language and verbal skills, and cognitive impairments can interfere with a person's ability to listen, remember, and respond to questions. Similarly, people who are actively delusional or hallucinatory, or who are not fully in touch with reality for any reason, may have difficulty attending to the conversation. Adverse medication effects that can interfere with communication

Barriers to Communication With Older Adults

Sociocultural Factors Relating to the Older Adult or the Interviewer
- Stereotypes
- Differences in age, language, or cultural background
- Biases to differences in race, cultural background, sexual orientation, religious or spiritual beliefs

Barriers Within Older Adults
- Sensory impairments
- Physical discomfort (e.g., pain, thirst, hunger)
- Medication effects or pathologic conditions
- Impaired psychosocial function secondary to dementia or depression
- Diminished contact with reality

Barriers Associated With the Interviewer
- Insensitivity
- Poor listening skills
- Use of trite remarks
- False reassurances
- Judgmental attitudes, expressed verbally or nonverbally
- Use of inappropriate or unacceptable names
- Inarticulate speech
- Obstructive mannerisms

Barriers in the Interview Environment
- Noise and distractions
- Presentation of too much information at one time
- Too many people speaking at the same time

include dry mouth, clouded mentation, and tardive dyskinesia (discussed in Chapter 23). Display 9-1 summarizes the barriers that nurses may need to address to facilitate communication, especially for effectively addressing psychosocial issues.

Techniques to Enhance Communication With Older Adults

The manner in which conversations are initiated establishes the basis for further communication. The exchanging of names is an important but simple ritual that is often overlooked by nurses. Even in social settings, the exchange of proper names is a first step in establishing a mutual relationship. Nurses generally have access to information about the older person's name before the older person has information about the nurse's name. In institutional settings,

nurses can simply look at a wristband or a name card to find out the patient's name. Although this method may be an efficient and reliable one for identifying patients, it does nothing to promote a sense of respect for the person as an individual. A more personal approach is to ask the person his or her name, after making sure you have given your own name, and to use the wristband only as a means of confirming information when necessary.

Nurses do not always take the time to introduce themselves to the people for whom they provide care, especially when nametags routinely are used for staff. A verbal exchange of names, however, can be an effective way of establishing rapport. People sometimes feel at a disadvantage if someone else knows their name when they do not know the other person's name. A simple exchange of names can remove this barrier and is especially important for older adults who either cannot read nametags or cannot remember names. Such an exchange is also important for those who need assistance because people generally feel more secure and more comfortable about asking for help when they can address someone by name. Therefore, the nurse should begin any initial contact by stating his or her own name and role, acknowledging the other person's name, and inquiring about the person's preference with regard to how he or she would like to be addressed. The following message is an example of this kind of introduction: "Good morning, my name is Carol Miller and I'm the charge nurse today. Are you Señor Juan Garcia? You can call me Carol. What do you like to be called? I have your morning pills for you to take. Do you mind if I check your wristband first?" This approach is more likely to foster a trusting relationship than a scenario in which the nurse walks into a room, silently checks the wristband to confirm that the person is Juan Garcia, and says, "Here are your morning pills."

At the time of initial contact, a handshake can be used to facilitate communication and to promote the development of a positive relationship. Although not all people are receptive to this form of nonverbal communication, no harm is done as long as a response has not been forced. In most instances, the handshake dispels some of the formality of the situation, and the person may then be more comfortable discussing psychosocial issues. A handshake also provides physical assessment information about skin temperature, the presence or absence of tremors, and other characteristics of one upper extremity. It also can provide clues about the person's social skills and awareness of others.

Physical touch can be used purposefully to enhance communication, provided the person is receptive to this approach. Older adults generally are quite receptive to touch, especially by a nurse whose responsibilities naturally entail much physical contact. However, the nurse should be aware of cultural influences and gender differences on a person's receptivity to different forms of touch because every culture has rules about appropriate use of touch. Nurses have recognized the importance and effectiveness of touch in their contacts with care recipients for decades, and touch is listed as a nursing intervention for many nursing diagnoses that are applicable to older adults (e.g., Hopelessness, Relocation Stress Syndrome, and Sensory/Perceptual Alterations: Kinesthetic). It also has been addressed in research, with many of the studies focusing on the use of touch with older adults, particularly in nursing home settings. For example, Butts (2001) explored the effects of comfort touch—defined as "skin-to-skin touch for the sole purpose of comfort" (p. 180)—on self-perceptions of older female nursing home residents, when a nurse used these interventions twice weekly for 4 weeks during 5-minute interactions. Positive effects of comfort touch identified in this study included improved self-perceptions of health status, self-esteem, well-being and social processes, life satisfaction and self-actualization, faith or belief, and self-responsibility.

The nurse begins a psychosocial assessment by explaining the purpose of the questions with a statement like one of the following: (1) "I'd like to get to know you better so we can make the best plans for follow-up after you leave the hospital"; (2) "I'd like to ask you some questions about your interests so we can plan for your care while you're here at the nursing home"; or (3) "I'd like to ask some questions about how you manage from day to day so we can identify any community services that might be helpful to you." Starting with questions about events of the remote past, such as where the person was born and grew up, is a nonthreatening way of introducing questions about psychosocial function. Nurses may believe that it is unprofessional to talk about themselves, but incorporating some personal information in conversations can facilitate the establishment of a trusting relationship. Offering a little information about their own pets or family, for instance, might encourage the older adult to share feelings that they might not mention otherwise and may help to establish a framework of mutual interest. Be aware, however, that older adults from some Asian and African cultures may not approve of dogs, cats, and other domestic animals being kept as pets, particularly when they are allowed indoors. Culturally, it may be considered inappropriate to keep these animals in one's home because they are considered unclean carriers of fleas, ticks, rabies, and other disease-causing

organisms. On the other hand, the nurse may find that these older adults consider birds or other types of pets to be entirely acceptable. Sharing information about ethnic background also can be an effective and nonthreatening way of obtaining information about possible cultural influences.

If formal mental status assessment questions are asked, they can be introduced after the older adult is more comfortable discussing psychosocial issues. Because questions about memory can be very threatening, the topic might be introduced as follows: "I notice you have a hard time remembering dates. Have you noticed any other problems with your memory? Is it okay with you if I ask some questions about your memory?" If no evidence of cognitive impairment is evident, but other people have expressed concern about the person's memory, a statement such as the following might be used: "Your daughter is concerned that you don't remember to keep appointments. Have you noticed any problems with your memory? Is it okay with you if I ask some questions about your memory?"

During discussions of psychosocial issues, attentive listening is the most effective communication skill. Usually, the best communication occurs when the nurse is verbally quiet and nonverbally responsive. Asking open-ended questions and nonverbally responding to indicate your interest in what the person is saying is usually effective in obtaining important information. Nonverbal responses, like sustained eye contact, and short verbal responses like, "And then what happened?" will encourage the person to elaborate on the information he or she considers most important.

During the early part of a psychosocial assessment, nurses can encourage older adults to choose the issues for discussion. Using this technique, the nurse can identify the issues that are least threatening and most dominant. Carefully listening as the older adult leads the conversation will help to identify appropriate questions. As an example, consider the case of Mrs. P. who, during an admission interview, gave the following response to a question about where she lives:

I moved to Sunnybrook Retirement Village after my last stroke. I couldn't stay in my own home because the bedrooms were on the second floor. The doctor told me I had to live where I could get help, and my daughter didn't want me with her. Now that I've fallen and broken my wrist, I'm not sure what the doctor will tell me. My daughter doesn't want to be bothered with me.

The nurse who is listening carefully will be able to identify several issues in this patient's response to a relatively simple question. In reply, the nurse might ask any of the following questions: (1) "What do you miss most since you moved?" (2) "You mentioned that your daughter didn't want you living with her. Is that something you had hoped you could do?" (3) "Do you worry that the doctor will suggest that you go to a nursing home?" and (4) "Do you see your daughter as often as you'd like?" Each question may lead to a discussion of significant issues. Answers to these questions might uncover some concerns that can be addressed by the nurse and may provide information that is helpful for discharge planning.

When communicating about psychosocial issues, it is important to clarify the messages periodically. One clarification technique is to repeat part of a prior answer when asking further questions. For example, saying to Mrs. P., "You mentioned that your daughter doesn't want you living with her . . ." gives feedback about what the nurse heard and also provides a basis for asking a question about the individual's underlying feelings. Feedback can also be helpful when discrepancies between verbal and nonverbal communication are observed. For example, Mrs. P. might begin to cry and clench her fists as she says, "My daughter has her own life to worry about. I can take care of myself. It doesn't bother me that I can't live with her." A statement like, "You look awfully sad. Are you sure it doesn't bother you?" might lead to an acknowledgment of feelings such as anger, rejection, and loneliness.

When communicating with older adults, nurses might hear information that is contrary to their own values or cultural expectations, such as the following examples:

- Older people may express feelings of racial prejudice.
- Older women may express attitudes of extreme passivity about their role in decisions.
- Older people may be in situations in which they are exploited by friends, family, or others.
- Older men may express attitudes about women that are not in accordance with the nurse's beliefs about women.

Nurses deal with these differences in many care situations, but they are even more likely to encounter anxiety-producing attitudes or responses when discussing psychosocial issues with older adults. In any such situation, it is important to be aware of one's own feelings and to deal with these feelings in appropriate ways. For example, during the psychosocial assessment, nurses must maintain a nonjudgmental attitude, but afterward they can share their feelings with colleagues. In some situations, however, it is appropriate for nurses to acknowledge their feelings or opinions during the

assessment. For instance, if the person describes an episode of extreme exploitation and expresses feelings of anger about the situation, the nurse can show empathy and understanding by a statement such as, "That sounds like a terrible situation to have been in."

Creating an Environment That Supports Good Communication

Face-to-face positioning facilitates verbal as well as nonverbal communication and is particularly important when visual or hearing impairments interfere with communication. Moreover, people usually feel more comfortable talking with others when they are at the same level of eye contact. Therefore, when conversing with someone in a bed or wheelchair, the nurse should sit in a chair. If possible, remove any physical barrier that interferes with direct face-to-face contact. For example, putting side rails down when talking with someone confined to bed, or moving a walker that is in the line of vision, can improve face-to-face contact. Before moving walkers or side rails, however, ask the older person's permission to do so; this demonstrates respect for the wishes of the individual.

Each person has his or her own "comfort zone" for communication, which is the physical space required for the person to feel at ease when communicating with others. This space varies according to the type of interactions and has been conceptualized as follows:

- Intimate distance is 0 to 18 inches.
- Personal distance is 1.5 to 4 feet.
- Social distance is 4 to 12 feet.

The provision of nursing care often requires that interactions take place in the intimate or personal zones, even though the relationship would normally dictate that interactions take place in the social distance zone. Thus, nurses need to be aware of the influence of personal space on the comfort level of the older person and consider this during communication interactions. Because cultural factors strongly influence perception of appropriate distance zones and many other aspects of nonverbal communication (e.g., touch, eye contact), it is essential to be sensitive to cultural differences that may affect communication. Culture Box 9-1 identifies some cultural influences on expressions of nonverbal communication.

During conversations with older adults, especially when discussing psychosocial issues, as much privacy as possible must be provided. This may be difficult in institutional settings, especially when patients or residents share rooms with others. Even in these situations, however, closing the door and pulling the bed curtain will increase the perception of privacy. In

CULTURE BOX 9-1 — Cultural Influences on Expressions of Nonverbal Communication

Perception of Personal Space

- Cultural groups that are likely to have a narrower comfort space for personal distance include Arabs, Hispanics, Japanese, East Indian, Latin Americans, and Middle Easterners.
- British, Canadians, and European North Americans are likely to require the most personal space.
- Men usually have larger personal space than women.

Touch

- Cultural groups that are likely to be most comfortable with physical touch are Jews, French, Spanish, Italians, Indonesian, and Latin Americans.
- Cultural groups that are likely to be uncomfortable with touch are British, Germans, and North Americans.
- Asians may believe that it is disrespectful to touch the head because it is thought to be a source of the person's strength.
- Vietnamese view the human head as the seat of life and highly personal; they may feel anxious if touched on their head or shoulders; if any orifice of the head is invaded, they may fear these procedures could provide an escape for the essence of life.
- Mexican Americans and Native Americans may view touch as a means for healing, preventing harm, or removing an evil spell.

Touch Between Men and Women

- Middle Eastern men and women do not touch outside the marital relationship.
- In many Hispanic and Middle Eastern cultures, male health care providers may be prohibited from touching or examining part or all of the female body.

- In some Asian cultures, touching between persons of the same sex (but not between those of the opposite sex) is common and acceptable.

Hand Shaking

- Middle Eastern women may not shake hands with men.
- Asian women may not shake hands with each other or with men.
- Native Americans may interpret vigorous handshaking as an aggressive action and are offended by a firm, lengthy handshake.

Eye Contact

- People from some Asian, Hispanic, Indochinese, Appalachian, Middle Eastern, and African American cultures may consider direct eye contact impolite, immodest, or aggressive, and they may avert their eyes when talking with health care professionals or when women are talking with men.
- Native Americans may direct their eye contact to the floor during conversations as an indication that they are paying close attention to the speaker.
- Hispanic cultures dictate appropriate deferential behavior in the form of downcast eyes toward others on the basis of age, sex, social position, economic status, and position of authority (e.g., elders expect respect from younger people).

Facial Expression

- Italians, Jews, Hispanics, and African Americans smile readily and use many facial expressions along with words and gestures to communicate pain, happiness, or displeasure.
- Irish, English, and northern Europeans generally do not use facial expressions or other nonverbal expressions.

(Data based partially on information from Andrews, M. M., & Boyle, J. S. [2003]. *Transcultural concepts in nursing care* [4th ed.]. Philadelphia: Lippincott Williams & Wilkins; and Giger, J. S., & Davidhizer, R. E. [1999]. *Transcultural nursing: Assessment and intervention* [4th ed.]. St Louis: Mosby.)

addition, nurses can take advantage of times that the roommate is out of the room; or, it may be appropriate for the nurse to ask the roommate to allow private use of the room. Eliminating distracting noises is also essential for establishing an environment that supports good communication. In institutional settings, closing the door to bedrooms not only increases privacy, but also eliminates noises from the hallway. Before closing a door or bed curtains, however, the nurse should ask permission from the older person. Asking permission shows respect for the person's territory and may be especially important when talking with people who become anxious when they are in closed spaces. Likewise, if a radio or television is on, the nurse can ask permission to turn it off.

All the environmental modifications related to improving hearing and vision (discussed in Chapters 12 and 13, respectively) may be appropriate interventions for enhancing the communication environment. One particularly easy and important consideration is the avoidance of background glare. In hospital or long-term care settings, people often stand in front of a window when talking to a patient in a bed near the window. When the sun is shining or lights are reflected in the window, the background glare may interfere with the older person's ability to see the person in front of the window. In these situations, simply closing the window curtains or sitting on the other side of the bed may significantly improve communication. In home settings, lack of lighting is a more common problem than glare. Asking the person's permission to turn on lights can be a very effective and easy way of improving communication. After finishing the conversation, the nurse must remember to ask whether the person wants the environment returned to the way it was before. Turning on radios and televisions,

Communication Strategies for Good Communication With Older Adults

- Arrange for face-to-face positioning whenever possible.
- Ensure as much privacy as possible.
- Provide good lighting and avoid background glare.
- Eliminate as much background noise as possible.
- Compensate as much as possible for vision or hearing impairments (e.g., make sure the person is using eyeglasses and hearing aid if appropriate).
- Begin contacts with an exchange of names and, if appropriate, a handshake.
- Use culturally appropriate titles of respect, such as Señor, Señora, Señorita, Mr., Mrs., Ms., Dr., Reverend, Elder, Bishop, and so forth.
- Before calling a person by his or her first name, obtain permission or wait until you have been invited to use this familiar form of address. In some cultures, it is considered inappropriate or disrespectful for anyone but family or close friends to use first names.
- Be sure to pronounce names correctly. When in doubt, ask the older adult to say his or her name. Names that are difficult to pronounce may be written phonetically on the chart for later reference.
- Be aware of subtle linguistic messages that may convey bias or inequality (e.g., using Mr. and the last name to call a white man but addressing an African American woman by her first name).
- Avoid slang expressions, such as "Pop," "Grandma," "dear," "chief," or similar terms, unless the older adult suggests that you do so.

- Never use slang, pejorative, or derogatory terms to refer to ethnic, racial, religious, or any other group (e.g., gays or lesbians).
- Use touch purposefully—providing the person is open to this—to reinforce verbal messages and as a primary method of nonverbal communication.
- In all interactions, be aware of cultural differences that influence the perception and interpretation of verbal and nonverbal communication.

Communication Strategies Specific to a Psychosocial Assessment

- Explain the purpose of the psychosocial assessment in relation to a nursing goal. Begin with questions about remote, nonthreatening topics.
- Use open-ended questions and learn to use silence effectively and comfortably.
- Periodically clarify the messages.
- Maintain good eye contact, use attentive listening, and encourage the person to elaborate on information.
- Remain nonjudgmental in your responses, but show appropriate empathy.
- Ask formal mental status questions, or the most threatening questions, toward the end of the interview.
- Gain the person's permission before asking formal assessment questions regarding memory and other cognitive abilities.

replacing walkers and side rails, and leaving bed curtains and doors the way they were found shows respect for the person's preferences. Display 9-2 summarizes verbal and nonverbal strategies to enhance communication with older adults and includes some strategies that are specific to communication during a psychosocial assessment.

CULTURAL ASPECTS OF CARING FOR OLDER ADULTS

Cultural Competence and Gerontological Nursing

For several decades, nurses have recognized the importance of transcultural nursing (i.e., the provision of nursing care across cultural boundaries), and in recent years, the importance of providing culturally competent nursing care is widely addressed by nurses and nursing organizations. For example, in the 1990s, both

the American Academy of Nurses and the American Nurses Association published statements about culturally competent care (American Academy of Nursing, 1992, 1993; American Nurses Association, 1994). In addition, the U.S. Department of Health and Human Services Office of Minority Health published 14 recommendations to be used as national standards to ensure cultural competence in health care (U.S. Department of Health and Human Services, 2001). Another federal initiative to promote cultural competence in health care is in the *Healthy People 2010* goal of eliminating disparities in health care for minority groups. In addition, regulatory, accrediting, and professional organizations (e.g., American Nurses Association, Joint Commission for Accreditation of Healthcare Organizations) are calling attention to the need to ensure that people of diverse cultural, racial, ethnic, and linguistic groups receive care that is culturally congruent and linguistically appropriate (Narayan, 2001). Organizations such as the Gerontological Society of America and the American Association of Retired

Persons (AARP) also are emphasizing the need to address cultural diversity in the aging population. Thus, there is a broad base of support for gerontological nurses to address cultural competence as an essential component of their care for older adults.

Cultural competence in nursing is defined as "a process, as opposed to an end point, in which the nurse continuously strives to work effectively within the cultural context of an individual, family, or community from a diverse cultural background" (Andrews, 2003b, p. 15). Similarly, *cultural care* in nursing is defined as "the subjectively and objectively learned and transmitted values, beliefs, and patterned lifeways that assist, support, facilitate, or enable another individual or group to maintain their health and well-being, to improve their human condition and lifeway, or to deal with illness, handicaps, or death" (Leininger & McFarland, 2002, p. 83). Cultural competence is often conceived as a continuum that indicates a progression from negative practices to positive approaches within an individual or organization. The continuum begins with the negative stage of cultural destructiveness; progresses through the stages of cultural incapacity, cultural blindness, cultural precompetence, and cultural competence; and ends with the positive stage of cultural proficiency (Luna, 2002).

An important initial step in achieving cultural competence is exploring one's own attitudes about people of different cultural backgrounds through a cultural self-assessment, also called a *cultural rooting exercise* (Zoucha, 2002). A cultural self-assessment provides insights that are essential for overcoming the ethnocentric tendencies and cultural stereotypes that perpetuate prejudice and discrimination against members of certain groups (Andrews, 2003b). Performing a cultural self-assessment also should improve one's level of comfort in assessing cultural aspects of function in older adults. Display 9-3 describes a brief cultural self-assessment that is particularly applicable for gerontological nurses.

In addition to performing a cultural self-assessment, other suggestions for providing culturally competent nursing care have been described by Narayan (2001):

- Cultivate attitudes associated with excellent transcultural care: caring, empathy, openness, and flexibility.
- Develop an awareness of the impact culture has on the beliefs, values, and practices of the patient and clinician and identify and avoid potential areas of cultural conflict (e.g., social values, communication patterns, and health beliefs and values).
- Become informed about cultural norms of the populations commonly served.

DISPLAY 9-3
Cultural Self-Assessment for Gerontological Nurses

What self-identity influences my world view?
- With what sociocultural and religious groups do I most closely identify?
- What does it mean to belong to these groups?
- Is there any stigma associated with any of these groups?
- What do I like and dislike about these groups and my sociocultural identity?

How has my cultural background influenced me?
- How has (does) the society in which I grew up (currently live in) influenced the dominant values that I now hold?
- What is my perception of concepts such as time, work, leisure, health, family, relationships?
- How do my perceptions differ from those of people who come from different cultural backgrounds?

What is my attitude toward people, especially older adults, . . .
- Who are immigrants?
- Who have difficulty with the English language?
- Who have difficulty communicating?
- Who have a cultural background different from my own?

What are my attitudes about and experiences with health practices that differ from my own?
- Do (did) my parents, grandparents, great-grandparents have health care practices that differed from conventional Western medicine practices (e.g., herbs, poultices, folk remedies)?
- Do (did) they consult with folk, indigenous, religious, or spiritual healers?
- How do I feel about alternative or complementary health care practices for myself and for older adults?

What do I do and how do I feel when I have difficulty understanding people whose accents and primary language are different from my own?

What have I learned about myself because of this self-assessment?

- Perform a cultural assessment and include questions that address cultural influences on nutrition, medication management, pain assessment, and psychosocial assessment.
- Individualize care plans that are culturally congruent.
- When unfamiliar with different cultural norms, avoid mistakes by taking cues from the other person and mirroring their behaviors; observe for cues that your actions or words are not culturally sensitive (e.g., discomfort, withdrawal).

In planning care for older adults, particularly with regard to health education and other health promotion interventions, it is important to understand their cultural perceptions of health, illness, aging, and coping. For example, cultural influences can significantly influence one's diet and eating patterns (as discussed in Chapter 14). Health education materials must not only be age-appropriate for older adults, but they must be culturally and linguistically appropriate. Increasingly, health education materials are available in languages other than English, and these materials often can be obtained from the Internet sites listed in the Educational Resources sections throughout this text.

Linguistic Competence in Care of Older Adults

Linguistic competence, which refers to health care services that are respectful of and responsive to a person's linguistic needs, is a form of cultural competence. This concept is important for gerontological nurses because they frequently work with older adults whose primary language differs from their own. Older adults may be particularly disadvantaged for English proficiency if they immigrated as adults and had few opportunities to learn English (Enslein et al., 2002). The challenge of communicating with people who do not speak the same language or dialect is magnified when the person also has dementia or sensory impairments, as is often the situation in long-term care settings. Gerontological literature describes interventions to address cultural differences and communication needs of residents of long-term care facilities (e.g., Burgio et al., 2000; Camp et al., 1996; Gorek et al., 2002). Interventions described by Camp and colleagues (1996) employ simple and cost-effective audio and visual aids to teach staff essential foreign-language skills to improve communication with residents who do not speak English.

Because the Civil Rights Act of 1964 upholds the rights of individuals with limited English proficiency to have equal access to health and social services programs, health care providers must ensure effective use of interpretation services. Some of the circumstances that indicate the need for using an interpreter to facilitate communication at all key decision-making points in health care encounters are as follows:

- When client and practitioner speak different languages
- When the client has limited understanding of the practitioner's language
- When the practitioner has only a rudimentary understanding of the client's primary language

- When cultural tradition prohibits the client from speaking directly to the practitioner (Enslein et al., 2002)

Gerontological nurses have developed an excellent evidence-based protocol, called *Interpreter Facilitation for Individuals with Limited English Proficiency*, that provides comprehensive guidelines to assist in facilitating the effective use of language interpretation services with older adults who have limited English proficiency (Enslein et al., 2002). Some nurses have found the AT&T Language Line Service to be a useful resource when interpreters are unavailable (see the list of Educational Resources at the end of this chapter). Display 9-4 summarizes guidelines for using interpreters in health care settings with older adults.

DISPLAY 9-4
Guidelines for Using Interpreters

Before the Interaction

- Whenever possible, use the services of a professional interpreter. Avoid using visitors or staff from auxiliary services unless permission to do so has been obtained from both the older adult and the interpreter.
- Given that there are more than 140 languages spoken in North America, be certain that the correct language and dialect have been identified before arranging for an interpreter. For example, does the person speak Cantonese or Mandarin Chinese?
- If an interpreter for the primary language is unavailable, determine whether the older adult speaks other languages. For example, many older adults from Vietnam and some African nations are also fluent in French.
- Be aware of age, gender, and socioeconomic class considerations in selecting an interpreter. In general, it is best to use an interpreter who is the same gender and of the same approximate age and socioeconomic class as the older adult.
- Organize your thoughts and plan ahead to ensure that the most important topics are covered.
- Allow sufficient time for the interaction and expect that it will take longer than an interaction with an older adult for whom English is the primary language.

During the Interaction

- Review the importance of confidentiality.
- Talk to the older adult, not the interpreter.
- Talk about only one topic at a time.
- Use short sentences and simple vocabulary.
- Use the active voice. Avoid vague modifiers.
- Avoid professional jargon, idioms, and slang.
- Be aware that many words do not translate into another language. For instance, the English word *depression* has no equivalent in many Asian and other languages.

Cultural Factors That Influence Psychosocial Function

Cultural considerations are important for assessing and addressing many aspects of function, but they are especially important in relation to psychosocial function because a person's cultural background significantly influences the way a person defines and perceives all aspects of psychosocial function. In assessing psychosocial function in older adults, for example, it is essential to recognize that every society has standards of "normal" or "abnormal" behaviors, and these standards provide guidelines for determining whether behaviors are healthy or unhealthy. Many societies, however, do not have the rigid distinctions between health and illness that are part of Western cultures, and concepts such as mental health have little meaning in many non-Western societies (Kavanagh, 2003). Cultural perceptions determine all of the following aspects of psychosocial function:

- Definition of mental health and mental illness
- Belief about the causes of mental health and illness
- Expression of symptoms or clinical manifestations
- Criteria for labeling or diagnosing someone as mentally ill
- Decisions concerning appropriate healers
- Choice of treatment to cure mental illness
- Determination that mental health has been restored following an illness episode
- Relative degree of tolerance for abnormal behavior by other members of society

Culture Box 9-2 identifies some of the cultural influences on psychosocial function and is particularly applicable to psychosocial nursing assessment.

CULTURE BOX 9-2   Cultural Influences on Psychosocial Function

Cultural Influences on Beliefs About the Cause of Mental Disorders

- In traditional Chinese culture, many diseases are attributed to an imbalance of yin and yang.
- Many Native American groups embrace a belief system in which balance and harmony are essential for mental and physical health.
- For some Hispanics, mental illness may be viewed as a punishment by a supreme being for past transgressions.
- Some African Americans, especially those of circum-Caribbean descent, may attribute the cause of mental illness to voodoo, sorcery, or other spiritual forces.
- Some European Americans believe that mental illness has physiologic origins related to chemical disturbances, genetic disturbances, or both.

Cultural Influences on the Manifestations of Mental Illness

- Cultural norms determine whether behaviors such as any of the following are viewed as either normal or abnormal: dreams, fainting, visions, trances, sorcery, delusions, hallucinations, intoxication, suicide, speaking in tongues, communicating with spirits, and the use of certain substances (e.g., alcohol, tobacco, peyote, marijuana, and other drugs) (Kavanagh, 2003).
- Posttraumatic stress disorders are relatively common in immigrants and refugees (Boyle, 2003a).
- Hispanic older adults define mental health problems as alcohol and other drug abuse (American Association of Retired Persons, 1997).
- Filipino Americans consider forgetfulness and anger to be mental health problems (American Association of Retired Persons, 1997).
- Although psychotic disorders (i.e., loss of contact with reality) occur in every society and are characterized by similar primary symptoms (e.g., insomnia, delusions, hallucinations, flat affect, and social or emotional withdrawal), the secondary features are highly influenced by cultural factors (Kavanagh, 2003).
- Whereas sadness, joylessness, anxiety, tension, and lack of energy are common manifestations of depression across cultures, feelings of guilt and suicidal ideation occur only in some groups (Kirmayer & Groleau, 2001).

Cultural Influences on Stress and Coping

- Cultural factors often create barriers to the use of formal support services by ethnic elders, and these barriers may increase the feelings of burden experienced by caregivers.
- African American families tend to use religion and spirituality to help them cope with caregiving stress, and religious organizations are a major source of social support for them (Boyle, 2003b).
- In Latino families, the stress of caregiving may be appraised in relation to the degree of disruption to the family rather than the degree of interference with a person's perceived control over life circumstances (Aranda & Knight, 1997).
- In Chinese families, cultural ideals promoting filial piety, family interdependence, veneration of elderly family members, and acceptance of family caregiving roles may affect the way families experience and cope with stress related to their roles as caregivers.

In some instances, people from diverse cultures may perceive or interpret physical symptoms and their interconnected psychological or emotional components in a manner that is unfamiliar to the nurse. For example, this is likely to occur with people who have a *culture-bound syndrome*, defined as a disorder that is "restricted to a particular culture or group of cultures because of certain psychosocial characteristics of those cultures" (Andrews, 2003a, p. 42). Because these conditions are unique to a particular culture, they may be unrecognized as a disease condition in the biomedical health care system and by professionals who do not share the same cultural background. Anthropologists have identified approximately 150 culture-bound syndromes, and some of these are listed as diagnoses in official diagnostic manuals, such as the *Diagnostic and Statistic Manual of Mental Disorders* (DSM-IV) and the *International Classification of Mental Disorders* (ICD-10), which was developed by the World Health Organization (Mezzich et al., 2001). Table 9-1 lists selected culture-bound syndromes found in specific cultural groups.

Professionals and folk or indigenous healers with the same cultural background usually are knowledgeable about interventions for culture-bound syndromes. Older adults may be reluctant to discuss culture-bound syndromes or folk treatments with health care professionals, especially if the care provider has a different cultural background. The reasons for withholding such information are complex and may include fears that the nurse or other health care provider will disapprove, ridicule, or fail to understand their folk or indigenous healing system. Because of these factors, nurses may consider asking the person's permission to include folk or indigenous healers in discussions about health-related issues. These healers frequently have considerable insight into the cultural and psychosocial aspects of human behavior, and they may be remarkably successful in treating culture-bound syndromes and other disorders that have psychological and emotional components. Because herbal remedies that sometimes are used to treat culture-bound syndromes may interact with prescription or over-the-counter medications,

TABLE 9-1 ● Selected Culture-Bound Syndromes

Group	Disorder	Remarks
Blacks, Haitians	Blackout	Collapse, dizziness, inability to move
	Low blood	Not enough blood or weakness of the blood that is often treated with diet
	High blood	Blood that is too rich in certain things because of the ingestion of too much red meat or rich foods
	Thin blood	Occurs in women, children, and old people; renders the individual more susceptible to illness in general
	Diseases of hex, witchcraft, or conjuring	Sense of being doomed by spell; gastrointestinal symptoms, e.g., vomiting; hallucinations; part of voodoo beliefs
Chinese, Southeast Asians	*Koro*	Intense anxiety that penis is retracting into body
Greeks	Hysteria	Bizarre complaints and behavior because the uterus leaves the pelvis for another part of the body
Hispanics	*Empacho*	Food forms into a ball and clings to the stomach or intestines, causing pain and cramping
	Fatigue	Asthma-like symptoms
	Mal ojo, "evil eye"	Fitful sleep, crying, diarrhea in children caused by a stranger's attention; sudden onset
	Pasmo	Paralysis-like symptoms of face or limbs; prevented or relieved by massage
	Susto	Anxiety, trembling, phobias from sudden fright
Japanese	*Wagamama*	Apathetic childish behavior with emotional outbursts
Koreans	*Hwa-byung*	Multiple somatic and psychological symptoms: "pushing up" sensation of chest, palpitations, flushing, headache, "epigastric mass," dysphoria, anxiety, irritability, and difficulty concentrating; mostly afflicts married women
Native Americans	Ghost	Terror, hallucinations, sense of danger
North India Indians	Ghost	Death from fever and illness in children; convulsions, delirious speech (or incessant crying in infants); choking, difficulty breathing; based on Hindu religious beliefs and curing practices
Whites	Anorexia nervosa	Excessive preoccupation with thinness; self-imposed starvation
	Bulimia	Gross overeating and then vomiting or fasting

(Andrews, M. M. [2003]. Cultural competence in the health history and physical examination [p. 43]. In M. M. Andrews & J. S. Boyle [Eds.], *Transcultural concepts in nursing care* [4th ed., pp. 36–72]. Philadelphia: Lippincott Williams & Wilkins.)

nurses need to make every effort to elicit information about such remedies as part of an assessment (see Chapter 23).

The following case study is based on a case described by Andrews and Boyle (2003):

> Mrs. Y. is a 79-year-old native of the Philippines. She moved to an urban area in California to be near her four children, who live in the same state. She had lived in the same town in the Philippines for her entire adult life and had stayed there to care for her husband and her sister, who both required care for chronic conditions. Although she was a much-needed and highly esteemed member of her household in the Philippines, Mrs. Y., like many other immigrants, experienced role reversal when she lost her once-dominant position in the family and became financially dependent on her adult children after her relocation.

Like many older immigrants from the Philippines, Mrs. Y. had a more active social network before her relocation. She, like many of her peers, spoke a dialect and did not speak Tagalog, the language spoken by many younger residents of the Philippines. After her relocation to the United States, her communication and interaction with others became restricted to her extended family because she did not feel confident using her limited English and could not find other speakers of her dialect.

To buffer the disequilibrium she felt as a result of her migration, Mrs. Y. sought comfort through prayer and regular attendance at the local Roman Catholic Church. She also began to care for her two daughters' children regularly.

You are the nurse at the local hospital who treated Mrs. Y. in the emergency department after she fractured her wrist. During your assessment, you noted that Mrs. Y.'s injury would place a strain on the family because they would temporarily be without their childcare provider.

 ## THINKING POINTS

> How would you involve the family members in the discharge plan for Mrs. Y. so that her recovery could be ensured, she would not lose respect, and she would not feel responsible to assume her usual duties until she felt better?

> What problems would you anticipate with communicating with Mrs. Y. in the emergency room? How would you handle these problems?

> What psychosocial repercussions did Mrs. Y.'s move to the United States have? Did she cope with these effectively? Would you have had any other suggestions for helping her to cope?

> How did Mrs. Y's culture influence her coping mechanisms?

CHAPTER SUMMARY

Identifying and addressing barriers to communication (e.g., sociocultural factors, sensory impairments or diminished contact with reality in the older person, and insensitivity and poor communication skills on the part of the nurse) is essential for effective communication with older adults. Nurses use verbal and nonverbal strategies to enhance communication with older adults, with particular attention on cultural factors that may influence communication patterns. Strategies include adapting the environment to facilitate optimal communication, using touch and other nonverbal communication purposefully, and using culturally appropriate titles of respect.

Gerontological nurses must provide culturally competent care, and some of the steps to achieve this goal are performing a cultural self-assessment, becoming knowledgeable about cultural norms of populations commonly served, and developing individualized care plans that are culturally congruent. Cultural factors can have a strong impact on many aspects of psychosocial function, and nurses need to recognize and address these influences. Nurses also need to address language barriers through appropriate communication strategies such as the use of interpreters.

 ## CRITICAL THINKING EXERCISES

1. Think of several different situations in the past few weeks in which you communicated with older adults.
   - What actual or potential barriers to communication may have affected these exchanges?
   - What factors hindered or enhanced interaction with these older adults?
   - Are there verbal or nonverbal techniques that may have improved the interactions?
2. Complete the cultural self-assessment in Display 9-3.
3. Think of the various settings in which you work with older adults and describe what you would do or whom you would call if you needed to communicate with an older adult who did not speak English.
4. Identify one culturally diverse group that you are likely to work with in your geographic area and use the Internet to find information about cultural factors that are likely to influence their perceptions of health and illness.

EDUCATIONAL RESOURCES

AT&T Language Line
1 Lower Ragsdale Drive, Bldg. 2, Monterey, CA 93940
(800) 752-0093, ext. 441
http://www.languageline.com

DiversityRx: Resources for Cross Cultural Health Care
8915 Sudbury Road, Silver Spring, MD 20901
(301) 588-6051
http://www.diversityrx.org

Transcultural Nursing Society
36600 Schoolcraft Road, Livonia, MI 48150-1173
(888) 432-5470
http://www.tcns.org

U.S. Department of Health and Human Services, Office of Minority Health
P.O. Box 37337, Washington, D. C., 20013-7337
(800) 444-6472
http://www.omhrc.gov

REFERENCES

American Academy of Nursing. (1992). AAN expert panel report: Culturally competent health care. *Nursing Outlook, 40,* 277–283.

American Academy of Nursing. (1993). *Promoting cultural competence in and through nursing education.* Subpanel on Nursing Education. New York: American Academy of Nursing.

American Association of Retired Persons (AARP). (1997). *Mental health issues for minority seniors.* Washington, DC: Author.

American Nurses Association. (1994). *Position statement on cultural diversity in nursing practice.* Washington, DC: American Nurses Association Board of Directors.

Andrews, M. M. (2003a). Cultural competence in the health history and physical examination. In M. M. Andrews & J. S. Boyle (Eds.), *Transcultural concepts in nursing care* (4th ed., pp. 36–72). Philadelphia: Lippincott Williams & Wilkins.

Andrews, M. M. (2003b). Culturally competent nursing care. In M. M. Andrews & J. S. Boyle (Eds.), *Transcultural concepts in nursing care* (4th ed., pp. 15–35). Philadelphia: Lippincott Williams & Wilkins.

Andrews, M. M. & Boyle, J. S. (2003). *Transcultural concepts in nursing care* (4th ed). Philadelphia: Lippincott Williams & Wilkins.

Aranda, M. P., & Knight, B. G. (1997). The influence of ethnicity and culture on the caregivers stress and coping process: a sociocultural review and analysis. *Gerontologist, 37,* 342–354.

Boyle, J. S. (2003a). Culture, family, and community. In M. M. Andrews & J. S. Boyle (Eds.), *Transcultural concepts in nursing care* (4th ed., pp. 315–360). Philadelphia: Lippincott Williams & Wilkins.

Boyle, J. S. (2003b). Transcultural perspectives in the nursing care of adults. In M. M. Andrews & J. S. Boyle (Eds.), *Transcultural concepts in nursing care* (4th ed., pp. 181–208). Philadelphia: Lippincott Williams & Wilkins.

Burgio, L. D., Allen-Burge, R., Roth, D.L., Bourgeois, M.S., Dijkstra, K., Gerstle, J., et al. (2000). Come talk with me: Improving communication between nursing assistants and nursing home residents during care routines. *Gerontologist, 41,* 449–460.

Butts, J. (2001). Outcomes of comfort touch in institutionalized elderly female residents. *Geriatric Nursing, 22,* 180–183.

Camp, C. J., Burant, C. J., & Graham, G. C. (1996). The InterpreCare System: Overcoming language barriers in long-term care. *Gerontologist, 36,* 70–75.

Enslein, J., Tripp-Remer, T., Kelley, L.S., Choi, E., & McCarty, L., (2002). Interpreter facilitation for individuals with limited English proficiency. *Journal of Gerontological Nursing, 28*(7), 5–11.

Giger, J. S., & Davidhizer, R. E. (1999). *Transcultural nursing: Assessment and intervention* (4th ed.). St Louis: Mosby.

Gorek, B., Martin, J., White, N., Peters, D., & Hummel, F. (2002). Culturally competent care for Latino elders in long-term care settings. *Geriatric Nursing, 23,* 272–275.

Kavanagh, K. H. (2003). Transcultural perspectives in mental health nursing. In M. M. Andrews & J. S. Boyle (Eds.), *Transcultural concepts in nursing care* (4th ed., pp. 272–314). Philadelphia: Lippincott Williams & Wilkins.

Kirmayer, L. J., & Groleau, D. (2001). Affective disorders in cultural context. *Psychiatric Clinics of North America, 24,* 465–478.

Leininger, M., & McFarland, M. R. (2002). *Transcultural nursing: Concepts, theories, research & practice.* New York: McGraw-Hill.

Luna, I. (2002). Diversity issues in the delivery of healthcare. *Lippincott's Case Management, 7*(4), 138–146.

McKenna, M. A. (2003). Transcultural nursing care of older adults. In M. M. Andrews & J. S. Boyle (Eds.), *Transcultural concepts in nursing care* (4th ed., pp. 209–246). Philadelphia: Lippincott Williams & Wilkins.

Mezzich, J. E., Berganza, C. E., & Ruiperez, M. A. (2001). Culture in DSM-IV, ICD-10, and evolving diagnostic systems. *Psychiatric Clinics of North America, 24*(3), 407–419.

Narayan, M. C. (2001). Six steps toward cultural competence: A clinician's guide. *Home Health Care Management & Practice, 14*(1), 40–48.

U.S. Department of Health and Human Services, OPHS Office of Minority Health. (2001). *National standards for culturally and linguistically appropriate services in health care: Final report* [On-line]. Available at http://www.omhrc.gov/omh/programs/2pgprograms/final report.pdf.

Zoucha, R. (2002). Understanding the cultural self in promoting culturally competent care in the community. *Home Health Care Management & Practice, 14,* 452–456.

Psychosocial Assessment

LEARNING OBJECTIVES

1. Describe the goals of and the procedure for psychosocial assessment of older adults.

2. List the criteria for assessing the following specific components of mental status: physical appearance, motor function, social skills, response to the interview, orientation, alertness, memory, speech characteristics, higher language skills, and decision making.

3. Identify questions and observations for assessing decision making and executive function.

4. Discuss guidelines for assessing affective function.

5. List the distinguishing characteristics of delusions, hallucinations, and illusions as they relate to the underlying causes (delirium, dementia, depression, and paranoid disorder).

6. List criteria for assessing the following components of social supports: social network, barriers to services, economic resources, and religion and spirituality.

Psychosocial assessment is a complex and challenging part of a multidimensional assessment. Although impaired psychosocial function may often be attributed to factors relating to normal aging or to untreatable conditions, a careful psychosocial assessment can identify the underlying causes of mental changes, many of which can then be reversed or addressed through interventions. A psychosocial assessment addresses the following indicators of psychosocial function, each of which is reviewed in this chapter: mental status, decision making, affective function, contact with reality, and sociocultural supports. Rather than addressing all components of the nursing process, this chapter focuses solely on assessment and is intended to be used in conjunction with information about other components of the nursing process in Chapters 7 and 8 on cognitive and psychosocial function. In addition, it can be used to supplement assessment information in other chapters of this text, particularly the chapters on dementia (Chapter 24), depression (Chapter 25), and elder abuse and neglect (Chapter 26).

OVERVIEW OF THE PSYCHOSOCIAL ASSESSMENT PROCESS

Psychosocial Assessment as a Nursing Responsibility

Traditionally, many aspects of psychosocial function have been viewed as the exclusive purview of psychologists, psychiatrists, social workers, and other mental health professionals. Physical assessment procedures are viewed as part of a routine evaluation of a person's physical health to detect illness in its early stages or to identify the underlying cause of troublesome symptoms. Psychosocial assessment procedures, however, may be perceived as measures that involve mysterious batteries of tests aimed at identifying people who are in need of psychiatric treatment. Consequently, they do not enjoy the same level of acceptance and are not routinely incorporated into overall health assessments. However, when applying a holistic approach to the care of older adults, a psychosocial assessment is a necessary component of comprehensive care provided by gerontological nurses.

Nurses often participate in physically intimate activities, such as bathing, as a normal part of caring for older adults and generally feel comfortable providing such care; however, they may be less comfortable participating in a psychosocial assessment. Many aspects of psychosocial assessment of older adults involve discussions of specific issues related to older adulthood, and some involve emotionally charged issues that would not normally be discussed with strangers. Thus, both the nurse and the older adult initially may feel uncomfortable during a psychosocial assessment. Because increased awareness of one's own attitudes is an important first step in becoming comfortable in performing a psychosocial assessment, nurses can use a self-assessment guide (Display 10-1) to examine their own attitudes about older adults and identify areas of discomfort.

In this chapter, the mental status assessment addresses all the aspects of psychosocial function that are assessed by nurses and that are important to the overall assessment of older adults. This comprehensive overview is like the emergency cart that is available in every hospital unit. The cart stands ready at all times and is equipped with any items that would be needed to handle medical emergencies. When a

serious medical problem arises, health care professionals quickly pull the cart to the patient's bedside and select the needed items. Similarly, gerontological nurses must have access to an array of skills for assessing psychosocial function as the need arises. In a few situations, their entire array of skills will be called into play, but in most situations, only a few of the examination tools will be necessary. Nurses can use the material in this chapter to "fill their mental status assessment carts" so that they are prepared to select the appropriate tools for each situation.

Goals of Psychosocial Assessment

From a nursing perspective, the psychosocial assessment provides the basis for identifying health promotion interventions to address psychosocial needs of older adults. Thus, the goals, like those of a physical health assessment, are to detect asymptomatic or unacknowledged health problems at an early stage and to address any existing symptoms of illness. In addition, one of the purposes of psychosocial assessment in the context of the functional consequences theory is to identify those risk factors (especially those that are amenable to interventions) that interfere with cognitive, emotional, or social function. Last, a good psychosocial assessment provides information about the person's usual personality, coping mechanisms, and cognitive abilities, as well as how those characteristics may have changed during older adulthood. This information is then used to plan interventions that are based on realistic expectations.

When the nursing assessment identifies mental changes in an older adult, a multidisciplinary approach is important for further assessment and implementation of effective interventions. A common mistake is to label the changes as "normal for the person's age." This not only is unfair to the older adult, but also can be detrimental, especially in cases in which a treatable underlying condition is overlooked or appropriate interventions to improve functional abilities are neglected. As should be clear from the discussion of cognitive function in Chapter 7, age-related cognitive changes are rarely brought to the attention of health care professionals. For example, an older adult would be unlikely to describe the following complaint: "I know I can learn new information, but I don't seem to be able to comprehend information as quickly as I used to." Mental changes that are noted by other people or brought to the attention of health care professionals are more likely to arise from a pathologic process than from age-related processes. Therefore, whenever changes in psychosocial function are identified, health care professionals must make every effort to identify the underlying cause.

Procedure for Psychosocial Assessment

The procedure for collecting psychosocial assessment information involves interviewing older adults and their caregivers and observing older adults in their environments. The tools for an effective psychosocial assessment are a trusting relationship, a listening ear, an intuitive mind, and a sensitive heart. The establishment of a trusting relationship and the use of good communication skills are prerequisites for performing an accurate psychosocial assessment and for obtaining emotionally charged information. In acute care settings, nurses perform an assessment at the time of admission to establish a baseline for planning nursing care. When patients are admitted to an acute care

facility, the focus of the assessment is necessarily on physical care related to their immediate needs, and it is not always appropriate to do a psychosocial assessment upon admission. However, this assessment should not be overlooked because it may provide clues to the causes of existing medical problems, in addition to providing a basis for discharge planning. As soon as the patient's condition is medically stable, the nurse begins addressing psychosocial issues.

Nurses working in long-term care settings usually have more time to collect psychosocial assessment information than do those working in hospitals. Nurses in home and community settings also have sufficient time to perform a psychosocial assessment, except in crisis situations. In these settings, nurses may have the additional advantages of observing the person's environment and meeting the caregivers who are involved in the daily routines of the older adult's life. Observations of interactions between older adults and their caregivers and environments provide valuable information for the psychosocial assessment.

In addition to interviewing and observing older adults, nurses obtain psychosocial assessment information from other sources. In situations in which the older person's cognitive functions have declined, it is essential to obtain information from family members and others who can provide a reliable history of the mental changes. In long-term care settings, nursing assistants, usually the health care workers who spend the most time with residents, are an important source of psychosocial information. Nursing assistants usually are not included in care plan conferences at which psychosocial problems are addressed, but nurses can obtain information from them at other times and incorporate the information in the care plans.

Approaches to Performing a Psychosocial Assessment

An important aspect of psychosocial assessment is identifying the meaning of events for each person, so that the nurse can better understand the psychosocial needs of the older adult. Initial questions might focus on events that occurred many years ago because the person is likely to be quite comfortable discussing such topics. For example, a question such as "What kind of work did you do?" may prompt a discussion of feelings about retirement. Since changes in living arrangements can precipitate feelings of loss, a non-threatening question such as "What were the circumstances of your moving here?" might lead to further discussion of the meaning of the living arrangement for that person. A question such as "Do you ever think about moving from this house?" encourages a discussion of concerns about living arrangements. People who have experienced the loss of a pet may be reluctant to acknowledge the depth of their feelings. When an older person asks the nurse a question such as "Do you have a dog?" he or she may be indirectly testing the nurse's feelings about pets. The astute nurse will use this opportunity to explore the person's feelings about the subject, perhaps responding, "No, but I have a cat. Have you ever had any pets?" Pets may be especially significant for older adults, and, indeed, may be the only meaningful relationships that remain in their life. In planning for hospital admissions and long-term care arrangements, consideration also must be given to the person's responsibilities for and relationship with pets. Therefore, even if the person does not initiate the topic, at least one question about pets is included in the psychosocial assessment of older adults.

People usually are very receptive to discussing concerns about their health with a nurse because they view the nurse as someone who possesses knowledge about health problems and is committed to helping people deal with these problems. For the purposes of the psychosocial assessment, however, it is important not only to address the physical aspects of health problems, but also to assess the meaning of medical conditions for the person because adjusting to and coping with medical problems and functional limitations is a common and very challenging task for many older adults. Nurses also try to identify the person's concerns about the functional consequences that are likely to be associated with illness and disability, which may be more significant to the person than the immediate medical diagnosis. For example, older adults with diabetes may be less interested in knowing how the pancreas functions than in learning to cope with the attendant visual impairment or their fear of increasing dependence on others. Therefore, rather than focusing the assessment on medically labeled problems, the nurse begins with open-ended questions about the person's self-perceptions of health and function. Rather than asking specifically about the identified problem of diabetes, the nurse might begin with a question such as "If you had to rate your health on a scale of 0% to 100%, what rating would you give it today?" After the person responds to this question, the nurse might ask additional questions, such as "What would have to be changed for you to feel 100% healthy?" or "What rating would you have given yourself a year ago?" Answers to these questions assist the nurse in assessing the impact of the illness on the person's life and in establishing realistic goals for interventions.

MENTAL STATUS ASSESSMENT

A mental status assessment is an organized approach to collecting data about a person's psychosocial function. Although the mental status assessment is very broad in scope, the discussion in this section focuses on the components associated with cognitive abilities; other aspects of psychosocial function (i.e., affective function, contact with reality, and social supports) are discussed in subsequent sections. Some indicators of psychosocial function that are included in this section on a mental status assessment are: physical appearance, psychomotor behavior, social skills, orientation, alertness, memory, and speech characteristics. Mental status assessments are performed by various health care professionals, with each discipline specializing in various components. For example, psychiatrists are skilled in assessing affective and cognitive components, whereas social workers are skilled in assessing family relationship components. In the framework of this text, gerontological nurses assess the aspects of psychosocial function that most directly influence the day-to-day activities of older adults.

Nurses and other gerontological health care workers frequently use standard screening tools, such as the Mini-Mental State Exam (MMSE), developed by Folstein (1975). Information regarding the MMSE is in the Educational Resources section. The MMSE assesses orientation, word recall, language skills, and attention and concentration. Although scoring 23 or fewer out of 30 points is often considered the cutoff score for dementia, gerontologists have recently suggested that scores of 25 or 27 or fewer points more accurately identify people who have dementia (Salmon & Lange, 2001). A major limitation of this tool is its inability to detect some of the cognitive deficits that occur early in dementia, including some of the abilities that are most important in daily function and decision making (e.g., insight, judgment, and problem solving) (Mathuranath et al., 2000). Another limitation of the MMSE is that performance on this test can be significantly influenced by cultural influences and level of education. Despite these limitations, the MMSE is useful as a screening tool and a measure of change in cognitive abilities over time. However, it is important to recognize that this tool can provide information about some aspects of cognitive function but does not provide a broad perspective of psychosocial function.

Physical Appearance

Physical appearance is readily observed and reveals many aspects of psychosocial function. Clothing, grooming, cosmetics, and hygiene provide many clues to psychological function, but they are only clues, and questions must be asked before any conclusions are drawn. For example, when assessing an older woman who has body odor, poor hygiene, and tattered clothing, the nurse considers that these conditions in an older person may be indicators of any of the following: depression, incontinence, impaired cognitive abilities, limited financial resources, overwhelming caregiving responsibilities, impaired vision or sense of smell, or lack of access to or inability to use bathing facilities.

Other observations about personal appearance can prompt similar considerations. For example, the person's weight, particularly a history of weight loss, may provide clues to depression, cognitive impairment, medical status, or other barriers to adequate nutrition. Observations about how the person's clothing fits provide clues to weight changes that might not be acknowledged by the person. For instance, nurses may gain important information about weight changes if they notice that a belt has extra buckle holes to make it smaller. Of course, before any conclusions are drawn, it is important to find out if the belt originally belonged to that person. An observation such as this gives the nurse a natural lead-in for a question such as "Your belt looks like it's pretty big for you now. Have you been losing weight?"

The nurse notes the person's apparent age as well as cosmetic and grooming practices that influence the apparent age. Some questions that might arise from the observation that an 85-year-old woman dyes her hair include the following: Is this a reflection of positive or negative self-esteem? Does she want to appear younger than her age because she believes that old age is not as socially acceptable as youth? Does she want to deny her age because she associates old age with negative images? High-heeled shoes may also reflect a woman's self-image and her desire to avoid looking like an "old lady." This is an important assessment issue because high-heeled shoes may also be a risk factor for falls and fractures.

Motor Function and Psychomotor Behaviors

Assessment of motor function (e.g., posture, movement, and body language) can provide clues to broader aspects of function. For example, stooped posture may be a clue to depression, whereas erect posture may indicate positive self-esteem. A shuffling, staggering, or uncoordinated gait could indicate neurologic deficits secondary to a disease process or adverse effects from alcohol or medications. Gait disturbances, as well as other abnormal movements, are possible signs of tardive dyskinesia or extrapyramidal

symptoms. Any evidence of tardive dyskinesia raises the question of past or present use of psychotropic medications, as discussed in Chapter 23. This information is particularly useful in assessing people who deny having any psychiatric illness or who cannot give an accurate psychiatric history.

Body language and movement provide clues to affective illnesses and behavioral disturbances. Slouching and head hanging, for example, are common manifestations of withdrawal and depression. Poor eye contact, especially looking at the floor, may be indicative of depression or the inability to answer questions, but nurses assess this in relation to cultural factors that influence the type and amount of eye contact considered to be appropriate (as described in Chapter 9). Depressed older adults frequently are very slow in their activities; if they are experiencing agitated depression, however, they may be excessively active. Repetitive body motions, especially of the extremities, could indicate anxiety, but these motions also can be manifestations of tardive dyskinesia. Agitation can be symptomatic of cognitive, affective, or other psychiatric disturbances; it also may be an adverse medication effect. In people with dementia, agitation is often an indicator of a physiologic disturbance (e.g., dehydration, electrolyte imbalance) or a pathologic condition (e.g., pneumonia, urinary tract infection).

Psychomotor behaviors are part of the mental status assessment because the ability to carry out simple motor skills purposefully is highly influenced by cognitive abilities. For example, observations of how someone navigates and avoids obstacles in the environment provide clues to the person's judgment (providing that the person has good vision). Nurses can assess psychomotor behaviors by asking the person to perform a simple activity of daily living (e.g., combing hair) and observing the person's ability to comprehend and perform the request.

Social Skills

Assessing the older adult's level of social skills helps nurses draw accurate conclusions about other aspects of psychosocial function. For example, friendly and cooperative people with good conversational skills may use social skills to hide their cognitive deficits, especially if they are motivated to do so. By contrast, people with long-standing patterns of hostility, social isolation, inadequate social skills, and lack of ambition are less likely to be motivated to perform well and are more likely to be viewed as psychosocially impaired. In addition, nurses need to keep in mind that the following social skills sometimes obscure cognitive deficits: humor, evasiveness, leading the conversation, and making up answers to questions. Some older adults with dementia maintain very good social skills, even in the later stages of dementia when other skills have declined long before. As discussed in Chapter 9, it is essential to be aware of cultural differences in social skills and to consider the cultural context of the relationship between the interviewer and the interviewee.

Response to the Interview

The nurse observes the person's initial response to the interview, as well as changes in attitude that occur during the interview, because these observations can give important assessment information. For example, the older adult may initially be very receptive to the questions, but become defensive or sarcastic when he or she is uncomfortable with the line of questioning. In addition, nurses assess the amount of effort expended in answering questions. Such observations are especially important when trying to differentiate between dementia and depression because cognitively impaired people may exert great effort in responding to questions but depressed people may fail to answer correctly because they lack the energy or motivation. Thus, two people may score the same on a formal mental status questionnaire, but one may miss the questions because of dementia and the other may miss them because of depression. When nurses suspect that lack of motivation is a reason for incorrect or missing answers, they might clarify this by asking, "Is it that you don't know the answers, or that you just don't feel like answering the questions?"

Assessing for confabulation, the process of making up information, is difficult when the nurse does not know the correct information. For example, the accuracy of answers regarding one's place of birth or childhood experiences cannot always be determined. Therefore, these kinds of questions are not good indicators of mental status unless the accuracy of the answers is confirmed. Circumstantiality, another cover-up technique, involves the use of excessive details and roundabout answers in responding to questions.

Hostility, resistance, and defensiveness also may be exhibited during an interview. Depressed people may be apathetic and may not want to expend the energy to answer the questions. Cognitively impaired people may be angry, hostile, or defensive, especially if they are trying to hide or deny the deficits. People who have always been reclusive or suspicious may not be receptive to a mental status assessment and may feel very defensive or refuse to answer the questions. Because these attitudes influence the responses to

mental status questions, assessing the person's underlying attitude is as important as assessing the actual responses, or lack of responses, to questions.

Finally, the person's attitudes and responses must be considered in relation to their usual (baseline) personality traits. For example, highly sociable people might always use humor, whereas talkative people might naturally use circumstantiality. The use of humor and circumstantiality by people who are normally quiet and serious might indicate a great effort to cover up cognitive deficits. On the other hand, people who are normally quiet and withdrawn may be perceived falsely as being depressed. Finding out about the usual personality of an individual is difficult; however, a question such as, "Would you describe what you were like when you were 40 years old?" might be asked. Family members and caregivers who have known the person for a long time are good sources of information about lifelong personality characteristics. Display 10-2 summarizes guidelines for assessing physical appearance, motor function, social skills, and response to the interview in relation to the person's psychosocial function.

Orientation

Because it is easy to measure, orientation to person, place, and time is the indicator of mental status that is most frequently assessed and documented. Often, however, orientation is inaccurately viewed as the primary indicator of cognitive function, rather than as one small piece of a larger picture—it is overused, or used simplistically, to the detriment of more meaningful standards of mental status. For example, the following questions are considered to be the standards for determining orientation: "What is your name?" "Where are you?" and "What time is it?" Based on whether each answer is correct or incorrect, the person is then labeled as "oriented times one," "oriented times two," or "oriented times three." The superficial use of orientation questions and the subsequent labeling of the person as oriented times one, two, or three, ignores important considerations, such as the following:

- Do sociocultural factors influence the person's response to these questions?
- Can the person name familiar people, such as a spouse or children, even if he cannot state his own name?
- If the person cannot give specific names of other people, can he describe the correct role of the other person?
- If the person cannot state the exact time, can he give the general time of day?

DISPLAY 10-2

Guidelines for Assessing Physical Appearance, Motor Function, Social Skills, and Response to the Interview

Observations Regarding Physical Appearance and Motor Function

- What is the person's apparent age in relation to his or her chronologic age?
- How do the following factors reflect psychological function: hygiene, grooming, clothing, cosmetics?
- Does the person's physical appearance provide clues to dementia or depression, or to other impairments of psychosocial function?
- What do the person's gait, posture, and body language indicate about his or her psychological function?
- Is there any evidence of tardive dyskinesia or other adverse medication effects?
- How does the person maneuver in the environment, and what does this reflect regarding judgment, vision, and other skills?

Observations Regarding Social Skills and Response to the Interview

- What are the person's lifelong patterns of social skills, and how do these influence the assessment process?

- How do the person's social skills influence the interviewer's interpretation of other aspects of psychosocial function?
- Is the person motivated to answer questions?
- What is the person's attitude about the interview?
- If the person does not answer the questions, or gives incorrect answers, is it because of inability, cultural factors, or lack of motivation?
- Does the person use any of the following in an attempt to hide possible cognitive deficits: humor, sarcasm, avoidance, evasiveness, confabulation, circumstantiality, or leading the conversation?
- Does the person manifest any of the following characteristics: anger, hostility, resistance, defensiveness, or suspiciousness?
- Do the person's underlying attitudes reflect his or her usual personality, or are they manifestations of cognitive or affective disturbances?

- Are any environmental clues available to the person to orient them to the time or place?
- Has the person been at the institution long enough to have learned its name?
- If the person cannot state the exact name of the facility, can he or she describe the type of facility or its general location?
- Does the person have medical problems that interfere with cognition?
- Is the person taking medications that can influence mental function?

A good assessment extends beyond the three classic questions and describes levels of orientation that are meaningful for the person in a particular setting. For example, the following description is far more useful than simply noting that the person is "oriented times one":

Mrs. S. could state her name, but did not remember the name of this hospital. She could not give her daughter's name, but was able to introduce her daughter to me, without stating her name. She thought that the month was December because of the Chanukah decorations in her room. She could not state the time because she did not have her watch with her, but she thought that it was afternoon because lunch had recently been served.

If the nurse had used only the standard questions of "What is your name?" "Where are you?" and "What time is it?" Mrs. S. would be judged to be "oriented times one." Most health care providers, after reading the results of that assessment, would have assumed that Mrs. S. had serious cognitive impairment, especially if she was 85 years of age or older. Mrs. S.'s actual responses, however, reflected various cognitive skills involved in organizing information, making associations, and using judgment. The more detailed description shows that Mrs. S. is probably a quite logical person who has not yet learned the name of the hospital and who might have some temporary memory impairment because of anxiety, medications, or acute medical problems.

Alertness

Along with orientation, level of alertness is the mental status indicator that health care providers most frequently assess and document. Level of alertness is measured along a continuum, which ranges from stupor to hyperalertness. The levels between these two extremes include drowsiness, somnolence, and intermittent alertness and drowsiness. An important aspect of assessing the person's level of alertness is the identification of any factors that can affect alertness, such as medications, caffeine, alcohol, and pathologic conditions (e.g., dementia, depression, medical disorders). For example, daytime somnolence is a common adverse effect of a hypnotic that has a long half-life (e.g., flurazepam); therefore, an older adult who has taken a medication for sleep may have diminished alertness during the following day. People commonly use caffeine to increase alertness, whereas they may use alcohol to diminish alertness and awareness.

Diminished alertness due to daytime somnolence raises many questions about potential causative factors. For example, undetected medical disturbances, such as electrolyte imbalances, may be manifested by drowsiness in their early stages, especially in older adults. As a practical consideration, people who are caregivers may be somnolent during the daytime because of nighttime caregiver responsibilities. Even if information about some of these influences is not readily available, it is important to identify any underlying factors that may contribute to diminished alertness. Therefore, if the person shows any sign of altered alertness, additional information must be obtained to identify potential causes, especially those that can be remedied through nursing measures.

Memory

Formal memory testing assesses remote events, recent past events, and immediate memory, which is further divided into retention, recall, and recognition. Memory is assessed during all conversations because all verbal communication depends to some degree on memory function. Thus, nurses assess memory by observing the person in daily activities and by interviewing older adults and their caregivers. Nurses pay particular attention to assessing memory in relation to activities that are important in daily life, such as remembering to pay bills, take medications, and shop for groceries. This assessment is made in relation to the expectations and demands of the person's usual environment. For example, if the person lives alone and manages finances independently, the ability to pay bills is quite important. By contrast, if the person lives with a daughter and her family, remembering the birth dates of grandchildren may be an important memory task.

Assessment of memory is especially challenging because although memory complaints are common among older adults, the complaints are not necessarily based on actual deficits in memory function. For example, memory complaints are often prominent in people who are depressed, even though their memory skills are good. Thus, the question "Do you ever have trouble remembering things?" may elicit a positive response, but the response is likely to tell you more about the person's perception of memory than about his or her actual memory function. Although this question may be quite useful in identifying any concerns that the older adult might have, it is not very useful in assessing memory function. This is particularly true for older adults who deny the deficits or attempt to hide their memory difficulties.

In addition to assessing memory directly, the nurse assesses the person's use of memory aids by posing a question like, "Is there anything you do to help you remember appointments or other things?" Assessment of the extent to which the person depends on memory aids is useful in setting goals and planning for improved memory function. For example, if the person's memory function is barely adequate and is based heavily on memory aids, then the potential for further improvement is minimal. On the other hand, if the person has some memory deficits but does not use any memory aids, then the potential for improvement is increased. Observations about the use of memory aids also may provide clues to unacknowledged memory deficits. For example, if the person denies any problems with memory, but repeatedly refers to written notes during an interview, he or she may be compensating for an impaired memory. In this situation, the person is quite willing to use memory aids but is unwilling to acknowledge the need for such aids. Display 10-3 summarizes guidelines for nursing assessment of orientation, alertness, and memory and includes examples of appropriate questions for assessing the different types of memory. Examples of direct questions are identified by quotation marks to distinguish them from the questions that are answered indirectly through observations.

Speech and Language Characteristics

Speech and language characteristics provide important information about many aspects of psychosocial function, such as the ability to organize and communicate thoughts. In addition, a good assessment of language skills helps the nurse identify words and language patterns that are most appropriate for use with the older person. Rather than using formal assessment questions, nurses can assess speech and language characteristics during any verbal interaction. Because speech and language skills are highly dependent on cultural, educational, and socioeconomic factors, it is important to consider these influences, especially when assessing foreign-born older adults. All of the following speech characteristics can be assessed during conversations: pace, quality, and the ability to organize and communicate thoughts. In addition, nurses observe for any abnormal speech or language characteristics or patterns.

Interview Questions to Assess Orientation

- *Person*: "What is your name?" "What is your wife's name?" If names can't be given, can the person describe roles?
- *Place*: "What is your address?" "What is the name of this place?" "What kind of place is this?" "What is the name of this city?" "What is the name of this state?"
- *Time*: "What time is it?" "What day of the week is today?" "What month and date is it today?" "What season is it?"

Observations to Assess Alertness

- What is the person's level of alertness on the following continuum: hyperalert, alert, drowsy, somnolent, stuporous?
- Does the person's level of alertness fluctuate? If so, is there any pattern to the fluctuations?
- Are there physiologic factors that might influence the person's level of alertness, such as medical conditions or effects of chemicals or medications?
- Are there psychosocial factors that might influence the person's level of alertness, such as anxiety, depression, nighttime caregiving responsibilities, or any other factor that might disrupt nighttime sleep?

Interview Questions to Assess Memory

- *Remote events*: "Where were you born?" "Where did you go to grade school?" "What was your first job?" "When were you married?"
- *Recent past events*: "Do you live with anyone?" "Do you have any grandchildren?" "What are the names of your grandchildren?" "When was the last time you went to the doctor?"
- *Immediate memory, retention*: State three unrelated words and ask the person to repeat the information, both immediately and again after 5 minutes.
- *Immediate memory, general grasp and recall*: Ask the person to read a short story and then to summarize the information presented in the story.
- *Immediate memory, recognition*: Ask a multiple-choice question and then ask the person to choose the correct answer.

Nurses use good listening skills to assess pace and quality of verbal communication, and they try to identify factors that may influence these speech characteristics. For example, rapidly paced verbal communication may arise from anxiety, agitation, or mental illness, whereas slow-paced or excessively brief verbal communication may indicate depression, cognitive impairment, or simple cautiousness. The quality of a person's speech includes a variety of characteristics, such as tone, volume, and articulation. Tone of voice can be a good indicator of indirectly expressed feelings, such as anger, hostility, and resentment. Abnormally low speech volume, called *hypophonia*, may be associated with depression, physical illness, low self-esteem, or long-standing speech habits. An abnormally loud volume may be indicative of a hearing impairment or prolonged experience communicating with someone who is hearing impaired. Poor articulation or slurred speech may be attributable to any of the following factors: ill-fitting dentures; lack of teeth or dentures; long-term hearing impairments; nervous system disorders, including dementia; or the effects of alcohol or medications.

The ability to organize speech sounds into words and sentences requires many cognitive skills, and this ability may be impaired for a number of reasons. Errors in pronunciation, called *phonemic errors*, can arise from hearing impairments, cognitive deficits, or educational and cultural influences. Misinterpretation of the meaning of words, or *semantic errors*, may result from cognitive deficits, but may also be attributable to hearing impairments that interfere with a person's ability to hear words accurately. The use of *neologisms* (i.e., self-created and meaningless words) usually occurs secondary to dementia or psychopathologic conditions (e.g., schizophrenia); however, their use may be attributable to the repetition of a word that was not heard accurately in the first place. Some of the factors that cause incoherent speech are dementia, aphasia, psychiatric disorders, and alcohol or medication effects.

Perseveration and agnosia are manifestations of neurologic disturbances, such as dementia. *Perseveration* is a repetitive or stuttering pattern of verbal or written communication. For example, the affected person may begin speaking or writing a sentence and remain stuck on the first few words or letters. *Agnosia* refers to difficulty finding the correct words, or the inability to name objects accurately. People with only small deficits in word-finding ability may be able to give correct answers about familiar objects with simple names. The deficit may be more apparent, however, if the person is asked to name parts of an object, such as the buttonhole of a shirt.

Aphasia often is associated with strokes or vascular dementia, and it may be the only persistent neurologic deficit following a stroke. *Expressive aphasia* occurs when comprehension abilities are not affected but word retrieval or word-finding abilities are impaired. *Receptive aphasia* occurs when verbal and comprehension abilities are impaired but some language skills are retained. *Global aphasia,* which is a combination of receptive and expressive aphasia, results from more extensive neurologic damage and is manifested in inconsistent and poorly controlled language skills.

Higher Language Skills

Reading, writing, spelling, and arithmetic are calculation and higher language skills that are assessed as indicators of cognition. As with the assessment of other cognitive skills, the person's education, occupation, and other influencing factors must be considered. Although formal psychometric tests rely heavily on measures of these skills to assess cognition, nurses can informally assess the skills involved with performing important daily activities. For example, for an older adult who lives alone, an assessment of the ability to pay utility bills and use money to purchase groceries is more valuable than a measurement of mathematical skills using a psychometric test. Likewise, a person's ability to comprehend the daily newspaper or the markings on a thermostat may be a more valid gauge of functional ability than a score on a formal reading test.

Written health education materials can be used to assess reading and comprehension skills informally, and they also have a practical purpose. For example, when collecting a clean voided urine sample, the nurse can give the person a list of instructions and ask him to read the instructions aloud. Observations of how well the person comprehends the instructions will provide an excellent assessment of the reading skills that are important in daily life. Another opportunity for assessing reading comprehension may arise if the nurse observes that an older adult has a newspaper nearby. A nonthreatening question, such as "What's new in the paper today?" can provide information about the person's interests in outside events and his or her ability to comprehend and remember written information.

Nurses can assess writing and other higher language skills by observing older adults during interactions that pertain to their care. For example, nurses can observe the way an older adult signs his or her name on documents, such as permission forms. Nurses can also observe the older adult during performance of more complex tasks, such as compiling a written medication list or a list of questions to discuss with the primary care provider. Difficulty with writing skills is a common sign of early stages of dementia. Of all the higher language skills, spelling is the least important in terms of daily function of most older adults, but it is a good indicator of changes in mental abilities.

With traditional psychometric testing, calculation is measured with the "serial 7s" test: the person is asked to subtract 7 from 100 and to continue subtracting 7s.

Because this test is highly influenced by level of education, it is not necessarily the most appropriate test for older adults. It may be more appropriate to ask the older person to add 3 plus 3, and to continue adding 3s. Older adults who are depressed may not answer correctly because they do not want to expend the energy to calculate serial 7s. Older adults who have dementia may be able to perform well on this task if they try hard and if they previously had highly developed mathematical skills. From the point of view of the functional approach, performance on formal tests is not as important as performance in daily activities. If people are able to manage money to meet their daily needs, then their ability to subtract 7 from 100 is not important, except as one small indicator of cognitive abilities. Display 10-4 summarizes the considerations that are important in assessing speech characteristics and calculation and higher language skills. Examples of direct questions are identified by quotation marks to distinguish these from other considerations and observations.

DISPLAY 10-4
Guidelines for Assessing Speech Characteristics and Calculation and Higher Language Skills

Observations to Assess Speech Characteristics

- Is the pace of speech normal, slow, or fast?
- Is the tone of voice suggestive of underlying feelings, such as anger, hostility, or resentment?
- Is the volume abnormally soft or loud?
- Do the sentences flow coherently and smoothly?
- Is there evidence of any problem with integrating speech sounds into words (e.g., neologisms, or phonemic or semantic errors)?
- Do any of the following factors affect the person's speech: dry mouth, poorly fitting dentures, absence of teeth or dentures, alcohol or medication effects, or neurologic or other pathologic processes?
- Does the person exhibit any of the following: agnosia; perseveration; or expressive, receptive, or global aphasia?

Observations to Assess Calculation and Higher Language Skills

- What is the person's ability to comprehend written materials encountered in the course of routine activities, such as the daily newspaper or instructions for medications?
- What is the quality of the person's handwriting (e.g., his or her signature)?
- Is the person able to perform mathematical computations necessary for daily activities?

DECISION MAKING AND EXECUTIVE FUNCTION

Decision making, one of the most important and complex of all cognitive abilities, is an important aspect of psychosocial function because health care practitioners are increasingly recognizing the rights of older adults, including those with dementia, to be involved in decisions about their care. Researchers have found that about 30% of people with dementia who live in institutional settings consistently make decisions about their health care (Feinberg & Whitlatch, 2001). Insight, learning, memory, reasoning, judgment, problem solving, and abstract thinking are some of the cognitive skills that are involved with decision making. Although no one assessment tool focuses specifically on decision making, nurses have numerous opportunities to assess this aspect of psychosocial function by observing the abilities of older adults to solve problems during the course of daily activities and by asking assessment questions such as the ones in Display 10-5.

Abstract thinking is difficult to assess because it is strongly influenced by other factors, such as education and affective state. People who are very anxious or depressed may lack the attention or motivation required to respond to the questions typically used for the assessment of abstract thinking patterns. Similarity questions, such as "How are apples and oranges alike?" are used to assess the person's ability to think abstractly. Asking someone to explain the meaning of an adage, such as "People who live in glass houses shouldn't throw stones," is another way to assess the person's level of abstract thinking.

During the course of an interview, opportunities for assessing abstract thinking may arise, and the nurse listens for clues to the person's level of abstract, versus concrete, thinking. The following exchange is an example of an unsolicited opportunity this author had to assess one older adult's concrete thinking pattern:

> *Nurse:* How did you feel about having to move from your home in Texas to live with your daughter and her family here in Ohio?
>
> *Mr. L.:* I don't know, how would you feel?
>
> *Nurse:* I'm not sure how I'd feel, that's never happened to me. I'm not in your shoes.
>
> *Mr. L.:* Well, here, put them on [stated emphatically while taking off his shoes to give to the nurse].

One interpretation of Mr. L.'s response is that his thinking pattern is very concrete, rather than abstract.

Nurses assess problem-solving abilities through observations about how older adults meet their needs in a particular situation. For instance, the nurse observes the way older adults use call lights to meet their needs when confined to bed, or the way they engage in the complex decisions related to discharge planning. Similarly, a very important problem-solving task for an older adult who lives alone may be meeting basic safety needs. Therefore, a question such as "What would you do if you woke up at night and smelled smoke?" might be an appropriate way of assessing judgment related to safety. For an older adult who lives in a nursing home, a very important but complex problem-solving task may involve dealing with a disruptive roommate. In this situation, the answer to a question such as "What would you do if your roommate started taking your belongings?" might provide the most pertinent information for assessing problem-solving skills.

Assessment of judgment is based on observations such as the following:

- Does the person pay bills on time?
- Does the person have enough food in the house?
- What resources does the person use in dealing with illness?
- Are the person's clothing and grooming appropriate for the situation?
- Does the person use memory aids to compensate for any deficits?
- Does the person know how to find phone numbers when help is needed?

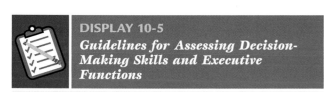

DISPLAY 10-5
Guidelines for Assessing Decision-Making Skills and Executive Functions

Abstract Thinking
- "How are apples and oranges alike?"
- "How are a table and chair alike?"

Reasoning and Judgment
- "What would you do if you woke up in the middle of the night and smelled smoke?"
- "If you received $100 as a gift, how would you spend it?"

Insight
- "What's the reason for your hospitalization?"
- "What kind of help do you think you might need when you leave the hospital?"

Cognitive Flexibility
- "Say as many words as you can that begin with the letter 'T' without using people's names."

- Can the person prepare food, or use resources such as a home-delivered meals program, to meet nutritional needs?

Insight is the ability to understand the significance of the present situation. This skill is an important component of the problem-solving process because it establishes a basis for planning care. Insight is influenced by psychosocial factors such as feelings, personality, and coping mechanisms. Denial is a defense mechanism that is often used to protect oneself from unpleasant realities; the stronger the denial, the more limited the insight. It is important to assess for denial because if the person refuses to acknowledge that he or she has a condition, it will be very difficult to plan interventions. Nursing assessment of insight concentrates on those areas of function that are the focus of the nurse's care plan and interventions. For example, in assessing the insight of an older adult who has been brought to the hospital with malnutrition and uncontrolled hypertension, the nurse may ask questions such as the following: What's the reason your daughter brought you to the hospital? How do you manage with grocery shopping and getting your meals? Do you take any medications? What are the medications for? What kinds of things does your daughter do for you? Answers to questions such as these allow the nurse to assess the person's understanding of the present situation and provide a basis for planning care.

When answers to questions indicate that the person has little or no insight, the nurse tries to identify the factors that interfere with insight. In the example just described, insight may be absent or limited because of feelings of depression and hopelessness, lack of information about the medication regimen, denial of a reality that is too threatening, inability to remember information, or fear of losing independence. An essential component of discharge planning is identifying both the level of insight and the factors that interfere with insight. In addition, the nurse attempts to identify factors that may improve the insight. For example, if insight is lacking because of denial that stems from exaggerated fears, then alleviating the fears may facilitate insight.

In recent years, gerontologists have emphasized the importance of assessing *executive function* abilities as important aspects of decision making (Cummings, 2000). The following cognitive abilities are identified as components of executive function:

- Insight
- Judgment
- Reasoning
- Attention
- Concept formation
- Cognitive flexibility

- Problem-solving skills
- Abstraction
- Self-evaluation
- Ability to plan and initiate activity with future goals in mind
- Ability to think, plan, initiate, sequence, monitor, and stop complex behavior

Executive function deficits can precede memory disturbances and can arise in the very early stages of dementia, especially if the frontal lobes are affected. Because people with executive cognitive dysfunction may perform well on the MMSE but still have severe functional limitations, it is imperative that a mental status assessment addresses executive function skills (Dubois et al., 2000; Juby et al., 2002). The following behaviors may be indicators of executive function deficits: reduced mental flexibility, inability to solve problems, decline in ability to conceptualize, difficulty adapting to new situations, diminished ability to think abstractly, and increased time required to shift thought processes from one idea to another (Piguet et al., 2002). Because it is important to assess these skills in relation to previous level of function, it may be necessary to ask family members, or the person being assessed, if they have noticed changes in these abilities in recent years. When families or health care providers have serious questions about the decision-making abilities of an older person, or when a major decision must be made and there is disagreement about it, a more comprehensive assessment using neuropsychological tests may be warranted. For example, if an older person who is cognitively impaired expresses a strong desire to live alone, but family members question the person's ability to function safely, a comprehensive geriatric assessment with particular emphasis on decision-making and executive function skills is likely to provide information on which to base recommendations. Nurses can use Display 10-5 as a guide to assessing decision-making skills and identifying deficits in executive functions.

AFFECTIVE FUNCTION

Affective function refers to a person's mood, emotions, and expressions of emotions. Happiness and sadness are feelings commonly associated with affective states, but all of the following have been identified as primary affects (also called discrete emotions): joy, awe, hope, fear, pain, rage, pride, guilt, shame, anger, regret, relief, hatred, surprise, interest, boredom, elation, confusion, jealousy, depression, suspicion, frustration, anxiety, bewilderment, amorousness, and lack of feelings. Self-esteem usually is not listed as a primary affect; rather, it is defined as the feelings one holds about oneself. Contrary to what many people believe, older adults experience a wide range of positive emotions, such as happiness, contentment, and gratitude, that are more common than negative emotions, such as sadness and frustration (Chipperfield et al., 2003).

The components of affective state that are reviewed in this section are general mood, anxiety, self-esteem, depression, and happiness. These five aspects were selected for the following reasons:

1. An assessment of general mood assists the nurse in determining appropriate goals based on the person's usual affective state.
2. Anxiety is a common factor in older adults that can often be alleviated or minimized through nursing interventions.
3. Self-esteem is a major determinant of feelings, especially depression and happiness.
4. Self-esteem is a particularly important affective consideration for older adults because old age and its accompanying problems present many threats to self-esteem.
5. Depression and happiness are two primary affects that have been the focus of much of the research regarding affective states in older people.
6. Nursing interventions are directed toward all of these affective components to improve the quality of life of older adults.

Guidelines for Assessing Affective Function

Affect is assessed both quantitatively and qualitatively in relation to expectations about appropriate expressions of emotions. For example, people are expected to show some expression of sadness when talking about sad events. When the quality of expressed feelings is not consistent with the external event, however, the affect is considered to be inappropriate. The quantity of affect also is assessed in relation to the personal meaning and the nearness in time of an event. People are expected to show greater feelings of sadness in response to tragic news than in response to neutral events. Likewise, people are expected to show a deeper affective response soon after experiencing a sad event than they would years after the event occurred.

The depth and duration of affect, which are important considerations in differentiating between dementia and depression in older adults, also are assessed. The affect of depressed people generally is sad and negativistic and is not influenced by external circumstances. By contrast, the affect of people who have dementia fluctuates more and changes in response to

distractions. Emotional lability is a characteristic of vascular dementia that is often seen in people who have had strokes.

Nonverbal behaviors provide a wealth of useful information about a person's affective state: anxiety, happiness, and sadness are readily manifested in observable behaviors. During a mental status assessment, nonverbal behaviors provide information that the person may not offer verbally. For example, despite a person's denial of feeling sad, he or she may exhibit the following nonverbal cues: crying, slouching over, looking at the ground, and having a mournful facial expression. The nurse uses this information as the basis for a leading comment, such as "You look like you're feeling sad."

Expressions of emotions are strongly determined by cultural norms and personality characteristics. In most Western societies, crying is more acceptable for women and children than for men and older boys, and showing anger and rage is more acceptable for men than for women. Cultural expectations also influence the way a person expresses feelings in certain circumstances. For example, a person may be expected to cry and loudly proclaim mournful feelings at a funeral, but may be prohibited from expressing any feelings in front of strangers or in a public place, such as a hospital. Because some emotions, such as anger or depression, are viewed as less acceptable than others, such as happiness, people learn to deny and hide some feelings. Older adults, especially, may have learned that certain feelings should not be expressed directly or verbally. Thus, it is especially important to observe for any indirect or nonverbal clues of anger, depression, and other less socially acceptable feelings.

In assessing the affective state of older adults, it is important to identify the terminology that is most acceptable. Many people will not admit to feeling anxious or depressed because they associate these terms with a serious mental illness or with a socially unacceptable state. Therefore, the nurse begins the assessment of affective state by focusing on feelings that are viewed positively or neutrally. If the person initiates the topic of feeling anxious or depressed, the nurse responds to those feelings and pursues a related line of questioning. In most circumstances, however, it is best to begin with open-ended questions. A simple question, such as "How are you feeling today?" when asked with sincerity, is a familiar and comfortable way of eliciting information.

Mood

Mood is closely associated with emotions but differs from them in that it is more pervasive, less intense, and longer lasting. People are usually quite comfortable describing their mood as either bad or good, and are more likely to refer to their mood than their emotions. Thus, during a mental status examination, a question such as "How would you describe your usual mood?" may be perceived as less threatening than the question, "How do you feel most of the time?" Nonverbal behaviors provide many clues about a person's mood and may be more accurate than verbal responses as an indicator of affective state. Joy, anger, anxiety, sadness, happiness, and depression are examples of moods that are expressed in nonverbal behaviors in everyday life by most people.

Anxiety

Anxiety is defined as a feeling of distress, subjectively experienced as fear or worry and objectively expressed through autonomic and central nervous system responses. Moderate anxiety is beneficial because it motivates protective behaviors, but extreme anxiety is detrimental because it channels personal energy into defensive behaviors. Therefore, it is important to assess the degree of anxiety and the extent to which the anxiety is beneficial or detrimental. In recent years, there has been increasing attention to generalized anxiety disorders, which are the most common psychiatric condition in older adults (Dada et al., 2001). Generalized anxiety disorder is characterized by excessive and uncontrollable worry accompanied by physiologic symptoms, including fatigue, irritability, restlessness, sleep disturbances, and difficulty concentrating.

In assessing anxiety, nurses must identify the terminology that is most acceptable to the older adult. Words like "worries" and "concerns" are readily understood and usually elicit responses about sources of anxiety. Older adults also often use the phrases "nerve trouble" or "trouble with my nerves" in reference to anxiety states. Asking questions such as "Do you ever have nerve trouble?" or "What kinds of things give you trouble with your nerves?" may elicit a response filled with information about sources of anxiety.

Observations of physical and nonverbal manifestations of anxiety can supplement the information obtained from verbal communication. In any adult, anxiety may be manifested in the following nonverbal ways: pacing, shakiness, restlessness, irritability, fidgeting, diaphoresis, tachycardia, hyperventilation, dry mouth, voice changes, smoking habits, urinary frequency, increased muscle tension, poor eye contact, poor attention span, inability to sit still, changes in eating patterns, rapid or disconnected speech, or repetitive motions of facial muscles or any extremities. Although any of these indicators may be observed in older adults, the presence of mobility limitations or pathologic conditions can interfere with some of them. For example, older adults who are confined to bed cannot pace but may experience subtle changes in eating or sleeping patterns because of anxiety. Older adults may be reluctant to report that they are worried or anxious and are more likely to focus on physiologic symptoms of anxiety. Any of the following complaints about physical discomfort may be indirect indicators of anxiety: pain, fatigue, anorexia, insomnia, or stomach distress.

Because anxiety is always a response to real or perceived threats, the nurse tries to identify sources of anxiety, even though they many not be readily apparent. Potential sources of anxiety (i.e., real or perceived threats) include health, assets, values, environment, self-concept, role function, needs fulfillment, goal achievement, personal relationships, and sense of security. People do not always recognize the source of their anxiety because it may arise from unconscious conflicts, unacknowledged fears, maturational crises, or developmental challenges. Even when people recognize the source of anxiety, they may be reluctant to discuss it, or they may refer to the threat only indirectly. For example, an older adult may have the perception that other people have the power to "put him away" in a nursing home simply because of a slight memory impairment. If the person knows other older adults who have been admitted unwillingly to a nursing home, this fear may be exacerbated. Further anxiety might arise from the person's fear of discussing the subject because of the perception that initiating the topic might precipitate actions leading to nursing home admission. Rather than directly talking about the fears, the person might provide vague clues, such as by stating, "I felt so sorry for Mildred when her son put her in the nursing home."

Interview questions aimed at identifying sources of anxiety must be phrased in the least threatening way possible. When older adults express feelings about other older people, it may be appropriate to ask questions aimed at determining whether they have the same worries about themselves. For example, in response to the statement "I felt so sorry for Mildred," the nurse might ask, "Do you ever worry that you'll have to go to a nursing home?" Open-ended questions that allow for a wide range of answers are used to identify sources of anxiety that might not otherwise be revealed. For example, nurses in institutional settings can ask, "What is your biggest worry about going home?" or "Do you have any worries about how you'll manage at home after you leave here?" In home settings, the nurse might ask an even broader question, such as "Do you have any concerns about the future?" or "What kinds of things do you worry about?" Answers to these questions usually are filled with clues to sources of anxiety and provide a basis for many additional questions.

Anxiety can be caused or exacerbated by physiologic conditions arising from disease processes or adverse chemical effects. Therefore, obtaining information about medical conditions, as well as about the person's use of herbs, caffeine, and medications, is an essential component of the assessment of anxiety. Anxiety is often an indicator of pathologic processes that diminish cerebral oxygen, such as pulmonary or cardiovascular diseases. In older adults, endocrine disorders, such as hyperthyroidism, may be manifested primarily by anxiety or other psychosocial symptoms. People with dementia may show signs of excessive anxiety when they are experiencing pain or physical discomfort, especially if their verbal communication skills are impaired. Pacing is a commonly observed manifestation of anxiety in ambulatory older adults who have dementia.

Chemicals or medications that stimulate the central nervous system or act on the autonomic nervous system may precipitate or exacerbate anxiety. Akathisia is a frequently reported extrapyramidal effect of some neuroleptics that may subjectively or objectively be interpreted as anxiety. *Akathisia* is defined as an inner sense of restlessness that is worsened by inactivity and is manifested by motor restlessness. It occurs early or late in the course of treatment with psychotropic medications. Akathisia is more common in women and older people. Therefore, if an older adult who is taking neuroleptics complains of certain feelings, such as "shaking on the inside," the possibility of adverse medication effects must be considered as a cause.

In addition to identifying sources and manifestations of anxiety, it is important to identify acceptable methods for reducing anxiety. Even if the sources of anxiety are not identified or cannot be changed, the experience of anxiety can be addressed through psychosocial and educational interventions that facilitate effective coping for management of anxiety (Frazier et al., 2002). To this end, the nurse asks questions about usual coping methods. Questions such as "What do you do when you have trouble with your nerves?" or "What do you find helpful when your nerves are bad?" may initiate a problem-solving process aimed at helping the person cope with the anxiety. If the person does not respond with concrete suggestions, the nurse offers suggestions in a nonjudgmental way and assesses the person's response to them. For example, any of the following questions can be asked: "Does it help to talk to someone about your worries?" "Have you ever tried any relaxation methods when you're nervous?" "Do you find that taking a walk outside helps you when your nerves are bad?" Incorporating questions such as these in the assessment sets the stage for planning interventions.

Self-Esteem

In much of the literature on mental health and aging, self-esteem is cited as one of the characteristics most highly associated with both depression and happiness. Self-esteem is defined as the feelings one has about one's self, or the extent to which one perceives oneself to be worthy or significant. It is the emotional component of self-concept and is based on one's perceptions of other people's opinions about oneself. Because self-esteem is influenced by the opinions held by others, and because industrialized societies generally hold negative opinions about old age, it is logical to conclude that the self-esteem of older adults may be lower than that of younger adults. However, studies suggest that self-esteem increases slightly from early adolescence through the remainder of the life course (Giarrusso et al., 2001). Self-esteem influences goals, values, desires, and thought processes and is the single most significant factor influencing behavior (Groh & Whall, 2001). Thus, it is a very important aspect of psychosocial assessment.

Although nurses often make judgments about self-esteem—describing it as low or high, good or bad, positive or negative—unlike high or low blood pressure, it cannot be measured numerically with standard equipment. Judgments about self-esteem are based on a compilation of verbal and nonverbal indicators of how a person views himself or herself. Verbal cues about self-esteem are revealed in self-initiated statements, such as "You're wasting your time on me, you have more important things to do." Nonverbal indicators of self-esteem include the way people dress, care for themselves, and present themselves to others.

Interpreting behaviors in relation to self-esteem must be done with caution, but the following behaviors may be associated with low self-esteem: rigidity, procrastination, unnecessary apologies, lack of confidence, expectations of failure, exaggeration of deficits, disappointment in self, self-destructive behaviors, constant approval-seeking, overemphasis on weaknesses, inability to accept compliments, minimizing of one's abilities, disregard for one's own opinions, inability to form close relationships, inability to accept help from others, and inability to say no when appropriate. In most situations, nurses do not ask formal questions to assess self-esteem, but do note the many behaviors that may reflect self-esteem. It may be appropriate to ask some questions, however, especially about the person's perception of positive qualities. For example, a question such as "What is the quality in yourself that other people admire the most?" is nonthreatening and is aimed at helping the person identify strengths. The answer can provide valuable information about self-esteem, especially if the person offers an answer such as "I can't think of anything."

In addition to identifying whether the older adult has high or low self-esteem, the assessment of self-esteem is aimed at identifying actual and potential threats to self-esteem. This is especially important when older adults are admitted to institutional settings because nurses may be able to identify environmental or other factors that can quickly and easily be modified to minimize or eliminate a threat to self-esteem. For example, in some institutional settings, staff members are accustomed to addressing residents or patients by their first names because they believe that this helps to establish a comfortable atmosphere. Some older people, however, may be insulted if they are addressed by any name other than their formal name. If, during the admission interview, the nurse asks the older adult about his or her preferences in this matter and explains the usual procedure in the institution, a potential threat to self-esteem may be averted.

Another potential threat to self-esteem that nurses can address as part of an admission process concerns what accommodations the person needs to maintain independence. For example, for the person with sensory or mobility limitations, the provision of good lighting and the assurance that assistive devices will be accessible may be the most important means of preserving self-esteem. For other people, a factor as simple as having a choice about food might be important to self-esteem. The identification of such factors is accomplished by asking open-ended questions, such as "Is there anything that we can do to help you manage better while you're here?" or "Is there anything you're worried about that I can help you with?" If the person has already identified potential threats to self-esteem, this question will provide an opportunity to discuss the threat and to plan interventions.

Because self-esteem is influenced by the person's perception of the opinions held by significant others, it is important to identify who the significant others are for any particular person (e.g., peers, spouse, or partner; authority figures; and people in the work, church, and social environments). Culture often defines who is the significant other. Some Chinese American older adults, for example, expect their oldest son to look after their affairs and make key decisions about their health and well-being. Widows in some Middle Eastern and African cultures expect one of their husband's brothers to take care of them, an arrangement that fosters social and economic security for women who have lost a spouse. Being cared for by a family member (rather than by strangers) enhances self-esteem for older adults from all cultural backgrounds and increases the likelihood that their needs will be met as they age.

In addition to the influence of significant others, self-esteem is affected by one's perceptions of the effect that one is able to exert on the environment. Therefore, the environment also must be assessed for sources of threats to self-esteem, especially in long-term care settings in which older adults view the institution as their home but have little control over the environment. Environmental factors that influence self-esteem include decor, social roles, perceived control, social interactions, architectural design, amount of space and privacy, and the extent to which the environment impedes or promotes an individual's ability to function.

For dependent older adults, the negative impact of disability and functional impairments on self-esteem is heightened by caregiver attitudes of infantilization (i.e., treating an adult in a way that is similar to the way infants are treated). Such attitudes may be reflected in remarks by caregivers, such as "He acts just like a baby" or "Now, now, dear, let's be a good girl." Infantilization also may be reflected in the use of diapers for incontinence, especially when used solely for the caregiver's convenience. Another threat to self-esteem arises when caregivers promote unnecessary dependence for their own convenience. For example, telling a bedridden person to wet the bed because it is easier to change the disposable bed pad than to assist with toileting is a tremendous blow to the person's self-esteem.

Depression

In this section, depression is discussed as one component of affective function that is routinely assessed during a psychosocial assessment. In Chapter 25, depression is comprehensively discussed as an aspect of impaired psychosocial function, and guidelines for assessing and addressing depression are reviewed. Thus, the assessment information in this section is intended to be used in conjunction with assessment information in Chapter 25, which also describes screening tools that are commonly used for identifying depression in older adults.

Like other indicators of affective state, depression is assessed by examining both verbal and nonverbal cues. Direct questions such as "Are you depressed?" usually are not effective in eliciting information because people may associate the word "depressed" with states of overwhelming grief. Older adults may be more comfortable responding to questions about whether they feel "sad," "blue," or "down in the dumps." Therefore, unless the older adult uses the term "depressed" to describe his or her feelings, other terminology is more likely to elicit an accurate response. As with other aspects of the mental status assessment, it is best to start with open-ended questions, such as "How are you feeling right now?" or "How have you been feeling this week?"

One of the purposes of an assessment of depression is to identify the person's usual patterns of coping with losses. For this reason, the nurse encourages older adults to express their feelings about significant changes in their lives. For instance, when an older adult talks about a change that might be experienced as a loss, nurses can ask nonthreatening questions that might lead to a discussion of feelings. Examples of this type of question are: "What's it like to live alone after 50 years of being married?" "How is life different since your friend moved away?" "Are there people you miss seeing since you retired?" If the open-ended questions do not elicit information about feelings, the nurse can comment on specific feelings that the person is likely to be experiencing. For example, a remark such as, "It seems like it would be pretty sad and lonely being here all by yourself after 55 years of marriage" allows the person to agree, disagree, or offer an alternative to the suggested feelings. Be aware that, for older adults from some Asian, Native American, and other cultures, expressing one's emotions overtly or discussing them with a stranger may be considered inappropriate.

Happiness and Well-Being

Happiness in relation to aging is often equated with morale, contentment, well-being, life satisfaction, successful aging, quality of life, and "the good life." Although these terms often are used interchangeably, happiness is an affective quality, whereas well-being and life satisfaction are cognitive qualities. The concept of quality of life, which also is the focus of much attention in gerontology, includes both affective and cognitive qualities (Ryff & Kwan, 2001). Researchers have tried for several decades to identify the factors that significantly affect happiness and life satisfaction in older adults. In recent years, they have agreed on the following key dimensions of psychological well-being in older adults (Blazer, 2002b; Ryff & Kwan, 2001):

- Positive relations with others
- A sense of identity
- Self-acceptance
- Self-efficacy
- Autonomy, self-determination, and the capacity to follow one's own convictions
- A unifying outlook and sense of meaning and purpose in life
- An accurate perception of reality and sensitivity to situations of others
- An investment in living and in realizing one's potential
- Personal growth
- Mastery of the environment, including the ability to solve problems, manage the demands of daily life, and create living contexts suitable to one's needs and capacities.

Although these characteristics are too wide-ranging to address comprehensively in a psychosocial assessment, it is important to include a few questions about happiness and well-being. Psychologists sometimes use the following question to assess happiness: "Taking all things together, how would you say things are today—would you say you're very happy, pretty happy, or not too happy these days?" Asking the person to rate his or her happiness is an effective way of eliciting information that provides a basis for further discussion. A question similar to the question about health can be used: "If you had to rate your present level of happiness on a scale of 0 % to 100 %, what rating would you give it?" Based on the response to this question, additional questions could be asked: "What would have to change to increase the rating by 10 %?" "What kinds of things interfere with your happiness?" "If you could change one thing to be happier, what would it be?" Older adults usually will respond to these questions in a realistic manner, and their answers will provide information for establishing appropriate goals.

It is particularly important to assess happiness and well-being in long-term care settings because these health care settings are likely to be the "home environment" for the residents. An assessment tool to identify psychosocial preferences of older adults in nursing homes has been developed and can serve as a guide for identifying the factors that influence happiness and well-being for older adults in these settings (Carpenter et al., 2000). This assessment tool also can be used by nurses to identify the factors that can be addressed to improve quality of life for nursing home residents. For example, the tool can be used to identify preferences regarding daily care routines, the way the person likes to spend time, and the degree of involvement they like to have in decision making.

DISPLAY 10-6
Guidelines for Assessing Affective Function

General Affective Function

- Are the quantity and quality of emotions appropriate for the objective reality?
- What is the depth and duration of emotions regarding a particular event?
- What are the nonverbal cues to the person's affective state?
- How do sociocultural or environmental factors influence the person's expression of emotions?
- What terminology is acceptable to this person, especially with regard to feelings such as anger, anxiety, and depression?
- Does the person have any pets, or has he or she lost any pets?

Observations/Questions to Assess Mood

- What is the person's usual affective state?
- What are the nonverbal indicators of the person's mood?

Observations/Questions to Assess Anxiety

- What are the nonverbal indicators of anxiety?
- What real or perceived threats are present that might be sources of anxiety for the person?
- Might any of the following factors be contributing to the person's anxiety: caffeine, pathologic conditions, medications, herbs, or interventions by folk or indigenous healers that act on the central or autonomic nervous systems?
- What methods of coping has the person tried, and what have been the effects of these interventions?
- "What kinds of things do you worry about?"
- "Do you have any worries that you'd be willing to discuss with me?"
- "Do you ever have trouble with your nerves?"

Observations/Questions to Assess Self-Esteem

- What verbal and nonverbal clues to self-esteem can be detected?
- What are the factors that influence self-esteem for this person?
- Does the environment present any real or potential threats to self-esteem?
- How are my actions as a nurse influencing the self-esteem of the older adults to whom I relate?
- Are caregiver attitudes, such as infantalization or the promotion of unnecessary dependence, influencing the person's self-esteem?

Observations/Questions to Assess Depression

- What are the verbal and nonverbal clues to depression?
- "Do you ever feel blue or down in the dumps?"
- "How has your life changed since your husband died?"
- "What do you miss the most since you moved from your family home?"

Observations/Questions to Assess Happiness and Life Satisfaction

- How is the person's happiness and life satisfaction influenced by the following: functional abilities, personal relationships, and socioeconomic resources?
- "On a scale of 0% to 100%, how happy would you say you are right now?"
- "If you could change one thing to increase your happiness rating, what would it be?"

Display 10-6 summarizes the considerations involved in assessing affective function in older adults. Examples of direct questions are identified by quotation marks to distinguish them from the questions that are answered indirectly through observations.

CONTACT WITH REALITY

Although a certain amount of fantasy is acceptable, people are expected to remain in contact with the world around them and to respond appropriately to the same realities that others perceive. People who deviate from this norm to a notable degree are labeled as "nuts" or "crazy" or are described as "off their rockers" or "a little bit touched in the head." People lose contact with reality for numerous reasons, ranging from schizophrenic disturbances to a transient denial of a threatening reality. In older adults, loss of contact with reality most frequently is associated with

dementia, depression, or delirium. Many causes of loss of contact with reality are amenable to interventions, and older adults are just as likely as younger adults to have a treatable reason for any disturbance in their contact with reality. When older people lose their contact with reality, however, a different set of labels may be applied to them. They may be viewed as "senile" or may be faced with the attitude of "it's what you'd expect at the age of 84." Families may explain the behavior of an older person as "always a little eccentric, but a little more so now." Because of stereotypes about older people, as well as the broad array of potential causes for loss of contact with reality, the assessment of an older person's contact with reality is an especially challenging aspect of the psychosocial evaluation.

Loss of contact with reality includes a wide range of behaviors ranging from simple and harmless misperceptions of reality to firmly held delusions or disturbing hallucinations. For example, in the early stages of dementia, people may conceal memory deficits or avoid acknowledging them by denying reality. In later stages of dementia, however, loss of contact with reality may progress to the point that the person's judgment is impaired, leading to behaviors that are inappropriate or even dangerous. For example, if someone believes that his belongings have been stolen, he may report the theft to the police or insist on going out to look for the robber. Delusions, hallucinations, and illusions are the three aspects of denial of reality discussed in the following sections. They are defined as follows:

1. *Delusions* are fixed false beliefs that have little or no basis in reality and cannot be corrected by appealing to reason.
2. *Hallucinations* are sensory experiences that have no basis in an external stimulus. Visual and auditory hallucinations are most common, but tactile, olfactory, and gustatory hallucinations also occur.
3. *Illusions* are misperceptions of an external stimulus. They may be mistaken for hallucinations, but differ in having some basis in reality, whereas hallucinations do not.

Delusions

Delusions arise from the need to preserve one's ego and maintain one's sense of power and control in threatening situations. In older adults, delusions provide a way of organizing information that is difficult to process, even though the delusions may be bizarre and implausible to others (Blazer, 1998). Just as a fever is one manifestation of a physical illness, delusions are one manifestation of a psychiatric illness. In older adults, delusions are associated most often with sensory impairment or pathologic conditions such as dementia, depression, delirium, and paranoid disorder. Delusions arising from each of these disorders are characterized in particular ways and are seen in combination with other clues to the specific underlying disorder, as discussed in the following sections.

Paranoia, one of the most common forms of delusions, is an extreme degree of suspiciousness. In older adults, paranoia is so commonly associated with delusions that the terms are sometimes used interchangeably, but inaccurately, in the geriatric literature. The following are typical paranoid complaints or behaviors of older adults:

- The accusation that others are stealing their money or belongings
- The perception that they are being cheated, observed, attacked, persecuted, or sexually harassed

- The accusation that others are coming in and taking things, or messing up their belongings
- The belief that they have been injured by medical interventions, such as pills or radiation

The onset of delusions or paranoia in later adulthood is associated with delirium, dementia, depression, persistent persecutory states, or sensory impairments.

Delusions Associated With Delirium

Delusions arising from delirium—also referred to as an acute confusional state—are only one manifestation of a complex pathologic process that is further characterized by physiologic disturbances, diminished attention, a clouded state of consciousness, and, possibly, hallucinations. Assessment of such delusions is relatively easy because they are commonly accompanied by the usual manifestations of delirium and will disappear once the delirium is resolved. Another characteristic of delusions associated with delirium is that they are likely to be poorly organized and persecutory in nature. Delusions as a manifestation of delirium are not unique to older adults, and they often accompany delirium in people of any age. Older adults, however, are more susceptible to delirium because the older brain is less able to adapt to metabolic disturbances, and the older person is more likely to have precipitating conditions, such as physiologic disturbances and adverse medication reactions. In addition to being associated with delirium, delusions may be the sole or primary manifestation of pathologic conditions (e.g., strokes, hypothyroidism, hyperthyroidism) and functional impairment (e.g., disability in daily life) (Ostling, 2002; Talbot-Stern et al., 2000). Some of the physiologic disorders that are likely to cause delusions in older adults are listed in Table 10-1.

TABLE 10-1 ● Physiologic Disorders Causing Delusions

Type of Disorder	Specific Examples
Metabolic disorders	Uremia, dehydration, electrolyte imbalance
Endocrine disorders	Hypoglycemia, hypothyroidism, hyperthyroidism
Neurologic disorder	Stroke, cerebral trauma
Deficiency states	Vitamin deficiencies (B$_{12}$, folate, niacin, thiamine)
Infections	Septicemia, penumonia, urinary tract infections, subacute bacterial endocarditis
Adverse medication effects	Anticholinergics, anticonvulsants, antidepressants, antiparkinsonian agents, benzodiazepines, cimetidine, clonidine, corticosteroids, digitalis toxicity, propranolol

Delusions Associated With Dementia

Studies indicate that delusions and hallucinations occur in up to 73% of people with dementia, with most studies reporting a prevalence between 30% and 40% (Sweet et al., 2000). Delusions occur more commonly than hallucinations, and some researchers suggest that delusions may be more common in vascular dementia than in Alzheimer's dementia (Paulsen et al., 2000; Rozzini et al., 2000). Delusions associated with dementia may be caused by impaired memory and an inability to integrate information. The psychiatric literature usually does not differentiate between delusions that are typical of people with dementia and those that are characteristic of people with psychotic disorders but without dementia. Despite the lack of published studies, however, gerontological nurses and other professionals who care for people who have dementia can describe many examples of delusions that are not typical psychotic delusions. In contrast to delusions arising from psychotic states, delusions arising from dementia are not fixed and well organized and are readily changed or forgotten. Common themes of delusions associated with dementia are fearfulness, theft of property, and concern about deprivation. Nurses may be reluctant to label these behaviors as delusions because they are probably misinterpretations of reality, rather than fixed false beliefs. Until the geropsychiatric literature suggests a better term, however, delusion is the most accurate label that can be used.

In one of the early studies that has specifically addressed delusions associated with dementia, Cummings (1985, p. 190) described the categories of complex delusions and simple persecutory delusions:

> *Simple persecutory delusions consisted of elementary, loosely structured, usually transient beliefs, such as believing that possessions or money were being stolen or that one's spouse was unfaithful. Complex delusions were characterized by a more complicated and intricate structure, rigidity, and stability and were supported by substantial, though distorted, "confirmatory" observations.*

The terms *simple delusion* and *complex delusion* are not widely used, but they could be used to distinguish delusions associated with dementia from those that are associated with psychosis. This distinction could be quite helpful because nursing interventions differ for people with psychosis or dementia. For example, a typical psychiatric nursing approach for dealing with delusions in people who are psychotic is to talk with the patient about the delusional thoughts as a problem in his or her life. In contrast, appropriate interventions for people with dementia include avoidance of arguing and provision of distractions.

Delusions regarding theft of personal belongings are one of the most common behavioral manifestations of dementia and are particularly problematic in home and long-term care settings. These delusions occur because the person with dementia forgets where an article is kept or was placed, then, in an attempt to deny the memory impairment, or as a defense against acknowledging the deficit to others, comes to believe that the article has been stolen and accuses someone else of stealing it. Caregivers, roommates, and family members are often the targets of such accusations for those who live with others. For people living alone, the accusations may be directed toward "strangers who come in when I'm gone." Assessment of this type of delusion is not difficult for the nurse, who often deals not only with the delusional person but also with the family, caregivers, and nursing staff who are the targets of the accusations.

Delusions associated with dementia commonly involve misidentification of, or false beliefs about, people or environments. These misidentifications arise from the person's inability to match his or her perceptions with the memory or recognition of people or environments that were once familiar. This type of delusion can lead to behaviors that are quite challenging. For example, in home settings, this false belief is especially problematic when a spouse or other devoted caregiver is accused of being a stranger intent on harming the person. Another common misidentification delusion is the belief that the person is not in his or her own home. These delusions can lead to troublesome behaviors such as wandering and agitation, with the person insisting on going out to "find my home." Another delusion associated with dementia is the belief that deceased parents or other close relatives are still alive. Delusions such as this precipitate agitation and searching behavior, typified by the person who insists that he or she "has to go take care of Mother." Another common type of delusion that is similar to the misidentification type is a false belief about spousal infidelity. In these situations, the person with dementia may firmly believe that his or her spouse is having sexual relationships with other people.

The assessment of delusions associated with dementia is facilitated by the comparative ease with which information generally is offered, which contrasts with the secretiveness and withholding of information that is typical of people who do not have dementia. In many cases, the nurse is given more information than is desired! The challenge in assessing these delusions, however, is to identify the possible reality of the situation. Just because people have serious cognitive impairments, it should not be assumed that all accusations are unfounded. Before labeling the thoughts as delusional, the nurse must be sure that there is no basis in reality. Even the most bizarre-sounding delusions may be based partially or entirely on reality.

Delusions Associated With Depression

Persecutory and other delusions can be one manifestation of a major depression, such as that commonly seen in patients admitted to psychiatric settings. When these manifestations are seen in older adults living in community or long-term care settings, however, they are often overlooked or attributed to other factors. For example, when dementia and depression coexist, the delusions may be attributed to the dementia, rather than considered as possible indicators of a treatable affective disorder. Likewise, when a person with a paranoid personality becomes depressed, the delusions may be falsely attributed to the personality, rather than to the affective disorder, especially if the delusions are persecutory in nature. When delusions arise from depression, other manifestations of depression usually are identified in a thorough depression assessment, as discussed in Chapter 25.

Delusional themes may provide clues to an affective disorder, especially if the focus is on a recent loss. Therefore, carefully listening to the content of the delusions is essential to an accurate assessment. In depressed older adults, delusional themes often revolve around an exaggerated emphasis on guilt, money, illnesses, self-reproach, foreboding of gloom, diminished self-esteem, or feelings of worthlessness. Although some basis may exist in reality, the feelings of being persecuted and deserving of punishment are grossly exaggerated. The following are some examples of delusions arising from depression:

- Mrs. N. believes that she is responsible for her husband's death; therefore, she believes she does not deserve help for her own illness.
- Mr. A. believes that his Medicare insurance has been canceled as punishment for his not cashing his Social Security check and insists that he cannot go to a doctor because of his lack of insurance.
- Ms. K. has an unshakable belief that she has undiagnosed cancer and begins to plan for her funeral even though numerous doctors have not found any disease process.
- Mr. M., who recently had surgery for prostate cancer, is convinced that his house is going to explode from a gas leak, and repeatedly calls the gas company to come check it.

Delusions Associated With Paranoid Disorder

Paranoid disorder—also called *paranoid ideation* or *paranoid symptom*—refers to a delusional disorder that is not associated with schizophrenia and is characterized by the tendency to view individuals or agencies with suspicion or as having harmful intentions (Bazargan et al., 2001). A similar term, *paraphrenia*, was first used in Germany in 1919 and is now being used by some geropsychiatrists in the United States to describe a disorder of late life that is characterized primarily by persecutory delusions and the absence of any cognitive impairments or affective manifestations (Blazer, 1998). Factors that increase the risk for developing a late-life paranoid disorder include depression, increased age, social isolation, medical illness, cognitive impairments, vision or hearing impairment, a sense of injustice and deprivation, a greater number of stressful life events, and a sense of loss of control over the environment (Bazargan et al., 2001; Ostling, 2002). Common themes of delusions include spies, noises, threats, obscenities, lethal gases, bodily harm, stolen belongings, sexual infidelity or molestation, poisoned food or water, and having people enter living quarters by mysterious means at night. The delusions may occur more often when the person is socially isolated or in a particular environment, such as the home. If the person takes action based on the delusions, such as moving to another apartment or living with a family member, the delusions may subside temporarily.

Many people who have a paranoid disorder function well in the community, with the exception of one or two functional areas that are influenced by the delusions. Sometimes, a delusional state that was previously well hidden may surface when the person is admitted to a long-term care facility, and the staff may think that the problem is new, rather than just newly discovered. In other situations, nurses will identify a paranoid disorder upon making a home visit or interviewing an older person who has been admitted to the hospital. If the person also suffers from dementia, the delusions may mistakenly be attributed to the dementia or be interpreted as evidence of advancing dementia. When this occurs, a recommendation for long-term institutional care may be made when other recommendations might be more appropriate. The importance of identifying this type of disorder in the assessment is that the disturbing symptoms can be alleviated with appropriate interventions. When left unattended or written off as eccentricities, these disorders cause anxiety and may progress to a point at which they seriously disrupt functional abilities. When delusions and cognitive impairments coexist, therefore, it is essential to determine whether the delusions existed before the dementia, and to what extent, if any, they interfered with daily activities. If the delusions are part of a long-term pattern that has not interfered with the person's ability to function in daily life, the person may be able to remain in the community with support services directed toward the cognitive impairment and without medical interventions for the delusions. When delusions interfere with daily activities, however, medical intervention (e.g., psychotropic medications) may be effective in eliminating the delusions or minimizing their effects so that the person can maintain an independent level of function. With interventions directed toward both the delusions and the cognitive impairment, the older person's functional abilities may prove to be adequate for community living.

Hallucinations and Illusions

In older adults, hallucinations and illusions are associated most often with dementia, depression, sensory deprivation, and physiologic disturbances, including adverse medication effects. Gerontological nurses deal less frequently with hallucinations than with delusions, but this is partially because hallucinations are more easily overlooked or hidden. People experiencing hallucinations may know that their behavior is not socially acceptable. They may not offer information about hallucinations; in fact, they may try to hide their hallucinatory experiences. Older adults who are socially isolated are especially successful in hiding hallucinatory experiences. As with delusions, it is important to identify the underlying cause of hallucinations and illusions because the selection of appropriate interventions depends on an accurate assessment.

Because hallucinations and illusions are abnormal sensory experiences, it is essential to consider the effect of the environment on sensory perception and to look for any external stimuli before determining that someone is hallucinating. Also, it is important to make sure that any sensory deficits are compensated for to the extent that this is feasible. Researchers found that when older adults with mild hearing impairment wore bilateral, functional hearing aids, their performance on mental status tests improved, and they were less likely to be diagnosed as having a psychopathologic condition (Kreeger et al., 1995).

Hallucinations and Illusions Associated With Delirium

As with delusions associated with delirium, hallucinations and illusions arising from delirium are relatively easy to assess because they are only one manifestation of a complex process. These hallucinations are characteristically vivid, visual, colorful, threatening, and accompanied by other signs of delirium. When illusions arise from a delirium, they are usually brief and poorly organized. Occasionally, hallucinations or illusions arise from altered physiologic states or adverse medication effects, and they may

TABLE 10-2 • Physiologic Disorders Causing Hallucinations	
Type of Disorder	**Specific Examples**
Adverse medication effects	Alcohol, anticholinergics, clonidine, corticosteroids, digitalis toxicity, levodopa, propranolol
Endocrine disorders	Thyrotoxicosis
Neurologic disease	Brain tumor or cortical ischemia
Deficiency state	Niacin deficiency
Drug or alcohol withdrawal	Alcohol, barbiturates, meprobamate

not be accompanied by overt signs of delirium in the early stages. When hallucinations or illusions are caused by adverse medication effects, they are likely to be overlooked, underreported, or attributed to some other cause. Hallucinations arising from withdrawal from drugs or alcohol may occur during the first days of admission to an acute care setting, or in any circumstance in which the person suddenly does not have access to the usual drugs or alcohol. The auditory hallucinations arising from alcohol-induced delirium are characterized as accusatory and threatening, and they are sometimes organized into a complete paranoid system. Table 10-2 summarizes the physiologic disorders, including some adverse medication effects, that are most likely to cause hallucinations.

The detection of alcohol-induced delirium is especially important in acute care settings because people who are dependent on alcohol are more likely to acknowledge the problem and agree to appropriate interventions when they are in a crisis situation. The following example illustrates such a situation.

Mr. K. is 73 years old and has been caring for his wife, who has Alzheimer's disease. He is a very proud man who has difficulty accepting help. One morning, Mr. K. begins vomiting coffee-ground emesis and is admitted to an acute care setting with the diagnosis of gastrointestinal bleeding. On admission, Mr. K. is very pleasant and expresses concern about his wife's care. The next morning, Mr. K. complains angrily to the nurses about the bars on the windows and is very belligerent about the fact that he has been put in jail. He develops additional manifestations of delirium and is treated for alcohol withdrawal.

When the delirium has subsided, the nurse initiates a conversation about the care of his wife and asks him how he copes with the responsibility. Mr. K. admits that he has difficulty coping with his and his wife's declining health and his increasing loneliness and responsibilities. He has always been a social drinker, but he has gradually increased his consumption of alcohol to three six-packs of beer a day. As part of the discharge plan, Mr. K. agrees to talk with a sponsor from Alcoholics Anonymous.

Visual hallucinations may occur in older adults who are visually impaired and have no additional functional or cognitive impairments (Teunisse et al., 1995). One review of the literature on visual hallucinations found that eye disease was the most common cause of visual hallucinations for people of all ages, and that one third of the people who underwent surgery for cataracts reported no further experience with visual hallucinations (Beck & Harris, 1994). Another finding of this review was that visual hallucinations were most prevalent among people 71 years of age or older.

Hallucinations and Illusions Associated With Dementia

Hallucinations and illusions may occur at any time in the course of a dementing illness and also are likely to occur during a transient ischemic attack, a condition associated with vascular dementia. Visual hallucinations occur more commonly than auditory hallucinations in people with dementia (Chung & Cummings, 2000). When illusions occur, they often are related to environmental conditions that can be modified. For example, visual illusions may be caused by poor lighting or reflections from glass or mirrors, and auditory illusions may be caused by background noises, especially for people with hearing aids.

The psychiatric literature usually addresses illusions only with regard to misperceptions of visual or auditory stimuli, but an illusion, by definition, is a misinterpretation of any external stimulus. Nurses who care for people with dementia can cite numerous examples of behaviors that fit this broader definition of an illusion: (1) mistaking the identity of caregivers, family members, or other familiar people; (2) perceiving an object as something other than what it really is; (3) taking an object under the mistaken belief that it belongs to them; and (4) refusing to believe that they are in their home when they really are. These experiences might be labeled as delusions or disorientation, but they are more accurately defined as illusions because they involve a misinterpretation of reality rather that a false perception that has no basis in reality.

Hallucinations Associated With Depression

Severely depressed older adults are more likely to experience delusions rather than hallucinations, but visual and auditory hallucinations of deceased loved ones commonly occur during periods of bereavement. When hallucinations occur as a manifestation of depression, they are likely to be auditory and derogatory, or they may involve visual perceptions of dead people. They also may take the form of false perceptions of smell, taste, touch, movement, or body sensation (Blazer, 2002a). The following examples are typical of hallucinations arising from depression:

- Ms. C. reports that at night she hears the people in the next apartment saying that she has cancer.
- Mr. T. reports hearing younger men say that he is sexually impotent and that he was not a good provider to his wife (who died within the past year).
- Ms. F. looks down from her second-floor window and sees a man, dressed in black, lying injured on the sidewalk.

Olfactory hallucinations are less common than other hallucinations associated with depressive states, but they can occur. When olfactory hallucinations accompany depression, they are likely to be associated with rotten smells, such as pervasive pollution, or with impending danger, such as a gas leak.

Hallucinations Associated With Paranoid Disorder

If hallucinations are a symptom of paranoid disorder, they are likely to be closely related to the theme of the delusions. The following examples are characteristic of hallucinations arising from paranoid states:

- Mr. F. says that he hears people in the next apartment talking about him. These are the same people whom he believes will come in and steal things when he leaves the apartment.
- Ms. J. reports seeing men observing her when she undresses or takes a bath. Moreover, when she goes to the grocery store, the man at the checkout always offers her money in exchange for sexual favors.

Table 10-3 summarizes the characteristics that distinguish delusions, hallucinations, and illusions according to their underlying causes.

Special Considerations for Assessing Contact With Reality

Goals of the nursing assessment of contact with reality are to identify any underlying causes that can be alleviated and to plan interventions for the management of disturbing behaviors. Based on these assessment goals, the previous sections addressed delusions,

TABLE 10-3 • Distinguishing Features of Delusions, Hallucinations, and Illusions

Underlying Cause	Accompanying Manifestations	Characteristics
Delirium	Diminished attention, a clouded state of consciousness, and other typical manifestations of delirium; metabolic disturbance, adverse medication effect, or other underlying cause	*Delusions:* poorly organized, persecutory. *Hallucinations:* vivid, visual, colorful, threatening; accusatory auditory hallucinations induced by alcohol withdrawal. *Illusions:* brief, poorly organized.
Dementia	Cognitive impairment (especially memory deficits); alert level of consciousness. Agitation, anxiety, or wandering may be associated with loss of contact with reality. Neurologic manifestations may accompany hallucinations, particularly when the underlying cause is vascular dementia.	*Delusions:* not fixed, loosely organized, readily changed or forgotten. Themes may include theft, fears, misidentification of places or people, and spousal infidelity. *Illusions:* occur more commonly than hallucinations; may be partially attributable to environmental factors. *Hallucinations:* more often visual than auditory; may be partially attributable to environmental factors.
Depression	Typical depressive symptoms, including anorexia, lack of energy, sleep disturbances, and weight loss	*Delusions:* Themes may include death, guilt, money, illnesses, self-reproach, foreboding of gloom, diminished self-esteem, and feelings of worthlessness. There may be some basis in reality, but perceptions are exaggerated. *Hallucinations:* typically auditory and derogatory.
Paranoid disorder	Absence of cognitive deficits or affective disorders; long-term social isolation or suspicious personality; may be well hidden for years	*Delusions:* fixed and well organized; may subside temporarily in different environments. Themes usually involve plots, noises, threats, obscenities, or sexual assaults. *Hallucinations:* If present, these are related to the delusional themes.

hallucinations, and illusions in terms of the characteristics that are likely to be associated with specific underlying disorders. During the assessment, nurses consider cultural factors that are likely to influence perceptions of reality and manifestations of mental illness, as discussed in Chapter 9. For example, older adults whose cultural identity is Irish Catholic are likely to include religious figures, such as Jesus, a saint, or the Virgin Mary, in their delusions and hallucinations. Similarly, delusions or hallucinations of Muslims with African, Near Eastern, or Middle Eastern cultural heritage may include the Prophet Mohammed.

Delusions, illusions, and hallucinations present a special assessment challenge for gerontological nurses for reasons such as the following:

- People may try to conceal delusions and hallucinations.
- When delusions and hallucinations arise from social isolation, opportunities for assessment are extremely limited.
- To determine whether a reported experience is delusional, the nurse needs information about the reality, which is difficult to obtain if a reliable and objective observer is not available.
- Even after delusions or hallucinations are identified as such, the underlying factors may be difficult to identify.

Delusions usually are more readily acknowledged than hallucinations, and the most effective way of detecting delusions is to listen carefully. Most older adults will confide their delusions to a nurse whom they perceive as interested, sympathetic, and nonjudgmental, especially if a trusting relationship has been established. Difficulty arises, however, when nurses hear information that may be delusional but that is based wholly or partially in reality. For example, financial exploitation, violation of rights, and other aspects of elder abuse are not uncommon, especially in older adults who are cognitively impaired or who live with family members who are psychosocially impaired. When older adults who have cognitive impairments or a lifelong suspicious personality describe abusive or exploitative situations, they are likely to be considered delusional or not to be taken seriously. In these situations, the assessment challenge is to determine what is real, what is distorted, and what is not based at all in reality.

Environmental and interpersonal factors influence a person's ability to maintain contact with reality. For example, poor lighting conditions may be a contributing factor in the development of visual hallucinations, and stressful interpersonal relationships may contribute to the development of paranoid ideations. Another factor that can obscure the assessment of contact with reality is the presence of cognitive impairments such as dementia. In general, the more severe the cognitive impairment, the more likely that behaviors such as delusions and hallucinations will be attributed, perhaps inaccurately, to the dementing process, rather than to reversible factors. Finally, in identifying factors that influence a person's contact

DISPLAY 10-7
Guidelines for Assessing Contact With Reality

General Principles

- In assessing any loss of contact with reality, the effects of alcohol, medications, and physiologic disturbances must always be considered as potential causative influences.
- People who are not cognitively impaired are usually more reluctant to talk about delusions and hallucinations than people who have dementia.
- When people talk about things that might be delusional, it is important to determine, through information provided by a reliable and objective observer, whether their perceptions have any basis in reality.
- When delusions are initially identified, it is important to determine whether they are of recent onset or have been long-standing but only recently discovered.
- When delusions are identified in someone who has dementia, it is especially important to consider the influence of treatable causative factors, such as depression or physiologic disturbances.
- People who have dementia are likely to have illusions rather than hallucinations.

- People who are socially isolated are usually quite successful in concealing hallucinations.
- In assessing hallucinations and illusions, it is especially important to consider the influence of the environment.

Interview Questions to Assess Delusions, Hallucinations, and Illusions

- "Do you have any thoughts that you can't seem to get rid of?"
- "People sometimes have thoughts that they're afraid to talk about because they believe others will think they're 'crazy.' Do you ever have thoughts like that?"
- "Do you sometimes hear voices when you're alone?"
- "Do you sometimes think you see things that other people don't see?"

Nonverbal Clues to Hallucinations

- Extreme withdrawal and isolation
- Contentment with social isolation, especially if the person previously had many social contacts
- Gestures and other actions that normally occur in response to perceived stimuli

---

with reality, it is important to assess whether a lack of assistive devices, such as eyeglasses and hearing aids, is contributing to the perceptual alteration. For example, if someone usually depends on eyeglasses, contact lenses, or a hearing aid for adequate visual or auditory function, the absence of these items may contribute to the development of illusions or hallucinations. The effects of lighting also are assessed as a potential influence. For example, in an institutional setting, the reflection of fluorescent lights on a highly polished floor can produce the illusion of water on the floor, and an older adult might be seen walking around the reflection. Display 10-7 summarizes guidelines for assessing an individual's contact with reality.

SOCIAL SUPPORTS

Social supports, which are categorized as *informal* and *formal*, refer to the services provided to address functional and psychosocial needs. Even the most independent people receive social supports (e.g., emotional support from family and friends), but social supports are usually discussed in relation to meeting the needs of people who have to depend on others in some way to provide assistance. Whereas informal social support is provided by friends, family, clergy, neighbors, or coworkers, formal social support is pro-

vided by workers who are paid by the older person or their family or by health and social service agencies or institutions.

Social supports significantly influence psychosocial function in older adults because they affect one's ability to cope with stressful life experiences. Researchers have consistently found that social supports protect older people against harmful effects of stress and promote physical and emotional well-being (Jang et al., 2002). Because the importance of social supports increases in relation to the degree of functional impairment of the older adult, it is essential to assess social supports for any older adults who have conditions that affect their functional abilities. Nurses have developed an excellent family assessment tool, which has been used effectively for improving care of hospitalized older adults (Salinas et al., 2002). Nurses also have developed guidelines for assessing friends as a major component of social support for people with dementia (Lilly et al., 2003). Nursing literature emphasizes the importance of assessing loneliness and social isolation as factors that affect social support for older adults (Hicks, 2000; Waterman et al., 2001).

The purposes of a nursing assessment of social supports are (1) to identify the resources that can help older adults function at their highest level, (2) to determine which of these resources are already available or being used, (3) to identify barriers to the use

DISPLAY 10-8
Guidelines for Assessing Social Supports

Interview Questions to Assess Social Supports

- "On whom do you rely for help?"
- "Is there anyone who helps you with grocery shopping? Getting to doctor appointments? Getting prescriptions filled? Managing your money and paying bills?"
- "Is there anyone you can talk to when you have worries or difficulties?"
- "Is there anything you would like help with that you don't have help with now?"
- "Is there anyone in the family who could help with grocery shopping?"
- "Have you ever received information about the transportation services (or meals, or other services) that are available through the senior center?"

Potential Barriers to the Use of Formal Supports

- Unwillingness to acknowledge, or lack of insight to recognize, the need for services
- Expectation that family members will provide the needed care
- Unwillingness to admit that family members cannot or will not provide the needed care
- Lack of financial resources to purchase services, or unwillingness to spend money for services
- Perceived correlation between formal services and "welfare"
- Lack of transportation to access services
- Mistrust of service providers, or an unwillingness to allow outsiders into the home

- Bad experiences with service providers, or hearsay about the bad experiences of others
- Fear that the home situation will be judged as socially unacceptable, or embarrassment because it is socially unacceptable
- Fear that having outsiders in the house will lead to admission to a nursing home
- Lack of time, energy, or problem-solving ability to obtain information about and select the appropriate services
- Fear that the service will be provided by someone about whom the care recipient holds prejudices
- Language and cultural barriers

Interview Questions to Assess Financial Resources

- "Do you have any money worries?"
- "Do you have any concerns about paying for services that you might need?"
- "Would you like to talk to someone about any financial concerns?"
- "Do you think you can afford the kind of help that your doctor recommended?"
- "Have you received any advice about financial planning for nursing home care?"

Interview Questions to Assess Religious Affiliation

- "Do you belong to any particular church or synagogue?"
- "Are you aware of any programs available at your church or synagogue that might be helpful to you?"

of appropriate resources, and (4) to plan interventions to meet unmet needs for social resources. For nurses in hospitals and nursing homes, the assessment of social supports is the basis for discharge planning; for nurses in home and community settings, it is the basis for planning long-term care. Specific aspects of social supports that are assessed include social network, barriers to obtaining social supports, economic resources, and religion and spirituality. Display 10-8 summarizes important questions and considerations involved in assessing social supports.

Assessment of social supports generally is viewed as a social work responsibility, but in gerontological care settings, nurses are often responsible for assessing social supports as an integral part of the assessment and care planning process. Likewise, when older adults are discharged from hospitals or nursing homes, nurses are involved with establishing and reviewing the plan for postdischarge care, and this plan often requires that arrangements be made for formal or informal support services. In institutional settings, nurses are the professionals who are most

available to observe and meet with visitors, and they are the professionals who are most likely to be approached when family members have questions or wish to discuss an issue. In home care settings, nurses have many opportunities to assess social supports, and they often observe relationships and environmental conditions that would not be discussed or discovered outside the home setting.

Social Network

Nursing assessment of the social network addresses the supports that are important for day-to-day functioning as well as those that affect the person's quality of life. The nurse can initiate the assessment by asking a broad question such as, "Whom do you rely on for help?" The nurse can then ask more specific questions about how the person accomplishes tasks that are most important for day-to-day function. For example, in discussing a follow-up appointment for medical care, the nurse may ask, "How do you get to your doctor appointments?" Because a relationship with a confidant is a significant predictor of quality of life for older adults, at least one question relating to this factor should be posed, such as "Is there anyone you can talk to about your worries?" The answer to this question may also be important if the nurse or health care team is assisting the older adult with a decision about long-term care because the older adult may want the confidant to be involved in the decision making process. In addition, the response to this question may provide important information as to whether the older person has recently experienced a loss, or change in the availability, of a confidant.

After identifying existing resources, the nurse identifies the resources that might be helpful in addressing unmet needs. Such questions as "Do you have any grandchildren or neighbors who could help with shoveling the snow?" are aimed at identifying informal supports that may be available but are not currently being used. A question such as "Are you aware that the senior center has a van that takes people to doctor appointments?" is aimed at identifying the person's awareness of formal supports that might not be in use.

Barriers to Obtaining Social Supports

In addition to assessing the number and types of social supports available, nurses try to identify the barriers that interfere with the use of social supports. Only 20% of older adults who are eligible for service programs use these resources, which are viewed as costly, impersonal, overly structured, and hard to arrange (Anetzberger, 2002). Groups of older adults who are least likely to use formal services include minority older adults; those who are blind, visually impaired, or have mental health problems; and those who have more complex needs that span both the aging network and other networks, such as mental health or mental retardation networks (Biegel, 2001).

Because older adults prefer to receive help from family and friends, negative attitudes about the use of formal social supports may be a source of resistance to their use. In the absence of adequate informal supports, or when conflicts exist between older adults and their informal supports, an increase in dependence can trigger less effective coping mechanisms. The following example is typical of such a situation:

Mr. and Mrs. S. always expected their children to care for them, but the children have moved to other cities and only visit several times a year. Mr. and Mrs. S. refuse to accept any of the formal services that are available because of their cost and also because they expect their children to provide the services out of filial responsibility. Furthermore, Mrs. S. cared for
her parents when they were old, so she expects her daughter to do the same for her.

Mr. and Mrs. S. frequently call their daughter and son-in-law to complain about their inability to get groceries and go to doctors' appointments. Rather than making use of transportation or other services available from the community, they neglect themselves. During the children's visit over the Christmas holiday, they find that their parents have not been eating adequately and are not taking their prescribed medications. When they mention these observations to their parents, Mr. and Mrs. S. tell their children, "If you loved us, you'd be taking care of us, and this wouldn't be happening."

In addition to some older people's preference for obtaining services from families rather than outside agencies, there are many other barriers to the use of formal services. Fears about outsiders coming into the home rank high among the barriers to the provision of in-home services. Financial barriers also often exist, because of either an inability or an unwillingness to pay for services. Additional barriers include unwillingness to accept help, lack of knowledge about types of services available, and not knowing where to go for specific services. The identification of these barriers is essential because counseling and educational interventions (e.g., providing information about services that are available) can address many of these issues. Issues that are not amenable to intervention may represent impenetrable barriers to the provision of social supports.

The assessment of barriers to support services is particularly challenging because direct questions about these issues often are inappropriate and usually are very threatening. Rather, identification of these barriers is best accomplished by carefully listening to older people and their caregivers and by asking non-threatening questions. For example, a caregiver might talk about a friend who had a home health aide who did nothing but watch television all day and got paid $12 an hour. In response to this, the nurse might ask, "Do you think that might happen if we arrange for a home health aide to care for your father?" Other attitudinal barriers, such as prejudices, may be identified through statements made by the caregiver about prior experiences.

Economic Resources

Financial issues are generally within the purview of social workers, and nurses usually prefer to avoid discussing money with older adults or their families. In planning for formal services for older adults, however, some assessment of financial assets is necessary, and the nurse is often the health care professional who obtains this information, especially in home or other community settings. If no long-term care or community-based services are needed, the nurse can forego the financial assessment.

Many older adults and their families are shocked to find out that Medicare does not cover the costs of long-term care, with the exception of skilled care. In addition, people are often appalled by the restrictive definition of skilled care, as well as many other restrictions that are applied to determine eligibility for services. Even if a social worker has explained these facts, it is usually the nurse who deals with the related anxiety and other emotional reactions of the older adult and their families. Because gerontological nurses are in a position to help older adults and their families address and cope with the financial issues of long-term care, they frequently become involved in assessing the financial resources of the person and family.

It is not always necessary to ask details about monthly income or the exact amount of savings and assets, but questions must be asked about the resources available for the purchase of services. Asking a question such as "Do you have any money worries?" might reveal some anxieties that can be dealt with or allayed through counseling or the provision of accurate information. When the nurse reviews with the older adult or caregiver the services that are available, information also can be provided about the cost of these services, at which time a question such as "Do you think you could afford this kind of help?" can be posed.

Religion and Spirituality

The biopsychosocial–spiritual model of care emphasizes that everyone has a spiritual history, and for many people, "this spiritual history unfolds within the context of an explicit religious tradition" (Sulmasy, 2002, p. 27). As discussed in Chapter 8, religion and spirituality become more important in older adulthood, and they are resources that should be identified as a part of a comprehensive psychosocial assessment. The person's religious affiliation is assessed as a component of his or her social supports, whereas spirituality is assessed as a separate component of the psychosocial assessment.

Identification of religious affiliation is a simple but important part of the psychosocial assessment because available religion-based programs for older adults may be perceived as more acceptable than those provided by a public or nonreligious agency. For example, an older Jewish person might be willing to go to the Jewish Community Center for a senior meal program, and an older Roman Catholic adult might be willing to accept mental health services from Catholic Social Services, but these people might refuse to avail themselves of the same kinds of services when they are offered by another organization. Often, religion-based services are viewed by the older adult as services that they deserve as a reward for years of attendance at or service to a church or synagogue. Although most religion-based programs serve older adults regardless of their religious affiliations, the programs often are perceived as more acceptable if the person is of the same faith.

In addition to being perceived as more acceptable, some religion-based services are not available elsewhere, and they often are provided by trained volunteers free of charge. Examples of programs or services that may be available to members of a particular church or synagogue include transportation, respite care, peer counseling, chore assistance, friendly visiting, and telephone reassurance. Older adults also can take advantage of any church- or synagogue-based program that is available for people of all ages. The Stephen Ministries, founded in 1975, is an example of a volunteer program that is available in many Christian denominations throughout the United States. This program offers peer counseling and other services, provided by volunteers with special training in ministering to older, depressed, shut-in, and grieving persons.

Identification of a specific place of worship is also important because attendance at religious services may be a significant factor in the older adult's social life. For many older adults, especially those with limited mobility or those who have full-time caregiving responsibilities, attendance at religious services is their only opportunity for social interaction and personal support. Most people who are unable to attend religious services can arrange for home visits by a clergy person or lay minister; indeed, these visits may be the only source of outside contact and emotional support that is acceptable to a home-bound older adult. Moreover, for people who are socially isolated, a visitor from their place of worship may be the only person monitoring the home situation. In these situations, health professionals who are concerned about homebound older adults may be able to monitor their status through these visitors, as in the following example:

Mr. S. was admitted to the hospital after a syncopal episode that resulted in a minor car accident. On admission, Mr. S. was slightly unkempt and showed some memory deficits, but his self-care abilities improved during his 2-day hospitalization. The nurse suggested that Mr. S. consider home-delivered meals and the use of other community resources, but he refused these services. His situation did not warrant a report to a protective services agency.

The nurse was concerned because Mr. S. lived alone and had no outside contacts other than Ms. C., a lay minister who had visited weekly for 2 years. The nurse asked for and received permission from Mr. S. to contact Ms. C. to inform her of available community services. Ms. C. was grateful for the information and said that she would contact the appropriate agencies if Mr. S.'s condition declined or if he agreed to accept help.

In this situation, information about the church affiliation enabled the nurse to implement a discharge plan that otherwise would not have been possible.

Nursing assessment of spiritual needs, like nursing assessment of sexual needs, is not routinely included in an assessment because it is not always relevant to the health issues being addressed. There are times, however, when a nursing assessment of the spiritual needs of older adults is warranted. When an older person provides clues about spiritual distress or discom-fort, the nurse must be willing to respond to the older person, rather than simply ignore the clues, as discussed in Chapter 8. Moreover, when a nurse is addressing quality-of-life issues, it is important to include questions about spirituality (Display 10-9). For example, when long-term care is being planned, it is especially important to assess and address spiritual needs. Assessment of spiritual needs is directed toward a discussion of sources of power and meaning in the older person's life and is not intended to evaluate whether a person is more or less spiritual or beholden to doctrinaire beliefs (Ortiz & Langer, 2002).

Nurses, like many people, may not be comfortable discussing spirituality, but they can increase their comfort level by recognizing their own feelings and acknowledging that spirituality is a universal human need (Display 10-9). Nurses might avoid discussion of spiritual needs because they believe that they are not skilled in meeting these needs. However, nurses routinely identify many needs that they are not

---

DISPLAY 10-9
Guidelines for Assessing Spiritual Needs

Guidelines for Nursing Assessment
- Be aware of your own feelings about spirituality so you can recognize and respond to the spiritual needs of others.
- Recognize that spiritual needs are a universal human phenomenon. Although not all people experience spiritual distress, all people have spiritual needs and the potential for spiritual growth.
- Recognize that it is within the realm of holistic nursing care to identify and plan interventions for spiritual growth as well as for spiritual distress.
- Convey a nonjudgmental, open-minded attitude when eliciting information about a person's spirituality and religious beliefs.

Questions to Assess Spiritual Health
- "What in your life is meaningful and important?"
- "What do you hope to accomplish in your life?"
- "What do you do that gives you pleasure and satisfaction?"
- "Who are the people you can turn to when you need someone to listen to you or to help you?"
- "Do you believe in a higher being?" (examples: God, Goddess, Divinity) "How do you describe this being?"
- "Do you participate in any activities (rituals) that foster a connection with a higher being?" (examples: prayer or other religious activities)
- "What activities are helpful in bringing you inner peace and relieving stress?" (examples: meditation, walking in the woods)
- "What are your beliefs about death?"
- "Do you see a connection between your body, your mind, your emotions, and your soul?"

- "Is there anything you need or would like to have to support your beliefs and your spiritual needs?" (example: Bible, sacred or revered object)
- "Would you like to arrange a visit from a spiritual leader?"
- "Are there any health practices that you would like to consider, even though our society may not consider them to be conventional?" (examples: therapeutic touch, guided imagery)

Observations/Questions to Assess Spiritual Distress
- During the psychosocial interview, listen for clues to spiritual distress, such as the following: suicidal ideation; anger toward God; inability to forgive others; feelings of hopelessness, uselessness, or abandonment; questions about the meaning of life, losses, or suffering.
- "Are there any conflicts between your beliefs or values and actions that you feel you should be taking?" (example: feeling entitled to some time to oneself, which may be in conflict with the demands of caregiving for a spouse)
- "Are there any conflicts between what you believe in and what society or health care professionals are encouraging or suggesting you do?" (example: questioning the wisdom of using a feeding tube for a spouse who is chronically and severely impaired and unable to participate in the decision)
- "Do you have any special religious considerations that are not being addressed?" (examples: dietary practices, observance of religious holidays)
- *For people in institutional settings:* "Is there anything here that interferes with your spiritual needs?" (examples: noisy environment, lack of privacy)

trained to meet directly. If nurses view the assessment of spiritual needs as one aspect of overall health, they may become comfortable addressing the spiritual needs of the older adults to whom they provide care. As with other broad health problems, nurses address the nursing aspects of those problems and refer the person to the appropriate resource for interventions that address the nonnursing aspects. In addition to providing direct nursing interventions to address spiritual needs, nurses suggest referrals to appropriate clergy or spiritual practitioners. Involvement with support groups can also be effective in dealing with spiritual distress when it arises from feelings of guilt, anger, or inadequacy. Assessment of spiritual needs includes not only the factors that cause spiritual distress but also the factors that are essential to spiritual growth, even in the absence of spiritual distress.

CHAPTER SUMMARY

Assessment of psychosocial function is a very complex process that involves the use of good communication skills, interview questions, purposeful observations, and assessment tools. Nurses can assess their own attitudes to increase their comfort level in performing a psychosocial assessment of older adults. An assessment of mental status involves an assessment of all of the following: physical appearance, motor function, social skills, response to the interview, orientation, alertness, memory, speech characteristics, and calculation and higher language skills. Assessment of cognitive skills, such as executive function, is particularly important for determining the ability of the older adult to participate in decision making. An assessment of affective function includes consideration of mood, anxiety, self-esteem, depression, and happiness and well-being. Assessment of a person's contact with reality is a very complex aspect of psychosocial function, and emphasis must be placed on identifying potential underlying causes of any loss of contact with reality. An assessment of social supports addresses all of the following: social network, barriers to social supports, economic resources, religious affiliation, and spirituality.

CRITICAL THINKING EXERCISES

1. Complete the psychosocial self-assessment in Display 10-1.
2. Think of several different situations in the past few weeks in which you worked with older adults and answer the following questions:

- What aspects of psychosocial function did you observe?
- What questions did you ask that would give you information about their psychosocial function?
- What information did you obtain about their social supports?
3. Name at least three things you would observe or determine in order to assess each of the following when you are working with older adults: physical appearance, social skills, orientation, alertness, memory, speech characteristics, calculation and higher language skills, decision-making skills, anxiety, self-esteem, depression, and contact with reality.
4. What questions would you ask an older adult to identify social supports and barriers to the use of services?
5. What approach would you use to assess an older adult's spiritual health and identify spiritual distress?

EDUCATIONAL RESOURCES

The Mini-Mental State Examination
Psychological Assessment Resources, Inc.
16204 North Florida Avenue, Lutz, FL 33549
(800) 331-8378
http://www.minimental.com

REFERENCES

Anetzberger, G. J. (2002). Community resources to promote successful aging. *Clinics in Geriatric Medicine, 18,* 611–626.

Bazargan, M., Bazargan, S., & King, L. (2001). Paranoid ideation among elderly African American persons. *Gerontologist, 41*(3), 366–373.

Beck, J., & Harris, M. J. (1994). Visual hallucinosis in non-delusional elderly. *International Journal of Geriatric Psychiatry, 9,* 531–536.

Biegel, D. E. (2001). Social supports (formal and informal). In M. D. Mezey (Ed.), *The encyclopedia of elder care* (pp. 610–612). New York: Springer.

Blazer, D. G. (1998). *Emotional problems in later life: Intervention strategies for professional caregivers* (2nd ed.). New York: Springer.

Blazer, D. G. (2002a). *Depression in late life* (3rd ed.). New York: Springer.

Blazer, D. G. (2002b). Self-efficacy and depression in late life: A primary prevention proposal. *Aging & Mental Health, 6*(4), 315–324.

Carpenter, B. D., Van Haitsma, K., Ruckdeschel, K., & Lawton, M. P. (2000). The psychosocial preferences of older adults: A pilot examination of content and structure. *Gerontologist, 40*(3), 335–348.

Chipperfield, J. G., Perry, R. P., & Weiner, B. (2003). Discrete emotions in later life. *Journal of Gerontology: Psychological Sciences, 58B,* P23–P34.

Chung, J. A., & Cummings, J. F. (2000). Neurobehavioral and neuropsychiatric symptoms in Alzheimer's disease: Characteristics and treatment. *Neurology Clinics, 18,* 829–846.

Cummings, J. L. (1985). Organic delusions: Phenomenology, anatomical correlations, and review. *British Journal of Psychiatry, 146,* 184–197.

Cummings, J. L. (2000). New tests for dementia. *Neurology, 55,* 1601.

Dada, F., Sethi, S., & Grossberg, G. T. (2001). Generalized anxiety disorder in the elderly. *Psychiatric Clinics of North America, 24.*

Dubois, B., Slachevsky, A., Litvan, I., & Pillon, B. (2000). The FAB: A frontal assessment battery at bedside. *Neurology, 55,* 1621–1626.

Feinberg, L. F., & Whitlatch, C. J. (2001). Are persons with cognitive impairment able to state consistent choices? *Gerontologist, 41,* 374–382.

Folstein, M. F., Folstein, S. E., & McHugh, P. R. (1975). Mini-Mental State: A practical method for grading the cognitive state of patients for the clinician. *Journal of Psychiatric Research, 12,* 189–198.

Frazier, L. D., Waid, L. D., & Fincke, C. (2002). Coping with anxiety in later life. *Journal of Gerontological Nursing, 28*(12), 40–47.

Giarrusso, R., Mabry, J. B., & Bengtson, V. L. (2001). The aging self in social contexts. In R. H. Binstock & L. K. George (Eds.), *Handbook of aging and the social sciences* (5th ed., pp. 295–312). San Diego: Academic Press.

Groh, C. J., & Whall, A. L. (2001). Self-esteem disturbance. In M. L. Maas, K. C. Buckwalter, M. D. Hardy, T. Tripp-Reimer, M. G. Titler, & J. P. Specht (Eds.), *Nursing care of older adults: Diagnoses, outcomes, and interventions* (pp. 593–600). St. Louis: Mosby.

Hicks, T. J. (2000). What is our Life like now? Loneliness and elderly individuals residing in nursing homes. *Journal of Gerontological Nursing, 26*(8), 15–19.

Jang, Y., Haley, W. E., Small, B. J., & Mortimer, J. A. (2002). The role of mastery and social resources in the association between disability and depression in later life. *Gerontologist, 42,* 807–813.

Juby, A., Tench, S., & Baker, V. (2002). The value of a clock drawing in identifying executive cognitive dysfunction in people with a normal mini-mental state examination score. *Canadian Medical Association Journal, 167,* 859–864.

Kreeger, J. L., Raulin, M. L., Grace, J., & Priest, B. L. (1995). Effect of hearing enhancement on mental status ratings in geriatric psychiatric patients. *American Journal of Psychiatry, 152,* 629–631.

Lilly, M. L., Richards, B. S., & Buckwalter, K. C. (2003). Friends and social support in dementia caregiving: Assessment and intervention. *Journal of Gerontological Nursing, 29*(1), 29–36.

Mathuranath, P. S., Nestor, P. J., Berrios, G. E., Rakowicz, W., & Hodges, J. R. (2000). A brief cognitive test battery to differentiate Alzheimer's disease and frontotemporal dementia. *Neurology, 55,* 1613–1620.

Ortiz, L. P. A., & Langer, N. (2002). Assessment of spirituality and religion in later life: Acknowledging clients' needs and personal resources. *Journal of Gerontological Social Work, 37*(2), 5–21.

Ostling, S. (2002). Psychotic symptoms and paranoid ideation in a nondemented population-based sample of the very old. *Archives of General Psychiatry, 59*(1), 53–59.

Paulsen, J. S., Salmon, D. P., Thal, L. J., Romero, R., Weisstein-Jenkins, C., Galasko, D., Hofstetter, C. R., Thomas, R., Grant, I., & Jeste, D. V. (2000). Incidence of and risk factors for hallucinations and delusions in patients with probable AD. *Neurology, 54,* 1965–1971.

Piguet, O., Grayson, D. A., Broe, A., Tate, R. L., Bennett, H. P., Lye, T. C., et al. (2002). Normal aging and executive functions in "old-old" community dwellers: Poor performance is not an inevitable outcome. *International Psychogeriatrics, 14*(2), 139–159.

Rozzini, L., Padovani, A., Borroni, B., & Trabucchi, M. (2000). Incidence of and risk factors for hallucinations and delusions in patients with probable AD. *Neurology, 55,* 1240–1241.

Ryff, C. D., & Kwan, C. M. L. (2001). Personality and aging: Flourishing agendas and future challenges. In J. E. Birren & K. W. Schaie (Eds.), *Handbook of the psychology of aging* (5th ed., pp. 477–499). San Diego: Academic Press.

Salinas, T. K., O'Connor, L. J., Weinstein, M., Lee, S. Y. V., & Fitzpatrick, J. J. (2002). A family assessment tool for hospitalized elders. *Geriatric Nursing, 23,* 316–319, 335.

Salmon, D. P., & Lange, K. L. (2001). Cognitive screening and neuropsychological assessment in early Alzheimer's disease. *Clinics in Geriatric Medicine, 17,* 229–254.

Sulmasy, D. P. (2002). A biopsychosocial-spiritual model for the care of patients at the end of life. *Gerontologist, 42*(Special Issue III), 24–33.

Sweet, R. A., Hamilton, R. L., Lopez, O. L., Klunk, W. E., Wisniewski, S. R., Kaufer, D. I., et al. (2000). Psychotic symptoms in Alzheimer's disease are not associated with more severe neuropathologic features. *International Psychogeriatrics, 12*(4), 547–558.

Talbot-Stern, J. K., Green, T., & Royle, T. (2000). Psychiatric manifestations os systemic illness. *Emergency Medicine Clinics of North America, 18,* 199–209.

Teunisse, R. J., Cruysberg, J. R. M., Verbeek, A., & Zitman, F. G. (1995). The Charles Bonnet syndrome: A large prospective study in the Netherlands. *British Journal of Psychiatry, 166,* 254–257.

Waterman, J. D., Blegen, M., Clinton, P., & Specht, J. P. (2001). Social isolation. In M. L. Maas, K. C. Buckwalter, M. D. Hardy, T. Tripp-Reimer, M. G. Titler, & J. P. Specht (Eds.), *Nursing care of older adults: Diagnoses, outcomes, and interventions* (pp. 651–663). St. Louis: Mosby.

4

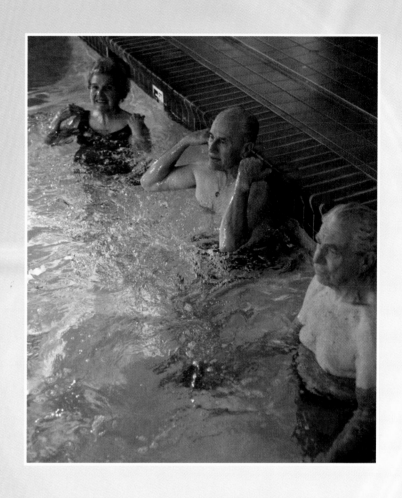

PHYSIOLOGIC ASPECTS
OF FUNCTION

Overall Functional Assessment

LEARNING OBJECTIVES

1. Discuss the purpose of functional assessment of older adults.

2. List the measurement criteria for the following activities of daily living (ADLs): bathing, dressing, mouth care, hair care, dietary intake, transfer mobility, ambulation, bed mobility, mental status, and bladder and bowel control.

3. List the measurement criteria for the following instrumental activities of daily living (IADLs): meal preparation, shopping, telephone use, transportation, medications, housekeeping, laundry, and money management.

The functional assessment approach, which is central to the functional consequences theory of gerontological nursing (discussed in Chapter 3), is used throughout this text in relation to specific aspects of functioning in older adults. In contrast to the commonly used assessment approach that emphasizes medical diagnoses, the functional assessment approach to planning care emphasizes specific aspects of functioning in daily life. For example, a functional assessment for a person with hemiparesis caused by a stroke would assess the limitations and abilities of the person in carrying out his or her usual activities so that goals could be identified and a care plan could be developed. In gerontological practice settings, the term *functional assessment* usually refers to the measurement of a person's ability to fulfill responsibilities and perform tasks for self-care.

Accordingly, this chapter provides guidelines for assessing an older adult's ability to perform activities of daily living (ADLs) and instrumental activities of daily living (IADLs). It is similar to Chapter 10 in that it does not address the age-related changes, risk factors, functional consequences, or interventions specific to one area of function. Rather, it focuses on assessing functional abilities and is meant to supplement information in other chapters. Functional assessment is discussed from a historical perspective as it has been used by health care professionals, with particular emphasis on the application of functional assessment to older adults. In addition, two models of functional assessment of ADLs and IADLs are presented.

HISTORY OF THE FUNCTIONAL ASSESSMENT

The concept of functional assessment was first used in relation to workers' compensation. In the 1920s, the primary purpose of such an assessment was to measure the loss of function in work activity in order to assign a cash value to an impairment (Frey, 1984). Initially, no standards were used, and the determination was based solely on a physician's opinion. In the 1940s, primarily as a result of World War II, the number of people with functional impairments increased dramatically; with this increase came a new emphasis on rehabilitation. Concomitantly, there was a surge of interest in functional assessment for rehabilitation. In 1954, the term *activities of daily living* was first coined (Frey, 1984).

Beginning in the late 1950s, a few forward-thinking gerontological practitioners published articles about the interrelationships between ADLs, chronic disease, and older people (e.g., Benjamin Rose Institute, 1959; Katz et al., 1963). During the 1960s, researchers developed functional assessment instruments that would be applicable to older people in a number of situations. For example, Lawton and Brody (1969) developed a point-system scale to measure six ADL items (toileting, feeding, dressing, grooming, bathing, and ambulation), as well as more complex tasks that they identified as IADLs, such as shopping and housekeeping. Another development during the 1960s was the broadening of the concept of functional assessment to assess person–environment interactions. This approach was used to identify the impact of environmental modifications and other rehabilitation interventions on the person's level of function.

Although gerontologists first used functional assessment measures to facilitate research and planning during the 1970s, not until the 1980s did gerontological practitioners recognize the clinical value of these assessment tools. This appreciation of the functional assessment approach was closely related to a growing recognition of the inadequacy of diagnostic labels for describing the health needs of people with chronic illnesses. At a special conference on functional assessment convened in 1983 by the National Institute on Aging, physicians were advised to use a functional assessment tool along with their traditional, disease-oriented, diagnostic evaluations. Geriatricians and gerontologists also emphasized (1) the importance of identifying functional impairments as early manifestations of active illness in older people (Besdine, 1983), and (2) the importance of assisting the patient and family in maintaining the greatest degree of functional independence possible (Williams, 1983). By the mid-1980s, geriatricians were applying the concept of functional assessment to rehabilitation programs.

CURRENT USE OF FUNCTIONAL ASSESSMENTS IN GERONTOLOGICAL PRACTICE

In 1987, the Omnibus Budget Reconciliation Act (OBRA) mandated that all Medicaid- and Medicare-funded nursing homes begin using a standardized assessment form, which was developed by the Health Care Financing Administration. This form, known as the Minimum Data Set (MDS) for Resident Assessment and Care Screening, included a Resident Assessment Instrument (RAI). The purpose of the RAI was "to improve assessment of residents by identifying strengths, preferences, and functional abilities, and improve the care planning process so resident needs would be addressed better by nursing home staff" (Rantz et al., 1999, p. 36). The value of the MDS/RAI has been internationally recognized; it has been translated and validated in more than 15 countries (Yamada & Ikegami, 2001). In 1995, a second version of the MDS replaced the initial assessment tool; subsequent nursing research has supported the reliability and clinical utility of this version as well (Morris et al., 1997). Currently, the MDS is viewed as an essential source of data related to quality indicators such as falls, dehydration, weight loss, and restraint use (Rantz et al., 1999).

Because the use of the MDS/RAI as an assessment instrument has been successful in improving care in nursing homes, the federal government and accrediting organizations (e.g., the Joint Commission on Accreditation of Healthcare Organizations) have promoted the use of standardized functional assessment tools in all gerontological health care settings. For example, a home version of the MDS (MDS-HC) is currently used in Medicaid- and Medicare-funded home care agencies. Positive outcomes of programs that use the MDS-HC include fewer hospital readmissions and shorter lengths of stay (Landi et al., 2001).

In recent years, gerontologists have broadened the concept of functional assessment to include the concept of "everyday competence." This term refers to "a person's ability to perform, when necessary, a broad array of activities considered essential for independent living, even though in daily life the individual may not perform these tasks on a regular basis or may only perform a subset of these activities" (Diehl, 1998, p. 422). Assessment of everyday competence expands on the functional assessment in the following ways:

- It emphasizes the person's potential to perform tasks rather than actual daily behaviors of the person.
- It emphasizes the interactions among physical, cognitive, emotional, and social functioning that affect the person's daily functioning.

- It emphasizes the need to be sensitive to cultural and contextual factors that influence a person's behaviors (Diehl, 1998).

A specific aspect of everyday competence that is addressed in gerontological literature is the interrelationship between functional abilities and environmental factors (Wahl, 2001). This is particularly important to consider in a functional assessment of older adults because environmental factors can significantly hinder or improve functional abilities. For example, environmental factors can significantly affect hearing, vision, and mobility (discussed in Chapters 12, 13, and 18). Fielo and Warren (2001) have developed an excellent guide for nursing assessment and interventions related to home environments of older adults. The actual or potential use of items such as mobility aids (e.g., canes and walkers) and adaptive equipment (e.g., grab bars) also should be assessed as environmental factors that can significantly affect everyday competence (Allen et al., 2001).

Another specific aspect of everyday competence that is addressed in gerontological literature is the influence of cognitive abilities on function (Njegovan et al., 2001; Tabbarah at al., 2002). Assessment scales have been developed to address the need for a functional assessment tool that is applicable to people with dementia in a variety of settings and at all levels of cognitive impairment. One such scale that has been used since the early 1990s, the Cleveland Scale for Activities of Daily Living (CSADL), divides ADLs into smaller components that may be affected by the underlying cognitive impairment (Patterson et al., 1992). Because this scale was developed specifically to evaluate the effect of dementia on a person's ability to perform ADLs, the items focus on potential effects of cognitive deficits (Patterson & Mack, 2001). Studies have found that this instrument, illustrated in Figure 11-1, is reliable and valid as a measurement of functional deficits in people with Alzheimer's disease (Patterson & Mack, 2001). The scale and accompanying manual, which includes instructions and percentile scores for comparison with other people with dementia, can be obtained by contacting the University Memory and Aging Center (listed in the Educational Resource section at the end of this chapter). The Alzheimer's Disease Activities of Daily Living International Scale (ADL-IS) was developed to fill the need for an ADL scale that is "useful for the earliest stages of AD, and which is simultaneously non-gender-biased and cross-nationally relevant" (Reisberg et al., 2001). The ADL-IS assesses 40 items, divided into the following categories: conversation, recreation, self-care, household activities, general activities, medication, social functioning, telephone use, reading, organization, food preparation, travel, and driving.

A current trend in gerontological health care related to functional assessment is the development of easy-to-use assessment guides and screening tools to identify target conditions that commonly occur in older adults (Sherman, 2001). Since the early 1990s, the Nurses Improving Care to the Hospitalized Elderly (NICHE) project of the John A. Hartford Foundation for Geriatric Nursing has been in the forefront of developing brief assessment guides for nurses to use in acute care settings. The first assessment guide, called SPICES, addressed the following target conditions: Skin impairment, Poor nutrition, Incontinence, Confusion, Evidence of falls or functional decline, and Sleep disorders (Fulmer, 1991). In recent years, the SPICES tool has been modified and expanded to include target conditions of pain, safety, restraints, bowel elimination, and elder mistreatment (Guthrie et al., 2002; Lee & Fletcher, 2002; Pfaff, 2002). NICHE recently expanded this model of care to include a family assessment guide, called FAMILY, that assesses the following: Family involvement, Assistance needed, Members' needs, Integration into care plan, Links to community support, and Your intervention (Salinas et al., 2002). Tools such as these are not substitutes for a functional assessment but are commonly used, especially in acute care settings, to increase the nurse's awareness of areas that need to be addressed in assessment of older adults. Thus, they can be used in conjunction with functional assessment tools and other assessments as a basis for planning care for older adults.

Currently, the functional assessment is viewed as a core component of a comprehensive geriatric assessment, which is performed by an interdisciplinary team of gerontological health care practitioners (Fillenbaum, 2001). Researchers and gerontological health care practitioners are increasingly supporting the use of comprehensive geriatric assessment programs for older adults with complex health and functional problems (Aminzadeh et al., 2002). For gerontological nurses, functional assessments serve the following purposes: measurement of outcomes, design of interventions, and prediction and prevention of functional disability (Bennett, 1999).

SAMPLE FUNCTIONAL ASSESSMENT TOOL

Functional assessment tools generally include a scale for measuring a person's level of independence in performing specific ADLs and IADLs. ADLs include activities that are essential to personal care, whereas IADLs comprise the more complex activities that are essential in community-living situations. The assessment of ADL performance is important in determining the

(text continues on page 219)

CLEVELAND SCALE FOR ACTIVITIES OF DAILY LIVING (CSADL)

Name or ID of Subject _____   Date _ _ / _ _ / _ _   Rater _____
                                                                    m m d d y y

Name of Informant _____

Relation of Informant to Subject (*Circle one.*)   Contact with Subject   Interview Type

1 Spouse   4 Friend or other family   1   2 days/week   1   Visit
2 Child   5 Professional: _____   2   3-4 days/week   2   Telephone
3 Sibling   6 Other: _____   3   5 or more days/week

To administer this scale, the rater must be thoroughly familiar with the Manual, which includes the full instructions. Place rating in blank after each item number. Several items have specific rating instructions. In particular, some require special questioning if the subject is rated as dependent (rating of 1, 2, or 3).

Rating	Meaning of Rating
0	**Never Dependent.** [S] does this effectively, quite independently, without any direction or help.
1	**Sometimes Dependent.** [S] usually does this independently, but sometimes or in some situations [S] needs direction or help.
2	**Usually Dependent.** [S] usually requires some direction or help, but sometimes or in some situations [S] does it independently.
3	**Always Dependent.** [S] always requires direction or help. [S] never does it independently.
9	Cannot rate because of insufficient information

Bathing

1. _____   Initiates bath or shower with appropriate frequency and at appropriate times

2. _____   Prepares bath/shower (draws water of proper temperature, ensures soap and towel are present, etc.)

3. _____   Gets in and out of tub or shower

4. _____   Cleans self

Toileting

5. _____   Able to physically control timing of urination

6. _____   Able to physically control timing of bowel movements

7. _____   Recognizes need to eliminate

8. _____   After toileting, cleans and re-clothes self appropriately

Personal Hygiene and Appearance

9. _____   Initiates personal grooming with appropriate frequency and at appropriate times

10. _____   Washes hands and face

11. _____   Brushes teeth

12. _____   Combs hair, shaves (as appropriate)

FIGURE 11-1 The Cleveland Scale for Activities of Daily Living (CSADL). This functional assessment form was specifically designed for use with people with Alzheimer's disease. (Used with permission from the University Memory and Aging Center, Case Western Reserve University, Cleveland, Ohio. Copyright 1994.)

Dressing

13. ____   Initiates dressing at appropriate time

14. ____   Selects clothes

15. ____   Puts on garments, footwear, etc.

16. ____   Fastens clothing (buttons, shoelaces, zippers, etc.)

Eating

17. ____   Initiates eating at appropriate times of day and with appropriate frequency

18. ____   Carries out physical acts of eating (including using utensils)

19. ____   Eats with acceptable manners, e.g. with appropriate speed, does not speak with food in mouth, etc.

20. ____   Prepares own meals (includes cooking on stove). *This item requires special questioning.*

Mobility

21. ____   Initiates actively moving about the environment, as opposed to sitting, not attempting to get about, etc.

22. ____   Actively moves about environment (with or without assisting device)

22a.   Does subject have physical limitations of mobility? *(Circle one of following codes.)*

    0   No physical limitations of mobility

    1   Yes, there are physical limitations of mobility. *(Circle all that apply.)*

Needs assistance of other persons to walk	Trouble getting in or out of bed	Other Mobility Problems
Needs cane	Trouble getting in or out of chair	*(describe):*
Needs walker	Trouble getting on or off toilet	
Needs wheelchair	Trouble climbing or descending stairs	

Medications

23. ____   Takes medications as scheduled and in correct dosages. *If subject has taken no medications during prior year, rate item as 9. This item requires questioning.*

Shopping

24. ____   Does necessary grocery shopping, buying appropriate items and quantities. *This item requires special questioning.*

25. ____   Does necessary clothes shopping, buying appropriate items and quantities. *This item requires special questioning.*

Travel

26. ____   Finds way about in familiar surroundings

27. ____   Orients to unfamiliar surroundings without undue difficulty

28. ____   Travels beyond walking distance (i.e., driving own vehicle or using public transportation)

29. ____   Drives motor vehicle. *This item requires special questioning.*

FIGURE 11-1 *(Continued)*

Hobbies, personal interests, employment

30. ____ Initiates activities of personal interest (e.g. card playing, woodworking, others). *This item requires special questioning.*

31. ____ Carries out such activities. *This item requires special questioning.*

32. ____ Does subject work for pay? *If subject does not work because of having reached an age appropriate to retirement from his or her occupation, rate 9. This item requires special questioning.*

Housework/home maintenance (as appropriate to individual situation)

33. ____ Initiates work around house as needed. *This item requires special questioning.*

34. ____ Carries out work effectively, e.g. cleanly, neatly, accurately, efficiently. *This item requires special questioning.*

Types of work done (*Don't score, just circle*)

Dish washing	Vacuuming	Mowing lawn
Sweeping	Scrubbing floors	Gardening
Personal laundry	Small home repairs	Minor car care
Other types of work (*Describe*):		

Telephone

35. ____ Looks up numbers

36. ____ Dials numbers

37. ____ Answers phone

38. ____ Takes messages

Money Management

39. ____ Pays for purchases (selecting appropriate amount and determining correct change). *This item requires special questioning.*

40. ____ Manages financial responsibilities beyond paying for immediate purchases (e.g., paying monthly bills, managing checking or savings account, etc.). *This item requires special questioning.*

Communication Skills

41. ____ Spontaneously expresses thoughts and needs to others

42. ____ Responds accurately to spoken instructions and conversation

43. ____ Reads and understands single words and short phrases (signs, lists, etc.)

44. ____ Reads and understands complex material (books, newspapers, etc.)

45. ____ Writes short phrases (lists, brief messages)

46. ____ Writes complex material (letters, diary, etc.)

FIGURE 11-1 (*Continued*)

Social Behavior

47. ____ Behaves in a socially appropriate manner. Socially inappropriate behaviors encompass a **wide** range of behavior, including but not limited to such things as making rude remarks, belching, touching private parts, showing little regard for personal privacy, etc. For this item, dependency refers to the extent to which other people must direct or manage the subject to ensure that he or she behaves in a socially appropriate fashion.

Other Problems — Are there any situations in which patient does not behave in an independent and responsible fashion that have not been covered by these questions? (*Circle one of following codes.*)

48.   0   No other dependent behaviors

         1   Yes, there are other dependent behaviors. (*Please provide details below.*)

QUALITY OF INTERVIEW (Rater's Judgment)

Interview appeared valid   0

Some questions about interview, but it is probably acceptable   1

Information from interview is of doubtful validity   2

Rater should record the basis for judging the interview of questionable or doubtful validity.

Comments:

FIGURE 11-1 *(Continued)*

level of assistance needed on a daily basis and is particularly helpful in planning long-term care for older adults. Likewise, an evaluation of IADLs is important in determining the level of assistance needed by people in independent or semi-independent settings. Functional assessment instruments are used to measure changes that occur over time, identify factors that influence functional abilities, and provide a basis for planning care. The functional assessment tool illustrated in Figure 11-2 was developed by nurses in a geriatric rehabilitation setting and can be used to measure a person's functional status at different times. An initial assessment can be done at the time of admission, and this information can then be used as a baseline for establishing goals for care. The form also includes a column for information about the person's reported level of function before admission, which is helpful in determining the person's potential level of function. At the time of discharge, the reassessment information enables the staff to determine whether the goals were met. In settings in which postdischarge follow-up is possible, or in settings in which the person is readmitted at different times, the same assessment form is used to measure changes over time. Each category of activity is assigned a numeric value based on the criteria listed in Displays 11-1 and 11-2. The numeric values are then used as a guide to measure progress toward goals as the person's level of function changes.

		Date	PTA	ADM	DISCH		
Personal Care	*Bathing* 5 completely dependent 4 dependent with some assist 3 heavy partial 2 light partial 1 independent with devices 0 independent						
	Dressing 5 complete assist 3 partial assist 1 compensated 0 independent						
	Mouth care 5 totally unable to do 3 some assist 1 independent with device 0 independent						
	Hair care 5 completely unable 3 some assist 1 independent with device 0 independent						
	Dietary intake 5 total assist 4 assist with feeding 3 supplements 2 set up/encouragement 1 independent with device 0 independent						
Mobility	*Transfer* 5 completely unable 4 3-person/portalift 3 2-person 2 1-person 1 independent with devices 0 independent						
	Ambulation 5 completely unable 4 3-person assist 3 2-person assist 2 1-person assist 1 independent with devices 0 independent						
	Bed 5 unable to move in bed 3 needs assist 1 independent with device 0 independent						
Mental Status	*Mental* 5 totally impaired 4 assist with simple tasks 3 assist with complex tasks 2 inconsistent 1 compensated 0 no impairment						

FIGURE 11-2 Functional assessment of older adults. This form allows for recording changes over time. The three time designations indicated on the form signify the period prior to admission *(PTA)*, the time of admission *(ADM)*, and the day of discharge *(DISCH)*. The unmarked columns may be used at any time after discharge, or upon readmission. (From Fairview General Hospital, Cleveland, OH 44111-5659. Used with permission.)

The functional assessment form in Figure 11-2 differs from many others in two ways. First, allowance is made for measurement of changes over time. The three time designations indicated on the form signify the period prior to admission (PTA), the time of admission (ADM), and the day of discharge (DISCH). The unmarked columns may be used at any time after discharge, or upon readmission. In a rehabilitative or long-term care setting, these measurements over time are particularly helpful

		Date	PTA	ADM	DISCH		
Elimination	*Bladder* 5 completely incontinent 3 occasionally incontinent 1 continent with assist/device 0 continent/independent						
	Bowel 5 completely incontinent 3 occasionally incontinent 1 continent with assist/device 0 continent/independent						
	Assist/device codes A bedside commode E ostomy I catheter, intermittent B bathroom F incontinence pads J verbal cuing/supervision C urinal G catheter, external K other_____ D bedpan H catheter, indwelling						
Instrumental Activities of Daily Living	*Meal preparation* 5 unable to do 3 assist/supervise 1 independent with resources 0 independent						
	Shopping 5 unable to do 3 assist/supervise 1 compensated 0 independent						
	Telephone 5 unable to do/doesn't have 3 assist 1 independent with device 0 independent						
	Transportation 5 completely homebound 3 assist 1 arranges own 0 independent						
	Medications 5 unable to take 3 assist 1 independent 0 doesn't use						
	Housekeeping 5 unable to do 3 assist 1 independent with resources 0 independent						
	Laundry 5 unable to do 3 assist 1 independent with resources 0 independent						
	Money management 5 unable to handle 3 assist 1 independent with resources 0 independent						
	Total Points						

FIGURE 11-2 *(Continued)*

in evaluating progress and reevaluating goals. Second, for each activity category, the number 1 rating is used to indicate that the person does not depend on others, but depends on some adaptive device or equipment for independent function in that area. The adaptive device might be as small as a shoehorn or as complex as an electric wheelchair. The importance of this designation is that the staff is then aware that the person has compensated for a deficit, but that the compensatory mechanism must be available for the person's use.

Nurses obtain assessment information for the functional assessment from several sources. When older adults are able to provide reliable information about

DISPLAY 11-1
Criteria for Assessing Activities of Daily Living (ADL)

Bathing

5 Unable to assist in any way
4 Able to cooperate but cannot assist
3 Able to wash hands, face, and chest with supervision; needs help with completing the bath
2 Able to wash face, chest, arms, and upper legs; needs help with completing the bath
1 Bathes self but requires devices (e.g., long-handled sponge)
0 Bathes self independently

Dressing

5 Needs total assistance
4 Needs total supervision, but is able to dress self if clothing articles are given one at a time or set out in the order they are needed
3 Needs reminding and encouragement and some assistance with clothing selection, but can dress with little supervision
2 Dresses self, but needs help with activities requiring fine motor skills (e.g., zippers, shoelaces)
1 Dresses self using assistive devices (e.g., zipper pullers, long-handled shoehorn)
0 Dresses independently

Mouth Care

5 Cannot perform oral hygiene, but requires that it be done by others
4 Needs total supervision; needs toothpaste put on brush
3 Needs reminding and some supervision
2 Needs reminding but is otherwise independent
1 Performs oral hygiene using devices (e.g., toothbrush with built-up handle)
0 Performs oral hygiene independently

Hair Care

5 Cannot perform hair care, but requires that it be done by others
4 Needs total supervision
3 Needs some assistance with daily care
2 Performs daily care independently, but needs assistance with washing hair
1 Performs hair care using devices (e.g., hairbrush with built-up handle)
0 Performs all hair care (including washing) independently

Dietary Intake

5 Cannot prepare or obtain food; cannot feed self; nutritional requirements would not be met without total assistance
4 Needs assistance in obtaining and preparing food; needs total supervision with eating, but can feed self; nutritional requirements would not be met adequately without assistance
3 Needs assistance in tasks that involve complex skills (e.g., cutting meat, opening packages, preparing and obtaining food), but feeds self; nutritional needs would be met partially without assistance
2 Requires some assistance with obtaining and preparing food, but eats independently; would maintain adequate nutrition with encouragement or a little assistance
1 Needs assistive devices for food preparation and consumption (e.g., plate rings, rocker knife); adequately maintains nutritional requirements
0 Requires no assistance

Transfer Mobility

5 Cannot transfer, except with extreme difficulty
4 Needs assistance of three people for transfers, or needs two people and a lifting device
3 Needs the assistance of two people
2 Needs the assistance of one person
1 Transfers independently with a device (e.g., sliding board)
0 Transfers independently

Ambulation

5 Completely unable to walk
4 Walks with the assistance of three people
3 Walks with the assistance of two people
2 Walks with the assistance of one person
1 Walks independently with device (e.g., walker, quad cane)
0 Walks independently

Bed Mobility

5 Unable to move in bed
4 Needs the assistance of two people
3 Needs the assistance of one person
2 Needs to be encouraged and supervised
1 Moves indepedently with device (e.g., uses side rails or trapeze)
0 Moves independently in bed

Mental Status

5 Has extremely poor memory function; cannot follow directions; has minimal ability to identify and express needs; requires a totally structured environment
4 Has obvious memory impairment that interferes with daily life; has poor judgment and may undertake inappropriate actions; may be aware of the deficit and, consequently, may be anxious or depressed; can participate in daily routine but needs supervision; requires a strong orientation and reminder program
3 Fluctuates between levels two and four; unpredictable on a routine basis; requires monitoring and some supervision; may engage in risky behaviors at times
2 Minimal short-term memory loss; able to perform most daily tasks with only minimal reminding or supervision; has good to fair judgment and occasionally needs assistance, but does not engage in any risky behaviors
1 Is dependent on self-initiated reminders and cues for daily activities
0 No observable impairment in memory; no cognitive or psychosocial impairment that interferes with daily activities

Bladder and Bowel Elimination

5 Consistently soils self
4 Needs supervision and assistance on a regular basis
3 Needs reminding on a regular basis
2 Generally controls elimination; has accidents no more than once a week
1 Maintains control of elimination with devices (listed in Fig. 11-1)
0 Fully continent without any assistance

DISPLAY 11-2
Criteria for Assessing Instrumental Activities of Daily Living (IADL)

Meal Preparation

5 Unable to prepare even simple meals
4 Can assist with meal preparation
3 Prepares meals, but cannot obtain groceries
2 Prepares meals with reminding or supervision
1 Prepares meals and obtains food using resources (e.g., specialized equipment, Meals on Wheels program, transportation to the grocery store)
0 Independent in obtaining and preparing food

Grocery Shopping

5 Cannot participate in shopping
4 Can accompany someone else and assist with food selection
3 Can shop and select appropriate food with some supervision
2 Can shop, but has difficulty obtaining transportation
1 Is able to arrange for necessary help with shopping
0 Shops independently

Telephone Use

5 Cannot dial or answer the phone, or carry on a routine phone conversation
4 Can talk on the phone, but cannot dial or answer it
3 Can use the phone with assistance (e.g., help in dialing)
2 Can use the phone with supervision
1 Depends on adaptive devices for telephone activities (e.g., automatic dialing system, speaker phone)
0 Independent in phone-related activities

Transportation

5 Does not leave home, even for medical care
4 Leaves home only for medical care or in rare circumstances
3 Needs assistance in arranging for transportation and needs special accommodations (e.g., wheelchair lift)
2 Needs assistance in arranging for transportation, but can get in and out of cars with little or no help
1 Arranges for own transportation, but depends on others for any transportation other than walking
0 Independent in traveling from one place to another (e.g., drives a car)

Medications

5 Unable to obtain or take medications without assistance or complete supervision
4 Cannot obtain medications, but can take them with assistance or supervision
3 Can obtain and take medications with reminders from others or with a system set up by others
2 Can obtain and take medications with a self-initiated reminder or set-up system
1 Safely takes and prepares all medications
0 Does not use medications

Housekeeping

5 Cannot perform any routine household tasks
4 Can assist with household tasks (e.g., bed making, dusting, vacuuming)
3 Can perform household tasks if supervised during the activity
2 Can perform household tasks if encouraged to do so
1 Arranges for housekeeping assistance
0 Is independent in all routine tasks

Laundry

5 Cannot perform any laundry tasks
4 Can assist with folding clothes; cannot wash or iron clothes
3 With assistance, can perform laundry tasks adequately
2 Can perform laundry tasks with supervision and reminding
1 Arranges for laundry to be done
0 Completes all laundry tasks independently

Money Management

5 Unable to manage any aspect of finances
4 Can handle simple cash transactions, but no other financial transactions (e.g., writing checks)
3 Can write checks with supervision or assistance; cannot handle any higher-level transactions (e.g., bank withdrawals)
2 Maintains checkbook, pays bills appropriately, and understands currency exchanges, but needs some assistance or supervision with these tasks
1 Arranges for someone else to handle financial matters
0 Handles all finances independently

---

their level of function before admission, data for the column marked "PTA" are obtained through an interview with the person within 24 hours of the admission to the care facility. When, as is often the case, older adults are not able to provide this information, the nurse interviews a family member or other person who is knowledgeable about the person's level of function before admission. Nurses use direct observation of the person's current level of function in performing ADLs to complete the columns marked "ADM" and "DISCH." Much of the information for the sections on IADLs must be obtained by questioning the older adult or his or her caregivers because

many of these activities pertain only to community-based settings. The source of information is noted on the chart, and any discrepancies between objective and subjective information also are noted.

In interviewing the older adult or caregiver, it is important to ask specific details about how tasks are accomplished, rather than open-ended questions such as "Do you have any difficulty with . . .?" Also, it is important to find out whether the task is meaningful to the person, rather than assuming that the person wants or needs to do the task. For example, in the IADL categories, a person who lives with other people might never have to participate in grocery shopping or money management. Therefore, assessment information, particularly regarding IADLs, must be considered in relation to the person's support system and living arrangements.

Assessment of Activities of Daily Living (ADLs)

The following areas of function are those generally considered in an assessment of ADLs: grooming, bathing, dressing, eating, elimination, and mobility. The assessment format illustrated in Figure 11-2 further specifies these activities as follows: bathing, dressing, mouth care, hair care, dietary intake, transfer mobility, ambulation, bed mobility, and bladder and bowel elimination. In addition, a brief mental status assessment is included on the ADL form. This approach is taken, rather than using a separate mental status assessment tool, because it reinforces the fact that cognitive function is an integral component of ADLs. In addition, it helps to determine whether ADL impairments are attributable, at least in part, to cognitive impairments, rather than primarily to physical limitations. See Display 11-1 for the functional assessment criteria for each of the ADLs as well as for mental status.

Assessment of Instrumental Activities of Daily Living (IADLs)

IADLs are less important in institutional settings than they are in community settings. In institutional settings, however, an assessment of IADLs is an important consideration in discharge planning. When older adults cannot perform IADLs independently, caregivers often provide the assistance that enables the person to remain in a community setting. When older adults cannot perform IADLs and have no caregiver to help with the task, community resources often are available to meet these needs. Home-delivered meals programs, for example, might be appropriate for older adults who have difficulty with shopping or meal preparation. Community resources often can be arranged with one or two phone calls, and they can be effective and efficient ways of improving an older adult's ability to perform IADLs. See Display 11-2 for the assessment criteria for the IADLs that are included in Figure 11-2.

CHAPTER SUMMARY

A functional assessment is a formal process of measuring a person's ability to fulfill responsibilities and perform self-care tasks. Functional assessments were first used in the 1920s for measuring loss of function in work activities for determining workers' compensation benefits. During the 1960s, gerontologists developed functional assessment tools for measuring ADLs and IADLs, but it was not until the 1980s that gerontological health care practitioners recognized the usefulness of such tools. In 1987, the federal government mandated the use of standardized assessment tools, which included functional assessment scales, in all nursing homes. Subsequently, the MDS was developed for use in nursing homes; this assessment tool has been revised and currently is widely used. Functional assessment tools focus primarily on the person's ability to perform ADLs and IADLs. In recent years, gerontological researchers and health care practitioners have recognized the need to assess the functional abilities of older adults in relation to both their environment and their cognitive abilities. The functional assessment tool discussed in this chapter can be used by nurses to measure a person's functional status at different times. Functional assessment tools provide a base for planning interventions aimed at improving the person's functional abilities.

 CRITICAL THINKING EXERCISES

1. Identify an older adult (in a clinical setting or someone you know personally) who has some functional impairment as well as some cognitive impairment and perform a functional assessment on them, using Figure 11-1.
2. Identify an older adult (in a clinical setting or someone you know personally) who has some functional impairment but no cognitive impairment and perform a functional assessment on them, using Figure 11-2.

EDUCATIONAL RESOURCE

University Memory and Aging Center
12200 Fairhill Road, Cleveland, OH 44120
(800) 252-5048
http://www.memoryandagingcenter.org

REFERENCES

Allen, S. M., Foster, A., & Berg, K. (2001). Receiving help at home: The interplay of human and technological assistance. *Journal of Gerontology: Social Sciences, 56B,* S374–S382.

Aminzadeh, F., Amos, S., Byszewski, A., & Dalziel, W. B. (2002). Comprehensive geriatric assessment: Exploring clients' and caregivers' perceptions of the assessment process and outcomes. *Journal of Gerontological Nursing, 28*(6), 6–13.

Benjamin Rose Institute. (1959). Multidisciplinary studies of illness in aged persons. II. A new classification of functional status in activities of daily living. *Journal of Chronic Disease, 9,* 55.

Bennett, J. A. (1999). Activities of daily living: Old-fashioned or still useful? *Journal of Gerontological Nursing, 25*(5), 22–29.

Besdine, R. W. (1983). The educational utility of comprehensive functional assessment in the elderly. *Journal of the American Geriatrics Society, 31,* 651–656.

Diehl, M. (1998). Everyday competence in later life: Current status and future directions. *Gerontologist, 38,* 422–433.

Fielo, S. B., & Warren, S. A. (2001). Home adaptation: Helping older people age in place. *Geriatric Nursing, 22,* 239–246.

Fillenbaum, G. G. (2001). Multidimensional functional assessment: Overview. In M. D. Mezey (Ed.), *The encyclopedia of elder care* (pp. 438–440). New York: Springer.

Frey, W. D. (1984). Functional assessment in the '80s: A conceptual enigma, a technical challenge. In A. S., Halpern & J. J. Fuhrer (Eds.), *Functional assessment in rehabilitation* (pp. 11–443). Baltimore: Paul H. Brookes.

Fulmer, T. T. (1991). The geriatric nurse specialist role: A new model. *Nursing Management, 22,* 91–93.

Guthrie, P. F., Edinger, G., & Schumacher, S. (2002). A NICHE program at North Memorial Health Care. *Geriatric Nursing, 23,* 133–138.

Katz, S., Ford, A. B., Moskowitz, R. W., Jackson, B. A., & Jaffee, M. W. (1963). Studies of illness in the aged: The index of ADL, a standardized measure of biological and psychosocial function. *Journal of the American Medical Association, 185,* 914–919.

Landi, F., Onder, G., Tua, E., Carrara, B., Zuccala, G., Gambassi, G., et al. (2001). Impact of a new assessment system, the MDS-HC on function and hospitalization of homebound older people: A controlled clinical trial. *Journal of the American Geriatrics Society, 49,* 1288–1293.

Lawton, M. P., & Brody, E. M. (1969). Assessment of older people: Self-maintaining and instrumental activities of daily living. *Gerontologist, 9,* 179–186.

Lee, V. K., & Fletcher, K. R. (2002). Sustaining the geriatric resource nurse model at the University of Virginia. *Geriatric Nursing, 23,* 128–132.

Morris, J. N., Nonemaker, S., Murphy, K., Hawes, C., Fries, B. E., Mor, V., & Phillips, C. (1997). A commitment to change: Revision of HCFA's RAI. *Journal of the American Geriatrics Society, 45,* 1011–1016.

Njegovan, V., Man-Son-Hing, M., Mitchell, S. L., & Molnar, F. J. (2001). The hierarchy of functional loss associated with cognitive decline in older persons. *Journal of Gerontology: Medical Sciences, 56A,* M638–643.

Patterson, M. B., & Mack, J. L. (2001). The Cleveland Scale for Activities of Daily Living (CSADL): Its reliability and validity. *Journal of Clinical Geropsychology, 7*(1), 15–28.

Patterson, M. B., Mack, J. L., Neundorfer, M., Martin, R. J., Smyth, K. A., & Whitehouse, P. J. (1992). Assessment of functional ability in Alzheimer's disease: A review and a preliminary report on the Cleveland scale for activities of daily living. *Alzheimer Disease and Associated Disorders, 6*(3), 145–163.

Pfaff, J. (2002). The geriatric resource nurse model: A culture change. *Geriatric Nursing, 23*(3), 140–144.

Rantz, M., Popejoy, L., Zwygart-Stauffacher, M., Wipke-Tevis, D., & Grando, V. T. (1999). Minimum Data Set and Resident Assessment Instrument: Can using standardized assessment improve clinical practice and outcomes of care? *Journal of Gerontological Nursing, 25*(6), 35–43.

Reisberg, B., Finkel, S., Overall, J., Schmidt-Gollas, N., Kanowski, S., Lehfeld, H., et al. (2001). The Alzheimer's Disease Activities of Daily Living International Scale (ADL-IS). *International Psychogeriatrics, 13*(2), 163–181.

Salinas, T. K., O'Connor, L. J., Weinstein, M., Lee, S. Y. V., & Fitzpatrick, J. J. (2002). A family assessment tool for hospitalized elders. *Geriatric Nursing, 23,* 316–319, 335.

Sherman, F. T. (2001). Functional assessment: Easy-to-use screening tools speed initial office work-up. *Geriatrics, 56*(8), 36–40.

Tabbarah, M., Crimmins, E. M., & Seeman, T. E. (2002). The relationship between cognitive and physical performance: MacArthur studies of successful aging. *Journals of Gerontology: Medical Sciences, 57A,* M228–M235.

Wahl, H-W. (2001). Environmental influences on aging and behavior. In J. E. Birren and K. W. Schaie (Eds.), *Handbook of the psychology of aging* (5th ed., pp. 215–237). San Diego: Academic Press.

Williams, T. F. (1983). Comprehensive functional assessment: An overview. *Journal of the American Geriatrics Society, 31,* 637–641.

Yamada, Y., & Ikegami, N. (2001). Multidimensional functional assessment: Instruments. In M. D. Mezey (Ed.), *The encyclopedia of elder care* (pp. 440–442). New York: Springer.

Hearing

LEARNING OBJECTIVES

1. Delineate age-related changes that affect the ability of older adults to hear.
2. Examine risk factors that influence the ability of older adults to hear.
3. Discuss the functional consequences of age-related changes and risk factors that affect hearing.
4. Describe nursing assessment techniques that are applicable to assessing hearing and identifying opportunities for health promotion in older adults.
5. Identify interventions to enhance the auditory abilities of older adults and address risk factors that interfere with hearing.

The auditory system receives and interprets verbal communications by converting sound waves into neural impulses. Auditory function influences the performance of many daily activities, particularly those that depend on understanding verbal instructions. Safe maneuvering in one's environment is highly dependent on the accurate perception of auditory cues. Also, one's quality of life is influenced significantly by the ability to hear sounds, such as voices, music, and sounds of nature.

 AGE-RELATED CHANGES THAT AFFECT HEARING

Auditory function takes place in the three compartments of the ear and the auditory cortex of the brain. Interpretation of sounds entails coding them according to intensity and frequency. Intensity, or amplitude, reflects the loudness or softness of the sound and is measured in decibels (dB). Frequency, which is measured in cycles per second (cps) or hertz (Hz), determines whether the pitch is high or low. Age-related changes that occur in the ear and the auditory nervous system affect the ability of older adults to perceive accurately the pitch of sounds. Perception of sound intensity is not significantly affected by age-related changes, but it can be impaired as a consequence of risk factors that are likely to be present in older adults. Thus, hearing impairments are a very common functional consequence for older adults.

External Ear

Hearing begins in the outer ear, which consists of the pinna and the external auditory canal. These cartilaginous structures control the discernment of resonance and provide the basis for sound localization, especially of higher-frequency sounds. Sound localization enables a person to identify the source of a sound. Although the pinna undergoes changes in size, shape, flexibility, and hair growth with increasing age, no evidence exists that these changes alter the conduction of sound waves in healthy older adults. The auditory canal is covered by skin and lined with hair follicles and cerumen-producing glands. Cerumen is a natural protective substance that is categorized as either dry (gray, flaky) or wet (dark brown, moist). Whites and African Americans are likely to have wet cerumen, whereas Asians and Native Americans are likely to have dry cerumen. Normally, cerumen is expelled through natural processes. But age-related changes such as an increased concentration of keratin, the growth of longer and thicker hair (especially in men), and thinning and drying of the skin lining the canal predispose the older adult to a build-up of cerumen. An age-related diminution in sweat gland activity further increases the potential for cerumen accumulation by making the wax increasingly dry and difficult to remove. A prolapsed or collapsed ear canal is another age-related change that may occur. This structural alteration of the canal may affect the localization and perception of sounds, particularly those in the highest frequency ranges.

Middle Ear

The tympanic membrane is a transparent, pearl-gray, slightly cone-shaped layer of flexible tissue separating the outer and middle ear. Its primary functions are to transmit sound energy and protect the middle and inner ear. With increased age, collagenous tissue replaces the elastic tissue, resulting in a thinner and less resilient eardrum. Sound vibrations pass through the tympanic membrane to the three auditory ossicles: the malleus, incus, and stapes. These bones are connected to each other but move independently, acting as a lever to amplify sound. Their primary function is to transmit vibrations across the air-filled middle ear, through the oval window, and to the fluid-filled inner ear. Transmission of sounds is influenced by the frequency of each sound and is most effective in the frequency range of normal voices and least effective at the lowest and highest frequencies. With advanced age, the ossicular bones become calcified and hardened, possibly interfering with the transfer of sound vibrations from the tympanic membrane to the oval window.

The middle ear muscles and ligaments contract in response to loud noises, stimulating the acoustic reflex, which protects the delicate inner ear and filters out auditory distractions originating from one's own voice and body movements. With increased age, the middle ear muscles and ligaments become weaker and stiffer; this may have a detrimental effect on the acoustic reflex. These degenerative changes also can compromise the resiliency of the tympanic membrane.

Inner Ear

In the inner ear, vibrations are transmitted to the cochlea, where they are converted to nerve impulses and coded for intensity and frequency. Nerve impulses stimulate fibers of the eighth cranial nerve and send the auditory message to the brain. This process transpires primarily in the sensory hair cells of the organ of Corti in the cochlea.

Age-related changes of the inner ear structures include loss of hair cells, reduction of blood supply, diminution of endolymph production, decreased basilar membrane flexibility, degeneration of spiral ganglion cells, and loss of neurons in the cochlear nuclei. These inner ear changes result in the degenerative hearing impairment termed *presbycusis*. One commonly used classification system for presbycusis is based on the specific structural source of the impairment, and can be delineated as follows:

1. *Sensory presbycusis,* which is associated with degenerative changes of the hair cells and the organ of Corti in the cochlea, is characterized by a sharp hearing loss at high frequencies, with little effect on speech understanding.
2. *Neural presbycusis* is related to widespread degeneration of nerve fibers in the cochlea and spiral ganglion; it is characterized by reduced speech discrimination.
3. *Metabolic* or *strial presbycusis* is caused by degenerative changes in the stria vascularis and a subsequent interruption in essential nutrient supply. Initially, these changes reduce the sensitivity to all sound frequencies; eventually, they interfere with speech discrimination.

4. *Mechanical presbycusis* results from mechanical changes in the inner ear structures and is characterized by a hearing loss that initially involves lower frequencies and gradually spreads to higher frequencies. When sensitivity to the higher frequencies becomes impaired, speech discrimination is diminished.

Although useful for analyzing the physiologic basis for various types of presbycusis, this classification is limited because presbycusis usually involves not one, but several, age-related processes.

Auditory Nervous System

From the inner ear, the auditory nerve fibers pass through the internal auditory meatus and enter the brain. Functions of the auditory nerve pathway include localizing sound direction, fine-tuning auditory stimuli, and transferring information from the primary auditory cortex to the auditory association area.

With increased age, the entire auditory nerve pathway undergoes atrophic changes, which combine with degenerative changes in related structures to cause hearing deficits in older adults. Hair cell atrophy in the organ of Corti, narrowing of the auditory meatus from bone apposition, and degeneration of the arterial blood vessels that supply the auditory nerve are age-related changes that affect the auditory nervous system. Age-related changes in the central nervous system, particularly those that affect speech-specific cognitive abilities, interfere with auditory processing. Although some researchers have suggested that age-related changes in cognitive abilities may be responsible for much of the increased difficulty that older adults experience with speech perception in noisy environments, Schneider and colleagues (2000) have concluded that speech comprehension difficulties of older adults primarily reflect declines in hearing rather than in cognitive ability.

RISK FACTORS THAT AFFECT HEARING

In addition to the age-related changes that interfere with hearing, other factors, such as lifestyle, heredity, environment, impacted wax, and disease processes, also can contribute to the development of hearing loss. Much research is being done on risk factors for hearing impairment, with emphasis on modifiable risk factors, such as noise, that can be addressed through health promotion. Research is also focusing on the interrelationship between risk factors, such as between noise and ototoxic substances and between heredity and ototoxic

substances. Future research on modifiable risk factors is likely to find that some hearing losses now attributed to age-related changes are the consequences of prolonged exposure to noise or ototoxic substances. This may lead to implementation of preventive strategies and more public health education about protection of hearing. Although modifiable risk factors ideally should be addressed beginning in childhood, it is never too late to begin health education about prevention of hearing loss (Display 12-1).

Lifestyle and Environmental Factors

The most well recognized risk factor for impaired hearing is exposure to noise, which can be viewed as both a lifestyle and environmental factor. Prolonged exposure to noise in occupational or avocational environments has long been identified as a primary risk factor for hearing impairment and permanent damage to the auditory system. Although for the past several decades most of the focus has been on the detrimental effects of prolonged exposure to noise, attention in recent years also includes the effects of brief intermittent exposure to high-decibel noise levels, such as those experienced by firefighters and other emergency workers (Kales et al., 2001).

Compared with whites, African Americans are less susceptible to noise-induced hearing loss (Overfield, 1995).

DISPLAY 12-1

Factors That Increase the Risk for Impaired Hearing

Genetic predisposition
Increased age
Recreational or occupational exposure to noise
Cigarette smoking
Ototoxic medications
    Aminoglycosides
    Aspirin and other salicylates
    Cisplatin
    Erythromycin
    Ibuprofen
    Imipramine
    Indomethacin
    Loop diuretics
    Quinidine
    Quinine
Ototoxic environmental chemicals
    Carbon monoxide
    Lead
    Mercury
    Tin
    Toluene

Healthy People 2010 has identified noise-induced hearing loss (NIHL) as the most common occupational disease and one of the most modifiable risk factors (USDHHS, 2000). People who may be at an increased risk for NIHL as a result of their occupation include miners, farmers, plumbers, musicians, carpenters, firefighters, and armed services members. Researchers have confirmed a significant association between hearing loss in farmers and long-term exposure to noisy equipment (Beckett et al., 2000; Hwang et al., 2001). Older adults are likely to have worked in settings where noise level recommendations that are now enforced by the National Institute of Occupational Safety and Health were not implemented. For instance, older people who were once employed as weavers or textile workers are likely to have been exposed to detrimentally noisy environments during their work years. Because the effects of NIHL and age-related changes are cumulative, the hearing loss may not be noticed until later adulthood. When it is noticed, it is likely to be falsely attributed to age-related changes.

Exposure to toxic chemicals in the workplace or the environment is another risk factor that has been under investigation since the 1990s as a potential cause of hearing loss. Pesticides and organic solvents are two types of chemicals that are being investigated as potentially ototoxic. For example, Morata and colleagues (2002) found that age, exposure to noise, and exposure to the organic solvent styrene were all risk factors for hearing loss, but styrene increased the risk to a greater degree than either age or noise exposure.

Leisure-time activities also can contribute to NIHL, especially if people engaging in these activities do not use protective ear devices. Researchers have found that the risk for developing a hearing loss in men who engaged in hunting or woodworking increased by 7% and 6%, respectively, for every 5-year period of participation in that activity (Dalton et al., 2001; Nondahl et al., 2000). Other activities that are likely to cause neurosensory damage unless protective mechanisms are used include listening to loud music; operating tractors, chain saws, or leaf blowers; and riding motorcycles, airplanes, snowmobiles, or motorboats. Figure 12-1 illustrates the noise levels of various activities. Sounds louder than 80 dB are considered potentially ototoxic.

Cigarette smoking, as well as living in a household with a smoker, is another lifestyle and environmental factor being investigated as a risk for hearing impairment. Nakanishi and colleagues (2000) found that the risk for high-frequency hearing loss increased over a 5-year period directly in proportion to numbers of cigarettes per day and number of pack-years of exposure.

Medication Effects

Medications can cause or contribute to hearing impairments by damaging the ear structures, particularly the cochlear and vestibular divisions of the auditory nerve. Despite the fact that quinine and salicylate ototoxicities were first observed more than a century ago, the ototoxic effects of medication have received little attention in clinical settings. Although age alone does not increase the risk for ototoxicity, older adults are more likely to be taking ototoxic medications, such as aspirin and furosemide. Other contributing factors that commonly occur in older adults and increase the risk for ototoxicity include renal failure, long-term use of ototoxic medications, and potentiation between two ototoxic medications, such as

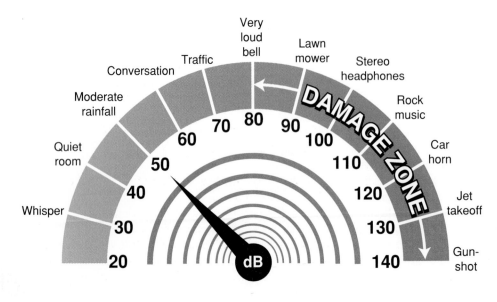

FIGURE 12-1 Noise levels associated with common activities are measured in decibels (dB). Sounds louder than 80 dB are potentially harmful to ears.

furosemide and aminoglycoside antibiotics. Medications that are likely to be ototoxic are listed in Display 12-1. Ototoxicity is often dose related, and hearing loss may be temporary if medications are discontinued or the dose is reduced. Although ototoxicity is potentially reversible, both professionals and nonprofessionals often mistakenly ascribe hearing loss in older adults to inevitable and irreversible degenerative changes.

Disease Processes

Otosclerosis is a hereditary disease of the auditory ossicles that causes ankylosis of the footplate of the stapes to the oval window. Although otosclerosis usually begins in youth or early adulthood, detection of the symptoms may be delayed until middle or later adulthood, when age-related middle ear changes compound the disease-related changes. Otosclerosis usually causes a conductive hearing loss, so the earliest symptom may be difficulty hearing soft and low-pitched sounds. The hearing loss progresses and may be accompanied by dizziness, tinnitus, or balance problems.

Atherosclerosis, hypertension, and hyperlipidemia are cardiovascular diseases that have been associated with increased risk for hearing impairment. Tomei and colleagues (2000) studied the relationship between noise and cardiovascular disease and found that noise may be the underlying factor that increases the risk for both hypertension and hearing loss. They suggest that chronic exposure to noise can detrimentally affect the cardiovascular system as well as the auditory system and that some people may be more susceptible to these effects, which often occur in the same person.

Ménière's disease and acoustic neuromas are examples of diseases that affect the auditory system and that may cause or contribute to hearing impairment. Examples of systemic diseases that cause or contribute to hearing impairment are syphilis, myxedema, diabetes, hypothyroidism, and Paget's disease. Other disorders that may cause hearing deficits are meningitis, head trauma, high fevers, and viral infections (e.g., measles and mumps).

Impacted Cerumen

Impacted cerumen is common in older adults and is the leading cause of conductive hearing loss. Age-related changes may cause wax to accumulate and occlude the auditory canal, and the use of hearing aids increases the possibility of impacted wax. About one third of community-living and hospitalized older adults and up to 42% of older adults in nursing homes have severe to complete cerumen impaction (Mahoney, 1996). Cerumen accumulation is the most easily preventable and treatable cause of hearing deficits; most importantly, it

is readily amenable to nursing interventions, as discussed later in this chapter.

Combinations of Risk Factors

Combinations of risk factors may be especially harmful. For example, people taking ototoxic drugs or exposed to ototoxic environmental chemicals may be even more susceptible to the damaging effects of noise exposure. Similarly, people with a genetic predisposition to hearing loss may be more susceptible to NIHL or hearing loss from ototoxic drugs. For example, Casano and colleagues (1999) found that some people may have a genetic predisposition to aminoglycoside-induced hearing loss. Because age-related changes increase the risk for hearing loss, it is especially important to identify modifiable risk factors in older adults so that those risks can be addressed through health promotion. See Display 12-1 for a list of the factors that increase the risk for impaired hearing, either alone or in combinations.

➤ Mr. H. is 60 years old and owns a small home-remodeling business. He has been a carpenter for 38 years, but in the past 9 years, he has spent most of his time in the office managing his business. He enjoys hunting and fishing on weekends. He smokes two packs of cigarettes a day and has smoked since he was 16 years old. His wife has been telling him she thinks he has "selective hearing" and only hears what he wants to hear. Mr. H. admits that he turns the television volume up louder than he used to but denies having any "real hearing problem."

 THINKING POINTS

➤ What age-related changes and risk factors contribute to Mr. H.'s hearing loss?

➤ Describe the hearing loss that Mr. H. is likely to be experiencing.

➤ What environmental conditions will contribute to Mr. H.'s hearing difficulty?

PATHOLOGIC CONDITIONS THAT CAN AFFECT HEARING

Tinnitus is the persistent perception of ringing, roaring, blowing, buzzing, or other types of noise that does not originate in the external environment. Tinnitus is a common pathologic condition in older adults and is often associated with both conductive and sensorineural hearing loss. It is also highly associated with ototoxic medications and with Ménière's disease. It may be caused by impacted wax, especially if the wax is attached to the tympanic membrane. Tinnitus may be exacerbated by caffeine, alcohol, or nicotine. Anyone with tinnitus should be evaluated for associated pathologic conditions or modifiable contributing factors such as alcohol, medications, impacted wax, or cigarette smoking.

FUNCTIONAL CONSEQUENCES ASSOCIATED WITH HEARING IN OLDER ADULTS

Although hearing loss is not exclusively a condition of older adulthood, 43% of hearing-impaired people are age 65 years of age or older (NAAS, 1999). About one third of adults between the ages of 65 and 75 years and about half of people older than 75 years of age have a hearing loss. Hearing impairment is most likely to occur in men, people of low economic status, and people exposed to prolonged job-related or recreational noise. Poor health is also associated with a higher risk for impaired hearing, with only 39% of people who are hearing impaired reporting excellent or very good physical health, compared with 68% of those without a hearing impairment reporting excellent health (NAAS, 1999). Whites are twice as likely as African Americans or Hispanic Americans to be deaf or hearing impaired. The probability of hearing impairment also increases with a family history of otosclerosis, which disproportionately affects white middle-aged women.

Hearing losses are categorized according to the site of the impairment. Abnormalities of the external and middle ear impair the sound-conduction mechanism and are classified as *conductive hearing losses*. Abnormalities of the inner ear interfere with the sensory and neural structures and are classified as *sensorineural hearing losses*. Sensorineural hearing loss often is age related or noise induced. Hearing losses that involve both conductive and sensorineural impairments are called *mixed hearing losses*.

The Impact of Hearing Changes on Speech Comprehension

It is not uncommon for older adults to experience several age-related changes, as well as contributing factors, that influence hearing ability. Accurate comprehension of speech depends on speech pace, sound frequencies, environmental noise, and internal auditory function. Structural changes in the ear and nervous system influence different sound frequencies, with high-frequency tones being affected first. Hearing acuity

begins to decline in early adulthood, and by the ages of 30 years in men and 50 years in women, there is a decline in hearing sensitivity at all frequencies. The rate of change in hearing level is more than twice as fast in men than in women, and the cumulative effects are usually noticed by men in their 50s and women in their 60s (Fozard & Gordan-Salant, 2001). Consequently, older adults typically experience changes in their ability to code sound frequencies precisely. Older adults with cognitive impairments will have increased difficulty with speech comprehension.

Speech comprehension is most directly influenced by the frequency of phonemes, the smallest units of sound. Each phoneme in a word has a different frequency, with vowels generally having lower frequencies and consonants generally having higher frequencies. Although most word phonemes have lower-range frequencies, sibilant consonants (those that have a whistling quality, such as *ch, f, g, s, sh, t, th,* and *z*) have higher-range frequencies. Because the earliest and most universal age-related changes affect one's ability to code higher-frequency sounds, words rich in sibilants will be most affected by age-related changes of the auditory system.

Presbycusis, as mentioned earlier, is the sensorineural hearing loss associated with an age-related degeneration of the auditory structures. Presbycusis usually occurs in both ears, but the degree of impairment in each ear may vary. An early functional consequence of presbycusis is the loss of ability to hear high-pitched sounds and sibilant consonants. When high-pitched sounds are filtered out, words become distorted and jumbled, and sentences become incoherent. A sentence like "I think she should go to the store" might be interpreted by a listener with presbycusis as "I wish we could go to the show." This characteristic, known as diminished speech discrimination, is influenced by the speaker's rate of speech: rapid, slow, or slurred speech patterns make it increasingly difficult for the older person to discern words. As the hearing loss progresses, explosive consonants, such as *b, d, k, p,* and *t,* also become distorted.

Older people with presbycusis have even greater difficulty with speech discrimination when background noises are present or when they are in a room with poor acoustics or echoing. The older adult in a hospital or long-term care facility, for example, may be particularly sensitive to background noises to which the staff may have become accustomed. Some hearing-impaired older adults experience hypersensitivity to high-intensity sounds, which makes these sounds disproportionately loud. This may cause amplified sound to feel unpleasantly harsh and difficult to tolerate.

A conductive hearing loss is characterized by an inability to hear vowels and low-pitched tones.

Intensity of sound is reduced, but sounds can be heard at all frequencies once the hearing threshold is reached. Background noise does not interfere with speech perception in the same way it does with presbycusis. Often, there is a history of otosclerosis, perforated eardrum, or other ear disease. In older adults, impacted cerumen is a common contributing factor. Depending on the causative factor, conductive hearing loss occurs in one or both ears. Table 12-1 summarizes the age-related changes affecting hearing as well as the functional consequences of these changes.

The ability to understand speech is also influenced by environmental conditions (e.g., competitive background noise) and the pace of the verbal messages. For older adults, any adverse environmental conditions, especially the presence of background noise, may compound the negative influence of age-related changes. In adverse listening situations, the speech comprehension of older people is disproportionately more impaired than that of younger people (Fozard & Gordon-Salant, 2001). Factors such as background noise and increased rates of speech, then, can be seen as risk factors for hearing impairment in older adults.

Implications of this are that an improvement in the listening conditions or the presentation has the potential to improve the hearing abilities of older adults.

Men report more difficulty with background noise than women, and a greater aversion to amplified sound (Fozard & Gordon-Salant, 2001).

The Impact of Hearing Changes on Quality of Life, Safety, and Functioning

Hearing is a primary component of communication for daily living in society: through it one enjoys humor, appreciates music, obtains information, and relates to others. Hearing deficits inevitably affect these and many other activities of daily life.

Communication impairments caused by an inability to understand spoken words often have a profoundly negative effect on self-confidence. People who are unable to discriminate words are afraid to respond to questions and may choose not to answer rather than risk feeling foolish. Performance on mental status examinations may be influenced negatively by a person's fear of not hearing the questions accurately as well as by the concomitant reduction of sensory stimuli. Poor performance on tests of cognitive abilities may mistakenly lead to a perception that the person has dementia when, in fact, the person simply has a hearing loss.

Hearing deficits may also lead to fear, boredom, apathy, depression, social isolation, and feelings of low self-esteem (Kramer et al., 2002). The psychosocial consequences of hearing impairment are influenced by the lifestyle of the person affected. For example, hearing impairments are relatively more detrimental for people whose occupations or avocations are highly dependent on good hearing. By contrast, hearing impairments may be less detrimental for people who have few social relationships and who do not depend on hearing for occupational or leisure activities. Older women were more likely than older men to report feelings of anger, anxiety, annoyance, and aggravation because of their hearing loss (Garstecki & Erler, 1999). Nursing home residents who have hearing impairments are likely to have low levels of social engagement and to spend little or no time in activities (Resnick et al., 1997). When hearing loss interferes with one's ability to perceive reality accurately, it can lead to suspiciousness, paranoia, and loss of contact with reality. When only parts of a conversation are heard, a person may come to believe that the conversation is about him or her, and persecutory delusions may develop.

TABLE 12-1 • Age-Related Changes Affecting Hearing		
	Change	Consequence
External Ear	• Longer, thicker hair • Thinner, drier skin • Increased keratin	Potential for impacted cerumen and subsequent impaired sound conduction
Middle Ear	• Diminished resiliency of tympanic membrane • Calcified, hardened ossicles • Weakened and stiff muscles and ligaments	Impaired sound conduction
Inner Ear and Nervous System	• Diminished neurons, endolymph, hair cells, and blood supply • Degeneration of spiral ganglion and arterial blood vessels • Decreased flexibility of basilar membrane • Degeneration of central processing systems	Presbycusis: diminished ability to hear high-pitched sounds, especially in the presence of background noise

In addition to impacting quality of life negatively, hearing deficits may affect the safety and functioning of older adults. For example, people with hearing impairments may have more difficulty negotiating the environment safely when warning signals are sounded for fires, ambulances, and other emergency situations. Besides creating actual safety hazards, the hearing deficit may lead to fear and anxiety about one's safety. Hearing impairment in older adults also is associated with functional decline. A 1-year study of more than 2400 adults between the ages of 50 and 102 years concluded that even mild hearing impairment is independently associated with a decline in physical performance and basic and instrumental activities of daily living (Wallhagen et al., 2001).

Negative societal attitudes about aging and hearing loss may result in a doubly negative effect on the person who is old as well as hard of hearing. The older person may be reluctant to acknowledge a hearing deficit, choosing to limit opportunities for communication rather than face the stigma associated with hearing impairments. These attitudes and accompanying behaviors may cause other psychosocial consequences such as loneliness and social isolation. Figure 12-2 summarizes age-related changes, risk factors, and negative functional consequences that influence an older adult's ability to hear.

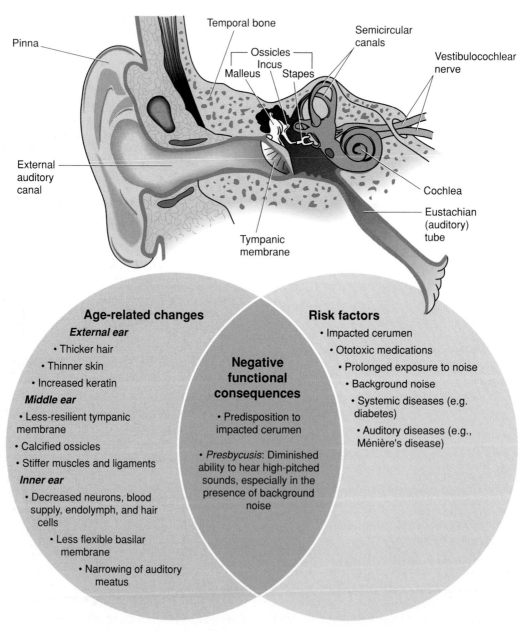

FIGURE 12-2 Age-related changes and risk factors intersect to negatively affect hearing in older adults.

➤ Mr. H. is now 69 years old and has been retired for several years. He spends several days a week hunting and fishing seasonally. He also spends time in his basement making small pieces of furniture and doing other woodworking. He continues to smoke, but has cut down to one pack per day. His wife and he attend the weekly "Lunch Bunch" group at the local senior center where you are the nurse. They make an appointment to talk with you because Mrs. H. is concerned about her husband's hearing. Mr. H., who blames his problem on "old age," refuses to have an evaluation for a hearing aid because he doesn't think an aid would do any good and "besides, it would stick out like a sore thumb."

THINKING POINTS

➤ What factors are likely to contribute to Mr. H.'s hearing loss?

➤ What environmental and other conditions might make the hearing loss worse?

➤ What myths or misunderstandings are likely to influence Mr. H.'s perception of his hearing problem and potential interventions for it?

NURSING ASSESSMENT OF HEARING

Nursing assessment of hearing is aimed at identifying: (1) the presence of any hearing deficit; (2) the impact of any hearing deficits on the person's safety and quality of life; and (3) opportunities for health promotion interventions. Each of these factors is important in helping older adults and their caregivers compensate for hearing deficits. Assessment is accomplished through interview questions, observation of behavioral cues, and administration of hearing tests.

Interviewing About Hearing Changes

Interview questions are used to acquire information about: (1) past and present risk factors; (2) the person's awareness and acknowledgment of a hearing impairment; (3) the psychosocial impact of any hearing deficit; and (4) attitudes that might influence health promotion interventions (Display 12-2). The hearing assessment interview begins with questions about family history of hearing impairments and a personal history of prolonged exposure to loud noises. Identification of ototoxic medications as a risk factor can be included as part of the hearing assessment or as part of the medication history. Questions about risk factors may prompt the older person to discuss a hearing problem.

If the older adult does not initiate a discussion of hearing problems, the nurse should ask direct questions about the person's discernment of any hearing deficit. If the older adult denies having a hearing problem but shows behavioral cues indicative of a hearing deficit, the nurse tries to elicit further information by asking leading questions such as, "I notice you turn your left ear toward me. Is your hearing better in that ear?"

Questions about any changes in the social activities of the older adult may reveal psychosocial consequences of hearing impairment that may be alleviated through interventions aimed at improving communication.

If no hearing impairment is present, questions about lifestyle do not necessarily have to be included as part of the hearing assessment. When a person acknowledges the existence of a hearing impairment, however, the nurse should ask about any associated changes in social and occupational activities.

> A study of gender differences in attitudes about, and adjustment to, hearing loss found that older women were more likely than men to admit to communication problems, perceive the problems as important, and use nonverbal strategies to compensate for the hearing deficits (Garstecki & Erler, 1999).

Identifying Opportunities for Health Promotion

The nurse must assess the older person's attitudes toward assistive listening devices because these will influence his or her acceptance of interventions. Identification of myths or misunderstandings may provide opportunities for health education that will improve the hearing of the older adult. Older adults may believe that hearing aids are too costly or of little use, or they may be embarrassed to use a device that is visible to others. They also may not know how to go about arranging for an evaluation and may distrust advertisements about hearing aids. Resistance toward hearing aids may also arise from lack of money, transportation, or motivation to communicate. A careful assessment of attitudes about hearing aids may identify barriers that can be addressed through health promotion interventions.

Using Hearing Screening Tools

The Hearing Handicap Inventory for the Elderly (HHIE-S) is a 10-item questionnaire (Figure 12-3) that can be administered to older adults in about

DISPLAY 12-2
Guidelines for Assessing Hearing

Questions to Identify Risk Factors for Hearing Loss
- Do you have a family history of hearing loss or deafness?
- Have you been exposed to loud noises in your job or leisure activities?
- Do you have a history of any of the following: diabetes, hypothyroidism, Ménière's disease, or Paget's disease?
- What medications do you take? (Refer to Display 12-1 to identify potentially ototoxic medications.)
- Have you ever had impacted wax in your ears?

Questions to Assess Awareness and Presence of Hearing Deficit
- Do you have any trouble with your hearing?
- Have you noticed any change in your ability to understand conversations or hear words?
- Are you bothered by any noises in your ears, such as ringing or buzzing?

Questions to Ask If Hearing Loss Is Acknowledged
- How long have you noticed a hearing loss?
- Do you notice differences in hearing in your left ear, versus your right ear?
- Has there been a progressive loss, or did the hearing problem begin suddenly?
- Describe your hearing difficulty.
- Are there any conditions, such as noisy environments or particular voices or sounds, that especially interfere with your hearing?
- Does your hearing loss interfere with your ability to communicate with others, either individually or in groups?
- Are there any activities that you would like to do, but feel you cannot because of hearing problems?

- Have you ever had, or thought about having, an evaluation for a hearing aid?
- Have you ever tried using a hearing aid?

Questions to Identify Opportunities for Education About Disease Prevention and Health Promotion
- Does the person engage in any activities that expose him or her to loud noises, such as woodworking or lawn mowing? If so, does he or she understand the importance of wearing ear protectors?
- If the person has a history of impacted wax, does he or she take preventive measures?
- Does the person smoke cigarettes or live in a household with a smoker? (If so, does the person realize that this is a risk factor for hearing loss?)
- What are the person's attitudes about hearing loss?
- Is hearing loss considered normal and untreatable?
- Is a hearing aid considered to be a stigma?
- If the person is resistant to an audiologic evaluation, what are the barriers? (For example, are there financial or transportation limitations that interfere with obtaining a hearing aid?)
- Does the hearing loss contribute to a sense of isolation, depression, paranoia, or low self-esteem?
- What are the person's usual communication opportunities, and how does the hearing loss influence these usual patterns? (For instance, does the person live in an environment where it is important to be able to use the phone?)
- Does the person live in a noisy environment and find relief in the hearing impairment?
- If the person lives in an environment where group activities are a large part of daily activities, does the person want to participate in these activities?

5 minutes. This tool was developed two decades ago for use with cognitively intact older adults in a variety of clinical and community settings. In 2001, the Hartford Institute for Geriatric Nursing identified this as the best tool for assessing the handicap effect of hearing impairment on the person's daily function. The HHIE-S is also useful for assessing the likelihood that someone will accept interventions (Demers, 2002) and for measuring the effects of hearing aids on hearing handicap. One study in which the HHIE-S was used found that 26% of the sample of 234 people between the ages of 65 and 74 years had a previously undiagnosed hearing handicap. Further assessment with the HHIE-S 6 months after hearing aids were prescribed

found that 79% of those who were fitted with a hearing aid had a reduction in hearing handicap (Hands, 2000).

Observing Cues to Hearing Function

Behavioral cues related to hearing loss provide important information about the presence of a hearing impairment, the psychosocial consequences of any such impairment, and the person's attitudes about assistive devices. If the older adult denies a hearing deficit that has been noticed by others, behavioral cues may be the primary source of assessment information. Denial of a hearing deficit may result from lack of awareness of the impairment because of gradual onset or, if the older

ITEM	YES (4 pts)	SOMETIMES (2 pts)	NO (0 pts)
Does a hearing problem cause you to feel embarrassed when you meet new people?	_____	_____	_____
Does a hearing problem cause you to feel frustrated when talking to members of your family?	_____	_____	_____
Do you have difficulty hearing when someone speaks in a whisper?	_____	_____	_____
Do you feel handicapped by a hearing problem?	_____	_____	_____
Does a hearing problem cause you difficulty when visiting friends, relatives, or neighbors?	_____	_____	_____
Does a hearing problem cause you to attend religious services less often than you would like?	_____	_____	_____
Does a hearing problem cause you to have arguments with family members?	_____	_____	_____
Does a hearing problem cause you difficulty when listening to TV or radio?	_____	_____	_____
Do you feel that any difficulty with your hearing limits or hampers your personal or social life?	_____	_____	_____
Does a hearing problem cause you difficulty when in a restaurant with relatives or friends?	_____	_____	_____

RAW SCORE_____(sum of the points assigned each of the items)

INTERPRETING THE RAW SCORE
0 to 8 = 13% probability of hearing impairment (no handicap/no referral)
10 to 24 = 50% probability of hearing impairment (mild-moderate handicap/refer)
26 to 40 = 84% probability of hearing impairment (severe handicap/refer)

FIGURE 12-3 The screening version of the Hearing Handicap Inventory for the Elderly (HHIES). (Reprinted with permission from Ventry, I., & Weinstein, B. [1983, July]. *Identification of elderly people with hearing problems* [pp. 37–42]. Rockville, MD: American Speech-Language-Hearing Association. Copyright American Speech-Language-Hearing Association.)

person is socially isolated, may result from a paucity of opportunities for communication. Feelings of embarrassment or misconceptions that the hearing loss is an inevitable and untreatable consequence of aging may also contribute to denial. Display 12-3 lists behavioral cues that should be observed by the nurse as part of the hearing assessment.

Using an Otoscope and Tuning Fork

Nursing assessment of hearing includes the use of a tuning fork to check hearing and examination of the external ear and tympanic membrane with an otoscope. The purpose of the tuning fork test is to detect hearing impairments and to differentiate between conductive and sensorineural losses. The purpose of

the otoscopic examination is to identify factors, such as cerumen accumulation, that might interfere with hearing. Display 12-4 describes the procedure for performing a nursing assessment of hearing using the otoscope and tuning fork. If any hearing deficits are reported by the older adult or identified as a result of this examination, the nurse should recommend that a further evaluation be conducted at a speech and hearing center or by a specialized physician, such as an otolaryngologist.

> Recall that Mr. H. is a 69-year-old participant in activities at the local senior center where you are the nurse. You are meeting with Mr. and Mrs. H. to discuss Mrs. H.'s concerns about her husband's hearing problem.

DISPLAY 12-3
Guidelines for Assessing Behavioral Cues Related to Hearing

Behavioral Cues to a Hearing Deficit
- Inappropriate or no response to questions, especially in the absence of opportunities for lip reading
- Inability to follow verbal directions without cues
- Short attention span, easy distractibility
- Frequent requests for repetition or clarification of verbal communication
- Intense observation of the speaker
- Mouthing of words spoken by the speaker
- Turning of one ear toward the speaker
- Unusual physical proximity to the speaker
- Lack of response to loud environmental noises
- Speech that is too loud or inarticulate
- Abnormal voice characteristics, such as monotony
- Misperception that others are talking about him or her

Behavioral Cues About Psychosocial Consequences
- Uncharacteristic avoidance of group settings
- Lack of interest in social activities, especially those requiring verbal communication or those that the person enjoyed in the past (e.g., bingo, card games)

Behavioral Cues About Assistive Devices
- Not using a hearing aid that has been purchased
- Failure to obtain batteries for a hearing aid
- Expression of embarrassment about using assistive devices

THINKING POINTS

➤ Which of the questions and considerations in Displays 12-2 and 12-3 would you use in assessing Mr. H.?

➤ Would you involve Mrs. H. in any part of the assessment? If so, how would you involve her?

➤ What health promotion advice would you give Mr. H. at this time?

NURSING DIAGNOSIS

Based on the focused nursing assessment, the nurse may identify an actual hearing deficit or risk factors for impaired hearing. The hearing impairment may or may not have psychosocial consequences such as social isolation. An appropriate nursing diagnosis for an older adult with a hearing impairment would be Disturbed Sensory Perception: Auditory. This is defined as "a state in which the individual/group experiences or is at risk of experiencing a change in the amount, pattern, or interpretation of incoming stimuli" (Carpenito, 2002, p. 845). If the focus of care is on the person's responses to the hearing loss, then the nursing diagnosis of Impaired Communication might be applicable. Impaired Communication is "the state in which the individual experiences, or is at high risk to experience, difficulty exchanging thoughts, ideas, wants, or needs with others" (Carpenito, 2002, p. 208). Related factors that are common in older adults are hearing loss, auditory nerve damage, ototoxic medications, and environmental conditions, such as background noise. If psychosocial consequences are identified, other pertinent nursing diagnoses might include Anxiety, Impaired Adjustment, Impaired Social Interaction, and Ineffective Individual Coping. When the hearing impairment is severe and uncompensated to the point that the person does not function safely, then Risk for Injury might be an applicable nursing diagnosis.

OUTCOMES

Nursing-sensitive outcomes that directly relate to the effectiveness of interventions to resolve or compensate for hearing loss include Loneliness, Self-Care, Information Processing Social Involvement, Communication Ability, Personal Safety Behavior, and Quality of Life (Swanson & Drury, 2001). Indicators of goal achievement include documentation of hearing status and improvement in hearing (Stevenson, 2001). An outcome for people with impacted wax is that this risk factor is eliminated through nursing and self-care interventions. An outcome for people with irreversible hearing loss is improved communication. This is accomplished through the use of appropriate sound amplification devices and compensatory communication techniques, as well as through the education of families and other caregivers about these techniques. The goal of improved quality of life for hearing-impaired older adults is addressed through health education interventions that foster increased safety and independent performance of activities of daily living and other desirable activities. Specific interventions to achieve these outcomes are discussed in the following section.

DISPLAY 12-4
Guidelines for Otoscopic and Tuning Fork Assessment

Using the Otoscopic to Assess Factors That Could Interfere With Hearing

- Hold the otoscope upside down, resting your hand on the person's head to stabilize the instrument.
- Before inserting the speculum, pull the pinna upward and backward, while tilting the person's head slightly back and toward the opposite shoulder.
- If cerumen has accumulated to the point of interfering with the examination or occluding the canal, follow the cerumen removal procedure described in the section on Nursing Interventions.
- Normal otoscopic findings in older adults include the following:

  Small amount of cerumen

  Pinkish-white epithelial lining, no redness or lesions

  Pearl-gray tympanic membrane, which is less translucent than in younger adults

  Light reflex anteroinferiorly from the umbo

  Visible landmarks

Using the Tuning Fork to Detect Hearing Impairment

- Use a tuning fork with frequencies of 512 to 1024 cps (Hz).
- Hold the tuning fork firmly at the stem.

- Strike the fork against the palm of your hand, or strike the fork with a rubber reflex hammer, to set it in motion.

Weber's Test

Procedure: Place the tip of a vibrating tuning fork at the center of the person's forehead. Ask where they hear the sound and whether it is louder in one ear than in the other.
Normal finding: The tuning fork is heard equally in both ears.
Abnormal finding: The tuning fork is heard better in one ear, indicating a possible hearing loss.

Rinne's Test

Procedure: Mask one ear, then place a vibrating tuning fork on the mastoid process of the opposite ear until the person indicates that it can no longer be heard. Then, quickly place the tuning fork in front of the ear canal with the top near the ear canal.
Normal finding: The length of time the tuning fork can be heard over the ear canal is about twice as long as the time it can be heard over the mastoid bone.
Abnormal finding: The length of time the tuning fork is heard in front of the ear is shorter than twice as long as the time it can be heard when placed on the mastoid process. In such a case, the person should undergo further tests for impaired hearing.

NURSING INTERVENTIONS TO IMPROVE HEARING

Preventing Disease and Promoting Health

Interventions to prevent hearing loss ideally begin early in life, but it is never too late to begin protecting ears from NIHL. One goal of *Healthy People 2010* is to reduce adult hearing loss in the noise-exposed public (USDHHS, 2000). Many older adults engage in recreational or occupational activities that can cause NIHL and may not realize that age-related changes increase their susceptibility to developing hearing loss. Nurses have many opportunities to educate older adults about protective interventions with regard to hearing (Display 12-5). It might also be necessary to challenge perceptions that all hearing loss is an inevitable consequence of growing older. Nurses can educate older adults about the potentiating effects of two or more risk factors, such as smoking and age-related changes, or medication effects and a genetic predisposition to ototoxicity. People who already experience a mild hearing impairment may be motivated to protect their hearing by avoiding hazardous noise and protecting their ears when they are exposed to noise. Similarly, if they are experiencing a hearing loss and recognize that nicotine can be ototoxic, they may be more motivated to quit smoking.

Another goal of *Healthy People 2010* is to "increase the proportion of persons who have had a hearing examination on schedule" (USDHHS, 2000). Although guidelines for audiology screening are not specific, *Healthy People 2010* recommends screening once every 10 years between the ages of 18 and 50, "with more frequent monitoring after age 50 years" (USDHHS, 2000). Whenever a nursing assessment identifies a hearing impairment, nursing interventions should include a referral for medical and audiology evaluations. Sometimes the nursing interventions also need to address barriers to obtaining a hearing aid, as discussed later in the section on Hearing Aids. Nurses in community or residential settings for older adults may be able to find an audiologist who is willing to provide screening programs at little or no cost. So long as the sponsors of these programs do not have a vested interest in promoting a particular type of hearing aid, they may be effective resources for screening programs.

A major aspect of health promotion is identifying risk factors during the nursing assessment and

Prevention and Early Detection of Hearing Loss

- Use ear protection devices when engaging in activities that emit loud noise.
- Have hearing screening done with questionnaire or audiometry when any change in hearing is noted.
- Have ears checked for impacted wax; use ceruminolytic agents if needed.

Interventions for Compensating for Hearing Loss

- Obtain evaluation at a Speech and Hearing Center for a hearing aid, assistive hearing device, or aural rehabilitation services.

Nutritional Considerations

- Adequate intake of zinc, magnesium, and vitamins A, D, and E

Complementary and Alternative Care Practices

- Herbs for tinnitus: ginkgo, sesame, goldenseal, black cohosh
- Herbs to improve circulation to the ear: ginger, ginkgo
- Homeopathic remedies for tinnitus: salicylic, carbonium sul, China sul, Kali iod, Kali carb, two drops of almond oil in each ear weekly
- Homeopathic remedies to reduce earwax: causticum
- Homeopathic remedy for earwax removal: warm one drop of German camomile oil in five drops of olive oil and instill in the ear

addressing these risks through health education. Heredity, disease processes, exposure to noise, and use of ototoxic medication are common risk factors for hearing impairment. Although the effects of most of these risk factors are irreversible, the use of ototoxic medication is one factor that can be addressed. Nurses should teach older adults and their professional and family caregivers about the potential ototoxicity of the medications listed in Display 12-1. When effective alternatives are available, or when the older adult is experiencing hearing difficulties, efforts should be made to avoid the use of these medications. As with other questions about medication, older adults and their caregivers should be advised to discuss their concerns about ototoxic medications with the prescribing health care practitioner. Cigarette smoking is another modifiable factor that can be addressed through health education.

Tinnitus and hearing impairment caused by impacted wax can be alleviated or prevented through nursing interventions and health education of older adults and their caregivers. Over-the-counter otic solutions

containing ingredients such as glycerin, hydrogen peroxide, mineral oil, carbamide peroxide, and propylene glycol may prevent cerumen accumulation when periodically instilled in the ear canal. Liquid forms of docusate sodium (but not syrup forms) have been found to be an effective ceruminolytic (Singer et al., 2000). This solution is inexpensive and readily available in many settings where older adults receive care. The schedule for instillation of otic drops varies from semi-weekly to monthly.

When an ear canal is impacted with cerumen, the nurse must determine whether there is a possible ruptured tympanic membrane or any other contraindication to irrigation. If any contraindications, such as pain, swelling, or a recent ear infection, are identified, the person should be instructed to seek medical care from an otolaryngologist or other qualified professional.

If there are no contraindications, the following procedure should clear the canal of cerumen:

1. Soften the cerumen with a ceruminolytic agent.
2. Irrigate the canal with body-temperature tap water using a syringe or dental irrigation device and gentle pressure.
3. Aim water at the sides of the canal, and allow drainage from the ear to collect in a basin.
4. Drain excessive fluid from the ear by tilting the head toward the affected side.
5. If the cerumen is difficult to remove, instill a softening preparation twice daily for several days, then attempt irrigation again.

After the wax buildup has been removed, teach the person to prevent the recurrence of impacted cerumen by using a ceruminolytic agent, as discussed earlier in this section.

Compensating for Hearing Deficits

Interventions for people who are hearing impaired should be considered only after a medical evaluation is done to identify medical and treatable causes of the hearing loss. Further testing and examination can then be done by an audiologist to determine the best approach for facilitating communication. People with irreversible hearing deficits who are interested in corrective measures can be encouraged to participate in an aural rehabilitation program. One goal of *Healthy People 2010* is to "increase access by persons who have hearing impairments to hearing rehabilitation services and adaptive devices, including hearing aids, cochlear implants, or tactile or other assistive or augmentative devices" (USDHHS, 2000). Individualized aural rehabilitation programs consist of counseling, together with any or all of the following services: amplification devices, auditory training, lip reading, and speech skills. These programs are available at speech and hearing centers, which are often affiliated with hospitals, medical centers, or universities. Internet resources, such as the National Association for Hearing and Speech Action web site and others listed in the Educational Resources section of this chapter, can provide information about local resources for the evaluation and treatment of hearing disorders. Nurses play an important role in suggesting referrals for aural rehabilitation, discussing such programs with older adults and their caregivers, and facilitating or encouraging the use of recommended sound amplification devices.

Sound amplification generally is achieved by using hearing aids or assistive listening devices. Hearing aids are individually prescribed and require audiology services, whereas assistive listening devices are not individualized and are available without professional assistance or recommendation. These two types of sound amplification are discussed in the following sections.

Surgical implantation of an electronic device, such as a cochlear implant, may be indicated to compensate for damaged or nonfunctional parts of the inner ear. Adults who have lost all or most of their hearing later in life are candidates for this type of surgery, but extensive evaluation of the person is necessary to determine the appropriateness of the procedure. As this procedure becomes more common, nurses will be caring for more older adults who have had cochlear implants. One nursing implication is that the implanted devices are not compatible with magnetic resonance imaging (MRI); hence, nurses need to make sure that MRIs are not ordered for people with cochlear implants.

Assistive Listening Devices

Any device that amplifies or replaces sounds for individual or group communication without being individualized is categorized as an *assistive listening device*. These devices are sometimes called *personal listening systems*. A stethoscope is an assistive listening device commonly used by health care workers. Megaphones and microphones are examples of amplification devices used for group communication. Closed-captioned television is an assistive device that substitutes visual cues for auditory cues. Catalogues and Internet sites describe various assistive listening devices that are available. Self Help for Hard of Hearing People (SHHH), listed in the Educational Resources section, provides consumer information about assistive listening devices. Local chapters of this organization distribute information about public buildings equipped with assistive listening devices.

Assistive listening devices, which consist of a small, battery-powered amplifier and headphones, can be used easily in any setting to improve communication temporarily. Advantages of assistive listening devices over hearing aids include lower cost and the fact that several people can share the device. In addition, most of these devices do not require as much manual dexterity as hearing aids, and some of them are more effective than hearing aids in filtering out background noise. Assistive listening devices can be used in conjunction with hearing aids, or they can be used by people who do not use hearing aids. Figure 12-4 shows one example of a very portable assistive listening device that can be used to enhance communication with someone who is hard of hearing.

Assistive listening devices are available for home use to amplify specific sounds, such as those from the radio, doorbell, television, or telephone. Telephone receivers with an amplifying device, called a *T-coil*, can be used in conjunction with the "T" position on a hearing aid. Other devices serve as substitutes for sound when amplification is impractical or ineffective, for example, flashing lights for doorbells or doormats, and alarm clocks that vibrate the pillow or flash a light. People with more serious hearing impairments but with adequate vision may benefit from closed-captioned television, which provides subscripts for many programs. Since 1990, all televisions with screens 13 inches or larger are required to include a closed-captioned option.

Portable assistive listening devices are available for use in public places. Churches, theaters, and

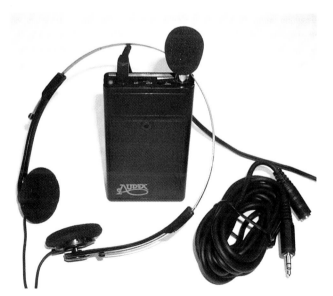

FIGURE 12-4 This assistive listening device (with extension cord) is very portable and can be used in a variety of settings to facilitate communication with hearing-impaired people. (Courtesy of Audex.)

government buildings sometimes equip their facilities with assistive devices to amplify sound, and hearing-impaired people can ask about arrangements for the use of these devices. Small, hand-sized amplifiers can be attached temporarily to pay phones and other telephones, and special devices are also available for mobile phones. In residential and institutional settings for older adults, having an assistive listening device available may be useful for nurses, especially when they are providing health education interventions. Nurses in a residential care facility identified the following benefits from using a small portable amplifier for nurse-resident communication: improved communication, fewer misunderstandings, fewer disruptions to conversation, and considerably less effort required for communication (Erber, 1994).

Hearing Aids

A hearing aid is a battery-operated device that consists of an amplifier, a microphone, and a receiver. Hearing aids can be classified by size, location worn, and technology. The largest are about the size of a deck of cards and are worn on the body, whereas the new smaller types fit completely in the ear canal. These can be seen only with close inspection of the ear and have a nylon string attached for insertion and removal. Preferred hearing aid locations include in the ear, in the canal, and completely in the canal. Body-worn and behind-the-ear hearing aids have become much less popular in recent years because of the availability of smaller, more powerful hearing aids made possible by newer technology.

Until recently, the amplifying power of a hearing aid was strongly associated with it size because most hearing aids used the same type of technology, and severely impaired people needed larger body-worn aids. New technology, however, has made available a variety of types of hearing aids that can be programmed and adjusted for individual differences. Currently, the effectiveness of a hearing aid is associated more with the type of technology used than with its size. Hearing aids are classified by whether they are analog or digital and according to the degree of individualized adjustments or programming possible. As discussed later, cost of hearing aids increases as the programming becomes more adjustable and individualized.

Conventional, or traditional, hearing aids use analog technology to amplify sound but they do not correct distortions. These aids are the simplest type and are adjusted by the manufacturer based on an evaluation by an audiologist. Although the person wearing the aid can adjust its volume and the audiologist can make some minor adjustments, the aid becomes less effective as the person's hearing changes and may need to be replaced if the hearing loss progresses. Because analog aids amplify all sounds equally, they tend to be unsatisfactory for people who have only a mild high-frequency hearing loss and may be more beneficial to people with impairments at multiple frequencies. This characteristic also makes them difficult to use in noisy environments, but older adults may find that they are satisfactory in quiet situations and one-on-one conversations. Nurses may need to encourage the selective use of analog aids in their appropriate environments. A major advantage of these aids is that they are the least expensive type: their cost ranges between $400 and $900. This is an important consideration because only the most comprehensive health insurance policies cover the cost of hearing aids and most people pay out-of-pocket for hearing aids. Until the cost of more sophisticated hearing aids decreases, these conventional hearing aids are likely to remain the most popular choice for older adults.

A variation of the conventional hearing aid is the recently developed disposable hearing aid, which lasts for about 30 to 40 days and costs about $40. These hearing aids were developed for people with a mild to moderate hearing loss and are about as effective as other analog hearing aids. Because they are not customized, they may not fit as well and are more likely to be associated with discomfort or feedback problems. These aids were approved by the Food and Drug Administration (FDA) in 2000 and cannot be obtained without a prescription from a qualified hearing specialist. If these hearing aids become more popular, it is likely that choices in size and amplification will increase.

Programmable analog hearing aids are more advanced than conventional hearing aids because they are selectively programmed to meet the needs of a hearing-impaired person. A major advantage of these hearing aids is that they are acoustically superior to conventional models and can be adjusted for different listening situations. Some programmable aids can automatically adjust their volume to the level of incoming sound by making soft sounds louder and loud sounds softer. Some programmable aids are equipped with a tiny remote-control device, so that the user can conveniently make adjustments for different environments. Remote devices are sometimes built into a wristwatch. Disadvantages include the need to train the wearer, the cost of up to $2000, and the need for frequent adjustments by the hearing health care professional.

Digital hearing aids use the most advanced technology and are the most flexible for individual needs because the audiologist uses a computer to program the aid to amplify specific frequencies for each person's hearing loss. The digital technology examines the incoming sounds and adapts the amplification without adding noise or distortion. In addition, some of these aids have directional microphones, enabling them to collect sounds from two directions and allowing the wearer to adjust the directionality. These aids can be programmed for different listening environments, and the wearer can use a remote control device to adjust the aid for various listening situations. The only disadvantage of these aids is their high cost, which is at least several thousand dollars.

Despite the major improvements in hearing aids in the past decade, this intervention is still underused by older adults, with only 20% of older hearing-impaired people purchasing and consistently using them (Fozard & Gordon-Salant, 2001). Hearing aid use by older Native Americans and Hispanic Americans who have impaired hearing is less than 10%, and hearing aid use by older African Americans is even lower, with one study finding that only 4.3% of the subjects reporting poor hearing were using a hearing aid (Bazargan et al., 2001; Bassford, 1995; Rousseau, 1995). Nurses can play an important role in helping older adults to explore the many options available in assistive listening devices and hearing aids. If the nursing assessment identifies barriers to obtaining an evaluation of hearing, attempts should be made to address these issues. For example, when misinformation or lack of information creates barriers, the nurse can suggest that the older person obtain accurate information from one of the organizations listed in the Educational Resources section. If financial or transportation limitations are problematic for an older person who is otherwise receptive to obtaining a hearing aid, interventions can be aimed at identifying community resources to address these concerns. Older adults and their families should be encouraged to obtain initial information about hearing aids from consumer and health care organizations, rather than primarily from a hearing aid dealer who is selling only one kind of device. Many web sites provide objective information about the various types of hearing aids. The International Hearing Society, for example, distributes a Hearing Aid Helpline consumer kit free of charge, and the Better Business Bureau provides information about local hearing aid dispensers.

In addition to the high cost of hearing aids, common barriers to obtaining and using them are the high levels of manual dexterity, fine motor movement, and good vision required to adjust the volume and other controls and to change batteries. Despite these limitations, older adults using hearing aids have reported significant improvements in communication ability and in social, cognitive, and emotional function (Tesch-Römer, 1997).

Nurses play an important role in encouraging the use of hearing aids. Nurses who work with older adults in residential or other institutional settings have many opportunities for health promotion education about the appropriate use of these aids in different environments. For example, the nurse can encourage the older person to use the aid for one-on-one conversations in his or her rooms, but to remove it in the dining area where there is a lot of background noise. Nurses also can provide health education about realistic expectations with regard to hearing aids and assistive listening devices. Older adults need to understand that a hearing aid generally improves hearing by about 50% and that the goal is not to restore normal hearing but to improve communication and quality of life (Karev & Bartz, 2001).

Although it is impossible to know about all the varieties of hearing aids available today, nurses need to keep up to date on various types available and their implications for older adults. For example, it is important for nurses to know whether a person has an analog-based or a digital hearing aid because the person with an analog aid may not be willing to use it in settings where background noise is problematic. It is also important for the nurse to know if the person has a remote-control device for the hearing aid, so that the nurse can assist with adjusting the settings and give special attention to keeping track of the device.

Nurses must be familiar enough with hearing aids to assist older adults and their caregivers with their use and care. Although nurses can expect that hearing aid dispensers will provide initial instructions regarding use and care of the aid, these instructions may have to be reviewed or revamped as dependency needs and caregiver roles change. Older adults who normally depend on family members for assistance with their hearing aid may not be able to use and care for it properly when they are in a hospital or nursing home. Likewise, nurses in home settings may have to teach caregivers about hearing aids if the older adult needs assistance that was not previously provided by that caregiver. This is likely to occur if the caregiver changes, or if the older adult becomes more dependent because of increased functional impairment. Display 12-6 summarizes the teaching points related to the use and care of hearing aids.

Communicating With Hearing-Impaired Older Adults

Good communication techniques are essential in assisting the older adult to compensate for hearing deficits. The primary functional consequence of presbycusis is a

DISPLAY 12-6
Use and Care of Hearing Aids

Guidelines for Insertion and Use

- With the volume of the device turned off and the canal portion pointing into the ear, insert the hearing aid.
- Make sure the aid fits snugly in the ear canal.
- The M, T, and O settings designate microphone, telephone, and off, respectively.
- Turn the M-T-O switch to M.
- Turn the volume up slowly, beginning at one-third to one-half volume, until a comfortable level is reached.
- If whistling (feedback) is heard, check the position of the device in the ear and the volume. The aid may not fit snugly enough, or the volume may be too high.
- Begin wearing the aid for short periods, in a familiar and quiet environment, and in one-on-one conversations.
- Gradually increase the length of time the aid is worn, the variety of environments, and the number of people included in conversations.
- Allow several months before expecting to feel totally comfortable with the hearing aid.
- Avoid noisy environments and eliminate background noise when possible (e.g., turn off televisions and radios; close doors to rooms).
- Use the appropriate setting (T) for telephone calls.

- Understand that hearing aids do not restore hearing to normal, but rather amplify sound, including all environmental noises.

Guidelines for Care and Maintenance

- Keep a fresh battery available (batteries can be expected to last for 70 to 85 hours), but do not purchase batteries more than 1 month in advance.
- Turn off the hearing aid before changing the battery.
- Remove the battery or turn off the aid when not in use.
- Clean the aid weekly, using warm, soapy water for the earmold and a toothpick or pipe cleaner for the channel.
- Never use alcohol on the earmold because this will cause drying and cracking.
- Check the earmold for cracks or scratches.
- Avoid extreme heat, cold, or moisture (e.g., do not leave the hearing aid near the stove, do not wear it while using a hair dryer, and do not wear it outside, unless it is protected well in rainy or extremely cold weather).
- Avoid exposure to chemicals, such as hairspray or permanent solutions.
- Avoid dropping the aid on a hard surface; when handling it, keep it over a soft or padded surface.

---

diminished acuity for high-frequency sounds, which is exacerbated by fast speech pace and environmental noise. Therefore, communication interventions must be aimed at improving the clarity of words, slowing the rate of speech, and eliminating environmental noise and distractions. Techniques that directly enhance auditory communication should be augmented by effective use of nonverbal and written communication techniques, and particular attention must be given to body language. Display 12-7 summarizes the communication techniques that should be used to enhance the hearing abilities of older adults with impaired hearing. Nurses should use these techniques and should teach professional and family caregivers to use them.

In recent years, increased attention has been directed toward planning or modifying environments to diminish background noise and to improve the ability of people to hear. Some noise-control modifications, such as using window draperies, are relatively simple and can be applied to many settings. Other noise-control measures, such as selection of building materials, need to be implemented while environments are being designed. Reference materials about noise-control measures are now available, and these can serve as

helpful resources in planning environments for people with hearing impairments (e.g., Brawley, 1997).

▶ Mr. H. is now 83 years old and has been a widower for 1 year. He has given up hunting and woodworking because he developed Parkinson's disease 11 years ago and cannot manage the necessary fine motor movements. He continues to fish seasonally, play poker monthly, and smoke one pack per day of cigarettes. In addition to Parkinson's disease, he has hypertension and coronary artery disease. He still lives in his own home and attends the local senior center for meals and social activities three times a week. His hearing loss has progressed to the point that he has difficulty with phone conversations and has to turn the television up loud. He cannot hear the doorbell. At the senior center, participants avoid conversations with him because he has difficulty hearing. You are the nurse at the senior center and you see him during your weekly Wellness Clinic for blood pressure checks. One week he tells you that his daughter is upset with him because he never answers his phone when she calls and she cannot have a decent phone conversation with him. She lives in another state and worries about him. She has offered to pay for a hearing aid evaluation for him, but he has told her "those things stick out like a sore thumb and they don't

DISPLAY 12-7
Communicating With Hearing-Impaired People

- Stand or sit directly in front of, and close to, the person.
- Talk toward the better ear, but make sure your lips can be seen.
- Make sure the person pays attention and looks at your face.
- Address the person by name, pause, and then begin talking.
- Speak distinctly, slowly, and directly to the person.
- Do not exaggerate lip movements because this will interfere with lip reading.
- Avoid chewing gum, covering your mouth, or turning your head away.
- If the person does not understand, repeat the message using different words.
- Avoid or eliminate any background noise.
- Do not raise the volume of your voice; rather, try to lower the tone while still speaking in a moderately loud voice.
- Keep all instructions simple and ask for feedback to assess what the person heard.
- Avoid questions that elicit simple yes or no answers.
- Keep sentences short.
- Use body language that is congruent with what you are trying to communicate.
- Demonstrate what you are saying.
- Use large-print written communication and pictures to supplement verbal communication.
- Make sure only one person talks at a time; arrange for one-on-one communication whenever possible.
- If eyeglasses normally are worn to improve vision, make sure they are clean.
- Provide adequate lighting so that the person can see your lips; avoid settings in which there is glare behind or around you.

do any good anyway. I can hear anything I want to hear and there's a lot I don't care to hear so why should you spend a lot of money for something that I won't use." He asks your opinion about this and is wondering if he should at least get a checkup to pacify his daughter. He expects he will be told that nothing can be done and that his daughter will have to be satisfied with the situation.

 THINKING POINTS

➤ Which information in Display 12-2 would be most pertinent to obtain at this time?

➤ What myths and misunderstandings influence Mr. H.?

➤ What nursing diagnosis would you apply to Mr. H.?

➤ Which information in Display 12-5 would be pertinent to this situation?

➤ What health promotion teaching would you do to address Mr. H.'s resistance to having his hearing evaluated?

➤ What additional health promotion advice would you give?

➤ Because you usually see Mr. H. weekly, you can develop a long-term teaching plan. How would you establish priorities for immediate and long-term goals?

EVALUATING EFFECTIVENESS OF NURSING INTERVENTIONS

Nurses observe compensatory behaviors of hearing-impaired older adults to evaluate the effectiveness of interventions for the nursing diagnosis of Disturbed Sensory Perception: Auditory. Some indicators of successful accomplishment include attention and concentration, correct use of hearing aid, appropriate response in conversation, demonstration of voice-hearing acuity, and appropriate response to auditory cues (Swanson & Drury, 2001). If goals address the psychosocial impact of hearing impairment and if social involvement is identified as a desired outcome, nurses could observe the extent to which interventions improve the person's ability to participate in social activities. For example, nurses could observe the impact of interventions such as sound amplification, effective communication techniques, and control of environmental noise. In residential facilities, an outcome might be to identify activities that the person would find satisfying despite a hearing deficit. For example, nurses could observe that hearing-impaired residents enjoy activities that take place in small, quiet rooms but dislike activities held in a large, noisy room.

Health promotion goals address the need for ongoing management of hearing deficits. Goals and interventions vary according to different health care settings. For example, one goal might be for the older adult to obtain an evaluation for a hearing aid. Nurses in short-term institutional settings would address such a goal through a discharge plan that includes information about resources for hearing evaluations and other relevant community services. Evaluation of the effectiveness of this health education intervention would be based on the patient's positive response to the nurse's suggestions. However, in short-term care settings, the nurse is not likely to have any opportunity to know whether the person followed through with the referral and had beneficial outcomes. In home, community, and long-term care settings, nurses address long-term goals more directly by assisting older adults and their caregivers in using additional services. In these settings, the evaluation of long-term goals might be based on the actual use of additional resources that improve the person's verbal communication abilities.

CHAPTER SUMMARY

Older adults experience an age-related hearing impairment called presbycusis. In its early stage, high-pitched sounds, as well as words with sibilants, become distorted. Eventually, speech comprehension becomes more impaired, and the older person has difficulty understanding verbal communication. This hearing deficit is exacerbated by the presence of background noise and by rapid-paced speech. Besides the age-related changes that can impair hearing, risk factors are common causes of hearing problems in older adults, and it is difficult to distinguish the effects of risk factors from those of age-related changes. Some risk factors, such as impacted cerumen, are modifiable. Other risk factors are associated with cumulative effects of lifestyle and environmental factors, such as noise and toxins.

Nursing assessment of hearing focuses on identifying any hearing deficits, modifiable risk factors, and barriers to the use of hearing aids. Nursing assessment can identify many areas for health teaching and health promotion interventions. Pertinent nursing diagnoses include Disturbed Sensory Perception and Impaired Communication. Nursing care plans are directed toward addressing risk factors and improving communication. Health promotion interventions regarding risk factors include raising questions about ototoxic medications and preventing and alleviating impacted cerumen. Nursing responsibilities regarding communication include addressing the need for a hearing evaluation and sound amplification, using techniques to enhance communication, and controlling or eliminating background noise. Nursing care is evaluated based on the improved ability of the older adult to understand verbal communication.

CONCLUDING CASE STUDY AND NURSING CARE PLAN

➤ Mr. H. is an 89-year-old widower who has had Parkinson's disease for 17 years. Presbycusis is listed as an additional diagnosis on his medical record. He is being admitted to a nursing home because his condition has declined to the point that his daughter, Ms. D., can no longer manage his care in her home, where he has lived for several years. He is medically stable but needs assistance in all activities of daily living.

■ Nursing Assessment

During the admission interview, you notice that Mr. H. has difficulty hearing your questions and that he frequently asks his daughter to give the requested information. He shows no significant cognitive deficits, but he seems to have difficulty understanding verbal communication. When you ask about any hearing impairment, Ms. D. tells you that her father has used hearing aids for 5 years and has been reevaluated periodically at a speech and hearing center. Two months ago, he obtained new hearing aids, but wears them only for one-on-one conversations with her. Because of Mr. H.'s tremors and difficulty with fine motor movements, Ms. D. cares for his hearing aids and assists with their insertion and removal.

Ms. D. has encouraged her father to wear his hearing aids during family gatherings, but he says the noise from small children is too annoying. Except for family gatherings, Mr. H. has very few opportunities for social interaction, and he has become more and more withdrawn. He used to enjoy playing poker but has not played in several years because all of his friends have died. Now he spends much of his time watching closed-captioned television programs. Ms. D. hopes that her father will respond to the opportunities for social interaction provided at the nursing home and that his quality of life will improve.

■ Nursing Diagnosis

In addition to nursing diagnoses related to Mr. H.'s chronic illness and self-care deficits, you identify a nursing diagnosis of Impaired Social Interaction related to the effects of hearing loss. You select this, rather than Disturbed Sensory Perception: Auditory as a nursing diagnosis because Mr. H.'s hearing impairment has already been evaluated, and sound amplification devices are available to him.

■ Nursing Care Plan

In your care plan (Display 12-8), you address the psychosocial consequences of Mr. H.'s hearing impairment. Your nursing care is directed toward improving his social interaction through the use of available devices and through other communication techniques that will enhance his social interaction skills.

DISPLAY 12-8 • NURSING CARE PLAN FOR MR. H.

EXPECTED OUTCOME	NURSING INTERVENTIONS	NURSING EVALUATION
Mr. H. will develop effective communication techniques for resident-staff interactions.	• During the initial interview, talk with Mr. H. and Ms. D. about the importance of good verbal communication with staff; emphasize the need for the staff to get to know Mr. H so his needs can be addressed. • Ask Mr. H. to wear his hearing aids during all one-on-one interactions with staff. • Use good communication techniques when talking with Mr. H (as in Display 12-7). • Make sure all staff members provide appropriate assistance with insertion and removal of Mr. H.'s hearing aids. • Include hearing aid maintenance as part of the daily responsibilities of the nursing aide.	• Mr. H. will wear his hearing aids during all one-on-one conversations with staff. • Mr. H. will report satisfactory verbal interactions with the staff. • Mr. H.'s hearing aids will be maintained in good operating condition.
Mr. H. will engage in social interaction with one other resident.	• During the initial care plan conference, identify several other residents who might converse with Mr. H. • Ask the staff to encourage one-on-one conversations between Mr. H. and the selected resident (e.g., suggest that they watch closed-captioned television programs together). • Ask Mr. H. to wear his hearing aids during one-on-one interactions with residents. • Provide assistance with inserting and removing hearing aids as needed. • Provide a quiet environment for one-on-one conversations with other residents.	• Mr. H. will wear his hearing aids at least once daily for a conversation with one other resident.
Mr. H. will engage in small group activities with other residents.	• During the first monthly care review conference, ask the activities staff to invite Mr. H. to a poker game with three other residents in the small-group room. • Make sure that environmental noise is controlled as much as possible.	• By the second month in this facility, Mr. H. will participate in weekly poker games with three other residents.

 ## CRITICAL THINKING EXERCISES

1. Answer the following questions with regard to Mr. H. at 89 years old:
   - What nursing responsibilities would you have with regard to addressing Mr. H.'s hearing impairment? How would you work with other staff to implement the care plan described in the concluding case example?
   - What are some of the advantages and disadvantages of hearing aids in a long-term care setting? How would you address the disadvantages?
   - How would you involve Ms. D. in the care plan to address Mr. H.'s hearing impairment?
   - If Mr. H. were in an acute care setting, how would you address his hearing problem?
2. Describe presbycusis and explain the functional consequences of this condition as it affects the everyday life of an older adult.
3. What risk factors would you consider in an 83-year-old person who complains of recent problems with hearing?
4. What advice would you give to someone who asks you about a brochure she received from a hearing aid company that offers free hearing screenings

describing a new high-powered hearing aid? The person has trouble hearing but has never had an evaluation.

5. Describe at least 10 ways in which you can adapt your communication for a hearing-impaired person.
6. Find at least one resource (*not* a hearing aid dealer) in your community that you could recommend to an older adult who needs a hearing evaluation.
7. Visit at least three Internet sites that provide educational materials about hearing impairment, and choose the one you think would be best for obtaining health information brochures.

Future Directions for Healthier Aging: Focus on Hearing

- Longitudinal and population-based studies are trying to identify modifiable health-related risk factors to lay the groundwork for aggressive programs of prevention, particularly for NIHL.
- Digital technology offers hope for further refinements of hearing aids and assistive listening devices, but cost factors are likely to remain a problem.
- Technology behind cochlear implants continues to develop rapidly, but these devices will continue to be interventions primarily for people who are profoundly deaf or severely hard of hearing.

RESEARCH INITIATIVES OF THE NATIONAL INSTITUTE ON AGING ACTION

- Continue identifying risk factors for age-related hearing loss.
- Develop strategies to improve functional independence of older adults with hearing loss.
- Encourage manufacturers to redesign products and develop new technologies to enhance hearing abilities.

EDUCATIONAL RESOURCES

American Speech-Language-Hearing Foundation (ASH Foundation)
10801 Rockville Pike, Rockville, MD 20852
(301) 897-5700
http://www.ashfoundation.org

American Tinnitus Association (ATA)
P.O. Box 5, Portland, OR 97207-0005
(800) 634-8787
http://www.ata.org

Better Hearing Institute (BHI)
515 King Street, Suite 420, Alexandria, VA 22314
(703) 684-3391
Toll-free: (800) 327-9355
http://www.betterhearing.org

Canadian Hard of Hearing Association
2435 Holly Lane, Suite 205, Ottawa, ON K1V 7P2
(613) 526-1584
http://www.chha.ca

Hear Now
4248 Park Glen Road, Minneapolis, MN 55416
Toll-free: (800) 648-4327

International Hearing Society (IHS)
16880 Middlebelt Road, Suite 4, Livonia, MI 48154
(734) 522-7200
Toll-free: (800) 521-5247
http://www.ihsinfo.org

National Campaign for Hearing Health (NCHH)
1050 17th Street, NW, Suite 701, Washington, DC 20036
(202) 289-5850
http://www.hearinghealth.net

National Institute on Deafness and Other Communication Disorders (NIDCD)
Office of Health Communication and Public Liaison
MSC 2320, 31 Center Drive, Bethesda, MD 20892-2320
(301) 496-7243
http://www.nidcd.nih.gov/

Self Help for Hard of Hearing People, Inc. (SHHH)
7910 Woodmont Avenue, Suite 1200, Bethesda, MD 20814
(301) 657-2248
http://www.shhh.org

REFERENCES

Bassford, T. L. (1995). Health status of Hispanic elders. *Clinics in Geriatric Medicine, 11*(1), 25–38.

Bazargan, M., Baker, R. S., & Bazargan, S. H. (2001). Sensory impairments and subjective well-being among aged African American person. *Journal of Gerontology: Psychological Sciences, 56B,* P268–278.

Beckett, W. S., Chamberlain, D., Hallman, E., May, J., Hwang, S. A., Gomez, M., Eberly, S., Cox, C., & Stark, A. (2000). Hearing conservation for farmers: Source apportionment of occupational and environmental factors contributing to hearing loss. *Journal of Occupational and Environmental Medicine, 42*(8), 806–813.

Brawley, E. C. (1997). *Designing for Alzheimer's disease: Strategies for creating better care environments.* New York: John Wiley & Sons.

Carpenito, L. J. (2002). *Nursing diagnosis: Application to clinical practice* (9th ed.). Philadelphia: Lippincott.

Casano, R. A., Johnson, D. F., Bykhovskaya, Y., Torricelli, F., Bigozzi, M., & Fischel-Ghodsian, N. (1999). Inherited susceptibility to aminoglycoside ototoxicity: Genetic heterogeneity and clinical implications. *American Journal of Otolaryngology, 20*(3), 151–156.

Dalton, D. S., Cruickshanks, K. J., Wiley, T. L., Klein, B. E., Klein, R., & Tweed, T. S. (2001). Association of leisure-time noise exposure and hearing loss. *Audiology, 40*(1), 1–9.

Demers, K. (2002). Hearing screening. *Home Healthcare Nurse, 20,* 132–133.

Erber, N. P. (1994). Communicating with elders: Effects of amplification. *Journal of Gerontological Nursing, 20*(10), 6–10.

Fozard, J., & Gordon-Salant, S. (2001). In J. E. Birren & K. W. Schaie (Eds.), *The psychology of aging* (5th ed., pp. 241–266). San Diego: Academic Press.

Garstecki, D., & Erler, S. F. (1999). Older adult performance on the Communication Profile for the Hearing Impaired: Gender difference. *Journal of Speech, Language, and Hearing Research, 42,* 735–796.

Hands, S. (2000). Hearing loss in over-65s: Is routine questionnaire screening worthwhile? *Journal of Laryngology and Otology, 114,* 661–666.

Hwang, S. A., Gomez, M. I., Sobotova, L., Stark, A. D., May, J. J., & Hallman, E. M. (2001). Predictors of hearing loss in New York farmers. *American Journal of Industrial Medicine, 40*(1), 23–31.

Kales, S. N., Freyman, R. L., Hill, J. M., Polyhronopoulos, G. N., Aldrich, J. M., & Christiani, D. C. (2001). Firefighters' hearing: A comparison with population databases from the international Standards Organization. *Journal of Occupational and Environmental Medicine, 43*(7), 650–656.

Karev, M., & Bartz, S. N. (2001). Hearing aids. In M. D. Mezey (Ed.), *The encyclopedia of elder care* (pp. 334–336). New York: Springer.

Kramer, S. E., Kapteyn, T. S., Kuik, D. J., & Deeg, D. J. H. (2002). The association of hearing impairment and chronic diseases with psychosocial health status in older age. *Journal of Aging and Health, 14,* 122–137.

Mahoney, D. F. (1996). Cerumen impaction and hearing impairment among nursing home residents: Nursing implications. In V. Burggraf & R. Barry (Eds.), *Gerontological nursing: Current practice and research* (pp. 159–168). Thorofare, NJ: SLACK.

Morata, R. C., Johnson, A-C, Nylen, P., Svensson, E. B., Cheng, J., Krieg, E. F., Lindblad, A-C., Emstgard, L., & Franks, J. (2002). Audiometric findings in workers exposed to low levels of styrene and noise. *Journal of Occupational and Environmental Medicine, 44,* 806–814.

Nakanishi, N., Okamoto, M., Nakamura, K., Suzuki, K., Tatara, K. (2000). Cigarette smoking and risk for hearing impairment: A longitudinal study in Japanese male office workers. *Journal of Occupational and Environmental Medicine, 42*(11), 1045–1049.

National Academy on an Aging Society (NAAS). (1999). *Hearing loss: A growing problem that affects quality of life.* Washington, DC: Author.

Nondahl, D. M., Cruickshanks, K. J., Wiley, T. L., Klein, R., Klein, B. E., & Tweed, T. S. (2000). Recreational firearm use and hearing loss. *Archives of Family Medicine, 9*(4), 352–357.

Overfield, T. (1995). *Biological variation in health and illness: Race, age, and sex differences.* Boca Raton, FL: CRC Press.

Resnick, H. E., Fries, B. E., & Verbrugge, L. M. (1997). Windows to their world: The effect of sensory impairments on social engagement and activity time in nursing home residents. *Journal of Gerontology: Social Sciences, 52B*(3), S135–S144.

Rousseau, P. (1995). Native-American elders: Health care status. *Clinics in Geriatric Medicine, 11*(1), 83–95.

Schneider, B. A., Daneman, M., & Murphy, D. R. (2000). Listening to discourse in distracting settings: The effects of aging. *Psychology and Aging, 15*(1), 110–125.

Singer, A. J., Sauris, E., & Viccellio, A. W. (2000). Ceruminolytic effects of docusate sodium: A randomized, controlled trial. *Annals of Emergency Medicine, 36*(3), 228–232.

Stevenson, J. S. (2001). Health seeking behaviors. In M. L. Maas, K. C. Buckwalter, M. D. Hardy, T. Tripp-Reimer, M. G. Titler, & J. P. Specht (Eds.), *Nursing care of older adults: Diagnoses, outcomes, and interventions* (pp.75–85). St. Louis: Mosby.

Swanson, E. A., & Drury, J. (2001). Sensory/perceptual alterations. In M. L. Maas, K. C. Buckwalter, M. D. Hardy, T. Tripp-Reimer, M. G. Titler, & J. P. Specht (Eds.), *Nursing care of older adults: Diagnoses, outcomes, and interventions* (pp.75–85). St. Louis: Mosby.

Tesch-Römer, C. (1997). Psychological effects of hearing and use in older adults. *Journal of Gerontology: Psychological Sciences, 52B*(3), P127–P138.

Tomei, F., Fantini, S., Tomao, E., Baccolo, T. P., & Rosati, M. V. (2000). Hypertension and chronic exposure to noise. *Archives of Environmental Health, 55*(5), 319–325.

U.S. Department of Health and Human Services (USDHS). (2000). *Healthy people 2010* (2nd ed). Washington, DC: U.S. Government Printing Office.

Wallhagen, M. I., Strawbridge, W. J., Shema, S. J., Kurata, J., & Kaplan, G. A. (2001). Comparative impact of hearing and vision impairment on subsequent functioning. *Journal of the American Geriatrics Society, 49,* 1086–1092.

Vision

LEARNING OBJECTIVES

1. Delineate age-related changes that affect the visual abilities of older adults.
2. Examine risk factors that influence the visual abilities of older adults.
3. Discuss the functional consequences of age-related changes and risk factors that affect vision.
4. Describe interview questions, behavioral cues, and tests of visual skills that can be used to assess vision in older adults.
5. Identify environmental modifications and other interventions designed to assist older adults in attaining and maintaining optimal visual performance.

Important daily activities, such as communicating, enjoying visual images, and maneuvering in the environment, are influenced by one's ability to see. Thus, a diminished ability to see can affect safety, performance of daily activities, and quality of life. Age-related changes to the structure of the eye, alone or in the presence of environmental factors or pathology, can negatively affect vision in older adults. Fortunately, there are many health promotion interventions within the scope of nursing to assist the older adult in maintaining optimal visual function and in compensating for visual limitations. This chapter explores age-related changes that affect vision as well as some common visual impairments and pathologic conditions. In addition, the role of the nurse in helping older adults to preserve vision and effectively cope with any visual impairment that does occur is discussed.

AGE-RELATED CHANGES THAT AFFECT VISION

Visual function depends on a sequence of processes, beginning with the visual perception of an external stimulus and ending with the processing of neural impulses in the cerebral cortex. Age-related changes affect all of the structures involved in visual function and alter visual perception for the older adult. In the absence of disease processes, these gradual changes have only a subtle impact on the daily activities of the older person. Unless compensatory actions are taken, however, age-related vision changes may interfere with the older person's quality of life and influence the enjoyment and safe performance of many activities.

General Eye Changes

Although age-related changes in the appearance of the eye do not affect visual performance, these changes may be a source of anxiety or discomfort and therefore can be addressed in health promotion activities. Changes are seen in the eye itself as well as in the associated structures (e.g., the eyelids and tear ducts). Education about age-related changes may alleviate anxiety, and interventions aimed at eye comfort may relieve bothersome symptoms. Thus, changes in eye appearance and tear production are briefly reviewed in this section on age-related changes.

As the eye ages, lipids accumulate in the outer part of the cornea, and a white or yellowish ring develops between the iris and the sclera. This phenomenon, termed *arcus senilis,* can be observed in most eyes by the ninth decade. Other changes in the eye's appearance include a loss of translucency of the cornea, a yellowing of the sclera, and fading of the pigment in the iris.

> Arcus senilis occurs in 90% of men between the ages of 70 and 80 years and in all men after the age of 80 years. In women, this pattern is delayed by about 10 years (Yanoff, 1999).

Changes in the eyelids and surrounding skin also affect the appearance of the eye, but they usually do not affect visual function. Certain changes, such as loss of orbital fat, development of wrinkles, decreased elasticity of the eyelid muscles, and accumulation of dark pigment around the eyes, contribute to the overall appearance of sunken eyes, called *enophthalmos.* If the loss of orbital fat and muscle elasticity progresses to the point that a lid fold develops, vision may be impaired. This condition, termed *blepharochalasis,* can be surgically treated. Relaxation of the lower lid

muscles to an extreme degree may result in the age-related conditions of ectropion or entropion. In *ectropion,* the lower lid falls away from the conjunctiva, blocking the flow of tears through the lower punctum and decreasing lubrication of the conjunctiva. In *entropion,* the lower lid becomes inverted and the eyelashes may irritate the cornea, eventually leading to infection.

Age-related diminution in tear production may lead to chronic dry eye syndrome. The older adult may complain of dryness, burning, or photosensitivity. Subsequent irritation and rubbing of the cornea may lead to infections. Contrary to what might be expected, dry eye syndrome can lead to excessive tearing because the lack of normal lubricating tears stimulates the production of reflex tears.

Cornea and Sclera

The cornea is a translucent covering over the eye that refracts light rays and provides 65% to 75% of the focusing power of the eye. As the eye ages, the cornea becomes more opaque and yellowed, interfering with the passage of light, especially ultraviolet rays, to the retina. Other corneal changes, such as the accumulation of lipid deposits, cause an increased scattering of light rays and may have a blurring effect on vision. In younger adults, the cornea is more highly curved and, therefore, has greater refractive power on the horizontal plane than on the vertical plane. With increased age, the corneal curvature changes, causing a reversal in this pattern and influencing the refractive ability.

Lens

The lens consists of concentric and avascular layers of clear, crystalline protein. Because the lens has no blood supply, it depends on the aqueous humor for all metabolic and support functions. The transparent lens fibers are continually forming new layers without shedding old layers. As new layers form peripherally, the old layers are compressed inward toward the center, where they eventually become absorbed into the nucleus. This process gradually increases the size and density of the lens, causing a tripling of its mass by the age of 70 years. Thus, the lens gradually becomes stiffer, denser, and more opaque.

Because of these age-related changes, the lens moves forward in the eye and responds less effectively to the ciliary muscle. These changes also interfere with the transmission of light rays, resulting in a scattering of the rays that pass through the lens and a reduction in the amount of light reaching the retina. These changes do not affect all wavelengths equally; rather, the most detrimental effect occurs with the shorter blue and violet wavelengths.

Iris and Pupil

The iris is a pigmented sphincter muscle that dilates and contracts to control pupillary size and to regulate the amount of light reaching the retina. With increasing age, the iris becomes more sclerotic and rigid, reducing the size of the pupil and interfering with its ability to respond to changes in light. The pupillary size begins to diminish during the third decade and levels off during the seventh decade. This condition, called *senile miosis,* causes a marked diminution in the amount of light reaching the retina.

Ciliary Body

The ciliary body is a mass of muscles, connective tissue, and blood vessels surrounding the lens. These muscles regulate the passage of light rays through the lens by changing the shape of the lens. The ciliary body controls the functions of *accommodation,* a process that controls one's ability to focus on near objects. In addition, the ciliary body is responsible for the production of aqueous fluid. Beginning in the fourth decade, the ciliary body gradually atrophies, and muscle cells are replaced with connective tissue. By the sixth decade, the ciliary body is smaller, stiffer, and less functional. With advanced age, less aqueous humor is secreted, which leads to diminished nourishment and cleansing of the cornea and lens.

Vitreous

The vitreous is a clear, gelatinous mass that forms the inner substance and maintains the spherical shape of the eye. During the fifth decade, this gelatinous substance begins to shrink, and the proportion of liquid increases. These age-related changes may cause the vitreous body to pull away from the retina, causing the older person to experience symptoms such as floaters, blurred vision, distortion of images, or light flashes without any external stimuli. Additionally, these changes may cause light to scatter more diffusely through the vitreous, reducing the amount of light reaching the retina.

Retina

The transformation of visual stimuli into neural impulses begins in the rods and cones of the retina. Rods and cones are photoreceptor cells that produce pigments and perform specific visual functions. Cones are responsible for acuity and color perception, and they require high levels of light to function effectively. Rods are responsible for vision under low light conditions, and they have no ability to perceive color. Cones are concentrated in the central and most sensitive part of the macula, called the *fovea,* whereas rods are distributed throughout the peripheral retina.

Age-related changes affect the photoreceptor cells, particularly the cones, beginning around the age of 20 years, when the number of cones begins to decrease. There is only a minimal loss of cones in the fovea, where they are most highly concentrated; most of the loss occurs in the peripheral part of the retina. Although the number of rods declines in the central retina, the remaining rods increase in size and are able to maintain their ability to capture light.

Additional retinal structures that undergo age-related changes include the pigment epithelium and the blood vessels, which become thinner and more sclerotic. Lipofuscin accumulates in the retinal pigment epithelium, and the choroid protrudes through it. Research on the effect of these changes on visual function is sparse. It is generally agreed, however, that these retinal changes do have functional consequences, as discussed later in this chapter.

Retinal–Neural Pathway

Photoreceptor cells converge in the ganglion cells that form the optic nerve. Neurosensory information is passed from the optic nerve, through the thalamus, to the visual cortex. Neurons in the visual cortex decline in quantity and quality with increased age. Age-related changes in the retinal–neural pathway affect the speed of processing visual information, particularly in conditions of low illumination. Additional age-related central nervous system changes that affect cognitive function also may contribute to declines in visual function in older adults.

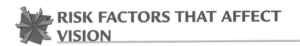

RISK FACTORS THAT AFFECT VISION

Environmental factors can exacerbate age-related vision changes in the lens and retina and detrimentally affect visual function. For example, long-term exposure to ultraviolet light (i.e., sunlight) has been associated with the development of cataracts and the loss of photoreceptor cells, particularly the cones. Furthermore, because age-related changes can diminish the protective response to harmful ultraviolet wavelengths, older adults may be more vulnerable to eye damage from sunlight. Warmer environmental temperatures have been associated with an earlier age of onset for *presbyopia* (i.e., loss of near vision). Dry eyes can be caused by environmental conditions such as wind, sunlight, low humidity, and cigarette smoke.

Certain pathologic conditions may adversely affect visual function in a variety of ways. People with Alzheimer's disease, even in the early stages, may have impaired contrast sensitivity and other visual impairments. People with diabetes are at increased risk for cataracts, glaucoma, and diabetic retinopathy. People with hypertension or hypercholesterolemia are at higher risk for age-related macular degeneration (AMD). Malnutrition has been associated with cataract development, and vitamin A deficiency has been associated with dry eyes from reduced tear production.

Cigarette smoking is a risk factor for cataracts and macular degeneration. Longitudinal studies have found that smoking cessation can reduce the risk for cataracts by limiting total dose-related damage to the lens, but the risk for cataracts remains higher among past smokers than among never smokers (Christen et al., 2000; Weintraub et al., 2002).

Medications that may be associated with adverse effects on vision include aspirin, haloperidol, nonsteroidal antiinflammatory agents, tricyclic antidepressants, digitalis, anticholinergics, phenothiazines, isoniazid, tamoxifen, amiodarone, sildenafil, and oral or inhaled corticosteroids. Cataracts are common in people with glaucoma because of the anticholinesterase drugs used in the treatment of this condition. Medications that can cause or contribute to dry eyes include estrogen, diuretics, antihistamines, anticholinergics, phenothiazines, ß-blockers, and antiparkinsonian medications. Systemic anticoagulants may precipitate intraocular hemorrhage in people with preexisting macular degeneration. In recent years, questions have been raised about statin drugs increasing the risk for cataracts, particularly when other drugs increase their bioavailability (Schlienger et al., 2001).

EFFECTS OF AGE-RELATED CHANGES ON VISION

All adults, regardless of race, gender, ethnicity, or socioeconomic status, notice some changes in their visual abilities by their fifth decade, and prescription glasses or contact lenses are almost universal by the eighth decade. Even the rare person who has 20/20 visual acuity at the age of 90 years experiences subtle changes in overall vision. However, despite the universal prevalence of age-related vision changes, most older adults can perform their usual activities if they use low-vision aids and modify their environment. Visual impairment, which is defined as vision loss that cannot be corrected by eyeglasses or contact lenses alone, ranges from mild impairment to blindness. Mild visual impairments are commonly associated with normal age-related changes and

may be significantly exacerbated by environmental conditions such as glare and poor lighting. Compensatory interventions are quite effective in improving visual function for people with age-related vision changes. For example, a person who uses reading glasses and bright nonglaring light to improve his or her ability to read would be compensating effectively for mild visual impairment. Consequences of age-related changes that cause mild visual impairment are discussed in the following sections. Consequences of the more significant visual impairments are discussed in the section that follows the section on pathologic conditions.

Loss of Accommodation

Loss of accommodation, or the ability to focus clearly and quickly on near objects and objects at various distances, is usually the earliest age-related vision change. Presbyopia usually begins during the fifth decade. This vision change is caused primarily by age-related changes in the lens, the structure that adjusts the eye's focus for different distances. Degenerative changes of the ciliary body may play a minor role in the development of presbyopia. Functionally, accommodative changes cause a gradual increase in the near point of vision, the closest point at which a small object can be seen clearly. Consequently, the person with presbyopia will hold reading materials farther from the eye to focus clearly on the print.

Diminished Acuity

Acuity is the ability to detect details and discern objects. This visual skill is customarily assessed using a Snellen chart, and it is measured against a normal value of 20/20. Visual acuity is best around the age of 30 years, after which it gradually declines with increasing age. Diminished acuity results from age-related ocular changes, including decreased pupillary size, scatter of light in the cornea and lens, opacification of the lens and vitreous, and loss of photoreceptor cells in the retina. These changes interfere with the passage of light to the retina, contributing to the threefold reduction in retinal illumination that occurs between the ages of 20 and 60 years.

Acuity is also influenced by extraocular factors, such as the size and movement of an object and the amount of light reflected off an object. Low or poor illumination compounds the effects of age-related ocular changes, particularly on visual acuity. Visual acuity for moving objects is more impaired than acuity for static objects, and acuity becomes more impaired as the speed of the object increases. This combination of age-related changes and external factors hinders the older person's ability to see moving objects and to perform tasks in low illumination. Consequently, older people require a relatively greater degree of illumination and may experience a marked decline in night driving competence.

Delayed Dark and Light Adaptation

The ability to respond to dim light is gauged by the level of vision achieved and the length of time needed to reach maximum visual perception. This visual capacity, called *dark adaptation,* begins to decline around the age of 20 years and diminishes more markedly after the age of 60 years. This decline is associated with decreased retinal illumination as well as age-related changes in retinal metabolism and retinal–neural pathways. The functional impact of these changes is that the older adult requires more time to adapt to decreased illumination when moving from a brighter to a darker environment. For instance, when entering a darkened movie theater, an older person needs extra time to adapt to the dim environment before proceeding down the aisle to find a seat.

The ability to respond to high levels of illumination is also affected by age-related changes in the lens and pupils. These changes reduce the amount of light reaching the retina. Functionally, this means that an older person has a decreased ability to respond to bright lights, such as the headlights of an oncoming car, and requires increased time to recover from exposure to glare and bright lights.

Increased Glare Sensitivity

Glare occurs when a scattering of light in the optic media reduces the clarity of visual images. Glare is experienced when light is reflected from shiny surfaces, when it is excessively bright or inappropriately focused, or when bright light originates from several sources at once. Glare is classified according to three types: veiling, dazzling, and scotomatic. *Veiling glare* is caused by the scattering of light over the retinal surface and results in diminished contrast of the viewed object. Veiling glare may occur, for example, when bright fluorescent lights in a grocery store reflect on the clear plastic covering over meat products in a white case. *Dazzling glare,* which is caused by bright visual displays, interferes with the ability to discern details. Glass-covered directories in brightly lit shopping malls may produce a dazzling glare that interferes with a person's ability to read the words in the directory, particularly if there is poor contrast between the letters and the background. *Scotomatic glare* is a blinding glare caused by loss of retinal sensitivity and overstimulation of retinal pigments after exposure to bright lights. On sunny or snowy days,

scotomatic glare may be noted when driving toward the sun.

Beginning in the fifth decade, age-related changes increase a person's sensitivity to glare and the time required to recover from glare. Glare sensitivity is influenced primarily by opacification of the lens; it also may be affected by age-related changes in the pupil and vitreous. Functionally, these changes may have a significant impact on night driving as well as on a person's ability to read signs, see objects, and maneuver safely in bright environments. In many modern buildings and shopping malls, the bright lights, large windows, and highly reflective floors generate glare that can lead to accidents and inaccurate perceptions.

Reduced Visual Field

A visual field is an oval-shaped area encompassing the total view that the person can perceive while keeping the eyes fixed on a constant point straight ahead. The scope of the visual field narrows slightly between the ages of 40 and 50 years and then declines steadily. Functionally, the visual field is important in the performance of tasks requiring a broad perception of the environment and moving objects. Walking in crowded places and driving a vehicle are examples of activities that depend on the field of vision.

Diminished Depth Perception

Depth perception is the visual skill responsible for localizing objects in three-dimensional space, for judging differences in the depth of objects, and for observing relationships among objects in space. As with many other visual skills, depth perception depends on interactions between ocular and extraocular factors. Stereopsis, or the disparity between retinal images that is caused by the separation of the two eyes, is the primary ocular characteristic that affects depth perception. Extraocular factors that influence depth perception include prior perceptual experiences of the observer; movement of the observer's head or body; and characteristics of the object, such as size, height, distance, texture, brightness, and shading.

Information about how age-related changes affect depth perception is limited by the complexity of the ocular and extraocular factors involved and by the fact that stereopsis has been the only factor studied. Researchers generally agree, however, that there is a decline in depth perception in older people, but the origins of these changes have not been identified. Functionally, depth perception enables people to use objects effectively and to maneuver safely in the environment. Thus, diminished depth perception may lead to falls and tripping following miscalculations about the distance and height of objects.

Altered Color Vision

Pigments in three types of cones absorb light in the red, blue, or green range of the visual spectrum. As with many other visual functions, color perception is influenced by the type and quantity of light waves reaching the retina. Consequently, any age-related changes that interfere with retinal illumination, such as lens opacification and pupillary miosis, can interfere with accurate color perception. Opacification and yellowing of the lens interferes most directly with shorter wavelengths, causing an altered perception of blues, greens, and violets. Age-related retinal or retinal–neural changes may also affect color perception, as can extraocular influences such as low levels of illumination.

Functionally, altered color perception is manifested as a relative darkening of blue objects and a yellowed perception of white light. Color perception is increasingly impaired in conditions of poor illumination. Accurate color perception is not essential in all daily activities, but it is important, for instance, in differentiating between medications that are similar in color or tone, especially those in the blue-green range and the yellow-white range. In addition, altered color perception may interfere with the detection of spoiled food.

Diminished Critical Flicker Fusion

Critical flicker fusion is the point at which an intermittent light source is perceived as a continuous, rather than flashing, light. The ability to perceive flashing lights accurately is a function of the retinal receptors and is influenced by extraocular factors, such as the size, color, and luminance of the object. Age-related changes in the retina and retinal–neural pathway, as well as the changes that decrease retinal illumination, interfere with critical flicker fusion. Low levels of illumination further exacerbate the effects of these changes. Functionally, diminished critical flicker fusion distorts the perception of a flashing light, making it appear to be a continuous light. Thus, diminished critical flicker fusion may interfere with the discernment of emergency vehicles and road construction lights, especially at night.

Slower Visual Information Processing

The retinal–neural pathway is responsible for processing visual information accurately and efficiently. Older adults need additional time to process visual information and to search their visual memory in the performance of everyday tasks, but age-related differences are minimal or negligible when the tasks are familiar or well practiced.

Table 13-1 summarizes age-related vision changes and their effects on vision.

➤ Mrs. F. is 60 years old and has used "readers" (reading glasses) for 15 years but has never needed glasses for anything other than reading and sewing. She recently noticed that when she is in the shopping mall she has trouble reading the directory that is enclosed in a glass case. She works in an office building with an atrium that has skylights, and she has trouble reading the signs on the office doors.

TABLE 13-1 ● Age-Related Changes Affecting Vision	
Change	**Consequence**
Appearance and Comfort	
• Decreased elasticity of the eyelid muscles	Potential for ectropion, entropion, blepharochalasis
• Enophthalmos	
• Decreased tears	Potential for dry eye syndrome
Structures	
• Yellowing and increased opacity of cornea	**Presbyopia:** diminished ability to focus on near objects
• Changes in the corneal curvature	
• Increase in lens size and density	Diminished accommodation
• Sclerosis and rigidity of the iris	Diminished acuity
• Decrease in pupillary size	Slower response to changes in illumination
• Atrophy of the ciliary muscle	Increased sensitivity to glare
• Shrinkage of gelatinous substance in the vitreous	Narrowing of the visual field
• Atrophy of photoreceptor cells	Diminished depth perception
• Thinning and sclerosis of retinal blood vessels	Altered color perception
• Degeneration of neurons in the visual cortex	Distorted perception of flashing lights
	Slower processing of visual information

THINKING POINTS

➤ What age-related changes contribute to the vision changes that Mrs. F. notices?

➤ What environmental factors are likely to contribute to Mrs. F.'s difficulty when she is in the shopping mall or at work?

➤ When Mrs. F. is in her home environment, what tasks might be more difficult because of age-related vision changes?

PATHOLOGIC CONDITIONS THAT CAN AFFECT VISION

Pathologic conditions leading to vision impairment occur very commonly in older adults. Functional consequences associated with three commonly occurring conditions are described in the following sections because nurses play an important health promotion role in both detection and management of these conditions. Nurses can identify clues to undiagnosed eye conditions by carefully assessing vision changes, as discussed later in the chapter. This is particularly important with glaucoma, which is the most readily treated of the common eye conditions but is often undiagnosed. Among older adults, the three most common pathologic eye conditions are cataracts, AMD, and glaucoma (Figure 13-1, Table 13-2).

Cataracts

Cataracts are the leading cause, as well as the most reversible cause, of visual impairment in older adults. About one fourth of noninstitutionalized people aged 70 years and older reported that they currently had cataracts, with a higher percentage of women than men reporting cataracts (Desai et al., 2001). Cataract formation is often viewed as an age-related change in an extreme degree because changes in the lens begin in everyone between the ages of 30 and 40 years and eventually can progress to the point of extreme opacification. When the cataracts cause the normally transparent lens to become cloudy, the transmission of light to the retina is diminished, and vision is impaired. For some older adults, the degree of opacification never progresses to the point of causing significant visual impairment, but many older adults experience significant visual impairments because of cataracts. In addition to being caused by age-related changes, cataracts may be caused by systemic disease, medications, and environmental factors, as discussed in the section on risk factors and summarized in

Table 13-2. Also, they are likely to occur more commonly after glaucoma surgery or other types of eye surgery.

Cataracts usually occur in both eyes, but they do not necessarily progress bilaterally at the same rate. Cataracts are classified according to their location: *cortical* cataracts occur in the cortex, *nuclear* cataracts occur in the nucleus, and *posterior subcapsular* cataracts occur on the back of the membrane that surrounds the lens. The location of the cataract significantly influences the impact on vision, with nuclear cataracts causing the most interference.

In their early stages, cataracts do not necessarily affect visual acuity, but as they progress, they can lead to complaints of glare, blurred vision, and decreased night vision. People with cataracts may complain of dimmed or blurred vision (see Figure 13-1), a need for increased illumination when reading, a lessened ability to discern contrast, the perception of halos around bright lights, an increased sensitivity to glare, distorted or double images, frequent changes in corrective lenses, the perception of a "film" over the eye, and distorted or diminished color perception (e.g., blue appears dulled, and red, yellow, and orange appear brighter). Activities such as reading and driving (particularly night driving) are often hindered by cataracts.

Cataracts cannot be treated medically, but in the early stages, they are managed by the prescription of stronger eyeglasses or contact lenses. When visual acuity declines to about 20/50 and cataracts interfere with important activities, cataract surgery is usually recommended. When surgery is required for both eyes, the procedure is usually done on one eye at a time, with the second surgery being done after the first one heals completely. Although cataracts can be diagnosed by an optometrist or ophthalmologist, only an ophthalmologist can perform cataract surgery, which is the most commonly performed operation in the United States today. Decisions about when to recommend cataract surgery are based on the impact of the progression of the visual loss on the person's safety and quality of life. During the past decade, many advances have been made with regard to cataract surgery, and the procedure is simpler and safer than it used to be.

Several surgical techniques are available to remove the affected lens. In one common technique, called *phacoemulsification,* ultrasound waves are used to break up the clouded lens, and then a suction device is used to aspirate the tiny particles. After the cataract is removed, an intraocular lens is implanted. The entire surgical procedure is done with local anesthesia, takes less than 1 hour, and has a very low rate of complications.

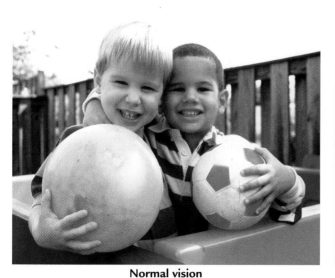

Normal vision

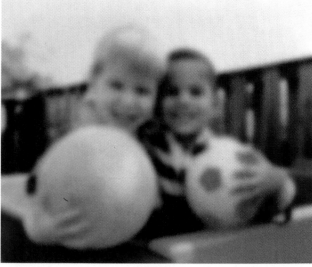

Cataracts

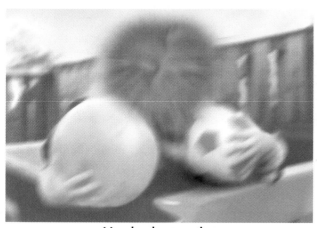

Macular degeneration

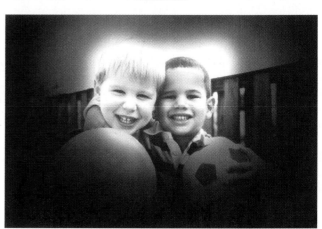

Glaucoma

FIGURE 13-1 Examples of normal vision, vision with cataracts, vision with age-related macular degeneration, and vision with glaucoma. (Courtesy of the National Eye Institute, National Institutes of Health.)

Nurses play an important role in dispelling myths that might interfere with older adults obtaining surgical treatment for cataracts. Many older adults may think that cataract surgery is more complicated or more risky than it actually is because they are familiar with experiences of older friends or relatives who had cataract surgery many years ago. In providing health promotion teaching about cataracts, it is important to emphasize that significant progress has been made in techniques for cataract surgery in recent years. Although nurses need not be thoroughly familiar with the surgical techniques, they can emphasize that the techniques used today are much simpler than those used a decade ago and that they have a very high success rate. Nurses also can encourage older adults to obtain reliable information from eye care practitioners and to have cataracts evaluated

periodically, rather than simply tolerating a loss of vision due to cataracts.

Age-Related Macular Degeneration

AMD is the leading cause of severe vision loss in older adults in the United States and other developed countries. AMD, in various stages, affects 18% of people between the ages of 70 and 74 years and 47% of people aged 85 and older. In younger adults, the prevalence of AMD does not differ significantly by gender or race, but in people 70 years of age and older, AMD affects women more than men and non-Hispanic whites more than African Americans. AMD is associated with the factors reviewed earlier in the section on risk factors and summarized in Table 13-2.

TABLE 13-2 • Common Disease Conditions Affecting Vision

	Risk Factors	Symptoms	Management
Cataract	Advanced age, exposure to sunlight, smoking, diabetes, malnutrition, trauma or radiation to the eye or head, medications (corticosteroids, phenothiazines, amiodarone, benzodiazepines, anticholinesterases)	Increased sensitivity to glare, decreased contrast sensitivity, blurred vision, distorted images, double vision, diminished color perception, frequent eyeglass prescription changes	Surgical removal of lens followed by implantation of an intraocular lens
Age-Related Macular Degeneration (AMD)	Advanced age, non-Hispanic white ethnicity, family history of AMD, smoking, hypertension, hyperlipidemia, medications (tamoxifen, phenothiazines, chloroquine)	Gradual progressive loss of central vision, distorted straight lines, blurred vision	Visual rehabilitation programs, argon laser therapy for wet type, experimental treatments under investigation for both types
Glaucoma	Advanced age, African American race, family history of glaucoma, diabetes, medications (anticholinergics, corticosteroids)	**Chronic:** Slow onset, diminished vision in dim light, increased sensitivity to glare, decreased contrast sensitivity, diminished peripheral vision **Acute:** sudden onset, intense pain, blurred vision, halos around lights, nausea and vomiting	**Chronic:** Medical therapy with miotics, adrenergic agonists, carbonic anhydrase inhibitors, β-blockers, and prostaglandins (administered as eye drops) **Acute:** immediate treatment with medications to reduce pressure, followed by laser surgery

The macula is the small area in the middle of the retina where visual acuity is best. Early in the disease, deposits of yellow byproducts of retinal pigment, called *drusen,* build up in the macula and can be seen on funduscopic examination. As the disease progresses, it is classified either as *dry type,* which accounts for 80 % to 90 % of cases, or *wet (exudative) type.* In the dry type, damage is caused by death of the photoreceptors, which is seen on fundoscopy as tiny areas of atrophy of the retinal pigment epithelium. In the wet type, the damage is caused by the formation of new blood vessels in the choroid, a process called *choroidal neovascularization,* followed by hemorrhage into the subretinal space. The dry type of AMD usually progresses slowly and does not cause total blindness. If the wet type develops, visual loss may be rapid and severe.

In the early stage, the person may have blurred vision and more difficulty reading in dim light. Like most other eye conditions, AMD occurs in both eyes, but it may initially appear only in one eye, and its course may differ in each eye. As AMD progresses, its effects on central vision significantly interfere with the visual skills necessary for reading, driving, watching television, recognizing people, and performing many other activities of daily living (see Figure 13-1). Laser photocoagulation and photodynamic therapy are two interventions that are effective in treating the choroidal neovascularization that occurs in the wet form. Not all people with the wet form of AMD meet the medical criteria for these two treatments, however. The primary treatment goal for patients with either type of AMD is to simply reduce the risk for further vision loss.

The nurse's role in the management of AMD is often that of a support person who encourages the older adult to take advantage of vision rehabilitation programs to learn the most effective ways of compensating for declining vision. Although there is no cure for AMD, much current research is focused on developing treatments for this condition. Older adults with AMD can be encouraged to keep up to date on new developments by obtaining information from organizations listed in the Educational Resources section at the end of this chapter. People with AMD are usually taught to test their eyes daily using Amsler's grid (Figure 13-2) so that they will be aware of sudden changes. In long-term care settings and for older adults with memory problems, nurses may have to incorporate daily reminders or assistance with carrying out this task. Nurses also need to encourage people with AMD to receive ongoing evaluation by eye care practitioners to detect treatable aspects of this disease.

Glaucoma

The term *glaucoma* refers to a group of eye diseases in which the ganglion cells of the optic nerve are damaged by an abnormal buildup of aqueous humor in the eye. Aqueous humor is a clear fluid that is produced in the anterior chamber of the eye and normally helps maintain eye pressure between 10 and 20 mm Hg. If

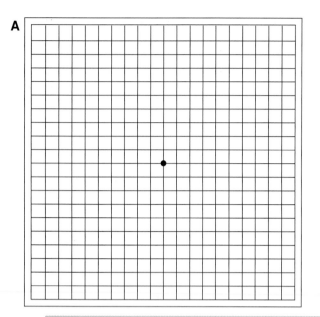

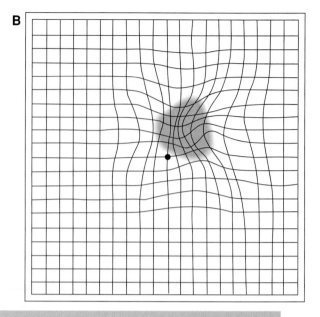

Instructions for Use

1. Tape this page at eye level where light is consistent and without glare.
2. Put on your reading glasses and cover one eye.
3. Fix your gaze on the center black dot.
4. Keeping your gaze fixed, try to see if any lines are distorted or missing.
5. Mark the defect on the chart.
6. TEST EACH EYE SEPARATELY.
7. If the distortion is new or has worsened, arrange to see your ophthalmologist at once.
8. **Always** keep the Amsler grid the **same distance** from your eyes each time you test.

FIGURE 13-2 Amsler grid. (A) People with age-related macular degeneration (AMD) use Amsler's grid to perform a simple daily test for sudden changes in their condition. (B) This is what the Amsler grid might look like to someone with AMD. (*Part A:* Reprinted with permission from American Macular Degeneration Foundation, 888-MACULAR, http://www.macular.org.)

the fluid is unable to flow out of the anterior chamber of the eye through the normal channel between the iris and the cornea, it accumulates and pushes the optic nerve into a cupped or concave shape. The resulting damage to the optic nerve causes a loss of peripheral vision. If left untreated, the damage can progress to blindness. About 8% of noninstitutionalized older adults have glaucoma, with a much higher prevalence among African Americans (15%) than whites (7%) (Desai et al., 2001). Glaucoma is the second leading cause of blindness in the United States and the leading cause of irreversible blindness in African Americans.

> African Americans have an earlier age of onset of glaucoma than do whites.

Chronic (open-angle) glaucoma, which accounts for as many as 90% of cases of glaucoma in the United States, occurs when the drainage canals become clogged. This condition has an insidious onset and does not cause vision changes until optic nerve damage occurs. Early signs include increased intraocular pressure, poor vision in dim lighting, and increased sensitivity to glare. If the condition progresses, manifestations include headaches, "tired eyes," impaired peripheral vision, a fixed and dilated pupil, the appearance of halos around lights, and frequent changes in the prescription for corrective lenses. Chronic glaucoma usually occurs in both eyes but may begin in only one eye and does not necessarily progress at the same rate in both eyes. Because chronic glaucoma progresses slowly and causes little or no visual impairments in the early stage, annual assessments of intraocular pressure are necessary to detect the condition before visual impairments occur. Chronic glaucoma is most commonly managed with medications, but surgical treatment options include argon laser surgery and other types of eye surgery. Medical management usually includes one or several types of eye drops administered one to four times daily. Miotics, prostaglandins, ß-blockers, adrenergic agonists, and carbonic anhydrase inhibitors are some of the types of drugs currently being used to treat chronic glaucoma.

Normal-tension glaucoma is another type of glaucoma that can occur in older adults. With this type of glaucoma, the intraocular pressure is within the normal range, but the optic nerve is damaged, and the visual field is narrowed (see Figure 13-1). Guidelines for the treatment of normal-tension glaucoma are not clear, but this condition is often managed with the same medications and surgical approaches that are used for chronic glaucoma.

Acute (closed-angle) glaucoma is caused by a sudden complete blockage of the flow of aqueous humor. This condition has an abrupt onset in one or both eyes and should be considered a medical emergency. People with acute glaucoma present with increased intraocular pressure, severe eye pain, clouded or blurred vision, dilation of the pupil, and nausea and vomiting. This condition may be precipitated by medications that cause pupil dilation, such as anticholinergics. Immediate treatment with medications may be effective for acute attacks, but surgical intervention is often needed.

Health education for older adults with glaucoma needs to focus on the importance of adherence to ongoing medication treatments as prescribed by the eye care practitioner. If older adults with glaucoma are admitted for institutional care, nurses need to ensure that eye drops for glaucoma are administered as ordered. In home care situations, nurses may need to develop a plan for administering eye drops on a daily or more frequent basis. If an older adult has memory problems, establishing a routine for administering eye drops can be quite challenging. Many times, complicated eye drop regimens can be simplified by working with the eye care practitioner to decrease the number of eye drops that are necessary or to prescribe a longer-acting medication that can be administered less frequently. Nurses play an important role in developing plans to ensure compliance with medication routines for people with glaucoma.

 Mrs. F. is now 72 years old and has been retired for several years. You are the nurse at her local senior center, and she makes an appointment to see you. A review of Mrs. F.'s medical history reveals that she has smoked a pack of cigarettes a day for 40 years. She reports that about 5 years ago, her doctor told her she had high blood pressure. She has also developed arthritis within the last 5 years. During a recent medical checkup, her doctor said he thought she had early cataracts, but he told Mrs. F. that he felt it was too early to do anything about them. She has never had an eye examination other than the checkup her regular doctor has done periodically. When asked about her symptoms, Mrs. F. tells you that she sometimes feels like there is a film over her eyes and that she has trouble seeing when she is

outside on sunny days. Mrs. F. says that she never liked wearing sunglasses and hopes she won't have to start wearing them now. She has recently purchased stronger reading glasses, and these help a little with reading and sewing.

 THINKING POINTS

➤ What factors likely contributed to the development of Mrs. F.'s cataracts?

➤ When Mrs. F. is driving during the day, what difficulties might she notice because of vision changes? Because of environmental conditions?

➤ When Mrs. F. is driving at night, what difficulties might she notice because of vision changes? Because of environmental conditions?

➤ When Mrs. F. is in her home, what changes in visual abilities might she notice because of cataracts and vision changes?

FUNCTIONAL CONSEQUENCES ASSOCIATED WITH VISION IN OLDER ADULTS

When the best-corrected visual acuity is 20/50 or worse, the person is said to have a "functional visual impairment" (Carter, 2001). The most serious visual impairments that affect older adults are generally caused by pathologic conditions, such as cataracts, glaucoma, or AMD, all of which are increasingly likely to occur with advanced age. People aged 65 years and older account for 30% of all visually impaired people in the United States and for almost 37% of all visits to physicians' offices for eye care. Trouble seeing, even with corrective lenses, affects 14% of people between the ages of 70 and 74 years and 32% of those 85 years of age and older (Desai et al., 2001). The following sections describe the functional consequences that are associated with the types of visual impairments that are most likely to occur in older adults.

> African Americans and Mexican Americans have a higher prevalence of blindness and visual impairment than do whites.

The Impact of Vision Changes on Safety and Function in Daily Activities

Because visual impairments are associated with many aspects of safety and independence, people who are visually impaired are likely to be more dependent on others for assistance with their activities of daily living. Wallhagen and colleagues (2001) studied the effects of vision and hearing impairments on more than 2400 adults between the ages of 50 and 102 years and found that vision impairments exerted a more wide-ranging impact on functional status, ranging from physical disability to social functioning (Wallhagen et al., 2001). The daily activities most directly influenced by age-related vision changes include getting outside; driving a vehicle; shopping for groceries; going up and down stairs; getting in and out of bed or a chair; maneuvering safely in dark or unfamiliar environments; seeing markings on clocks, radios, thermostats, appliances, and televisions; and reading newspapers, directories, small-print signs and posters, and labels on food items and medication containers. Most of these daily activities are affected by alterations in several visual skills. In addition, the ability to perform these activities is influenced significantly by glare, lighting, and other environmental factors.

Visual impairments also are associated with postural instability, gait and balance problems, and an increased risk for falls and fractures in older adults. Lord and Dayhew (2001), in a 1-year study of 156 community-living people between the ages of 63 and 90 years, found that impaired vision is an important and independent risk factor for falls. These researchers identified depth perception and distant-edge contrast sensitivity as two visual skills that were particularly important for maintaining balance and detecting and avoiding environmental hazards (Lord & Dayhew, 2001). Age-related vision changes that increase the risk for falls include diminished acuity, reduced visual field, impaired contrast sensitivity, and increased sensitivity to glare. West and colleagues (2002) found a significant association between mobility limitations and impaired acuity and contrast sensitivity. Additionally, delayed processing of visual information may interfere with the quick responses necessary for preventing falls. Cataracts and AMD also are likely to increase further the risk for falls. Visual impairments can interfere with the perception of environmental hazards and increase the likelihood of trip-related falls. Visual impairment may also increase the risk for serious injury secondary to falling.

The Impact of Vision Changes on Driving

Examination of the impact of age-related changes on the ability to drive safely illustrates the complex functional consequences of altered visual skills on the performance of daily activities. Because driving is an aspect of daily life associated with considerable safety and independence concerns for the individual who drives (as well as for his or her family), and because unsafe drivers can place others at risk, there has been increasing and intense interest in recent years in the

relationship between age-related visual changes and driving skills of older adults.

Visual dimensions that influence driving abilities are near vision, visual search, dynamic vision, light sensitivity, and visual processing speed. In older adults, slower dark and light adaptation creates problems when driving in and out of tunnels and when driving at night on streets with inconsistent lighting. Decreased peripheral vision interferes with the wide visual field that is important for avoiding collisions. Decreased acuity interferes with the perception of moving objects, especially vehicles moving at fast speeds. Diminished accommodation and acuity create problems when the older adult tries to read the speedometer or other dashboard instruments after focusing on the road. If the car has tinted windows, the diminished illumination further interferes with visual skills. Glare interferes with the perception of objects and is heightened by rainy, snowy, or sunny conditions. Bright sunlight shortly after sunrise or before sunset may significantly interfere with the perception of red and green traffic lights because of the older adult's increased sensitivity to glare. The consequences of visual impairment with regard to driving include increased difficulty with reading signs, adjusting to glare, seeing dimly lit display panels, accurately determining vehicle speed, and perceiving and responding to unexpected vehicles or obstructions.

The Impact of Vision Changes on Quality of Life

Age-related vision changes develop gradually and often go unnoticed for many years. As the changes progress to the point of interfering with activities of daily living, the older adult may withdraw from usual activities rather than acknowledge a vision problem or adjust to the changes. In a study of the impact of sensory impairment on older African American men and women, visual impairments were associated with a lower level of psychological well-being even after other factors such as functional limitations were controlled for (Bazargan et al., 2001). Visual impairments in residents of long-term care facilities are associated with disruptive behaviors, low levels of social engagement, and little or no involvement with activities (Horowitz, 1997; Resnick et al., 1997). Rovner and Casten (2002) found a high incidence of depression in older adults with AMD, with the level of depression increasing in relation to decreased participation in valued activities. In addition, depression contributed to excess disability by exacerbating visual limitations beyond what would be explained independently by the severity of visual loss (Rovner & Casten, 2002).

Of course, a person's usual lifestyle influences the extent of any psychosocial impact related to vision changes. If the leisure activities chosen by the older adult require good visual skills, such as with reading, sewing, or needlework, the older adult may become bored and even depressed when vision changes interfere with these endeavors. If artistic pursuits and entertainment events are important activities for the older adult, diminished visual function may interfere with the person's quality of life. By contrast, if the person prefers music or other activities that are less dependent on visual skills, the effect of vision impairment on the adult's usual lifestyle may be minimal.

One's living environment and support systems are other determinants of the psychosocial consequences of vision changes. Good visual skills are more important for people who live alone or who provide care for others than they are for people who live with, or have frequent contact with, others who have good vision. Also, if visually impaired people can modify their living environment to compensate for the impairments, the psychosocial consequences will be minimized. By contrast, people who live in institutional settings may experience relatively greater negative consequences because of unalterable environmental conditions.

Many older adults who notice declines in their vision develop fears that negatively impact their quality of life. For example, many people may mistakenly fear going blind because they think they have a serious and progressive disease. Fear of blindness may be based on myths, inaccurate information, or the experiences of friends who have serious visual impairments. Negative or hopeless attitudes about vision changes may deter the older person from acknowledging the problem or seeking help. Fear of falling is another serious concern for many older adults who notice visual changes. Inaccurate depth perception may lead to frequent bumping into objects, and the older adult may feel insecure and unsafe, even in familiar environments. If the person has experienced falls or tripping or knows someone who suffered a fracture as a result of falling, the fears may be magnified.

Figure 13-3 summarizes some of the important age-related changes, risk factors, and negative functional consequences that may affect vision in older adults.

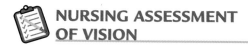

NURSING ASSESSMENT OF VISION

Nursing assessment of vision is aimed at identifying (1) risk factors for vision impairment that might be amenable to interventions, (2) existing visual disorders that might be amenable to interventions, (3) the impact of any vision changes on safety, independ-

ence, or quality of life, (4) opportunities for health promotion activities and other interventions, and (5) barriers to carrying out these activities and interventions. Nursing assessment of visual function is not a substitute for an examination by an eye care specialist. Whereas the purpose of an eye examination by an eye care specialist is to detect and initiate appropriate treatment of vision problems, the goal of the nursing assessment is to assist the older adult in minimizing the negative consequences of vision changes. Nursing assessment also aims at identifying modifiable risk factors that can be addressed in health promotion. Nurses assess visual abilities by interviewing the older adult (or, if the older adult is dependent, by interviewing his or her caregivers), by observing the older adult's ability to perform activities of daily living, and by testing the older adult's visual skills.

Interviewing About Vision Changes

Interview questions are used to elicit the following information: past and present risk factors for vision impairment, the person's awareness of any vision changes, the impact of these changes on daily activities and quality of life, and the person's attitudes about interventions (Display 13-1). The interview begins with direct questions about the person's awareness of any changes in vision. If the person acknowledges a visual impairment, additional details about the onset and progression of vision changes are elicited. Questions about symptoms that cause discomfort or that indicate the possible presence of disease processes also are asked.

Subsequent questions focus on the person's awareness of any differences in his or her usual activities that might be associated with vision changes. If the person has acknowledged vision changes, specific questions may be asked about how these changes have influenced everyday activities. If the person has denied that any vision changes have occurred, the nurse inquires about any changes in the performance of complex activities, such as driving, shopping, and meal preparation. Questions about leisure interests are incorporated into the interview to obtain additional information about the psychosocial consequences of vision impairments. Although the older adult may not associate lifestyle changes with vision impairments, questions about changes in hobbies and leisure activities may reveal a need for interventions to improve visual function.

Identifying Opportunities for Health Promotion

Nurses can identify opportunities for health promotion interventions by asking questions about the person's usual eye care practices and about potential

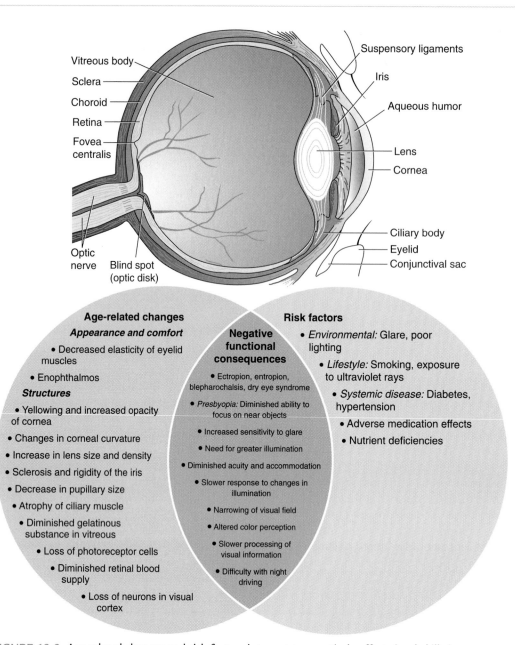

FIGURE 13-3 Age-related changes and risk factors intersect to negatively affect visual skills in older adults.

risk factors for eye disorders. Responses to questions about the source, frequency, and dates of the person's last eye examinations will provide information about his or her usual eye care practices. Answers to these questions are important in planning health promotion interventions that address the early detection of eye disease. Answers also might help the nurse identify myths or misunderstandings that should be addressed through health education. If visual impairment has been acknowledged, questions are asked to ascertain the person's attitude toward eye examinations and ongoing management of chronic conditions such as glaucoma. If a visual impairment has been denied, questions are directed toward identifying attitudes about early detection of treatable conditions.

Lastly, the identification of modifiable risk factors will provide an opportunity for health education. If the person has cataracts, AMD, or a family history of AMD, it is especially important to ask about cigarette smoking. If the older person is likely to spend time outdoors in sunny climates, an inquiry is made about exposure to sunlight. Placing this question toward the end of the interview sets the stage for educating the older adult about protective measures, such as the use of sunglasses. The nurse can then

Questions to Assess Awareness and Presence of Vision Impairment

- Have you noticed any changes in your vision during the past few years?
- Do you experience any uncomfortable symptoms, such as dry eyes?
- Do you have difficulty managing any of your usual activities because you have trouble seeing? (For instance, ask about the following: sewing, reading, driving, grooming, hobbies, preparing meals, watching television, managing money, writing letters, using the telephone, using dials on appliances, shopping for groceries, and going up and down stairs.)
- Have you ever tripped or fallen because you had trouble seeing?
- Have you stopped doing any activities because of vision problems? (For example, have you stopped driving at night because of difficulty seeing?)
- Are there things you would do if you could see better?

Questions to Ask if Vision Loss Is Acknowledged

- When did you first notice a loss of vision or a change in your ability to see?
- Have the changes been gradual, or did you notice sudden changes at any particular time?

- How would you describe the changes in your ability to see?
- Have you noticed pain, blurred vision, burning or itching, halos around lights, intolerance to bright light, a difference between day and night vision, or spots or flashing lights in front of your eyes?
- What kind of medical evaluation and care, if any, have you had for this problem?

Questions to Identify Opportunities for Education About Disease Prevention and Health Promotion

- When was the last time you had your eyes checked?
- Where do you go for eye care?
- Have you ever had your eyes checked for cataracts, glaucoma, and other eye conditions?
- What do you think about going for regular checkups for glaucoma and other eye problems?

Questions to Identify Risk Factors for Vision Loss

- When you spend time outdoors in the sun, do you use sunglasses or a hat to protect your eyes from bright light?
- Do you smoke cigarettes?
- Do you have a history of diabetes or hypertension?
- What medications do you take? (Refer to Table 13-2 to identify medications that may increase the risk for vision loss.)

incorporate education about corrective and adaptive measures to prevent eye disease and promote optimal visual health.

Observing Cues to Visual Function

Reliable information about a person's visual function can be obtained simply by being observant. The nurse begins by looking at the older person's eyes— are there any abnormalities, such as serious lid lag, that might interfere with visual function? Other, more subtle, indications that visual function is impaired may be detected by observing the person's appearance and ability to perform daily activities. Finally, observation of the person's home environment, if possible, may enable the nurse to identify environmental conditions that could be interfering with the person's ability to see.

Observations are judged in relation to the person's usual patterns of personal care and daily activities. For example, observation of spots and soiled marks on the person's clothing would be interpreted differently for someone known to be meticulous about his or her clothing than for an individual who had never showed much concern about personal

appearance. Observation of a person's ability to carry out activities of daily living are best made in the person's home or usual environment. When observing older people who are not in their usual environment, any circumstances that might influence their visual performance, either positively or negatively, are noted. An example of a positive influence might be the presence of good overhead lighting and good color contrast. Negative influences, such as glare from fluorescent lights reflecting on highly polished floors, are more likely to exist in an institutional setting than a home setting. Observations of the person's visual performance outside the home setting also must take into account the influences of factors such as illness, medication effects, psychological stress, changes in routines, and unavailability of corrective lenses. These influences are of particular concern in institutional settings and are likely to have a negative impact on the older person's performance of daily activities. In these settings, nurses can ask the older person and caregivers for information about the person's abilities in the home setting. Suggestions for observing behavioral and environmental cues related to visual function are listed in Display 13-2.

DISPLAY 13-2

Guidelines for Assessing Behavioral and Environmental Cues Related to Visual Performance

Behavioral Cues

- Is clothing spotted, soiled, or mismatched, in contrast to a former pattern of neatness and sense of style?
- Is makeup applied in heavy quantities, in contrast to the usual manner of application?
- Does the person rely heavily on nonvisual cues in performing usual activities, especially maneuvering in the environment (e.g., using the hands to find objects or to probe for obstacles)?

Environmental Cues

- What kind of lighting is used for various tasks? If the lighting is not adequate, can adjustments be made to improve the person's visual abilities?
- Does the person try to economize at home by using dim lights or no lights at all? If so, does this interfere with visual abilities or safe functioning?
- Where does the person usually sit in relation to light sources? Does glare from a facing window interfere with vision? Do shadows from lamps interfere with vision? Do overhead lights cause glare? Are light bulbs of sufficient wattage?
- What are the sources of light on stairways and hallways?
- Is there sufficient color contrast in the following areas: walls and floors; stairs and landings; furniture, walls, and floors; eating utensils and place settings; cooking utensils and counter tops; markings and background on appliance dials?
- Are nightlights used in hallways and bathrooms?

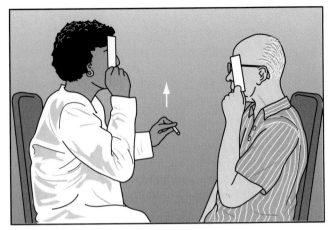

FIGURE 13-4 Performing the confrontation test to assess visual fields. The nurse and the patient sit approximately 2 feet apart. The patient covers his left eye, while the nurse covers her right eye. To test the inferior visual field, the nurse extends her left arm and slowly moves a pencil upward until the patient sees the pencil. The test is repeated for each of the remaining three visual fields (i.e., superior, temporal, and nasal), and then the four visual fields are tested for the other eye. With normal peripheral vision, the patient will see the pencil at the same time the nurse sees it.

Using Standard Vision Tests

Peripheral vision and acuity for near and distant objects can be measured using both formal and informal tests. These tests are not a substitute for a complete eye examination, but they can provide objective information that will assist the nurse in planning care and identifying the need for further evaluation. Some tests, such as checking distance vision with the Snellen chart, assessing visual fields with the confrontation test, and evaluating near vision by asking the person to read small-print text, require minimal equipment (Figure 13-4). Nursing assessment of these three parameters provides information about visual functions that often are affected by age-related changes and that influence the safe performance of daily activities.

For accurate assessment of visual skills, place a good light source above the person's head to provide lighting and to avoid shadows. If the person normally wears corrective lenses, make sure that they are clean and in place. Test each eye separately, using an appropriate eye cover; avoid using a hand as a cover.

To assess near acuity, the nurse can ask the person to read a newspaper or other printed material of various type sizes. An informal assessment of near acuity can also be made in cases in which the signature of an older person is required on a form. The nurse can ask the person to read a line or two of the form, subsequently observing his or her ability to find the signature line. Other opportunities for assessment may be created by providing written educational materials and asking the older person to read a specific part, such as a phone number to call.

The Snellen chart, described in Display 13-3, is a standard test for measuring distance acuity. An informal assessment of distance acuity, however, can also be accomplished by asking the older person to look out a window or down a hallway and to describe certain details, such as the words on a sign. This test is based on the assumption that the nurse's distance acuity is normal. When performing any distance vision tests in older adults, eliminate all sources of glare and make sure that color contrast for the viewed object is adequate.

A standard confrontation test provides a gross estimate of the peripheral visual fields of the examinee, as measured against the examiner's peripheral vision. As with informal distance acuity tests, the results of the confrontation test are based on a comparison with the examiner's visual skill, which must be normal for an accurate comparison to be made. Instructions for performing the confrontation test are given in Display 13-3.

DISPLAY 13-3
Guidelines for Using Vision Screening Tests

Using the Snellen Chart to Assess Distance Acuity

- Position the chart 20 feet away from the person, at eye level.
- If space does not permit a 20-foot distance, the distance between the person and the chart should be either 15 or 10 feet, with final measurements adjusted for distance. Alternatively, a scaled-down Snellen card can be used, if available.
- If the person usually wears corrective lenses, test the corrected vision.
- Ask the person to start reciting the letters in the line that can be read most easily; then ask him or her to read as many letters as possible in the lines directly below that line.
- Document the findings for each eye by noting the figure at the end of the last line on which at least half of the letters were read correctly.
- The upper figure denotes the distance of the person from the chart, whereas the lower figure denotes the distance from the chart at which a person with normal vision would be able to read the line. (That is, a vision measurement of 20/50 indicates that the person being tested can see things at a distance of 20 feet that a person with normal vision would be able to see at a distance of 50 feet.)
- Normal Snellen chart test results for older adults are as follows:
  - A corrected vision of 20/20 is considered to be normal.

- If a distance of 10 feet is used, the corrected vision should be 10/10.
- The average corrected vision for older adults ranges from 20/20 to 20/50.

Performing the Confrontation Test to Assess Peripheral Vision

- Sit directly across from the older person, about 2 feet away.
- Cover your left eye and have the examinee cover his or her right eye.
- Instruct the examinee to focus on your right eye while you focus on the examinee's left eye.
- Fully extend your right arm midway between you and the examinee.
- Slowly move your right hand, with the fingers wiggling, from the outer periphery toward the center, testing visual fields from top to bottom.
- While maintaining continuous eye contact, ask the examinee to report the point at which your fingers are visualized.
- Repeat these steps, covering your right eye and the examinee's left eye and using your left arm.
- Normal confrontation test results for older adults: your wiggling fingers should be seen simultaneously by both you and the older person in all quadrants.

➤ Recall that you are the nurse at the senior center in Mrs. F.'s neighborhood. During a recent visit, the 72-year-old Mrs. F. has mentioned to you that it is as if there is a "film" over her eyes and that she has trouble seeing when she is outside on sunny days. Her doctor believes that she may be in the early stages of cataract development, but he has told Mrs. F. that it is too soon for surgical intervention.

 THINKING POINTS

➤ Which questions from Display 13-1 would you ask Mrs. F. at this time?

➤ What sort of information might you be able to glean from behavioral or environmental cues about Mrs. F.'s ability to see (Display 13-2)?

➤ Would assessing Mrs. F.'s vision using vision screening tests be appropriate (Display 13-3)? Is so, which tests would you perform?

➤ What health promotion education would you give Mrs. F. at this time?

NURSING DIAGNOSIS

The nursing assessment is designed to identify both actual visual impairments and risk factors for poor visual function (e.g., a dimly lit environment). In addition, the nurse may be able to determine whether visual problems interfere with safety, self-care, or quality of life. An appropriate nursing diagnosis for an older adult with a visual impairment would be Disturbed Sensory Perception: Visual. This is defined as a "state in which the individual/group experiences or is at risk of experiencing a change in the amount, pattern, or interpretation of incoming stimuli" (Carpenito, 2002, p. 845). Related factors that commonly affect older adults include age-related vision changes (e.g., presbyopia), sensory organ alterations (e.g., glaucoma), and environmental factors (e.g., glare, dim lighting, or poor color contrast). The care plan in this chapter is based on a nursing diagnosis of Disturbed Sensory Perception: Visual related to age-related changes, sensory organ alterations, and environmental factors. Other nursing diagnoses might be addressed if the visual impairment interferes with the older adult's safety, quality of life, or performance of activities of daily living. Possible diagnoses to address these functional consequences include Anxiety, Activity Intolerance, Self-Care Deficit, Impaired Social Interaction, Impaired Physical Mobility, and Risk for Injury.

OUTCOMES

Nursing-sensitive outcomes that directly relate to the effectiveness of interventions to resolve or compensate for vision loss include Self-Care, Mobility Level, Anxiety Control, Cognitive Orientation, Social Involvement, Communication Ability, Personal Safety Behavior, and Quality of Life (Swanson & Drury, 2001). Indicators of health promotion goals that address eye health focus on maintaining vision at optimal level for the individual (Stevenson, 2001). The goal of attaining and maintaining optimal visual function is addressed by offering health education about early detection of vision disorders, managing conditions that affect vision, and providing eye comfort and protection measures. The goal of compensating for deficits in visual skills is addressed through health education about the use of low-vision aids and modifications of the living environment. The goal of improved quality of life for older adults who are visually impaired is addressed through health education interventions that foster increased safety and independent performance of activities of daily living and other desirable activities. Specific interventions to achieve these outcomes are discussed in the following section.

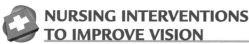 ## NURSING INTERVENTIONS TO IMPROVE VISION

Preventing Disease and Promoting Health

Prevention strategies include health education about reducing or eliminating risk factors that may cause visual impairments (Display 13-4). Because prolonged exposure to ultraviolet light (especially UV-B) may lead to visual impairment, nurses should teach older adults about the importance of protecting their eyes when they are out in sunlight. Broad-rimmed hats and close-fitting sunglasses with UV-B–absorbing lenses have the long-range effect of protecting the eyes from harmful rays; they also have the immediate benefit of screening out sun glare that can interfere with visual function. Older adults, as well as their caregivers, need to be educated about the benefits of these simple measures. Another modifiable risk factor for eye disease is smoking. People who have a

 DISPLAY 13-4
Health Promotion Teaching about Vision

Nurses can educate the older adult in the following areas:

Prevention and Early Detection of Disease
- The damaging effects of UV light and how to minimize exposure (broad-brimmed hats, close-fitting sunglasses with UV-absorbing lenses)
- The importance of annual eye examinations, including screening for glaucoma, cataracts, and retinal disease
- Eye care practitioners and what they do (see Display 13-5)
- The importance of managing diabetes and hypertension
- Smoking cessation
- The importance of timely evaluation of any changes in vision

Nutritional Considerations
- Include foods high in antioxidants (fruits and vegetables) and B-complex vitamins daily.
- Vitamins A, C, and E may have a protective role in preventing cataracts.
- People who have AMD may benefit from a daily supplement containing the following antioxidants and minerals: 500 mg vitamin C, 400 IU vitamin E, 15 mg beta-carotene, 80 mg zinc oxide, and 2 mg cupric oxide (copper).
- Avoid coffee, alcohol, artificial sweeteners, and excessive doses of riboflavin (i.e., more than 10 mg/day).

Compensating for Visual Impairments
- Referrals for vision rehabilitation if appropriate
- Bright, nonglare lighting and environmental modifications (see Displays 13-6 and 13-7)
- Low-vision aids (see Displays 13-8 and 13-9)

Complementary and Alternative Care Practices
- Herbs for prevention of cataracts: catnip, ginger, purslane, bilberry, rosemary, turmeric
- Homeopathic remedies for prevention of cataracts: silica, calcerea, phosphorus

diagnosis or family history of AMD should be taught about the relationship between smoking and AMD and should be encouraged to quit smoking. Strategies for encouraging older adults to quit smoking are discussed in Chapter 17. To reduce the risk for eye disease, people should be encouraged to include foods that are high in antioxidants. Display 13-4 provides additional details about nutritional considerations.

Because most eye diseases progress very slowly, disease prevention must also focus on regular vision examinations to detect the leading causes of visual impairment: cataracts, AMD, glaucoma, and diabetic retinopathy. Three objectives of *Healthy People 2010* are directed toward the early detection of cataracts, glaucoma, and diabetic eye disease; this is the first time vision objectives have been included in Healthy People initiatives (USDHHS, 2000). Nurses play an important role in achieving these objectives when they educate older adults and their caregivers about the importance of early detection of glaucoma and about treatments available for cataracts, glaucoma, and other eye disorders.

> About half of people with glaucoma do not know they have it, but Quigley and colleagues (2001) found that 62% of Hispanic Americans with glaucoma were undiagnosed.

It is recommended that people 35 years of age and older undergo biannual measurements of intraocular pressure to screen for glaucoma and that people 65 years of age and older undergo such measurements annually. Annual dilated eye examinations are rec-ommended for people with diabetes. Nurses can encourage older adults to take advantage of vision screening tests that might be available in the community through nonprofit organizations such as the Lions Club International. Even in the absence of disease conditions, annual eye examinations are an important tool for identifying people who would benefit from changes in eyeglasses. Munoz and colleagues (2000) studied Americans between the ages of 65 and 84 years and found that one third of the subjects with impaired vision improved to an acuity of 20/40 with refraction. In this same study, more than half of the subjects with visual impairment or blindness had conditions that were treatable or potentially preventable with interventions.

In providing health education, it may be helpful to review the differences between opticians, optometrists, and ophthalmologists (Display 13-5) with the person. Educational materials describing the scope of services of these eye care providers are distributed by some of the organizations listed in the Educational Resources section at the end of this chapter. The older adult may also benefit from the

---

DISPLAY 13-5
Eye Care Practitioners

Practitioners

Ophthalmologists are licensed doctors of medicine (M.D.) or osteopathy (D.O.) who are trained to diagnose and treat diseases and conditions of the eye. Ophthalmologic services include:

- Comprehensive eye examinations
- Diagnosis of eye diseases and disorders of the eye
- Prescription medications for eye problems (e.g., glaucoma)
- Eye surgery and postoperative care (e.g., cataracts)
- Laser treatments (e.g., retinopathy)
- Prescriptions for eyeglasses and contact lenses
- Prescriptions for low-vision aids
- Referrals for low-vision aids and training
- Medical referrals for diseases of the body that affect the eyes

Optometrists are licensed doctors of optometry (O.D.), not physicians, who are trained to examine eyes, screen for common eye problems, and prescribe eye exercises or corrective lenses. Optometrists use diagnostic medications, and in more than half the states in America, they can prescribe certain therapeutic drugs for eye diseases. Optometric services include:

- Comprehensive eye examinations
- Eye refractions to determine the need for corrective lenses

- Prescriptions for eyeglasses, contact lenses, and low-vision aids
- Vision therapy to improve certain skills, such as tracking and focusing the eyes
- Referrals for low-vision aids and training
- Referrals to physicians for surgery, medication, or further evaluation
- Diagnosis of eye disorders (in some states)
- Postoperative care (in some states)

Opticians are eye care practitioners who are trained to fit, adjust, and dispense eyeglasses and contact lenses that have been prescribed by an optometrist or ophthalmologist. In many states, opticians are licensed. They do not perform eye examinations or refractions, and they cannot prescribe corrective lenses or medications.

Health Insurance Coverage

Medicare and other health insurance programs cover many optometric and ophthalmologic services for the diagnosis and treatment of eye diseases. Routine eye examinations and corrective lenses usually are not covered, except by some supplemental or managed care plans. Beginning in 2002, Medicare covers annual dilated eye examinations for all people at high risk for glaucoma. After cataract surgery, eyeglasses and contact lenses are usually covered by health insurance if they are considered part of the cataract treatment. Optician services are not covered by Medicare.

many educational brochures that are available on the subjects of eye diseases, common vision problems, age-related eye changes, and low-vision aids. Nurses can use these publications to supplement and reinforce the health education components of their care plans. Local sight centers, or the organizations listed in the Educational Resources section at the end of this chapter, provide these materials at little or no cost, and some brochures are available in Spanish and other languages. Additionally, much of the information can be obtained and printed directly from these organizations' websites. The National Association for the Visually Handicapped (NAVH) is an excellent resource for information about interventions for older adults with visual impairments. In contrast to publications from organizations that focus primarily on blindness, materials from the NAVH are written for people with gradual and partial visual losses. The American Academy of Ophthalmology and the American Optometric Association also are good sources of free pamphlets about eye problems that commonly affect older adults. Do-it-yourself eye test kits are available from Prevent Blindness America. These kits enable people to determine whether they are seeing as well as they should and provide guidelines for obtaining further evaluation.

Teaching About Comfort Measures for Dry Eyes

If pertinent, simple measures to relieve dry eyes can be discussed. Use of over-the-counter artificial tears or ocular lubricants, especially before reading or other activities that require frequent eye movements, usually will afford symptomatic relief. People who use eye drops more frequently than every 3 hours should be advised to use preservative-free solutions to prevent any adverse effects from the preservatives. Other comfort measures, such as applying cold compresses or wearing wraparound glasses, are designed to prevent evaporation of tears. Maintenance of adequate environmental humidity, especially during the winter months or in dry climates, also decreases evaporation of eye moisture and adds to eye comfort. People who experience discomfort from dry eyes should avoid irritants, such as smoke and hairspray, as well as adverse environmental conditions, such as hot rooms and high wind. People who are bothered by dry eyes and are taking a medication that might exacerbate the discomfort should be encouraged to discuss the problem with their primary care practitioner.

Improving Safety and Function Through Environmental Adaptations

Simple environmental modifications can improve the older person's safe performance of activities of daily living, thereby reducing the risk for falls and accidents. Because many functional consequences result from the age-related reduction in retinal illumination, proper lighting is the single most important intervention that improves an older adult's vision. Increased illumination is one of the easiest and least costly modifications that can be made in any setting (Display 13-6). Both the quality and quantity of light are important when providing illumination for optimal visual performance. For example, selection of broad-spectrum fluorescent lights and daylight-simulating lamps may be particularly beneficial in compensating for age-related vision changes.

Another important consideration in adapting the environment for optimal visual function is color contrast. Appliances and other items, such as ovens, irons, radios, thermostats, and televisions,

DISPLAY 13-6
Considerations for Optimal Illumination

- Older adults need at least three times as much light as younger people do.
- Older adults function best in environments with bright, broad-spectrum, nonglaring, indirect sources of light.
- Place sources of illumination 1 to 2 feet away from the object to be viewed.
- Flickering light, such as that generated by a single fluorescent tube, will cause fatigue and decreased visual performance.
- Light bulbs should be kept clean.
- Replace light bulbs when they become dim, rather than waiting for them to burn out.
- The amount of light decreases fourfold when the distance is doubled.
- Increased illumination has a greater positive effect on impaired vision than it does on normal vision.
- A gradual decrease in illumination from foreground to background is better than sharp contrasts in lighting.
- Moderate overhead lighting can be used to enhance brighter foreground lighting and prevent sharp contrasts.
- To reduce glare from reading material, place the light source to the left side of right-handed readers and to the right side of left-handed readers.
- Avoid glossy paper for reading materials.

may be difficult to use because of poor color contrast around the control mechanisms. Modifications can easily be made to improve the older person's ability to use these items safely and accurately. For example, two dots of red nail polish can be used to mark the most commonly used temperature settings, and the older adult can be instructed to turn the dial above or below the dots for different settings.

Architectural designs and institutional constraints may limit the extent of environmental adaptations that nurses can implement in hospitals and nursing homes. In most settings, however, nurses can improve the visual abilities of older adults by using appropriate colors to enhance contrast, by using curtains to control light and glare, and by placing chairs in positions that enhance illumination and avoid glare. Nurses have many opportunities to teach older adults and their caregivers about the environmental modifications that are most effective for optimal visual function. Display 13-7 summarizes some environmental adaptations that may compensate for deficits in visual skills and improve safety. All older adults can benefit from these environmental modifications,

even in the absence of diagnosed eye disorders, because they are effective ways of improving vision for all people.

Improving Safety and Function Through the Use of Low-Vision Aids

People with visual impairments can improve their safety and quality of life through the use of low-vision aids that improve focus, contrast, magnification, or illumination (Display 13-8). Low-vision aids are most beneficial when used in conjunction with environmental modifications. For example, magnifiers are most effective when combined with measures that improve illumination and control glare. Reading glasses and other optical aids that magnify an image for visual tasks are available with or without a prescription. Nonoptical aids are devices that enhance contrast, reduce glare, improve lighting, or enlarge the image. Printed and Internet catalogues with illustrations of low-vision aids are available through many organizations (see the Educational Resources section). Also, local sight centers are good sources of low-vision aids and of training related to their use.

DISPLAY 13-7
Environmental Adaptations for Improving Visual Performance

Illumination, Glare Control, and Dark/Light Adaptation
- Position a 60- or 75-watt soft-white light bulb above and close to the head of the older person.
- Use a clear plastic shower curtain, rather than solid colors or printed curtains, for the tub or shower.
- Use light-colored, sheer curtains to eliminate glare from windows.
- Place nightlights in hallways and bathrooms, or keep a high-intensity flashlight at the bedside.
- Use illuminated light switches.
- Provide good lighting in stairways and hallways.
- Use illuminated or magnified mirrors.

Color Contrast
- Use brightly colored tape or paint on the edges of stairs, especially on the top and bottom steps.
- Use light-colored and dark-colored cutting boards to contrast with dark and light foods.
- Use contrasting, rather than matching, colors for china, placemats, and napkins.
- Use a toilet seat that contrasts with the bathroom walls and floor. Use colored bars of soap on white sinks and tubs.
- Use utensils with brightly colored handles.

- Place pillows of contrasting colors on stuffed furniture.
- Use decorative or lighted plates over light switches and wall sockets; avoid light switch plates that blend in with the wallpaper or paint.
- Place decorative items of contrasting colors, such as plants and ceramics, on tables to provide clues to depth, especially on light-colored furniture that is in a room with light-colored walls.
- Use brightly colored grooming utensils, such as combs, brushes, and razors.
- Use pens with black ink rather than blue ink.

General Adaptive Measures and Environmental Modifications
- Do not rearrange furniture without informing or showing the older person.
- Advise older adults to pause in doorways when going from light to dark rooms (or vice versa) to allow time for their eyes to adjust to the light change.
- Teach older people to use their feet and hands as probes to feel for curbs, steps, edges of chairs, and the like.
- When walking with an older person, stop when necessary to allow a change in focus from near to far and from light to dark.

DISPLAY 13-8
Low-Vision Aids for Improving Visual Performance

Enlargement Aids
- Microscopic spectacles
- Hand-held or standing magnifiers
- Binoculars and hand-held or spectacle-mounted telescopes
- Magnifying sheets
- Field expanders for diminished peripheral vision
- Large-print books, magazines, and newspapers
- Photocopy machines or laser printers (used to enlarge print)
- Telephones with enlarged letters and numbers, or a pad with enlarged letters and numbers designed to fit over rotary-dial or push-button phones
- Large numbers on rulers, playing cards, and other items
- Thermometers with good color coding and enlarged numbers
- Large-eye needles

Illumination Aids
- High-intensity lights
- Gooseneck lamps
- Floor or table lamps with three-way light bulbs

Contrast Aids
- Use of broad-tipped felt markers in dark, yet bright, colors and colored construction paper for making signs
- Red print on a yellow background or white letters on a green background
- Reading and signature guides (typoscopes)
- Clip-on yellow lenses

Glare Control Aids
- Sunglasses with UV-absorbing lenses
- Sun visors and broad-rimmed hats
- Nonglare (antireflective) coating on eyeglasses
- Yellow and pink acetate sheets
- Pinhole occluders

Although special low-vision aids must be ordered through catalogues or obtained at sight centers, everyday items, if used advantageously, can serve as low-vision aids. An example of a low-vision aid that may be available to nurses is a photocopy machine that can be used to convert regular-print materials into large-print materials. Likewise, household lamps, placed in the correct position and equipped with the right wattage bulb, can also serve as low-vision aids. Lighthouse International (listed in the Educational Resources section) provides educational materials that illustrate examples of effective color contrast and effective ways of making text legible. These free materials, which can be obtained through the mail or from the Internet, can be used as guides for developing more readable printed materials for signage, health education, and other purposes.

Training in the use of low-vision aids should be provided to maximize the beneficial effects on visual performance. For example, the likelihood that an illumination aid is placed in the most effective position may be increased if the person understands that halving the distance of a light source increases the illumination fourfold. As an illustration of this principle, a light bulb that is 1 foot away from someone will provide four times as much illumination as one that is 2 feet away. To teach others how to adapt to visual limitations, nurses should be familiar with the basic principles of illumination (see Display 13-6) and magnification (Display 13-9). Local sight centers provide detailed training in the use of low-vision aids, and the NAVH publishes a helpful guide regarding their use. *Healthy People 2010* objective 28-10 is to "increase the use of vision rehabilitation services and adaptive devices by people with visual impairments" (USDHHS, 2000). Nurses have an important role in meeting this objective by becoming familiar with local vision rehabilitation services and suggesting that older adults and their families use these resources.

Maintaining and Improving Quality of Life

As discussed earlier, the psychosocial consequences of impaired vision can be quite significant for older adults. Many of the interventions that help older adults

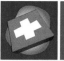

DISPLAY 13-9
Guidelines for Using Magnifying Aids

Using a Hand-Held Magnifier
- Begin with the magnifier close to the reading material.
- Slowly move the magnifier toward the face until the image totally fills the lens.
- For optimal focus, move the magnifier back toward the print about a distance of 2 cm.

Using a Stand Magnifier
- Rest the stand flat against the reading material.
- Do not move the stand.

Using a Spectacle-Mounted Magnifier
- Begin with the reading material close to the nose.
- Slowly move the material away until it becomes clear.

compensate for visual deficits and function at their highest level also will improve their quality of life and address the psychosocial consequences of impaired vision. For example, the use of appropriate reading glasses and good environmental lighting may enable older adults to read books, newspapers, and magazines. Subsequently, they may experience an improvement in their quality of life because they have more satisfying social interactions and increased intellectual stimulation.

> Mrs. F. is now 81 years old. She had cataract surgery and an intraocular lens implant in her left eye when she was 76 years old, and in her right eye when she was 77 years old. Her vision was good until a year ago when she developed macular degeneration. She knows this condition will be progressive, but she continues to drive and live alone. Her current medical conditions are arthritis, hypertension, and coronary artery disease. She quit smoking several years ago after she was hospitalized for her coronary artery disease. You are the nurse at the senior center where Mrs. F. comes for lunch several times a week. During a conversation with you, Mrs. F. confides that she is terrified of becoming totally blind and of losing her independence. Her grandmother went blind several years before she died and had to move to a nursing home.

 THINKING POINTS

> Which nursing diagnosis or diagnoses would you apply to Mrs. F. at this time?

> Which information in Displays 13-4 through 13-9 might be appropriate for Mrs. F.?

> What health promotion advice would you give?

> Would you suggest any referrals for information or community resources?

> What interventions would address Mrs. F.'s fear of becoming blind and losing her independence?

EVALUATING EFFECTIVENESS OF NURSING INTERVENTIONS

Nurses observe compensatory behaviors of visually impaired older adults to evaluate the effectiveness of interventions for Disturbed Sensory Perception: Visual. Two indicators of success include wearing correct eyeglasses or contact lenses and reading newsprint (Swanson & Drury, 2001). Outcomes that address self-care or personal safety behavior could be measured according to improved ability of the older adult to perform other tasks, such as dressing, personal care, using appliances, and managing medications. Assessment of

abilities before interventions and reassessment after interventions provides objective criteria for evaluating the effectiveness of nursing interventions. If goals address the psychosocial impact of visual impairment and improved quality of life is identified as a desired outcome, nurses could observe the extent to which interventions improve the person's ability to participate in enjoyable activities. Specifically, nurses could assess the impact of interventions such as environmental adaptations and low-vision aids. For example, better lighting and the use of a large-print *Reader's Digest* may enable someone to enjoy reading again.

Health promotion goals are long term and focus on maintaining vision at optimal level. Goals and interventions vary according to different health care settings. For example, one goal might be for an older adult to obtain an evaluation of vision problems. Nurses in institutional settings would address these goals through a discharge plan that includes information about local resources for further evaluation. Also, the discharge plan might include suggestions for obtaining educational materials from a local sight center or one of the resources listed at the end of this chapter. Evaluation of the effectiveness of this health education would be based on the person's indication of his or her intent to follow through with the recommended referral or course of action. In home, community, and long-term care settings, nurses may be able to facilitate referrals for vision screening or other vision care services. In these settings, the evaluation of the effectiveness of interventions could be based on feedback from the older adults or their caregivers about the actual use of suggested resources.

CHAPTER SUMMARY

Beginning at about the age of 40 years, adults experience the earliest effects of age-related vision changes when they notice they need reading glasses for small print. Additional age-related vision changes include diminished depth perception, a narrower visual field, difficulty seeing objects clearly, an increased sensitivity to glare, and delayed adaptation to dark and light. Older adults are also likely to have visual impairments as a result of common eye conditions such as cataracts, AMD, and glaucoma. Visual impairments can have a significant impact on the performance of daily activities, such as reading, shopping, walking safely, and seeing markings on objects such as clocks and appliances. Also, older adults are at increased risk for falls and injuries because of difficulty maneuvering safely in stairways and unfamiliar or dimly lit environments.

Nursing assessment of vision focuses on identifying risk factors (e.g., dimly lit environments), problems with visual skills (e.g., increased glare sensitivity), opportunities for health promotion (e.g., reduction of risk factors), and the psychosocial consequences of impaired vision (e.g., impaired social interaction). Relevant nursing diagnoses include Sensory-Perceptual Alterations: Visual; Activity Intolerance; Self-Care Deficit; and High Risk for Injury. Nursing care is directed toward assisting the older adult to attain and maintain optimal visual function and to compensate for any visual limitations. Interventions focus on environmental modifications, use of low-vision aids, and health education about interventions. Nursing care is evaluated according to the degree of improvement in level of function, the use of low-vision aids, the effectiveness of environmental modifications, and the response of the older adult to the suggested resources. Numerous patient education resources are readily available from the resources listed at the end of this chapter.

CONCLUDING CASE STUDY AND NURSING CARE PLAN

➤ Mrs. F. is now 86 years old and is recovering from a recent fractured hip, which occurred when she fell while getting out of bed to go to the bathroom at night. After a brief hospitalization for surgical repair of the fractured hip and a 2-week period of skilled rehabilitation, Mrs. F. was referred to a home care agency for further rehabilitation therapy, assessment and monitoring of her medical status, and evaluation of her ability to manage at home.

In addition to AMD, Mrs. F.'s current medical diagnoses include arthritis, hypertension, coronary artery disease, and congestive heart failure. Mrs. F.'s medical conditions had been stable for several years, but during her hospitalization for the fractured hip, she was started on oxygen, and her medications were changed. Current medications are furosemide, 40 mg daily; digoxin, 0.125 mg daily; and enalapril, 10 mg twice daily. A 2-g sodium diet has been prescribed, and she has been discharged with an order for oxygen per nasal cannula at a rate of 2 L/min as needed.

Before her accident, despite the visual limitations from macular degeneration, Mrs. F. had lived alone in her own home, but her daughter has become increasingly concerned about her mother's safety. Now Mrs. F.'s daughter is convinced that her mother should not remain in her own home but should instead move to an assisted-living facility. Mrs. F. is adamant in her desire to stay in her own home and says the only reason she fell and broke her hip was because she was rushing to get to the bathroom. She says she has learned a lesson and will not hurry when she gets up at night. Furthermore, she says, she gave up driving to satisfy her daughter last year—now she's to give up her home, too? Mrs. F.'s daughter is staying with her mother

for a couple of weeks until her mother regains her mobility to the point of independence. The daughter hopes that in the interim, she will be able to convince her mother to make arrangements to move to an assisted-living facility. You are the home care nurse working with Mrs. F. in her home.

Nursing Assessment

During your initial nursing assessment, you determine that Mrs. F. is motivated to regain her mobility and manage her medical conditions, but she has difficulty reading small-print instructions because of poor vision. When you review Mrs. F.'s medications with her, you observe that she cannot read the labels on the bottles. You also observe that Mrs. F. keeps her medications on the shelf above the kitchen counter, where the lighting is very dim. When you review the proper use of the oxygen, you note that she has difficulty seeing the markings on the flowmeter. Her daughter has been helping her with these regimens, but Mrs. F. hopes to perform these activities independently so that she can remain in her own home.

Mrs. F. tells you that she is not concerned about falling because she knows she will not hurry when she gets up during the night to go to the bathroom. She now uses a walker and says she feels safe. Her daughter expresses concern about her mother managing the oxygen and the walker when going to the bathroom. Mrs. F. uses the oxygen when she sleeps, and her daughter is skeptical about her ability to get to the bathroom without rushing.

You observe that the hallway between the bedroom and bathroom is dark and that the bedroom has an overhead light, but no bedside lamp. The bathroom has a narrow doorway, and the toilet is at the other side of the sink. You assess the home for safety and determine that the pathways are clear and there is good lighting on the stairway and in the living areas. You identify no additional risks (e.g., throw rugs) to Mrs. F.'s safe mobility, but you do have concerns about Mrs. F.'s ability to safely navigate to the toilet with a walker.

When questioned about her vision problems, Mrs. F. gives her history of successful cataract surgery and a diagnosis of AMD at the age of 80 years. She sees her ophthalmologist every year, and he has told her that her vision will get worse and there's nothing to be done about it. He had mentioned that the local sight center provides some rehabilitation services for people with low vision, but he told her that those services are mostly for "younger blind people." Also, she is concerned that the sight center will suggest she purchase items that cost a lot of money, which she wouldn't be able to afford anyway. She says her daughter got her a subscription for the large-print *Reader's Digest*, which she enjoys, and that she's not interested in reading the newspaper because she watches the news on television. She has an appointment to see her eye doctor next month.

■ Nursing Diagnosis

In addition to the nursing diagnoses related to Mrs. F.'s medical condition, you identify a nursing diagnosis of Disturbed Sensory Perception: Visual, related to age-related changes, sensory organ alterations, and environmental factors. Supporting evidence for this diagnosis can be found in Mrs. F.'s inability to read labels, instructions, or the flowmeter markings, and in the environmental factors that contribute to unsafe mobility. The nursing diagnoses of Anxiety, Self-Care Deficit, and Risk for Injury might also be applicable. The diagnosis of Sensory-Perceptual Alterations: Visual, however, addresses the source of Mrs. F.'s anxiety, risk for injury, and inability to perform her instrumental activities of daily living and therefore is probably the most comprehensive diagnosis. Also, this diagnosis prompts you to include a long-term goal of encouraging further evaluation and management of the visual impairments.

■ Nursing Care Plan

The nursing care plan you develop for Mrs. F. is given in Display 13-10.

 CRITICAL THINKING EXERCISES

1. Consider the following questions in relation to Mrs. F. at 86 years of age:
   - How would you address concerns about Mrs. F. living alone? What aspects of her safety and quality of life would you consider?
   - How would you use any of the displays in this chapter for health promotion teaching?
   - What additional nursing diagnoses and outcomes would you identify for Mrs. F.?
   - What additional interventions and referrals would you consider for Mrs. F.?
   - Identify at least one resource in your community that might provide help or information for Mrs. F. Call that agency to obtain information about their services.
2. Describe presbyopia and explain the functional consequences of this condition in the everyday life of an older adult.
3. What environmental factors are likely to interfere with the visual function of older adults?

4. Describe the specific effects of glaucoma, cataracts, or AMD on one's ability to see a television program.
5. How would you assess the visual abilities of an older adult?
6. Explain the differences between opticians, optometrists, and ophthalmologists.
7. List at least 10 adaptations that might be implemented to improve the visual function of older adults.

Future Directions for Healthier Aging: Focus on Vision

- A goal of the National Institute on Aging Action Plan for Aging Research for 2001–2005 is to work with the National Eye Institute to continue identifying risk factors for age-related vision decline. Current research is focusing on improving functional independence of visually impaired older adults and on redesigning products and developing new technologies to make reading easier (National Institute on Aging, 2001).
- Longitudinal and population-based studies are being used to identify modifiable health-related risk factors to lay the groundwork for aggressive programs of prevention, particularly for cataracts, glaucoma, and AMD.
- Researchers are examining the complex relationships between neural function and vision changes, with practical implications for prevention of falls. Visual abilities in relation to falls, gait, balance, stumbles, and proprioception are being addressed (Fozard & Gordon-Salant, 2001).
- Because of the intense interest in the impact of vision changes on one's ability to drive safely and the lack of adequate standardized criteria for evaluating driver safety, tools are being developed to determine whether people are safe drivers.
- The National Eye Institute has funded bioengineering research with the goal of developing new optical and electronic devices to improve visual function, with particular emphasis on visual skills involved in safe driving. Bioptic telescopes are available to help compensate for some of the visual loss that interferes with safe driving; other bioptic techniques are under investigation for their role in improving driving safety for people with visual impairments. Updated information on new developments in these areas can be found on the websites of Lighthouse International and the National Eye Institute.

DISPLAY 13-10 • NURSING CARE PLAN FOR MRS. F.

EXPECTED OUTCOME	NURSING INTERVENTIONS	NURSING EVALUATION
Mrs. F. will manage her medication regimen accurately and independently.	• Print simplified medication instructions on large index cards using black felt-tip marker. • Use colored dots to match pill bottles with instruction cards. • Establish a medication management system using pill organizer boxes with markings that are bold and have good color contrast. • Teach Mrs. F. how to fill the pill boxes weekly, using the index cards you prepared for her. • Suggest that Mrs. F. fill the pill boxes at the kitchen table during daylight hours while using overhead light.	• Mrs. F. will demonstrate that she can accurately fill the pill boxes. • Mrs. F. will take her medications correctly. • Mrs. F.'s daughter will observe that her mother follows the prescribed regimen.
Mrs. F. will self-administer oxygen as needed.	• Use a copy machine to enlarge the small-print instructions for the oxygen equipment. • Place a colored dot at the 2-L mark on the flowmeter. • Keep the oxygen tank in a well-lit location and suggest using a flashlight to help illuminate the flowmeter setting.	• Mrs. F. will demonstrate the safe and independent operation of the oxygen equipment. • Mrs. F.'s daughter will observe that her mother administers her oxygen correctly.
Mrs. F. will be able to use a commode safely and independently.	• Ask Mrs. F. to use a bedside commode during the night; emphasize the importance of preventing another fall. • Work with physical and occupational therapists to (1) evaluate the feasibility of installing grab bars or other devices that will assist Mrs. F. in safely using the toilet; (2) identify a safe way for Mrs. F. to use the bathroom during the daytime; (3) teach Mrs. F. to transfer between the bed and commode for nighttime use; (4) teach her to empty the bedside commode. • Place a lamp on the nightstand and make sure that Mrs. F. can turn it on easily while in bed. Teach Mrs. F. to turn the bedside lamp on and sit at the edge of the bed for a few minutes before getting up at night.	• Mrs. F. will demonstrate that she safely uses the bathroom during the day and a bedside commode at night. • Mrs. F. will be able to empty the commode independently. • Mrs. F. will have no further falls in the bathroom.
Mrs. F. will compensate as much as possible for her progressive visual loss.	• Educate Mrs. F. and her daughter about the services provided at the local sight center for people with low vision; emphasize that these services address the needs of older adults and people with recent and progressive visual loss. The services are for anyone with low vision, and there are many low-vision aids available to improve the visual function of people with macular degeneration. • Suggest that Mrs. F. ask her eye doctor for a referral to the sight center when she sees him next month. • Include Mrs. F.'s daughter in the discussion about these services, and ask her to assist with following through once a referral is obtained.	• Mrs. F. will make and keep an appointment for an initial evaluation at the sight center. • Mrs. F. will use low-vision aids to improve visual function.

EDUCATIONAL RESOURCES

American Academy of Ophthalmology
P.O. Box 7424, San Francisco, CA 94120-7424
(415) 561-8500
http://www.aao.org/news/eyenet

American Foundation for the Blind
11 Penn Plaza, Suite 300, New York, NY 10001
(800) 232-5463
http://www.afb.org

American Optometric Association
243 North Lindbergh Blvd., St. Louis, MO 63141
(314) 991-4100
http://www.aoanet.org

Canadian National Institute for the Blind
1929 Bayview Avenue, Toronto, ON M4G 3E8
(416) 486-2500
http://www.cnib.ca

The Glaucoma Foundation
116 John Street, Suite 1605, New York, NY 10038
(212) 285-0080
http://www.glaucoma-foundation.org

Lighthouse International
111 East 59th Street, New York, NY 10022
(212) 821-9200
Toll-free: (800) 829-0500
http://www.lighthouse.org

Lions Clubs International
300 West 22nd Street, Oak Brook, IL 60523-8842
(630) 571-5466
http://www.lionsclubs.org

National Association for Visually Handicapped (NAVH)
22 West 21st Street, New York, NY 10010
(212) 889-3141
http://www.navh.org

National Eye Institute (NEI)
31 Center Drive, MSC 2510, Building 31, Room 6A32
Bethesda, MD 20892-2510
(301) 496-5248
http://www.nei.nih.gov

Prevent Blindness America
500 East Remington Road, Schaumburg, IL 60173
(800) 331-2020
http://www.preventblindness.org

REFERENCES

Bazargan, M., Baker, R. S., & Bazargan, S. H. (2001). Sensory impairments and subjective well-being among aged African American person. *Journal of Gerontology: Psychological Sciences, 56B,* P268–278.

Carpenito, L. J. (2002). *Nursing diagnosis: Application to clinical practice* (9th ed.). Philadelphia: Lippincott Williams & Wilkins.

Carter, T. L. (2001). Vision changes and care. In M. D. Mezey (Ed.), *The encyclopedia of elder care* (pp. 673–676). New York: Springer.

Christen, W. G., Glynn, R. J., Ajani, U. A., et al. (2000). Smoking cessation and risk of age-related cataract in men. *Journal of the American Medical Association, 284*(6), 713–716.

Desai, M., Pratt, L. A., Lentzner, H., & Robinson, K. N. (2001). *Trends in vision and hearing among older Americans. Aging Trends, No. 2.* Hyattsville, MD: National Center for Health Statistics.

Fozard, J., & Gordon-Salant, S. (2001). In J. E. Birren & K. W. Schaie (Eds.), *The psychology of aging* (5th ed., pp. 241–266). San Diego: Academic Press.

Horowitz, A. (1997). The relationship between vision impairment and the assessment of disruptive behaviors among nursing home residents. *Gerontologist, 37*(5), 620–628.

Lord, S. R., & Dayhew, J. (2001). Visual risk factors for falls in older people. *Journal of American Geriatrics Society, 49,* 508–515.

Munoz, B., West, S. K., Rubin, G. S., Scheim, O. D., Quigley, H. A., Bressler, S. B., & Bandeen-Roche, K. (2000). Causes of blindness and visual impairment in a population of older Americans: The Salisbury Eye Evaluation Study. *Archives of Ophthalmology, 118,* 819–825.

National Institute on Aging. (2001). *Action plan for aging research: Strategic plan for fiscal years 2001–2005.* Washington, DC: U.S. Department of Health and Human Services. HIH Publication No. 01-4961.

Quigley, H. A., West, S. K., Rodriguez, J., Munoz, B., Klein, R., & Snyder, R. (2001). The prevalence of glaucoma in a population-based study of Hispanic subjects: VER. *Archives of Ophthalmology, 119,* 1819–1826.

Resnick, H. E., Fries, B. E., & Verbrugge, L. M. (1997). Windows to their world: The effect of sensory impairments on social engagement and activity time in nursing home residents. *Journal of Gerontology: Social Sciences, 52B,* S135–S144.

Rovner, B. W., & Casten, R. J. (2002). Activity loss and depression in age-related macular degeneration. *American Journal of Geriatric Psychiatry, 10,* 305–310.

Schlienger, R. G., Haefelia, W. E., Jick, H., & Meier, C. R. (2001). Risk of cataract in patients treated with statins. *Archives of Internal Medicine, 161,* 2021–2026.

Stevenson, J. S. (2001). Health seeking behaviors. In M. L. Maas,, K. C. Buckwalter, M. D. Hardy, T. Tripp-Reimer, M. G. Titler, & J. P. Specht (Eds.), *Nursing care of older adults: Diagnoses, outcomes, and interventions* (pp. 75–85). St. Louis: Mosby.

Swanson, E. A., & Drury, J. (2001). Sensory/perceptual alterations. In M. L. Maas, K. C. Buckwalter, M. D. Hardy, T. Tripp-Reimer, M. G. Titler, & J. P. Specht (Eds.), *Nursing care of older adults: Diagnoses, outcomes, and interventions* (pp. 476–491). St. Louis: Mosby.

U.S. Department of Health and Human Services (USDHHS). (2000). *Healthy people 2010* (2nd ed). Washington, DC: U.S. Government Printing Office.

Wallhagen, M. I., Strawbridge, W. J., Shema, S. J., Kurata, J., & Kaplan, G. A. (2001). Comparative impact of hearing and vision impairment on subsequent functioning. *Journal of the American Geriatrics Society, 49,* 1086–1092.

Weintraub, J. M., Willett, W. C., Rosner, B., Colditz, G. A., Seddon, J. M., & Hankinson, S. E. (2002). Smoking cessation and risk of cataract extraction among US women and men. *American Journal of Epidemiology, 155,* 72–79.

West, C. G., Gildengorin, G., Haegerstrom-Portnoy, G., Schenck, M. E., Lott, L., & Brabyn, J. A. (2002). Is visual function related to physical functional ability in older adults? *Journal of the American Geriatrics Society, 50,* 136–145.

Yanoff, M. (1999). *Ophthalmology.* St. Louis: Mosby.

Digestion and Nutrition

LEARNING OBJECTIVES

1. Delineate age-related changes that affect eating patterns and digestive processes.

2. List the age-related changes in nutritional requirements for calories, protein, carbohydrates and fiber, fats, and water.

3. Discuss risk factors that affect the digestion and nutrition of older adults.

4. Identify the functional consequences of age-related changes and risk factors affecting digestion and nutrition.

5. Describe interview questions, behavioral cues, physical assessment and laboratory data, and assessment tools that may be useful in assessing digestion and nutrition in older adults.

6. Identify nursing interventions to address risk factors that interfere with digestion and nutrition, to promote good oral and dental care, and to promote optimal nutrition in older adults.

Digestion of food and maintenance of nutrition are influenced to a small degree by age-related gastrointestinal changes and to a large degree by risk factors that commonly occur in older adulthood. Older adults can easily adjust their eating habits to compensate for age-related changes in the digestive tract, but they have more difficulty compensating for the consequences of the many factors that interfere with their ability to obtain, prepare, and enjoy food.

Age-related changes and functional consequences are discussed in relation to digestion, eating patterns, and nutritional requirements.

 ## AGE-RELATED CHANGES THAT AFFECT DIGESTION AND EATING PATTERNS

Age-related changes affect the senses of smell and taste and all the organs of the digestive tract. These changes have very few functional consequences for healthy older adults, but they increase the vulnerability of older adults to risk factors.

Smell and Taste

Although the senses of both taste and smell affect food enjoyment, the sense of smell has a more significant influence and declines more than does the sense of taste in older adults. The ability to smell depends on the perception of odorants by the sensory cells in the olfactory mucosa and on central nervous system processing of that information. The ability to detect and identify odors is best around the age of 30 years, then gradually declines. Age-related changes in the central nervous system contribute to this decline, as do other factors such as cigarette smoking, vitamin B_{12} deficiency, medications (e.g., antihistamines, diltiazem, streptomycin), periodontal disease and oral infections, upper respiratory diseases (e.g., sinusitis), systemic diseases (e.g., dementia, diabetes, hypothyroidism), and occupational experiences (e.g., working in a factory) (Bromley, 2000; Finkel et al., 2001; Morley, 2002).

A survey of adults in America and Africa found that African respondents reported better olfactory function than did American respondents (Barber, 1997).

The ability to taste depends primarily on receptor cells in the taste buds, which are located on the tongue, palate, and tonsils. Characteristics of taste sensation are measured according to the ability to perceive intensity of taste, which diminishes with aging, and the ability to identify different tastes. Although taste cells can regenerate and are replaced every few days, a small decline in the number of taste cells—and a concomitant decrease in the ability to identify food based on taste—occurs with aging. Because these age-related changes do not affect all taste sensations equally, healthy older adults maintain the ability to detect sweet taste but have more

difficulty detecting sour, salty, and bitter tastes. Older adults who are malnourished, use dentures, take medications, or have medical conditions are likely to experience significant difficulty in detecting tastes.

Oral Cavity

Digestion begins when food enters the mouth and is acted on by the teeth, saliva, and neuromuscular structures responsible for mastication. Age-related changes in the teeth and support structures influence digestive processes and food enjoyment. With increased age, the tooth enamel becomes harder and more brittle, the dentin becomes more fibrous, and the nerve chambers become shorter and narrower. Because of these age-related changes, the teeth are less sensitive to stimuli and more susceptible to fractures. These changes, along with decades of abrasive and erosive action, also cause a gradual flattening of the chewing cusps. The bones supporting the teeth of older adults diminish in height and density, and teeth may loosen or fall out, particularly in the presence of pathologic conditions (e.g., periodontal disease).

Saliva and the oral mucosa play important roles in digestion. Saliva is essential for promoting chewing and swallowing and for maintaining a moist oral mucosa. Saliva facilitates digestion by supplying digestive enzymes, regulating oral flora, remineralizing the teeth, cleansing the taste buds, lubricating the soft tissue, and preparing food for chewing. Saliva production does not significantly diminish in healthy older adults, but about 30% of older adults experience xerostomia (dry mouth) because of medications and disease processes, as discussed in the section on risk factors (Ghezzi et al., 2000; Ship et al., 2002). Age-related changes of the oral mucosa include loss of elasticity, atrophy of epithelial cells, and diminished blood supply to the connective tissue. Age-related changes can be exacerbated by conditions common in older adults (e.g., xerostomia, vitamin deficiencies), making the oral mucosa more friable and susceptible to infection and ulceration.

Age-related neuromuscular changes that can affect mastication and swallowing include diminished muscle strength and slower swallowing. Although these age-related changes do not have a major impact on healthy older adults, they may increase the probability that older adults will develop dysphagia and other swallowing problems (Nicosia et al., 2000). Problems with chewing and swallowing in older adults are generally attributable to risk factors, such as tooth loss or neurologic conditions, rather than to age-related changes alone.

Esophagus

The second phase of digestion occurs when a combination of propulsive and nonpropulsive waves propels food through the pharynx and esophagus into the stomach. In older adults, the intensity of propulsive waves decreases, and the frequency of nonpropulsive waves increases. This condition is called *presbyesophagus*. Researchers disagree about whether presbyesophagus is caused by age-related or pathologic processes, and whether it slows the transit time or affects the esophageal sphincter. They do agree, however, that the functional impact of presbyesophagus is minimal, and that most esophageal dysfunction is attributable to pathologic conditions such as diabetes mellitus or neurologic disease (Jensen et al., 2001; Shaker & Staff, 2001).

Stomach

After passing through the esophageal sphincter, food enters the stomach, where gastric enzymes liquefy it and gastric action transforms it into chyme. As with esophageal changes, researchers disagree about the cause, extent, and consequences of gastric changes, but they agree that aging is associated with a modest slowing of gastric emptying, particularly when larger amounts of food are consumed (Horowitz, 2000; Jensen et al., 2001; Morley, 2002). Delayed gastric emptying may explain the early satiation (feeling full with less food intake) common in older adults.

Some earlier studies, which mostly focused on people with gastrointestinal symptoms, suggested that gastric secretions diminished in older adults; however, recent studies have not found any significant age-related decline in secretion of acid and pepsin by the stomach (Jensen et al., 2001). More than 80% of older adults maintain normal gastric acid secretion, and secretions may even increase in some older people (Linder & Wilcox, 2001). Diminished gastric acid secretion (achlorhydria) in older adults is likely to be caused by pathologic conditions such as atrophic gastritis or *Helicobacter pylori* infection (Horowitz, 2000; Jensen et al., 2001).

Small Intestine

After the chyme passes into the small intestine, digestive enzymes from the small intestine, liver, and pancreas convert the food substances into usable nutrients. A process of segmentation moves the chyme backward and forward, facilitating the digestion of food and the absorption of nutrients through the villi in the walls of the small intestine. Age-related changes that occur in the small intestine include atrophy of muscle fibers and mucosal surfaces; reduction in the number of lymphatic follicles; gradual reduction in the weight of the small intestine; and shortening and widening of the villi, which gradually form parallel ridges rather than finger-like projections. These structural changes do not significantly affect small intestine motility, permeability, or transit time; however, they may affect immune function and absorption of some nutrients (e.g., calcium and vitamin D).

Liver, Pancreas, and Gallbladder

The liver assists in digestion by producing and secreting bile, which is essential for the utilization of fats. It also plays an important role in the metabolism and storage of medications and nutrients (e.g., vitamins and carbohydrates). With increasing age, the liver becomes smaller and more fibrotic, lipofuscin (a brown pigment) accumulates, and blood flow to the liver decreases by about one third. However, some of these changes may be pathologic, rather than age-related, in origin. Despite any age-related or pathologic changes, the liver has an enormous regenerative and reserve capacity, which allows it to compensate for such changes without significantly affecting digestive function.

A primary digestive function of the pancreas is the secretion of enzymes essential for neutralizing acids in the chyme and breaking down fats, proteins, and carbohydrates in the small intestine. The pancreas also functions as an endocrine gland and produces insulin and glycogen, which are essential for glucose metabolism. Age-related changes of the pancreas include decreased weight, hyperplasia of the duct, fibrosis of the lobe, and decreased responsiveness of pancreatic B cells to glucose. Although these changes have little or no direct impact on digestive functioning, diminished insulin secretion increases the susceptibility of older adults to develop glucose intolerance and type II diabetes (Horowitz, 2000).

Age-related changes that affect the gallbladder and biliary tract include diminished bile acid synthesis, widening of the common bile duct, and increased secretion of cholecystokinin, a peptide hormone that contracts the gallbladder and relaxes the biliary sphincter. Effects of these age-related changes include biliary stasis, increased biliary bacterial flora, and increased incidence of cholelithiasis (gallstones) in older adults (Horowitz, 2000; Ross & Forsmark, 2001). In addition, the higher level of cholecystokinin that occurs in older adults may suppress the appetite and reduce food intake (Morley, 2002).

Large Intestine

After nutrients are absorbed in the small intestine, the chyme passes into the large intestine, where water and electrolytes are absorbed and waste products are expelled. Age-related changes in the large intestine include reduced secretion of mucus, decreased elasticity of the rectal wall, and diminished perception of rectal wall distention. These age-related changes have little or no impact on motility of feces through the bowel, but they may predispose the older person to constipation because larger rectal volumes are needed before the urge to defecate is perceived (Prather, 2000).

AGE-RELATED CHANGES IN NUTRITIONAL REQUIREMENTS

Until recently, little attention was focused on age-related changes in nutritional requirements for older adults, especially in relation to healthy older adults. A review of studies of nutrient intakes across the adult life span found some evidence that older adults require an increased intake of several nutrients because of diminished absorption and utilization, but "nutrition research is urgently needed to determine metabolic changes and nutrient needs of older people" (Wakimoto & Block, 2001, p. 79). Until the late 1990s, the Recommended Dietary Allowances (RDA) of the National Academy of Sciences (introduced in 1941) was the primary reference standard for measuring the intake levels of essential nutrients that were considered adequate for meeting the nutrient needs of healthy people. An important limitation of the RDA is that a single standard applied to all people age 51 years and older. In January 2001, a major revision of the RDA—called the Dietary Reference Intakes (DRIs)—was published jointly by the Food and Nutrition Board, the Institute of Medicine, the National Academy of Sciences, and Health Canada. The DRIs set standards for meeting the basic nutrient needs of healthy adults, and they include indicators for preventing chronic disease and avoiding the harmful effects of consuming too much of a nutrient. In addition to focusing on the role of nutrients in health promotion, the DRIs address specific age groups (e.g., adults aged 51 to 70 years of age and those 70 years of age and older). Because these standards apply only to healthy older adults, they need to be adjusted to compensate for conditions such as nutrient deficiencies and medical conditions. In addition, adjustments for food and drug interactions may be necessary for people who take one or more medications. For example, people with gastroesophageal reflux disease are likely to need significantly increased intake or supplements of vitamin B_{12} because the condition and many medications used for it interfere with this vitamin's absorption.

Calories

The energy-producing potential of food is measured in units called *calories*. Caloric requirements are determined by a combination of factors, including height, weight, gender, body build, health–illness state, and usual level of physical activity. Because energy requirements gradually decrease throughout adulthood—owing to decreased physical activity and the decline in basal metabolic rate that is associated with diminished muscle mass—nutritional guidelines recommend a gradual reduction in calories beginning at about 40 to 50 years of age. Surveys of the nutritional status of older adults indicate that mean daily energy intake declines by 1000 to 1200 calories in men and by 600 to 800 calories in women between the ages of 20 and 80 years (Wakimoto & Block, 2001). Distribution of calories also changes, with older adults consuming a higher percentage of calories in carbohydrates and a lower percentage in fats, while maintaining a relatively stable protein intake (Wakimoto & Block, 2001). Any decrease in caloric intake requires a proportionate increase in the quality of calories (nutritional density) to meet minimal nutritional requirements. Thus, nutritional deficiencies will occur unless a reduced caloric intake is accompanied by an increased intake of foods with a high nutritional value and a concomitant decrease in the intake of foods containing little or no nutrients.

Mean caloric intake for groups in the United States is highest in whites, lower in Mexican Americans, and lowest in African Americans (Wakimoto & Block, 2001).

Protein

Protein provides the essential components for new tissue growth in the human body. Age-related changes, such as decreased lean body mass and muscle tissue and decreased plasma albumin and total body albumin levels, may influence protein requirements in older adults, but little is known about the specific effects of these changes in healthy older adults. A minimum daily protein intake of 1 g/kg of body weight is recommended for older adults, and this can be achieved if about 10% to 20% of the daily caloric intake is derived from protein. Older adults with acute medical conditions may need a daily protein intake of 1.5 g/kg of body weight (Jensen et al., 2001).

Carbohydrates and Fiber

Carbohydrates provide an essential source of energy and fiber. Without an adequate intake of carbohydrates, energy will be derived from fat and protein, causing an increase in serum cholesterol and triglyceride levels and a depletion of water, electrolytes, and amino acids. Fiber has received much attention in recent years, primarily for its role in disease prevention, as an essential food component. Soluble fibers, found in oats and pectin, are beneficial in lowering serum cholesterol levels and improving glucose tolerance in people with diabetes. Insoluble fibers, found in most grains and many vegetables, are important for maintaining good bowel function and for preventing constipation. Definitions recently proposed by the National Academy of Sciences (2002) recommend that fiber be categorized as dietary fiber when it is an intrinsic component of food and as functional fiber when it is an isolated or extracted nondigestible carbohydrate that has beneficial physiologic effects in humans. Some fibers, such as cellulose, can be either dietary (when it occurs naturally in foods) or functional (when it is added to foods). The average daily intake of fiber for Americans is 10 to 15 g, which is significantly less than the 25 to 38 g/day recommended by the National Cancer Institute and other health authorities (DeBusk, 2002; National Academy of Sciences, 2002). Dietary guidelines suggest a daily intake of five to nine servings of fruits and vegetables, with at least 55 % of the total calories consumed derived from complex carbohydrates.

Fats

The primary functions of fat are to assist in temperature regulation, provide a reserve source of energy, facilitate the absorption of fat-soluble vitamins, and reduce acid secretion and muscular activity of the stomach. Fats are also useful in providing a feeling of satiety and improving the taste of foods. Fats are categorized according to their source. Saturated fats are derived from animals, whereas unsaturated fats are found in vegetables. Although either type of fat can meet nutritional needs, only the saturated fats are associated with the detrimental accumulation of serum cholesterol. Adults in most industrialized societies consume far more calories in fats than is healthy or necessary. Because excessive fat intake is associated with harmful effects, such as hyperlipidemia, fat should constitute no more than 10 % to 30 % of a person's daily caloric intake. Those fats that are consumed should be polyunsaturated and monounsaturated fatty acids, rather than cholesterol and saturated fats (see Chapter 16 for further discussion of types of fat).

Water

Water is such a commonly available substance that it is often overlooked as a nutritional requirement. However, it is essential for all metabolic activities and must be consumed in adequate amounts for proper physiologic performance. The functions of water include regulating body temperature, maintaining a suitable metabolic environment, diluting water-soluble medications, and facilitating renal and bowel excretion. Potential consequences of reduced body water include decreased efficiency of thermoregulation, increased susceptibility to dehydration, and increased concentrations of water-soluble medications in the body.

Throughout life, the proportion of total body water as a percentage of body weight gradually decreases. Whereas water constitutes about 80 % of a newborn infant's weight, it represents 60 % of a younger adult's weight and about 50 % or less of an older adult's weight. This decrease in total body water is associated with a loss of lean body mass and is influenced by gender and degree of leanness, with women and obese people having a lower percentage of body water than men and lean, muscular people. In older adults, total body water may be further diminished by poor fluid intake secondary to age-related factors, such as diminished thirst sensation. It is recommended that older adults consume 1500 to 2000 mL (6 to 8 glasses) of noncaffeinated fluid daily to maintain adequate hydration.

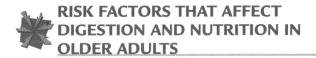

RISK FACTORS THAT AFFECT DIGESTION AND NUTRITION IN OLDER ADULTS

Certain behaviors and common disease processes are likely to interfere with nutrition and digestion in older adults. Behaviors that are detrimental to nutrition and digestion, such as limiting fluid intake and avoiding fresh fruit, may be based on myths and misconceptions. Although these conditions can create risks for people at any age, they are more typical in older adults, and the potential for harm is much greater in older adults than in other age groups because of the collective effects of risk factors and age-related changes. Risk factors affect every phase of digestion and nutrition and can significantly influence eating patterns and nutritional intake. A recent review of assessment data on newly admitted nursing home residents identified the following risks as predictors of poor nutrition: recent weight loss, psychiatric diagnosis, missing all or some teeth, living alone before admission, using a diuretic or antidepressant, and having a decline in

TABLE 14-1 • Causes and Consequences of Nutrient Deficiencies

Nutrient	Possible Causes of Deficiency	Functional Consequences of Deficiency
Calories	Anorexia, depression, mental or physical impairments	Weight loss, lethargy, edema, anemia
Protein	Lack of teeth or dentures, anorexia, depression, dementia, high alcohol or carbohydrate consumption	Poor tissue healing, hypoalbuminemia, reduced protein binding of drugs
Fat	Neomycin, phenytoin, laxatives, alcohol, colchicine, cholestyramine	Inability to absorb vitamins A, D, E, and K
Vitamin A	Mineral oil, neomycin, alcohol, cholestyramine, aluminum antacids, liver disease	Dry skin and eyes, photophobia, night blindness, hyperkeratoses
Thiamine (B_1)	High consumption of alcohol or caffeinated tea, pernicious anemia, diuretics	Neuropathy, muscle weakness, heart disease, dementia, anorexia
Riboflavin (B_2)	Malabsorption syndromes, chronic diarrhea laxative abuse, alcoholism, liver disease	Cheilitis, glossitis, photophobia, blepharitis, conjunctivitis
Niacin (B_3)	Poor dietary habits, diarrhea, cirrhosis, alcoholism	Dermatitis, stomatitis, diarrhea, dementia, depression
Pyridoxine (B_6)	Diuretics, hydralazine	Dermatitis, neuropathy
Folate (B_9)	Anticonvulsants, triameterene, sulfonamides alcohol, smoking	Macrocytic anemia, elevated levels of homocysteine
Vitamin B_{12}	Malabsorption syndrome, H_2-receptor blockers, proton pump inhibitors, colchicine, oral hypoglycemics, potassium supplements, vegetarian diet	Pernicious anemia, weakness, dyspnea, glossitis, numbness, dementia, depression
Vitamin C	Aspirin, tetracycline, lack of fruits and vegetables in diet	Lassitude, irritability, anemia, ecchymosis, impaired wound healing
Vitamin D	Phenytoin, mineral oil, phenobarbital, sunlight deprivation	Muscle weakness and atrophy, osteoporosis, fractures
Vitamin E	Malabsorption syndromes	Peripheral neuropathy, gait disturbance, retinopathy
Vitamin K	Mineral oil, warfarin sodium (Coumadin), antibiotics, cholestyramine, phenytoin	Ecchymosis; hemorrhage involving the gastrointestinal, urinary, or central nervous system
Calcium	Phenytoin, aluminum-based antacids, laxatives, tetracycline, corticosteroids, furosemide, high intake of fiber or caffeine	Osteoporosis, fractures, low back pain
Iron	Achlorhydria; neomycin; aspirin; antacids; low intake of animal protein; high consumption of fiber, caffeine, or tannic acid (contained in some teas)	Anemia, weakness, lassitude, pallor
Magnesium	Alcohol, diuretics, diarrhea, bulk-forming laxatives	Cardiac arrhythmias, neuromuscular and central nervous system irritability, disorientation
Zinc	Penicillamine, aluminum-based antacids, bulk-forming laxatives, high consumption of fiber	Poor wound healing, hair loss
Potassium	Laxatives, furosemide, antibiotics, corticosteroids, diarrhea	Weakness, cardiac arrhythmias, digitalis toxicity
Water	Diuretics, laxatives, immobility, incontinence, diarrhea	Dry skin and mouth, dehydration, constipation
Fiber	Poor dietary habits	Constipation, hemorrhoids

functional status from morning to evening (Crogan & Corbett, 2002). Risks that can cause specific nutrient deficiencies are listed in Table 14-1, along with the related functional consequences.

Inadequate Oral Care

Inadequate oral care practices have been cited as a very common cause of oral health problems that contribute to poor nutrition and interfere with digestion,

particularly for older adults in institutional settings. Studies in Europe and North America have found widespread occurrence of poor oral health in nursing home residents, and one survey cited routine oral hygiene as the greatest single need among older nursing home residents (Coleman, 2002). Poor oral hygiene causes or contributes to stomatitis, xerostomia, tooth loss, dental caries, and periodontal disease—conditions that can interfere with nutrition and food selection and enjoyment. Although inadequate oral care is a common and serious risk factor for problems associated with nutrition and digestion, nursing home staff generally do not recognize it as a serious problem, nor do they consider it a priority for nursing care (Chung et al., 2000; Wardh et al., 2000). Thus, attitudes and behaviors of nurses related to provision of oral care for dependent older adults is a common risk factor that needs to be addressed through interventions (Ship, 2002).

Xerostomia and tooth loss are common among older adults, but both conditions are attributable to risk factors rather than to age-related changes. For example, medications have been cited as the most common cause of decreased saliva production and complaints of xerostomia in older people (Ship et al., 2002). A recent review of data concluded that 95% of older adults have dental caries, with the highest risk being associated with mental confusion, physical frailty, and dependency on others for oral care (Ettinger, 2001). Until recently, tooth loss was so common among older people that it has been inaccurately viewed as a normal consequence of aging; but the oral health of older people has improved in the past few decades so that older adults today are less likely to be edentulous (without any teeth). In the late 1990s, about half of all nursing home residents 75 years of age and older and one third of noninstitutionalized people aged 65 years or older were edentulous (Ritchie, 2002). Tooth loss in older adulthood is often attributable to inadequate dental care, xerostomia and periodontal disease, and other pathologic conditions that occur with increasing frequency in later years. Women and people who smoke have higher rates of tooth loss (Randolph et al., 2001). Factors that contribute to inadequate dental care include low income, low education, lack of transportation, lack of dental insurance, the high cost of dental services, and inaccessibility of services as a result of distance or environmental barriers, such as stairs to dental offices.

> African Americans, American Indians, and Alaska Natives are more likely than white Americans to have fewer natural teeth (USDHHS, 2000).

Negative attitudes on the part of dentists or older adults also may interfere with the provision of dental services. For example, if a dentist or an older adult views tooth loss as an inevitable concomitant of old age, restorative and preventive dental services may not be offered by the dentist or not requested by the patient. Additionally, many older adults have been fully or partially edentulous since the 1930s and 1940s because of the dental practices of that era, which espoused the removal, rather than the preser-

vation, of teeth. Because preventive dental care is a recent trend, older adults may believe that they should visit a dentist only when a toothache does not respond to home remedies.

Functional Impairments and Disease Processes

Functional impairments are strongly associated with poor nutrition and difficulty procuring food, particularly in community-living older adults (Sharkey, 2002). For example, mobility or visual impairments can interfere with the ability to procure and prepare food. In community settings, however, the extent to which functional impairments affect nutrition depends to a large degree on the availability of social supports, such as family, friends, or agencies that assist with provision of food. As many as 60% of nursing home residents have some degree of dysphagia (difficulty swallowing), a functional impairment that can significantly affect nutrition (Lewis, 2001). Dysphagia in older adults most commonly is caused by neurologic disorders, such as stroke and dementia. Chronic gastritis (an inflammation of the gastric mucosa) is common in older adults and is a leading cause of vitamin B_{12} deficiency (Andres et al., 2002). Pernicious anemia, peptic ulcers, and stomach cancer occur more often in older adults, and these conditions may be associated with diminished capacity of the gastric mucosa to resist damage (Horowitz, 2000). Other pathologic conditions interfere with appetite and enjoyment of food in many ways. For example, infections, hyperthyroidism, hypoadrenalism, and congestive heart failure are associated with anorexia, and rheumatoid conditions and chronic obstructive pulmonary disease (COPD) are associated with both decreased appetite and increased energy expenditure. Alzheimer's disease and other dementias, especially in later stages, often have serious negative effects on eating and nutrition.

Medication Effects

Medications create risk factors for impaired digestion and inadequate nutrition through their effects on digestion, eating patterns, and utilization of nutrients (Table 14-2). Although these medication effects are not uniquely age-related, they are more likely to occur in older adults because of their increased use of prescription and over-the-counter medications. Moreover, because medication effects can exacerbate and interact with age-related changes and other risk factors, they are likely to be more detrimental in older adults.

Medications can interfere with digestion and eating through adverse effects such as anorexia, xerostomia,

TABLE 14-2 • Potential Effects of Medications on Digestion and Nutrition

Medications	Potential Effect on Digestion and Nutrition
Digoxin, theophylline, fluoxetine, antihistamines (including over-the-counter cold or sleep preparations)	Anorexia
Anticholinergics, narcotics, iron sulfate, antidepressants, antipsychotics, aluminum- and calcium-based antacids	Constipation
Cimetidine, laxatives, antibiotics, iron sulfate, cardiovascular drugs, antidementia drugs	Diarrhea, nausea, vomiting
Diuretics, ibuprofen, hypnotics, antipsychotics, antidepressants, antihistamines, decongestants, antiadrenergic agents (e.g., clonidine), any medication that has anticholinergic effects	Dry mouth
Ibuprofen, phenylbutazone, indomethacin, aspirin, phenobarbital, corticosteroids	Gastric irritation
Anticholinergics, potassium-depleting medications (e.g., furosemide)	Paralytic ileus
Bulk-forming agents (e.g., psyllium, methylcellulose), when taken before meals	Early satiety
Diuretics, vasodilators, antihistamines, antimicrobials, antihypertensives, hypoglycemic agents, psychotropic medications	Diminished smell and taste sensations
Mineral oil, cholestyramine	Diminished absorption of vitamins A, D, E, and K
Anticonvulsants	Diminished storage of vitamin K, decreased absorption of calcium
Aluminum- or magnesium-based antacids	Diarrhea; decreased levels of calcium, fluoride, and phosphorus
Products containing sodium bicarbonate	Sodium overload, water retention
Gentamicin and penicillin	Hypokalemia
Tetracyclines	Diminished absorption of zinc, iron, calcium, and magnesium
Neomycin	Diminished absorption of fat, iron, lactose, nitrogen, calcium, potassium, and vitamin B_{12}
Aspirin	Gastrointestinal bleeding; decreased levels of iron, folate, and vitamin C
Corticosteroids	Increased need for calcium, phosphorus, B vitamins, and vitamins C and D
Cimetidine, potassium supplements	Diminished absorption of vitamin B_{12}
Nonsteroidal anti-inflammatory drugs (NSAIDs)	Nausea, vomiting, gastrointestinal ulcers and bleeding, diminished absorption of iron

early satiety, and impaired smell and taste perception. In addition to being a common cause of xerostomia, medications are a common cause of eating or chewing discomfort. For example, gum hyperplasia is associated with phenytoin, nifedipine, diltiazem, and cyclosporine. Medications can alter chemosensory perceptions through their action at peripheral receptors, neural pathways, and the brain. More than 250 medications are associated with abnormal or dulled taste sensation (Staveren et al., 2002).

Constipation is another common adverse effect of many medications, especially agents that act on the central nervous system. Paralytic ileus, which has a serious impact on digestive function, may arise from anticholinergic medications or from hypokalemia caused by potassium-wasting diuretics. Medications also cause adverse effects that interfere with the ability to procure, prepare, eat, and enjoy food. For example, medications that cause confusion, depression, and other mental changes can indirectly but significantly affect the older person's eating patterns.

Medications can affect nutrition by interfering with the absorption and excretion of nutrients. Nutrient synthesis, for example, may be impaired by alterations in the intestinal flora caused by broad-spectrum antibiotics. Medications and vitamins that are similar in chemical structure may compete at sites of action, altering their excretion pattern. Other medications, such as tetracycline, bind to particular ions, such as iron and calcium, to form compounds that cannot be absorbed. Diuretics can interfere with the transport of water, sodium, glucose, and amino acids. Nutritional supplements and herbal preparations also can have detrimental effects. For example, the long-term use of beta-carotene supplements can cause a vitamin E deficiency. Food, herb, and medication interactions are discussed in Chapter 23.

Lifestyle Factors

Alcohol and smoking may alter an older person's nutritional status in several ways. Alcohol has a high caloric content but low nutrient value; hence, it provides empty calories. In addition, it interferes with the absorption of the B-complex vitamins and vitamin C. Alcoholism is often unrecognized and undertreated in older adults and may be a common contributing factor to nutritional disorders (Meyyazhagan & Palmer, 2002). Smoking diminishes the ability to smell and taste food and interferes with absorption of vitamin C and folic acid.

Psychosocial Factors

Psychosocial factors are likely to affect an older person's appetite and eating patterns. Any changes in mealtime companionship, as may occur through loss or disability of a spouse, are likely to have a negative impact on eating patterns. Eating alone has been associated with a 30% decline in caloric intake when compared with caloric intake of people who eat in the company of others, and loneliness has been identified as a risk factor for anorexia in older adults (de Castro, 2002; Staveren et al., 2002). When a long-term pattern of preparing meals for family and spouse has been established, it may be especially difficult for the older adult to adjust to purchasing, preparing, and eating food for just one person. Similarly, older adults who have never participated in the purchase or preparation of foods may have great difficulty assuming these tasks after the loss of a spouse or other person who performed these tasks. If the older adult depends on others for assistance in procuring food, any factors that limit the availability of support resources may affect the older adult's ability to obtain food.

Stress and anxiety affect digestive processes through their influence on the autonomic nervous system. Although stress-related effects on digestion are not unique to older adults, any alteration of the autonomic nervous system may compound age-related effects that otherwise would not have much effect. Depression, which is common in older adults, typically is accompanied by anorexia and loss of interest in food. Confusion, memory problems, and other cognitive deficits may significantly interfere with eating patterns and the ability to prepare food.

Cultural and Socioeconomic Factors

Ethnic background, religious beliefs, and other cultural factors strongly influence the way people define, select, prepare, and eat food and beverages. Cultural factors also can influence eating patterns and selection of food in relation to health status. For example, Asian and Hispanic people may classify foods, beverages, and medicines as hot or cold, and they may select a particular food based on their belief that their illness would respond to warm, hot, cool, or cold types of remedies. According to this health belief model, illnesses are caused by an imbalance between hot and cold and must be treated with substances that have the opposite characteristics.

Cultural dietary customs usually are not detrimental for healthy older adults, as long as essential nutrients are included in the diet and extremes are avoided. However, for the older adult with a medical condition that requires diet modification (e.g., diabetes or hypertension), cultural food patterns may aggravate the condition and create barriers to nutritional therapy. For example, the use of large amounts of soy sauce may contribute to hypertension. Culture Box 14-1 summarizes some of the food habits that are associated with major cultural and religious groups in the United States. It is usually not necessary to try to change culturally influenced eating patterns, but it is important to recognize any cultural factors that may affect an older adult's nutritional status.

A person's present and past economic status also influences food choices. If nutrient intake has been inadequate because of long-standing financial limitations, the progressive effects of poor nutrition may precipitate new problems in older adults, especially in combination with age-related changes in nutrient intake and utilization. People of low socioeconomic status usually have a narrower selection of foods than do people of higher socioeconomic status. Edentulism is almost twice as common in people with incomes below the poverty line than in those with incomes at or above the poverty line (Vargas et al., 2001). Education may also affect nutritional status, with limited education being associated with poor nutrition and less use of dental services. For example, people who have more than a high school education are twice as likely to have visited a dentist in the past year as people with less than a high school education (Vargas et al., 2001).

> Edentulism is higher among African Americans than among whites (Kramarow et al., 1999).

Environmental Factors

Environmental factors affect the enjoyment of food as well as the ability to obtain and prepare it. Many barriers to food enjoyment have been identified in the dining environments of nursing homes and other institutional settings. Limited food selection and low staffing levels are two of the most commonly identified

African Americans

- "Soul food" is common, particularly in the southern United States.
- Common main courses: wild game, fried fish and poultry, pork and all parts of the pig
- Common vegetables and side dishes: corn, rice, okra, greens, legumes, tomatoes, hot breads, sweet potatoes
- Methods of food preparation: stewing, barbecuing, and frying with lard or saltpork
- Low consumption of milk (possibly owing to lactose intolerance)
- Low calcium dietary intake

Asian Americans

- Common foods: rice, wheat, pork, eggs, chicken, soybean products, and a variety of vegetables
- Methods of food preparation: stir-frying with lard, peanut oil, or sesame oil; seasoning with ginger, soy sauce, sesame seeds, and monosodium glutamate
- Beverages: green tea; rare use of milk products because lactose intolerance is common

Hispanic Americans

- Common main courses: eggs, tacos, chicken, corn tortillas, pinto or calico beans
- Common vegetables and side dishes: rice, corn, squash, bread, tomatoes
- Methods of food preparation: frying with lard; seasoning with garlic, onions, and chili powder
- Beverages: herbal teas, carbonated soda, milk in hot beverages

Native Americans

- May obtain foods from their natural environment (e.g., fish, roots, fruits, berries, wild greens, and wild game)
- May rely on nonperishable foods because of lack of refrigeration
- May depend on commodity foods provided by the U.S. Department of Agriculture
- May be influenced by tribal culture
- May have limited use of dairy products because of lactose intolerance

Religious Influences

- Orthodox Jews follow prescribed rules for preparing and serving foods (e.g., they eat only kosher meat and poultry and do not eat shellfish or any pork products).
- Mormons do not drink tea, coffee, or alcohol.
- Hindus are vegetarians.
- Seventh Day Adventists are lacto-ovovegetarians.
- Roman Catholics do not eat meat on Ash Wednesday or Good Friday.

barriers to nutrition care in nursing homes (Crogan et al., 2001; Simmons et al., 2001). Older adults in congregate housing and long-term care facilities may find it difficult to adjust to unfamiliar environments. Moreover, they may not desire the opportunity for mealtime social interaction that is part of the institutional environment. A noisy or crowded dining room may have a negative impact on food enjoyment and consumption. Such an environment may be particularly stressful for an older adult who uses a hearing aid or who is accustomed to eating alone. The potential outcomes of a move to a new environment include poor nutrition and loss of interest in eating, particularly during the initial adjustment period.

Older adults who live in their own homes and have functional impairments may be particularly affected by environmental influences, such as inclement weather conditions. For example, an older person who walks to the store or depends on public transportation may be unable or unwilling to obtain groceries in snowy or rainy weather. Likewise, the older adult may not be able to tolerate hot or sultry conditions, especially if car transportation is not readily available. People who depend on others for transportation or who have difficulty maneuvering in adverse weather conditions are likely to shop for groceries less frequently and to purchase their groceries at smaller convenience stores, where prices are higher and selection is limited. The additional cost and limited selection may interfere with food intake and lead to nutrient deficiencies. Finally, environmental conditions and packaging trends in the grocery store may create additional difficulties for older people, especially those who are functionally impaired. For example, the combined glare of fluorescent lights, highly polished floors, cellophane wrappers, and white freezer cases often make it extremely difficult, if not impossible, for the older adult with vision changes to read labels, especially when the print is small and contrasts poorly against the background.

Behaviors Based on Myths and Misunderstandings

Myths and misunderstandings may have a detrimental effect on food intake and behaviors related to bowel function. For example, during the 1950s and 1960s, a widely held belief was that roughage and raw fruits or vegetables were harmful to the older person. It is now known that lack of roughage in the diet and consumption of only cooked fruits and vegetables are eating patterns that contribute to constipation by slowing the transit time of feces through the large intestine. Another commonly held belief is that a daily bowel movement is the norm for good digestive function. Rigid adherence to this standard may, in fact, lead to the unnecessary and detrimental use of laxatives. This false belief has been further reinforced by advertisements implying that daily bowel movements should be attained through medication. Although recent advertising trends emphasize the achievement of healthy bowel patterns through the ingestion of high-fiber food items, the negative impact of long-term beliefs may be difficult to overcome.

Misunderstandings about fluid intake also may interfere with digestion and nutrition. Many older adults reduce the amount of liquids they consume with the expectation that this practice will decrease the incidence of urinary incontinence. Fluid intake also may be restricted if functional limitations, such as impaired mobility or manual dexterity, interfere with either the ability to obtain liquids or the ease of urinary elimination. Reduced fluid intake can have a number of detrimental consequences, such as constipation, xerostomia, and diminished food enjoyment.

PATHOLOGIC CONDITIONS ASSOCIATED WITH DIGESTION AND NUTRITION

Constipation—the "subjective interpretation of a real or imagined disturbance of bowel function" (Wald, 2000, p. 1231)—is one of the most common pathologic conditions associated with digestion. Up to 80% of institutionalized older adults and 45% of community-living older adults report constipation problems (Frank et al., 2001). Prevalence of constipation is highest among women, African Americans, people older than 60 years, and people who have low incomes, less education, and lower levels of physical activity (Hinrichs, et al., 2001).

Definitions of constipation usually are based on characteristics of bowel movements, including frequency and difficulty passing the stool. The normal frequency for bowel movements, which shows significant individual variation but does not necessarily change with aging, ranges from three times daily to once or twice weekly. Constipation is characterized by all of the following conditions:

- The stool is excessively hard.
- There is a decrease in the person's normal frequency pattern.
- The stool is difficult to pass (i.e., straining with bowel movements).
- The person experiences a feeling of incomplete evacuation after a bowel movement.

Although constipation is a common complaint of older adults, it is caused by risk factors rather than age-related changes. It is often associated with functional impairments (e.g., diminished mobility), pathologic conditions (e.g., hypothyroidism), adverse medication effects (including long-term laxative abuse), and poor dietary habits (e.g., inadequate intake of bulk, fiber, and fluid). Because constipation occurs so commonly in older adults, nurses assess for

risk factors and initiate health promotion interventions, as discussed in the sections on Nursing Assessment and Nursing Interventions.

> Mr. and Mrs. D., who are 71 and 72 years old, respectively, attend the senior center where you provide monthly group health education sessions and weekly one-on-one "Counseling for Wellness" sessions. Mrs. D. makes an appointment to see you because her bowels get "bound up" and she always feels "bloated." When you ask about her bowel patterns she reports that she has a bowel movement "about every other day" and has to "sit on the commode for a good half-hour before anything happens." She has taken magnesium hydroxide (Milk of Magnesia) every night for about 20 years, but "it doesn't seem to be any help anymore." She avoids fresh fruits and vegetables because her mother always told her that canned fruits and vegetables were easier to digest. She rarely eats cereal and uses white bread. Her weight is about 125% of her ideal body weight, and she does not walk often because of trouble with arthritis. She takes levothyroxine sodium (Synthroid), 100 μg once daily, and an over-the-counter generic calcium supplement that contains 500 mg calcium carbonate twice daily.

 THINKING POINTS

- Identify at least five risk factors that are likely to contribute to Mrs. D.'s constipation.
- Describe how you would begin addressing one of these risk factors in health education.

 ## FUNCTIONAL CONSEQUENCES ASSOCIATED WITH DIGESTION AND NUTRITION IN OLDER ADULTS

Functional consequences affect the following aspects of digestion and nutrition of older adults: (1) procurement, preparation, and enjoyment of food; (2) mastication and digestion of food; (3) nutritional status, and (4) psychosocial function. Negative functional consequences occur primarily because of risk factors, rather than because of age-related changes alone.

The Impact of Changes on Procurement, Preparation, and Enjoyment of Food

Activities involved in procuring, preparing, consuming, and enjoying food depend on the skills of cognition, balance, mobility, and manual dexterity as well as on the five senses. Food procurement depends on getting to the grocery store, pushing a shopping cart, reaching for food items on high shelves, reading the small print on shelves and food packages for cost and nutrition information, and coping with the glare of bright lights, especially in the frozen food sections. Age-related changes and conditions that may interfere with these activities include vision impairments and any illness, such as arthritis, that limits mobility, balance, or manual dexterity.

Food preparation activities that are likely to be more difficult for older adults include cutting food items, measuring ingredients accurately, carrying food and liquid without spilling, standing for long periods in the kitchen, reaching for items on high shelves and in cupboards, safely using the oven or stove, and reading the temperature controls correctly. Impairments of vision, balance, cognition, mobility, or manual dexterity are likely to cause difficulties in the performance of these tasks.

Food enjoyment is likely to be affected by sensory changes, which may interfere with the accurate perception of color, taste, or smell. Impaired sense of smell can cause poor appetite and dulled sensation of hunger (DeJong, 1999). Diminished gustatory and olfactory skills may lead to excessive use of condiments and seasonings, such as salt and sugar. Visual and olfactory impairments may make it difficult to detect spoiled food. Moreover, food choices are influenced by the condition of the oral cavity and teeth as well as by the quantity and quality of natural or replacement teeth.

The Impact of Changes on Oral Function and Digestion of Food

Digestive processes in healthy older adults are not significantly affected by age-related changes, but older adults often have digestive complaints (e.g., "heartburn," constipation), which are caused by commonly occurring risk factors. For example, many negative functional consequences are associated with medications (see Table 14-2). Xerostomia causes negative functional consequences because it can interfere with oral comfort, food enjoyment, and taste sensitivity. It also interferes with food digestion because diminished saliva production makes it more difficult to chew food and increases the susceptibility of the teeth and tongue to bacterial action. Other consequences of impaired salivary function include gingivitis, dry lips, dental caries, excessive plaque, periodontal disease, difficulty swallowing, speech dysfunction, poorly fitting dentures, decreased nutritional intake, inflammation of the mucous membrane, oral mucosal infections (e.g., candidiasis), and traumatic oral lesions (Ghezzi et al., 2000; Ship et al., 2002). The functional consequences of being edentulous or using dentures include avoidance of certain foods, decreased chewing efficiency, and increased susceptibility to accidental choking from ineffective mastication. Because edentulous people tend to avoid meats, salads, fresh fruits, and raw vegetables, they may be at risk for nutritional deficiencies (Hutton, 2002; Vargas et al., 2001). Weight loss is another consequence of being edentulous (Ritchie et al., 2000).

The Impact of Changes on Nutritional Status

Because older adults need fewer calories, a deficiency of essential minerals or vitamins is likely to occur if the quantity of calories is reduced without a corresponding increase in the quality of the food consumed. In addition, risk factors (e.g., medications and pathologic conditions) that commonly occur in older adults often cause nutrient deficiencies. For example, iron deficiency is associated with chronic diseases and low socioeconomic status. Other minerals and vitamins that commonly are deficient in older adults are zinc, calcium, most B vitamins, and vitamins D and E. See Table 14-1 for examples of nutrient deficiencies and associated risk factors and functional consequences that are likely to affect older adults.

Some researchers have identified the prevalence of specific nutritional deficits among older adults, but conclusions of the studies are clouded by a lack of common definitions. The following findings from two research reviews (Johnson et al., 2002; Meyyazhagan & Palmer, 2002) are indicative of significant concerns about nutritional intake among older adults:

- Half of older adults have a vitamin and mineral intake less than the recommended dietary allowance.
- Undernutrition occurs in 5% to 12% of community-living older adults, in up to 55% of hospitalized elderly, and in 52% to 85% of older adults in nursing homes.
- Ten to 30% of older adults have abnormally low serum levels of vitamins and minerals.
- Vitamin D deficiency occurs in 5% to 25% of community-living older adults and in 48% to 80% of older adults in nursing homes.
- Vitamin B_{12} deficiency occurs in 12% to 14% of community-living older adults and in up to 25% of older adults in nursing homes.

A type of malnutrition that is common in frail older adults is *protein-energy* (also called *protein-calorie*) *undernutrition*, which occurs when the intake of calories and protein is less than the amount required to meet daily needs. This condition is associated with a high-carbohydrate, low-protein diet, which often results from one or several of the risk factors already discussed (e.g., depression, loss of appetite, pathologic conditions). Characteristics of mild or moderate protein-energy undernutrition (called *marasmus*) include weakness, lethargy, unintentional weight loss, diminished muscle mass, marked decrease in subcutaneous fat, and impaired ability to respond to physiologic stresses (e.g., surgery, infection). If the condition progresses and becomes severe (a state called *kwashiorkor*), it is characterized by edema and loss of visceral protein. In a study of patients between the ages of 65 and 99 years, Liu and colleagues (2002) found that protein-energy undernutrition is a significant independent factor for increased mortality within the year following hospitalization. Additional consequences of protein-calorie undernutrition are poor wound healing, increased risk for infection, and decline in cognition and functioning.

The Impact of Changes on Quality of Life

Good food and nutrition are essential components of health-related quality of life, particularly for older adults (Amarantos et al., 2001). In day-to-day life, many food-related activities are associated with pleasurable events, and mealtime activities often are associated with caring, comfort, nurturing, and social interaction. For example, in certain circumstances, food is a focal point of celebrations, religious rituals, or gatherings to share significant events. Thus, when mealtime enjoyment is affected in any way, the psychosocial aspects of eating are also affected. Older adults who enjoyed participating in family meals or eating in restaurants may withdraw from these activities if food is no longer enjoyable. Consequently, they may lose the social interaction that occurs in these settings.

Perhaps even more detrimental than the psychosocial consequences of diminished food enjoyment are the psychosocial effects of inadequate nutrition. When fluid or nutrient intake is inadequate, older adults are likely to develop malnutrition and dehydration because of impaired homeostatic mechanisms. Changes in mental status, including memory impairment, are among the early signs of malnutrition, dehydration, and electrolyte imbalance in older adults. Sometimes these mental changes are attributed to irreversible conditions (e.g., dementia) rather than to a treatable and reversible metabolic imbalance. For example, folate and vitamin B_{12} deficiencies are two of the most common nutritional causes of mental changes.

Finally, negative psychosocial consequences are associated with loss of teeth and poor oral health. Edentulism, dental caries, and periodontal disease are factors that contribute to diminished self-esteem (Vargas et al., 2001). Figure 14-1 illustrates some of the age-related changes, risk factors, and negative functional consequences that can influence digestion and nutrition.

 NURSING ASSESSMENT OF DIGESTION AND NUTRITION

Nursing assessment of digestion and nutrition is aimed at identifying (1) the effects of age-related changes on digestion, nutrition, and eating patterns; (2) the presence of risk factors that interfere with optimal nutrition; (3) cultural factors that influence eating patterns; (4) the nutritional status and usual eating patterns of the older adult; and (5) any negative functional consequences of altered digestion or inadequate nutrition. Nurses use the assessment information to identify opportunities for health promotion, particularly with regard to education about risk factors that interfere with optimal nutrition.

Identifying Opportunities for Health Promotion

Nurses use an assessment interview to identify opportunities for health promotion by asking about the following information: usual eating patterns and nutrient intake; age-related changes and risk factors that affect nutritional needs or digestive processes; environmental or social support factors that affect the procurement, preparation, and enjoyment of food; and symptoms of gastrointestinal dysfunction. A dietary history is important in assessing the adequacy of nutrient intake. If the assessment does not need to be completed immediately, the older adult or caregiver can be asked to keep a 7-day diary of nutrient intake and eating patterns. If time does not allow for this, the person can be asked to describe foods and beverages consumed during an average day or during the past 24-hour period. If the older person is unable to convey this information accurately, the nurse can obtain the information from caregivers. A logical sequence for assessment questions is to begin with information about the oral cavity and end with information about bowel elimination. A major goal for assessing patterns of bowel elimination is to identify opportunities for health education about constipation. Hinrichs and colleagues (2001) developed an excellent research-based protocol for nursing assessment and management of constipation. Display 14-1 summarizes interview questions for a nursing assessment of nutrition and digestion in older adults.

Observing Cues to Digestion and Nutrition

Observations are important for assessing eating patterns and chewing and swallowing abilities. Nurses also observe for indicators of cultural factors that influence eating and nutrition.

Behavioral cues to digestion and nutrition can be observed by staff in institutional settings, and similar

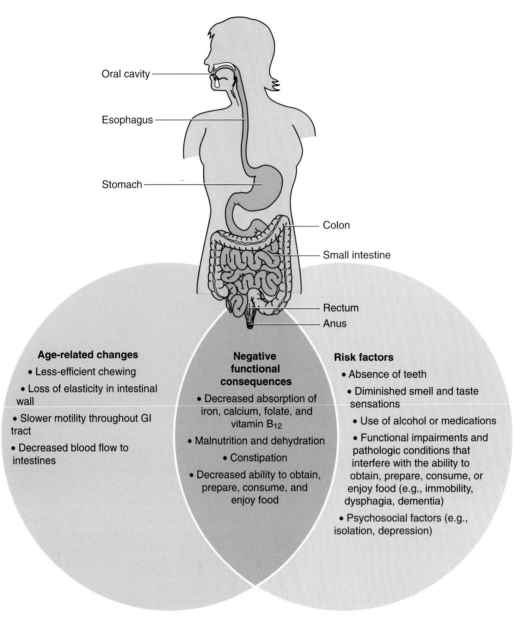

FIGURE 14-1 Age-related changes and risk factors intersect to negatively affect digestion and nutrition in older adults.

information can be obtained from caregivers or through a home visit assessment. Nursing assessment of chewing and swallowing is especially important for older adults at risk for dysphagia, which often develops gradually and eventually can cause serious complications such as aspiration pneumonia. Nurses in institutional settings are responsible for observing older adults at mealtime to identify any difficulties with chewing and swallowing. If dysphagia is suspected, a bedside or mealtime swallowing evaluation can be performed by a speech therapist. Shanley and O'Loughlin (2000) provide a comprehensive protocol for assess-

ment and management of dysphagia in nursing home residents. Display 14-2 summarizes behavioral cues to nutrition and digestion, including cultural considerations, observations related to eating patterns and the eating environment, and indicators of dysphagia.

Using Physical Assessment and Laboratory Information

Physical assessment and laboratory data provide important additional information for assessing the older adult's nutritional and hydration status.

Assessing Oral Comfort and Chewing Ability

- Do you have any difficulty with soreness or bleeding in your mouth?
- Do you have any teeth that hurt, are loose, or are sensitive to hot or cold temperatures?
- Do your gums bleed?
- Do you have any problems chewing or swallowing food or liquids? *If yes, ask about particular types of food or liquids that are problematic.*
- Are there foods you avoid because of problems with chewing or swallowing?
- Does your mouth or tongue ever feel dry?

Assessing Dental Habits and Attitudes Toward Dental Care

- How often do you see a dentist?
- When is the last time you had dental care?
- Where do you go for dental care?
- *If the person does not seek dental care at least once per year:* What prevents you from seeing the dentist?
- How do you care for your teeth?
- Do you use dental floss? *If yes:* How often? *If no:* Have you ever been taught to use dental floss?

Assessing Nutritional Needs

- Do you have diabetes, heart disease, or any condition that requires dietary modifications?
- Do you have any food allergies?
- What medications do you take?
- What is your usual daily activity pattern?

Identifying Patterns of Food Procurement

- How do you get your grocery shopping done?
- Do you have any help getting to the store?

- Where and how often do you do your grocery shopping?
- What is your usual food budget?
- Do you have any difficulty getting food because of problems with vision, walking, or transportation?

Identifying Patterns of Food Preparation and Consumption

- Where do you eat your meals?
- With whom do you eat?
- Does anyone help you prepare your meals?
- Do you have any trouble fixing your meals (e.g., difficulty opening containers)?
- Do you have any difficulties getting around your kitchen, using appliances, or reaching the cupboards?
- Have there been recent changes in your eating or food preparation patterns (e.g., loss of eating companion or change in caregiver situation)?

Assessing Patterns of Bowel Elimination

- How often do you have a bowel movement?
- Have you noticed any recent changes in your pattern of bowel movements?
- Do you have any difficulty with your bowel movements? (e.g., Do you strain with bowel movements? or Is the stool hard, dry, or difficult to pass?)
- Do you ever have problems with loose stools or diarrhea?
- Do you take laxatives or any other products to help you move your bowels?
- Do you ever have pain or bleeding when you move your bowels?

Height, weight, and body mass index (BMI) provide important clues to nutritional status. Ideal body weight based on a standardized table is not necessarily the most realistic or appropriate goal for older adults; maintenance of a stable weight may be more important (Lewis, 2001). Patterns of weight loss and gain are important indicators of the older person's overall health condition. Weight loss is considered in relation to percentage of loss, which is calculated by subtracting current weight from usual weight and dividing that by the usual weight, for example: (160 pounds – 120 pounds) / 160 pounds = 40 pounds, or a 25 % weight loss. An unintentional weight loss of more than 5 % of body weight in 1 month, more than 7.5 % in 3 months, or more than 10 % in 6 months is considered a significant indicator of poor nutrition

(Omran & Salem, 2002). The BMI—a measure of body composition related to body fatness—is commonly used as an indicator of malnutrition. Normal BMI (weight [kg]/height [m]^2) is between 22 and 27, and an older person with a BMI lower than 19 should be considered at risk for malnutrition (Lewis, 2001). A BMI of 24 for adults older than 70 years of age is considered to be healthiest because it is associated with the lowest risk for morbidity and mortality (Russell, 2001).

Physical assessment of hydration in older adults is particularly challenging because typical manifestations of dehydration may either be caused by or masked by age-related changes or pathologic conditions. For example, younger adults who are dehydrated are likely to have dry mucous membranes

DISPLAY 14-2
Behavioral Cues to Nutrition and Digestion

Cultural Considerations That May Influence Nutrition and Eating Patterns

- What are the usual patterns of meals eaten (e.g., content, frequency, timing)? What is the usual social context of meals?
- Are there any culturally influenced food taboos or preferences? (Refer to Culture Box 14-1.)
- Are there any special foods that are important because of religious or cultural factors? (If yes, are they accessible to the older adult?)
- Are certain foods or beverages avoided or preferred in relation to an illness or chronic condition (e.g., foods or beverages that are considered yin and yang foods)?
- Is there a preference for the temperature of beverages (e.g., use of iced or heated beverages)?
- Is the person's ethnic background likely to increase his or her chance of being lactose intolerant? (Prevalence is highest among Asians, American Indians, and African and American blacks; high among Hispanics; and lowest among whites of northern European descent.)

Observations To Assess Eating Patterns

- Does the person seem to enjoy eating meals with others, or does the presence of other people seem to interfere with mealtime enjoyment?
- If the person has dentures, are they worn at meals? If not, why not?

- What are the person's between-meal food and fluid consumption patterns?
- Are enjoyable noncaffeinated liquids readily available for between-meal fluid intake?
- What cultural influences affect the person's food preferences and preparation?

Observations To Assess the Eating Environment

- Do environmental or social influences negatively affect mealtime enjoyment (e.g., a noisy dining room or disruptive mealtime companions)?
- If the person eats alone, is this the best arrangement, or should consideration be given to providing mealtime social interaction?

Indicators of Dysphagia

- Drooling
- Slurred speech
- Incomplete lip closure
- Nasal regurgitation of food
- Pocketing of food in cheeks
- Refusing or resisting food or drink
- Increased congestion or secretions after eating
- Wet, hoarse, or gurgly voice after swallowing
- Slow chewing or slow or delayed swallowing
- Coughing or choking (while or soon after drinking thin liquids or chewing and swallowing food)

---

and complain of being thirsty, but older adults are likely to have dry mucous membranes because of medication effects and may have a dulled thirst sensation. Assessment of skin turgor in older adults may be more accurate on the forehead and over the anterior chest wall because these areas are less affected by age-related skin changes. Orthostatic hypotension, oliguria or anuria, changes in mental status, and dry tongue and mucous membranes are common manifestations of dehydration in older adults. Urinalysis provides clues to a person's hydration status, with highly concentrated urine being an indicator of dehydration. Blood values that may be altered in dehydration include elevations in sodium, hematocrit, creatinine, osmolality, and blood urea nitrogen. In addition, a sudden loss of body weight also might be an indicator of dehydration. Laboratory data are especially useful components of the nutritional assessment of older adults because abnormal biochemical blood values often offer the first clues to nutritional deficiencies, even before any clinical signs are evident. Questions have

been raised about the effect of age-related changes and pathologic conditions on the range of normal laboratory values, particularly regarding some of the indicators used to assess nutritional status. For example, serum albumin is commonly used as a marker of nutritional status, but low serum albumin levels are not necessarily an accurate indicator of poor nutrition (Covinsky et al., 2002). Serum albumin levels are elevated in people who are dehydrated and are likely to be decreased under the following conditions: trauma, edema, infection, neoplasm, overhydration, nephrotic syndrome, and malabsorption syndromes (Lewis, 2001). Despite these limitations, however, serum albumin and other laboratory test results provide important clues to nutritional status, especially when they are evaluated in relation to the person's overall health status. For instance, dehydration may cause false elevations in the hemoglobin and hematocrit. Display 14-3 summarizes information about physical assessment indicators and laboratory values that are especially important in assessing the nutritional status of

DISPLAY 14-3
Physical Assessment and Laboratory Data

Examination of the Oral Cavity
- Inspect the oral cavity using a tongue depressor and a light.
- Observe for evidence of oral disease, including pain, lumps, soreness, bleeding, swelling, loose teeth, and abraded areas.
- Note the presence or absence of teeth, dentures, and partial bridges.

Normal Findings
- Lips: pink, moist, symmetrical
- Teeth: intact, without cavities or tartar
- Gums: pink, no bleeding
- Mucous membranes: pink, moist
- Tongue: pink, moist; presence of numerous varicosities on undersurface
- Pharynx: soft palate rises slightly when "ahh" is vocalized

Indicators of Nutritional Deficiency
- Lips: dry, fissured, cracked at corners
- Teeth: decayed or missing
- Gums: red, swollen, recessed, spongy or prone to bleeding
- Mucous membranes: dry, ulcerated, inflamed, bleeding, white patches
- Tongue: dry, swollen, reddened, or very smooth

Examination of the Abdomen and Rectum
- Examine the abdomen with the person lying comfortably in the supine position.
- Perform a rectal examination with the person in the side-lying position.

Normal Findings
- Symmetrical, soft abdomen that moves with respirations
- Audible bowel sounds (heard through the diaphragm of a stethoscope) occurring at irregular intervals (5 to 15 seconds apart)

- Smooth skin around anus; no evidence of hemorrhoids, fissures, inflammation, or rectal prolapse
- Soft, brown stool that tests negative for occult blood

Indicators of Nutritional Deficiency
- Swollen abdomen
- Stool that tests positive for occult blood

General Physical Assessment Indicators of Malnutrition
- Weight loss
- Lack of subcutaneous fat
- Diminished size and strength of muscles
- Skin that is dry, rough, or tissue thin
- Abnormal pulse or blood pressure
- Edema, especially in the face or lower extremities
- Hair that is dry, dull, thin, brittle, or sparse
- Dry or dull-looking eyes
- Listless, apathetic, or depressed mood
- Difficulty with walking or maintaining balance

Laboratory Data
- Biochemical data that will provide information about nutritional status: serum ferritin; serum or red blood cell folate and vitamin B_{12}; complete lipid profile; and serum albumin, glucose, sodium, and potassium levels
- Urinalysis results should be within the normal adult range, except for a slight decrease in the upper limit for specific gravity

Indicators of Nutritional Deficiency
- Anemia
- Lymphocytopenia
- Serum albumin level of less than 3.5 g/dL
- Cholesterol levels of less than 160 mg/dL
- Total iron-binding capacity less than 250 μg/dL

older adults. Additional indicators of nutrient deficiencies are listed in Table 14-1 in the column describing functional consequences.

Using Assessment Tools

In recent years, nutrition assessment tools have been promoted for identifying people at risk for dehydration and nutritional problems so that preventive and treatment interventions can be implemented (Patterson, 2002; Thomas et al., 2000; Vellas & Lauque, 2001; Zembrzuski, 2000). The parameters most frequently included in nutrition assessment tools are diet history,

clinical presentation, anthropometric measurements, and laboratory and immunologic assessments (Wakefield, 2001). The Mini Nutritional Assessment and the Nutritional Form for the Elderly are widely used in a variety of settings as reliable and validated assessment tools for identifying older adults who are malnourished or at risk for poor nutrition (Bleda et al., 2002; Delahunt, 2002; Salva & Pera, 2001; Soderhamn, 2002). A short six-item form, which can be administered in 5 minutes, has also been found to be reliable as a first-step screening process for identifying older adults who should be assessed further for poor nutrition (Figure 14-2).

NESTLÉ NUTRITION SERVICES

Nestlé

Mini Nutritional Assessment
MNA®

Last name:		First name:		Sex:		Date:
Age:	Weight, kg:		Height, cm:		I.D. Number:	

Complete the screen by filling in the boxes with the appropriate numbers.
Add the numbers for the screen. If score is 11 or less, continue with the assessment to gain a Malnutrition Indicator Score.

Screening

A Has food intake declined over the past 3 months due to loss of appetite, digestive problems, chewing or swallowing difficulties?
0 = severe loss of appetite
1 = moderate loss of appetite
2 = no loss of appetite ☐

B Weight loss during the last 3 months
0 = weight loss greater than 3 kg (6.6 lbs)
1 = does not know
2 = weight loss between 1 and 3 kg (2.2 and 6.6 lbs)
3 = no weight loss ☐

C Mobility
0 = bed or chair bound
1 = able to get out of bed/chair but does not go out
2 = goes out ☐

D Has suffered psychological stress or acute disease in the past 3 months
0 = yes   2 = no ☐

E Neuropsychological problems
0 = severe dementia or depression
1 = mild dementia
2 = no psychological problems ☐

F Body Mass Index (BMI) (weight in kg)/(height in m)^2
0 = BMI less than 19
1 = BMI 19 to less than 21
2 = BMI 21 to less than 23
3 = BMI 23 or greater ☐

Screening score (subtotal max. 14 points) ☐ ☐
12 points or greater Normal–not at risk–no need to complete assessment
11 points or below   Possible malnutrition–continue assessment

Assessment

G Lives independently (not in a nursing home or hospital)
0 = no   1= yes ☐

H Takes more than 3 prescription drugs per day
0 = no   1= yes ☐

I Pressure sores or skin ulcers
0 = no   1= yes ☐

Ref: Guigoz Y, Vellas B and Garry PJ. 1994. Mini Nutritional Assessment: A practical assessment tool for grading the nutritional state of elderly patients. *Facts and Research in Gerontology.* Supplement #2:15-59.

Rubenstein LZ, Harker J, Guigoz Y and Vellas B. Comprehensive Geriatric Assessment (CGA) and the MNA: An Overview of CGA, Nutritional Assessment, and Development of a Shortened Version of the MNA. In: "Mini Nutritional Assessment (MNA): Research and Practice in the Elderly". Vellas B, Garry PJ and Guigoz Y, editors. Nestlé Nutrition Workshop series. Clinical & Performance Programme, vol. 1. Karger, Bâle, in press.

J How many full meals does the patient eat daily?
0 = 1 meal
1 = 2 meals
2 = 3 meals ☐

K Selected consumption markers for protein intake
• At least one serving of dairy products (milk, chesse, yogurt) per day? yes☐ no☐
• Two or more servings of legumes or eggs per week? yes☐ no☐
• Meat, fish or poultry every day? yes☐ no☐
0.0 = if 0 or 1 yes
0.5 = if 2 yes
1.0 = if 3 yes ☐ ☐

L Consumes two or more servings of fruits or vegetables per day?
0 = no   2 = yes ☐

M How much fluid (water, juice, coffee, tea, milk...) is consumed per day?
0.0 = less than 3 cups
0.5 = 3 to 5 cups
1.0 = more than 5 cups ☐ ☐

N Mode of feeding
0 = unable to eat without assistance
1 = self-fed with some difficulty
2 = self-fed without any problem ☐

O Self view of nutritional status
0 = views self as being malnourished
1 = is uncertain of nutritional state
2 = views self as having no nutritional problem ☐

P In comparison with other people of the same age, how does the patient consider his/her health status?
0.0 = not as good
0.5 = does not know
1.0 = as good
2.0 = better ☐ ☐

Q Mid-arm circumference (MAC) in cm
0.0 = MAC less than 21
0.5 = MAC 21 to 22
1.0 = MAC 22 or greater ☐ ☐

R Calf circumference (CC) in cm
0 = CC less than 31   1 = CC 31 or greater ☐

Assessment (max. 16 points) ☐ ☐ ☐

Screening score ☐ ☐

Total Assessment (max. 30 points) ☐ ☐ ☐

Malnutrition Indicator Score
17 to 23.5 points   at risk of malnutrition ☐

Less than 17 points   malnourished ☐

FIGURE 14-2 The Mini Nutritional Assessment (MNA). (From Nestlé Nutrition Services. © Nestlé, 1994. Available at http://www.mna-elderly.com.)

> Recall that you are the nurse at the senior center attended by Mr. and Mrs. D., who now are 75 and 76 years old, respectively. During a "Counseling for Health" session, Mrs. D. asks your advice about her gradual unintended weight loss over the past few months. Although Mrs. D. continues to cook meals because her husband enjoys eating, she states that food no longer appeals to her. You notice that her mouth is very dry and her teeth are in poor condition. She had a stroke 2 years ago and recovered well except for some dysphagia and right-sided weakness. She takes an antidepressant and two blood pressure medications, but does not know the names of the pills. She asks what she can do about the weight loss.

 THINKING POINTS

> What risk factors are likely to be contributing to Mrs. D.'s weight loss?

> Make a list of assessment questions you would use with Mrs. D. Select applicable questions from Display 14-1 and list any additional questions that you would use for further assessment.

> What would you ask Mrs. D. to do to provide additional assessment information so that you can plan some teaching interventions?

NURSING DIAGNOSIS

The nursing assessment may identify problems related to nutrition, digestion, or oral health. If nutritional deficits are identified, a pertinent nursing diagnosis is Imbalanced Nutrition: Less Than Body Requirements. This is defined as "the state in which an individual who is not NPO experiences or is at risk of experiencing reduced weight related to inadequate intake or metabolism of nutrients for metabolic needs" (Carpenito, 2002, p. 610). Related factors that may affect older adults include medications, anorexia, depression, chewing difficulties, social isolation, and inability to procure or prepare food. If the nursing assessment identifies constipation or risks for constipation, the applicable nursing diagnosis is Constipation. The nursing assessment may also identify certain oral health problems that are common in older adults. These include xerostomia, medication effects, chewing difficulties, periodontal disease, diminished taste sensation, ill-fitting dentures, inadequate oral hygiene, and broken or missing teeth. A relevant nursing diagnosis to address these problems would be Impaired Oral Mucous Membrane.

OUTCOMES

Nursing-sensitive outcomes for Altered Nutritional Status: Less Than Body Requirements include the following indicators of Nutritional Status: Weight, Energy, Body Mass, Nutrient Intake, Biochemical Measures, and Food and Fluid Intake (Wakefield, 2001). Nursing interventions are directed toward alleviating the factors that interfere with food procurement, preparation, and enjoyment. Another goal of nursing interventions is to assist the older adult to attain and maintain the highest possible level of nutrition and digestive function. The outcome criteria for this goal would be that the older adult: (1) consumes food and fluids that meet his or her daily nutritional needs; (2) maintains stable body weight; (3) establishes a bowel routine that achieves regular bowel movements; and (4) maintains moist oral mucous membranes. A nursing goal for older adults with psychosocial consequences might be to improve their health-related quality of life.

 ## NURSING INTERVENTIONS TO PROMOTE HEALTHY DIGESTION AND NUTRITION

Nursing interventions to promote healthy digestion and nutrition in older adults include health education about optimal nutrition and disease prevention and direct interventions to eliminate risk factors that interfere with digestion, nutrition, and oral health.

Addressing Risk Factors That Interfere With Digestion and Nutrition

Nursing interventions may be needed to address functional consequences of age-related changes even in healthy older adults. For example, if older adults experience early satiety during meals, they may benefit from eating five smaller meals a day, rather than the customary three meals a day. Similarly, older adults can be encouraged to maintain a sitting or upright position during eating and for $1/2$ to 1 hour after eating to compensate for any effects of presbyesophagus.

When functional limitations interfere with the activities involved in procuring, preparing, and enjoying food, interventions focus on improving the person's access to palatable and nutritious meals. For the community-living older adult, this may involve identifying resources that offer assistance in obtaining food. Home-delivered meal programs may be available to older adults at minimal cost, and group meal programs are available in almost every community through the federally funded National Nutrition

Program for the Elderly, established under the Older Americans Act. In addition to providing inexpensive and nutritionally balanced meals, these programs provide opportunities for social interaction. Local offices on aging may provide assistance with transportation or grocery shopping and are an excellent source of information about group and home-delivered meal programs. When environmental barriers, such as high cupboards, interfere with the older adult's ability to prepare meals safely, environmental modifications can be made. Many of the environmental adaptations suggested in the chapters on vision (Chapter 13) and mobility (Chapter 18) can be applied to improve the ability of the older person to prepare meals.

In institutional settings, environmental factors may interfere with food enjoyment. Although modifying large institutional environments is often difficult or impossible, nurses may be able to identify simple interventions that will increase food enjoyment, particularly in nursing homes. For example, the seating arrangement in a dining room might be planned to improve social interaction and to minimize the negative effects of disruptive people. In some long-term care settings, two mealtimes are scheduled for each meal to allow increased flexibility in seating arrangements. Additional examples of environmental modifications that nurses can implement to improve nutrition and eating in nursing home settings are described in gerontological journals (e.g., Brush et al., 2002; Roberts & Durnbaugh, 2002).

In long-term care settings, inadequate access to enjoyable beverages is a common barrier to optimal fluid intake that can be addressed through nursing interventions. For example, one nursing home used a colorful beverage cart and colorful pitchers and glasses to serve a variety of hot and cold beverages twice daily to the residents. This intervention was cost-effective because outcomes of improved hydration for the residents included reduction in laxative use, increased frequency of bowel movements, and a decline in the number of falls and other negative outcomes of dehydration (Robinson & Rosher, 2002).

Food additives can be used to enhance food flavors for people with diminished smell and taste sensations. Although the use of monosodium glutamate as a flavor enhancer has been discouraged because it contains sodium, the use of very small amounts of flavor enhancers that contained monosodium glutamate can improve food palatability and increase nursing home residents' dietary intake without significantly increasing their sodium intake (Mathey et al., 2001). Nurses can encourage the use of low- or no-sodium food additives and flavor enhancers, such as herbs and lemon, and can teach older adults and their caregivers how to check the sodium content of food additives.

Nursing interventions also address smoking and poor oral care when these are risk factors that interfere with food enjoyment. Good oral hygiene, especially before meals, can be effective in enhancing food flavors. If older adults smoke, encourage them to abstain from smoking for 1 hour before meals.

When the older adult is misinformed about constipation, or when other risk factors (e.g., a low-fiber diet) interfere with good bowel function, nursing interventions are directed toward education. Examples of effective programs for the prevention and management of constipation are found in nursing and medical literature (e.g., Hinrichs et al., 2001; McLane & McShane, 2001). Daily use of bran cereals or bran mixed with other foods is a common and effective strategy for preventing constipation. Howard and colleagues (2000) found that daily use of a mixture of applesauce, wheat bran, and unsweetened prune juice resulted in decreased use of medications for constipation and improved predictability of bowel movements so that patients could be toileted more accurately. Display 14-4 identifies some of the foods and other interventions that aid in preventing constipation.

When medications affect nutrition and digestion, the nurse, caregiver, or older adults can discuss this problem with the prescribing health care practitioner to identify ways of alleviating this risk or addressing the consequences. If over-the-counter medications have a detrimental effect on nutrition or digestion, the nurse educates the older adult about medication–nutrient

DISPLAY 14-4
Health Education Regarding Constipation

- A bowel movement every day is not necessarily the norm for every adult.
- Each adult has an individual pattern of bowel regularity, with the normal range varying from 3 times a day to 2 times a week.
- Include several portions of the following high-fiber foods in your daily diet: fresh, uncooked fruits and vegetables; bran and other cereal products made from whole grains.
- Drink 8 to 10 glasses of noncaffeinated liquid, including fruit juices, every day.
- Avoid laxatives and enemas.
- If medication is needed to promote bowel regularity, a bulk-forming agent (e.g., psyllium or methylcellulose) is least likely to have detrimental effects, especially if fluid intake is adequate.
- Do not ignore the urge to defecate; try to respond as soon as you feel the urge.
- Exercise regularly.

interactions and discusses ways of addressing the negative effects. Pharmacists may be helpful in suggesting interventions that will compensate for, or minimize, the effects of both prescription and over-the-counter medications on nutrition and digestion.

When consumption of alcohol interferes with nutrition, interventions might address the potential problem of alcoholism, or they may be aimed at compensating for the detrimental effects on nutrition. Vitamin supplementation for people with a history of alcoholism can be recommended after a medical evaluation has been performed and any underlying conditions, such as pernicious anemia, have been identified.

Promoting Oral and Dental Health

In its goals related to oral health conditions, *Healthy People 2010* includes the objective of improving access to dental care for older adults, particularly for residents of long-term care facilities (USDHHS, 2000). This goal is addressed through dental services and good daily oral care; nurses have important responsibilities in implementing interventions to achieve this goal. If the older adult has avoided dental care because of resignation to poor oral health or a poor understanding of the need for preventive dental care, the nurse attempts to change these attitudes through education. Nurses also emphasize the importance of obtaining dental care every 6 months and, if appropriate, facilitate referrals for dental care. For homebound older adults, home dental services are often available, especially in large urban communities. In addition, low-cost dental services and dentures may be available through schools of dentistry. Nurses need to be familiar with local resources so that they can teach older adults and their caregivers about the dental services that are available in their community. In long-term care settings, nurses are usually responsible for facilitating referrals for dental care every 6 months. For older adults in any setting, if xerostomia interferes with digestion or nutrition, the nurse may suggest or facilitate a referral for a medical evaluation to identify disease processes or medication effects that may be contributing factors.

Daily oral care as an essential, but often overlooked, component of nursing care for dependent older adults is gaining increased attention in the nursing literature (e.g., Charteris & Kinsella, 2001; Coleman, 2002; Reese, 2001; Stiefel et al., 2000). An important initial intervention in institutional settings may be educational strategies to develop a culture "that promotes, values, and communicates oral health caregiving as fundamental to geriatric nursing practice as are restraint reduction and skin care practices" (Coleman, 2002, p. 193). An intervention that has been found to be effective in nursing homes is the use of specially trained aides whose only responsibility is to provide oral care to residents. Because the cost of implementing this model is offset by reducing the cost of care related to consequences of poor oral hygiene (e.g., aspiration pneumonia), this model may be associated with measurable cost savings (Terpenning & Shay, 2002). Nurses also facilitate referrals for occupational therapists for assisting functionally impaired older adults in self-care oral hygiene activities.

Nurses and researchers also are trying to identify cost-effective oral care products that improve oral hygiene and are easy to use. For example, Simons and colleagues (2002) found that older residents of residential homes who had some natural teeth and chewed sugar-free gum containing xylitol alone or xylitol and chlorhexidine for 15 minutes after the morning and evening meals had significant increases in saliva flow rates and reductions in denture stomatitis, angular cheilitis, and denture debris scores compared with a control group that did not chew gum. A recent nursing review of oral care products suggested that ultrasonic oral care devices or specially designed manual brushes (e.g., the Collis-curve brush, available at www.colliscurve.com) are more effective and convenient than traditional manual brushes for use with dependent older adults (Coleman, 2002). Nurses can adapt handles of toothbrushes, or obtain specially designed brushes, to increase the self-care abilities of people with functional limitations that interfere with normal use of a toothbrush. Battery-operated brushes are effective, easy to use, and relatively inexpensive. Although foam swabs have been commonly used in institutional settings for several decades, they are not effective for cleaning teeth or removing plaque. Similarly, lemon and glycerin swabs, which have been available since the 1940s, are no longer recommended because they reduce the oral pH and dehydrate oral mucous membranes. Mouth rinses containing chlorhexidine (e.g., Peridex, PerioGard) are effective in inhibiting plaque and treating periodontal disease, and they have been used as an alternative to mechanical plaque removal for frail or dependent older adults (MacEntee, 2000).

Display 14-5 can be used as a guide to health education about interventions for oral care and alleviation of xerostomia.

Promoting Optimal Nutrition and Preventing Disease

Therapeutic diets have long been recognized as essential interventions for some diseases (e.g. diabetes, renal or liver failure), and in recent years, the

DISPLAY 14-5
Health Education Regarding Oral and Dental Care

Health Education Regarding Care of the Teeth and Gums

- Oral care should include daily use of dental floss as well as twice daily brushing of all tooth surfaces.
- Use a soft-bristled toothbrush and fluoridated toothpaste.
- If you have any limitations that interfere with your ability to use a regular toothbrush, you may benefit from using an electric or battery-powered brush or a brush with a specially designed handle (available where medical supplies are sold).
- Easy-to-use floss aids are inexpensive and widely available for facilitating dental flossing; they are especially helpful for people with any limitations in manual strength or dexterity or limited range of motion in the upper extremities.
- Some mouth rinses have cleansing, antimicrobial, and moisturizing effect, but they are used in conjunction with, not instead of, brushing.
- Avoid the use of alcohol-containing mouthwashes because of their drying effect.
- Because sugar is a major contributing factor to tooth decay, it is important to limit the intake of sugary substances, especially substances that are kept in the mouth for long periods (e.g., gum, hard candy).
- After eating sugar-containing foods, rinse your mouth or brush your teeth.
- Visit a dentist every 6 months for regular oral care.

- If partial or complete dentures are worn, remove them at night, keep them in water, and clean them before placing them back in your mouth.

Health Education Regarding Dry Mouth

- Excessive dry mouth may be caused by medical conditions or medication effects and should be evaluated before symptomatic treatment is initiated.
- Drink at least 10 to 12 glasses of noncaffeinated fluid during the day, and drink sips of water at frequent intervals.
- Suck on xylitol-flavored fluoride tablets or sugar-free hard candies to stimulate saliva flow.
- Chew sugar-free gum with xylitol for 15 minutes after meals to stimulate saliva flow and promote oral hygiene.
- Try using one of the many brands of saliva substitutes available at drugstores, but avoid those that contain sorbitol because this can worsen the condition.
- Avoid sucking lozenges containing citric acid because of their detrimental effects on tooth enamel.
- Avoid alcohol, alcohol-containing mouthwashes, and highly acidic drinks (e.g., orange or grapefruit juice) because these tend to exacerbate the condition.
- Avoid smoking because this exacerbates the symptoms and further irritates the oral mucous membranes.
- Pay particular attention to oral hygiene because a dry mouth increases the risk for gum and dental diseases.
- Maintain optimal room humidity, especially at night.

role of nutrients is increasingly being supported as an important health promotion and disease prevention intervention for people of all ages. For example, a goal of *Healthy People 2010* is to "promote health and reduce chronic disease associated with diet and weight" (USDHHS, 2000), p. 19-9). Specific objectives address food and nutrient consumption of fruit, grains, sodium, calcium, vegetables, and total and saturated fats. Gerontologists and gerontological health care practitioners currently emphasize the role of nutrition as a secondary prevention intervention that can contribute to improved health and longer life expectancy for older adults (Chernoff, 2001). Nutritional interventions for older adults are specifically directed toward conditions such as diabetes, obesity, hypertension, osteoporosis, cardiovascular disease, and age-related macular degeneration.

Recent attention also is focused on nutritional interventions for healthy aging, with many recommendations emphasizing the inclusion of foods containing antioxidants and other nutrients that may play a protective and preventive role. Researchers are exploring the role of nutrients as primary prevention interventions for age-associated conditions such as dementia, cataracts, cardiovascular disease, and age-related macular degeneration (Smeeding, 2001), but results of studies are not likely to be available in the near future. In analyzing information about potential benefits of nutrients as preventive interventions, distinctions must be made between nutrients obtained from foods and those that are found in supplements. For example, a high dietary intake of a particular nutrient (e.g., carotenoids) may be beneficial in health promotion or disease prevention, but a dietary supplement product with the same nutrient may not necessarily have the same beneficial effects. Thus, nurses need to educate older adults about the importance of obtaining nutrients from food sources rather than relying primarily on dietary supplements.

Nurses teach older adults about basic nutritional requirements, using easy-to-understand educational materials. Healthy older adults generally maintain optimal nutritional status through the daily intake of

DISPLAY 14-6
Guidelines for Daily Food Intake for Older Adults

- Nutrient requirements do not diminish with age, but caloric needs decrease gradually in older adulthood. Therefore, it is important to select a variety of high-quality foods.
- Use salt, sugar, and sodium only in moderation.
- The amount of each type of food will vary according to the caloric needs of each older person, with men generally needing a greater number of servings than women.
- Basic nutritional requirements will be met if the daily diet includes at least the minimum number of servings from each food group listed below and if it includes complex carbohydrates and high-fiber foods. Basic nutritional requirements are as follows:

Servings	Food Group
6–9	Bread, rice, pasta, and cereal
3–4	Vegetables
2–3	Fruits
2–3	Meat, fish, poultry, or legumes (dried peas and beans, lentils, nut butters, soy products)
2–3	Milk, cheese, yogurt, and dairy desserts
8 or more	8-ounce glasses of noncaffeinated liquid

the foods listed in Display 14-6 and illustrated in Figure 14-3. If the older adult has any illness or takes any medications or chemicals that interfere with homeostasis, digestion, or nutrition, the daily diet will have to be modified to compensate for these effects. If, for any reason, the food intake is inadequate to meet daily nutritional requirements, the older adult can be encouraged to use a broad-spectrum vitamin and mineral supplement. Display 14-7 summarizes health education guidelines regarding nutritional supplements and complementary and alternative practices related to digestion and nutrition.

Nutrition education can be provided on an individual basis or in group settings, perhaps in conjunction with registered dietitians. In acute care settings, registered dietitians are usually available, but their services are often limited to people who have special dietary needs or an identified nutritional problem. In long-term care settings, a registered dietitian generally assesses the nutritional needs and usual eating patterns of older adults and establishes a plan of care aimed at attaining and maintaining optimal nutrition. In community settings, nurses sometimes provide nutrition education to groups of older adults. Nurses making home visits include nutrition education in

their health teaching, make referrals for registered dietitian assessment and recommendations, and use available community resources to supplement these interventions. Nurses can use the Transtheoretical Model (discussed in Chapter 4) as an effective approach to working with older adults toward improved nutrition and changes in eating patterns (Burkholder & Evers, 2002).

Determining the appropriate role of nutritional supplements is becoming increasingly difficult, despite their burgeoning availability and variety, because much of the information about them is provided by groups that benefit from their sale. Thus, nurses need to keep abreast of scientifically based research and resources relating to this topic by using the Educational Resources section at the end of this chapter.

➤ Mrs. D. returns for a "Counseling for Health" follow-up session with a 7-day diet history and a list of her medications, as you requested. You review the diet history and find that in response to your previous health education about constipation, Mrs. D. now uses whole wheat bread instead of white and eats more fresh fruits and vegetables. You assess that her daily intake is only about 800 calories, of which pastries account for a high percentage. She rarely eats meat, perhaps because of the poor condition of her teeth. Her medications include citalopram (Celexa), 20 mg daily; clonidine (Catapres), 0.2 mg daily; and triamterene 37.5 mg/hydrochlorothiazide 25 mg (Dyazide), daily.

 THINKING POINTS

➤ What specific risk factors do you address in your health teaching interventions?
➤ What health teaching would you give about alleviating risk factors?
➤ What interventions would you suggest to improve Mrs. D.'s nutrition?
➤ What interventions would you suggest to address Mrs. D.'s dry mouth (which you noticed during Mrs. D.'s last visit)?
➤ What health teaching would you provide about oral and dental care?

EVALUATING EFFECTIVENESS OF NURSING INTERVENTIONS

Nursing care for older adults with Imbalanced Nutrition: Less Than Body Requirements is evaluated by determining whether the older adult has a daily

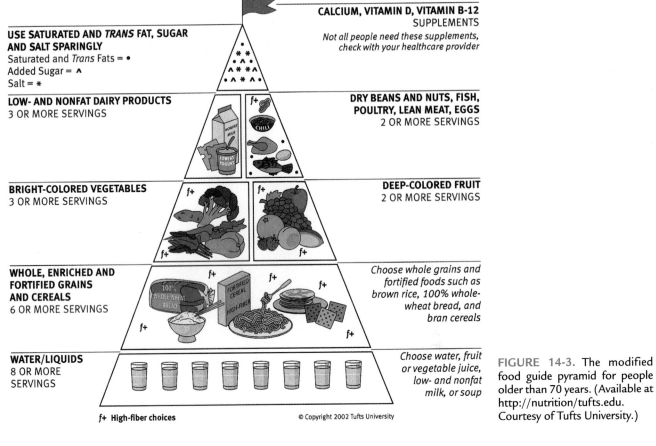

CALCIUM, VITAMIN D, VITAMIN B-12
SUPPLEMENTS
Not all people need these supplements, check with your healthcare provider

USE SATURATED AND *TRANS* FAT, SUGAR AND SALT SPARINGLY
Saturated and *Trans* Fats = •
Added Sugar = ∧
Salt = ∗

LOW- AND NONFAT DAIRY PRODUCTS
3 OR MORE SERVINGS

DRY BEANS AND NUTS, FISH, POULTRY, LEAN MEAT, EGGS
2 OR MORE SERVINGS

BRIGHT-COLORED VEGETABLES
3 OR MORE SERVINGS

DEEP-COLORED FRUIT
2 OR MORE SERVINGS

WHOLE, ENRICHED AND FORTIFIED GRAINS AND CEREALS
6 OR MORE SERVINGS

Choose whole grains and fortified foods such as brown rice, 100% whole-wheat bread, and bran cereals

WATER/LIQUIDS
8 OR MORE SERVINGS

Choose water, fruit or vegetable juice, low- and nonfat milk, or soup

f+ High-fiber choices

© Copyright 2002 Tufts University

FIGURE 14-3. The modified food guide pyramid for people older than 70 years. (Available at http://nutrition/tufts.edu. Courtesy of Tufts University.)

nutrient intake that corresponds with metabolic needs and by the older adult's achieving a body weight within 110% of the ideal body weight for that individual. For older adults with Constipation, or risks for constipation, evaluation criteria would depend on the older adult's verbalizing accurate information about constipation, identifying the factors that contribute to constipation, and reporting that he or she passes soft stools on a regular basis without any straining or discomfort.

DISPLAY 14-7
Health Education About Nutritional Supplements and Complementary and Alternative Practices

Guidelines for Vitamin Supplementation in Older Adults
The following daily vitamin supplements are recommended for older adults (Johnson et al., 2002):

- One multivitamin
- A total of 800 IU vitamin D for people with osteoporosis or risks for osteoporosis or vitamin D deficiency (e.g., sunlight deprivation)
- A total of 1 mg folate for people with cardiovascular risk factors (especially smoking) and for people with alcoholism
- Up to a total of 10 mg thiamine for people with alcoholism
- Up to a total of 2000 IU vitamin E for people with dementia (but observe for signs of toxicity—e.g., malaise, headache, gastrointestinal disturbances—in doses of 1000 IU or higher)

Guidelines Regarding Complementary and Alternative Practices

- Moderate amounts of the following herbs may be effective for constipation: flax, aloe, senna, fennel, rhubarb, buckthorn, cascara, psyllium, fenugreek, and licorice.
- Avoid large amounts of herbal laxatives (including teas) because these may adversely affect the gastrointestinal tract.
- Homeopathic remedies that may be helpful for constipation include graphites, bryonia, alumina, nux vomica, and natrum muriaticum.
- Complementary and alternative practices that may be helpful for treating constipation include yoga, acupuncture, acupressure, reflexology, gentle massage of the abdomen, and hot compresses to the abdomen.

CHAPTER SUMMARY

Digestion and nutrition in older adults is often affected by risk factors, such as tooth loss, medication effects, functional impairments, pathologic conditions, and cultural, environmental and socioeconomic influences. Risk factors can directly affect digestion and nutrition, and can also interfere with the activities involved with obtaining, preparing, and enjoying food. Poor nutrition is a common consequence of risk factors. In the absence of risk factors, the primary consequence of age-related changes is a reduction in caloric requirements. Thus, older adults need to consume higher-quality foods and beverages to achieve adequate nutrient intake with fewer calories. Nursing assessment focuses on identifying risk factors that interfere with optimal nutrition and bowel elimination, determining the nutritional status and usual eating patterns of the older adult, and recognizing any detrimental effects associated with risk factors. Relevant nursing diagnoses include Imbalanced Nutrition, Constipation, and Impaired Oral Mucous Membrane. Nursing interventions focus on alleviating risk factors that interfere with nutrition and digestion. Health promotion interventions focus on good oral care and dental health and on preventing disease and promoting optimal nutrition. Effectiveness of nursing care is evaluated by the degree of improvement in the older adult's eating patterns, nutritional status, or bowel elimination.

CONCLUDING CASE STUDY AND NURSING CARE PLAN

➤ Mr. D. is an 85-year-old widower who was referred for home care following a hospitalization in the Acute Care for the Elderly (ACE) unit for congestive heart failure. During the hospitalization, the geriatric assessment team diagnosed protein-energy undernutrition because Mr. D.'s weight (116 pounds) is only 75% of his ideal body weight (155 pounds). In addition, laboratory work revealed the following abnormal values: hemoglobin, 11%; hematocrit, 35%; and serum albumin, 3.2 g/dL. Mr. D.'s congestive heart failure is stable, and he ambulates with a walker but is very weak. In addition to orders pertaining to assessment and management of the newly diagnosed congestive heart failure, home care orders include nursing assessment of his home situation, nutrition education, and monitoring of weight. The geriatric assessment team in the ACE unit, which included a registered dietitian, recommended that Mr. D. have a daily intake of 1600 calories, including a minimum of 60 g of protein (240 calories). Mr. D. could meet this goal if his daily intake included the minimum number of servings from each food group as listed in Display 14-6.

■ Nursing Assessment

Mr. D. lives alone in a senior high-rise apartment and, until recently, participated in social activities and took advantage of van transportation to get to medical appointments and the grocery store. He used to prepare his own meals and shop for his groceries once a week but has not been out of his apartment in the past month because of gradually increasing weakness, shortness of breath, and swelling in his legs. After his health began declining, a neighbor began doing his grocery shopping. Typical meals are toast and coffee for breakfast; canned soup, a lunchmeat sandwich, and cookies for lunch; and a "Budget Gourmet" entree for supper. Mr. D. says that he never really learned to cook very well, but that he got along "well enough for a man my age." He says that he does not particularly enjoy the convenience foods that he eats, but states, "They sure are easy to fix, even if they are boring." Mr. D. acknowledges that he has thought about going to the daily noon meal offered at a nearby church, but has not followed through because "the senior van doesn't go there, but it does go to the grocery store. Besides, I'm never very hungry because food just doesn't interest me the way it used to when I had Magda's good Hungarian cooking." Mr. D. reports a gradual weight loss of about 50 pounds since his wife died 2 years ago. He says that he was too heavy when his wife used to do the cooking, so he is not concerned about his weight loss. He has full dentures but has not used them for the past year because they do not fit well anymore. He has not done anything about his dentures because he manages to chew the kinds of food he buys. In addition, his dentist retired 2 years ago, and he has not considered going to a new one.

■ Nursing Diagnosis

One of the nursing diagnoses that you address in your home care plan is Altered Nutrition: Less Than Body Requirements, related to social isolation, declining health, ill-fitting dentures, and lack of enjoyment of food. You also question whether depression may be a contributing factor. Evidence comes from his low body weight, laboratory data consistent with poor nutritional status, and his descriptions of his eating and food preparation patterns.

■ Nursing Care Plan

The nursing care plan you devise for Mr. D. is shown in Display 14-8.

DISPLAY 14-8 • NURSING CARE PLAN FOR MR. D.

EXPECTED OUTCOME	NURSING INTERVENTIONS	NURSING EVALUATION
Mr. D. will state what his daily needs are for each food group.	• Give Mr. D. a copy of Display 14-6 and use it as a basis for teaching about daily nutrient requirements.	• Mr. D. will describe an eating pattern that meets his daily nutritional needs.
Mr. D. will identify a method for meeting his nutrient needs.	• Gain Mr. D.'s permission to arrange for home health aide assistance three times weekly for meal preparation and grocery shopping. • Explore with Mr. D. various options for broadening his food selection to improve his nutritional intake (e.g., including dairy products and more fruits and vegetables). • Develop a meal plan with Mr. D. that includes foods that he enjoys but are not currently part of his diet. Discuss the nutritional value of these foods and suggest that he add new food items in each of the food group categories in which he is deficient.	• Mr. D. will describe an acceptable plan for meeting his nutritional needs. • Mr. D. will gain between 1 and 2 pounds weekly until he reaches the goal of 150 to 155 pounds.
Mr. D. will have his dentures evaluated and modified or replaced.	• Discuss with Mr. D. the importance of dentures in chewing efficiency and food enjoyment. • Discuss the long-term detrimental effects of lack of dentures. • Explore ways of obtaining a dental evaluation.	• Mr. D. will chew his food with dentures that fit properly.

 CRITICAL THINKING EXERCISES

1. Discuss specific ways in which each of the following conditions might influence the eating patterns of older adults: depression, medications, sensory changes, cognitive impairments, functional impairments, economic factors, social circumstances, and oral health factors.
2. Describe at least three characteristics of eating patterns for each of the following cultural groups: Native Americans, Hispanic Americans, African Americans, and Asian Americans.
3. How would you assess digestion and nutrition for an older adult in each of the following settings: home, nursing home, and acute care facility?
4. Outline a health education plan for teaching older adults about constipation. Include the following points: definition of constipation, risk factors for constipation, and interventions to prevent and address constipation.
5. Outline a health education plan for teaching older adults about oral and dental care.

Future Directions for Healthier Aging: Focus on Digestion and Nutrition

Research priorities of the National Institute on Aging for 2001 to 2005 include the following:
• Ideal body weight for older adults
• Adverse medication–nutrient interactions
• Mechanisms that underlie age-related changes in nutritional requirements
• Special dietary concerns related to age-related changes in digestion and absorption of nutrients
• Promotion of healthy eating habits, especially in frail older adults
• Interventions for flavor enhancement of food
• Nutritional interventions for primary and secondary prevention of cancer, diabetes, hypertension, hypercholesterolemia, and other conditions that occur commonly in older adults

EDUCATIONAL RESOURCES

American Dietetic Association
120 South Riverside Plaza, Suite 2000, Chicago, IL 60606-6995
(800) 366-1655
http://www.eatright.org

Canadian National Institute of Nutrition
408 Queen Street, 3rd Floor, Ottawa,
Ontario KIR 5A7 Canada
(613) 235-3355
http://www.nin.ca

Food and Drug Administration
5600 Fishers Lane, Rockville, MD 20857
(888) 463-6332
http://www.fda.gov

Food and Nutrition Information Center
National Agriculture Library
10301 Baltimore Avenue, Beltsville, MD 20705-2351
(301) 504-5755
http://www.nal.usda.gov/fnic

Mini Nutritional Assessment
http://www.mna-elderly.com

National Dairy Council
10255 W. Higgins Road, Suite 900, Rosemont, IL 60018
(800) 426-8271
http://www.dairyinfo.com

National Oral Health Information Clearinghouse
1 NOHIC Way, Bethesda, MD 20892-3500
(301) 402-7364
http://www.nohic.nidcr.nih.gov/

Nutrition Screening Initiative
1010 Wisconsin Avenue, NW, Suite 800,
Washington, DC 200007
(202) 625-1662
http://www.aafp.org/nsi.xml

REFERENCES

Amarantos, E., Martinez, A., & Dwyer, J. (2001). Nutrition and quality of life in older adults. *Journal of Gerontology: Series A, 56A*(Special Issue II), 54–64.

Andres, E., Kaltenbach, G., Perrin, A. E., Kurtz, J. E., Schlienger, J. L. (2002). Food-cobalamin malabsorption in the elderly. *American Journal of Medicine, 13*(4), 351–352.

Barber, C. E. (1997). Olfactory acuity as a function of age and gender: A comparison of African and American samples. *International Journal of Aging and Human Development, 44*, 317—334.

Bleda, M. J., Bolibar, I., Pares, R., & Alava, A. (2002). Reliability of the mini nutritional assessment (MNA) in institutional elderly people. *Journal of Nutrition, Health & Aging, 6*, 134–137.

Bromley, S. M. (2000). Smell and taste disorders: A primary care approach. *American Family Physician, 61*(2), 427–436.

Brush, J. A., Meehan, R. A., & Calkins, M. P. (2002). Using the environment to improve intake for people with dementia. *Alzheimer's Care Quarterly, 3*(4), 330–338.

Burkholder, G. J., & Evers, K. A. (2002). Application of the Transtheoretical Model to several problem behaviors. In P. M. Burbank, & D. Riebe (Eds.), *Promoting exercise and behavior change in older adults: Interventions with the Transtheoretical Model* (pp. 85–145). New York: Springer.

Carpenito, L. J. (2002). *Nursing diagnosis: Application to clinical practice* (9th ed.). Philadelphia: Lippincott Williams & Wilkins.

Charteris, P., & Kinsella, T. (2001). The Oral Care Link Nurse: A facilitator and educator of maintaining oral health for patients at the Royal Hospital for Neuro-Disability. *Special Care Dentistry, 21*, 68–71.

Chernoff, R. (2001). Nutrition and health promotion in older adults. *Journal of Gerontology: Series A, 56A*(Special Issue II), 47–53.

Chung, J-P., Mojon, P., & Budtz-Jorgensen, E. (2000). Dental care of elderly in nursing homes: Perceptions of managers, nurses, and physicians. *Special Care Dentistry, 20*, 12–17.

Coleman, P. (2002). Improving oral health care for the frail elderly: A review of widespread problems and best practices. *Geriatric Nursing, 23*, 189–197.

Covinsky, K. E., Covinsky, M. H., Palmer, R. M., & Sehgal, A. R. (2002). Serum albumin concentration and clinical assessments of nutritional status in hospitalized older people: Different sides of different coins? *Journal of the American Geriatrics Society, 50*, 631–637.

Crogan, N. L., & Corbett, C. F. (2002). Predicting malnutrition in nursing home residents using the minimum data set. *Geriatric Nursing, 23*, 224–226.

Crogan, N. L., Shultz, J. A., Adams, C. E., & Massey, L. K. (2001). Barriers to nutrition care for nursing home residents. *Journal of Gerontological Nursing, 27*(12), 25–31.

DeBusk, R. M. (October 2002). Oats vs. wheat for heart health. *Integrative Medicine Consult, 108*, 117–118.

De Castro, J. M. (2002). Age-related changes in the social, psychological and temporal influences on food intake in free living, healthy, adults humans. *Journal of Gerontology: Medical Sciences, 57A*, M368–M377.

De Jong, N., de Mulder, I., de Graaf, C., & van Staveren, W. A. (1999). Impaired sensory functioning in elders: The relation with its potential determinants and nutritional intake. *Journal of Gerontology: Biological Sciences, 54A*, B324–331.

Delahunt, A. (2002). The use of the mini nutritional assessment tool for older people attending a day hospital. *Irish Journal of Medical Science, 170*(3), 106–126.

Ettinger, R. (2001). Oral health. In E. A. Swanson, T. Tripp-Reimer, & K. Buckwalter (Eds.), *Health promotion and disease prevention in the older adult* (pp. 81–101). New York: Springer.

Finkel, D., Pedersen, N. L., & Larsson, M. (2001). Olfactory functioning and cognitive abilities: A twin study. *Journal of Gerontology: Psychological Sciences, 56B*, P226–P233.

Frank, L., Flynn, J., & Rothman, M. (2001). Use of a self-report constipation questionnaire with older adults in long-term care. *Gerontologist, 41*, 778–786.

Ghezzi, E. M., Wagner-Lange, L. A., Schork, M. A., Meter, E. J., Baum, B. J., Streckfus, C. F., & Ship, J. A. (2000). Longitudinal influence of age, menopause, hormone replacement therapy, and other medications on parotid flow rates in healthy women. *Journal of Gerontology: Medical Sciences, 55A*, M34–M42.

Hinrichs, M., Huseboe, J., Tang, J., & Titler, M. G., (2001). Research-based protocol: Management of constipation. *Journal of Gerontological Nursing, 27*(2), 17–28.

Horowitz, M. (2000). Aging and the gastrointestinal tract. In M. H. Beers & R. Berkow (Eds.), *The Merck manual of geriatrics* (3rd ed., pp. 1000–1006). Whitehouse Station, NJ: Merck Research Laboratories.

Howard, L.V., West, D., & Ossip-Klein, D. J. (2000). Chronic constipation management for institutionalized older adults. *Geriatric Nursing, 21*, 78–81.

Hutton, B. (2002). Is there an association between edentulism and nutritional state? *Journal of the Canadian Dental Association, 68,* 182–187.

Jensen, G.L., McGee, M., & Brinkley, J. B. (2001). Gastrointestinal disorders in the elderly. Nutrition in the elderly. *Gastroenterology Clinics, 30,* 313–334.

Johnson, K. A., Bernard, M. A., & Funderburg, K. (2002). Vitamin nutrition in older adults. *Clinics in Geriatric Medicine, 18,* 773–801.

Kramarow, E., Lentzner, H., Rooks, R., Weeks, J., & Saydah, S. (1999). *Health and aging chartbook. Health United States, 1999.* Hyattsville, MD: National Center for Health Statistics.

Lewis, M. M. (2001). Long-term care in geriatrics. Nutrition in long term care. *Clinics in Family Practice, 3,* 627–651.

Linder, J. D., & Wilcox, C. M. (2001). Gastrointestinal disorders in the elderly. Acid peptic disease in the elderly. *Gastroenterology Clinics, 30,* 363–376.

Liu, L., Bopp, M. M., Roberson, P. K., & Sullivan, D. H. (2002). Undernutrition and risk of mortality in elderly patients within 1 year of hospital discharge. *Journal of Gerontology: Medical Sciences, 57A,* M741–M746.

MacEntee, M. (2000). Oral care for successful aging in long-term care. *Journal of Public Health Dentistry, 60,* 326–329.

Mathey, M-F., Siebelink, E., de Graaf, C., & Van Staveren, W. A. (2001). Flavor enhancement of food improves dietary intake and nutritional status of elderly nursing home residents. *Journal of Gerontology: Medical Sciences, 56A,* M200–M205.

McLane, A. M., & McShane, R. E. (2001). Constipation. In M. L. Maas, K. C. Buckwalter, M. D. Hardy, T. Tripp-Reimer, M. G. Titler, & J. P. Specht (Eds.), *Nursing care of older adults: Diagnoses, outcomes, and interventions* (pp. 220–226). St Louis: Mosby.

Meyyazhagan, S., & Palmer, R. M. (2002). Nutritional requirements with aging. *Clinics in Geriatric Medicine, 18*(3), 557–576.

Morley, J. E. (2002). Pathophysiology of anorexia. *Clinics in Geriatric Medicine, 18,* 661–674.

National Academy of Sciences. (2002). Dietary, functional, and total fiber. In *Dietary reference intakes for energy, carbohydrates, fiber, fat, protein and amino acids (macronutrients)* (pp. 265–334). Washington, DC: Author.

Nicosia, M. A., Hind, J. A., Roecker, E. B., Carnes, M., Doyle, J., Dengel, G. A., & Robbins, J. (2000). Age effects on the temporal evolution of isometric and swallowing pressure. *Journals of Gerontology: Medical Sciences, 55A,* M634–M640.

Omran, M. L., & Salem, P. (2002). Diagnosing undernutrition. *Clinics in Geriatric Medicine, 18,* 719–737.

Patterson, A. J. (2002). Relationship between nutrition screening checklist and the health and well-being of older Australian women. *Public Health Nutrition, 5*(1), 65–71.

Prather, C. M. (2000). Constipation, diarrhea, and fecal incontinence. In M. H. Beers & R. Berkow (Eds.), *The Merck manual of geriatrics* (3rd ed., pp. 1080–1095). Whitehouse Station, NJ: Merck Research Laboratories.

Randolph, W. M., Ostir, G. V., & Markides, K. S. (2001). Prevalence of tooth loss and dental service use in older Mexican Americans. *Journal of the American Geriatrics Society, 49,* 585–589.

Reese, J. L. (2001). Altered oral mucous membrane. In M. L. Maas, K. C. Buckwalter, M. D. Hardy, T. Tripp-Reimer, M. G. Titler, & J. P. Specht (Eds.), *Nursing care of older adults: Diagnoses, outcomes, and interventions* (pp. 172–182). St. Louis: Mosby.

Ritchie, C. S. (2002). Oral health, taste, and olfaction. *Clinics in Geriatric Medicine, 18*(4), 709–718.

Ritchie, C. S., Joshipura, K., Silliman, R. A., Miller, B., & Douglas, C. W. (2000). Oral health problems and significant weight loss among community-dwelling older adults. *Journal of Gerontology: Medical Sciences, 56A,* M366–M371.

Roberts, S., & Durnbaugh, T. (2002). Enhancing nutrition and eating skills in long-term care. *Alzheimer's Care Quarterly, 3,* 316–329.

Robinson, S. B., & Rosher, R. B. (2002). Can a beverage cart improve hydration? *Geriatric Nursing, 23,* 208–211.

Ross, S. O., & Forsmark, C. E. (2001). Gastrointestinal disorders in the elderly. *Gastroenterology Clinics, 30,* 531–545.

Russell, C. (2001). Caloric intake. In M. D. Mezey (Ed.), *The encyclopedia of elder care* (pp. 105–108). New York: Springer.

Salva, A., & Pera, G. (2001). Nutrition and ageing. Screening for malnutrition in dwelling elderly. *Public Health and Nutrition, 4,* 1375–1378.

Shaker, R., & Staff, D. (2001). Gastrointestinal disorders in the elderly: Esophageal disorders in the elderly. *Gastroenterology Clinics, 30,* 335–361.

Shanley, C., & O'Loughlin, G. (2000). Dysphagia among nursing home residents: An assessment and management protocol. *Journal of Gerontological Nursing, 26*(8), 35–48.

Sharkey, J. R. (2002). The interrelationship of nutritional risk factors, indicators of nutritional risk, and severity of disability among home-delivered meal participants. *Gerontologist, 42,* 373–380.

Ship, J. A. (2002). Improving oral health in older people. *Journal of the American Geriatric Society, 50,* 1454–1455.

Ship, J. A., Pillemer, S. R., & Baum, B. J. (2002). Xerostomia and the geriatric patient. *Journal of the American Geriatrics Society, 50,* 535–543.

Simmons, S. F., Osterseil, D., & Schnelle, J. F. (2001). Improving food intake in nursing home residents with feeding assistance: A staffing analysis. *Journals of Gerontology: Medical Sciences, 56A,* M790–M794.

Simons, D., Brailsford, S. R., Kidd, E. A. M., & Beighton, D. (2002). The effects of medicated chewing gums on oral health in frail older people: A 1-year clinical trial. *Journal of the American Geriatrics Society, 50,* 1348–1353.

Smeeding, S. J. W. (2001). Nutrition, supplements, and aging. *Geriatric Nursing, 22,* 219–224.

Soderhamn, U. (2002). Reliability and validity of the nutritional form for the elderly (NUFFE). *Journal of Advanced Nursing, 37*(1), 28–34.

Staveren, W. A., de Graaf, C., & de Groot, L. C. P. G. M. (2002). Regulation of appetite in frail persons. *Clinics in Geriatric Medicine, 18,* 675–685.

Stiefel, K., Damron, S., & Sowers, N. (2000). Improving oral hygiene for the seriously ill patient: Implementing research-based practice. *Medsurg Nursing, 9,* 40–43, 46.

Terpenning, M., & Shay, K. (2002). Oral health is cost-effective to maintain but costly to ignore. *Journal of the American Geriatrics Society, 50,* 584–585.

Thomas, D. R., Ashmen, W., & Morley, J. E., for the Council for Nutritional Strategies in Long-Term Care. (2000). Nutritional management in long term care: Development of a clinical guideline. *Journal of Gerontology: Medical Sciences, 55A,* M725–M734.

U.S. Department of Health and Human Services (USDHHS). (2000). *Healthy people 2010* (2nd ed). Washington, DC: U.S. Government Printing Office.

Vargas, C. M., Kramarow, E. A., & Yellowitz, J. A. (2001). *The oral health of older Americans. Aging Trends (3).* Hyattsville, MD: National Center for Health Statistics.

Vellas, B. C., & Lauque, S. (2001). Nutritional assessment. In M. D. Mezey (Ed.), *The encyclopedia of elder care* (pp. 456–458). New York: Springer.

Wakefield, B. (2001). Altered nutrition: Less than body requirements. In: M. L. Maas, K. C. Buckwalter, M. D. Hardy, T. Tripp-Reimer, M. G. Titler, & J. P. Specht (Eds.), *Nursing care of older adults: Diagnoses, outcomes, and interventions* (pp.145–157). St. Louis: Mosby.

Wakimoto, P., & Block, G. (2001). Dietary intake, dietary patterns, and changes with age: An epidemiological perspective. *Journal of Gerontology, 56A*(Special Issue II):65–80.

Wald, A. (2000). Advances in gastroenterology. *Medical Clinics of North America, 84,* 1231–1246.

Wardh, I., Hallberg, L., Beggren, U., Andersson, L., & Sorensen, S. (2000). Oral health care: Low priority in nursing. *Scandinavian Journal of Caring Sciences, 14,* 137–142.

Zembrzuski, C. (2000). Nutrition and hydration. *Journal of Gerontological Nursing, 26*(12), 6–7.

Urinary Function

The primary function of urinary elimination is the excretion of water and chemical wastes, such as metabolic and pharmacologic by-products, that would become toxic if allowed to accumulate. Efficient urinary excretion depends on renal blood flow, filtering activities within the kidneys, good functioning of the urinary tract muscles, and nervous system control over voluntary and involuntary mechanisms of elimination. Control of urinary elimination also depends on ambulatory and sensory abilities and on social, emotional, cognitive, and environmental factors.

In the absence of risk factors, healthy older adults experience very few negative functional consequences affecting urinary elimination. In the presence of risk factors, however, negative functional consequences, such as urinary incontinence, can readily occur. An important risk factor—and one that can be alleviated through health education interventions—is the false belief that urinary incontinence is an inevitable part of old age. Nursing interventions such as addressing environmental risk factors and teaching about pelvic muscle exercises can be effective in promoting urinary continence. Because urinary incontinence can seriously interfere with one's daily routines, nursing interventions directed toward eliminating risk factors can be quite effective in improving the quality of life for older adults.

 ## AGE-RELATED CHANGES THAT AFFECT URINARY FUNCTION

Age-related changes in the kidneys, bladder, urethra, and nervous system affect the physiologic processes related to urinary elimination. In addition, any age-related change that interferes with the skills involved in socially appropriate urinary elimination may interfere with urinary control and contribute to the development of incontinence. The next two sections discuss the age-related changes that affect the physiologic processes of urinary elimination and the skills involved in socially appropriate urinary elimination.

Homeostasis and Urinary Elimination

Urinary excretion is a complex process that begins in the kidneys with the filtering and removal of chemical wastes from the blood. Blood circulates through glomeruli, where liquid wastes, collectively termed the *glomerular filtrate*, pass through Bowman's capsule and the renal tubules to the collecting ducts. During this process, substances needed by the body (such as water, glucose, and sodium) are retained, and waste products are excreted in the urine. These functions play important roles in maintaining homeostasis and in the excretion of many medications. Excretory function, which is measured by the glomerular filtration rate (GFR), depends on the number and efficiency of nephrons and on the amount and rate of renal blood flow.

The kidney increases in weight and mass from birth until early adulthood, when the number of functioning nephrons begins to decline, particularly in the cortex, where the glomeruli are located. This decline continues throughout life, resulting in about a 25% decrease in kidney mass by the age of 80 years. The remaining glomeruli undergo various age-related changes, such as increased size, diminished lobulation, and thickened basement membrane. In addition,

the proportion of sclerotic glomeruli increases from fewer than 5% at the age of 40 years to 35% by the age of 80 years. Beginning in the fourth decade, renal blood flow gradually diminishes, particularly in the cortex, at a rate of 10% per decade.

An average decline in renal function of 1% per year has been widely accepted since the 1970s as an age-related change that begins between the ages of 30 and 40 years. However, recent results of longitudinal studies indicate that there is a great deal of individual variation in renal function among healthy older adults, and about one third of older people show no decrease in renal function (Lindeman, 2000). Any decline in renal function that occurs in older adults is probably associated with common pathologic conditions, such as hypertension, rather than being caused by age-related changes alone.

Dilution and concentration of urine, and subsequent excretion of water from the body, are regulated in the renal tubules and have a diurnal rhythm. The physiologic processes responsible for urine concentration and water excretion are influenced by the following factors:

- The amount of fluid in the body
- Resorption of water through, and transport of substances across, the tubular membrane
- Osmoreceptors in the hypothalamus, which regulate the level of circulating antidiuretic hormone (ADH) according to plasma water concentration
- Substances and activities that influence ADH secretion, such as caffeine, medications, alcohol, pain, stress, and exercise
- The concentration of sodium in the glomerular filtrate

Normally, production of ADH is stimulated by hemorrhage, dehydration, and other conditions that affect plasma volume or osmolality. This physiologic protective mechanism helps to maintain plasma volume and conserve fluid and sodium under conditions of water or sodium deprivation.

Many age-related changes affect the renal tubules and thereby affect dilution and concentration of urine. These changes include fatty degeneration, the presence of diverticula, a loss of convoluted cells, and alterations in the composition of the basement membranes. Functionally, the renal tubules in older adults are less efficient in the exchange of substances, the conservation of water, and the suppression of ADH secretion in the presence of hypoosmolality. Age-related changes also decrease the ability of the older kidney to conserve sodium in response to salt restriction. These age-related changes may predispose healthy older adults to hyponatremia and other fluid and electrolyte imbalances, especially in the presence of any condition that alters renal circulation, water or sodium balance, or plasma volume or osmolality.

After being filtered by the kidneys, liquid wastes pass through the ureters into the bladder for temporary storage. The bladder is a balloon-like structure composed of collagen, smooth muscle (called detrusor), and elastic tissue. Liquid wastes are eliminated from the bladder through a complex physiologic process that depends on the following mechanisms:

- The ability of the bladder to expand for adequate storage and to contract for complete expulsion of liquid wastes
- The maintenance of higher urethral pressure relative to intravesical pressure
- Regulation of the lower urinary tract through autonomic and somatic nerves
- Voluntary control of urination (micturition) through the cerebral centers

Age-related changes alter each of these mechanisms, affecting the process of urination in older adults. In younger adults, the bladder is able to store 350 mL to 450 mL of urine before the person experiences sensations of fullness and discomfort. However, with increasing age, hypertrophy of the bladder muscle and thickening of the bladder wall interfere with the bladder's ability to expand, and the amount of urine that can be stored comfortably diminishes to about 200 to 300 mL.

As urine flows into the bladder, the smooth muscle expands without increasing intravesical pressure, and the urethral pressure increases, to the point that it is slightly higher than the intravesical pressure. As long as the volume of urine does not rise above 500 to 600 mL, this balance can be maintained, and urination can be controlled voluntarily. If the volume rises above this level, or if the detrusor muscle contracts involuntarily, the intravesical pressure will exceed the urethral pressure, and incontinence is likely to occur.

In addition to being influenced by the amount of urine in the bladder, the balance between intravesical and urethral pressure is influenced by the following factors: abdominal pressure; thickness of the urethral mucosa; and tone of the pelvic, detrusor, urethral, and bladder neck muscles. With increasing age, connective tissue replaces some of the smooth muscle in the bladder and urethra. This age-related change alters the balance between the intravesical and urethral pressures and contributes to urinary incontinence.

Internal and external sphincters regulate urine storage and bladder emptying. The internal sphincter is part of the base of the bladder and is controlled by autonomic nerves. The external sphincter is part of the pelvic floor musculature and is controlled by the pudendal nerve. When urination takes place, the detrusor and abdominal muscles contract, and the perineal and external sphincter muscles relax. When necessary, the external sphincter contracts to inhibit or interrupt voiding and to compensate for sudden surges in abdominal pressure. Age-related changes, such as loss of smooth muscle in the urethra and relaxation of the pelvic floor muscles, reduce the urethral resistance and diminish the tone of the sphincters. As the bladder fills with urine, sensory receptors in the bladder wall send a signal to the sacral spinal cord. Motor impulses in the spinal cord control urination, but higher centers in the brain are responsible for detecting the sensation of bladder fullness, for inhibiting bladder emptying when necessary, and for stimulating bladder contractions for complete emptying. In healthy older adults, degenerative changes in the cerebral cortex may alter both the sensation of bladder fullness and the ability to empty the bladder completely. In younger adults, a sensation of fullness begins when the bladder is about half full. This sensation occurs at a later point for older adults, so that the interval between the initial perception of the urge to void and the actual need to empty the bladder is shortened, which may trigger an episode of incontinence.

Many structures involved in urination contain estrogen receptors and are affected by hormonal changes, especially those that occur in menopausal women. For example, diminished estrogen can cause a loss of collagen support in the urogenital tissues and a loss of tone and strength in the smooth muscles of the bladder and urethra. These changes contribute to a decrease in urethral closure pressure, which predisposes to urinary leakage problems. Decreased estrogen levels also can lower the sensory threshold and cause the bladder to be more responsive to irritating stimuli because nerve endings contain estrogen receptors. This, in turn, leads to an increased urge to void. The decline in estrogen associated with menopause may partially account for the increased prevalence and earlier onset of incontinence in women.

Diminished thirst perception is another age-related change that can affect homeostasis and urinary function. Healthy older adults who are deprived of fluid do not sense thirst, experience discomfort from dry mouth, or drink enough water to rehydrate themselves. In the presence of conditions that place additional demands on fluid and electrolyte balance, such as infection or elevated body temperature, reduced thirst sensation may interfere with the mechanisms that normally compensate for these physiologic stresses. Consequently, older people are likely to be at increased risk for dehydration because of inadequate fluid intake.

Control Over Socially Appropriate Urinary Elimination

Control over urination depends not only on satisfactory functioning of the urinary tract and nervous system but also on other functional aspects, such as adequate cognition and mobility, that significantly affect the skills needed for socially appropriate urinary elimination. The following factors affect a person's capacity for socially appropriate urinary elimination:

- Identification of a designated receptacle in a private area
- Accessibility and acceptability of toilet facilities
- Ability to get to and use a suitable receptacle
- The interval between the perception of the urge to void and the actual need to empty the bladder
- Voluntary control over the urge to void from the time of its perception until the person is able to use an appropriate receptacle

These factors are influenced by age-related changes that directly affect urinary elimination as well as by those changes that affect the ability to identify and reach appropriate toileting facilities. Thus, balance, mobility, visual impairments, manual dexterity, and age-related vision changes are some of the factors that may influence urinary control. Older adults often experience an increase in postural sway, an age-related change that can interfere with one's ability to stand still. With increasing postural sway, older men may find it more difficult to maintain a standing position for urination. If urinary incontinence does occur, a diminished ability to smell may interfere with the older adult's perception of offensive odors. Although this does not have a functional impact on urinary elimination, the presence of urinary odors is viewed as socially inappropriate and may lead to isolation and rejection of the older adult.

Standards for socially appropriate urinary elimination may vary according to different social environments. For example, an independent, community-living older adult is expected to remain free of urinary odors or wetness and to urinate in private, designated places; however, a dependent or institutionalized older adult may not be expected to adhere so strictly to these standards. In any setting, attitudes and

behaviors of caregivers can significantly influence patterns of urinary elimination, as discussed in the following section on Risk Factors.

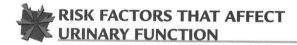

RISK FACTORS THAT AFFECT URINARY FUNCTION

As with many other areas of functioning, risk factors play a more significant role than age-related changes in causing negative functional consequences. Types of risk factors that can significantly affect urinary function include behaviors based on myths and misunderstandings, functional impairments, pathologic conditions, medications, and environmental and lifestyle influences.

Behaviors Based on Myths and Misunderstandings

Attitudes based on myths or lack of knowledge about urinary function can have a detrimental effect on the behavior of older adults and their caregivers. Older adults and their health care providers commonly accept urinary incontinence as an inevitable, irreversible, and normal part of aging; this perception can interfere with the older person seeking and getting help (Locher et al., 2002). Dugan and colleagues (2001) found that the perception of urinary incontinence as a normal consequence of aging was a major reason that fewer than 30% of older adults with bladder control problems report their condition to their health care professional. Health care professionals may reinforce these misperceptions and may even discourage patients from seeking treatment for incontinence. Much evidence indicates that incontinence is frequently ignored as a health care problem by patients as well as health care providers, and this is particularly problematic for older adults (Schnelle & Smith, 2001).

Because of such attitudes of resignation, early signs and symptoms of urinary dysfunction may be managed inappropriately, and the problem may progress. For example, older adults often underestimate the interval between the perception of the urge to void and the actual need to empty the bladder. When incontinence occurs because of this, they may compensate by decreasing their fluid intake or urinating at more frequent intervals. However, these compensatory actions can lead to further urgency and incontinence, which, in turn, may reinforce the myth that incontinence is an inevitable problem of aging.

Attitudes, behaviors, and expectations of caregivers also interfere with the ability of the older adult to maintain continence. For example, when episodes of incontinence are noted soon after admission of an older adult to a long-term care facility, nursing staff members are likely to view the resident as having chronic incontinence, and their subsequent behaviors may reinforce the expectation of incontinence. In reality, the episode of incontinence may have occurred because the toilet is too far away or the older adult could not readily locate it. When staff members assume that incontinence is the norm for that person, they might initiate use of absorbent pads by the resident, giving the older adult the message that voluntary control over urination is not expected.

In acute and long-term care settings, staff attitudes and nursing procedures strongly influence the standards for urinary elimination. In acute care facilities, indwelling catheters might be used because of patient illness, surgical procedures, or staff convenience. Once an indwelling catheter is inserted, it frequently remains in place until the person is discharged, and little or no time may be available to reestablish normal voiding patterns during the hospitalization. In long-term care facilities, heavy workloads, poor communication, lack of teamwork, or inadequate knowledge about appropriated interventions are barriers to continence care (Mather & Bakas, 2002). In any setting, caregivers may believe that the use of pads or other incontinence products for the management of incontinence is easier and more convenient than preventing incontinence by assisting with toileting activities at the necessary intervals. For example, an older adult who needs a great deal of assistance with mobility may be encouraged to use incontinence products and avoid the need for going to the bathroom because this is less time consuming for the caregiver. In these situations, dependent older adults are likely to behave according to the expectations of the caregivers, and incontinence will be the inevitable consequence. Medicare policies also may influence the caregiver's approach to urinary management; for example, reimbursement for skilled care services is provided for people with indwelling catheters, but not for those who manage incontinence by other methods.

Limited fluid intake in response to the fear or onset of incontinence—or for any reason—is another behavior that can unintentionally exacerbate incontinence. Johnson and colleagues (2000) found that almost 37% of incontinent older adults limited their fluid intake as a self-care practice. If bladder fullness is not adequately achieved, as in states of dehydration or limited fluid intake, the neurologic mechanism that controls bladder emptying will not

function effectively, and incontinence can occur because the person does not perceive the urge to void. Dehydration and inadequate hydration also cause increased bladder irritability, with subsequent uninhibited contractions and incontinence.

Functional Impairments

Functional impairments are a major risk factor for the development of incontinence in older adults because they can interfere with the ability to recognize and respond to the urge to void in a timely manner. In the presence of age-related changes that shorten the interval between the perception of the urge to void and the actual need to empty the bladder, any delay in reaching an appropriate receptacle may result in incontinence. Thus, dependency in performing activities of daily living (ADLs) for any reason is strongly associated with incontinence. For example, conditions such as arthritis or Parkinson's disease may slow the ambulation of older adults as well as their ability to manipulate clothing. Likewise, dementia and other conditions that impair cognitive abilities can interfere with the timely processing of information that is necessary for maintaining voluntary control over urination. Finally, restraints can cause significant functional limitations and increase the risk for incontinence.

Disease Processes

Disease processes that commonly increase the risk for urinary incontinence in older adults can be divided into those that directly involve the urinary tract and those that affect other systems and indirectly cause incontinence. Most of the conditions that affect the urinary tract are gender specific, whereas those that affect other systems can affect all older adults.

Conditions of the Genitourinary Tract

Weakening of pelvic floor muscles in women, which may be secondary to postmenopausal estrogen depletion or to pregnancy, increases the risk for incontinence. With weakening of the pelvic muscles, any sudden increase in abdominal pressure may cause the involuntary expulsion of small amounts of urine. A cystocele, rectocele, or urethrocele may develop because of extreme pelvic muscle stretching or relaxation. These disorders frequently coexist with uterovaginal prolapse and are often identified as causes of urinary incontinence. Pelvic muscle weakness also interferes with complete emptying of the bladder, resulting in residual urine and increased risk for bacteriuria. In addition to causing degenerative changes in the pelvic floor muscles, decreased estrogen levels cause atrophy of the vaginal and trigonal tissue with subsequent diminished resistance to pathogens. Vaginitis and trigonitis may develop and cause urinary urgency, frequency, and incontinence.

Benign prostatic hyperplasia is a common cause of voiding problems in older men, and prostatic carcinoma is a less common cause. In its early stage, prostatic hyperplasia obstructs the vesical neck and compresses the urethra, causing a compensatory hypertrophy of the detrusor muscle and subsequent outlet obstruction. With progressive hypertrophy, the bladder wall loses its elasticity and becomes thinner. Subsequently, urinary retention occurs, increasing the risk for bacteriuria and infection. Eventually, the ureter and kidney are affected, and hydroureter, hydronephrosis, diminished GFR, and uremia may develop. Men with prostatic hyperplasia may experience nocturia, decreased urine flow, incomplete bladder emptying, and urinary urgency and frequency. Another cause of decreased urethral resistance in men is the residual effect of transurethral surgery or radical prostatectomy.

Urinary tract infections are a common cause of incontinence in older adults, with an annual incidence of 10%. The female-to-male ratio for urinary tract infections is 2:1, and they have been identified as the most common nosocomial infection in older people who have indwelling catheters (Yoshikawa, 2000). Older adults also are likely to have chronic bacteriuria, a condition characterized as 10^5 or more colony-forming units without symptoms of urinary tract infection. Manifestations of urinary tract infections in older adults may be very subtle; urinary incontinence may be the initial or primary sign. A change in behavior or level of functioning may be the presenting sign, especially in people with dementia.

Other Conditions That Cause Urinary Incontinence

Many pathologic conditions affecting either the central or peripheral nervous system increase the risk for incontinence. Dementia is strongly associated with urinary incontinence, but the relationship between these two conditions is complex, and incontinence should not be viewed as an inevitable and untreatable component of dementia (Ostbye et al., 2002). For example, older adults with dementia may lack the perceptual abilities that are necessary for finding and using appropriate facilities, but they may be able to maintain continence when given appropriate cues and reminders. When urinary incontinence develops in people with dementia, it often is associated with

functional declines such as impaired mobility. Interventions that address the contributing factors (e.g., mobility or cognitive impairment) often are effective in alleviating incontinence (Specht et al., 2002).

Conditions of the gastrointestinal tract that can cause incontinence include gastroenteritis, constipation, and fecal impaction. The mass of stool that is present with constipation or fecal impaction places pressure on the bladder and diminishes its storage capacity. In turn, this causes urinary frequency, urgency, and incontinence. Fecal impaction also can obstruct the bladder outlet, causing bladder distention and urinary retention or incontinence. Other conditions that are highly associated with incontinence are diabetes, alcoholism, multiple sclerosis, Parkinson's disease, cerebrovascular accident, and chronic obstructive pulmonary disease (COPD).

Many conditions that affect physiologic processes can cause or exacerbate incontinence. For example, delirium and other acute illnesses may be manifested or accompanied by urinary incontinence. Metabolic disturbances that induce diuresis, such as diabetes and hypercalcemia, also may contribute to incontinence. Any acute illness or surgical intervention that temporarily limits mobility or compromises mental abilities also represents a risk factor for urinary incontinence. Hip fracture has been identified as a common cause of hospital-acquired incontinence, and the risk is exacerbated in cognitively impaired older adults and those who had mobility limitations before the hip fracture (Palmer et al., 2002).

Medication Effects

Medications influence urinary function in a number of ways and are common risk factors in the development of urinary incontinence. For example, loop diuretics increase urinary output, placing additional demands on the urinary system and compounding the effects of an age-related decrease in bladder capacity. Many medications, especially those that act on the central or autonomic nervous system, directly affect the urinary tract and cause incontinence. Older adults with other urinary tract conditions may be particularly susceptible to adverse medication effects. For example, men with prostatic hyperplasia may be especially prone to developing urinary retention when they take an adrenergic or anticholinergic agent (even those in over-the-counter decongestants and antihistamines). Similarly, menopausal women who are not taking estrogen are more likely to develop stress incontinence if they are taking α-adrenergic blocking agents (commonly used for hypertension). Some of the medications that are used to treat some types of incontinence also can cause incontinence. For example, terazosin is used for benign prostatic hyperplasia, but it can cause urethral relaxation and stress incontinence. Thus, it is imperative that causes of incontinence be identified accurately before treatment is initiated.

In addition to causing incontinence through their direct effects on the urinary tract, medications can cause incontinence through their effects on functional abilities. For example, anticholinergics (including those in over-the-counter agents) are commonly associated with cognitive and other functional impairments, which can interfere with the older adult's voluntary control over urination. Anticholinergics also cause dry mouth, and the subsequent increased fluid intake and diuresis can precipitate incontinence. Many medications cause constipation, which is a causative factor for incontinence. This adverse effect may be especially detrimental in the presence of prostatic hyperplasia or weakened pelvic floor muscles. Table 15-1 summarizes some types and examples of medications that commonly cause incontinence in older adults.

In addition to creating risk factors for incontinence, medications can compromise kidney function through the overstimulation of ADH secretion, which may compound age-related effects that predispose older adults to hyponatremia. Medications that stimulate ADH secretion include aspirin, narcotics, acetaminophen, antidepressants, barbiturates, chlorpropamide, clofibrate, fluphenazine, and haloperidol.

Dietary and Lifestyle Factors

Obesity (i.e., weight that exceeds average weights by more than 20%) increases the risk for incontinence, particularly for women. Deficiencies of zinc, calcium, magnesium, protein, and vitamins C and B_{12} predispose to incontinence through their effects on the detrusor and other urinary tract muscles (Bottomley, 2000). Smoking of cigarettes and other nicotine-containing products may increase the risk for urinary urgency, frequency, and urge incontinence. Certain foods (e.g., chocolate and spicy or acidic foods), food additives (e.g., aspartame and other artificial sweeteners), and caffeinated or carbonated beverages can cause incontinence. Specific effects of these substances that lead to incontinence and urinary urgency and frequency include increased diuresis, irritation of the bladder mucosa, and involuntary bladder contractions (Bottomley, 2000).

Environmental Factors

Environmental factors may impede or prevent older adults from reaching and using the toilet in home, public, and institutional settings. When these environmental obstacles are accompanied by mobility limitations and age-related changes that affect urinary function, incontinence may result. Examples of environmental obstacles include stairs, an absence of grab bars and railings, and toilet seats that are not the appropriate height. Display 15-1 summarizes some

TABLE 15-1 • Medications That Can Cause Urinary Incontinence

Medication Type	Examples	Mechanism of Action
Loop diuretics	Furosemide, bumetanide	Increased diuresis can cause urinary urgency, frequency, and polyuria
Anticholinergic agents	Antihistamines, antipsychotics, antidepressants, antispasmodics, anti-parkinsonian agents	Decreased bladder contractility and relaxed bladder muscle can cause urinary retention, frequency, and incontinence
Adrenergics (alpha-adrenergic agonists)	Decongestants	Decreased bladder contractility and increased sphincter tone can cause urinary retention, frequency, and incontinence
Alpha-adrenergic blockers	Prazosin, terazosin, doxazosin	Decreased urethral and internal sphincter tone can cause leakage and stress incontinence
Calcium channel blockers	Nifedipine, nicardipine, isradipine, felodipine, nimodipine	Decreased bladder contractility can cause urinary retention, frequency, nocturia, and incontinence
Angiotensin-converting enzyme inhibitors	Captopril, enalapril, lisinopril	Can cause chronic cough, which precipitates or exacerbates stress incontinence
Hypnotics and antianxiety agents	Benzodiazepines	Can interfere with voluntary control over urination by causing sedation, delirium, and cognitive impairments
Alcohol	Wine, beer, hard liquor	Can interfere with voluntary control over urination by causing sedation, delirium, increased diuresis, and cognitive impairments

environmental risk factors that may contribute to the incidence of incontinence in older adults.

PATHOLOGIC CONDITIONS ASSOCIATED WITH URINARY FUNCTION

Although age-related changes alone do not cause urinary incontinence, they predispose older adults to it, making it the most commonly occurring pathologic condition associated with the urinary tract in older adults. Between 15% and 35% of older adults in community settings, one third of those in acute care settings, and at least 50% of nursing home residents are incontinent of urine (Schnelle & Smith, 2001; Resnick & Yalla, 2002).

> Most studies find that women have a higher prevalence and earlier age at onset of incontinence than men (Lose et al., 2001; Maggi et al., 2001).

Urinary incontinence is defined by the International Continence Society as "the complaint of any involuntary leakage of urine" (Abrams et al., 2002, p. 118). In recent years, urinary incontinence has gained much attention as a medical condition and quality-of-life issue; in 2002, the International Continence Society promulgated major recommendations on standard-

ized terminology in reference to urinary incontinence and lower urinary tract function. Display 15-2 summarizes these recommendations, which are available in full at www.icsoffice.org. The International Continence Society notes that the current definition does not address the quality-of-life issues associated with urinary incontinence; however, they emphasize that instruments have been and are being developed to assess the psychosocial impact of incontinence (Abrams et al., 2002).

Urinary incontinence is categorized according to the signs and symptoms. *Urge incontinence* is characterized by urinary leakage due to the inability to hold urine long enough to reach a toilet after perceiving the urge to void. *Stress incontinence* is characterized by a sudden leakage of urine as a result of an activity that increases abdominal pressure (e.g., lifting, coughing, sneezing, laughing, or exercise). *Mixed incontinence* is characterized by leakage of urine due to a combination of increased abdominal pressure and the inability to delay voiding after perceiving the urge. *Functional incontinence* refers to urinary leakage that occurs because of functional impairments, environmental barriers, or other factors that interfere with the person's ability to reach the toilet in a timely manner. If urinary incontinence develops, a comprehensive assessment can usually identify causes and risk factors, and interventions can be implemented, as discussed later in this chapter.

FUNCTIONAL CONSEQUENCES ASSOCIATED WITH URINARY ELIMINATION IN OLDER ADULTS

Despite the many age-related changes in the urinary tract, the elimination of wastes is not significantly affected in healthy, nonmedicated, older adults. However, in the presence of any unusual physiologic demands, such as those that occur with medications or disease conditions, the older adult is increasingly likely to experience functional consequences affecting homeostatic mechanisms and urinary control. Age-related changes and risk factors also cause functional consequences in patterns of urinary elimination and predispose older adults to incontinence. When incontinence occurs, additional functional consequences, especially psychosocial effects, can be quite serious.

The Impact of Urinary Function Changes on Homeostasis and Urinary Elimination

In healthy older adults, age-related changes have only a limited effect on renal function, but functional consequences include impaired absorption of

---

DISPLAY 15-2

Recommendations of the International Continence Society on Standardized Terminology for Lower Urinary Tract Function

---

Terms Related to the Urinary Tract and Micturition (Urination)

Urinary bladder: the entire vesica urinaria organ

Detrusor: the smooth muscle structure that controls micturition

- *Normal detrusor function:* allows bladder filling with little or no change in pressure
- *Detrusor overactivity:* involuntary detrusor contractions during the filling phase
- *Detrusor underactivity:* a contraction of reduced strength and/or duration, resulting in prolonged bladder emptying and/or failure to achieve complete bladder emptying within a normal time span

Bladder sensation

- *Normal:* awareness of bladder filling and increasing sensation up to a strong urge to void
- *Increased:* sensation of an early and persistent desire to void
- *Reduced:* awareness of bladder filling but no sensation of a definite desire to void
- *Absent:* no sensation of bladder filling or desire to void
- *Nonspecific:* no specific bladder sensation, but perception of bladder filling as abdominal fullness, vegetative symptoms, or spasticity

Urinary flow pressures

- *Urethral:* the fluid pressure needed to just open a closed urethra

- *Intravesical:* pressure within the bladder
- *Abdominal:* pressure surrounding the bladder

Post void residual (PVR): the volume of urine left in the bladder at the end of micturition

Urgency (with or without urge incontinence, usually with frequency and nocturia): the overactive bladder syndrome, urge syndrome, or urgency–frequency syndrome

Terms Related to Incontinence

Stress urinary incontinence: involuntary leakage on effort or exertion, or on sneezing or coughing

Urge urinary incontinence: involuntary leakage accompanied by or immediately preceded by urgency

Detrusor overactivity incontinence: leakage due to an involuntary detrusor contraction

Urethral relaxation incontinence: leakage due to urethral relaxation in the presence of raised abdominal pressure or detrusor overactivity

Mixed urinary incontinence: involuntary leakage associated with urgency and also with exertion, effort, sneezing, or coughing

Enuresis: any involuntary loss of urine

Continuous urinary incontinence: continuous leakage

Terms That Should No Longer Be Used

- *Dysuria*
- *Detrusor instability*
- *Reflex incontinence*
- *Overflow incontinence*

---

calcium and a predisposition to developing hyponatremia and hyperkalemia. Age-related changes in the kidney and in aldosterone secretion interfere with compensatory mechanisms that maintain fluid and electrolyte balance, so that older adults have a delayed and less effective response to variations in sodium intake. Similarly, declines in renal function increase the time needed for pH imbalances to be corrected in older adults. Even with normal states of hydration, a decrease in GFR delays water excretion and may lead to hyponatremia in healthy older adults. Likewise, even routine daily activities can challenge the renal function of older adults because of diminished renal efficiency. For example, when older adults perspire during exercise, they may tire easily because of age-related delays in the mechanisms controlling water and sodium conservation.

With increasing age, the kidneys become less responsive to ADH and are less able to concentrate urine, causing a decrease in the maximal urinary concentration. Age-related changes also cause a doubling of urine production at night in older adults as compared with younger adults, even in the absence of pathologic factors (Miller, 2000).

Older adults who take medications or have medical conditions are likely to experience serious functional consequences, as the following examples illustrate:

- Diuretics are more likely to cause hypovolemia and dehydration in older adults than in younger people.
- Under conditions of physiologic stress (e.g., surgery, infection, or excessive fluid loss), older adults are likely to develop dehydration, volume depletion, and other fluid and electrolyte imbalances.
- Volume depletion may occur soon after the onset of fever-producing illnesses because of the inability to compensate for insensible fluid losses.
- Any condition or medication that stimulates ADH secretion, such as pneumonia or chlorpropamide, is likely to cause water intoxication

and hyponatremia in older adults because of their diminished ability to compensate for excessive levels of ADH.

Age-related changes in kidney function are most likely to affect water-soluble medications that are highly dependent on GFR (e.g., digoxin, cimetidine, and aminoglycoside antibiotics) or renal tubular function (e.g., penicillin and procainamide). Diminished renal function contributes to the increased incidence of drug interactions and adverse medication reactions in older adults. These adverse medication effects can significantly impair physical and mental abilities and have profound functional consequences. Unless medication doses are adjusted to account for age-related changes in GFR and renal tubular function, excretion may be delayed, and toxic substances are likely to accumulate. As a rule, older adults require a 50% higher urine volume to excrete the same solute load as their younger counterparts.

The Impact of Urinary Function Changes on Voiding Patterns

Older adults frequently experience changes in their voiding patterns because of age-related changes. Day and night urine volumes for older adults are 50 mL/hour and 70 mL/hour, compared with 75 mL/hour and 35 mL/hour in young adults (Miller, 2000). Consequently, nocturia may occur several times nightly. Because of age-related changes, the bladder of the older adult has a smaller capacity, empties incompletely, contracts during filling, and retains up to 50 mL of residual urine. Functionally, these age-related changes result in shorter intervals between voiding and less time between the perception of the urge to void and the actual need to empty the bladder. In addition, chronic residual urine is likely to cause symptomatic or asymptomatic bacteriuria, which does not necessarily have a direct effect on urinary elimination but predisposes older adults to develop urinary tract infections.

The Impact of Urinary Function Changes on Quality of Life

Urinary incontinence can negatively affect an older adult's quality of life through both physical and psychosocial consequences. Physical consequences of incontinence include a predisposition to falls, fractures, urosepsis, perineal rashes, pressure ulcers, and urinary tract infections (Resnick & Yalla, 2002). Consequences of limited fluid intake, a commonly used compensatory action, include increased risk for dehydration, bacteriuria, incontinence, constipation, adverse drug effects, and impaired homeostatic mechanisms.

Psychosocial consequences associated with urinary incontinence include shame, anxiety, depression, social isolation, and loss of self-confidence. Older adults who have experienced episodes of incontinence may become preoccupied with covering up any evidence of wetness or urinary odors so that they can avoid embarrassment or social rejection. In addition to being embarrassed about their incontinence, older adults may be embarrassed about having to use toilet facilities more frequently than might be considered socially appropriate. Psychosocial consequences also arise if caregivers have infantilizing attitudes and behaviors toward the older person who is incontinent (e.g., unnecessarily using "diapers" rather than providing assistance with toileting) because this can have a devastating effect on the older adult's dignity and self-esteem.

Psychosocial consequences can occur even for older adults who are not incontinent but experience urinary urgency because this sensation may lead to fears, restricted activity, and feelings of insecurity and powerlessness. In addition, older adults who do not understand age-related changes may have exaggerated fears of progressive incontinence, triggered by the mere onset of urgency or frequency. When urinary incontinence interferes with performance of their daily activities, older adults—especially those who are homebound—are likely to experience loneliness, depression, and other manifestations of psychological distress (Bogner et al., 2002; Engberg et al., 2001). Psychosocial consequences are more directly linked with the volume of urine lost than with the frequency of incontinence episodes (Fultz & Herzog, 2001; Iglesias et al., 2000). Finally, psychosocial consequences may be associated with nocturia because this has been cited as the most frequently reported cause of sleep disturbance in older people (Lose et al., 2001).

For caregivers of dependent older adults in home settings, the onset of urinary incontinence may create additional stress, especially if urinary incontinence is compounded by environmental barriers or functional limitations. Caregivers report that tasks related to incontinence are some of the most difficult aspects of providing care and represent a major source of stress. Langa and colleagues (2002) found that caregivers of community-living older adults spent an additional 1 hour daily for care specifically related to incontinence. Because urinary incontinence adds to the burden of caregiving stress, it is a major factor influencing the decision to seek institutional care for the dependent person.

Caregivers in home settings are likely to feel angry, guilty, frustrated, or inadequate when dealing with incontinence on a daily basis. Lifelong attitudes about control over urination may contribute to feelings of disgust about the care demands, which may be further compounded by guilt feelings regarding this initial reaction to caregiving tasks. If the caregiver perceives intentionality on the part of the dependent person in his or her failure to control urination, these feelings will likely be intensified. In institutional settings, nursing staff and other caregivers may experience these same feelings to a lesser degree.

Figure 15-1 illustrates the age-related changes, risk factors, and negative functional consequences that can affect urinary elimination.

➤ Mr. and Mrs. U., who are 69 and 68 years old, respectively, attend the senior center where you provide monthly group health education sessions, weekly blood pressure checks, and one-on-one "Counseling for Wellness" sessions. During a recent health counseling session, Mrs. U. confided that she does not know what to do about her husband's "smelly dribbling" and that she worries that he has prostate problems. She has perceived a strong odor of urine and has noticed yellow stains on his clothing when she does the laundry. Even their children have mentioned the odor to her, but when she tries to discuss it with her husband, he changes the topic. She says that he will not

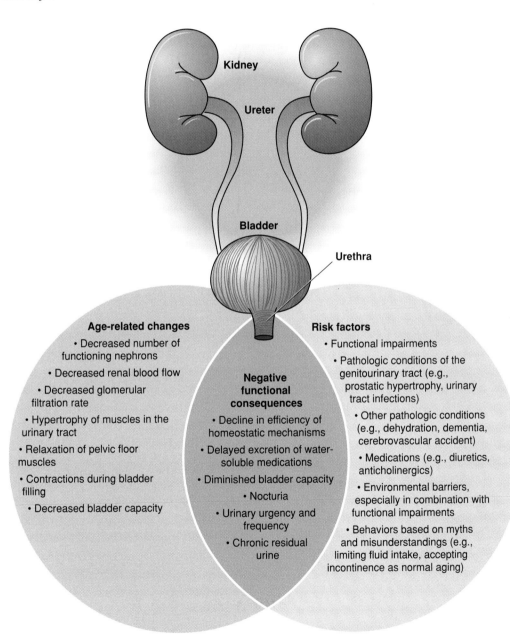

FIGURE 15-1 Age-related changes and risk factors intersect to negatively affect urinary function in older adults.

talk with his doctor about it because he "hears so much about prostate cancer and he's afraid that he has an untreatable condition." She asks your advice about this and asks if you would talk with him when he comes to see you next week. Your next group health education session is entitled "Control of Urine: What's Normal With Aging?" and you plan do have separate group discussions for the men and women. Since Mr. and Mrs. U. usually attend these sessions, you see this as an opportunity to initiate health education about this sensitive topic.

THINKING POINTS

What information would you include in the group session about each of the following topics:

➤ What can older men (women) expect of their urinary tract?

➤ What factors increase the risk for problems with urinary control in older men (women)?

NURSING ASSESSMENT OF URINARY FUNCTION

Numerous opportunities for health promotion interventions can be identified through nursing assessment of (1) risk factors that influence overall urinary function; (2) risk factors that increase the potential for incontinence; (3) signs and symptoms of any dysfunction involving urinary elimination; (4) fears and attitudes about urinary dysfunction; and (5) psychosocial consequences of incontinence. The nurse obtains most of this information by interviewing older adults and the caregivers of dependent older adults. In addition, the nurse obtains objective data from laboratory tests and by observing behaviors, behavioral cues, and environmental influences.

Interviewing the Older Adult About Urinary Function

Because urinary elimination is associated with certain social expectations, discussion of this topic may especially be influenced by a person's attitudes and feelings. Although nurses usually learn to discuss urinary elimination with relative ease, older adults may feel uncomfortable with the topic, especially if there are gender or age differences between the older person and the nurse, or if a communication barrier, such as a hearing impairment, exists.

Terminology related to urinary elimination presents further difficulties in interviewing older adults. In social settings, euphemisms are commonly used to avoid directly discussing urination (e.g., "I'm going to the powder room," "I'm going to take a leak," "I have to use the john"). Even the sounds associated with urinary elimination may be viewed as embarrassing; hence, people may run the faucet or flush the toilet to disguise the sound of urination when others are present. Because of this social context, successful interviewing about urinary elimination and incontinence depends on identifying the terms that are least embarrassing and most understandable to the older adult. Thus, an initial task in a nursing assessment of urinary function is to discover and use the terms that are most acceptable and comprehensible to the person. If any hearing impairment is present, a term such as "urinate," which is not used in everyday social language, or a one-syllable word like "pee" may be difficult to understand or may be misinterpreted. Although phrases like "use the toilet" and "go to the bathroom" are not specific to urinary elimination, they may prove to be acceptable, especially if additional questions are asked in order to distinguish between urinary and bowel elimination. Similarly, the term "incontinence" may be problematic for people who may not be familiar with this term. Hearing impairments, if present, may further interfere with comprehension of this word. Rather than referring to incontinence, it may be more acceptable to older adults to discuss "trouble holding their water." Older adults may tend to use phrases, such as "accidents," "leaking," "weak kidneys," or "bladder trouble," to describe incontinent episodes.

The nurse can set the stage for direct questions about urinary elimination by focusing initial questions on risk factors. Assessment of attitudes about urinary incontinence and its psychosocial consequences can be accomplished indirectly by evaluating the responses to the interview questions. If incontinence has been acknowledged, questions about what the person has done about it may help to identify fears and attitudes that contribute to psychosocial consequences or interfere with interventions. If depression and social withdrawal were first noted at the time of onset of incontinence, this can be a clue that the person's self-esteem and usual activities have been affected by the condition. If older adults show a willingness to discuss their incontinence, direct questions can be asked about its impact on their daily activities and social life.

Identifying Opportunities for Health Promotion

Display 15-3 summarizes interview questions related to urinary elimination. If information is already available from other parts of an assessment (e.g., medication use and medical history), the nurse can incorporate it

DISPLAY 15-3
Guidelines for Assessing Urinary Elimination

Interview Questions to Assess Risk Factors Influencing Urinary Elimination

- *(Men)* Have you had any surgery for prostate or bladder problems?
- *(Men)* Have you ever been told you had prostate problems? (or, Do you think you have prostate problems?)
- *(Women)* Have you had any children? (If yes, ask about the number of pregnancies and any problems with childbirth.)
- *(Women)* Have you had any surgery for pelvic, bladder, or uterine disorders?
- *(Women)* Have you had any infections in your vaginal area?
- Do you have any pain, burning, or discomfort when you urinate (pass water)?
- Have you had any urinary tract infections?
- Do you have any chronic illnesses?
- What medications do you take?
- Do you have any problems with your bowels?
- How much water and other liquids do you drink during the day? (Ask for details about timing and the amount of alcoholic, carbonated, and caffeinated beverages consumed.)

Interview Questions to Assess Risk Factors for Socially Appropriate Urinary Elimination

- Do you have any trouble walking or any difficulty with balance?
- Do you have any trouble reading signs or finding restrooms when you're in public places?

Interview Questions to Assess Signs and Symptoms of Urinary Dysfunction

- Do you ever leak urine?
- Do you ever wear pads or protective garments to protect your clothing from wetness?
- Do you ever have difficulty holding your urine (water) long enough to get to the toilet? (or, How long can you hold your urine after you first feel the need to go to the bathroom?)
- Do you have trouble holding your urine (water) when you cough, laugh, or make sudden movements?
- Do you wake up at night because you have to go to the bathroom to urinate (pass water)? (If the response is affirmative, try to differentiate between this symptom and the habit of going to the bathroom after waking up for some other reason.)
- Immediately after urinating (passing your water), does it feel like you haven't emptied your bladder completely?
- Do you have to exert pressure during urination to feel like your bladder is being completely emptied?
- *(Men)* When you urinate (pass water), do you have any difficulty starting the stream or keeping the stream going?

Interview Questions If Incontinence Has Been Acknowledged

- When did your incontinence begin?
- What have you done to manage the problem? (Have you cut down on the amount of liquids you drink? Do you empty your bladder at frequent intervals as a precautionary measure?)
- Are there certain things that make the problem worse or better?
- Does it happen all the time, or just at certain times?
- Do you have any pain when you urinate (pass water)?
- *(Women)* Do you feel any pressure in your pelvic area?

Interview Questions to Assess Fears, Attitudes, and Psychosocial Consequences of Incontinence

- Have you ever sought help or talked to a primary care provider or other health care professional about this problem?
- Have you changed any of your activities because you need to stay near a toilet?
- Do you avoid going to certain places because of difficulty holding your urine (water)?

into the assessment of urinary elimination rather than repeating questions. Nurses supplement their assessment interview by obtaining information about the person's patterns of urinary elimination and by assessing environmental factors that may interfere with control over urinary elimination.

A bladder diary—also called a bladder record, incontinence chart, or voiding or urinary diary—is one method of obtaining information about patterns of urinary elimination. This widely recommended assessment tool is used to document information about pad usage, fluid intake, the degree of urgency, the times and volumes of urinations, and times and degree of incontinence episodes (Dowling-Castrono-

vo, 2001; Locher et al., 2001). Although the length of time for keeping a bladder diary varies between 3 and 14 days, a 1-week period of data collection provides stable and reliable assessment information (Locher et al., 2001). Information from the bladder diary is used to identify potential causes of and interventions for incontinence and is particularly helpful in identifying opportunities for health education. Figure 15-2 is an example of a voiding diary.

Older adults who are cognitively impaired or dependent on others for their care may not be able to keep a bladder diary. In these situations, or when incontinence is an unacknowledged problem, observations about patterns of urinary elimination are

How to Use a "Uro-Log" (Voiding Diary)

Complete one form each day for four days before your appointment with a health professional. Each time you eat or drink during the day, write down the type of food and drink and the time of day it was consumed. Then record when you go to the bathroom and the approximate amount *(in ounces)* voided. If you have any leakage during the day, mark down the time it occurred, the amount *(small,* *medium, large),* the activity you were engaged in at the time of leakage, and whether or not an urge to urinate was present.

Use a new line on the "Uro-Log" for each entry *(when you eat, drink, void, leak, etc.)* and record the time of day the event occurred. Take the completed forms with you when you go to the doctor.

Time	Fluids		Foods		Did You Urinate?		ACCIDENTS		
	What kind?	How much?	What kind?	How much?	How many times?	How much? (in ounces)	Leakage How much? (sm, med, lg)	Did you feel an urge to urinate?	What were you doing at the time? Sneezing, exercising, etc.
Sample	Coffee	1 cup	Toast	1 slice	✓ ✓	6 oz.	sm	Yes	No (No)	Running
6-7 a.m.								Yes	No	
7-8 a.m.								Yes	No	
8-9 a.m.								Yes	No	
9-10 a.m.								Yes	No	
10-11 a.m.								Yes	No	
11-12 noon								Yes	No	
12-1 p.m.								Yes	No	
1-2 p.m.								Yes	No	
2-3 p.m.								Yes	No	
3-4 p.m.								Yes	No	
4-5 p.m.								Yes	No	
5-6 p.m.								Yes	No	
6-7 p.m.								Yes	No	
7-8 p.m.								Yes	No	
8-9 p.m.								Yes	No	
9-10 p.m.								Yes	No	

FIGURE 15-2. Example of a voiding diary. (Courtesy of the National Association for Continence [NAFC].)

particularly important. In long-term care facilities and other institutional settings, nurses have many opportunities to observe behavioral cues to incontinence. In home settings, caregivers of dependent older adults may observe behavioral cues and provide valuable information about urinary elimination patterns. Display 15-4 summarizes specific observations that may yield important assessment information.

Home environments are assessed for barriers that might interfere with the quick performance of urinary elimination (refer to Display 15-1). Stairways, long hallways, poor lighting, and cluttered surroundings may increase the time needed to get to the toilet, especially if the older adult has any functional impairment or uses assistive devices, such as a walker. Also, it is important to assess the environment for the presence of safety and assistive devices or their potential benefit to the individual. For instance, an elevated toilet seat, grab bars near the toilet, and grab bars on the walls leading to the toilet may improve the person's ability to urinate safely. See Display 15-4 for specific environmental factors that are assessed for their influence on socially appropriate urinary elimination.

Using Laboratory Information

Data from urinalysis and blood chemistry tests contribute important information to the assessment of urinary elimination. A midstream or second-void specimen is the best type of sample for a urinalysis. At the age of 80 years, the normal upper limit for specific gravity is 1.024, and slight proteinuria is normal in

DISPLAY 15-4
Guidelines for Assessing Behavioral Cues To and Environmental Influences On Incontinence

Behavioral Cues

- Does the older adult use disposable or washable pads or products?
- Is there an odor of urine on clothing or furniture (especially couches and stuffed chairs)?
- Has the older adult withdrawn from social activities, especially those held away from home?

Environmental Influences

- Where are the bathroom facilities located in relation to the older adult's usual daytime and nighttime activities?
- Does the person have to go up or down stairs to use the toilet at night or during the day?
- Are there any grab bars or other aids in, near, or on the way to the bathroom?
- Would the person benefit from using an elevated toilet seat?
- Does the person use a urinal or other aid to cut down on the number of trips to the bathroom?
- How many people share the same bathroom facilities?
- Is privacy ensured?

older adults. Other than these two variations, the urinalysis results should be within the normal range for healthy older adults.

Blood chemistry values that may be helpful in assessing renal function include the following: electrolyte level, creatinine level, creatinine clearance, nonprotein nitrogen level, and blood urea nitrogen level. In older adults, the serum creatinine may not be an accurate indicator of the GFR, but a 24-hour urine collection for creatinine clearance may have greater value as an indicator of renal functioning. Renal function in older adults is best assessed according to the Crockcroft-Gault formula for predicting creatinine clearances from serum creatinine concentrations. This formula, which uses a person's age and weight to calculate creatinine clearance, is as follows (for men):

$$\text{Creatinine clearance} = \frac{(140 - \text{age}) \times \text{weight [kg]}}{72 \times \text{serum creatinine [mg/100 mL]}}$$

The same calculation applies to women, except that the resulting value must be multiplied by 0.85.

➤ Recall that you are the nurse at the senior center attended by Mr. and Mrs. U. After your class ("Control of Urine: What's Normal With Aging?"), Mr. U. schedules an appointment for a "Counseling for Wellness" session. He

tells you that he has a "little dribbling" problem but has ignored it because it did not bother him very much. He has not talked with any doctor about this because he thought it was "to be expected," but now that he attended your session, he thinks that maybe he should have the problem evaluated and wants further information from you. During other health counseling sessions with Mr. U., he has told you that he is taking medications for hypertension and Parkinson's disease.

THINKING POINTS

➤ What risk factors are likely to be contributing to Mr. U.'s problems with urinary control?

➤ Make a list of assessment questions that you would use with Mr. U. (Use applicable questions from Display 15-3 and any additional questions that might be appropriate.)

➤ What observations would you make as part of your assessment?

➤ What would you teach Mr. U. about filling out the voiding diary (see Figure 15-2)?

NURSING DIAGNOSIS

When the nursing assessment identifies any risk factors for incontinence or any complaints about or evidence of incontinence, an applicable nursing diagnosis would be Urinary Elimination, Impaired. This is defined as the "state in which the individual experiences or is at risk for experiencing urinary elimination dysfunction" (Carpenito, 2002, p. 949). Major defining characteristics commonly found in older adults include urgency, frequency, dribbling, nocturia, hesitancy, and incontinence. Additional nursing diagnoses are addressed when negative functional consequences are identified in older adults or their caregivers. Nursing diagnoses that might address the consequences of incontinence in older adults include Anxiety, Social Isolation, Disturbed Body Image, Disturbed Sleep Pattern, and Impaired Skin Integrity. Caregiver Role Strain (or risk for such) is a nursing diagnosis that addresses consequences for caregivers.

OUTCOMES

Nursing care plans are directed toward preventing, minimizing, or compensating for the negative functional consequences that affect urinary elimination. Specific outcomes related to urinary elimination include maintenance of homeostasis and prevention of adverse medication effects. Outcomes for incontinent older adults include achieving continence and preventing negative consequences of incontinence. Initial outcomes should focus on controlling and alleviating, rather than simply managing, incontinence.

A nursing-sensitive outcome for urge incontinence is Urinary Continence, as indicated by the person having adequate time to reach the toilet between the urge and urination (Specht & Maas, 2001). An indicator for the nursing-sensitive outcome for Urinary Continence related to stress incontinence is "no urine leakage with increased abdominal pressure" (Specht & Maas, 2001, p. 254). Indicators for Urinary Continence due to mixed incontinence are "adequate time to reach toilet between urge and evaluation of urine" and "free of urine leakage between voidings" (Specht & Maas, 2001, p. 257). For functional urinary incontinence, indicators of Urinary Continence are "able to manage clothing independently" and "able to manage toilet independently" (Specht & Maas, 2001, p. 256). When urinary incontinence cannot be alleviated, Tissue Integrity: Skin and Mucous Membranes would be an applicable nursing-sensitive outcome, as indicated by intact skin and color in the expected range (Specht & Maas, 2001).

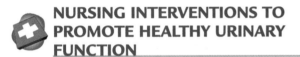

NURSING INTERVENTIONS TO PROMOTE HEALTHY URINARY FUNCTION

Preventing Disease and Promoting Health

Healthy older adults will not be greatly affected by age-related kidney changes during normal activities; but under conditions of physiologic stress, such as exercise, compensatory actions must be taken to prevent detrimental effects on homeostasis. Nurses provide health education about functional consequences affecting homeostasis so that older adults can take appropriate compensatory actions. For example, nurses can explain that exercising in a cool (rather than hot) environment and increasing one's fluid intake before exercise may compensate for the age-related diminished ability to conserve water and sodium. Nurses also can suggest that older adults can take protective measures when they are in very hot and humid environments. Examples of appropriate protective measures are using fans and air conditioners; increasing fluid intake; and avoiding alcoholic, carbonated, and caffeinated beverages.

Older adults taking normal doses of water-soluble medications are likely to experience adverse medication effects because of diminished renal function. Therefore, when water-soluble medications are prescribed for older adults, dose adjustments should be based on an accurate assessment of kidney function and serum drug levels. Nurses need to be aware of the increased potential for adverse medication effects, especially when the older adult is taking more than one medication. Further information about adverse medication effects and interventions for medication management is provided in Chapter 23.

Perhaps the risk factor most amenable to nursing interventions is the false perception of incontinence as an inevitable effect of aging for which nothing can be done. Because this attitude is based on myths or a lack of information, it can be changed through education. Nurses can teach older adults and their caregivers about normal age-related changes and risk factors that contribute to incontinence and about the need for a comprehensive evaluation of any problems with urinary elimination. They can emphasize that many factors increase the risk for incontinence and that many of these risks can be alleviated. For example, teaching older adults the rationale for maintaining adequate fluid intake as a means of preventing incontinence and maintaining good urinary function is a simple but important intervention. Older adults may be more willing to increase their fluid intake if they understand that concentrated urine due to fluid restriction can cause incontinence by stimulating bladder contractions. Nurses also can explain that because older adults often do not experience a sensation of thirst, even in the presence of dehydration, if they depend on their thirst sensation to indicate a need for fluids, their intake of liquids may be inadequate. Interventions to promote adequate fluid intake include the identification of nonalcoholic, noncaffeinated, and noncarbonated beverages that are most acceptable to the older adult and that will be consumed readily, even in the absence of thirst sensation.

When a risk factor contributes to incontinence or otherwise interferes with normal urinary elimination, interventions are directed toward optimal management of the precipitating factor. For example, if postmenopausal estrogen depletion leads to vaginitis and trigonitis, health education is directed toward encouraging the older woman to seek medical treatment for the underlying condition. When fecal impaction or chronic constipation are risk factors for urinary incontinence, interventions are aimed at attaining and maintaining good bowel function, as discussed in Chapter 14. Pelvic muscle exercises (PMEs), as discussed in the next section, are another health promotion intervention that can be performed by men and women who are at increased risk for developing, or who have developed, urinary incontinence. Display 15-5 summarizes teaching points about self-care activities that promote optimal overall urinary function and help older adults maintain continence.

DISPLAY 15-5
Health Education Related to Urinary Elimination

Health Promotion Activities for Good Urinary Function

- Drink 8 to 10 glasses of noncaffeinated liquid every day, with limited intake during the evening hours.
- Do not depend on thirst sensation as an accurate indicator for adequate fluid intake—drink liquids even if you do not feel thirsty.
- Avoid excessive use of alcoholic, caffeinated, or carbonated beverages, especially before bedtime.
- Avoid foods and beverages that can irritate the bladder (e.g., sugar, caffeine, alcohol, chocolate, artificial sweeteners, and spicy and acidic foods).
- Drink 1or 2 glasses of fluid before, and every 15 minutes during, periods of sweat-producing exercise or activity.
- Avoid smoking.
- Maintain ideal body weight and good physical fitness.
- Take steps to prevent constipation (refer to Chapter 14, Display 14-4).
- Practice pelvic muscle exercises (refer to Display 15-6).

Correction of Myths About Incontinence

- Incontinence is not an inevitable age-related change.

- Normal age-related changes affecting urination include a shortened interval between the perception of the urge to void and the actual need to empty the bladder, an increased frequency of voiding, and the need to get up to urinate several times during the night.
- Nocturia, urgency, and frequency do not necessarily lead to total incontinence.
- If incontinence occurs, a pathologic condition or other influencing factor can usually be identified through a comprehensive evaluation.
- One of the requirements for voluntary control over urination is the signal of the need to void because of a full bladder. Restricting fluid intake interferes with this signal.
- Highly concentrated urine, from inadequate fluid intake, will stimulate involuntary bladder contractions and may lead to incontinence.
- Consistently emptying the bladder at intervals of less than 1 or 2 hours may contribute to problems with incontinence.
- Seek medical advice from a knowledgeable practitioner about any difficulties with urinary continence.

Achieving Continence and Alleviating Incontinence

In some situations, urinary incontinence can be alleviated through health promotion interventions, such as PMEs. However, whenever incontinence is a persistent problem, a comprehensive evaluation must be done to determine the underlying cause of the incontinence so that appropriate interventions can be initiated. Nurses can facilitate referrals to specialty clinics, primary care practitioners, or a geriatric assessment program for an evaluation. Interventions also address contributing factors such as environmental conditions, resources and abilities of caregivers, functional and cognitive abilities of the older adult, and negative effects and social acceptability of the intervention. Recent nursing literature provides guidelines for nursing assessment and interventions of incontinence in older adults (e.g., Lekan-Rutledge, 2000; Lyons, et al., 2000; Mueller & Cain, 2002; Specht et al., 2002).

The following types of interventions are used singly or in combination for control of incontinence: PMEs, continence training, environmental modifications, biofeedback, medications, surgery, and a variety of urinary control devices. A combination of pharmacologic and nonpharmacologic interventions may be necessary, especially for urge incontinence (Burgio et al., 2000). Burgio and colleagues (2001)

found that a combination of behavioral interventions (i.e., health education, PMEs, and biofeedback) significantly reduced urge incontinence in 81% of community-living older women. Other studies have found that health education provided by nurses is an important component of behavioral interventions (Borrie et al., 2002; Dougherty et al., 2002). If incontinence cannot be alleviated, aids and equipment can be used to minimize the functional consequences.

Pelvic Muscle Exercises

When weakening of the pelvic floor musculature contributes to incontinence, exercises to strengthen these muscles can cure or improve incontinence. PMEs were first advocated in the late 1940s by A. H. Kegel, an American gynecologist, for postpartum therapy. Since then, many variations of these exercises have been promoted, both for control of incontinence and for enhancement of sexual pleasure. Since the 1980s, PMEs have been promoted as an intervention for alleviating or reducing stress, urge, and mixed incontinence. This intervention is sometimes used in combination with biofeedback, behavioral training, or pelvic floor electrical stimulation for improved effectiveness. Studies support the effectiveness of PMEs, either alone or in combination with other interventions, for incontinent people who are motivated and cognitively intact (Schnelle & Smith, 2001). These research results are strongest and most consistent in adult women with stress or mixed incontinence (Hay-Smith et al., 2002).

The goal of PMEs, also known as *pelvic muscle rehabilitation*, is improvement of urethral resistance through active exercise of the pubococcygeal muscle. There are no contraindications for or negative effects of these exercises, which can be initiated by any motivated person. They are recommended for women with stress incontinence and for men and women as adjuncts to bladder training and other interventions for urge and mixed incontinence (Schnelle & Smith, 2001). A very important aspect of teaching about PMEs is to help the person accurately identify the pubococcygeal muscle. Once the pubococcygeal muscle is identified, the person must practice contracting and relaxing this muscle, gradually increasing the ability to hold the contraction. It is important to emphasize that improvement is very gradual, and full effects are not noticed until 3 to 6 months of regular exercise have been completed. Even after full effects are achieved, daily maintenance exercises must be continued. Display 15-6 summarizes the points to cover when teaching adults to do these exercises.

In recent years, devices and equipment have become available as PME training aids, many of which are available without prescription. For example, weighted vaginal cones can be used gradually to improve the strength of contractions. A pelvic floor muscle exerciser, consisting of a vaginal probe connected to a hand-held indicator, can be used to monitor the strength of contractions. Educational materials are available from the organizations listed in the Educational Resources section of this chapter.

Continence Training

Continence training can be categorized as: (1) methods that are self-directed by motivated and cognitively intact people; or (2) methods that are directed by motivated caregivers of cognitively impaired people. The goal of continence training is to achieve a continent interval of 2 to 4 hours between voidings. These intervals will not necessarily be equal and will usually be longer during the night. In self-directed programs, the person hopes to regain voluntary urinary control, whereas in caregiver-directed programs, the caregiver hopes to reduce the episodes of incontinence. Self-directed continence training, alone or in combination with biofeedback or medications, is most successful with urge incontinence. Continence training cannot be effective if the bladder capacity is less than 150 mL.

DISPLAY 15-6
Instructions for Performing Pelvic Muscle Exercises

Purpose: To prevent the involuntary loss of urine by strengthening the pelvic floor muscles

Frequency: Minimum of 60 times daily for at least 6 weeks; ideally working up to 150 contractions daily in several sessions of at least 15 exercises per session (e.g., 3 to 10 sets of 15 exercises, or 4 to 6 sets of 20 exercises), continued indefinitely

Position: Lying, sitting, or standing

Identifying the Pubococcygeal Muscle

- Identify the pubococcygeal muscle by contracting the muscle that stops the flow of urine. Do NOT do this regularly when urinating
- *(Women)* Lie down and insert a finger about three quarters of the way up your vagina. Squeeze the vaginal wall so you feel pressure on your finger and a sensation in your vagina.
- *(Men)* Stand in front of a mirror and try to make your penis move up and down without moving the rest of your body.
- Biofeedback, weighted vaginal cones, or a perineometer (a balloon-like device that is placed in the vagina) can be used to assist in identifying the pubococcygeal muscle and in measuring the strength of the contraction.

Method

- Tighten your pubococcygeal muscle and hold for a period of 3 seconds.
- Relax this muscle for an equal period.
- Repeat the contraction—relaxation cycle (one exercise) for your scheduled number of times.
- Breathe normally during these exercises and do NOT tighten other muscles at the same time. Be careful not to contract your legs, buttocks, or abdominal muscles while you are contracting your pubococcygeal muscle.
- Repeat this exercise daily in several sessions for a total of 60 to 150 exercises.
- For each of the daily sessions, vary your position (e.g., perform the exercise while lying down in the morning, standing in the afternoon, and sitting in the evening).
- Gradually increase the duration of each exercise up to a count of 10 for a contraction and 10 for a relaxation.

Additional information: The National Association for Continence, (800) 252-3337, has audiotapes and written materials available about pelvic muscle exercises.

Although specific techniques may vary, essential elements of any continence training program include motivation, an assessment of voiding patterns, an individualized and carefully timed intake of about 2000 mL of fluid per day, timed voiding in the most appropriate place, methods of reinforcing expected behaviors, and ongoing monitoring. During the initial assessment, diaries are used to record times and circumstances of toileting and times of and reasons for any episode of incontinence. After the usual voiding pattern has been identified, the older adult is encouraged to resist the sensation of urgency and to postpone voiding rather than responding immediately to an urge.

With caregiver-directed methods—often referred to as *prompted voiding programs*—the caregiver uses the initial assessment of voiding patterns to establish a schedule for assisting with voiding. The caregiver gradually increases the interval between voidings until the person can maintain continence for 2 to 4 hours. These methods are most successful when the timed intervals are flexible and are based on a good assessment of the person's needs and voiding patterns. For example, caregivers need to adjust schedules for diurnal variations. Ouslander and colleagues (2001) found that prompted voiding is not effective between the hours of 10:00 PM and 6:00 AM; they suggest that routine nighttime checking of nursing home residents be done only when the residents are already awake. Caregiver-directed programs may include the use of electronic alarm devices or behavior modification techniques. These programs also incorporate social feedback (e.g., praising the person for behaviors such as staying dry between scheduled trips to the bathroom and self-initiating requests to toilet) (Lyons et al., 2000). Display 15-7 identifies some of the terms used for and the general principles of continence training programs.

Environmental Modifications

When incontinence is primarily caused by the inability to reach an appropriate receptacle after perceiving the need to void, interventions are directed toward modifying the environment and improving functional abilities. If environmental adaptations cannot be made, as in public places, older adults are encouraged to become familiar with the location and arrangement of the bathroom facilities before the need to urinate is imminent. In home and institutional settings, the provision of bedside commodes and privacy may be an effective intervention. If space is limited, however, or if privacy cannot be assured, bedside commodes may not be acceptable. Display 15-8 lists environmental modifications that can be implemented to prevent incontinence when functional limitations are a contributing factor. Interventions discussed in chapters on vision (see

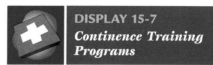

DISPLAY 15-7
Continence Training Programs

Goal Of Programs: To achieve voluntary control over urination at intervals of 2 to 4 hours

Terminology

Terms used for self-directed programs: bladder drill, bladder training, bladder retraining, bladder exercise, bladder retention exercise

Terms used for caregiver-directed programs: scheduled toileting, routine toileting, prompted voiding, timed voiding, habit training

Method

Step 1: Identify the usual voiding pattern, noting the times of incontinence and information about fluid intake. During the first few days, keep a diary to record the following information at hourly intervals: dry or wet, amount voided, place of voiding, fluid intake, and sensation and awareness of need to void.

Step 2: Using information from the voiding diary, establish a schedule that allows for emptying of the bladder before incontinence is likely to occur.

Step 3: Provide the equipment and assistance necessary for optimal voiding at scheduled times.

Step 4: Provide 2000 mL of noncaffeinated liquids per day for liquid intake. Consume the largest amounts during the early part of the day, and limit fluid intake about 2 to 4 hours before bedtime.

Step 5: Gradually increase the length of time between voidings until the interval is 2 to 4 hours long.

Chapter 13) and mobility (see Chapter 18) can be implemented to address functional limitations that can contribute to incontinence.

Medications

Medications have been used with varying degrees of success for treatment of incontinence, but their effectiveness is highly dependent on identifying and addressing the specific type of incontinence. Medications also can be effective in the treatment of an underlying condition that contributes to incontinence (e.g., vaginitis and benign prostatic hyperplasia). If medications are prescribed, nurses are responsible for knowing their expected positive effects as well as their potentially negative side effects.

Medications that act on the autonomic nervous system are most often used for control of incontinence. α-Adrenergic agents are used to control stress incontinence by increasing bladder outlet resistance through stimulating receptors at the trigone and internal sphincter. Anticholinergic medications may be used to control the uninhibited or unstable bladder by

DISPLAY 15-8
Environmental Modifications for Preventing Incontinence

Modifications to Enhance Visibility of Facilities
- Use contrasting colors for the toilet seat surroundings.
- Provide adequate lighting in and near toilet areas, but avoid creating glare.
- Use nightlights in the pathway between the bedroom and bathroom.

Modifications to Improve the Ability to Use the Toilet in Time
- Encourage the use of chairs or beds that are designed to help the person arise unaided after sitting or lying.
- Install handrails in the hallway(s) leading to the bathroom.
- Make sure the pathway to the bathroom is safe and uncluttered.

Modifications to Improve the Ability to Use the Toilet
- Place grab bars at appropriate places to facilitate getting on and off the toilet and to assist men in maintaining their balance when standing at the toilet.
- Use elevated toilet seats or an over-the-toilet chair to compensate for any functional limitations of the lower extremities.
- If the person has functional limitations involving the upper extremities, clothing for the lower body should feature easy-open closures, such as Velcro or elastic waistbands.

blocking the transmission of nerve impulses. Cholinergic medications are used to prevent urinary retention by stimulating bladder contractions or increasing intravesical pressure. α-Adrenergic blocking agents may be used, either alone or in combination with cholinergic agents, to decrease bladder outlet resistance in the treatment of incontinence. Table 15-2 summarizes the specific types and modes of actions for medications used in the treatment of incontinence.

Biofeedback and Stimulation Devices

Biofeedback and various methods of nerve stimulation are sometimes used as interventions for stress, urge, or mixed incontinence. Most nurses are not directly involved with administering these therapies, but all gerontological nurses are responsible for being familiar with the range of treatment options for incontinence. Nurses can emphasize that many effective and noninvasive therapies are available, and they can encourage incontinent older adults to obtain information about these therapies from knowledgeable health care practitioners.

Biofeedback is sometimes used as an intervention for urge or stress urinary incontinence, either alone or in conjunction with other treatment modalities, such as PMEs. This technique involves the use of monitoring devices to provide information about the physiologic activity involved in urination. Typically, a sensor is placed in the vagina of women or in or around the anus of men and connected to a computer that feeds back information about how the pelvic floor muscles are relaxing and contracting. The person uses this information to monitor the strength of muscle contractions to improve the effectiveness of PMEs.

Various electrical stimulation methods also are used, either alone or in conjunction with PMEs and other interventions, for stress and urge incontinence. Pelvic floor electrical stimulation, which can be done in office and home settings, uses an electrode to deliver small amounts of electrical stimulation to the nerves and muscles of the bladder and pelvic floor. This improves continence by increasing the sphincter tone and strengthening the levator and periurethral muscles. Devices that deliver pulsed magnetic fields to the pelvic floor muscles also are used as noninvasive methods of treating incontinence. Pulsed magnetic therapy is a passive treatment that is not dependent on the person's ability to perform PMEs. Sacral nerve stimulation therapy is effective for urge incontinence and involves the surgical implantation of a neurostimulator under the abdominal skin. The neurostimulator, which is about the size of a stopwatch and can be adjusted nonsurgically, sends mild electrical pulses to the sacral nerves that control bladder function. This improves continence by inhibiting involuntary bladder contraction and promoting an increase in bladder volume.

Urinary Control Devices

A variety of intravaginal or intraurethral devices are available for resolving stress incontinence. Pessaries have been used for many decades to treat cystocele in women. These pelvic organ support devices are placed in the vagina to support the bladder, compress the urethra, or both. They are available in many sizes and shapes and are individually fitted by a primary care practitioner. Pessaries need to be removed and reinserted at intervals ranging from nightly to once every few months, depending on the type that is used.

In recent years, many urinary control devices have become available or are in clinical trials for self-insertion into the urethra. One type of device controls urination through the inflation and deflation of a small balloon that rests at the bladder neck. Recent developments for stress incontinence in women include urethral plugs and intraurethral catheters with unidirectional valves. Another recent development is the external occlusive device, which covers the external

TABLE 15-2 • Medications for Treating Urinary Incontinence

Type of Incontinence	Medication Action	Examples
Urge incontinence associated with detrusor overactivity	Anticholinergic action relaxes bladder muscle and inhibits uncontrolled contractions	Oxybutynin (Ditropan) Tolterodine (Detrol) Propantheline (Pro-Banthine) Tricyclic antidepressants (Tofranil)
Stress incontinence associated with urethral sphincter insufficiency	Alpha-adrenergic stimulation increases strength of bladder muscle contractions	Phenylpropanolamine (Entex LA) Psuedoephedrine (Sudafed)
Incontinence associated with estrogen deficiency	Estrogen	Oral conjugated estrogens (Premarin) Oral estradiol (Entrace) Vaginal cream (Dienestrol) Vaginal ring (Estring) Transdermal (FemPatch)
Incontinence and retention associated with prostatic hyperplasia	Anti-adrenergic action relaxes smooth muscle of the urethra and prostatic capsule	Doxazosin (Cardura) Terazosin (Hytrin) Tamsulosin (Flomax)
Urinary retention with incontinence	Cholinergic action stimulates bladder contractions	Bethanecol (Urecholine)

urinary meatus and provides a watertight seal to prevent leakage. Foam-cushioned penile clamps with compression mechanisms are available for men. Because the availability of urinary control devices for both men and women is rapidly evolving, people with urinary incontinence should be encouraged to obtain current information from a qualified health care provider or from the National Association for Continence, listed in the Educational Resources at the end of this chapter.

Indwelling catheters have been widely used for decades as a urinary control device for incontinence. However, in recent years, many questions have been raised about their use because of the high rate of associated urinary tract infections and other complications. Their use in long-term care facilities has come under particular scrutiny, and currently the number of residents who have indwelling catheters is viewed as an indictor of quality of care in long-term care facilities (with lower numbers of indwelling catheters being associated with better quality of care). Indwelling catheters are recommended only for short-term use or when no other option is effective for urinary retention or total incontinence (Schnelle & Smith, 2001). Intermittent clean catheterization is sometimes used as a self-care or caregiver-administered intervention for some types of incontinence.

Surgical and Minimally Invasive Procedures

Surgical procedures have been used for many decades to control incontinence when structural abnormalities, such as a cystocele, are identified as the underlying cause. For example, several types of bladder suspension surgery or sling procedures are used for stress incontinence. The goal of bladder suspension surgery is to reposition the urethra so that the pelvic floor

muscles can squeeze it more effectively. When urinary incontinence is caused by loss of sphincter control, it may be treated successfully by surgical implantation of an artificial urinary sphincter, a device with an inflatable cuff that is placed around the urethra to hold it closed. To operate the artificial urinary sphincter, men squeeze a pump in the scrotum, whereas women press a valve in the labia to deflate the cuff, which automatically reinflates after voiding is completed. About 70 % of men who have intrinsic sphincter deficiency following prostatectomy regain continence with this procedure (Resnick, 2000).

In recent years, several minimally invasive surgical procedures have been developed for the treatment of incontinence. For example, periurethral injections of a bulking agent (e.g., collagen) may be effective in treating stress incontinence in men and women with intrinsic sphincter deficiency; however, several injections may be required, especially in men. A recent development in treatment of stress incontinence in women is the tension-free vaginal tape system. This procedure involves the surgical insertion of a mesh-like tape through the vagina to support the bladder neck and midsection of the urethra. Minimally invasive surgical procedures, such as visual laser ablation and transurethral needle ablation, are also being used to treat benign prostatic hyperplasia. Another minimally invasive treatment for men is the placement of a wire mesh stent in the urethra to maintain the flow of urine through an enlarged prostate.

Methods of Managing Incontinence

When incontinence cannot be alleviated, it may be managed with the use of various aids and equipment, including disposable and washable incontinence products; and collecting devices, such as urinals and commodes. When used in conjunction with environmental modifications to increase accessibility of toilet facilities, such equipment usually has beneficial effects; however, when aids and equipment are used by caregivers of dependent older adults as substitutes for other methods of achieving continence, they are beneficial only to the caregiver and are detrimental to the older adult. For example, if protective products are used to manage incontinence, the positive effect for the caregiver may be that this method facilitates ease of care; however, the negative effects for the older adult include the likelihood of skin breakdown and decreased self-esteem. Because continence aids can be beneficial as well as detrimental, they should be used only after careful evaluation of all contributing factors.

When an older adult depends on a caregiver for assistance with urinary elimination, the needs, limitations, and abilities of the caregiver must be considered in planning interventions. In institutional settings, different demands may be placed on caregivers, who are expected and trained to care for incontinent patients or residents using the most appropriate interventions. In home settings, the total caregiving situation must be considered, and the needs of the caregiver may take precedence over the needs of the older adult, especially if the caregiver has functional limitations.

Numerous products are available for managing incontinence, and selection of a product depends on factors such as cost, convenience, and effectiveness of different products. Economic considerations are particularly important because disposable incontinence products can be quite expensive, especially if used on a daily basis. Initial and periodic cost of reusable products also needs to be considered, as does the time and expense of laundering. Many types of products are available, and many are designed and fashioned for either male or female incontinence. Products are available according to degrees of absorbency, ranging from light to heavy protection. Absorbency of some disposable products is enhanced by the addition of gel or fiber materials. Often different products will be needed to address incontinence under particular circumstances. For example, a person may need a product with light protection during the day and heavy protection during night. Display 15-9 lists factors to be considered in selecting and using various types of aids and equipment for managing urinary incontinence. Nurses can keep up-to-date on new developments in incontinence products by visiting the Internet sites listed in the Educational Resources section of this chapter.

DISPLAY 15-9
Considerations Regarding Continence Aids and Equipment

Assessment Considerations

- What are the costs of various disposable and washable products, both initially and over a period of time? (Include the time and expense of laundry when considering costs of washable products.)
- What are the preferences of the incontinent person? (e.g., Is a "brief" or "pull-up" style garment more acceptable than a "diaper" style product? Also, how much noise a product makes when the person is walking or moving around in social settings may influence acceptability of a product.)
- What level of absorbency is appropriate for different circumstances?
- What are the needs and abilities of the caregivers of dependent older adults in home settings? (Can the caregiver manage the tasks involved in toileting?)
- What are the secondary benefits of various aids? (For example, in home settings, if the care of an individual with an indwelling catheter is covered by Medicare as skilled care, will additional services, such as home health aide assistance, also be covered?)
- What are the consequences if the incontinence cannot be managed in the home setting? (For example, will the older adult be institutionalized?)

Teaching Related to Aids and Equipment

- Many types of external collecting devices are available for men and women (e.g., male or female urinals, condom catheters, retracted penis pouches, and bedside urinals with attached drainage bags).
- An elevated toilet seat with rails can be used to increase safety and transfer mobility.
- Commodes are useful in diminishing the distance between the place of usual activities and toilet facilities.
- A variety of commodes are available and can be selected according to needs and preferences of the dependent person.
- If commodes are viewed as socially unacceptable, measures can be taken to ensure privacy and increase their social acceptability. Privacy can be ensured by placing an attractive screen around the commode.
- Commodes are now available that are attractively designed to resemble normal furniture items.
- A bedpan can be placed on a regular chair, especially in the bedroom, and removed when not in use.

Mr. and Mrs. U. are now 73 and 72 years old, respectively, and continue to attend the senior center where you are the nurse. Mr. U. has been under the care of a urologist for 3 years and has been taking terazosin for prostatic hyperplasia. Until recently, he had been able to maintain urinary continence, but lately his Parkinson's has worsened, and 1 month ago, he started taking furosemide, 80 mg daily, for congestive heart failure. He makes an appointment to ask your advice about incontinence products that would be best for him because "it's just hopeless to get to the toilet on time because our only bathroom is upstairs and I like to be downstairs during the day." He reports that he limits his fluid intake to 4 cups of liquid daily, which includes 2 cups of black coffee. Because of his Parkinson's disease, he has trouble standing at the toilet and usually sits down; however, he is "slow and clumsy" in managing his clothing. His son bought him some "jogging" outfits with elastic waists, but he does not wear them because he prefers to "dress up" when he goes to the senior center, so he wears trousers with belts.

Mrs. U. also makes an appointment to see you to discuss her recent problem with incontinence. She tells you that for several years she has been wearing "light days pads" because "I have trouble holding my water whenever I sneeze or cough." In the past few months, she notices that she has to go to the bathroom every hour or two and is reluctant to be away from her house for more than an hour at a time. Her health has been good overall, but her arthritis has been getting worse and she is very slow in her mobility, especially when she needs to go up and down stairs. She drinks about 6 cups of liquid daily, consisting mostly of tea and coffee. She's heard some of her friends talking about "those Kegel exercises we had to do when we had our babies." One friend even talked about having some "cones she puts in to help her with exercises."

THINKING POINTS WITH REGARD TO MR. U.

- What risk factors are likely to be contributing to Mr. U.'s incontinence, and which factors might be alleviated with interventions?
- What environmental modifications might be helpful in addressing the incontinence?
- What health education would you give about alleviating risk factors?
- What health education would you give about incontinence products?

THINKING POINTS WITH REGARD TO MRS. U.

- What risk factors are likely to be contributing to Mrs. U.'s incontinence?
- What environmental modifications might be helpful in addressing the incontinence?
- What health education would you give about alleviating risk factors?
- What health education would you give about Kegel exercises?
- What health education would you give about incontinence products?

EVALUATING EFFECTIVENESS OF NURSING INTERVENTIONS

Nursing care for older adults with urinary incontinence is evaluated by measuring the extent to which the person is able to achieve periods of continence that are as long as possible. When older adults attribute incontinence to aging processes, the effectiveness of nursing interventions may be evaluated by the person verbalizing accurate information about age-related changes and risk factors that affect urinary elimination. Another measure of the effectiveness of nursing interventions in such cases would be that the person seeks evaluation for his or her incontinence, rather than accepting this condition as inevitable.

If incontinence cannot be resolved, nursing care is directed toward managing urinary elimination in such a way as to maintain the dignity of the older adult and prevent negative consequences. In these situations, nursing care might be measured by the extent to which the person maintains his or her daily activities. For example, if older adults restrict their social activities because of incontinence, a measure of the success of nursing interventions might be that they begin using incontinence products to permit them to be away from their home for 4 hours at a time. For people with total incontinence, a measure of the effectiveness of nursing interventions would be the absence of skin irritation and breakdown.

CHAPTER SUMMARY

Older adults have altered patterns of urinary elimination associated with the following age-related changes: diminished bladder capacity, bladder contractions during filling, incomplete bladder emptying, urinary urgency and frequency, and relaxation of the pelvic floor musculature. Additional consequences of age-related changes that affect urinary elimination include delayed excretion of water-soluble medications and decreased efficiency of homeostatic mechanisms.

Older adults, as well as professional and nonprofessional caregivers, commonly blame incontinence on age-related processes, and these myths and misunderstandings may interfere with older adults' seeking and receiving help for their incontinence. When urinary incontinence is not addressed, older adults are likely to restrict their social activities and experience additional negative consequences. Risk factors that can cause urinary incontinence include impaired physical function (e.g., limited mobility), pathologic conditions (e.g., dementia, prostatic hyperplasia, fecal impaction), adverse medication effects, dietary and lifestyle factors, and environmental barriers (e.g., a long distance to the bathroom).

Nursing assessment of urinary elimination focuses on the identification of any factors that influence overall urinary elimination or increase the risk for urinary incontinence. Nurses also assess signs and symptoms of urinary incontinence and identify any negative consequences. Applicable nursing diagnoses include Urinary Elimination, Impaired and specific types of urinary incontinence. Nursing care addresses the identified risk factors and is directed toward achieving continence and extending the time between incontinence episodes. When incontinence cannot be resolved or prevented, nursing goals address the actual and potential negative consequences (e.g., social isolation, impaired skin integrity). Evaluation of nursing care is measured by the extent to which the person achieves continence or, if continence cannot be achieved, by the success with which negative consequences are prevented.

CONCLUDING CASE STUDY AND NURSING CARE PLAN

➤ Mrs. U., who is now 79 years old, is being transferred to a nursing home for rehabilitation after sustaining a hip fracture. An indwelling catheter was inserted before her surgery 7 days ago, and it was removed yesterday. She is ambulating with a walker but needs one-person assistance. The discharge summary describes her as incontinent of urine. Mrs. U. hopes to regain her independence in performing ADLs so that she can return to her own home, where she lives with her husband.

Nursing Assessment

During your functional assessment, Mrs. U. tells you she has had "trouble holding her water" since they removed the catheter yesterday. She is quite embarrassed about this and has not discussed it with any other health care practitioner. She says that she had too many other questions to discuss with her orthopedic surgeon and states that the nurses kept a large absorbent pad on her bed so that she wouldn't have to walk to the bathroom. When she went to physical therapy, she used sanitary napkins, which her friend

brought to her. She limited her fluid intake to a cup of coffee with each meal and a few sips of water with her pills.

Further assessment of Mrs. U's incontinence reveals that, for many years, she has had difficulty with "leaking," particularly when she coughs, sneezes, or exercises. Also, she gets up to urinate about 4 to 5 times nightly. It was during one of these trips to the bathroom that she tripped and fractured her hip. She says that she wakes up a lot during the night and goes to the bathroom because she's afraid of wetting the bed. She does not feel the need to urinate every time she wakes up, but goes to the bathroom to prevent any leakage. She limits her fluid intake to 6 glasses per day and does not drink anything after 5:00 PM. A few years ago, a nurse taught her how to do "Kegel's and they helped for a couple years, but I don't bother to do them anymore." She tearfully confides that she thinks that the orthopedic surgeon damaged a nerve in her bladder, which she believes is the reason she has such little control over urination since the surgery. She thinks that the hospital staff inserted the catheter because she has "weak kidneys." She states, "Before I had this fractured hip, I just had the usual problems holding water like all my friends have, but now it's really bad and I'll probably never be able to hold my water. I wish you'd just put that tube back in me so I can go home again and not worry about accidents."

Nursing Diagnosis

In addition to the nursing diagnoses that are related to Mrs. U.'s impaired mobility, you address her problem with urinary incontinence. In deciding which type of urinary incontinence to include in your nursing diagnosis, you conclude that both Stress Incontinence and Functional Incontinence are appropriate because of the combination of long-term and recent factors that contribute to her incontinence. Your nursing diagnosis is Stress/Functional Incontinence related to limited mobility, recent indwelling catheter, and insufficient knowledge of normal urinary function and pelvic muscle exercises. Evidence for this diagnosis can be found in Mrs. U.'s statements reflecting misconceptions and lack of information and in her description of current and past problems with incontinence. Evidence also is derived from your observations that she needs one-person assistance for walking and that she uses sanitary napkins and bedpads for urinary incontinence.

Nursing Care Plan

A nursing care plan for Mrs. U. is given in Display 15-10.

DISPLAY 15-10 • NURSING CARE PLAN FOR MRS. U.

EXPECTED OUTCOME	NURSING INTERVENTIONS	NURSING EVALUATION
Mrs. U.'s knowledge of normal urinary function will increase.	• Discuss and describe normal urinary function, using a balloon partially filled with water and a simple illustration of the female urinary tract. • Emphasize the relationship between adequate fluid intake and the maintenance of continence.	• Mrs. U. will be able to describe normal urinary function and the mechanisms involved in maintaining continence.
Mrs. U.'s knowledge about causative factors for incontinence will increase.	• Describe age-related changes that contribute to incontinence, using the information contained in Display 15-5. • Discuss the effects of frequent bladder emptying and limited fluid intake on the maintenance of continence. • Discuss the relationship between limited mobility and urinary incontinence.	• Mrs. U. will describe age-related changes that influence urinary elimination. • Mrs. U. will identify risk factors that contribute to her incontinence.
Mrs. U.'s misconceptions about her urinary incontinence will be corrected.	• Emphasize that as Mrs. U. regains her mobility, she will regain her ability to maintain continence. • Emphasize that urinary incontinence is not an inevitable consequence of aging. • Explain that the orthopedic surgeon was not operating on or near her bladder or urinary tract. • Explain that the Foley catheter probably contributed to her current incontinence, but that this is a temporary situation that will resolve with proper interventions. • Emphasize that the nursing home staff will work with her to improve or alleviate her incontinence.	• Mrs. U. will state correct information about the relationship between her hip surgery and her incontinence. • Mrs. U. will express confidence in regaining urinary control.
The factors that contribute to Mrs. U.'s functional incontinence will be eliminated.	• Provide a bedside commode for Mrs. U.'s use until she regains her ability to walk to the bathroom without assistance. • Work with the physical therapy staff to teach Mrs. U. a proper technique for independent transfer to the commode. • The nursing and dietary staff will provide 2000 mL of fluids/day, taking into consideration Mrs. U.'s preferences. • The nursing and dietary staff will work with Mrs. U. to schedule her fluid intake at acceptable times of the day, with minimal intake in the evening. • Talk with Mrs. U. about eliminating the bedpads as soon as she feels confident about maintaining continence.	• Mrs. U. will be continent of urine, except for stress incontinence

(continued)

DISPLAY 15-10 • NURSING CARE PLAN FOR MRS. U. (Continued)		
EXPECTED OUTCOME	*NURSING INTERVENTIONS*	*NURSING EVALUATION*
Mrs. U. will regain full control over urination.	• Suggest that Mrs. U. seek a comprehensive assessment of her urinary incontinence. • Give Mrs. U. a copy of Display 15-6 for use as a guide for performing pelvic muscle exercises. • Emphasize the need to perform pelvic muscle exercises on an ongoing basis for alleviation of stress incontinence. • Give Mrs. U. information about educational resources that might be helpful for her.	• Mrs. U. will report a reduction in or elimination of her stress incontinence.

CRITICAL THINKING EXERCISES

1. Describe how each of the following age-related or risk factors might influence urinary function in older adults: medications, renal function, functional abilities, environmental conditions, altered thirst perception, changes in the urinary tract and nervous system, and myths and misunderstandings on the part of older adults, their caregivers, and health care professionals.
2. What are the psychosocial consequences of urinary incontinence for older adults and their caregivers?
3. Describe how you would address the following statement made by a 74-year-old woman: "Of course I have to wear pads all the time, just like when I was a teenager. I haven't talked to the doctor because I figured this was pretty normal at my age."
4. Describe the nursing assessment, with regard to urinary elimination, for a 75-year-old man and a 75-year-old woman.

Future Directions for Healthier Aging: Focus on Urinary Function

• The National Institute on Aging is promoting research on underlying causes of urinary incontinence and on health education of older adults and health care professionals.
• The National Institute on Aging is supporting research on the causes of and treatments for prostatic hyperplasia in older men.
• The National Institute on Aging and pharmaceutical companies are focusing on new medications and new methods of delivering medications for treating urinary incontinence.
• Medical device companies are focusing on new minimally invasive or noninvasive methods for treating urinary incontinence.

EDUCATIONAL RESOURCES

American Foundation for Urologic Disease
300 West Pratt Street, Suite 401, Baltimore, MD 21201
(800) 242-2383
http://www.afud.org

American Geriatrics Society (AGS) Foundation for Health in Aging
350 Fifth Avenue, Suite 802, New York, NY 10118
(212) 755-6810
http://www.healthinaging.org

The Canadian Continence Foundation
P.O. Box 30, Victoria Branch Westmount
Quebec CANADA H3Z 2V4
(800) 265-9575
http://www.continence-fdn.ca

International Continence Society
Southmead Hospital
Bristol BS10 5NB, United Kingdom
http://www.icsoffice.org

National Association for Continence (NAFC)
P.O. Box 1019, Charleston, SC 29402-1019
(800) 252-3337
http://www.nafc.org

National Bladder Foundation
P.O. Box 1095, Ridgefield, CT 06877
(203) 431-0005
http://www.bladder.org

The Simon Foundation for Continence
P.O. Box 835F, Wilmette, IL 60091
(800) 237-4666
http://www.simonfoundation.org

**U.S. Department of Health and Human Services
Agency for Healthcare Research and Quality**
AHCPR Publications Clearinghouse
P.O. Box 8547, Silver Spring, MD 20907
(800) 358-9295
http://www.ahcpr.gov

REFERENCES

Abrams, P., Cardozo, L., Fall, M., Griffiths, D., Rosier, P., Ulmsten U., et al. (2002). The standardisation of terminology of lower urinary tract function: Report from the Standardisation Sub-committee of the International Continence Society. *American Journal of Obstetrics and Gynecology, 187*(1), 116–126.

Bogner, H. R., Gallo, J. J., Sammel, M. D., Ford, D. E., Armenian, H. K., & Eaton, W. W. (2002). Urinary incontinence and psychological distress in community-dwelling older adults. *Journal of the American Geriatrics Society, 50,* 489–495.

Borrie, M. J., Bawden, M., Speechly, M., & Kloseck, M. (2002). Interventions led by nurse continence advisers in the management of urinary incontinence: A randomized controlled trial. *Journal of the Canadian Medical Association, 166*(10), 1267–1273.

Bottomley, J. M. (2000). Complementary nutrition in treating urinary incontinence. *Topics in Geriatric Rehabilitation, 16*(1), 61–77.

Burgio, K. L., Locher, J. L., & Goode, P. S. (2000). Combined behavioral and drug therapy for urge incontinence in older women. *Journal of the American Geriatrics Society, 48,* 370–374.

Burgio, K. L., Locher, J. L., Roth, D. L., & Goode, P. S. (2001). Psychological improvements associated with behavioral and drug treatment of urge incontinence in older women. *Journal of Gerontology: Biological Sciences, 56B,* P46–P51.

Carpenito, L. J. (2002). *Nursing diagnosis: Application to clinical practice* (9th ed.). Philadelphia: Lippincott Williams & Wilkins.

Dougherty, M. C., Dwyer, J. W., Pendergrast, J. F., et al. (2002). A randomized trial of behavioral management for continence with older rural women. *Research in Nursing and Health, 25,* 3–13.

Dowling-Castronovo, A. (2001). Urinary incontinence assessment. *Journal of Gerontological Nursing, 27*(5), 5–8.

Dugan, E., Roberts, C. P., Cohen, S. J., Preisser, J. S., Davis, C. C., Bland, D. R., & Albertson, E. (2001). Why older community dwelling adults do not discuss urinary incontinence with their primary care physicians. *Journal of the American Geriatrics Society, 49,* 462–465.

Engberg, S., Sereika, S., Weber, E., Engberg, R., McDowell, J., & Reynolds, C. F. (2001). Prevalence and recognition of depressive symptoms among homebound older adults with incontinence. *Journal of Geriatric Psychiatry and Neurology, 14,* 130–139.

Fultz, N. H., & Herzog, A. R. (2001). Self-reported social and emotional impact of urinary incontinence. *Journal of the American Geriatrics Society, 49,* 892–899.

Hay-Smith, E. J., Bo Berghmans, L. C., Hendriks, H. J., de Bie, R. A., & van Waalwijk van Doorn, E. S. (2002). Pelvic floor muscle training for urinary incontinence in women. *Cochrane Review, 4.*

Iglesias, F. J. G., Ocerin, C., Martin, J. P., Gama, E. V., Perez, M. L., Lopez, M. R., Aranguren, M. V. P., & Muno, J. B. G. (2000). Prevalence and psychosocial impact of urinary incontinence in older people of a Spanish rural population. (2000). *Journals of Gerontology: Medical Sciences, 55A,* M207–M214.

Johnson, T. M., Kincade, J. E., Bernard, S. L., Busby-Whitehead, J., & Defriese, G. H. (2000). Self-care used by older men and women to manage urinary incontinence: Results for the national follow-up survey on self-care and aging. *Journal of the American Geriatrics Society, 48,* 894–902.

Langa, K. M., Fultz, N. H., Saint, S., Kabeto, M. U., & Herzog, R. (2002). Informal caregiving time and cost for urinary incontinence in older individuals in the United States. *Journal of the American Geriatrics Society, 50,* 733–737.

Lekan-Rutledge, D. (2000). Diffusion of innovation: A model for implementation of prompted voiding in long term care. *Journal of Gerontological Nursing, 26*(4), 25–33.

Lindeman, R. H. (2000). Aging and the kidney. In M. H. Beers & R. Berkow. *The Merck manual of geriatrics* (pp. 9951–9954). Whitehouse Station, NJ: Merck Research Laboratories.

Locher, J. L., Burgio, K. L., Goode, P. S., Roth, D. L., & Rodriguez, E. (2002). Effects of age and causal attribution to aging on health related behaviors associated with urinary incontinence in older women. *Gerontologist, 42,* 515–521.

Locher, J. L., Goode, P. S., Roth, D. L., Worrell, R. L., & Burgio, K. L. (2001). Reliability assessment of the bladder diary for urinary incontinence in older women. *Journal of Gerontology: Medical Sciences, 56A,* M32–M35.

Lose, G., Alling-Moller, L., & Jennum, P. (2001). Nocturia in women. *American Journal of Obstetrics and Gynecology, 185*(2), 514–521.

Lyons, S. S., Specht, P., Mentes, J. C., & Titler, M. G. (2000). Prompted voiding protocol for individuals with urinary incontinence. *Journal of Gerontological Nursing, 12*(6).

Maggi, S., Minicuci, N., Langlois, J., Pavan, M., Enzi, G., & Crepaldi, G. (2001). Prevalence rate of urinary incontinence in community-dwelling elderly individuals: The Veneto study. *Journal of Gerontology: Medical Sciences, 56A*(1), M14–M18.

Mather, K. F., & Bakas, T. (2002). Nursing assistants' perceptions of their ability to provide continence care. *Geriatric Nursing, 23,* 76–82.

Miller, M. (2000). Nocturnal polyurias in older people: Pathophysiology and clinical implications. *Journal of the American Geriatrics Society, 48,* 1321–1329.

Mueller, C., & Cain, H. (2002). Comprehensive management of urinary incontinence through quality improvement efforts. *Geriatric Nursing, 23,* 82–87.

Ostbye, T., Hunskaar, S., & Sykes, E. (2002). Predictors and incidence of urinary incontinence in elderly Canadians with and without dementia. *Canadian Journal on Aging, 2*(1), 95–102.

Ouslander, J. G., Ai-Samarrai, N., & Schnelle, J. F. (2001). Prompted voiding for nighttime incontinence in nursing homes: Is it effective? *Journal of the American Geriatrics Society, 49,* 706–709.

Palmer, M. H., Baumgarten, M., Langengerg, P., & Carson, J. L. (2002). Risk factors for hospital-acquired incontinence in elderly female hip fracture patients. *Journal of Gerontology: Medical Sciences, 57A,* M672–M678.

Resnick, N. M. (2000). Urinary incontinence. In M. H. Beers & R. Berkow. *The Merck manual of geriatrics* (pp. 965–980). Whitehouse Station, NJ: Merck Research Laboratories.

Resnick, N. M., & Yalla, S. V. (2002). Geriatric incontinence and voiding dysfunction. In W. C. Walsh (Ed-in-Chief), *Campbell's urology* (pp. 1218–1223). St Louis: WB Saunders.

Schnelle, J. C., & Smith, R. L. (2001). Quality indicators for the management of urinary incontinence in vulnerable community-dwelling elders. *Annals of Internal Medicine, 135,* 752–758.

Specht, J. K. P., Lyons, S. S., & Maas, M. L. (2002). Patterns and treatments of urinary incontinence on special care units. *Journal of Gerontological Nursing, 28*(5), 13–21.

Specht, J. P., & Maas, M. L. (2001). Urinary incontinence: Functional, iatrogenic, overflow, reflex, stress, total, and urge. In M. L. Maas, K. C. Buckwalter, M. D. Hardy, T. Tripp-Reimer, M. G. Titler, & J. P. Specht (Eds.), *Nursing care of older adults: Diagnoses, outcomes, & interventions* (pp. 252–278). St Louis: Mosby.

Yoshikawa, T. T. (2000). Urinary tract infections. In M. H. Beers & R. Berkow. *The Merck manual of geriatrics* (pp. 980–987). Whitehouse Station, NJ: Merck Research Laboratories.

Cardiovascular Function

LEARNING OBJECTIVES

1. Delineate age-related changes that affect cardiovascular function.
2. Delineate risk factors for cardiovascular disease and hypotension.
3. Identify the functional consequences of age-related changes and risk factors that affect cardiovascular function.
4. Describe the assessment of cardiovascular function and risks for cardiovascular disease in older adults.
5. Identify interventions directed toward achieving optimal cardiovascular performance, reducing risk factors for cardiovascular disease, and preventing and managing hypertension, dyslipidemia, and hypotension in older adults.

Cardiovascular function is responsible for the life-sustaining activities of maintaining homeostasis, circulating blood cells, removing carbon dioxide and other waste products, and delivering oxygen, nutrients, and other substances to all of the body organs and tissues. Like many other physiologic systems, the cardiovascular system has a tremendous adaptive capacity to compensate for age-related changes. Healthy older adults, therefore, will not notice any significant change in cardiovascular performance because of age-related changes. In the presence of risk factors, however, the cardiovascular system is less efficient in performing life-sustaining activities, and serious negative functional consequences can occur.

AGE-RELATED CHANGES THAT AFFECT CARDIOVASCULAR FUNCTION

As with many other aspects of physiologic function, determining whether the changes in cardiovascular function that commonly affect older adults are attributable to age, disease, or lifestyle is difficult. Knowledge about distinct age- or disease-related changes in cardiovascular function is confounded by the fact that, until recently, no medical technology existed to detect asymptomatic pathologic cardiovascular processes (e.g., occlusion of a major coronary artery). Thus, early studies provided more information about common cardiovascular changes that affect older people and less information about age-related changes. Currently, researchers focus on subjects who have been carefully screened for cardiovascular disease.

In addition to differentiating between age- and disease-related changes in cardiovascular function, researchers are trying to distinguish between changes that are age related and those that can be linked to risk factors. Perhaps more than any other aspect of physiologic function, lifestyle factors significantly influence cardiovascular performance. Smoking, dietary habits, some medical conditions, and physical exercise, for example, are all known to have long-term effects on cardiovascular function. Less is known about how the long-term effects of lifestyle factors can be differentiated from age-related processes, particularly when entire societies are affected by these factors. Blood pressure, for example, has been found to increase gradually in adulthood in people who live in Western societies but not in people from less industrialized societies. Therefore, changes that are thought to be age related because they occur consistently in large population samples may be found to be related to lifestyle when cross-cultural studies are done. Lifestyle and environmental influences are important factors in explaining the wide range of variability in cardiovascular function among older adults, even for changes that are not disease related.

Myocardium and Neuroconductive System

Some of the commonly identified changes of the myocardium are amyloid deposits, lipofuscin accumulation, basophilic degeneration, myocardial atrophy or hypertrophy, valvular thickening and stiffening, and increased amounts of connective tissue. Researchers currently are investigating the extent to which these changes are age related or disease related, but they agree that myocardial atrophy is disease related and that a slight, but not marked, increase in

left ventricular wall thickness is the primary age-related change (Lakatta, 2000). In addition, the left atrium enlarges, even in healthy older adults. Other age-related changes include thickening of the atrial endocardium, thickening of the atrioventricular valves, and calcification of at least part of the mitral annulus of the aortic valve. These changes interfere with the ability of the heart to contract completely. With less effective contractility, more time is required to complete the cycle of diastolic filling and systolic emptying. In addition, the myocardium becomes increasingly irritable and less responsive to the impulses from the sympathetic nervous system.

Age-related changes in cardiac physiology are minimal, and the changes that do occur affect cardiac performance only under conditions of physiologic stress. Even under stressful conditions, the heart in healthy older adults is able to adapt, although the adaptive mechanisms may differ from those of younger adults or be slightly less efficient. The age-related changes that cause functional consequences primarily involve the electrophysiology of the heart (i.e., the neuroconductive system). Age-related changes in the neuroconductive system include a decrease in the number of pacemaker cells; increased irregularity in the shape of pacemaker cells; and increased deposits of fat, collagen, and elastic fibers around the sinoatrial node.

Vasculature

Age-related changes affect two of the three vascular layers, and functional consequences vary, depending on which layer is affected. For example, changes in the tunica intima, the innermost layer, have the most serious functional consequences in the development of atherosclerosis, whereas changes in the tunica media, the middle layer, are associated with hypertension. The outermost layer (the tunica externa) does not seem to be affected by age-related changes. This layer, composed of loosely meshed adipose and connective tissue, supports nerve fibers and the vasa vasorum, the blood supply for the tunica media.

The tunica intima consists of a single layer of endothelial cells on a thin layer of connective tissue. It controls the entry of lipids and other substances from the blood into the artery wall. Intact endothelial cells allow blood to flow freely without clotting; however, when the endothelial cells are damaged, they function in the clotting process. With increasing age, the tunica intima thickens because of fibrosis, cellular proliferation, and lipid and calcium accumulation. In addition, the endothelial cells become irregular in size and shape. These changes cause the arteries to become dilated and elongated, and as a result, the arterial walls are more vulnerable to atherosclerosis (discussed in the section on Pathologic Conditions).

The tunica media is composed of single or multiple layers of smooth muscle cells surrounded by elastin and collagen. The smooth muscle cells are involved in the tissue-forming functions of producing collagen, proteoglycans, and elastic fibers. Because it provides structural support, this layer controls arterial expansion and contraction. Age-related changes that affect the tunica media include an increase in collagen and a thinning and calcification of elastin fibers, resulting in stiffened blood vessels. These changes are particularly pronounced in the aorta, where the diameter of the lumen increases to compensate for the age-related arterial stiffening. Although these changes are viewed as age related, longitudinal and cross-cultural studies are beginning to raise questions about the impact of lifestyle variables on arterial stiffness.

Age-related changes in the tunica media cause increased peripheral resistance, impaired baroreceptor function, and diminished ability to increase blood flow to vital organs. These changes do not cause serious consequences in healthy older adults but do interfere with cardiac function by altering the resistance to blood flow from the heart. In addition, age-related vascular changes impair the pulsatile flow of blood and increase the pulse wave velocity. Consequently, the left ventricle is forced to work harder, and the baroreceptors in the large arteries lose their effectiveness in controlling blood pressure, especially during postural changes. This increased vascular stiffness causes a slight increase in the systolic blood pressure.

Veins undergo changes similar to those affecting the arteries, but to a lesser degree. Veins become thicker, more dilated, and less elastic with increasing age. Valves of the large leg veins become less efficient in the return of blood to the heart. Peripheral circulation is further influenced by an age-related reduction in muscle mass and a concurrent reduction in the demand for oxygen.

Baroreflex Mechanisms

Baroreflex mechanisms regulate blood pressure by increasing or decreasing the heart rate and peripheral vascular resistance to compensate for transient decreases or increases in arterial pressure. Age-related changes that alter baroreflex mechanisms include arterial stiffening and reduced cardiovascular responsiveness to adrenergic stimulation. These changes cause a blunting of the compensatory response to both hypertensive and hypotensive stimuli in older adults, so that the heart rate does not increase or decrease as

efficiently as in younger adults. Researchers currently are studying the effects of obesity, hypertension, and cardiovascular disease as factors that alter baroreflex mechanisms in older adults (Piccirillo et al., 2001).

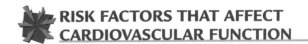

RISK FACTORS THAT AFFECT CARDIOVASCULAR FUNCTION

Because healthy older adults are affected by age-related cardiovascular changes only under conditions of physical stress, physical deconditioning (i.e., lack of exercise) is a risk factor for diminished cardiovascular function. Unfortunately, it is an almost universal risk factor among older adults because as people age they spend a smaller percentage of time performing physical activities (Messinger-Rapport & Sprecher, 2002). The most significant risk factors that contribute to cardiovascular disease are the same for both younger and older adults, but the cumulative effects of these risks are likely to cause more serious consequences for older adults. Gender-related differences in risk factors can significantly affect women beginning at menopause, and factors that increase the risk for hypotension begin affecting all older adults after the age of about 70 or 75 years.

Physical Deconditioning

Because physical deconditioning significantly influences many aspects of cardiovascular function, including blood pressure, heart rate, and oxygen consumption, it "influences every known heart disease risk factor except family history" (Gibbons & Clark, 2001, p. 348). Gerontologists and exercise physiologists have suggested that physical deconditioning, rather than age-related changes, is the major causative factor for many of the cardiovascular changes that affect older adults (Lakatta, 2000). A particular focus of current research is to identify the extent to which physical deconditioning affects cardiovascular response to exercise. There is increasing and irrefutable evidence that physical conditioning can improve the aerobic capacity of older adults by increasing cardiac output and oxygen utilization (Lakatta, 2000). Thus, it is likely that a sedentary lifestyle may be the major contributing, and potentially reversible, risk factor that affects the cardiovascular response to exercise in older adults. Factors that contribute to physical deconditioning include acute and chronic illnesses, a sedentary lifestyle, mobility limitations, cardiac disease or other diseases that interfere with physical activity, and psychosocial influences, such as depression or lack of motivation.

Risks for Cardiovascular Disease

Atherosclerosis and other cardiovascular diseases are associated with race, gender, obesity, diabetes, heredity, hypertension, dyslipidemia, increased age, dietary habits, physical inactivity, cigarette smoking, and environmental tobacco smoke. In addition, low socioeconomic status is widely recognized as a risk factor for cardiovascular disease. Tobacco smoking is the most powerful preventable risk factor for cardiovascular disease; evidence about the causal relationship between even a few cigarettes daily or exposure to environmental tobacco smoke is indisputable.

Dyslipidemia is a risk factor when low-density lipoprotein (LDL) cholesterol levels are high or when high-density lipoprotein (HDL) cholesterol levels are low. In contrast, high levels of HDL are considered protective against atherosclerosis and are associated with a lower risk for cardiovascular disease. Several recent studies identified subclinical hypothyroidism as a strong and independent risk factor for elevated LDL cholesterol levels and cardiovascular disease (Hak et al., 2000; Mya & Aronow, 2002).

Hypertension as a risk factor is usually defined as a blood pressure greater than or equal to 140/90 mm Hg, or a blood pressure that requires treatment with an antihypertensive medication. Researchers have found that blood pressure even at the high end of normal (i.e., 130 to 139/85 to 89 mm Hg) is a risk factor for cardiovascular disease (Prospective Studies Collaboration, 2002; Vasan et al., 2001). Until recently, diastolic blood pressure was considered a stronger risk factor for cardiovascular disease than systolic blood pressure, and some questions were raised about the value of treating isolated systolic blood pressure, especially in older adults. Recent studies, however, have confirmed the importance of both diastolic blood pressure and systolic blood pressure (Benetos et al., 2002; Mancia et al., 2002). Risk factors for hypertension include obesity, physical inactivity, and high-sodium diets. Older adults and African Americans may have a heightened salt sensitivity and therefore may be more likely than other groups to develop hypertension in response to sodium intake (Vollmer et al., 2001).

The heart disease death rate is consistently higher in African Americans than in whites, and heart disease mortality in rural Africans Americans in the United States is among the highest ever recorded anywhere in the world (Taylor et al., 2002).

Psychosocial risk factors that may increase the risk for cardiovascular disease include anxiety, depression, job strain, social isolation, poor social supports, high anger and hostility indices, stressful family relationships, and physical or emotional stress reaction (Eaton & Anthony, 2002; Williams et al., 2002). Chaput and colleagues (2002) found that hostility was an independent and potentially modifiable risk factor for recurrent myocardial infarctions in postmenopausal women.

Because cardiovascular disease has long been viewed as a disease of middle-aged men, early research focused primarily, or exclusively, on men. In the early 1990s, researchers began recognizing that the prevalence of cardiovascular disease in women increased dramatically after the age of 50 years and continued to increase until it surpassed that of men by the eighth decade. In early and middle adulthood, however, male gender is a risk factor because women tend to get cardiovascular disease about 10 years later than men with similar risk factor profiles (Keevil et al., 2002).

Many questions were raised about gender-specific risk factors for cardiovascular disease, and several major research initiatives were developed to address these questions, with particular emphasis on estrogen as an influencing factor. Many of the longitudinal studies are ongoing, and several of the studies address the influence of hormonal therapy for postmenopausal women. Eaton and Anthony (2002) reviewed recent research and identified the following characteristics that contribute to the increased risk for cardiovascular disease in postmenopausal women:

- An atherogenic lipid profile (i.e., low HDL cholesterol, high LDL cholesterol, and elevated triglycerides)
- Increased abdominal fat
- Increased incidence of obesity
- Increased incidence of hypertension, including isolated systolic hypertension
- Increased incidence of diabetes and insulin resistance

Hormonal therapy for menopausal women has been the focus of many studies since the 1960s. Initial studies with mostly observational data suggested that hormonal therapy reduced the risk for cardiovascular disease in postmenopausal women, but many of these studies did not adjust for confounding variables such as socioeconomic status (Humphrey et al., 2002; Laine, 2002). More recent randomized trials have shown no benefit of hormonal therapy for either primary or secondary prevention of cardiovascular disease, and there is some indication that hormonal therapy may actually increase the risk (Humphrey et al., 2002; Women's Health Initiative, 2002).

The death rate for heart disease is almost twice as high in men as in women, but the death rate for older women within a few weeks of a heart attack is twice as high as that in men.

Researchers currently are investigating the potential roles of antioxidants, alcohol intake, diet and nutrition, and nonsteroidal antiinflammatory drugs as factors that can positively or negatively influence the risk for cardiovascular disease. For example, researchers are investigating the role of dietary sodium and potassium in increasing or reducing the risk for stroke, hypertension, and other cardiovascular diseases (Aviv, 2001; Hajjar et al., 2001). Researchers also are investigating whether a wider pulse pressure (i.e., the difference between diastolic and systolic pressures) increases the risk for cardiovascular disease, particularly in people with hypertension (Blacher et al., 2000; Williams et al., 2002).

Risks for Hypotension

Increased age is a risk factor for hypotension because the incidence of both orthostatic and postprandial hypotension rises significantly after the age of 75 years. When hypotension occurs, it is usually due to a combination of age-related changes and risk factors. Pathologic conditions that affect the autonomic or central nervous systems increase the risk for orthostatic and postprandial hypotension. Similarly, medications that act on the nervous system can interfere with control of blood pressure and cause hypotension. Parkinson's disease increases the risk for orthostatic hypotension through its effects on the nervous system and through the effects of medications (e.g., levodopa) used to treat this condition. Examples of pathologic conditions and medications that increase the risk for hypotension are listed in Display 16-1. Additional risk factors that can cause orthostatic hypotension include prolonged immobility, surgical sympathectomy, and the Valsalva maneuver during voiding.

PATHOLOGIC CONDITIONS ASSOCIATED WITH CARDIOVASCULAR FUNCTION

Cardiovascular diseases most common in older adults are stroke (cerebrovascular accident), hypertension, atherosclerosis, heart failure, and coronary heart disease. Atherosclerosis (also called *atherosclerotic cardiovascular disease*) includes coronary artery disease, cerebrovascular disease, and peripheral vascular disease. Hypertension is the most prevalent cardiovascular disease, but coronary heart disease accounts for the most cardiovascular deaths (Messinger-Rapport

& Sprecher, 2002). Because hypertension is a significant risk factor for additional cardiovascular disease, it is discussed in the section on Assessing Risks for Cardiovascular Disease.

Atherosclerosis is a "disorder affecting medium and large arteries in which patchy subintimal deposits of lipids and connective tissue (atherosclerotic plaques) reduce or obstruct blood flow" (Vokonos, 2000, p. 849). Atherosclerosis is caused by a combination of risk factors and age-related vascular changes, but the physiologic changes of atherosclerosis begin in early adulthood, and the effects are cumulative. The "reaction to injury" theory, first described by Ross and Glomset (1976), is a widely accepted explanation for the development of athero-

---

DISPLAY 16-1
Risk Factors for Hypotension

Risks for Orthostatic Hypotension
Pathologic Processes
- Hypertension, including isolated systolic hypertension
- Parkinson's disease
- Cerebral infarct
- Diabetes
- Anemia
- Peripheral neuropathy
- Arrhythmias
- Volume depletion (e.g., dehydration)
- Electrolyte imbalances (e.g., hyponatremia, hypokalemia)

Medications
- Antihypertensives
- Anticholinergics
- Phenothiazines
- Antidepressants
- Levodopa
- Vasodilators
- Diuretics
- Alcohol

Risks for Postprandial Hypotension
Pathologic Processes
- Systolic hypertension
- Diabetes mellitus
- Parkinson's disease
- Multisystem atrophy

Medications
- Diuretics
- Antihypertensive medications ingested before meals

sclerosis. According to this theory, atherogenesis is a cyclical process that proceeds as follows:

1. The integrity of the intimal endothelium is injured because of repeated or continuing insults.
2. Circulating blood platelets arrive and aggregate at the site.
3. Compensatory processes eventually lead to migration of medial smooth muscle cells into the intima and the proliferation of these cells at the site of injury.
4. Lipids and connective tissue accumulate.

The initial injury may be caused by chemicals (as in hypercholesterolemia), mechanical stress (as with hypertension), or immunologic factors (as with renal transplantation). With repeated or chronic injury, this process continues; the intima becomes thicker, and blood flow over the injured sites is altered, thereby increasing the risk for further injury. Although the sequence of events is a vicious cycle that eventually leads to serious pathologic conditions (e.g., myocardial infarction or cerebrovascular accidents), the process can be halted by eliminating the cause of injury. This theory has been used to explain: (1) how age-related changes in the intima might contribute to atherosclerosis; (2) how risk factors might enhance lesion formation; (3) how inhibitors of platelet aggregation could interfere with lesion formation; and (4) how the process might be interrupted or retarded (Bierman, 1985).

FUNCTIONAL CONSEQUENCES ASSOCIATED WITH CARDIOVASCULAR FUNCTION IN OLDER ADULTS

Older adults who have no pathologic conditions experience no significant cardiovascular effects in the resting state, but their cardiovascular performance is less efficient during exercise. In addition, they are likely to develop orthostatic or postprandial hypotension because of a combination of age-related changes and risk factors. However, older adults who have hypertension, atherosclerosis, or other pathologic cardiovascular conditions are likely to experience negative functional consequences.

The Impact of Cardiovascular Changes on Cardiac Output, Heart Rate, and Rhythm

Cardiac output, the amount of blood pumped by the heart per minute, is an important measure of cardiac performance because it represents the heart's ability to meet the oxygen requirements of the body. Although reduced cardiac output is common in older adults, it is associated primarily with pathologic, rather than age-related, conditions. With the exception of a slight decrease in cardiac output at rest in older women, healthy older adults do not experience any decline in cardiac output.

The heart rates of healthy older people decrease gradually, from an average intrinsic sinus rate of 104 beats/minute at the age of 20 years to 92 beats/minute between the ages of 45 and 55 years (Lakatta, 2000). Age-related changes in cardiac conduction mechanisms are likely to cause harmless ventricular and supraventricular arrhythmias, even in healthy older adults. Atrial fibrillation—a more serious arrhythmia—commonly occurs in older adults, but this is more likely to be caused by pathologic conditions (e.g., hypertension, coronary artery disease) than by age-related changes alone.

The Impact of Cardiovascular Changes on the Response to Exercise

A negative functional consequence that affects cardiovascular performance in healthy older adults is a blunted adaptive response to physical exercise. Physiologic stress, such as that associated with exercise, increases the demands on the cardiovascular system by 4 to 5 times the basal level. The adaptive response involves many aspects of physiologic function, including the respiratory, cardiovascular, musculoskeletal, and autonomic nervous systems. The maximum heart rate achieved during exercise is markedly decreased, and the peak exercise capacity and oxygen consumption decline in older adults, but physical deconditioning and other risk factors account for some of this decline. Whereas a younger adult's heart rate speeds up to 180 to 200 beats/minute under stress (e.g., physical exercise), the heart rate of an 80-year-old person accelerates to only 135 to 150 beats/minute. Likewise, oxygen consumption during exercise diminishes by 50% between the ages of 20 and 80 years (Lakatta, 2000).

The Impact of Cardiovascular Changes on Blood Pressure

Age-related changes affecting blood pressure can be summarized as follows:

- In men, diastolic blood pressure increases steadily at a rate of 1 mm Hg per decade without any plateau or decline.
- In women, diastolic blood pressure increases significantly between the ages of 40 and 60 years,

then stabilizes, and may decline slightly after the age of 70 years.

- Systolic blood pressure gradually increases by 5 to 8 mm Hg per decade beginning around the age of 50 years in men and 40 years in women.
- Beginning around the age of 30 years, systolic blood pressure increases to a greater degree than diastolic blood pressure, so that the pulse pressure gradually widens.
- In older adults, the increase in systolic blood pressure that occurs in response to aerobic exercise is sustained for a longer period of time than in younger adults.

Because people in non-Western societies do not experience gradual increases in blood pressure, these changes cannot be viewed solely as age related. Rather, it is likely that blood pressure increases are associated with factors such as increased weight, dietary habits (e.g., high sodium intake), and lifestyle factors, such as cigarette smoking and physical inactivity.

Age-related changes that affect autonomic regulation of blood pressure predispose older adults to orthostatic hypotension and postprandial hypotension. These two distinct conditions are both associated with dysregulation of the autonomic nervous system and other risk factors; they tend to occur in older people who have hypertension, but do not necessarily occur together (O'Mara & Lyons, 2002). Researchers are currently trying to identify the relationships among these three types of blood pressure dysregulation.

Orthostatic hypotension (also called *postural hypotension*) is defined as a reduction in systolic blood pressure and diastolic blood pressure of at least 20 mm Hg or 10 mm Hg, respectively, that occurs within 1 to 3 minutes of standing after being recumbent for at least 5 minutes. Orthostatic hypotension occurs in about 20% of all adults older than 65 years of age and in more than 50% of older adults in nursing homes (Mukai & Lipsitz, 2002). In older adults, prevalence of orthostatic hypotension is lowest during the evening, and diastolic orthostatic hypotension is more common than systolic (Weiss et al., 2002). Orthostatic hypotension can occur in healthy older adults as a result of age-related changes but is more likely to occur in older adults who have additional risk factors (as discussed earlier).

Although some people with orthostatic hypotension have no symptoms, most experience such symptoms as weakness, headaches, dizziness, faintness, vertigo, lightheadedness, blurred vision, abnormal sweating, cognitive impairment, and urinary incontinence. Although orthostatic hypotension might seem to be relatively harmless, it can affect the safety and

quality of life of older adults and lead to serious negative functional consequences. For example, it can contribute to difficulty walking and maintaining balance and increase the risk for falls and fractures, particularly in the presence of additional risk factors, such as impaired vision and environmental barriers. In addition, people with orthostatic hypotension are at increased risk for strokes, coronary events, and transient ischemic attacks (Weiss et al., 2002).

Postprandial hypotension, a blood pressure reduction of 20 mm Hg within 75 minutes of eating a meal (particularly breakfast), occurs in 20% to 40% of healthy older adults, 36% of nursing home residents, and 82% of older adults with parkinsonism (Mehagnoul-Schipper et al., 2001; O'Mara & Lyons, 2002; Puisieux et al., 2000). Physiologic changes that are likely to cause postprandial hypotension include impaired baroreflex mechanisms, quicker rate of gastric emptying, the release of vasoactive gastrointestinal hormones, and impaired autonomic regulation of gastrointestinal perfusion. It is likely that postprandial hypotension is due to the combined effect of age-related changes, especially in autonomic cardiovascular control, and additional adverse effects of concomitant pathologic processes (Oberman et al., 2000). Postprandial hypotension is associated with the consumption of carbohydrates, particularly glucose, and is more likely to occur after a consumption of warmer foods that are high in carbohydrate content (Maurer et al., 2000; Vloet et al., 2001). Postprandial hypotension is now considered an important geriatric condition because it contributes to falls, syncope, hip fractures, myocardial infarction, stroke-related dizziness, and frailty and malnutrition (Morley, 2001; Puisieux et al., 2000). Geriatricians recommend that any older adult who falls, has syncope, or loses consciousness be evaluated for postprandial hypotension (O'Mara & Lyons, 2002).

The Impact of Cardiovascular Changes on the Circulation

Functional consequences also can affect circulation to the brain and the lower extremities. For example, age-related changes in cardiovascular and baroreflex mechanisms can reduce cerebral blood flow to some extent in healthy older adults and to a greater extent in older adults who have diabetes, hypertension, dyslipidemia, and heart disease. In addition, increased tortuosity and dilation of the veins, along with decreased efficiency of the valves, lead to impaired venous return from the lower extremities. Consequently, the older adult may have stasis edema of the feet and ankles and an increased susceptibility to certain diseases or conditions, such as venous stasis ulcers.

Figure 16-1 summarizes the age-related changes, risk factors, and negative functional consequences that affect cardiovascular performance.

➤ Mr. C. is a 64-year-old African American who frequently comes to your Senior Wellness Clinic for a blood pressure check. He has been taking hydrochlorothiazide, 25 mg, and verapamil, 120 mg, every morning, and his blood pressures range between 126/80 mm Hg and 130/84 mm Hg. Mr. C. sees his primary care provider once a year and obtains additional health care through community resources, such as health fairs. Mr. C.'s

86-year-old mother recently died from a cerebrovascular accident, and his father died in his early 50s from a heart attack. Mr. C. has had hypertension since the age of 24 years, and both of his daughters have high blood pressure as well. Neither Mr. C. nor anyone in the household smokes tobacco. He gets very little exercise and weighs 210 pounds, about 30 pounds more than his ideal weight. He reports that he "gets winded easily" when walking up or down a flight of steps or when he has to walk "a long distance" (which he defines as the distance across the parking lot to the senior center). He attributes this to "getting old."

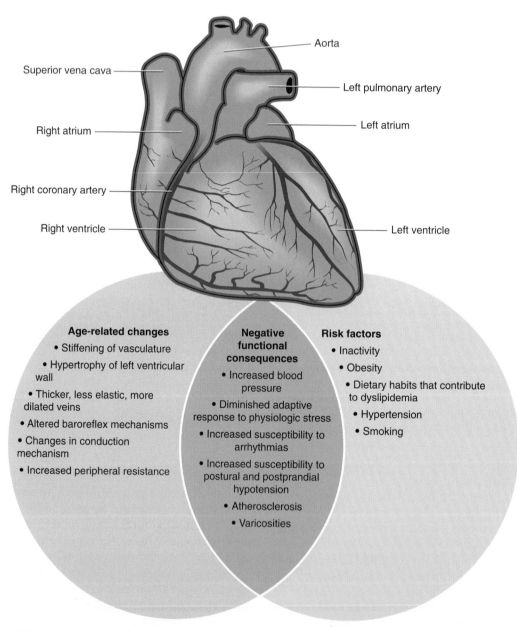

FIGURE 16-1 Age-related changes and risk factors intersect to negatively affect cardiovascular function in older adults.

THINKING POINTS

➤ What age-related changes in cardiovascular function is Mr. C. likely to be experiencing?

➤ What risk factors are likely to be contributing to Mr. C.'s experience of "getting winded?"

➤ What risk factors does Mr. C. have for cardiovascular disease?

➤ What further information would you want to obtain for assessing his risk for cardiovascular disease?

NURSING ASSESSMENT OF CARDIOVASCULAR FUNCTION

For adults of any age, identification of risks for cardiovascular disease is one of the most important aspects of the nursing assessment of cardiovascular function. It is especially important to identify the risk factors that can be addressed through interventions. Assessment of physical aspects of cardiovascular function (e.g., heart rate, blood pressure) is similar in older and younger adults, but nurses need to include an assessment of postural hypotension because this commonly occurs in older adults. Another difference that needs to be considered when assessing cardiovascular function in older adults is that they are more likely than younger adults to have asymptomatic myocardial ischemia or atypical manifestations of a heart attack. The following sections discuss the facets of assessment specific to older adults; these can be used in conjunction with the usual methods of assessing cardiovascular function in any adult.

Assessing Heart Rate, Rhythm, and Sounds

The normal range for heart rate in older adults is the same as or slightly lower than that for all adults, but heart sounds may differ in older and younger adults. The following changes may be observed on auscultation in healthy older adults, but they are insignificant in the absence of symptoms or other abnormal findings: (1) a fourth heart sound may be heard; (2) short systolic ejection murmurs are commonly heard; (3) heart borders may be difficult to percuss; and (4) heart sounds may be diminished or distant. Electrocardiographic changes observed in healthy older adults include arrhythmias, left axis deviation, bundle branch blocks, ST-T wave changes, and prolongation of the P-R interval. Other than these variations, physical assessment criteria are the same for younger and older adults.

Assessment of peripheral pulses does not differ in older and younger adults because peripheral circulation is not significantly affected by age-related changes. However, venous stasis and other disease-related conditions occur more commonly in older adults; thus, nurses take this into consideration when assessing peripheral circulation.

If a murmur, arrhythmia, or any other unusual finding is detected, it is important to determine whether it reflects a new development, a preexisting but previously unidentified condition, or a preexisting condition that has already been evaluated. The nurse asks questions to determine the person's awareness of such abnormal findings. Any of the following terms might be used by older adults to describe arrhythmias: fluttering, palpitations, skipped beats, extra beats, or flip-flops. It is advisable to ask the older person about a history of arrhythmias before auscultation because asking immediately after auscultation could cause undue concern. Arrhythmias may be caused by cardiac diseases, electrolyte imbalances, physiologic disturbances, or adverse medication effects; alternatively, they may be harmless manifestations of age-related changes. Likewise, murmurs may be caused by age- or disease-related conditions. Therefore, when murmurs or arrhythmias are detected, their significance is assessed in relation to the person's history, as well as in relation to the potential underlying causes. It is also important to find out the date of the person's last electrocardiogram because this may provide baseline information regarding the duration of asymptomatic or unrecognized changes.

Assessing Blood Pressure

Although only a few nurses have primary responsibility for medical management of blood pressure, all nurses are responsible for accurate assessment of blood pressure and for decisions regarding the implications of these findings. Thus, all nurses need to be familiar with the most current guidelines for detection of hypertension so that health promotion efforts can be directed toward interventions. Despite mounting medical evidence that the identification and management of hypertension has important health benefits for people of any age—including the "oldest old"—only about one fourth of community-living older adults with hypertension have adequately controlled blood pressure (Hajjar et al., 2002). Nurses are in a key position to detect hypertension, provide health education, and refer older adults for further medical evaluation and treatment.

It may be more difficult to assess blood pressure accurately in older adults because their blood pressure is more variable and has an increased tendency to fluctuate in response to postural changes and other factors. Another aspect of blood pressure assessment that may differ in older adults is the common occurrence of "pseudohypertension," which is the phenomenon of elevated systolic blood pressure readings that result from the inability of the external cuff to compress the arteries in older people with arteriosclerosis. This phenomenon explains the finding of extremely elevated systolic blood pressure readings in people without any evidence of end-organ damage and with normal diastolic blood pressure readings. Another assessment consideration is the common occurrence of "white coat hypertension" (also called "isolated office hypertension"), which is the phenomenon of blood pressure readings being high during office visits to a primary care practitioner but normal when self-assessed at home.

The practice of self-measurement of blood pressure, called *home blood pressure monitoring*, has become increasingly more accepted, and even encouraged, by primary care practitioners. Because older adults and people with hypertension are particularly susceptible to white coat hypertension, self-measurement of blood pressure in the home environment can provide additional assessment information that is important in management of hypertension (Frazier, 2002; Yarows et al., 2000). In addition, self-monitoring provides important assessment information for older adults whose blood pressure fluctuates significantly.

Assessment of blood pressure in older adults is aimed at detecting not only hypertension but also hypotension, a condition that often is overlooked. Because an older adult may have hypertension, orthostatic hypotension, and postprandial hypotension, nurses need to assess for all three of these conditions, particularly in frail older adults. Display 16-2 summarizes guidelines for accurate assessment of blood pressure in older adults, including the technique for assessing for orthostatic and postprandial hypotension.

Assessing Risks for Cardiovascular Disease

The assessment of risks for cardiovascular disease, with emphasis on identification of modifiable risk factors, provides a basis for health promotion interventions directed toward preventing negative functional consequences. Hypertension, dyslipidemia, and smoking cessation (discussed in Chapter 17) have been identified as the most important remediable factors for older adults who have these risks. Obesity, physical inactivity, and dietary habits are important lifestyle factors that can significantly affect the risk for cardiovascular disease. Many easy-to-use assessment tools are available to identify risk factors and provide a basis for health education; Figure 16-2 is an example of one. Display 16-3 provides guidelines for nursing assessment of risks.

Identifying Hypertension as a Risk

In the United States, about 60% of people between the ages of 65 and 75 years and 70% of those aged 75 years and older have hypertension, defined as blood pressure greater than 140/90 mm Hg (Aronow, 2002b). The Joint National Committee on Detection, Evaluation, and Treatment of High Blood Pressure (JNC) has published seven reports, most recently in 2003. Because each of these reports revised the classification of hypertension, a blood pressure measurement that was considered "normal" in 1980 could be deemed pathologic in later reports. Similarly, until recently, parameters for judging the significance of elevated blood pressure were determined at least in part by age. For example, "100 plus your age" was the "normal upper range" for systolic blood pressure, so an 84-year-old person could have a systolic blood pressure of 184 and not be diagnosed as having hypertension. This perspective has gradually changed, so that the same standards for determining hypertension apply to adults of all ages.

The 2003 JNC report establishes the cutoff for normal blood pressure as less than 120 mm Hg systolic and 80 mm Hg diastolic; it also establishes a new category of *prehypertension* to identify people who are at risk for developing hypertension. To clarify various terms, Table 16-1 defines some of the criteria used regarding blood pressure.

Prevalence of hypertension increases with age and is greater in women than men and in African Americans than in whites or Mexican Americans (Laucka & Trotter, 2001).

Identifying Dyslipidemia as a Risk

Public awareness of the importance of addressing dyslipidemia as a risk factor for cardiovascular disease has been gradually increasing since the early 1980s when saturated fat and polyunsaturated fat became household words. By the late 1980s, mass screening programs for serum cholesterol levels were as popular as the mass blood pressure screenings of the 1970s. During the 1990s, there was much debate about the value of cholesterol screening for older adults and little consensus about treatment of dyslipidemia in older adults, particularly those older than 75 years of age. During the early 2000s, observational studies supported the value of identifying and treating dyslipidemia in older adults, even in nonagenarians (Aronow, 2002a). In 2001, the National Cholesterol Education Program published Adult Treatment Panel (ATP) III, updated guidelines for identifying and treating dyslipidemia, with particular emphasis on people aged 50 years and older (Expert Panel, 2001). This report emphasizes the importance of considering

DISPLAY 16-2
Guidelines for Assessing Blood Pressure

For Accurate Blood Pressure Measurement in Older Adults

- Recognize that blood pressure readings are likely to vary, particularly in response to external factors (e.g., meals or postural changes).
- Blood pressure measurements may be lower in hot weather or at very warm indoor temperatures.
- Blood pressure measurements are likely to have a diurnal variation, with lowest levels during the night and highest levels after rising in the morning.
- The person should wait 1 hour after eating to have his or her blood pressure checked.
- The person should not have ingested caffeine or smoked a cigarette within ½ hour before having his or her blood pressure checked.
- The person should be seated and resting for 5 minutes before having his or her blood pressure checked.

For Assessment of Orthostatic Hypotension

- Obtain initial blood pressure reading after the person has been in a sitting or lying position for at least 5 minutes.
- Obtain second blood pressure reading after the person has been standing for 1 to 3 minutes.

For Assessment of Postprandial Hypotension

- Obtain initial blood pressure reading before a meal.
- Obtain second and third reading at 15-minute intervals after the meal is completed.

Method of Assessing Blood Pressure

- The person should be seated with arm bared and feet flat on the floor.
- Support the person's arm as near to the heart level as possible.
- Ask the person to refrain from talking while you check his or her blood pressure.
- Use a sphygmomanometer that has been checked for accuracy.
- Use an appropriate-sized cuff (i.e., the length of the cuff bladder should be at least 80% of the circumference of the arm, and the width should be 20% wider than the diameter of the arm).

- Record the cuff size that is used. (Cuffs that are too small will yield falsely high readings, whereas cuffs that are too large will yield falsely low readings.)
- Fit the deflated cuff firmly around the upper arm, with the center of the cuff bladder over the brachial artery and the bottom of the cuff about 1 to 1½ inches above the bend of the arm.
- Inflate the cuff to 20 or 30 mm Hg above the palpated systolic blood pressure.
- Deflate the cuff at a rate of 2 to 3 mm Hg per second.
- Measure systolic blood pressure at the first sound and diastolic blood pressure at the onset of silence.
- If auscultatory gaps are heard, estimate the systolic blood pressure by applying the cuff, palpating the radial pulse, and inflating the cuff until the pulse is no longer felt.
- Record the magnitude and range of the gap (e.g., 184/82 mm Hg, auscultatory gap 176–148).
- If a very low diastolic blood pressure is heard, record the onset of Korotkoff phases IV and V (e.g., 138/72/10 mm Hg). Also, be sure not to press too hard on the stethoscope.
- Measure blood pressure in both arms the first time it is assessed, then measure it in the arm with the higher reading on subsequent determinations.
- If sounds are difficult to auscultate, support the person's arm above his or her head for 30 seconds. Then inflate the cuff, have the person lower the arm, and measure the blood pressure.
- If it is necessary to recheck the blood pressure in the same arm, deflate the cuff fully before reinflating it and wait at least 2 minutes before taking another measurement.

Normal Findings

- Normal blood pressure is less than 120 mm Hg systolic blood pressure, and less than 80 mm Hg diastolic blood pressure.
- The normal difference between lying/sitting and standing systolic blood pressure is 20 mm Hg or less after standing for 1 minute.
- The normal difference between lying/sitting and standing diastolic blood pressure is 10 mm Hg or less after standing for 1 minute.

---

all of the following risk factors in assessing the additional risk posed by dyslipidemia:

- Cardiovascular disease (e.g., angina, angioplasty, bypass surgery)
- Cerebrovascular conditions (e.g., ischemic stroke, transient ischemic attacks, symptomatic carotid artery stenosis)
- Peripheral vascular conditions
- Diabetes mellitus

The report categorizes three levels of risk and recommends acceptable lipoprotein ranges according to the person's numbers of risk factors. For example, treatment is recommended for people with cardiovascular disease if their LDL cholesterol is higher than 130 mg/dL, but it is recommended for healthy people without any risk factors only if their LDL cholesterol is higher than 160 mg/dL (Expert Panel, 2001). The Expert Panel recommends that at least once every

What Is Your Risk of Developing Heart Disease or Having a Heart Attack?

In general, the higher your LDL level and the more risk factors you have (other than LDL), the greater your chances of developing heart disease or having a heart attack. Some people are at high risk for a heart attack because they already have heart disease. Other people are at high risk for developing heart disease because they have diabetes (which is a strong risk factor) or a combination of risk factors for heart disease. Follow these steps to find out your risk for developing heart disease.

Step 1 **Check the table below to see how many of the listed risk factors you have; these are the risk factors that affect your LDL goal.**

Major Risk Factors That Affect Your LDL Goal

- ○ Cigarette smoking
- ○ High Blood Pressure (140/90 mmHg or higher or on blood pressure medication)
- ○ Low HDL cholesterol (less than 40 mg/dL)*
- ○ Family history of early heart disease (heart disease in father or brother before age 55; heart disease in mother or sister before age 65)
- ○ Age (men 45 years or older; women 55 years or older)

If your HDL cholesterol is 60 mg/dL or higher, subtract 1 from your total count.

Even though obesity and physical inactivity are not counted in this list, they are conditions that need to be corrected.

Step 2 **How many major risk factors do you have? If you have 2 or more risk factors in the table above, use the risk scoring tables on the opposite page (which include your cholesterol levels) to find your risk score. Risk score refers to the chance of having a heart attack in the next 10 years, given as a percentage.**
(Use the Framingham Point Scores on the opposite page.)

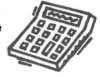

My 10-year risk score is _____%.

Step 3 **Use your medical history, number of risk factors, and risk score to find your risk of developing heart disease or having a heart attack in the table below.**

If You Have	You Are in Category
Heart disease, diabetes, or risk score more than 20%*	I. Highest Risk
2 or more risk factors and risk score 10-20%	II. Next Highest Risk
2 or more risk factors and risk score less than 10%	III. Moderate Risk
0 or 1 risk factor	IV. Low-to-Moderate Risk

Means that more than 20 of 100 people in this category will have a heart attack within 10 years.

My risk category is _____.

FIGURE 16-2 Example of an easy-to-use assessment tool for identifying risk factors for cardiovascular disease. (From U.S. Department of Health and Human Services, Public Health Service, National Institutes of Health, National Heart, Lung, and Blood Institute. [May 2001]. *What is your risk of developing heart disease or having a heart attack?* [NIH Publication No. 01-3290]. Rockville, MD: Author.)

Estimate of 10-Year Risk for Men

(Framingham Point Scores)

Age	Points
20-34	-9
35-39	-4
40-44	0
45-49	3
50-54	6
55-59	8
60-64	10
65-69	11
70-74	12
75-79	13

Total Cholesterol	Points				
	Age 20-39	Age 40-49	Age 50-59	Age 60-69	Age 70-79
<160	0	0	0	0	0
160-199	4	3	2	1	0
200-239	7	5	3	1	0
240-279	9	6	4	2	1
≥280	11	8	5	3	1

	Points				
	Age 20-39	Age 40-49	Age 50-59	Age 60-69	Age 70-79
Nonsmoker	0	0	0	0	0
Smoker	8	5	3	1	1

HDL (mg/dL)	Points
≥60	-1
50-59	0
40-49	1
<40	2

Systolic BP (mmHg)	If Untreated	If Treated
<120	0	0
120-129	0	1
130-139	1	2
140-159	1	2
≥160	2	3

Point Total	10-Year Risk %
<0	< 1
0	1
1	1
2	1
3	1
4	1
5	2
6	2
7	3
8	4
9	5
10	6
11	8
12	10
13	12
14	16
15	20
16	25
≥17	≥ 30

10-Year risk _____%

Estimate of 10-Year Risk for Women

(Framingham Point Scores)

Age	Points
20-34	-7
35-39	-3
40-44	0
45-49	3
50-54	6
55-59	8
60-64	10
65-69	12
70-74	14
75-79	16

Total Cholesterol	Points				
	Age 20-39	Age 40-49	Age 50-59	Age 60-69	Age 70-79
<160	0	0	0	0	0
160-199	4	3	2	1	1
200-239	8	6	4	2	1
240-279	11	8	5	3	2
≥280	13	10	7	4	2

	Points				
	Age 20-39	Age 40-49	Age 50-59	Age 60-69	Age 70-79
Nonsmoker	0	0	0	0	0
Smoker	9	7	4	2	1

HDL (mg/dL)	Points
≥60	-1
50-59	0
40-49	1
<40	2

Systolic BP (mmHg)	If Untreated	If Treated
<120	0	0
120-129	1	3
130-139	2	4
140-159	3	5
≥160	4	6

Point Total	10-Year Risk %
< 9	< 1
9	1
10	1
11	1
12	1
13	2
14	2
15	3
16	4
17	5
18	6
19	8
20	11
21	14
22	17
23	22
24	27
≥25	≥ 30

10-Year risk _____%

U.S. DEPARTMENT OF HEALTH AND HUMAN SERVICES
Public Health Service
National Institutes of Health
National Heart, Lung, and Blood Institute

NIH Publication No. 01-3290
May 2001

Questions to Identify Risk Factors for Cardiovascular Disease

- Do you have, or have you ever had, any heart or circulation problems (e.g., stroke, angina, heart attack, blood clots, or peripheral vascular disease)? *If yes, ask the usual questions about type of therapy, and so on.*

- When was the last time you had an electrocardiogram done?

- What is your normal blood pressure? Have you ever been told that you have high blood pressure, or borderline high blood pressure?

- Do you take, or have you ever taken, medications for heart problems or blood pressure? *If yes, ask the usual questions about type, dose, duration of therapy, and the like.*

- Do you smoke, or have you ever smoked? *If yes, ask additional questions, such as those appropriate for assessing respiratory function, Chapter 17.*

- Do you know what your cholesterol levels are? When was the last time you had your cholesterol checked?

- Do you have diabetes? When was the last time you had your blood sugar (glucose) level checked?

- What is your usual pattern of exercise?

Additional Considerations Regarding Risk Factors

- Compare the person's ideal weight to his or her present weight.

- Determine usual dietary habits, paying particular attention to the person's intake of sodium, fiber, and types of fat. (This information is usually obtained during the nutritional assessment.)

5 years, healthy older adults have their triglyceride, total cholesterol, HDL cholesterol, and LDL cholesterol levels checked. In contrast to previous reports that determined risk based partially on the ratio between LDL and HDL cholesterol, the updated report recognizes that HDL cholesterol should be maintained

Adult BP	Systolic (mm Hg)		Diastolic (mm Hg)
Normal	<120	and	<80
Prehypertension	120–139	or	80–89
Hypertension, Stage I	140–159	or	90–99
Hypertension, Stage II	≥160	or	≥100

TABLE 16-1 • Criteria for Normal Blood Pressure and Stages of Hypertension

(JNC. [2003]. The seventh report of the Joint National Committee on Prevention, Detection, Evaluation, and Treatment of High Blood Pressure. *Journal of the American Medical Association, 289*, 2560–2577.)

above 60 mg/dL and that LDL cholesterol should be low regardless of any ratio (Eidelman et al., 2002).

African Americans and Mexican Americans are less likely than whites to be screened for dyslipidemia (Nelson et al., 2002).

Assessing Signs and Symptoms of Heart Disease

Assessment of older adults for cardiac disease is complicated by the fact that the primary symptom often differs from the expected manifestations of cardiac disease. Congestive heart failure, for example, often begins very subtly, and the early manifestations may be mental changes secondary to the physiologic stress. Thus, older adults are likely to be in more advanced stages of heart failure before an accurate diagnosis is made. Likewise, older people with angina and acute myocardial infarctions are likely to have subtle and unusual manifestations, rather than the classic symptom of chest pain. Researchers have found that between 25% and 68% of all myocardial infarctions are not clinically recognized as such, and the incidence of these unrecognized episodes is higher in women and older adults (Aronow, 2003; Sheifer et al., 2001). In comparison with younger adults, older adults are more likely to have dyspnea or neurologic symptoms, rather than chest discomfort, as a primary sign of myocardial ischemia or acute myocardial infarction (Aronow, 2003; Williams et al., 2002). Canto and colleagues (2002) found that only 48% of people with unstable angina have typical manifestations, such as chest pain, and that factors associated with atypical manifestations included older age and a history of dementia. In this study, the predominant presenting atypical symptoms included nausea; shortness of breath; sharp, burning, or pleuritic chest discomfort; and pain or discomfort localized to an area of the upper body. Rather than complaining of chest pain, older adults are likely to have vague symptoms, such as fatigue, dyspnea, syncope, indigestion, and mental or behavioral changes. In addition, older adults who have mobility impairments or other functional limitations may not be active enough to experience exertion-related symptoms. Therefore, the absence of chest pain in older adults is not a good indicator of the absence of coronary artery disease.

Myocardial infarction is more likely to be unrecognized in African Americans (23%) than in whites (19%) (Boland et al., 2002).

When manifestations of myocardial ischemia or other cardiac disturbances are subtle or differ from what is expected, they may be attributed to a noncardiac cause, such as indigestion or arthritis in the shoulder. Therefore, any complaints about digestion, respiration, or pain or discomfort in the arms, shoulders, or upper trunk can be indicators of cardiac disease. Assessment of these complaints is complicated by the fact that older adults often have more than one underlying condition that could be responsible for these symptoms. It is not unusual, for example, for an older person to have an esophageal reflux disorder as well as a history of ischemic heart disease. Therefore, in addition to asking questions specifically related to cardiovascular function, the nurse must consider assessment information regarding other functional areas in relation to cardiovascular function. In addition, a baseline electrocardiogram is helpful in establishing the possibility of silent or atypical myocardial ischemia. Display 16-4 summarizes the guidelines for assessing cardiovascular function and detecting cardiovascular disease in older adults. This guide emphasizes the assessment components that are unique to older adults, and includes additional assessment components that apply to adults in general.

NURSING DIAGNOSIS

If the nursing assessment identifies risks for impaired cardiovascular function in a healthy older adult, a nursing diagnosis of Ineffective Health Maintenance may be applicable. This is defined as "the state in which an individual or group experiences or is at risk of experiencing a disruption in health because of an unhealthy lifestyle or lack of knowledge to manage a condition" (Carpenito, 2002, p. 442). Related factors common in older adults include lack of regular exercise; cultural influences on patterns of food intake and preparation; and insufficient knowledge about low-sodium diets, dietary measures to control cholesterol levels, and the effects of tobacco use.

For older adults with impaired cardiovascular function, applicable nursing diagnoses may include Activity Intolerance, Decreased Cardiac Output, and Ineffective Tissue Perfusion (Cardiopulmonary). The nursing diagnosis of Risk for Injury may be appropriate for older adults with orthostatic or postprandial hypotension, particularly in the presence of additional risk factors for falls and fractures (e.g., osteoporosis, neurologic disorders, and medication side effects).

OUTCOMES

A nursing-sensitive outcome for Altered Health Maintenance for someone with risks for cardiovascular disease would be Health Orientation, as indicated

DISPLAY 16-4
Guidelines for Assessing Cardiovascular Function in Older Adults

Questions to Assess for the Presence of Cardiovascular Disease

- Do you ever have chest pain or tightness in your chest? *If yes, ask the usual questions to explore the type, onset, duration, and other characteristics.*
- Do you ever have difficulty breathing? *If yes, ask the usual questions regarding onset and other characteristics.*
- Do you ever feel lightheaded or dizzy? *If yes, ask about specific circumstances, medical evaluation, and methods of dealing with symptoms and ensuring safety.*
- Do you ever feel like your heart is racing, is irregular, or has extra or skipped beats? *If yes, ask about any prior medical evaluation.*
- Have you ever been told that you had a heart murmur? *If yes, ask about any prior medical evaluation.*

Information Obtained During Other Portions of an Assessment That May Be Useful in Assessing Cardiovascular Function

- Do you tire easily or feel that you need more rest than is ordinarily required?
- Do you have any problems with indigestion?
- Do your feet or ankles ever get swollen?
- Do you wake up at night because of difficulty breathing or because of any other discomfort? Have you made any adjustments in your sleeping habits because of difficulty breathing (e.g., do you use more than one pillow or sleep in a chair)?
- Do you have any pain in your upper back or shoulders?

Interview Questions to Assess for Postural Hypotension

- Do you ever feel lightheaded or dizzy, especially when you get up in the morning or after you've been lying down?
- *If yes:* Is this feeling accompanied by any additional symptoms, such as sweating, nausea, or confusion?
- *If yes:* Do any of the risks listed in Display 16-1 apply to you? *If yes, ask about any prior medical evaluation.*

by a focus on wellness, a focus on disease prevention and management, or the perception that health is a high priority in making lifestyle choices (Glick & Ressler, 2001). Additional nursing-sensitive outcomes for health promotion related to cardiovascular function are Knowledge: Health Behaviors (as indicated by description of healthy nutritional practices and benefits of activity and exercise) and Health Promoting Behavior (as indicated by correct performance of health habits and monitoring of personal behavior for risks) (Glick & Ressler, 2001). In particular, outcomes to reduce risks for cardiovascular disease in older adults focus on blood pressure control, healthy serum cholesterol levels, maintenance of ideal body weight, incorporation of adequate physical exercise into daily routine, and smoking cessation, if applicable. Additional outcomes include maintenance of blood pressure within the normal range and prevention of negative consequences of hypotension (e.g., falls and fractures) when hypotension cannot be prevented.

NURSING INTERVENTIONS TO PROMOTE HEALTHY CARDIOVASCULAR FUNCTION

Nursing interventions to promote healthy cardiovascular function focus on primary and secondary prevention of cardiovascular disease. These nursing interventions address *Healthy People 2010's* goal of improving cardiovascular health and quality of life through the prevention, detection, and treatment of risk factors; early identification and treatment of heart attacks and strokes; and prevention of recurrent cardiovascular events" (USDHHS, 2000, p. 12–15). For primary or secondary prevention of cardiovascular disease in older adults with risk factors, highest priority is given to interventions for smoking, hypertension, and dyslipidemia (i.e., abnormal serum lipoprotein levels). Medications and other medical interventions are often used to reduce risk factors, but health promotion education is a nursing intervention that is appropriate in almost all situations, either alone or in conjunction with medical and other interventions. Nursing interventions can effectively prevent or manage orthostatic or postprandial hypotension, and they can also be used to prevent functional consequences, such as falls and fractures. Preventive measures are particularly important in young-old adults but should not be overlooked even in nonagenarians.

Addressing Risks Through Nutrition and Lifestyle Interventions

Nutrition interventions can be effective in reducing the risk for cardiovascular disease in all adults and are particularly important for prevention or management of hypertension and dyslipidemia (discussed in more detail in other sections on Interventions). Recently, there has been increasing recognition of the importance of fiber, folic acid, and vitamins B_6, B_{12}, C, D, and E in prevention of cardiovascular disease. For example, consuming more than eight servings a day of fruits and vegetables, particularly green leafy vegetables and vitamin C–rich fruits and vegetables, may diminish the risk for cardiovascular disease (Joshipura et al., 2001). Other nutrients that may be protective against cardiovascular disease include calcium, potassium, magnesium, and fiber and soy protein (e.g., legumes) (Bazzano et al., 2001). Studies also suggest that light-to-moderate consumption of alcohol (i.e., one to two drinks daily) and daily intake of green or black tea may have beneficial cardiovascular effects (Hodgson et al., 2001; DiCastelnuovo, 2002; Hirano et al., 2002). Nutritional interventions also are important in helping older adults to achieve and maintain their ideal body weight; nurses can encourage any person who is greater than or equal to 20% of the ideal body weight or has a body mass index (BMI) greater than or equal to 27 to lose weight.

Lifestyle interventions that are effective for prevention of cardiovascular disease in healthy older adults include remaining physically active, refraining from smoking, and maintaining ideal body weight (Figure 16-3). In recent years, there is increasing evidence supporting the importance of physical exercise as an intervention for improving cardiovascular performance in healthy older adults and in those with cardiovascular disease (Burke et al., 2001). Specific cardiovascular benefits include lower body fat ratios, lower blood pressure measurements, lower resting heart rates, improved physical working capacity, and lower rates of myocardial infarction. Fahlman and

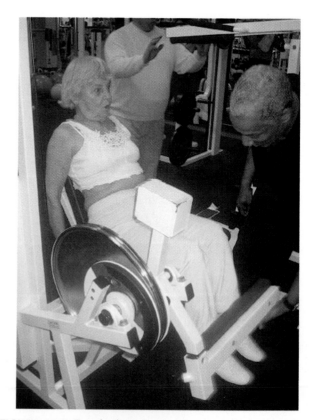

FIGURE 16-3 Exercise is an important preventive intervention. *Photo courtesy of Monte Unetic.*

colleagues (2002) found that a regular program of resistance or endurance exercise significantly improved the serum lipoprotein profiles of healthy women between the ages of 70 and 87 years. Similarly, researchers have concluded that aerobic exercise is an important component of lifestyle modification for primary and secondary prevention of hypertension (Whelton et al., 2002). Additional positive effects of exercise in other functional areas are noted throughout this text, and this information can be used in educating older adults about the many positive functional consequences of regular physical exercise.

Smoking is a major risk factor for cardiovascular disease, and quitting smoking has cumulative beneficial effects for people at any age. Williams and colleagues (2002) found that the benefits of smoking cessation as a secondary prevention intervention begin during the first year following myocardial infarction and are as effective in people older than 70 years of age as they are in younger people. People who cease smoking for 3 years after a myocardial infarction decrease their risk for recurrent coronary events to the equivalent of a nonsmoker's risk (Rea et al., 2002). An important nursing responsibility is to provide health education regarding smoking cessation, as discussed in Chapter 17.

Addressing Risks Through Medication Interventions

In recent years, some attention has focused on the use of hormonal therapy for menopausal women and low-dose aspirin therapy as measures for preventing cardiovascular disease. In the 1990s, hormonal therapy was recommended for menopausal women as primary and secondary prevention of cardiovascular disease, but this recommendation was reversed in 2002 because of longitudinal and large-scale investigations showing that risks outweighed the benefits as a preventive intervention (U.S. Preventive Services Task Force, 2002). The use of low-dose aspirin to reduce the risk for coronary events also has been somewhat controversial because aspirin therapy, even when administered in low doses, is accompanied by increased risks for gastrointestinal bleeding and hemorrhagic stroke. In 2002, the U.S. Preventive Task Force and the American Heart Association concluded that the balance of benefit and harm is most favorable in people with a high risk for, or a history of, cardiovascular disease and recommended doses of 75 to 160 mg aspirin daily for people who are at high risk and can tolerate this dose (Pearson et al., 2002). Display 16-5 summarizes health education interventions regarding risk for cardiovascular disease in older adults.

DISPLAY 16-5

Health Promotion Activities to Reduce the Risks for Cardiovascular Disease

Detection of Risks
- Have blood pressure checked annually.
- If the total serum cholesterol level is less than 200 mg/dL, have it rechecked every 5 years. If the total serum cholesterol level is between 200 and 239 mg/dL, follow dietary measures to reduce it and have it rechecked annually. If the total serum cholesterol level is 240 mg/dL or more, obtain a further medical evaluation.

Reduction of Risks
- Give high priority to smoking cessation, if you smoke.
- Avoid passive smoking (i.e., inhaling smoke from other people's cigarettes).
- Maintain weight at a level less than 110% of ideal weight.
- Exercise daily, and engage in aerobic exercise (i.e., exercise that increases the pulse rate) several times weekly for 30 to 45 minutes each time.
- Avoid foods that are high in sodium, and follow dietary measures to reduce serum cholesterol levels.
- Discuss with your primary care provider the use of low-dose aspirin therapy as a preventive measure, particularly if there is any history of coronary artery disease or cerebrovascular events.

Preventing and Managing Hypertension

Although relatively few nurses prescribe medications for hypertension, all nurses have a great deal of decision-making responsibility regarding the management of hypertension because they are responsible for taking appropriate steps when they assess blood pressure. Thus, nurses need to understand current guidelines and recommendations for management of hypertension so that they can make appropriate decisions about discussing blood pressure findings with primary care providers. Nurses also are responsible for evaluating the response of an older person to prescribed medications and for educating older adults and their caregivers about interventions for hypertension.

The stepped-care approach to management of hypertension was introduced in the first JNC report, published in the 1970s, and has been consistently recommended in subsequent reports. This approach recommends that lifestyle modifications might be tried initially, followed by pharmacologic interventions to achieve ideal blood pressure. Weight reduction and regular physical exercise can be effective first-line interventions for hypertension in people who are overweight or sedentary (Hinderliter et al., 2002). Because reduced sodium intake can effectively reduce blood pressure, especially in older adults, maintaining a daily sodium intake of less than 2.4 g is a nutrition intervention that is widely recommended (JNC, 2003). The National Institutes of Health have encouraged people to follow a nutrition plan called the "Dietary Approaches to Stop Hypertension" (DASH), health promotion materials for which are available at www.nih.gov. Although there is much support worldwide for the implementation of public health policies aimed at reducing sodium intake in most populations, the U.S. Department of Agriculture's Dietary Guidelines for Americans allow for more than 10 times the daily requirement of sodium intake (Labarthe & Ayala, 2002).

Many types of medications are used for treating hypertension, and selection of the best medication is based on a consideration of variables such as therapeutic effectiveness and the presence of concomitant conditions. Diuretics, either alone or in combination with β-blockers or angiotensin-converting enzyme (ACE) inhibitors, are commonly used as initial therapy for hypertension, and calcium channel blockers are used as adjunct therapy when needed (Moser, 2001). In recent years, there is increasing emphasis on selecting a medication that is effective not only in treating hypertension but also in addressing coexisting cardiovascular disease. For example, β-blockers are indicated for people with hypertension and a history of myocardial infarction and ACE inhibitors are recommended for treatment of hypertension in people with diabetes or heart failure (Kudzma, 2001). Another consideration is the potential for preventing cardiovascular events. Studies indicate that treatment of hypertension with a thiazide diuretic reduces the risk for ischemic stroke (Klungel et al., 2001). In addition, selection of medication is based on consideration of potential adverse effects, which is particularly important for older adults with functional impairments because the degree of risk from adverse effects is at least partially related to the type of functional impairment that exists. For example, if orthostatic hypotension is an adverse effect of a medication, this is potentially more detrimental to a frail but ambulatory 85-year-old woman than to a nonambulatory older adult.

Increasing attention also is focused on the influence of genetic factors and variations of different ethnic and cultural groups in response to drugs. For example, current research is attempting to identify variations in response to antihypertensive agents in whites, Asians, Hispanics, and African Americans (Kudzma, 2001). Sareli and colleagues (2001) found that calcium channel blockers are more effective than thiazides in African Americans for initial treatment of hypertension. Researchers also are addressing questions about age and gender differences in

---

CULTURE BOX 16-1

Cultural Considerations in Medication Management of Hypertension

- African Americans tend to respond best to thiazide diuretics or calcium channel blockers.
- Whites may respond best to β-blockers and angiotensin-converting enzyme (ACE) inhibitors.
- Asian Americans tend to respond best to calcium channel blockers, diuretics, and β-blockers.
- Asian Americans may need lower doses of β-blockers.
- Arab Americans may respond to lower doses of antihypertensive agents.
- Chinese Americans and some other cultural groups are likely to use herbal medicines for hypertension.

---

response to hypertensive medications. For example, women and older people experience greater antihypertensive effects from the extended-release form of the calcium channel blocker verapamil compared with men and younger people (White, 2001). Some cultural aspects of hypertension prevalence and treatment are summarized in Culture Box 16-1. Display 16-6 summarizes guidelines for interventions for hypertension and includes health education information about nutrition and lifestyle interventions.

➤ Mr. C. is now 70 years old, and his blood pressure fluctuates between 130/88 mm Hg and 146/94 mm Hg. He continues to take hydrochlorothiazide, 25 mg, and verapamil, 120 mg, every morning. Mr. C. and his wife live with their daughter and her teenage children. Mr. and Mrs. C. usually do the family grocery shopping, and Mrs. C. and daughter prepare the family meals. A diet history reveals that the family usually eats fried fish or chicken about four times a week and pig's feet or ham hocks for the other main meals. Common side dishes are corn, okra, grits, cornbread, sweet potatoes, black-eyed peas, and fried greens. For cooking, the family uses lard, saltpork, or bacon drippings. Their usual beverage is decaffeinated coffee with sugar and cream. The family generally has cereal and toast for breakfast, but they have bacon and eggs on Saturdays and Sundays. Mr. and Mrs. C. eat their noon meal at the senior center 5 days a week. Mr. C.'s weight is still about 30 pounds over his ideal weight. For the past several years he has participated in the exercise program at the senior center, but he gets little additional exercise and continues to complain of "getting winded" when he walks across the parking lot.

 THINKING POINTS

➤ What additional information would you obtain for further assessment of Mr. C.'s cardiovascular status?

DISPLAY 16-6

Guidelines for Nursing Management of Hypertension

Health Promotion Interventions

The following lifestyle modifications are recommended for all people with hypertension:

- Avoidance of tobacco
- Weight reduction when appropriate (i.e., when the person weighs more than 110% of his or her ideal weight)
- 30 to 45 minutes of exercise, such as brisk walking, at least 5 times weekly
- Limitation of alcohol intake to 1 drink per day (e.g., 2 ounces of 100-proof whiskey, 8 ounces of wine, or 24 ounces of beer)

The following nutritional interventions are recommended for all people with hypertension:

- Intake of no more than 2.4 g sodium daily
- Avoidance of processed foods
- Daily intake of 7 to 8 servings of grains and grain products and 8 to 10 servings of fruits and vegetables

Considerations Regarding the Treatment of Hypertension

- Risks from and definitions of hypertension apply to all age categories (refer to Table 16-1 for criteria).
- A person's blood pressure should be measured at least three times before making any decisions about treatment.

- The safety of antihypertensive agents is improved by carefully selecting the medication, starting with low doses, and changing the medication regimen gradually, in small increments, if necessary.

Treatment Goals

- The goals of hypertensive treatment are to control blood pressure by the least intrusive means and to prevent cardiovascular morbidity and mortality.
- Treatment is directed toward achieving and maintaining a systolic blood pressure of less than 140 mm Hg and a diastolic blood pressure of less than 90 mm Hg ($<$ 130/80 mm Hg in people with diabetes or chronic kidney disease).
- Blood pressure reduction to 130/85 mm Hg is recommended if this can be achieved without compromising cardiovascular function.
- For older adults with isolated systolic hypertension or systolic blood pressure levels of 140 to 160 mm Hg, lifestyle modifications should be the first treatment step.
- The initial goal of therapy for those with a systolic blood pressure of greater than 180 mm Hg is to reduce the systolic blood pressure to less than 160 mm Hg.
- For older adults with systolic blood pressure measurements of between 160 and 179 mm Hg, the initial goal is to reduce the systolic blood pressure by 20 mm Hg. If initial treatment is well tolerated, further reduction of the systolic blood pressure should be considered.

➤ What nutritional and lifestyle interventions would you discuss with Mr. C. regarding his hypertension?

➤ What teaching materials would you use for health education with Mr. C.?

Preventing and Managing Dyslipidemia

Nurses do not usually prescribe medications for treatment of dyslipidemia, but they do frequently have information about serum lipid levels of their patients, and often are responsible for providing health education about prevention and management of dyslipidemia. Thus, they need to be familiar with guidelines, such as the Adult Treatment Panel (ATP) III. This revised report paid particular attention to people aged 50 years and older and encouraged health care providers to consider a number of risk factors for people of any age when evaluating the need for interventions. Thus, goals for lipid profiles vary depending on the number of risk factors. For example, the LDL goal for healthy people with no risk factors is less than 160 mg/dL,

but the LDL goal for someone with multiple risks is less than 100 mg/dL. The Expert Panel (2001) identifies the following conditions as risk factors:

- Cardiovascular disease (e.g., angina, angioplasty, bypass surgery)
- Cerebrovascular conditions (e.g., ischemic stroke, transient ischemic attacks, symptomatic carotid artery stenosis)
- Peripheral vascular conditions
- Diabetes mellitus

As with treatment of hypertension, nutrition and lifestyle interventions are the first-line approach, and medications (e.g., statins) are used as necessary if goals are not achieved with nonpharmacologic interventions. The nutrition and lifestyle interventions that are essential interventions for dyslipidemia include dietary modifications, maintenance of ideal body weight, and incorporation of regular exercise in one's daily routine. Nutrition interventions focus on dietary fat intake, with emphasis on limiting foods containing saturated fats and trans fatty acids and increasing foods that are high in polyunsaturated and monounsaturated fats.

DISPLAY 16-7
Nutritional Interventions for People With High Cholesterol

Dietary Measures to Promote a Healthy Lipid Profile
- Include foods that are high in fiber content in your daily diet (e.g., whole grains).
- Include soy proteins in your daily diet (e.g., tofu, soy milk).
- Eat a minimum of two servings of fatty fish weekly.
- Limit total fat intake to less than 30% of your total daily calorie intake.
- Limit total daily cholesterol intake to between 250 and 350 mg.
- Use nonfat or low-fat dairy desserts.
- Limit consumption of butter or margarine.
- Limit consumption of egg yolks, including those in food, to two or three per week.
- Use egg whites or egg substitutes instead of whole eggs.
- Limit consumption of lean meats to five or fewer 3- to 5-ounce servings per week. Trim fat off meats and the skin off poultry.
- Avoid eating processed meats (e.g., bacon, bologna, sausage, hot dogs).
- Avoid gravies, fried foods, and organ meats.

Guide to Types of Fats

Type of Fat	Sources	Examples	Effect on Lipid Profile
Saturated fatty acids	Animal fats and some vegetable oils (usually solid at room temperatures)	Meat, poultry, butter, lauric and palm oils	Negative: increases LDL and total cholesterol
Trans fatty acids	Vegetable oils that are processed into margarine or shortening	Dairy products, baked goods, snack foods	Negative: increases LDL cholesterol and lowers HDL cholesterol
Monounsaturated fatty acids	Vegetable oils (usually liquid at room temperatures)	Olive, peanut, and canola oils	Positive: decreases LDL
Polyunsaturated fatty acids	Seafood and vegetable oils (soft or liquid at room temperatures)	Corn, sunflower, safflower, canola, and linoleic oils	Positive: decreases LDL
Omega-3 fatty acids	Fatty fish	Tuna, salmon, herring, mackerel	Positive: decreases LDL cholesterol and triglycerides

LDL, low-density lipoprotein; HDL, high-density lipoprotein.

Recent large-scale epidemiologic studies support the intake of foods containing omega-3 fatty acids (e.g., fish, seafood), which are also called *polyunsaturated fatty acids*, and food and oils containing α-linoleic acids (e.g., walnuts, soybeans, flaxseeds, and canola oil) (Harper & Jacobson, 2001; Kris-Etherton et al., 2002). Daily supplementation with 1 g of elemental calcium is another nonpharmacologic intervention that may increase serum HDL cholesterol and reduce serum LDL cholesterol (Reid et al., 2002). Display 16-7 summarizes health education interventions for prevention and management of dyslipidemia in older adults.

> Nutrition and exercise interventions may be particularly effective in American Indian populations (Kudzma, 2001).

Preventing and Managing Orthostatic and Postprandial Hypotension

Interventions aimed at preventing orthostatic and postprandial hypotension can be initiated as health measures for older adults who either have hypotension or have any of the risk factors listed in Display 16-1. For older adults with symptomatic orthostatic hypotension, interventions to alleviate the problem are important for maintaining quality of life and preventing serious consequences. When symptomatic orthostatic hypotension cannot be alleviated, interventions must be directed toward ensuring the individual's safety, particularly by preventing falls and fractures.

For older adults with postprandial hypotension, interventions can be implemented around mealtimes. In institutional or home care settings, registered

Prevention and Management of Both Orthostatic and Postprandial Hypotension

- Maintain adequate fluid intake (i.e., eight glasses of noncaffeinated beverages daily).
- Eat five or six smaller meals daily, rather than large meals.
- Avoid excessive alcohol consumption.
- Avoid sitting or standing still for prolonged periods, especially after meals.

Health Promotion Measures Specific to Orthostatic Hypotension

- Change your position slowly, especially when moving from a sitting or lying position to a standing position.
- Before standing up, sit at the side of the bed for several minutes after rising from a lying position.
- Maintain good physical fitness, especially good muscle tone, and engage in regular, but not excessive, exercise. (Swimming is an excellent form of exercise because the hydrostatic pressure prevents blood from pooling in the legs.)
- Wear a waist-high elastic support garment or thigh-high elastic stockings during the day, and put them on before getting out of bed in the morning.
- Sleep with the head of the bed elevated on blocks.
- During the day, rest in a recliner chair with your legs elevated.

- Take measures to prevent constipation and avoid straining during bowel movements.
- Avoid medications that increase the risk for orthostatic hypotension, particularly if additional risk factors are present (refer to Display 16-1).
- Avoid sources of intense heat (e.g., direct sun, electric blankets, and hot baths and showers) because these cause peripheral vasodilation.
- If taking nitroglycerin, do not take it while standing.

Health Promotion Measures Specific for Postprandial Hypotension

- Minimize the risk for postprandial hypotension by taking antihypertensive medications 1 hour after meals rather than before meals.
- Eat small, low-carbohydrate meals.
- Avoid alcohol consumption.
- Avoid strenuous exercise, especially for 2 hours after meals.

Safety Precautions if Hypotension Cannot Be Prevented

- Reduce the potential for falls and other negative functional consequences of postprandial hypotension by remaining seated (or by lying down) after meals.
- Call for assistance if help is needed with walking.
- Adapt the environment to minimize the risk and consequences of falling (e.g., ensure good lighting, install grab bars, keep pathways clear).

dietitians may be helpful in developing a plan for addressing postprandial hypotension, but in any setting, nurses assume responsibility for health education about interventions. In older adults with postprandial hypotension, low-carbohydrate meals are associated with significantly shorter periods of hypotension, significantly smaller declines in systolic blood pressure, and less frequent and less severe symptoms compared with normal and high carbohydrate meals (Vloet et al., 2001). Xylose (found in gum) and guar gum (a natural food supplement) may slow the rate of gastric emptying and be effective in alleviating postprandial hypotension (Jones et al., 2001). Additional interventions are summarized in Display 16-8, which can be used as a tool for health education about orthostatic and postprandial hypotension.

EVALUATING EFFECTIVENESS OF NURSING INTERVENTIONS

Goals that address the risk factors for impaired cardiovascular function would be evaluated by the extent to which the older adult verbalizes correct

information about the risks. Also, the older adult may verbalize an intent to change or eliminate the lifestyle factors that increase the risk for impaired cardiovascular function. For example, the older adult may agree to join an exercise program for seniors and to follow dietary measures to reduce serum cholesterol levels. Achievement of health promotion goals also can be measured by determining the actual reduction in risk factors. For example, the person's serum cholesterol level may decrease from 238 to 198 mg/dL after 6 months of regular exercise and dietary modifications. For older adults with impaired cardiovascular function, the nurse would evaluate the extent to which the person's signs and symptoms are alleviated and the extent to which the older adult verbalizes correct information about their impaired cardiovascular status.

CHAPTER SUMMARY

Age-related changes in cardiovascular function increase the susceptibility of older adults to atherosclerosis, cardiac arrhythmias, and orthostatic and postprandial hypotension. Age-related changes also interfere with their adaptive response to intense exercise. Factors that increase the risk for impaired cardiovascular function include obesity, hypertension, tobacco use, physical inactivity, and dietary habits that contribute to dyslipidemia. Risk factors that contribute to orthostatic hypotension include systemic diseases and adverse medication effects. Functional consequences associated with cardiovascular function in older adults include diminished ability to respond to physiologic stress, an increased susceptibility to cardiac arrhythmias, and increased susceptibility to orthostatic and postprandial hypotension.

Nursing assessment focuses on identifying remediable factors that increase the risk for cardiovascular disease. Cardiovascular assessment of older and younger adults does not differ significantly, but the manifestations of heart disease may be more subtle and less predictable in older adults. Relevant nursing diagnoses include Ineffective Health Maintenance, Decreased Cardiac Output, and Ineffective Cardiopulmonary Tissue Perfusion. Nursing interventions focus on the risk factors that actually or potentially interfere with cardiovascular function. For healthy older adults, nursing care is evaluated according to their increased knowledge of factors that influence cardiovascular function and their expressed intent to address the identified risk factors. For older adults with impaired cardiovascular function, nursing care is evaluated according to their improved cardiovascular function.

■ CONCLUDING CASE STUDY AND NURSING CARE PLAN

Mr. C. is now 74 years old and continues to come to the Senior Wellness Clinic for monthly blood pressure checks. He reports that his doctor recently started him on a medication for high cholesterol and told him to "watch my diet" but gave no further information or educational materials about what to do about his cholesterol.

■ Nursing Assessment

Mr. C. has no knowledge about dietary sources of cholesterol and is unaware that his diet, which he terms "soul food," is high in cholesterol. Although he says that he has heard a lot about "good and bad cholesterol" in the news, he does not know which foods are good or bad. He tries to buy foods that say "no

cholesterol" on the label, but says that the labels are too confusing about the different kinds of fats.

■ Nursing Diagnosis

Your nursing diagnosis is Ineffective Health Maintenance related to lack of regular exercise, dietary habits that contribute to hyperlipidemia, and insufficient information about lifestyle factors that increase the risk for cardiovascular disease. Evidence of these risk factors comes from Mr. C.'s inactivity, eating patterns, history of hypertension, and family history of cardiovascular disease. Also, Mr. C. has verbalized insufficient information about the relationship between exercise and cardiovascular function and about dietary measures to control cholesterol.

■ Nursing Care Plan

A nursing care plan for Mr. C. is given in Display 16-9.

 CRITICAL THINKING EXERCISES

1. Discuss how each of the following factors influences cardiovascular function, including orthostatic hypotension: lifestyle, medications, age-related changes, and pathologic conditions.
2. Demonstrate how you would teach a home health aide to assess blood pressure and orthostatic hypotension correctly.
3. Describe the questions and considerations that you would include in an assessment of cardiovascular function in an older adult who has no complaints of heart problems, but who has a history of falling twice in the past month and who has not been evaluated by a primary care provider in the past year.
4. You are asked to give a health education talk entitled "Keeping Your Heart Healthy" at a senior center. What information would you include in the presentation? What local resources (i.e., specific addresses and phone numbers of agencies or organizations in your area) would you suggest your audience contact for further information? What audiovisual aids would you use? How would you involve the participants in the discussion?
5. You are working in an assisted-living facility in which several of the residents have orthostatic hypotension. What would you include in your health education regarding management of orthostatic hypotension?

DISPLAY 16-9 • NURSING CARE PLAN FOR MR. C.

EXPECTED OUTCOME	NURSING INTERVENTIONS	NURSING EVALUATION
Mr. C.'s knowledge of risk factors for cardiovascular impairment will increase.	• Discuss the risk factors for impaired cardiovascular function, using Figure 16-2 and information from Display 16-3. • Emphasize the risk factors that can be addressed through lifestyle modifications (e.g., exercise, weight loss, and dietary measures to control cholesterol levels).	• Mr. C. will be able to describe his risk factors for cardiovascular disease. • Mr. C. will identify those risk factors that he can address through lifestyle changes.
Mr. C.'s knowledge of the relationship between diet and serum cholesterol levels will increase.	• Use teaching materials obtained from the American Heart Association to illustrate the relationship between diet and serum cholesterol levels. Provide a copy of these pamphlets for Mr. C. to take home. • Suggest that Mr. C. discuss the information in the pamphlets with his wife and daughter. • Ask Mr. C. to bring his wife to the nursing clinic next month so that you can talk with both of them about dietary measures to control cholesterol.	• Mr. C. will accurately describe the relationship between food intake and cholesterol levels. • Mr. C. will identify family eating habits that contribute to his elevated serum cholesterol level.
Mr. C. will modify one dietary habit that contributes to his high cholesterol level.	• Work with Mr. C. to make a list of the foods associated with high cholesterol levels (e.g., fried foods, ham hocks, lard, bacon, and eggs). • Give Mr. C. a copy of Display 16-7 and use it to discuss dietary measures to reduce cholesterol. • Ask Mr. C. to select one change in dietary habits that will have a positive effect on his cholesterol level (e.g., switching from lard to vegetable oil for frying foods).	• Mr. C. will state that he is willing to change one eating habit that contributes to his high cholesterol level. • Next month, Mr. C. will report that he has changed one eating pattern that contributes to high cholesterol levels.
Mr. C. will increase his knowledge about the relationship between exercise and cardiovascular function.	• Use pamphlets from the American Heart Association to teach about the effects of aerobic exercise on cardiovascular function. • Review information about the relationship between exercise and weight.	• Mr. C. will describe the beneficial effects of regular aerobic exercise.
Mr. C. will begin exercising on a regular basis.	• Discuss ways in which Mr. C. can incorporate regular exercise into his daily activities • Invite Mr. C. and his wife to participate in the daily Eldercise program that is offered following the noon meal at the senior center.	• Mr. C. will verbalize a commitment to perform 30 minutes of exercise 3 days a week.
Mr. C. will eliminate lifestyle factors that increase the risk for cardiovascular disease.	• Ask Mr. C. to invite his wife to your monthly appointments so that she can also receive important health education. • Identify a plan that will enable Mr. and Mrs. C. to incorporate additional dietary measures aimed at reducing cholesterol gradually into the family meal plans. • Identify a plan that will enable Mr. and Mrs. C. to include 30 minutes of exercise 5 times a week. • Discuss weight reduction with Mr. C. and emphasize that dietary modifications and regular exercise are interventions that should facilitate weight loss.	• Mr. C.'s total cholesterol level will be ≤200 mg/dL at the end of 6 months. • Mr. C.'s serum cholesterol level will remain below 200 mg/dL. • Mr. C. will report that he engages in 30 minutes of exercise 5 times weekly. • Mr. C. will report that he follows the dietary measures presented in Display 16-7. • Mr. C.'s weight will be reduced to between 180 and 198 pounds, and he will maintain that weight.

Future Directions for Healthier Aging: Focus on Cardiovascular Conditions

RESEARCH PRIORITIES OF THE NATIONAL INSTITUTE ON AGING ACTION PLAN FOR 2001–2005

- Address genetic and environmental risk factors for stroke, hypertension, and heart disease.
- Determine the causes of age-associated increases in vascular stiffness and identify the age-related changes in the structure and function of the cardiac conduction system.
- Reduce the progression of early atherosclerotic disease.
- Delineate the relationship between cardiac enlargement and aging and disease development.
- Determine the reasons for gender and racial differences in the aging cardiovascular system.

EDUCATIONAL RESOURCES

American Heart Association
7272 Greenville Avenue, Dallas, TX 75231-4596
(800) 242-8721
http://www.americanheart.org

American Stroke Association
7272 Greenville Avenue, Dallas, TX 75231-4596
(888) 478-7653
http://www.strokeassociation.org

Heart and Stroke Foundation of Canada
222 Queen Street, Suite 1402
Ottawa, ON K1P 5V9
(613) 569-4361
http://www.heartandstroke.ca

National Heart, Lung, and Blood Institute Information Center
31 Center Drive, MSC-2486, Bethesda, MD 20892
(301) 592-8573
http://www.nhlbi.nih.gov

National Stroke Association
9707 East Easter Lane, Englewood, CO 80112-5112
(800) 787-6537
http://www.stroke.org

REFERENCES

Appel, L. J., Espeland, M. A., Easter, L., Wilson, A. C., Folmar, S., & Lacy, C. R. (2001). Effects of reduced sodium intake on hypertension control in older individuals. Results for the trial of nonpharmacologic interventions in the elderly (TONE). *Archives of Internal Medicine, 161,* 685–693.

Aronow, W. S. (2002a). Should hypercholesterolemia in older persons be treated to reduce cardiovascular events? *Journal of Gerontology: Medical Sciences, 57A,* M411–M413.

Aronow, W. S. (2002b). What is the appropriate treatment of hypertension in elders? *Journal of Gerontology, 57A,* M483–M486.

Aronow, W. S. (2003). Silent MI: Prevalence and prognosis in older patients diagnosed by routine electrocardiograms. *Geriatrics, 58*(1), 24–40.

Aviv, A. (2001). Salt and hypertension: The debate that begs the bigger question. *Archives of Internal Medicine, 161,* 507–510.

Bazzano, L. A., He, J., Ogden, L. G., Loria, C., Vupputuri, S., Myers, L., & Whelton, P. K. (2001). Legume consumption and risk of coronary heart disease in US men and women. *Archives of Internal Medicine, 161,* 2573–2578.

Benetos, A., Thomas, F., Bean, K., Gautier, S., Smulyan, H., & Guize, L. (2002). Prognostic value of systolic and diastolic pressure in treated hypertensive men. *Archives of Internal Medicine, 162,* 577–581.

Bierman, E. L. (1985). Arteriosclerosis and aging. In C. E. Finch & E. L. Schneider (Eds.), *Handbook of the biology of aging* (pp. 842–868). New York: Van Nostrand Reinold.

Blacher, J., Staessen, J. A., Girerd, X., Gasowski, J., Thijs, L., Liu, L., et al. (2000). Pulse pressure not mean pressure determines cardiovascular risk in older hypertensive patients. *Archives of Internal Medicine, 160,* 1085–1089.

Boland, L. L., Folsom, A. R., Sorlie, P. D., Taylor, H. A., Rosamond, W. D., Chambless, L. E., & Copper, L. S. (2002). Occurrence of unrecognized myocardial infarction in subjects aged 45 to 65 years (the ARIC study). *American Journal of Cardiology, 90,* 927–931.

Burke, G. L., Arnold, A. M., Bild, D. E., Cushman, M., Fried, L. P., Newman, A., Nunn, C., & Robbins, J., for the Collaborative Research Group. (2001). Factors associated with healthy aging: The cardiovascular health study. *Journal of the American Geriatrics Society, 49,* 254–262.

Canto, J. G., Fincher, C., Kiefe, C. L. Allison, J. J., Li, Q, Funkhouser, E., et al. (2002). Atypical presentation among Medicare beneficiaries with unstable angina pectoris. *American Journal of Cardiology, 90,* 248–253.

Carpenito, L. J. (2002). *Nursing diagnosis: Application to clinical practice* (9th ed.). Philadelphia: Lippincott Williams & Wilkins.

Chaput, L. A., Adams, S. H., Simon, J. A., Blumenthal, R. S., Vittinghoff, E., Lin, F., et al. (2002). Hostility predicts recurrent events among postmenopausal women with coronary heart disease. *American Journal of Epidemiology, 156,* 1092–1099.

DiCastelnuovo, A. (2002). Meta-analysis of wine and beer consumption in relation to vascular risk. *Circulation, 105,* 2836–2844.

Eaton, C. B., & Anthony, D. (2002). Cardiovascular disease and the maturing woman. *Clinics in Family Practice, 4*(1), 71–88.

Eidelman, R. S., Lamas, G. A., & Hennekens, C. H. (2002). The new National Cholesterol Education Program guidelines. *Archives of Internal Medicine, 162,* 2033–2036.

Expert Panel on Detection, Evaluation, and Treatment of High Blood Cholesterol in Adults. (2001). Executive summary of the Third Report of the National Cholesterol Education Program (NCEP) Expert Panel on Detection, Evaluation, and Treatment of High Blood Cholesterol in Adults (ATP III). *Journal of the American Medical Association, 285,* 2486–2497.

Fahlman, M. M., Boardley, D., Lambert, C. P., & Flynn, M. G. (2002). Effects of endurance training and resistance training on plasma lipoprotein profiles in elderly women. *Journal of Gerontology: Biological Science, 57A,* B54–B60.

Frazier, L. (2002). Resting and reactive blood pressure: Predictors of ambulatory blood pressure in adults with hypertension. *Journal of Gerontological Nursing, 28*(9), 6–13.

Gibbons, L. W., & Clark, S. M. (2001). Exercise in the reduction of cardiovascular events: Lessons for epidemiologic trails. *Cardiology Clinics, 19*(3), 347–355.

Glick, O. J., & Ressler, C. (2001). Altered health maintenance. In M. L. Maas, K. C. Buckwalter, M. D. Hardy, T. Tripp-Reimer, M. G. Titler, & J. P. Specht (Eds.), *Nursing care of older adults: Diagnoses, outcomes, & interventions* (pp. 6–22). St Louis: Mosby.

Hajjar, I. M., Grim, C. E., George, V., & Kotchen, T. A. (2001). Impact of diet on blood pressure and age-related changes in blood pressure in the US population. *Archives of Internal Medicine, 161,* 589–593.

Hajjar, I., Miller, K., & Hirth, V. (2002). Age-related bias in the management of hypertension: A national survey of physicians' opinions on hypertension in elderly adults. *Journal of Gerontology: Medical Sciences, 57A,* M487–M491.

Hak, A. E., Pols, H. A. P., Visser, T. J., Drexhage, H. A., Hofman, A., & Witteman, J. C. M. (2000). Subclinical hypothyroidism is an independent risk factor for atherosclerosis and myocardial infarction in elderly women: The Rotterdam Study. *Annals of Internal Medicine, 132,* 270–278.

Harper, C. R., & Jacobson, T. A. (2001). The fats of life: The role of omega-3 fatty acids in prevention of coronary heart disease. *Archives of Internal Medicine, 161,* 2185–2192.

Hinderliter, A., Sherwood, A., Gullette, E. C. D., Babyak, M., Waugh, R., Georgiades, A., & Blumenthal, J. A. (2002). Reduction of left ventricular hypertrophy after exercise and weight loss in overweight patients with mild hypertension. *Archives of Internal Medicine, 162,* 1333–1339.

Hirano, R., Momiyama, Y., Takahashi, R., Taniguchi, H., Kondo, K., Nakamura, H., & Ohsuzu, F. (2002). Comparison of green tea intake in Japanese patients with and without angiographic coronary artery disease. *American Journal of Cardiology, 90,* 1150–1153.

Hodgson, J. M., Puddey, I. B., Mori, T. A., Baker, R. I., & Beilin, L. J. (2001). Effects of regular ingestion of black tea on haemostasis and cell adhesion molecules in humans. *European Journal of Clinical Nutrition, 55,* 881–886.

Humphrey, L. L., Chan, B. K. S., & Sox, H. C. (2002). Postmenopausal hormone replacement therapy and the primary prevention of cardiovascular disease. *Annals of Internal Medicine, 137,* 273–284.

Joint National Committee on Prevention, Detection, Evaluation, and Treatment of High Blood Pressure (JNC). (2003). The seventh report of the Joint National Committee on Prevention, Detection, Evaluation, and Treatment of High Blood Pressure (JNC IV). *Journal of the American Medical Association, 289,* 2560–2577.

Jones, K. L., MacIntosh, C., Su, Y. C., Wells, F., Chapman, I. M., Tonkin, A., & Horowitz, M. (2001). Guar gum reduces postprandial hypotension in older people. *Journal of the American Geriatrics Society, 49,* 162–167.

Joshipura, K. J., Hu, F. B., Manson, J. E., Stampfer, M. J., Rimm, E. B., Speizer, F. E., et al. (2001). The effect of fruit and vegetable intake on risk for coronary heart disease. *Annals of Internal Medicine, 134,* 1106–1114.

Keevil, J. G., Stein, J. H., & McBride, P. E. (2002). Cardiovascular disease prevention. *Primary Care: Clinics in Office Practice, 29*(3), 667–777.

Klungel, O. H., Heckbert, S. R., Longstreth, W. T., Furberg, C. D., Kaplan, R. C., Smith, N. L., et al. (2001). Antihypertensive drug therapies and the risk of ischemic stroke. *Archives of Internal Medicine, 161,* 37–43.

Kris-Etherton, P. M., Harris, W. S., & Appel, L. J. (2002). Fish consumption, fish oil, omega-3 fatty acids, and cardiovascular disease. *Circulation, 106,* 2747–2757.

Kudzma, E. C. (2001). Cultural competence: Cardiovascular medicine. *Progress in Cardiovascular Nursing, 16*(4), 152–160, 169.

Labarthe, D., & Ayala, C. (2002). Nondrug interventions in hypertension prevention and control. *Cardiology Clinics, 20,* 249–263.

Laine, C., (2002). Postmenopausal hormone replacement therapy: How can we be so wrong? *Annals of Internal Medicine, 137,* 290.

Lakatta, E. G. (2000). Cardiovascular aging in health. *Clinics in Geriatric Medicine, 16*(3), 419–444.

Laucka, P. V., & Trotter, J. M. (2001). Medication management of hypertension. *Topics in Geriatric Rehabilitation, 17*(2), 61–82.

Lindeman, R. H. (2000). Aging and the kidney. In M. H. Beers & R. Berkow. *The Merck manual of geriatrics* (pp. 9951–9954). Whitehouse Station, NJ: Merck Research Laboratories.

Mancia, G., Bombelli, M., Lanzarotti, A., Grassi, G., Ceasana, G., Zanchetti, A., & Sega, R. (2002). Systolic vs diastolic blood pressure control in the hypertensive patients of the PAMELA population. *Archives of Internal Medicine, 162,* 582–586.

Maurer, M. S., Karmally, W., Rivadeneira, H., Parides, M. K., & Bloomfield, D. M. (2000). Upright posture and postprandial hypotension in elderly. *Annals of Internal Medicine, 133,* 533–536.

Mehagnoul-Schipper, D. J., Boerman, R. H., Hoefnagels, W. H. L., & Jansen, R. W. M. M. (2001). Effects of levodopa on orthostatic and postprandial hypotension in elderly parkinsonian patients. *Journal of Gerontology: Medical Science, 56A,* M749–M755.

Messinger-Rapport, B. J., & Sprecher, D. (2002). Prevention of cardiovascular disease: Coronary artery disease. *Clinics in Geriatric Medicine, 18*(3), 463–484.

Morley, J. E. (2001). Postprandial hypotension: The ultimate Big Mac attack. *Journal of Gerontology: Medical Science, 56A,* M741–M743.

Moser, M. (2001). Is it time for a new approach to the initial treatment of hypertension? *Archives of Internal Medicine, 161,* 1140–1144.

Mukai, S., & Lipsitz, L. A. (2002). Orthostatic hypotension. *Clinics in Geriatric Medicine, 18,* 253–268.

Mya, M. M., & Aronow, W. S. (2002). Subclinical hypothyroidism is associated with coronary artery disease in older persons. *Journal of Gerontology: Medical Science, 57A,* M658–M659.

Nelson, K., Norris, K., & Mangione, C. M. (2002). Disparities in the diagnosis and pharmacologic treatment of high serum cholesterol by race and ethnicity. *Archives of Internal Medical, 162,* 929–935.

Obermen, A. S., Gagnon, M. M., Kiely, D. K., & Lipsitz, L. A. (2000). Autonomic and neurohumoral control of postprandial blood pressure in healthy aging. *Journal of Gerontology: Medical Science, 55A,* M477–M483.

O'Mara, G. O., & Lyons, D. (2002). Postprandial hypotension. *Clinics in Geriatric Medicine, 18,* 307–321.

Pearson, T. A., Blair, S. N., Daniels, S. R., Eckel, R. H., Fair, J. M., Fortmann, S. P., et al. (2002). AHA Guidelines for primary prevention of cardiovascular disease and stroke: 2002 update. *Circulation, 106,* 388–391.

Piccirillo, G., Di Giuseppe, V., Nocco, M., Lionetti, M., Moise, A., Naso, C., Tallarico, D., Marigliano, V., & Cacciafesta, M. (2001). Influence of aging and other cardiovascular risk factors on baroreflex sensitivity. *Journal of the American Geriatrics Society, 49,* 1059–1065.

Prospective Studies Collaboration. (2002). Age-specific relevance of usual blood pressure to vascular mortality: A meta-analysis of individual data for one million adults in 61 prospective studies. *Lancet, 360,* 1903–1913.

Puisieux, F., Bulckaen, H., Fauchais, A. L., Drumez, S., Salomez-Granier, F., & Dewailly, P. (2000). Ambulatory blood pressure monitoring and postprandial hypotension in elderly persons with falls or syncopes. *Journal of Gerontology: Medical Science, 55A,* M535–M540.

Rea, T. D., Heckbert, S. R., Kaplan, R. C., Smith, N. L., Lemaitre, R. N., & Psaty, B. M. (2002). Smoking status and risk for recurrent coronary events after myocardial infarction. *Annals of Internal Medicine, 137,* 494–500.

Reid, I. R., Mason, B., Horne, A., Ames, R., Clearwater, J., Bava, U., et al. (2002). Effects of calcium supplementation on serum lipid concentrations in normal older women: A randomized controlled trial. *American Journal of Medicine, 112,* 343–347.

Ross, R., & Glomset, J. (1976). The pathogenesis of atherosclerosis. *New England Journal of Medicine, 295,* 369, 420.

Sareli, P., Radecski, I. V., Valtchanova, Z. P., Lighaber, E., Candy, G. P., Hond, E. D., et al. (2001). Efficacy of different drug classes used to initiate antihypertensive treatment in black subjects. *Archives of Internal Medicine, 161,* 965–971.

Sheifer, S. E., Manolio, T. A., & Gersh, B. J. (2001). Unrecognized myocardial infarction. *Annals of Internal Medicine, 135,* 801–811.

Taylor, H. A., Hughes, G. D., & Garrison, R. J. (2002). Cardiovascular disease among women residing in rural America: Epidemiology, explanations, and challenges. *American Journal of Public Health, 92,* 548–551.

U.S. Department of Health and Human Services (USDHHS). (2000). *Healthy people 2010* (2nd ed.). Washington, DC: U.S. Government Printing Office.

U.S. Preventive Services Task Force. (October 2002). *Hormone replacement therapy for primary prevention of chronic conditions: Recommendations and rationale.*

Rockville, MD: Agency for Healthcare Research and Quality. www.ahrq.gov/clinic/3rduspstf/hrt/hrtr.htm

Vasan, R. S., Larson, M. G., Leip, E. P., Evans, J. C., O'Donnell, C. J., Kannel, W. B., & Levy, D. (2001). Impact of high-normal blood pressure on the risk of cardiovascular disease. *New England Journal of Medicine, 345,* 1291–1297.

Vloet, L. C. M., Mehagnoul-Schipper, J., Hoefnagels, W. H. L., & Jansen, R. W. M. M. (2001). The influence of low-, normal-, and high-carbohydrate meals on blood pressure in elderly patients with postprandial hypotension. *Journal of Gerontology, 56A*(12), M744–M748.

Vokonos, P. S. (2000). Atherosclerosis. In M. H. Beers & R. Berkow. *The Merck manual of geriatrics* (pp. 849–853). Whitehouse Station, NJ: Merck Research Laboratories.

Vollmer, W. M., Sacks, F. M., Ard, J., Appel, L. J., Bray, G. A., Simons-Morton, D. G., Conlin, P. R., Svetkey, L. P., Erlinger, T. P., Moore, T. J., & Karanja, N. (2001). Effects of diet and sodium intake on blood pressure: Subgroup analysis of the DASH-sodium trial. *Annals of Internal Medicine, 135,* 1019–1028.

Weiss, A., Grossman, E., Beloosesky, Y., & Grinblat, J. (2002). Orthostatic hypotension in acute geriatric ward. Is it a consistent finding? *Archives of Internal Medicine, 162,* 2369–2374.

Whelton, S. P., Chin, A., Xin, X., & He, J. (2002). Effect of aerobic exercise on blood pressure: A meta-analysis of randomized, controlled trials. *Annals of Internal Medicine, 136,* 493–503.

White, W. B. (2001). Gender and age effects on the ambulatory blood pressure and heart rate responses to antihypertensive therapy. *American Journal of Hypertension, 14,* 1239–1247.

Williams. M. A., Fleg, J. L., Ades, P. A., Chairman, B. R., Miller, N. H., Mohiuddin, S. M., et al. (2002). Secondary prevention of coronary heart disease in the elderly (with emphasis on patients ≥ 75 years of age). *Circulation, 105,* 1735–1743.

Women's Health Initiative Investigators (WHI). (2002). Risks and benefits of estrogen plus progestin in healthy postmenopausal women: Principal results from the Women's Health Initiative randomized controlled trial. *Journal of the American Medical Association, 288*(3), 321–333.

Yarows, S. A., Steva, J., & Pickering, T. G. (2000). Home blood pressure monitoring. *Archives of Internal Medicine, 160,* 1251–1257.

Respiratory Function

LEARNING OBJECTIVES

1. Delineate age-related changes that affect respiratory function.
2. Describe risk factors that interfere with optimal respiratory function in older adults.
3. Discuss the functional consequences of age-related changes and risk factors that affect respiratory performance.
4. Describe methods of identifying risk factors and assessing respiratory function in older adults.
5. Identify nursing interventions to reduce the risks of impaired respiratory function and lower respiratory infections in older adults, with emphasis on preventing disease and promoting health.

The primary functions of respiration are to supply oxygen to and remove carbon dioxide from the blood. Adequate respiratory performance is essential to life because all body organs and tissues need oxygen. For these reasons, it is noteworthy that the respiratory system shows less age-related decline than other body systems in healthy, nonsmoking, older adults. Studies of respiratory function in older adults show great individual variation; much of this variability is attributable to genetic effects. The age-related changes that do affect respiratory performance are subtle and gradual, and healthy older adults are able to compensate for these changes. When a complicating factor, such as illness or anesthesia, places extraordinary demands for oxygen on the body, age-related respiratory changes may influence the overall function of the older adult.

AGE-RELATED CHANGES THAT AFFECT RESPIRATORY FUNCTION

As with other body functions, it is difficult to separate the effects of age-related changes from those caused by disease processes and external influences, such as tobacco smoking. These influences occur throughout the life span, but because their effects are cumulative, their impact is more pronounced in older adults. In addition, their cumulative effect may cause negative functional consequences only when they interact with age-related changes, such as diminished immune response, or with risk factors, such as diminished mobility.

Upper Respiratory Structures

Although the nose is often overlooked in discussions of respiratory function, age-related changes of the upper respiratory structures can influence both comfort and function. Age-related connective tissue changes cause the nose in older persons to have a retracted columella (the lower edge of the septum), and a poorly supported, downwardly rotated tip. Although these changes may be viewed as having consequences that are more cosmetic than functional, they can cause small septal deviations that can interfere with the flow of air through the nasal cavity. These changes also may contribute to mouth breathing during sleep, causing snoring and obstructive apnea.

With increasing age, blood flow to the nose diminishes, causing the nasal turbinates to become smaller. Age-related changes also affect the submucosal glands, causing diminished secretions, even in healthy older adults. Because the secretions from the submucosal glands are thin and watery, their function is to dilute the thicker mucous secretions from the goblet cells. With diminished submucosal gland secretions, the mucus in the nasopharynx is thicker and more difficult to remove. This combination of age-related changes in turbinates, blood flow, and submucosal glands results in the presence of thicker and dryer secretions and a perception of nasal stuffiness. It also may lead to stimulation of the cough reflex and a persistent tickle in the throat.

The epiglottis and upper airway structures expel mucus and unwanted material from the lungs and protect the lower airway from harmful substances, ranging in size from microorganisms to large pieces of food. One of the age-related changes that affects these structures is calcification of the cartilage, which causes the trachea to stiffen. Another is blunting of the cough and laryngeal reflexes, with a concomitant decrease in coughing in older adults. Age-related reductions in the number of laryngeal nerve endings also have been noted, and these may contribute to diminished efficiency of the gag reflex.

Chest Wall and Musculoskeletal Structures

Together, the chest wall and lungs function like a bellows, with the chest expanding outward in relation to lung expansion. The rib cage and the vertebral musculoskeletal structures are affected by the same kind of age-related changes that affect other musculoskeletal tissue: the ribs and vertebrae become osteoporotic, the costal cartilage becomes calcified, and the respiratory muscles become weaker. As a result of these age-related processes, the following structural changes, which can affect respiratory performance, occur: kyphosis, shortened thorax, chest wall stiffness, and increased anteroposterior diameter of the chest. The overall impact on respiratory performance includes diminished respiratory efficiency and reduced maximal inspiratory and expiratory force. To compensate for age-related changes, older adults depend increasingly on accessory muscles, particularly the diaphragm; thus, they are increasingly sensitive to any changes in intraabdominal pressure. In summary, although older adults expend more energy to achieve the same respiratory efficiency as younger adults, the overall functional consequences for healthy older people are minimal.

Lungs

Even in healthy older adults, lungs become smaller and flabbier, and their weight diminishes by about 20%. The age-related changes that have the most significant functional consequences are those that occur in the lung parenchyma, or the part of the respiratory system where gas exchange takes place. The affected structures include the terminal bronchioles, alveolar ducts, alveoli, and capillaries. Beginning at about 20 to 30 years of age, the alveoli progressively enlarge, and their walls become thinner. This process of ductectasia continues throughout adulthood, causing about a 4% loss of alveolar surface area per decade. As a result of this loss of alveolar surface, the amount of anatomic dead space increases. Age-related changes also affect the pulmonary vasculature. The trunk of the pulmonary artery becomes thickened and less extensible, and its diameter widens. The number of capillaries also diminishes, and pulmonary capillary blood volume decreases. Finally, the mucosal bed, where diffusion takes place, thickens.

Elastic recoil enables lung tissue to resist expansion as it fills with air and assists in maintaining a positive pressure across the lung surface during inspiration, to hold the small airways open. During expiration, elastic recoil keeps the airways open until the pressure placed on them by the respiratory muscles forces them to collapse. If the airways close prematurely, air is trapped, and the lungs cannot expire to their maximum capacity. In healthy older adults, elastic recoil diminishes by a small degree, owing to a combination of age-related changes in the parenchyma and alterations in the elastic fibers. The end result is early airway closure, the mechanism that is primarily responsible for age-related changes in lung volumes and airflow rates.

Air Volumes and Airflow Rates

Specific aspects of lung function, such as air volumes and airflow rates, are measured by pulmonary function tests. In older adults, air volumes are altered because of the age-related changes in the chest wall and in lung elastic recoil. Because various air volumes are interrelated, however, the total lung capacity remains essentially the same owing to compensatory mechanisms. Airflow rates are affected to a small degree by age-related changes and to a greater degree by additional variables, such as height, gender, and air volumes. Overall, there is an age-related decline in all airflow rates, but because of the many additional factors, there is a wide range of normal levels. Table 17-1 summarizes the age-related changes of some lung function parameters.

Gas Exchange

Because gas exchange is the primary function of the respiratory system, it is the most important functional aspect to consider. Oxygen–carbon dioxide exchange depends on a close match between ventilation (i.e., the amount of air in the lungs) and perfusion (i.e., the amount of blood flowing into the lungs). Because of age-related changes, particularly early airway closure, gas exchange is more likely to be compromised in the lower, rather than in the upper, lung regions. As a consequence, inspired air is preferentially distributed in the upper regions, and ventilation–perfusion mismatch results. The end result of this mismatch is a gradual decrease in arterial oxygen pressure (PaO$_2$) of about 4 mm Hg per decade.

Response to Hypoxia and Hypercapnia

Compensatory changes in respiratory rate are made under conditions of hypercapnia (too much carbon dioxide) or hypoxia (too little oxygen). The response mechanism varies, depending on the stimulus. The

TABLE 17-1 • Age-Related Changes in Indicators of Lung Function

Indicator	Definition	Age-Related Change
Tidal volume	Amount of air moved in and out during a normal breath	Slight decrease
Residual volume	Amount of air left in the lungs after a forced expiration	Increases by 5%–10% per decade
Forced expiratory volume	Amount of air expelled within 1 second after a maximum inspiration	Decreases 23–32 mL/yr in men, 19–26 mL/yr in women
Forced inspiratory volume	Maximum volume of air that can be inhaled in addition to tidal volume	Decreases
Forced vital capacity	Maximum volume of air that can be expelled following a maximum inspiration	Decreases 14–30 mL/yr in men, 14–24 mL/yr in women
Total lung capacity	Amount of air that can be held in the lungs after a maximum inspiratory effort	Unchanged, as a result of compensatory mechanisms
Diffusing capacity	Ability of lungs to transfer gases between the lungs and blood	Declines 2.03 mL/minute/mm Hg per decade in men, and 1.47 mL/min/mm Hg in women
Arterial oxygen pressure (PaO$_2$)	Amount of oxygen in arteries	Declines 0.3% per year or 4 mm Hg per decade, but remains stable after age 75 years at 83 mm Hg

response to hypercapnia is initiated by the central chemoreceptor, located in the medulla, whereas the response to hypoxia is initiated by peripheral chemoreceptors, located in the carotid and aortic bodies. When these mechanisms operate efficiently, the respiratory rate and depth increase in response to either low levels of oxygen or high levels of carbon dioxide. Although there has been some controversy about age-related changes in respiratory response to hypoxia and hypercapnia, it is now widely believed that the ventilatory response to both hypoxia and hypercapnia is reduced by 40% to 50% between the third and eighth decades. As a result of this diminished response to hypoxia or hypercapnia, older adults are more likely to show mental changes rather than breathlessness when blood gases are abnormal.

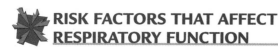

RISK FACTORS THAT AFFECT RESPIRATORY FUNCTION

For people of any age, tobacco smoking, particularly cigarette smoking, is the single most important risk factor for lung disease and impaired respiratory function. For smokers who have not succumbed to the detrimental effects before later adulthood, the risks of smoking are both immediate and cumulative. Other risks are mentioned because, particularly for nonsmokers, they can be addressed through health promotion interventions to improve respiratory function. For smokers, however, these other risks are of minimal importance, and attention must be focused on the serious negative consequences of smoking.

Smoking

Tobacco smoking causes detrimental effects through heat and chemical actions on the respiratory system. Toxic gases released from burning cigarettes include carbon monoxide, hydrogen cyanide, and nitrogen dioxide. In addition, burning cigarettes release tobacco tar, which contains nicotine and many other harmful chemicals. Harmful physiologic effects on the respiratory system include but are not limited to: (1) bronchoconstriction; (2) inflammation of the mucosa throughout the respiratory tract; (3) early airway closure (which is also an age-related change); and (4) inhibited ciliary action, leading to increased coughing and mucous secretions and diminished protection from harmful organisms. Risks in older adults are compounded by age-related changes and the cumulative effects of cigarette smoking. Even in otherwise healthy people, smokers have a doubled or tripled rate of decline, compared with nonsmokers, in the forced expiratory volume at 1 second (FEV$_1$). This reduced FEV$_1$ is an accelerated and exacerbated age-related change that increases the risk for diseases, such as chronic obstructive pulmonary disease (COPD). In addition to being associated with detrimental effects on lung functioning, cigarette smoking is strongly associated with increased risk for serious diseases of the lungs, cardiovascular system, and many other systems. Also, tobacco use is strongly associated with cancers of the head, neck, lung, larynx, stomach, kidney, bladder, pancreas, and esophagus (Kuper, 2002).

Smoking prevalence ranking among various groups in the United States, from highest to lowest, is: American Indians/Alaska Natives, African Americans, whites, Hispanics, Asians/Pacific Islanders (USDHHS, 2000).

Until recently, pipes and cigars were viewed as safer smoking alternatives than cigarettes because these types of tobacco are not inhaled. Iribarren and colleagues (1999), however, however, found that cigar smoking was associated with increased relative risk, in a dose-dependent pattern, of cardiovascular disease, chronic obstructive lung disease, and smoking-related cancers (Iribarren et al., 1999). Regardless of whether the person inhales when smoking pipes or cigars, the effects of the environmental tobacco smoke can be harmful to everyone who is exposed to sidestream smoke. Smokeless tobacco also has been falsely viewed as harmless, but its use is highly associated with increased risk for gingivitis, tooth loss, and cancers of the mouth; its only advantage is that it does not contribute to environmental tobacco smoke.

The negative effects of environmental tobacco smoke, also called sidestream, passive, or secondhand smoke, were first reported to the public in the 1972 Surgeon General's Report. Although this report was initially viewed with some skepticism, the National Institutes of Health are very clear about the cause-and-effect relationship between exposure to smoke and human cancer incidence. For instance, environmental tobacco smoke causes 3,000 lung cancer deaths annually and as many as 62,000 deaths from coronary heart disease among adult nonsmokers in the United States (CDC, 2001). Environmental smoke contains the same chemical compounds as mainstream smoke, but the particles are smaller and can be inhaled more deeply in the lungs. In fact, some of the harmful chemical compounds are in greater concentrations than in mainstream smoke (Nurminen & Jaakkola, 2001). Since the early 1990s, the Centers for Disease Control and Prevention (CDC), the National Institutes of Health, and other governmental health agencies have emphasized the importance of diminishing environmental tobacco smoke. An objective of *Healthy People 2010* is to eliminate exposure to environmental tobacco smoke through laws, policies, and regulations requiring smoke-free environments in schools, work sites, and public places (USDHHS, 2000). Because older adults are likely to be less knowledgeable than younger populations about the health hazards of active and passive smoking (Brownson et al., 1992), gerontological nurses have opportunities for health education not only about smoking but also about environmental tobacco smoke.

Environmental Factors

Along with the skin, the respiratory system is the area of physiologic function most directly influenced by environmental factors, such as air quality. Dry air can affect the upper airway by further drying the nasal secretions, causing them to be thicker and more difficult to remove. Another environmental risk factor that can lead to negative functional consequences is the inhalation of air pollutants. Like the effects of cigarette smoking, the effects of air pollution are cumulative over many years and, therefore, have an increased impact on older adults who have been exposed to air pollutants over much of their lifetime. For example, older adults who have lived their entire lives in urban environments may have been exposed to air pollutants for as many as seven or eight decades.

Older adults who previously worked in occupations such as mining and firefighting may have been exposed to toxic substances with long-term effects. Because hazards in the workplace were largely unregulated before the 1970s, many older people never benefited from the protections enforced under the Occupational Safety and Health Act. In addition, much of the information now available on the harmful effects of certain chemicals was not widely available when these older adults were part of the workforce. Therefore, older adults are more likely than younger adults to experience the long-term effects of occupational exposure to harmful substances. Occupational lung disease may not be identified until later adulthood when the cumulative effects present signs and symptoms. Some of the job categories that may be associated with an increased risk for respiratory disease are listed in Display 17-1.

Additional Risk Factors

A unique characteristic of respiratory performance is that the maximum level of function in middle and later adulthood is significantly influenced by the maximum level of function reached during the third decade of life, which is largely determined by factors that affected respiratory development in early life. Because respiratory complaints develop when pulmonary function is reduced to half of the maximally attained level, older adults can tolerate a relatively greater degree of age-related changes and exposure to risk factors before experiencing respiratory dysfunction if they attained a higher peak level of respiratory function. Conversely, if the maximum level attained was low, the impact of age-related changes and risk factors may be experienced sooner.

In addition to the age-related changes that involve the respiratory system, age-related changes affecting other aspects of functioning can also affect respiratory performance. For example, both kyphosis, which is caused by age-related skeletal changes, and poor posture can interfere with maximum respiratory performance. A decline in immune response and host defense mechanisms is an age-related change that is thought to contribute to the increased morbidity and mortality noted in older adults with pneumonia and other lower respiratory infections.

Any condition or chronic illness that interferes with mobility or activity increases the risk for impaired respiratory function. Restricted activity levels and a recumbent position exacerbate the effects of age-related changes and result in compromised respiratory performance in older adults. The function of the respiratory muscles, for example, is compromised by assuming a recumbent position or by any condition that contributes to shallow breathing. Therefore, any older adult who is on bed rest, even for short periods of time, is at increased risk for impaired respiratory function. The negative functional consequences of bed rest are also attributable, at least in part, to the fact that the recumbent position interferes with chest wall expansion, which is already compromised by age-related changes.

Obesity is another health-related risk factor that can interfere with respiratory function through its impact on an individual's overall activity level. Obesity also affects the ability to take deep breaths and to ventilate the lower lobes of the lung. Even minor changes in body weight have a significant effect on the ventilatory capacity, with weight gain and loss being associated with a decline or improvement in annual measurement of the forced expiratory volume (Morgan & Reger, 2000).

Medications are another risk factor that can influence respiratory function in several ways. Anticholinergic-based medications and sedatives can affect upper airway function by causing further drying of mucus. Medications also may impact on cough reflexes. Angiotensin-converting enzyme inhibitors, for example, can cause persistent dry cough.

DISPLAY 17-1

Workforces With an Increased Risk for Harmful Respiratory Effects

Firefighters
Miners
Traffic controllers
Shipyard workers
Rubber workers
Aluminum workers
Iron and steel foundry workers
Tunnel and street repair workers
Asbestos workers
Quarry workers
Farmers, agricultural workers, grain handlers
Construction workers
Paper mill workers
Workers exposed to the following: dust, fumes, gases, nickel, arsenic, beryllium, chromium, or radiation

PATHOLOGIC CONDITIONS THAT CAN AFFECT RESPIRATORY FUNCTION

COPD is a group of diseases, including emphysema and chronic bronchitis, characterized by chronic airflow obstruction. The prevalence of COPD in people between the ages of 55 and 85 years in North America is estimated at 10%, with the incidence increasing more rapidly in the past 15 years than that of any of the other nine leading causes of death (Terry, 2000). Studies suggest that there is significant underdiagnosis and misdiagnosis of COPD because simple spirometry testing is underused. Underdiagnosis is most likely to occur in women, in people with mild to moderate disease, and in people aged 45 years and older (Chapman et al., 2001; Petty, 2000). COPD is highly associated with a genetic predisposition and tobacco smoking. Other associated factors include increased age, low socioeconomic status, exposure to environmental toxins, and history of significant childhood respiratory disease. The most common manifestations of COPD are cough, dyspnea, wheezing, and increased sputum production. The condition is progressive, and its cumulative effects become more disabling as the person ages. Mental changes are likely to occur in older adults because of hypoxemia or hypercapnia. Older adults who have COPD are more likely than younger people to have longer hospitalizations and a greater likelihood of being discharged to an institutional setting (Terry, 2000).

> Although COPD is thought to be more prevalent among men than women, some of this disparity may be due to significant underdiagnosis of COPD, particularly in women (Chapman et al., 2001). Mortality rates for COPD are similar for men and women at age 55 years, but by age 85 years, mortality rates are 3.5 times higher among men (Terry, 2000).

FUNCTIONAL CONSEQUENCES ASSOCIATED WITH RESPIRATORY FUNCTION IN OLDER ADULTS

In the absence of smoking and other risk factors, healthy older adults will not experience any significant negative functional consequences related to their respiratory performance when performing ordinary activities. Age-related respiratory changes do not significantly affect exercise capacity, which is more likely to be altered by deconditioning and risk factors. Under conditions of physical stress, however, older adults may become dyspneic and fatigued because their respiratory system is less efficient in gas exchange. However, even this effect may be at least

TABLE 17-2 • Age-Related Changes Affecting Respiratory Function

Change	Consequence
Upper airway changes: calcification of cartilage, altered neuromuscular function and reflexes	Snoring, mouth breathing, diminished cough reflex, decreased efficiency of gag reflex
Increased anteroposterior diameter, chest wall stiffness, weakened muscles and diaphragm	Increased use of accessory muscles, increased energy expended for respiratory efficiency
Enlargement of alveoli, thinning of alveolar walls, diminished number of capillaries	Diminished efficiency of gas exchange, decreased arterial oxygen pressure (PaO$_2$)
Decreased elastic recoil and early airway closure	Changes in lung volumes, slight decrease in overall efficiency
Tidal volume unchanged or slightly diminished, increased residual volume, decreased vital capacity	Total lung capacity unchanged

partially compensated for through physical conditioning. The overall functional consequences of age-related changes are summarized in Table 17-2.

Even in the presence of risk factors, such as cigarette smoking, older adults experience the same negative consequences as younger adults. That is, they will have higher rates of cancer, cardiovascular disease, COPD, and other diseases than those without risk factors. In fact, people who smoke cigarettes during their early adult years are less likely to live long enough to experience any age-related changes because they tend to die at a younger age than do nonsmokers. For example, life expectancy at age 35 years for men and women who smoked and continued smoking until death was 69.3 and 73.8 years, respectively; for men and women who quit at age 35 years, life expectancy was 73.8 and 79.9 years. Men and women who quit smoking at age 65 years can expect an increase in life expectancy of 2.0 and 3.7 years, respectively, compared with people who continue to smoke (Taylor et al., 2002).

The only negative functional consequence of age-related changes and risk factors that is unique to older adults is an increased susceptibility to lower respiratory infections. Respiratory infections have more serious consequences in older adults and are more likely to lead to death or cause a decline in functional status (Barker et al., 1998). The combination of age-related changes in respiratory function and age-related changes in immunity contributes to an increased risk for acquiring pneumonia and influenza in older adulthood. Mortality rates from pneumonia show an age-related increase from a rate of 24 per 100,000 for people aged 60 to 64 years to 1032 per 100,000 for people aged 85 years and older (Callahan & Wolinsky, 1996).

In addition to being increasingly susceptible to pneumonia and influenza, older adults are also more susceptible to tuberculosis than their younger counterparts. The most common reason for this is the reactivation of dormant tuberculosis, particularly in the presence of risk factors such as smoking, diabetes, malnutrition, a debilitating illness, or long-term use of corticosteroids. The incidence of tuberculosis in community-living older adults is twice that of the general population; for older adults in nursing homes, the incidence is four times higher than that in the general population. Some of the cases of tuberculosis that affect nursing home residents are attributable to the ease with which this disease can spread among residents. Moreover, identification and treatment of tuberculosis may be delayed in older adults because disease manifestations are altered and usually more subtle in this population (as discussed in the Nursing Assessment of Respiratory Function section). Mortality rates for older adults with tuberculosis are higher than those for younger populations. Figure 17-1 summarizes age-related changes, risk

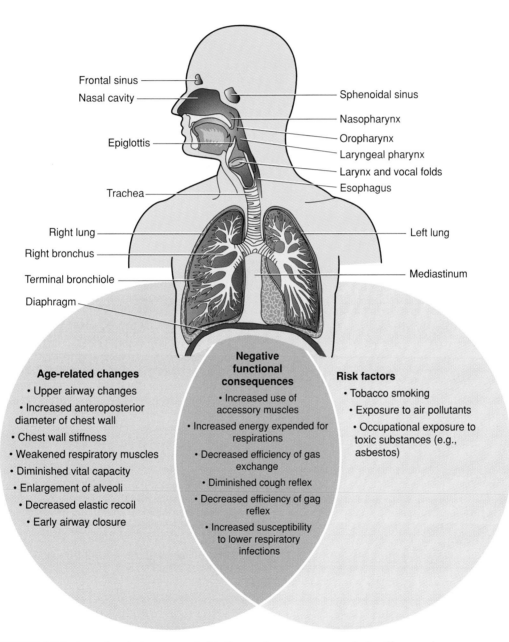

FIGURE 17-1 Age-related changes and risk factors intersect to negatively affect respiratory function in older adults.

factors, and negative functional consequences that influence an older adult's respiratory function.

Tuberculosis is more prevalent in African Americans, Hispanics, Native Americans, and Asian Americans than in whites.

NURSING ASSESSMENT OF RESPIRATORY FUNCTION

Nursing assessment of respiratory function differs only slightly in younger and older adults. Assessment of opportunities for health promotion must consider the different life experiences of older adults, particularly with regard to exposure to environmental toxins and attitudes about tobacco use. Other differences include the manifestations and effects of lower respiratory infections in older adults and minor variations in the physical assessment of their respiratory systems.

Identifying Opportunities for Health Promotion

Nurses interview the older adult, or their caregivers, to identify risk factors that can affect respiratory function because these factors can be addressed through health promotion activities. Cigarette smoking is the risk factor that contributes most to impaired respiratory function and lung diseases; thus, nurses must view this risk factor as potentially reversible, even in older adults. Information obtained through interview questions about smoking will provide the base for health education approaches. Interview information also will provide information about other preventive aspects, such as influenza and pneumonia vaccinations. It is important to identify attitudes of older adults about these preventive interventions so that nurses can plan appropriate health promotion approaches. Lastly, interview questions assess overall respiratory function to identify respiratory problems that should be addressed in the nursing care plan. Display 17-2 presents an interview format that may be used to assess risk factors, overall respiratory function, and opportunities for health education.

Detecting Lower Respiratory Infections

The term *detection* is more accurate than assessment with regard to lower respiratory infections because when older adults have pneumonia, they do not always meet the typical assessment criteria. Rather than presenting with a cough, chills, elevated temperature, and

---

DISPLAY 17-2
Guidelines for Assessing Respiratory Function

Questions to Identify Risk Factors for Respiratory Problems

- Have you had any respiratory problems, such as asthma, chronic lung disease, pneumonia, or other infections?
- Do you have a family history of chronic lung disease?
- Have you ever had tuberculosis?
- Have you ever worked in a job where you were exposed to dust, fumes, smoke, or other air pollutants (e.g., in mining, farming, or any of the occupations listed in Display 17-1)?
- Have you lived in neighborhoods where there was a lot of pollution from traffic or factories?
- Do you smoke now, or have you ever smoked? (If yes, continue with the questions in Display 17-3.)
- Have you been exposed to passive smoke in home, work, or social environments?

Questions to Identify Opportunities for Education About Disease Prevention and Health Promotion

- Have you ever had a pneumonia vaccination? (If yes, ask about when the vaccination was administered and whether a booster was ever given.)
- Do you get annual influenza vaccinations?

Questions to Assess Overall Respiratory Function

- Do you have any problems with breathing?
- Do you have any wheezing?
- Do you have spells of coughing? *If yes:* When do they occur? How long do they last? What brings them on? Are they dry or productive? Does the phlegm come from your throat or lungs? What does the phlegm look like?
- Do you ever have trouble getting enough air during any particular activities or when you lie down at night?
- Have you stopped doing any particular activities because of problems breathing? For example, have you stopped going up or down stairs, or have you limited the amount of walking you do? (For people with mobility limitations, this question might not be relevant.)
- Do you ever have any chest pain, or feelings of heaviness or tightness in your chest?
- Do you use more than one pillow at night, or make any other adjustments, because of trouble with breathing?
- Do you wake up at night because of coughing or difficulty with breathing?
- Do you ever feel as though you can't catch your breath?
- Do you have trouble breathing when the weather is hot, cold, or humid?
- Do you tire easily?

elevated white blood count, older adults are more likely to have subtler and nonspecific disease manifestations that must be detected. Even an initial chest radiograph may not provide accurate diagnostic information. Manifestations of pneumonia most commonly seen in older adults, particularly during the early stages of the disease, are headache, weakness, anorexia, lethargy, dehydration, changes in mental status, and a decline in overall function. An analysis of studies of presentation of pneumonia found that although both younger and older adults often present with nonspecific symptoms, older adults with dementia are most likely to present with nonspecific symptoms, the most common nonspecific manifestation in older adults being delirium (Johnson et al., 2000).

Tachypnea (a respiratory rate greater than 26 breaths/minute) may be the most reliable sign of a lower respiratory infection in an older adult (Feldman, 2001). Temperature elevations may occur later in the disease process rather than earlier. The changes in lung sounds that typically occur with pneumonia may not be present; in fact, the only respiratory sign may be tachypnea. Dyspnea or breathlessness is likely to have a later onset, or it may be absent if the older adult restricts his or her activities to avoid dyspnea on exertion. In older adults with pneumonia, the most significant finding on physical assessment of the lungs may be a diminished intensity of lung sounds or the presence of rales and rhonchi, which are very nonspecific findings.

Nurses must keep in mind that, although older adults may exhibit the typical manifestations of pneumonia, the absence of these manifestations is not as significant in older adults as it is in younger adults. In older adults, a change in mental status or another alteration in functional status, such as falls or incontinence, may be the major clue to a diagnosis of pneumonia. Thus, an important nursing responsibility is to detect nonspecific manifestations of pneumonia and collect additional information. This is especially important because the delay in diagnosis of pneumonia in older people, which may be due to the nonspecific manifestations, may partially explain the higher mortality rate of pneumonia in older people (Feldman, 2001).

In addition to being aware of the different manifestations of pneumonia in older adults, nurses also must be aware of the increased rates and varied manifestations of tuberculosis in this population. As with pneumonia, manifestations of tuberculosis in this age group are likely to be subtle and nonspecific. In contrast to younger adults, older adults with tuberculosis are less likely to have fever, hemoptysis, and night sweats and are more likely to have dyspnea, diminished serum albumin, and at least one other concomitant condition

(Perez-Guzman et al., 1999). Another reason that tuberculosis is more difficult to detect in older adults is that 30% to 40% of older adults have false-negative tuberculin skin test reactions. Because tuberculosis often occurs as a reactivation of dormant disease, nurses must be particularly alert for manifestations of this disease in older adults who have a history of tuberculosis. Despite the relatively high rate of false-negative results in older adults, giving a two-step tuberculin test with tuberculin purified protein derivative (PPD) using the Mantoux method is the recommended method of assessing for previous exposure to tuberculosis.

Assessing Smoking Behaviors

Although smoking affects all people, regardless of age, some aspects of smoking behaviors differ according to age cohorts. Therefore, an assessment of smoking as a risk factor must address the age-related factors that affect these behaviors. The cohort of people born between 1910 and 1930, for example, is the first age group to be exposed to the social pressures that encouraged smoking without knowing about its detrimental effects. As a result, people who began smoking in the early 1920s, when it became a popular habit for men in the United States, may have smoked for four or five decades before finding out that smoking is harmful. For women in the United States, smoking was not socially acceptable until the mid-1940s. Thus, the cohort of smoking women who are now in their 60s is the first group of women who have smoked throughout their adulthood. Not until 1964 was the first report on the detrimental effects of cigarette smoking, *Smoking and Health,* issued by the United States Surgeon General. By this time, men had been smoking for four decades and women had been smoking for two decades. The long-term consequences of smoking for older women are just now beginning to be recognized, as evidenced by the recent increase in lung cancer rates among older women. For example, between 1960 and 1990, lung cancer deaths among women increased by more than 400% (USDHHS, 2001). Because some people who are now in their 70s or 80s have a long history of smoking, they may be likely to adopt the attitude, "If I've smoked this long and am still alive, why should I quit now?"

In addition to assessing attitudes about smoking, nurses should assess past and present smoking patterns. Frequency of smoking and type of tobacco smoked are important determinants of the relative risk of smoking. Smokeless tobacco, for example, is not as detrimental to respiratory and cardiovascular function as cigarette smoking, but it does increase the risk for oral cancer. Cigarettes vary in the amount of nicotine they contain, and this variable influences the degree of risk associated with a particular type of cigarette. In contrast to younger adults, who began smoking when cigarettes had filters and were lower in nicotine, older adults began smoking when cigarettes had no filters and contained greater amounts of tar and nicotine. Older adults, therefore, are more likely than younger adults to smoke cigarettes that have higher nicotine levels and thus are more harmful. Older adults, in fact, may still roll their own cigarettes using loose tobacco.

For older adults who smoke, questions should be asked to determine their readiness to consider quitting smoking as well as their knowledge base about the health impact of smoking. Nurses also should assess the older adult's perception of cigarette smoking as a manifestation of his or her rights and autonomy. As with other health care decisions, adults are entitled to make decisions about their health-related behaviors, but these decisions should be based on full knowledge of the benefits and risks of their choices. Many beliefs and attitudes about smoking may arise primarily from lack of information. Wolfsen and colleagues (2001) found that elderly nursing home residents do not hold strong antismoking views and lack information about the relationships between smoking and health. Residents viewed smoking as "the singular remaining vestige of their former life as competent independent adults" (p. 10). The authors of this study suggested that educational interventions for nursing home residents might be a step toward reducing the prevalence of smoking in this population.

Nurses may need to examine their own attitudes about smoking, especially in relation to older adults. For example, it is important to identify ageist influences that can lead to the view that smoking cessation would not be beneficial for older adults. Similarly, although it is important to respect the rights of older adults who choose to smoke, health care professionals should not exclude older adults from health promotion interventions about smoking simply because they are old. Assessment questions designed to help determine smoking habits and attitudes about smoking are included in Display 17-3.

Identifying Other Risk Factors

Risk factors that have less significant effects on respiratory function than smoking does should also be assessed. As mentioned previously, maximum respiratory function is attained by early adulthood. Information about factors that may have influenced respiratory development in early life, such as nutrition, respiratory infections, and chronic exposure to cigarette smoke, may be helpful in assessing the older

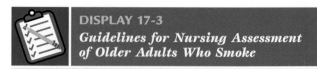

DISPLAY 17-3
Guidelines for Nursing Assessment of Older Adults Who Smoke

Questions to Assess Smoking Behaviors
- How long have you smoked?
- How much do you smoke?
- What do you smoke?
- Have you smoked other types of tobacco in the past?

Questions to Assess Knowledge of the Risk From Smoking
- Do you think there are any harmful effects of smoking for people in general?
- Do you think you are at risk for any harmful effects from smoking?
- Do you think there are any benefits to quitting smoking?

Questions to Assess Attitudes Toward Smoking
- Have you ever thought about quitting smoking?
- Has any health professional ever talked to you about quitting smoking?
- What do you think about the idea of quitting smoking?
- Have you ever tried to quit? *If yes:* What was your experience with the attempt?
- Would you be interested in finding out information about quitting smoking now?

adult's maximum respiratory function and in providing information about the person's vulnerability to the effects of age-related changes and risk factors.

For this reason, questions about exposure to sidestream smoke and harmful air pollutants should be incorporated in the assessment. Occupational exposure to certain harmful substances is particularly important for smokers because the risk for either one of these factors is compounded when the other factor is present. Information about the person's level of activity and about any factors that may interfere with mobility or routine activities will be helpful in assessing the degree to which additional exercise can be encouraged. If, for example, the person has severe mobility impairments as a result of arthritis, the potential for vigorous physical exercise may be quite limited. However, these individuals may benefit greatly from water exercises. Finally, information about the older adult's understanding of influenza and pneumonia vaccinations will provide a basis for education about these preventive measures. See Display 17-2 for the information that must be included in a nursing assessment of respiratory function in older adults.

Physical Assessment Findings

The normal respiratory rate of older adults may be slightly increased, ranging from 16 to 24 respirations per minute. The usual methods of inspection, palpation, percussion, and auscultation are used to evaluate respiratory performance in both younger and older adults. Some minor differences in assessment findings that may be observed in healthy older adults include: (1) increased anteroposterior diameter; (2) altered appearance (i.e., leaning forward) secondary to kyphosis; (3) increased resonance on percussion; (4) diminished intensity of lung sounds; and (5) an increased tendency for adventitious sounds to be auscultated in the lower lungs.

Assessment of respiratory function begins with observations about the person's breathing pattern when he or she is walking, changing position, or even sitting. Asking the older person to cough before auscultation of the lungs and having the person sit upright and breathe as deeply as possible with his or her mouth open will facilitate auscultation of breath sounds. When nurses have an opportunity to observe respirations in a sleeping older adult, they may see frequent but brief periods of apnea. This phenomenon is common in older adults and is highly associated with sleep problems, as discussed Chapter 20. With the exceptions of pneumonia and tuberculosis, the manifestations of most respiratory diseases, such as influenza and COPD, do not differ in older and younger adults.

➤ Mr. R. is 70 years old and comes with his wife to the senior center where you provide weekly nursing services. Both Mr. and Mrs. R. smoke 1 to 2 packs of cigarettes a day. Mr. R. has mild COPD, and Mrs. R. has hypertension and coronary artery disease. Every October, the senior center offers flu shots for anyone over the age of 65 years. As you are preparing to give flu shots, Mr. and Mrs. R. come to you and ask, "Is this the shot that takes care of pneumonia? Our daughter said we should get a pneumonia shot every year, but we don't want a flu shot because our friend says she got the flu from one of those shots and she'll never get a shot again. Can you just give us the pneumonia shot today? We got one from the doctor last year but it's too expensive to get it from him."

 THINKING POINTS

➤ What myths and misunderstandings are expressed by Mr. and Mrs. R.?

➤ What further assessment questions would you ask?

➤ What health promotion teaching would you do?

NURSING DIAGNOSIS

The nursing diagnosis of Ineffective Breathing Pattern would be applicable when the nursing assessment identifies factors that may impair the older adult's respiratory function. This diagnosis is defined as "the state in which the individual experiences an actual or potential loss of adequate ventilation related to an altered breathing pattern" (Carpenito, 2002, p. 765). Defining characteristics include cough, dyspnea, shortness of breath, and changes in respiratory rate or pattern from baseline. If impaired respiratory function interferes with activities of daily living, a nursing diagnosis of Activity Intolerance might be appropriate. Debilitated or chronically ill older adults who live in group settings may be at risk for infections, particularly pneumonia, influenza, and tuberculosis. For example, if a nursing home resident has active tuberculosis, the nursing staff might address the nursing diagnosis of Risk for Infection Transmission for the affected resident and the nursing diagnosis of Risk for Infection for all other residents. Likewise, when influenza affects one or more residents or staff of a nursing home or group living facility, the same nursing diagnoses may be applicable. Ineffective Health Maintenance is a nursing diagnosis that may be used for older adults who have insufficient knowledge about the detrimental effects of active or passive smoking. When nurses provide pneumonia or influenza immunizations for older adults, a nursing diagnosis of Health-Seeking Behaviors may be appropriate.

OUTCOMES

A nursing-sensitive outcome for the nursing diagnosis of Ineffective Breathing Pattern is Respiratory Status: Ventilation, as indicated by case of breathing and respiratory rate and rhythm in the expected range (Wakefield, 2001). These indicators can be assessed by nurses in any setting without the use of special equipment. Goals of treatment for patients with Ineffective Breathing Pattern include enhancing well-being, increasing endurance time, managing or avoiding dyspnea, and improving activities of daily living abilities and exercise tolerance (Wakefield, 2001). These outcomes would address the needs of older adults who have some chronic or acute impairment of respiratory function.

For most older adults who have adequate respiratory function, outcomes focus on disease prevention and health promotion by addressing their increased vulnerability to pneumonia, influenza, and tuberculosis. The nursing-sensitive outcome of Risk Control includes the following indicators that are pertinent to reducing the risk for pneumonia, tuberculosis, and influenza in older adults: prevents or detects infection, prevents resistant organism transmission, and monitors for environmental and personal behavior risk factors (Carter & Pottinger, 2001). For older adults who lack knowledge about how infections are transmitted, an appropriate outcome would be Knowledge: Health Behaviors. A specific and easily measured outcome of successful health education might be that older adults obtain immunizations against pneumonia and influenza.

For older adults who smoke and express a wish to change their behaviors, an appropriate outcome would be to decrease or eliminate tobacco use (Carpenito, 2002). Some of the nursing-sensitive outcomes that would be relevant to this type of situation are: (1) knowledge about risks, conditions, and self-care; (2) beliefs, attitudes, and values regarding health and lifestyle issues; and (3) health behavior that minimizes risk and that supports or advances health (Glick & Ressler, 2001). Because smoking is the most important factor that influences respiratory function, nurses working with older adults who smoke should always consider the possibility of identifying and working toward a goal of reducing or eliminating tobacco use.

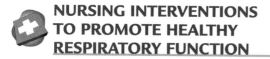

NURSING INTERVENTIONS TO PROMOTE HEALTHY RESPIRATORY FUNCTION

Preventing Disease and Promoting Health

It is widely acknowledged that smoking is the single most preventable cause of disease and death in the United States and therefore should be a major target of disease prevention activities. Because most older smokers already have at least minor smoking-related conditions affecting respiratory function and other systems, smoking cessation will address secondary or tertiary prevention rather than primary prevention. Smoking cessation is more cost-effective as a health promotion activity than other common preventive services including mammography, Pap tests, colon cancer screening, or treatment of hypercholesterolemia or mild to moderate hypertension (CDC, 2000).

Healthy People 2010 addresses 21 national health objectives related to tobacco smoking and several additional objectives related to tuberculosis, pneumonia, occupational lung disease, and COPD (USDHHS, 2000). Disease prevention and health promotion interventions related to respiratory function that are particularly applicable to older adults include pneumonia and influenza vaccinations and education about the importance of stopping smoking and avoiding environmental tobacco smoking. Numerous educational materials are available for use in disease prevention and health promotion interventions, some of which are available in languages other than English. These interventions are discussed in the following sections and summarized in Displays 17-4 and 17-5.

Preventing Lower Respiratory Infections

Interventions to prevent pneumonia and influenza are particularly important because these two conditions collectively constitute the fourth leading cause of death in people older than 65 years. Moreover, of all the leading causes of death in older adults, pneumonia and influenza are the only ones that can be prevented with investment of very little time, money, or motivation. Therefore, education about pneumonia and influenza vaccinations is an essential nursing intervention in caring for older adults. Although annual influenza immunizations are well accepted and well publicized, pneumonia vaccinations have received less attention. Pneumococcal vaccine is effective against 23 types of infections that cause 85% to 90% of all cases of pneumonia in the United States. The vaccine's effectiveness in immunocompetent adults aged 65 years and older is 75% (Gross, 2001). The CDC recommends pneumonia vaccinations for all people aged 65 years and older. Since 1997, the CDC has recommended a one-time booster dose for all people aged 65 years or older if they received an initial pneumonia vaccination 5 or more years earlier and if they were younger than 65 years at the time of initial vaccination. Pneumonia vaccinations are also recommended for older adults who are uncertain about their vaccination status.

Although influenza vaccinations are less effective in preventing influenza in older adults than in younger adults, they are very effective in reducing influenza-related death, hospitalizations, and other complications in older adults who do develop influenza (Gross, 2001; McElhaney, 2002). Despite the efficacy of influenza vaccinations, fewer than half of all older adults in the United States receive them each year. Current geriatric literature promotes the use of standing orders in institutional settings for influenza vaccination to increase the rate of vaccinations for older adults (Lawson et al., 2000). Gerontological nurses play a primary role in implementing annual influenza vaccination programs in community, residential, and institutional settings. Health care workers who work with older adults in any setting should also be encouraged to have annual influenza vaccinations because this reduces mortality from influenza in the older population. See Display 17-4 for a summary of current information about influenza and pneumonia immunizations along with information about risk factors for these illnesses.

DISPLAY 17-4

Health Promotion Teaching About Respiratory Problems

Factors That Increase the Risk for Pneumonia and Influenza

- Diabetes or any chronic lung, heart, or kidney disease
- Hospitalization within the past year for heart or lung diseases
- Severe anemia or a debilitating condition
- Confinement to bed or very limited mobility
- Residence in a nursing home or other group living setting
- Immunosuppressive medications

Preventing Respiratory Infection

- Wash your hands frequently with an antibacterial soap or hand sanitizer.
- Avoid hand-to-mouth and hand-to-eye contact.
- Avoid inhaling air that has been contaminated with particles from the cough or sneeze of someone with an infection.
- Avoid crowds during the flu season.
- Be sure that influenza and pneumonia vaccinations are up to date.

Information About Influenza Vaccinations

- New vaccinations are developed every year, based on information about the strains of viruses that are most likely to affect people during the influenza season.
- Vaccines are made from inactivated viruses and, therefore, should have few or no side effects.
- People who are allergic to eggs and egg products should NOT receive influenza immunizations.
- Immunizations do not offer immediate protection because there is a 2- to 3-week delay in developing an antibody response.
- Every year, the manufacturers of the influenza vaccination provide recommendations as to the best time for administering the immunizations for optimal effectiveness. The best time is during the late fall, but the exact time period will vary slightly from year to year.
- Vaccines are not 100% effective, but they are helpful for most older people.

- Influenza immunizations provide protection against the most serious viruses but not against all types of respiratory infections.
- The duration of effectiveness of vaccinations may be shorter than 6 months in some older people; therefore, one vaccination might not protect the person through the entire season.
- In 1993, Medicare began paying for flu shots.

Information About Pneumonia Vaccinations

- Pneumonia vaccinations are recommended for people older than 65 years of age.
- Pneumonia vaccinations were considered one-time-only immunizations, but boosters are now being recommended for older adults who received their initial immunization 5 or more years ago.
- Side effects, if they occur, are not serious and will subside within a few days.
- Common side effects include a slight fever accompanied by pain, redness, or tenderness at the injection site.
- Pneumonia vaccinations are covered by Medicare and other health insurance.

Nutritional Considerations

- Include foods high in zinc and vitamins A, B-complex, C, and E.

Complementary and Alternative Care Practices

- Humidifier, vaporizer, air filter, mustard poultice, steam therapy
- Herbs for colds or coughs: thyme, yarrow, garlic, hyssop, coltsfoot, licorice, peppermint, Echinacea, marsh mallow, slippery elm, red sage
- Homeopathic remedies for colds or coughs: aconite, bryonia, drosera, pulsatilla, nux vomica, antimonium tartaricum
- Aromatherapy: thyme, lemon, menthol, camphor, eucalyptus, lavender, tea tree
- Acupuncture may be used for coughs, influenza, upper respiratory infections, nasal allergic conditions, and chronic respiratory conditions

Nurses working in long-term care or other group living facilities commonly are responsible for implementing programs to detect and address tuberculosis. Nursing models of prevention and intervention programs in long-term care facilities can be found in gerontological nursing references (e.g., Brennan & Morgan, 2001; Gubser, 1998) and on the CDC web site (http://www.cdc.gov). These references provide guidelines for screening and diagnostic methods, such as skin testing. They also provide information about interventions for residents with tuberculosis and pre-

vention of the spread of the infection among staff and residents. Any nurse or direct-care staff member working with older adults should undergo periodic skin testing to screen for exposure to tuberculosis.

Eliminating the Risk From Smoking

An assessment of attitudes about smoking provides a basis for planning educational interventions that will help older smokers eliminate this risk factor. If the assessment reveals an "I'm too old to change" attitude,

DISPLAY 17-5
Health Promotion Teaching About Cigarette Smoking

Attitudes About Smoking

Stopping smoking at any age is more beneficial than continuing to smoke.

- Many of the harmful effects of smoking are reversed once the smoker quits.
- Although some of the effects of past smoking are irreversible, all of the harmful effects of future smoking can be avoided by quitting now.
- Smoking is a major risk factor for lung and heart disease, including high blood pressure and heart attacks.
- Smoking is a major risk factor for many cancers, including those of the lung, head, stomach, kidney, and pancreas.
- Passive smoking (inhaling smoke from the air) is associated with an increased risk for many diseases.

Type of Tobacco

- The lower the tar and nicotine content of cigarettes, the less harmful the effects. Many cigarettes with lower tar and nicotine levels, however, have additional chemical additives that can be harmful.
- Pipe and cigar smokers are at a higher risk for chronic lung disease than nonsmokers, just as cigarette smokers are.
- The harmful effects of tobacco use on the mouth and upper respiratory tract are equal for all types of tobacco, including smokeless tobacco. All smokers have the same risk for developing cancer of the mouth and upper respiratory tract. Snuff, chewing tobacco, and smokeless tobacco contain nicotine and many other harmful chemicals. The only advantage of smokeless tobacco is that it does not affect other people nearby.

Approaches to Quitting

- Any reduction in present tobacco use is better than maintaining the current level. The negative effects of smoking are directly proportional to the number of cigarettes inhaled.
- Various forms of prescription and over-the-counter nicotine substitutes (e.g., gum, skin patches, and nasal sprays) are available and may be helpful, especially when used in conjunction with counseling and self-help techniques.
- Besides nicotine substitutes, some nonnicotine prescription medications and over-the-counter products may be effective as a component of a smoking cessation program.
- People who are trying to quit smoking should discuss their goals with a health care professional to identify the methods that might be most effective.
- Many self-help programs are available for support and education regarding quitting smoking.
- Information about group programs can be obtained on the Internet or by calling the local office of any of the following organizations: American Lung Association, American Heart Association, or American Cancer Society.

Complementary and Alternative Care Practices to Help Quit Smoking

- Herbs: combination of coltsfoot and plantain
- Homeopathic remedies: plantain, nox vomica
- Citric acid throat spray
- Exercise, music, imagery, massage, meditation, affirmations, deep breathing, stress reduction, social support, individual or group counseling

the initial intervention might be to explore the older adult's understanding of his or her ability to change behavioral patterns. Using information about psychosocial development in older adulthood, the nurse might challenge such an attitude and encourage the older person to consider the possibility of a behavioral change.

Closely related to the "I'm too old to change" attitude is the "It's too late to do any good" attitude. Whenever older adults express such an attitude, nurses must challenge its underlying assumptions. This attitude might be prevalent among older adults because smokers older than 50 years of age are less likely than younger smokers to think that smoking affects their health now, and less likely to believe that there is a strong likelihood of serious health problems from smoking (Clark et al., 1997). Nurses can inform older adults that substantial health benefits are derived from quitting smoking, not only in terms of improved respiratory function, but also in terms of the reduced risk for heart disease and lung cancer, as compared with the risk from continuing to smoke.

Studies indicate that the benefits of smoking cessation in later life are proportionately less than they are in younger adults and may take longer to manifest; however, smoking cessation is the most effective method of reducing disease risk in older adults (Burns, 2000). Al-Delaimy and colleagues (2002) found that diabetic women who had quit smoking for 10 years decreased their risk for developing coronary heart disease to the same level as that of people who had never smoked. Similarly, Rea (2002) found that the risk for recurrent coronary events in people who quit smoking for 3 years after a myocardial infarction was equal to that of the nonsmokers who had a myocardial infarction. Health education about the many beneficial effects of quitting smoking may enhance the older adult's motivation to quit smoking.

Smokers are most likely to quit smoking after a smoking-related illness develops, as evidenced by a 50% quit rate among smokers who survive heart attacks (Timmreck & Randolph, 1993). Recently updated clinical practice guidelines emphasize the importance of nurses and other health care providers initiating the topic of smoking cessation and routinely identifying and intervening with all tobacco users at every opportunity (AHCPR, 2000). Guidelines for nursing interventions for smoking cessation can be found in nursing literature (e.g., O'Connell, 2001; Wynd, 1997). The transtheoretic model for health promotion (discussed in Chapter 4) has been widely studied as a model for smoking cessation programs and can be used effectively in health promotion for older adults who smoke (Burbank & Riebe, 2002).

Health education should include information about the variety of approaches to smoking cessation, including various prescription or over-the-counter pharmacologic therapies that can help treat nicotine addiction. Several new prescription and over-the-counter smoking cessation products have recently been approved for use in the United States. Available methods for delivering nicotine substitutes include gum, patches, inhalants, and nasal sprays. These products have all been found to be effective in significantly increasing the cessation rate, and some people may benefit from combining different types of products (Prochazka, 2000). In addition to nicotine substitution products, a sustained-release form of buproprion has been available since 1997 as the first nonnicotine medicinal aid to smoking cessation. A citric acid aerosol product is available as a smoking cessation product. Regardless of the methods that are used, it is widely agreed that counseling from a health professional is an important component of any smoking cessation efforts. Educational materials about group and individual self-help programs are available through the organizations listed in the Educational Resources section. See Display 17-5 for a summary of educational interventions that may be effective in helping older adults quit smoking.

> Mr. R. is now 77 years old and attends the senior center with his wife three times a week for meal and social programs. During your weekly Wellness Clinic he comes to have his blood pressure checked and says that he is thinking about quitting smoking, but that his son just quit and gained a lot of weight and had a lot of trouble sleeping. He's not sure if quitting smoking is worth the effort, especially because his son has been so miserable since he quit. Also, at his age, it probably won't do any good to quit now.

 THINKING POINTS

> What further questions would you ask to assess Mr. R.'s readiness to discuss quitting smoking?

> What health promotion teaching would you do?

> What would your response be if you determine that Mr. R. is not ready to consider quitting?

EVALUATING EFFECTIVENESS OF NURSING INTERVENTIONS

Measuring the effectiveness of interventions for the nursing diagnosis of Ineffective Breathing Pattern is based on a reassessment of subjective indicators such as ease of breathing and objective indicators such as lung sounds and respiratory rate and rhythm. An indicator of successful health education interventions for older adults with Ineffective Breathing Pattern is that they can accurately identify factors that can be addressed to improve their respiratory function. Disease prevention interventions for the nursing diagnosis of Risk for Infection could be documented on a record of the person's history of immunizations for pneumonia and influenza. For older adults who smoke and are willing to address this risk factor, effectiveness of interventions would be measured by the person's increased knowledge about the detrimental effects of smoking and by his or her willingness to develop a plan to stop smoking. Long-term effectiveness would be evaluated by the person's successful participation in the smoking cessation plan.

CHAPTER SUMMARY

Under normal circumstances, healthy, nonsmoking, older adults compensate well for any age-related changes that affect respiratory function. Respiratory performance may be compromised, however, by risk factors such as illness, tobacco use, or exposure to environmental pollutants. Older adults are more likely than younger adults to have lower respiratory infections, such as pneumonia, influenza, and tuberculosis. When lower respiratory infections occur in older adults, the manifestations are more subtle, and the consequences are likely to be serious or life-threatening.

Nursing assessment of respiratory function in older adults focuses on identifying risk factors, such as cigarette smoking and inadequate immunizations against pneumonia and influenza. Nursing assessment of smokers concentrates on gathering information about the person's knowledge of the harmful effects of active and passive smoking and about the person's attitudes about smoking cessation. For older adults who are at risk for lower respiratory infections, nursing assessment focuses on detecting the subtle manifestations of pneumonia or tuberculosis. Relevant nursing diagnoses include Ineffective Breathing Pattern and Risk for Infection.

Nursing care is directed toward alleviating risk factors that interfere with optimal respiratory function. Health education includes information about quitting smoking and obtaining pneumonia and influenza vaccinations. Nursing care may be directed toward the prevention and early detection of respiratory infections, especially in nursing homes and other group settings. Nursing care is evaluated by documented improvement in respiratory function, elimination of risk factors (e.g., cigarette smoking), and prevention of respiratory infections.

CONCLUDING CASE STUDY AND NURSING CARE PLAN

➤ Mr. R. is now 83 years old and recently moved into an assisted living complex where you are employed as the nurse. When he comes in for his flu shot, he asks you how he can get some nicotine gum because he has heard that this is a good way to cut down on cigarettes. Now that he lives in the assisted living complex, he can't smoke in the dining room, and he'd like to chew nicotine gum before and after he eats. He admits that he smokes a pack of cigarettes every day, but denies having experienced any bad effects from smoking. Mr. R. sees his doctor for COPD and takes Flovent, 2 puffs twice daily, and Serevent, 2 puffs twice daily.

Nursing Assessment

You begin your nursing assessment by exploring Mr. R.'s attitudes about smoking and ascertaining his knowledge about the harmful effects of cigarette smoking. Mr. R. says he thought about quitting smoking many times but never actually tried to quit because his wife smoked even more than he did until she died a few months ago. He felt it would be too hard to quit as long as she was smoking two packs per day, and it wouldn't do him any good to quit as long as he had to be around the smoke from her cigarettes. He states that he's been smoking for 40 years, and if he hasn't gotten lung cancer by now, he's not going to get it at his age. He also states that he's heard a lot about passive smoking and he figured it wasn't worth trying to quit as long as he was around his wife who smoked. To comply with the rules in the assisted-living facility, Mr. R. says he plans to chew nicotine gum when he can't smoke cigarettes, but he sees no reason to quit.

In assessing Mr. R.'s knowledge about the effects of cigarette smoking, you determine that he is aware of some of the harmful effects of passive smoking but has very little information about the detrimental effects of cigarette smoking. He relates that his wife died of lung cancer, but he attributes her death to a history of breast cancer, which she had 10 years before the lung cancer. Mr. R. has no knowledge about cigarette smoking as a risk factor for cardiovascular disease, nor does

he realize that his hypertension poses an additional risk. Mr. R. reports that he has experienced no ill effects from cigarette smoking, but when you ask about his history of respiratory infections, he admits he had pneumonia 3 years ago. He says that he received a pneumonia shot 2 years ago, so he doesn't have to worry about getting pneumonia again, and that he's had bronchitis several times, but now that he won't be out shoveling snow, he doesn't worry about getting any lung infections.

Nursing Diagnosis

Based on the assessment findings, an appropriate nursing diagnosis would be Ineffective Health Maintenance, related to insufficient knowledge about the effects of tobacco use and self-help resources. Some of Mr. R.'s statements reflect a lack of accurate information about the harmful effects of cigarette smoking, particularly regarding risks for respiratory infections and impaired cardiovascular function. Other statements probably reflect an intellectualization of his continued smoking. You intuit that, with some education and support, he may be willing to quit smoking. The nursing care plan you develop for Mr. R. is presented in Display 17-6.

 CRITICAL THINKING EXERCISES

1. Answer the following questions in relation to Mr. R.:
   • How would you assess Mr. R.'s readiness and motivation to quit smoking?
   • What health education approach would you take with Mr. R.?
   • What additional interventions or health education points would you use for Mr. R.?
2. What will a healthy, nonsmoking, 83-year-old person experience in his or her daily life with regard to respiratory function?
3. What would you include in a health education program, designed for older adults, on the prevention of pneumonia and influenza?
4. How would you address the following statement made by a 71-year-old person: "I've lived this long and don't have lung cancer; why should I start worrying now?"
5. Find the names, addresses, and phone numbers of local agencies that would be appropriate resources for someone interested in quitting smoking. Contact at least one of these organizations to find out specific information about support groups, written materials, and other resources.

DISPLAY 17-6 • NURSING CARE PLAN FOR MR. R.

EXPECTED OUTCOME	NURSING INTERVENTIONS	NURSING EVALUATION
Mr. R. will increase his knowledge about the harmful effects of cigarette smoking.	• Give Mr. R. brochures and illustrations provided by the Office on Smoking and Health and use them to discuss the effects of cigarette smoking. • Use brochures from the American Heart Association to discuss the risk factors for cardiovascular disease. • Discuss cigarette smoking as a risk factor for respiratory infections. • Give Mr. R. a copy of Display 17-5 and discuss the immediate and long-term benefits of quitting smoking.	• Mr. R. will verbalize correct information about the risks of cigarette smoking. • Mr. R. will describe the benefits derived from quitting smoking.
Mr. R. will be knowledgeable about techniques for quitting smoking.	• Using information from the American Lung Association, discuss some of the strategies for quitting smoking (e.g., quitting cold turkey, using nicotine substitutes, participating in self-help groups).	• Mr. R. will describe the advantages and disadvantages of the various methods of quitting smoking.
Mr. R. will quit smoking.	• Identify the method Mr. R. prefers for quitting smoking. • Emphasize the importance of nutrition, exercise, and adequate fluid intake. • Agree on realistic goals for smoking cessation. • Discuss supportive resources. Set up weekly appointments at the Senior Wellness Clinic for support and further discussions.	• Mr. R. will report that he has stopped or significantly reduced his smoking.

EDUCATIONAL RESOURCES

Agency for Health Care Policy and Research, U.S. Department of Health and Human Services
AHCPR Publications Clearinghouse
2101 Jefferson Street, Suite 501, Rockville, MD 20852
(301) 594-1364
http://www.ahcpr.gov

American Cancer Society
1599 Clifton Road, NE, Atlanta, GA 30329
(800) 227-2345
http://www.cancer.org

American Heart Association
7272 Greenville Avenue, Dallas, TX 75231-4596
(800) 242-8721
http://www.americanheart.org

American Lung Association
61 Broadway, 6th floor, New York, NY 10006
(212) 315-8700
http://www.lungusa.org

Lung Association of Canada
3 Raymond Street, Suite 300, Ottawa, ON K1R 1A3
(613) 569-6411
http://www.lung.ca

National Heart, Lung, and Blood Institute Information Center
P.O. Box 30105, Bethesda, MD 20824-0105
(301) 592-8573
http://www.nhlbi.nih.gov/health/index.htm

Office on Smoking and Health Centers for Disease Control and Prevention
Publications Catalog, Mail Stop K-50
4770 Buford Highway, NE, Atlanta, GA 30341-3717
(800) 232-1311
http://www.cdc.gov/tobacco

REFERENCES

Agency for Health Care Policy and Research (AHCPR). (2000). *Clinical practice guideline: Treating tobacco use and dependence.* U.S. Department of Health and Human Services. Washington, DC: U.S. Government Printing Office.

Al-Delaimy, W. K., Manson, J. E., Solomon, C. G., Kawachi, I., Stampfer, M. J., Willett, W. C., et al. (2002). Smoking and risk of coronary heart disease among women with type 2 diabetes mellitus. *Archives of Internal Medicine, 162,* 273–279.

Barker, W. H., Borisute, H., & Cox, C. (1998). A study of the impact of influenza on the functional status of frail older people. *Archives of Internal Medicine, 158,* 645–650.

Brennan, P. J., & Morgan, A. (2001). Tuberculosis. In M. D. Mezey (Ed.), *The encyclopedia of elder care* (pp. 648–652). New York: Springer.

Brownson, R. C., Jackson-Thompson, J., Wilkerson, J. C., Davis, J. R., Owens, N. W., & Fisher, E. B. (1992). Demographic and socioeconomic differences in beliefs about the health effects of smoking. *American Journal of Public Health, 82,* 99–103.

Burbank, P. M., & Riebe, D. (2002). *Promoting exercise and behavior change in older adults: Interventions with the transtheoretical model.* New York: Springer.

Burns, D. M. (2000). Cigarette smoking among the elderly: Disease consequences and the benefits of cessation. *American Journal of Health Promotion, 14,* 357–361.

Callahan, C. M., & Wolinsky, F. D. (1996). Hospitalization for pneumonia among older adults. *Journal of Gerontology: Medical Sciences, 51A,* M276–282.

Carpenito, L. J. (2002). *Nursing diagnosis: Application to clinical practice* (9th ed.). Philadelphia: Lippincott Williams & Wilkins.

Carter, C., & Pottinger, J. M. (2001). Risk for infection. In M. L. Maas, K. C. Buckwalter, M. D. Hardy, T. Tripp-Reimer, M. G. Titler, & J. P. Specht (Eds.), *Nursing care of older adults: Diagnoses, outcomes, and interventions* (pp. 47–63). St. Louis: Mosby.

Centers for Disease Control and Prevention (CDC). (2000). Reducing tobacco use: A report of the surgeon general. *Morbidity and Mortality Weekly Report, 16*(RR-16), 1–27.

Centers for Disease Control (CDC). (2001). *Exposure to environmental tobacco smoke and cotinine levels: Fact sheet.* CDC National Tobacco Control Program at http://www.cdc.gov.

Chapman, K. R., Tashkin, D. P., & Pye, D. J. (2001). Gender bias in the diagnosis of COPD. *Chest, 199,* 1691–1695.

Clark, M. A., Rakowski, W., Kviz, F. J., & Hogan, J. W. (1997). Age and stage of readiness for smoking cessation. *Journal of Gerontology: Social Sciences, 52B*(4), S212–S221.

Feldman, C. (2001). Pneumonia in the elderly. *Medical Clinics of North America, 85*(6), 1441–1459.

Glick, J. G., & Ressler, C. (2001). Altered health maintenance. In M. L. Maas, K. C. Buckwalter, M. D. Hardy, T. Tripp-Reimer, M. G. Titler, & J. P. Specht (Eds.), *Nursing care of older adults: Diagnoses, outcomes, and interventions* (pp. 6–22). St. Louis: Mosby.

Gross, P. A. (2001). Vaccines for pneumonia and new antiviral therapies. *Medical Clinics of North America, 86*(6), 1531–1544.

Gubser, V. L. (1998). Tuberculosis and the elderly: A community health perspective. *Journal of Gerontological Nursing, 24*(5), 36–41.

Iribarren, C., Tekawa, I. S., & Friedman, S. S. (1999). Effect of cigar smoking on the risk of cardiovascular disease, chronic obstructive pulmonary disease, and cancer in men. *New England Journal of Medicine, 340,* 1773–1780.

Johnson, J. C., Jayadevappa, R., Baccash, P. D., & Taylor, L. (2000). Nonspecific presentation of pneumonia in hospitalized older people: Age effect of dementia? *Journal of the American Geriatrics Society, 48,* 1316–1320.

Kuper, H. (2002). Tobacco use and cancer causation: Association by tumour type. *Journal of Internal Medicine, 252,* 206–224.

Lawson, F., Baker, V., Au, D., & McElhaney, J. E. (2000). Standing orders for influenza vaccination increased vaccination rates in inpatient settings compared with community rates. *Journal of Gerontology: Medical Sciences, 55A*(9), M522–M526.

McElhaney, J. E. (2002). Influenza: A preventable lethal disease. *Journal of Gerontology: Medical Sciences, 57A,* M627–M628.

Morgan, W. K. C., & Reger, R. B. (2000). Rise and fall of the FEV_1. *Chest, 118,* 1639–1644.

National Institute on Aging (NIA). (2001). *Action plan for aging research: Strategic plan for fiscal years 2001–2005.* Washington, DC: U.S. Department of Health and Human Services. NIH Publication No. 01-4961.

Nurminen, M. M., & Jaakkola, M. S. (2001). Mortality from occupational exposure to environmental tobacco smoke in Finland. *Journal of Occupational and Environmental Medicine, 43*(8), 687–693.

O'Connell, K. A. (2001). Smoking cessation among older clients. In E. A. Swanson, T. Tripp-Reimer, & K. Buckwalter (Eds.), *Health promotion and disease prevention in the older adult* (pp. 102–118). New York: Springer.

Perez-Guzman, C., Vargas, M. H., Torres-Cruz, A., & Villarreal-Velarde, H. (1999). Does aging modify pulmonary tuberculosis? A meta-analytical review. *Chest, 116,* 961–967.

Petty, T. L. (2000). Early studies of prevalence and NHANES III data: Basis for early identification and intervention. *Chest, 117*(5 Suppl. 2), 3265–3315.

Prochazka, A. V. (2000). New developments in smoking cessation. *Chest, 117*(4 Suppl. 1), 1695–1755.

Rea, T. D. (2002). Smoking status and risk for recurrent coronary events after myocardial infarction. *Annals of Internal Medicine, 137,* 494–500.

Taylor, D. H., Hasselblad, V., Henley, S. J., Thun, M. J., & Sloan, F. A. (2002). Benefits of smoking cessation for longevity. *American Journal of Public Health, 92,* 990–996.

Terry, P. B. (2000). Chronic obstructive pulmonary disease. In M. H. Beers & R. Berkow (Eds.), *The Merck manual of geriatrics* (3rd ed.). Whitehouse Station, NJ: Merck & Co., Inc.

Timmreck, R. C., & Randolph, J. F. (1993). Smoking cessation: Clinical steps to improve compliance. *Geriatrics, 48*(4), 63–70.

U.S. Department of Health and Human Services (USDHHS). (2000). *Healthy People 2010* (2nd ed.). Washington, DC: U.S. Government Printing Office.

U.S. Department of Health and Human Services (USDHHS). (2001). *Women and smoking: A report of the surgeon general.* Washington, DC: U.S. Government Printing Office.

Wakefield, B. (2001). Ineffective breathing pattern. In M. L. Maas, K. C. Buckwalter, M. D. Hardy, T. Tripp-Reimer, M. G. Titler, & J. P. Specht (Eds.), *Nursing care of older adults: Diagnoses, outcomes, and interventions* (pp. 313–323). St. Louis: Mosby.

Wolfsen, C., Barker, J. C., & Mitteness, L. S. (2001). Smoking and health: Views of elderly nursing home residents. *Journal of Gerontological Nursing, 27*(8), 6–12.

Wynd, C. A. (1997). Smoking cessation. In B. M. Dossey (Ed.), *Core curriculum for holistic nursing* (pp. 220–225). Gaithersburg, MD: Aspen.

Mobility and Safety

LEARNING OBJECTIVES

1. Delineate age-related changes that affect mobility and safety.
2. Examine risk factors that increase the risk for osteoporosis and influence the safety and mobility of older adults.
3. Discuss the following functional consequences: diminished musculoskeletal function, increased susceptibility to fractures, and increased susceptibility to falls.
4. Discuss the psychosocial and long-term consequences of falls, fractures, and osteoporosis.
5. Describe methods of assessing overall musculoskeletal performance and risks for falls and osteoporosis.
6. Identify interventions directed toward safe mobility and the elimination of risks for falls and osteoporosis.

Mobility is one of the most important aspects of physiologic function because it is essential for maintaining independence and because serious consequences occur when independence is lost. For older adults, mobility is influenced by age-related changes to some extent, but risk factors play a much larger role. Because of the many risks that threaten mobility, falls are an unfortunately common occurrence in old age. Older adults, then, have the dual challenge of maintaining mobility skills and avoiding falls. For these reasons, safety is considered an integral aspect of mobility.

 AGE-RELATED CHANGES THAT AFFECT MOBILITY AND SAFETY

The bones, joints, and muscles are the body structures most closely associated with mobility, but many additional functional aspects are involved in safe mobility.

Neurologic function, for example, influences all facets of musculoskeletal performance, and visual function influences the ability to interact safely with the environment. Within the musculoskeletal system, osteoporosis is the age-related change that has the most significant overall impact, has been studied the most, and is most amenable to interventions aimed at prevention and management. For these reasons, a separate section of this chapter is devoted to osteoporosis, and this section discusses other age-related changes that affect mobility.

Bones

Bones provide the framework for the entire musculoskeletal system and work in conjunction with the muscular system to facilitate movement. Additional functions of bone in the human body include storage of calcium, production of blood cells, and support and protection of body organs and tissues. Bone is composed of a hard outer layer, called cortical or compact bone, and an inner, spongy meshwork, called trabecular or cancellous bone. The proportion of cortical to trabecular components varies according to bone type. Long bones, such as the radius and femur, may be as much as 90% cortical, whereas flat and vertebral bones are composed primarily of trabecular cells. Both cortical and trabecular bone components are affected by age-related changes, but the rate and impact of age-related changes differ in the two types of bone. These changes are discussed in the separate section on osteoporosis as an age-related change.

Bone growth reaches maturity in early adulthood, but bone remodeling continues throughout one's lifetime. Age-related changes that affect this remodeling process include increased bone resorption, diminished calcium absorption, increased serum parathyroid hormone, impaired regulation of osteoblast activity, impaired bone formation secondary to reduced osteoblastic production of bone matrix, and a decreased number of functional marrow cells as a result of replacement of marrow with fat cells. These age-related changes affect both men and women and account for the age-dependent type of osteoporosis. In addition, diminished secretion of estrogen in women and testosterone in men is associated with an accelerated rate of bone loss. These factors are discussed in greater detail in the section on Osteoporosis as an Age–Related Change. The following factors also can affect bone remodeling and are common in older adults: hyperthyroidism, decreased activity levels, chronic obstructive pulmonary disease (COPD), deficiencies of calcium and vitamin D, and consumption of certain medications, such as glucocorticoids and anticonvulsants.

Muscles

All activities of daily living (ADLs) are directly influenced by the function of the skeletal muscles, which are controlled by motor neurons. The age-related changes that have the greatest impact on muscle function are: (1) a loss of muscle mass as a result of decreases in the size and number of muscle fibers; (2) deterioration of muscle fibers with subsequent replacement by connective tissue and, eventually, by fat tissue; and (3) deterioration of muscle cell membranes and a subsequent escape of fluid and potassium. By the age of 80 years, about 30% of the muscle mass is lost, although evidence indicates that some of this loss could be delayed by exercise (Westerterp & Meijer, 2001). In addition, an age-related loss of motor neurons occurs, and this, too, affects muscular function. The end result of these age-related changes is a decline in motor function and a loss of muscle strength and endurance. Although these are considered to be age-related changes, exercise programs to increase strength and endurance may help to prevent negative functional consequences.

Joints and Connective Tissue

Numerous age-related changes affect the tissues responsible for the function of all musculoskeletal joints, including non–weight-bearing joints. In contrast to the bones or muscles, which benefit from exercise, the joints are harmed, rather than helped, by continued use and show the effects of wear and tear, even in early adulthood. In fact, degenerative processes that affect the functional efficiency of the joints begin in the third decade, before skeletal maturity is reached, and affect the tendons, ligaments, and synovial fluid.

Some of the most significant age-related joint changes include the following:

1. Diminished viscosity of synovial fluid
2. Degeneration of collagen and elastin cells
3. Fragmentation of fibrous structures in connective tissue
4. Outgrowths of cartilaginous clusters in response to continuous wear and tear
5. Formation of scar tissue and areas of calcification in the joint capsules and connective tissue
6. Degenerative changes in the arterial cartilage resulting in extensive fraying, cracking, and shredding, in addition to a pitted and thinned surface

Some of the consequences of these changes include impaired flexion and extension movements, decreased flexibility of the fibrous structures, diminished protection from forces of movement, erosion of the bones underlying the outgrowths of cartilage, and diminished ability of the connective tissue to transmit the tensile forces that act on it.

Nervous System

Age-related changes of the nervous system affect gait, balance, body sway, and reaction time, which, in turn, affect safe mobility. Even in healthy older adults, combinations of age-related changes in vision, somatosensory function, and vestibular function affect balance control (Woollacott, 2000).

Maintenance of balance in an upright position is a complex skill that is affected by the following age-related changes: a decline in the righting reflex; impaired proprioception, particularly in women; and diminished vibratory sensation and joint position sense in the lower extremities. Body sway is a measure of the motion of the body when a person is standing still. Studies have found that age-related changes can have detrimental effects on postural control, causing an increase in body sway (Gill et al., 2001). Finally, age-related decreases in reaction time and speed of performance can influence mobility and safety. Diminished reaction time is one of the most widely acknowledged age-related changes, but there is disagreement about the mechanisms underlying this change. Regardless of the causative factors, the end result is slowed performance in walking and other ADLs. Also, decreased reaction time may interfere with cognitive and perceptual processes; indeed, older people have been found to respond more slowly to unexpected environmental stimuli than their younger counterparts. Therefore, older adults are at an increased risk for falls in unfamiliar environments or when encountering the unexpected.

OSTEOPOROSIS AS AN AGE-RELATED CHANGE

Osteoporosis is a process of gradual loss of bone mass that affects all adults to some degree and predisposes older adults to fractures. Geriatricians emphasize that the association between osteoporosis and low-trauma fractures (i.e., osteoporotic fractures) is so strong that "any meaningful definition of osteoporosis must include fracture" (Walker-Bone et al., 2001, p. 1). Of all the age-related changes, therefore, osteoporosis is the one that is most likely to cause serious negative functional consequences, even in the absence of additional risk factors.

Since the 1880s, primary care providers have been aware of the increased frequency of hip and forearm fractures in older women. However, it was not until the 1940s that estrogen deficiency was recognized as a major risk factor for osteoporosis and fractures in older women. By the 1960s, primary care providers suspected that many fractures in older women were associated with moderate or no trauma. During the 1970s and 1980s, the use of noninvasive methods for measuring bone density allowed much progress to be made in the understanding of osteoporosis. During the 1990s, pharmaceutical companies focused on developing safe and effective treatments for both the prevention and treatment of osteoporosis. By the early 2000s, the widespread availability and low cost of noninvasive measurements of bone density and the development and availability of several medication interventions for osteoporosis focused attention on the diagnosis, prevention, and treatment of osteoporosis in men as well as women. Emphasis also is currently being placed on lifestyle factors that reduce the risk for developing osteoporosis. Until the mid-1990s, most research focused on women, but current research and recommendations are attempting to address osteoporosis in older men and high-risk groups such as residents of long-term care facilities and people who use certain medications for long periods. A national consensus statement on osteoporosis was published by the National Institutes of Health in 2001 to report findings from an independent panel of experts (NIH, 2001). The statement addresses the following questions: (1) What is osteoporosis and what are its consequences? (2) How do risks vary among different segments of the population? (3) What factors influence skeletal health throughout life? (4) What is the optimal evaluation and treatment of osteoporosis and fractures? and (5) What are the directions for future research? (NIH, 2001). Current information about osteoporosis is reviewed in the following sections, and prevention and treatment approaches are discussed in section on Nursing Interventions to Prevent and Treat Osteoporosis.

Gender differences account for the relatively higher rate of osteoporosis among women compared with men. Both men and women reach peak bone mass in their mid-30s, but there are significant differences in patterns of bone loss between men and women. Women have a period of bone mass stability between peak level and the onset of menopause, when declining estrogen levels significantly impact bone mass. During the first decade after the onset of menopause, the annual rate of bone loss may be as much as 7%, but after menopause, it is between 1% and 2%. By contrast, the annual rate of bone loss in men is only about 1% after peak bone mass has been reached. Another gender difference is that men have more cortical bone than women and gain cortical bone through periosteal bone deposition until the age of 75 years

(Kenny & Prestwood, 2000). Consequently, bone diameter increases in men and confers a mechanical advantage in protecting from fractures (Shreyasee & Felson, 2001). In summary, primary osteoporosis occurs in both men and women, but women have a much greater percentage of bone loss over their lifetime and experience greater bone loss at an earlier age.

> Lifetime bone loss in women and men, respectively, is 35% and 23% (cortical bone) and 50% and 33% (trabecular bone).

With the wide availability of methods to assess bone mineral density (BMD), the diagnosis of osteoporosis has been defined according to standard deviation below peak bone mass. The World Health Organization's operational definition of osteoporosis is bone density that is at least 2.5 standard deviations below the mean for young white adult women (NIH, 2001). Because this definition applies only to white women, professional organizations, such as the World Health Organization and the National Osteoporosis Foundation, are currently addressing questions about how this definition applies to men and to younger and ethnically diverse populations (Kenny & Prestwood, 2000; NIH, 2001). Researchers have suggested several possibilities for defining osteoporosis in men, such as more than 2.5 standard deviations below the mean for young normal men (Shreyasee & Felson, 2001).

Traditionally, osteoporosis has been classified as primary when it is associated with age-related and menopause-related changes and as secondary when it is caused by medications or pathophysiologic disturbances. About 20% of women and between 40% and 50% of men with osteoporosis have a secondary cause (Kenny & Prestwood, 2000). Glucocorticoids, most commonly used for rheumatoid arthritis and COPD, are the medications that are most commonly associated with secondary osteoporosis. In recent years, attention has been paid to the potential relationship between inhaled glucocorticoids, a commonly used treatment for asthma, and diminished BMD. Israel and colleagues (2001) found that inhaled glucocorticoids are associated in a dose-dependent relationship with loss of BMD at the hip in premenopausal women. Researchers are addressing the potential relationship between inhaled glucocorticoids and lowered BMD for all gender and age categories. Antiepileptic agents, such as phenytoin and valproic acid, also are associated with osteoporosis (Sato et al., 2001). Pathologic conditions that are associated with secondary osteoporosis are osteomalacia, hyperthyroidism, hyperparathyroidism, and multiple myeloma. In men, hypogonadism is a common risk factor for secondary osteoporosis.

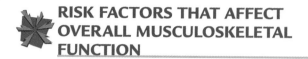

RISK FACTORS THAT AFFECT OVERALL MUSCULOSKELETAL FUNCTION

The risk factors for safe mobility that are of greatest concern are those that contribute to falls, fractures, and osteoporosis. These risks are of particular importance to gerontological nurses because health promotion interventions are appropriate for addressing many of the risk factors. In addition, when the risks are eliminated or minimized, the serious functional consequences are likely to be prevented.

Although it is difficult to differentiate between factors that increase the risk for falls, fractures, and osteoporosis and those that affect overall musculoskeletal function, some nutritional and lifestyle factors have been identified that have a detrimental effect on general musculoskeletal function. Lack of exercise is a well-known risk factor for diminished musculoskeletal performance, and evidence is mounting that various types of exercise are beneficial in slowing or preventing the age-related decline in muscle power (Evans, 2000). One review of studies indicated that a pattern of high physical activity is a critical factor in maintaining the structure and function of skeletal muscle and suggested that exercise training may delay age-induced declines in mobility that are associated with reduced physical activity (Westerterp & Meijer, 2001). Nutritional factors also are associated with overall musculoskeletal function; Campbell and colleagues (2001) concluded that the Recommended Dietary Allowance of 0.8 g/kg/day of protein may not be adequate for maintaining optimal skeletal muscle function in older adults. Another analysis suggested that low levels of vitamin D contribute to diminished muscle strength, impaired muscular function, and increased disability in community-living older women (Zamboni et al., 2002).

RISK FACTORS FOR THE DEVELOPMENT OF OSTEOPOROSIS AND FRACTURES

The development of primary osteoporosis is significantly influenced by gender differences, as discussed earlier, and by other factors, such as ethnicity. Both estrogens and androgens influence bone development in men and women. The role of estrogen in relation to osteoporosis in women has been studied for several decades, but studies are just beginning to address the role of testosterone in relation to osteoporosis in men. Late menarche, early menopause, and low endogenous estrogen levels have been associated with low BMD in women (NIH, 2001). Current studies are investigating the role of other hormones in osteoporosis as well as the role of estrogen as a risk factor in men. A discussion of hormonal influences in men concluded that healthy skeletal development of pubertal boys is strongly influenced by serum estradiol and testosterone levels, but that in older men, low BMD is associated more strongly with low estradiol levels than with either low testosterone or low adrenal androgens (Shreyasee & Felson, 2001).

> Rates of osteoporosis, ranging from highest to lowest are as follows:
> - Asians, Eskimos, Native Americans
> - White non-Hispanic women
> - Hispanic groups
> - White men and African American women
> - African American men

Additional risk factors associated with low BMD include increased age, family history, and low weight and body mass index (BMI). Daily intake of less than 1000 to 1500 mg of calcium and 400 to 600 IU of vitamin D also increases the risk for osteoporosis. High intakes of dietary protein, caffeine, sodium, and phosphorus can negatively affect calcium balance and may increase the risk for osteoporosis for people with inadequate calcium intakes (NIH, 2001). Lifestyle factors, such as cigarette smoking and inadequate amounts of weight-bearing activity, also can increase the risk for osteoporosis. The most widely acknowledged risks for developing osteoporosis are summarized in Display 18-1, along with the few factors that have been found to decrease the risk for osteoporosis.

In recent years, researchers have tried to identify those factors that increase the risk for fractures in people with osteoporosis. These studies attempt to differentiate between the risks for fracture and the risks for osteoporosis. Hip fracture is the more frequently studied type of fracture. Factors that consistently have been associated with increased fracture risk include impaired vision, impaired cognition, history of falls, the presence of environmental hazards, and diminished physical function, such as slow gait (NIH, 2001). Baron and colleagues (2001) found a strong association between the risk for hip fracture and duration of cigarette smoking in women, with more deleterious effects from smoking after menopause as compared with smoking before menopause. These researchers also found that the impact of smoking was reversible, with no increase in risk for hip fracture after 15 years of cessation. Studies of the effects of smoking in men also found an

DISPLAY 18-1
Factors Influencing the Risk for Osteoporosis

Factors That Increase the Risk for Osteoporosis
- Female gender
- Increased age
- Small bones
- Thinness, less-than-normal weight
- White or Asian race
- Genetic predisposition
- Low calcium intake, both past and current
- Inadequate vitamin D intake
- Prolonged immobility
- Lack of weight-bearing activity
- Estrogen deficiency (women)
- Decreased testosterone levels (men)
- Cigarette smoking
- Excessive alcohol intake
- Long-term use of certain medications (e.g., corticosteroids, anticonvulsants, thyroid hormones)
- Excessive use of antacids, particularly those that contain aluminum

Factors That Reduce the Risk for Osteoporosis
- Obesity
- Thiazide diuretics
- Hormonal therapy
- Medications approved for osteoporosis
- African American or Hispanic race

association between duration of smoking and lower BMD (Shreyasee & Felson, 2001). Wu and colleagues (2002) found that a history of a fracture between the ages of 20 and 50 years was associated with a 74% increase in the risk for fractures after the age of 50 years. Other studies suggest that a history of osteoporotic fracture at any site (even vertebrae) was predictive of developing additional osteoporotic fractures in older adults but not necessarily in younger adults (Walker-Bone et al., 2001).

Researchers have tried to identify gender and racial differences in risk factors for falls and fractures. For example, two specific gender differences relating to hip fractures are that men tend to be older than women when fractures occur and that men have more protection against fractures, such as that conferred by greater bone mass at maturity. Investigations of risk factors in older Mexican Americans found that hip fractures in women were associated independently with advanced age, history of a stroke, and living alone/not being married. These factors did not increase the risk for

Mexican American men in the study, but limitations in ADLs and instrumental ADLs increased the risk for hip fracture for both men and women (Espino et al., 2000). Ottenbacher and colleagues (2002) found that diabetes was associated with an increased risk for hip fracture in older Mexican Americans.

> Ms. M. is 55 years old and works as the secretary in the Senior Circle of Care program where you do health screening and educational programs. This program is a "senior wellness program" sponsored by one of the nonprofit hospitals in Minneapolis, Minnesota. Ms. M.'s responsibilities include finding and organizing health education materials under the direction of the nurses. You often go to lunch with her and discuss social and health-related topics. Ms. M. has always been inquisitive about health-related concerns, and one day she asks your advice about osteoporosis. She says that both she and her mother, who is 83 years old, have been receiving fliers about getting a bone density test, and that her mother asked if she would go with her so they could both be tested. You know from past conversations that Ms. M.'s mother fractured her wrist a long time ago but otherwise is relatively healthy. Ms. M. is pretty healthy, although she admits that she "could stand to lose a little weight." You also know from previous discussions that Ms. M. has been taking hormonal therapy for 5 years because you have had more than one lunchtime conversation with her about the pros and cons of estrogen. In your work as the senior wellness nurse, you have developed and presented several health education programs about osteoporosis and are fairly familiar with recent literature on osteoporosis.

 THINKING POINTS

> Based on what you know about Ms. M., what would you tell her about factors that influence her risk for osteoporosis?

> Based on what you know about Ms. M.'s mother, what additional information would you want to know before advising her about a test for her mother?

> How would you answer Ms. M.'s inquiry?

> What suggestions would you make to help Ms. M. become more knowledgeable about osteoporosis?

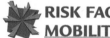 **RISK FACTORS FOR UNSAFE MOBILITY AND FALLS**

Falling is an age-related functional consequence that has been the focus of a great number of studies in Great Britain and the United States and continues to

be a major concern today. Almost a half century ago, an article entitled "On the Natural History of Falls in Old Age" began with the following declaration: "The liability of old people to tumble and often to injure themselves is such a commonplace of experience that it has been tacitly accepted as an inevitable aspect of ageing, and thereby deprived of the exercise of curiosity" (Sheldon, 1960, p. 1685). In the past decade, geriatricians and gerontologists have challenged this view that falls are a normal consequence of aging or are accidental or random events. It is now widely agreed that falls and mobility problems are caused by multiple, diverse, and interacting factors. The current clinical approach is to identify the most likely causes and contributing conditions and to plan interventions that address these factors (Morley, 2002).

Risk factors for falls can be categorized according to their origin as follows: age-related changes, common pathologic conditions and functional impairments, medication effects, and environmental factors (Display 18-2). Falls are the result of a combination of these factors, rather than one isolated risk factor, and the risk for falls increases in proportion to the number of fall risk factors. The many studies conducted to identify the underlying causes of falling in older adults have identified different underlying causes in different age groups. Falls in older adults younger than 75 years of age are often the consequence of trips and slips, predominantly attributable to a combination of age-related changes, such as vision changes, and unfavorable environmental conditions, such as poor lighting. A study of falls following a trip in healthy older adults found that walking quickly may be the greatest cause of this type of fall (Pavol et al., 2001). By contrast, falls in people older than 75 years of age are predominantly the result of a combination of disease- and medication-related factors (Tideiksaar, 1997).

Researchers also have identified different risks for falls according to the environment in which the older person lives. For example, falls in institutionalized older people are most often associated with weakness, dizziness, and gait and balance disorders, whereas falls in community-living populations tend to be associated with environmental factors (Rubenstein & Josephson, 2002). Basante and colleagues (2001) reviewed 21 studies of fall risks for older adults in long-term care facilities and identified medications (e.g., psychotropics), deconditioning (e.g., lower extremity weakness and gait and balance disorders), and physical restraints (e.g., vests, pelvic restraints, lap trays), or any combination of these factors as the major contributing factors. Harrison and colleagues (2001) studied risks for falls in 67 nursing home residents with a documented fall during a 3-month period and varying levels of cognition and found that the

---

DISPLAY 18-2
Examples of Risk Factors for Falls and Fractures

Age-Related Changes
- Vision and hearing changes
- Osteoporosis
- Slowed reaction time
- Altered gait, increased sway
- Postural hypotension
- Nocturia

Pathologic Conditions and Functional Impairments
- Cardiovascular diseases (e.g., arrhythmias or myocardial infarction)
- Respiratory diseases (e.g., chronic obstructive pulmonary disease [COPD])
- Neurologic disorders (e.g., parkinsonism, cerebrovascular accident [CVA])
- Metabolic disturbances (e.g., dehydration, electrolyte imbalances)
- Musculoskeletal problems (e.g., osteoarthritis)
- Transient ischemic attack (TIA)
- Vision impairments (e.g., cataracts, glaucoma, macular degeneration)
- Cognitive impairments (e.g., dementia, confusion)
- Psychosocial factors (e.g., depression, anxiety, agitation)

Medication Effects and Interactions
- Anticholinergics, including ingredients in over-the-counter products (e.g., diphenhydramine)
- Diuretics
- Benzodiazepines and other hypnotics
- Antipsychotics
- Antidepressants
- Antihypertensives
- Nonsteroidal antiinflammatory agents (NSAIDs)
- Alcohol

Environmental Factors
- Physical restraints, including bedrails
- Glare
- Inadequate lighting
- Lack of handrails on stairs
- Slippery floors
- Throw rugs
- Cords or clutter
- Unfamiliar environments
- Highly polished floors
- Improper height of beds, chairs, or toilets

---

number of falls increased as the level of cognition declined in residents with dementia. A study of 98 patients in a geriatric rehabilitation setting found that a primary diagnosis of cerebrovascular accident (CVA) was the only variable that increased the risk for falling (Patrick & Blodgett, 2001).

Age-Related Changes and Common Conditions in Older Adults

Age-related changes that can contribute to falls have been discussed throughout this text and were reviewed in the first section of this chapter. Nocturia, osteoporosis, vision changes, gait changes, orthostatic hypotension, decreased muscle strength, and central nervous system changes, such as decreased reaction time, may increase the risk for falls in older adults. Also, osteoporosis may increase the risk for serious injury when falls occur. Age-related changes alone rarely cause falls; rather, falls are usually attributable to interactions between the multiple risk factors that commonly affect older adults.

In addition to the age-related changes that increase the risk for falls, common pathologic conditions can also increase the risk for falls. Impaired vision caused by common pathologic conditions such as cataracts

and retinopathy is an important and independent risk factor for falls in older adults (Lord & Dayhew, 2001). Hearing impairments also influence safe mobility, particularly when older people are in unfamiliar or institutional environments. Hearing and vision, discussed comprehensively in Chapters 12 and 13, must be considered in any discussion of safe mobility.

Medical conditions are associated with falls in older adults in all of the following ways:

1. Medical conditions may be treated with medications that create risks for falling.
2. Illnesses can cause functional impairments, such as vision or mobility limitations.
3. Illnesses may cause metabolic or other physiologic disturbances that create risks for falls.
4. Falls may be one manifestation of an acute illness or a change in a chronic illness.
5. Chronic illnesses interfere with optimal exercise and other health practices that are important in promoting safe mobility.

A change in health status, such as a decline in a chronic condition or the onset of an acute medical condition, has been found to increase the risk for falls, especially when additional risk factors are present.

Considering all of these possible associations, it is not surprising that most falls resulting in injuries occur in people who have functional impairments and multiple, chronic medical problems.

Impairments in cognition or other areas of psychosocial function also can increase the risk for falls in older adults. Both dementia and depression may contribute to falls in that they diminish a person's awareness of the environment. Dementia can also interfere with the person's ability to process information regarding environmental stimuli. The following combination of factors is likely to increase the risk for falls in people with dementia: medications, concurrent conditions, decreased level of awareness, diminished ability to cope with environmental surroundings, and the severity of associated functional disabilities, such as mobility impairments (Shaw, 2002). Older adults who are depressed are at increased risk for falls secondary to gait changes, medication effects, and a diminished ability to concentrate on and respond to environmental factors. Sleep problems, also, have been found to be an independent risk factor for falls in community-living older adults (Brassington et al., 2000).

Medication Effects

Numerous studies have identified hundreds of medications that can contribute to falls, and some studies have looked at the relationship between falls, medications, and diagnosis. Not all conclusions are consistent with regard to specific medications or diagnoses, but the key to identifying an association between medications and falls is to consider the underlying mechanism of the medication action as well as the medical condition and the potential interactions between various factors. For example, orthostatic hypotension can be caused by medical conditions, age-related changes, or adverse medication effects. If an 80-year-old person has a medical condition (e.g., hypertension) that may cause orthostatic hypotension, and if the person is taking a medication (e.g., a vasodilator) that causes orthostatic hypotension, the risk for falls is significantly increased. Therefore, rather than memorizing all of the medications that have been found to increase the risk for falls, gerontological nurses can focus their attention on the underlying mechanisms that increase the risk for falls.

The following medication effects can increase the risk for falls: confusion, depression, sedation, arrhythmias, hypovolemia, orthostatic hypotension, delayed reaction time, diminished cognitive function, and changes in gait and balance (e.g., ataxia, decreased proprioception, and increased body sway). Thus, any medication that has one or more of these adverse effects may increase the risk for falls. Benzodiazepines have been widely studied in relation to an increased fall risk, and evidence suggests that a primary mechanism by which they contribute to falls is their effect on psychomotor function. This is just one of the adverse effects of benzodiazepines; others include sedation and impaired cognitive function.

Other medication-related considerations that influence the risk for falls include medication–disease interactions, medication–medication interactions, and medication–alcohol interactions. Also, the risk for falls can be affected by the dose, half-life, and administration time of the medication. For example, an association has been found between benzodiazepines with long half-lives (e.g., flurazepam) and an increased risk for falls and fractures and other fall-related injuries. Ray and colleagues (2000) found that the rate of falls among nursing home residents who were current users of benzodiazepines (versus the rate of falls in residents not using benzodiazepines) was increased 44% and that the risk for falls increased with higher doses, recent onset of use, and longer elimination half-life. In recent years, zolpidem has become a widely used nonbenzodiazepine sedative-hypnotic for older people because of the high association between benzodiazepines and falls. Wang and colleagues (2001), however, found that the use of zolpidem was associated with a 90% increased risk for hip fracture in a sample of older nursing home residents (mean age, 82 years), even after controlling for potential confounding effects.

Studies have focused primarily on prescription medications, but over-the-counter medications also can create risks for falls through their adverse effects on psychomotor function. For example, many over-the-counter preparations for pain, colds, and insomnia contain alcohol or anticholinergics. These ingredients may themselves pose risks, or may interact with other medications to increase the risk for falls. In recent years, the adverse effects of diphenhydramine, a widely used ingredient in over-the-counter products for sleep, colds, and allergies, have received much attention in the media and medical literature. Diphenhydramine has been associated with significant adverse effects on psychomotor skills involved in safe driving, and many states include this and other over-the-counter agents in laws pertaining to driving while impaired. Studies have found adverse effects of diphenhydramine on mood, speed, attention, vigilance, working memory, and level of activity. These effects may persist through the next day after an evening dose (Kay, 2000). The effects of even these over-the-counter medications on frail older adults can be a risk factor for falls and fall-related injuries. Some of the types of medications that are likely to increase the risk for falls are listed in Display 18-2.

Environmental Factors

Some environmental hazards were discussed in Chapter 13, but additional environmental influences must be considered specifically in relation to falls. In hospitals and nursing homes, for example, the first and second most common sites of falls are the bedroom and bathroom. In the bedroom, most falls occur while the person is getting in or out of bed, whereas some are related to climbing over side rails or footboards. In the bathroom, falls generally occur while transferring on or off of toilet seats or while hurrying to urinate or defecate. In community settings, most falls occur in the home, particularly in stairways, bedrooms, and living rooms. Activities that have been associated with falling in home settings include slipping on wet surfaces, slipping while descending stairs, getting in and out of beds and chairs, and tripping over floor coverings or objects on the floor. Studies have also revealed that the influence of some environmental factors differs depending on the setting. For example, assistive devices have been associated with falls in hospitals and nursing homes, but not in community settings (Tideiksaar, 1997). A nursing study of rural older adults found an association between a rural lifestyle and episodes of falling. For example, more than 50% of the falls occurred outdoors, and 44% of the falls occurred during tasks related to support or maintenance of the home (Baldwin et al., 1996).

Physical Restraints

Since the mid-1960s, physical restraints have commonly been used in institutional settings with the intent of protecting impaired people from injury and reducing staff work load. Historically, the belief that the use of physical restraints protects vulnerable people from falls and protects the institution from liability was widespread. Starting in the mid-1980s, however, the validity of this belief began to be questioned. Since the 1990s, there has been growing evidence that restraints not only do not reduce the risk of falls, but that when they are used older adults are more likely to experience serious injury from falls (Twersky, 2001). Dunn (2001) found no significant difference in the number of falls, but a decrease in severity of fall-related injuries, after a restraint-free environment was established in a long-term care facility. In addition to being associated with fall-related injuries, restraints have been found to cause agitation, strangulation, deconditioning, and pressure ulcers (Shorr et al., 2002).

Since the late 1980s, bedrails have been considered a form of restraint, except when they are used to facilitate bed mobility. In recent years, many questions have been raised about their safety and effectiveness, particularly for people who are cognitively impaired and unable to understand the intent of bedrails. As with other restraints, little evidence supports their use, and reducing the use of bedrails has not been associated with increased risk for falls. One study found that reducing the use of bedrails in hospitalized patients did not alter the number of falls but was associated with fewer serious injuries (Hanger et al., 1999). Another study of residents of a short-term rehabilitation unit found that bedrails did not enhance safety and that serious injuries were not associated with removal of bedrails (Si et al., 1999). Capezuti and colleagues (2002) concluded that bilateral bedrail use in nursing home residents does not significantly reduce the likelihood of falls, recurrent falls, or serious injuries.

During the 1990s, agencies such as the Food and Drug Administration (FDA), the Health Care Financing Administration, and the Joint Commission on Healthcare Organizations challenged the use of restraints in hospitals and nursing homes and urged the use of less restrictive safety measures. The American Nurses Association also has stated that physical restraints should be used only when no other viable option is available (American Nurses Association, 1999). In 2001, the American Geriatrics Society, the British Geriatrics Society, and the American Academy of Orthopaedic Surgeons Panel on Falls Prevention (2001) concluded that there is no evidence to support the use of restraints for fall prevention and, in fact, that restraints can contribute to serious injuries. These efforts have resulted in a 50% to 75% decrease in use of restraints in nursing homes since the late 1980s (Weintraub & Spurlock, 2002).

In summary, falls must be viewed as complex events that occur more commonly in older adults who have several contributing factors. The risk for falls increases as the number of contributing factors increases. Contributing factors can be intrinsic or extrinsic, and the risk can often be reduced through interventions, as discussed later in this chapter.

> Ms. M. is now 67 years old and has retired from her secretarial job. She attends weekly social and lunch gatherings at the local senior center, where you are the wellness nurse. One day she comes to the center with a cast on her left wrist and reports that she fractured her wrist when she slipped and fell on ice in her driveway. You know from prior conversations with her that she stopped taking hormonal therapy several years ago because she had been on it for more than 10 years and was concerned about long-term effects. You also know that she takes medications for arthritis, hypertension, and depression and that she self-monitors her

blood pressure. In the past 10 years, she has gradually gained "a little weight every year," and her current height/weight is 5'3"/172 pounds. She participates in the weekly "mall walkers" exercise program but does not often exercise independently. She says that "my housework is enough exercise" and that the weekly group exercise activity is "as much as my arthritis will tolerate." She lives in a small one-floor house. Although Ms. M. says she is not really concerned about sustaining any more fractures because she views the recent fall as a "fluke of bad winter luck," she makes an appointment to talk with you. During the appointment, she reports that she is a "little concerned about osteoporosis."

 THINKING POINTS

➤ What risk factors for osteoporosis can you identify from what you already know about Ms. M.?

➤ What risk factors for falls and fall-related injuries can you identify from what you already know about Ms. M.?

➤ Can you identify any factors that diminish her risk for falls or fractures?

➤ What additional information about Ms. M. would be helpful in identifying additional risks for osteoporosis?

➤ What additional information would be helpful in identifying additional risks for falls and fractures?

PATHOLOGIC CONDITIONS THAT CAN AFFECT MUSCULOSKELETAL FUNCTION

Osteoarthritis, a degenerative disease affecting joints, occurs almost universally in older adults. Although it is often viewed as an extreme progression of age-related changes, it is not necessarily an inevitable consequence of aging. Age-related changes of bones and cartilage are almost universally present after the age of 60 years, but not all older adults will have symptoms of osteoarthritis (Loeser, 2000). Osteoarthritis is now considered a very complex disease process that results from the interplay of factors such as trauma, genetics, obesity, and age-related changes. Diminished estrogen also may be a contributing factor in postmenopausal women. Preventive measures for osteoarthritis include regular, moderate exercise; weight loss if appropriate; avoidance of high-impact activities; and adequate intake of vitamins C and D.

Whites and African Americans have similar rates of arthritis, but African Americans have a higher rate of arthritis-related activity limitation.

Treatment measures include losing weight if appropriate; wearing good shock-absorbing shoes; using analgesics and moist heat for pain; balancing rest periods and weight-bearing activities; participating in a supervised exercise program that focuses on improving musculoskeletal strength, balance, and endurance; and using walkers and other assistive devices as appropriate for relief of weight-bearing, improved balance, or independent functioning. Complementary therapies commonly used for osteoarthritis include acupuncture; magnetic therapy; therapeutic touch; glucosamine and chondroitin; and vitamins C, D, and E. A care plan for management of osteoarthritis involves an interdisciplinary approach including medicine, nursing, physical therapy, and occupational therapy. Because self-care is an important aspect of management, nurses focus much of their interventions on health education.

 ## FUNCTIONAL CONSEQUENCES ASSOCIATED WITH MUSCULOSKELETAL CHANGES IN OLDER ADULTS

Musculoskeletal function is affected to some degree by age-related changes, but the functional consequences have little impact on healthy older adults and can be compensated for, at least in part, through exercise. Age-related changes in joint function slightly impact mobility and range of motion, but in the absence of osteoarthritis and other disease-related processes, the functional consequences are not serious. The functional consequences of osteoporosis, however, are quite serious, as are the functional consequences that occur as a result of the combination of age-related changes and the hundreds of risk factors that contribute to falls in older adults. As with many other aspects of function in older adulthood, cumulative and interacting effects of risk factors rather than age-related changes most significantly affect function and quality of life.

The Impact of Musculoskeletal Changes on Overall Musculoskeletal Function

Muscle strength, endurance, and coordination are affected to some extent by age-related changes, even in the absence of risk factors. Beginning at about the age of 40 years, muscle strength declines gradually, resulting in an overall decrease of 30% to 50% by the age of 80 years, with a greater decline in muscle strength in the lower extremities than in the upper extremities. Diminished muscle strength is attributed primarily to age-related loss of muscle mass. In addition, a person's current level of activity and lifelong patterns of exercise can influence muscle strength at any age. Muscle endurance and coordination diminish as a result of age-related changes in the muscles and central nervous system. As a consequence of these changes, older adults experience muscle fatigue after shorter periods of exercise compared with their younger counterparts.

Joint function begins to decline in the third decade and diminishes gradually throughout one's lifetime. The outcome of these degenerative changes is a diminished range of motion, resulting in the following changes: (1) decreased motion in the upper arms, potentially causing difficulty with activities such as writing, eating, and grooming; and (2) decreased lower back flexion, hip flexion and external rotation, knee flexion, and foot dorsiflexion, causing potential difficulties with putting shoes and socks on and climbing stairs and curbs. The overall impact of diminished joint function is that an older person's ability to respond to environmental stimuli and perform ADL is slowed.

Gait changes, which differ in men and women, are one of the more noticeable functional consequences that occur after the age of 75 years. A waddling gait and a narrower base of walking and standing develop in older women. In addition, women have less muscular control, and bowlegged-type changes develop that affect the lower extremities and alter the angle of the hip. In contrast to the narrower gait of older women, the walking and standing gait of older men becomes wider with age. Older men develop a walking pattern characterized by less arm swing, a shorter stride, decreased step height, and a more flexed position of the head and trunk than when they were younger. The overall impact of these changes is that older men and women have a slower walking speed and spend more time in the support phase of gait than in the swing phase. These changes are thought to contribute to the increased susceptibility of older adults to falls. For example, studies indicate that elderly persons who fall tend to have a slower walking speed, shorter stride length, and a greater variability in step length (Tideiksaar, 1997). Although many older adults have gait disorders, significant gait changes should not be considered an inevitable result of aging. Exercise and an active lifestyle can significantly improve gait in older adults.

The Impact of Musculoskeletal Changes on Susceptibility to Fractures

One of the most significant of all age-related functional consequences is the increased susceptibility to fractures that is the direct result of osteoporosis. Even in the absence of additional risk factors, this age-related change contributes to the high incidence of fractures in older adults. Fractures are not unique to older adults, but they do differ in many respects from those that occur in younger populations. First, bones of older adults may be fractured with little or no trauma, whereas bones of healthy children and younger adults are usually fractured in response to a forceful impact. Fractures are classified as osteoporotic, or fragility fractures, when they occur as the result of even minimal trauma—that is, trauma that is no more severe than that resulting from falling to the floor from a standing position. Second, the risk for fractures increases in direct relation to age (in older women, the number of years since menopause may be a more accurate risk indicator than chronologic age). Third, it is more likely that fractures in older adults, particularly hip fractures, will have serious consequences affecting independence and quality of life, as discussed later in this section.

There is little doubt that the functional consequences of age-related changes affecting the musculoskeletal system differ between men and women. In children and younger adults, men sustain fractures more often than women, but after the age of 35 years, the overall fracture incidence in women increases sharply to the point that the rates become twice those in men at about sixth decade (Walker-Bone et al., 2001). Whites and Asians have a much higher rate of osteoporotic fractures than do African Americans, but the reasons for this are not clear. Factors that may contribute to this discrepancy include the higher bone mass of African Americans at skeletal maturity, the greater bone density and thicker bone cortex of African Americans, and the slower rate of age- or menopause-related bone loss in the African American population.

The Impact of Musculoskeletal Changes on Susceptibility to Falls

Numerous age-related changes and risk factors contribute to the high incidence of falls among older adults, particularly older women. A review of studies regarding the frequency of falls in older adults revealed the following (Tideiksaar, 1997):

- In community settings, 25% of people aged 65 to 74 years and 33% of those aged 75 years and older fall every year. Fifty percent of these older adults who fall experience multiple falls.
- In acute care settings, about 20% of older patients fall during their hospital stay, with as many as 50% of those patients who fall experiencing multiple falls.
- In nursing homes, up to 50% of residents fall each year, with at least 40% of those who fall experiencing multiple falls.

The combination of age-related changes and multiple interacting risk factors doubly jeopardizes older adults by increasing the probability of both falls and fractures.

One of the reasons that falls, fractures, and osteoporosis have been the focus of so many studies is that these events have a tremendous impact on health care expenditures for older adults, and much of this financial impact is borne by the health care system and by society at large. This concern is warranted because falls are the most costly injury among older people in the United States and are the leading cause of injury-related hospitalizations for older people (Ellis & Trent, 2001). Additional financial implications include the following (Tideiksaar, 1997):

- Twenty percent of hospital admissions and up to 40% of nursing home admissions of older adults are related to falling.
- The average length of hospital stay for an individual who has fallen is nearly twice that of an individual who has not fallen.
- By the age of 90 years, 33% of women and 17% of men have had a hip fracture.
- The number of new hip fractures per year doubles during each decade beyond the age of 50 years.

Even more important than the financial consequences are the quality-of-life consequences associated with falls and fractures. Many studies confirm that falls and fractures contribute to long-term functional decline and impairment in older adults, but the impact on level of functioning cannot be measured in dollars and cents. The following statistics from several literature reviews reflect some of the long-term consequences of falls and fractures (Ellis & Trent, 2001; Magaziner et al., 2000):

- Eighteen percent to thirty-three percent of older people who fracture a hip die within a year.
- Forty-five percent of older adults who live at home at the time of their fracture are discharged to long-term care, and 15% to 25% remain in a long-term care setting for a year after the fracture.
- Nearly 67% of people aged 85 years or older admitted to a hospital for fall injuries are transferred to a long-term care facility.
- As many as 75% of those who are independent before a hip fracture can neither walk independently nor achieve their previous level of independent living within 1 year of the fracture.

Both men and women who fracture a hip have an increased risk for dying within 2 years, but this outcome is significantly greater for men (Fransen et al., 2002).

These statistics underscore the importance of health promotion interventions to prevent osteoporosis and the occurrence of falls in older adults. Health promotion interventions also can be directed at minimizing the risk for serious fall-related injuries.

The Impact of Musculoskeletal Changes on Quality of Life

Two decades ago, the phrase *postfall syndrome* was used to describe a distinct gait pattern that is adopted by older people who have fallen and have been admitted to the hospital for postfall injuries (Murphy & Isaacs, 1982). People who have this syndrome do not have any neurologic or orthopedic problems that could account for the gait, and the characteristic gait pattern was not present before the fall. Postfall syndrome is composed of the following characteristics: an expressed fear of falling when standing erect, a tendency to grab and clutch at objects within view, and marked hesitancy and irregularity in walking attempts (Murphy & Isaacs, 1982). Maki (1997) found that some gait changes, such as prolonged double support (i.e., longer time on both feet) and reduced speed and stride length, are more common in older people who are afraid of falling than those who are not. The author of this study suggested that these fear-related gait changes might increase stability and serve to protect against falls.

Beginning in the mid-1980s, the term *fallaphobia* was used to describe the following sequence of events: (1) older people fall, lose their balance, or feel at risk for falling; (2) they lose confidence in their ability to perform the activity that led to or created a risk for falling; (3) they stop performing the activity; and (4) they eventually become homebound or chair bound (Tideiksaar & Kay, 1986). During the 1990s, fear of falling was identified as "the most commonly reported anxiety among older people, exceeding even fear of robbery or financial difficulties" (Yardley & Smith, 2002, p. 17). Situational fear of falling occurs when fear of falling is associated with the performance of a particular activity (e.g., bathing, toileting, climbing stairs, or walking outside). People with situational fear of falling usually avoid the associated activity or become quite anxious when forced to participate in the feared activity. This fear and avoidance of activities may eventually extend to activities other than the one originally associated with fear of falls (Tideiksaar, 1997).

Fear of falling is often associated with the occurrence and severity of previous falls, but some studies have found that even nonfallers can develop a fear of falling (Murphy et al., 2002). Additional variables that are associated with a fear of falling include pain, frailty, anxiety, depression, poor health and balance, lower levels of mobility and activity, poorer quality of life, and use of prescription medications (Drozdick & Edelstein, 2001; Yardley & Smith, 2002). Cumming and colleagues (2000) found that fear of falling was a serious health problem even for nonfallers and that being afraid of falling was predictive of being admitted to a long-term nursing facility among fallers, but not among nonfallers. These researchers also found a strong relationship in both fallers and nonfallers between low fall-related self-efficacy and a decline in functional abilities.

Fear of falling can have a protective effect when it helps older adults avoid hazards, but it also is likely to have detrimental effects such as shame, anxiety, depression, social isolation, loss of confidence, and diminished quality of life. Fear of falling kindles the development of additional fears about physical harm, long-term functional disability, loss of independence, social embarrassment and indignity, and damage to personal confidence and identity (Yardley & Smith, 2002). Also, it often causes older people—especially those who are frail and have had an injurious fall—to restrict excessively their activities (Murphy et al., 2002). Fear of damage to one's identify may be the factor that explains the strong relationship between fear of falling and avoidance of situations in which falling may be publicly witnessed (Yardley & Smith, 2002).

Family caregivers of older adults also may be quite anxious about potential falls, and they may experience excessive worry about the possibility that the older person might fall. This fear can lead to decisions that restrict an older adult's activities unnecessarily or that result in a move to a setting that provides a greater level of assistance or supervision than the older person desires. Although a move to an unfamiliar environment will not necessarily protect the person from falls and may even increase the risk for falls, the caregivers who encourage or make such a decision may derive some peace of mind because they perceive that the older person is safer. Although there is now agreement that restraints do not prevent falls and are likely to contribute to more serious fall-related injuries, many families and some health care workers may continue to believe that restraints and restricted activity are safe and effective fall prevention interventions. Gerontological nurses are in a good position to provide health education about this most important aspect of care. Because of the current emphasis on providing restraint-free environments, more attention is being paid to identifying and addressing fall risks and to providing restraint-free methods of ensuring safe mobility for people who are at risk for falls.

Figure 18-1 illustrates the age-related changes and risk factors that are most likely to interact to cause negative functional consequences. Fig. 18-1

NURSING ASSESSMENT OF MUSCULOSKELETAL FUNCTION

Nursing assessment of musculoskeletal function focuses on identifying risk factors for falls and osteoporosis as well as identifying the functional consequences of age-related musculoskeletal changes that affect ADLs. Assessment of risks for falls and osteoporosis should pay particular attention to those factors that can be modified or alleviated through health promotion and other nursing interventions. Also, it is important to identify the degree of risk for either osteoporosis or falls so that appropriate preventive interventions can be planned and implemented based on the degree of risk. Although even a low risk for falls or osteoporosis creates numerous opportunities for health promotion interventions, a higher risk is associated with greater nursing responsibility for health education and preventive interventions.

Assessing Overall Musculoskeletal Performance

For healthy older adults, the primary effects of age-related changes on musculoskeletal performance are a change in gait and slower performance of some ADLs. Older adults who have osteoarthritis, neurologic conditions, or other conditions that can affect gait, balance, or joint function are likely to have additional functional consequences that affect their musculoskeletal function. In assessing overall musculoskeletal performance, it is important to identify whether the changes are due to age-related changes or a pathologic condition because interventions may vary depending on the underlying cause. Assessment of overall musculoskeletal performance begins with observation of the person's mobility and activities. In addition to watching the person walk, it is especially important to observe the person getting up from a hard-back chair without arms.

Additional assessment information is obtained by asking questions about the person's ability to perform ADLs. In addition, when any limitations are identified, it is important to find out whether the older adult is using assistive devices to improve mobility, balance, or overall function; safety; and independence. If the person is not using such devices and may benefit from them, the nurse should assess both the person's knowledge about the availability of such devices as well as his or her attitude about using them because attitudes are likely to influence the

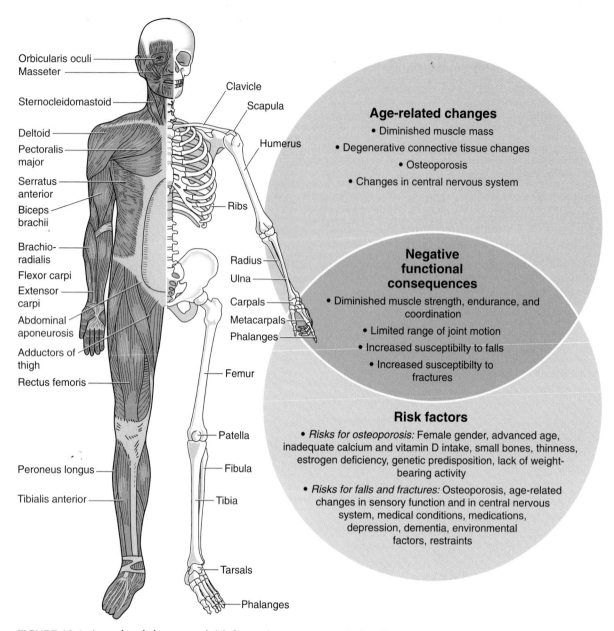

Orbicularis oculi
Masseter
Sternocleidomastoid
Deltoid
Pectoralis major
Serratus anterior
Biceps brachii
Brachio-radialis
Flexor carpi
Extensor carpi
Abdominal aponeurosis
Adductors of thigh
Rectus femoris
Peroneus longus
Tibialis anterior

Clavicle
Scapula
Humerus
Ribs
Radius
Ulna
Carpals
Metacarpals
Phalanges
Femur
Patella
Fibula
Tibia
Tarsals
Phalanges

Age-related changes
- Diminished muscle mass
- Degenerative connective tissue changes
- Osteoporosis
- Changes in central nervous system

Negative functional consequences
- Diminished muscle strength, endurance, and coordination
- Limited range of joint motion
- Increased susceptibilty to falls
- Increased susceptibilty to fractures

Risk factors
- *Risks for osteoporosis:* Female gender, advanced age, inadequate calcium and vitamin D intake, small bones, thinness, estrogen deficiency, genetic predisposition, lack of weight-bearing activity
- *Risks for falls and fractures:* Osteoporosis, age-related changes in sensory function and in central nervous system, medical conditions, medications, depression, dementia, environmental factors, restraints

FIGURE 18-1 Age-related changes and risk factors interact to negatively affect musculoskeletal function in older adults.

acceptability of using recommended aids. Criteria for the functional assessment of all ADLs are provided in Chapter 11 and can be used in conjunction with the assessment information in this chapter.

In addition to experiencing minor changes in performance of ADLs, older adults experience changes in posture and diminished height. Older adults may be concerned about loss of height or may not even be aware of this change; in any case, height changes do not significantly affect the usual activities of older adults. A height loss of about 2 to 4 cm per decade is normal, owing to osteoporosis and other age-related changes. Including a question about the person's usual height and any noticeable loss of height will give the nurse an opportunity to assess the older adult's awareness of this change. Although the functional consequences of decreased height are minimal, older people who never were very tall may experience increased difficulty performing activities that depend on height. In these situations, they may find that it is safer and more effective to use assistive devices, such as long-handled reachers. They also may need encouragement to rearrange cupboards so that the most frequently used items are accessible.

DISPLAY 18-3
Guidelines for Assessing Overall Musculoskeletal Function and Risks for Falls and Osteoporosis

Questions to Assess Overall Musculoskeletal Performance

- Do you have any trouble performing your usual activities because of joint limitations?
- Do you have any pain or discomfort in your joints?
- Do you ever feel like you are losing your balance?
- Do you have any trouble walking or getting around?
- Do you use any assistive devices (e.g., a walker, quad cane, or reaching devices) to help you do things?

Questions to Assess Risks for Osteoporosis
Questions to Ask All Older Adults

- Do you know of any blood relatives who have had osteoporosis or who have sustained fractures late in life?
- Have you sustained any fractures during your adult years? (If yes, ask additional questions regarding age at the time, type, location, circumstances, treatment, and so on.)
- Do you take any calcium or vitamin D supplements?
- Have you ever had your bone density measured?
- Have you ever talked with your primary care practitioner about prevention of osteoporosis?
- Do you take any medications for osteoporosis?

Questions to Ask Women

- When did you begin menopause?
- Do you take, or have you ever taken, estrogen or other hormonal therapy? (If yes, ask additional questions regarding type, dose, duration, and so on.)

Questions to Assess Risk for Falls and Fear of Falling

- Have you had any falls in the past few years? (If yes, ask additional questions about the circumstances and ask about pertinent risk factors as summarized in Display 18-2.)
- Are you afraid of falling? (If yes, ask additional questions about specific fears, such as, *What do you think might happen if you were to fall?*)
- Are there any activities you would like to do, but do not do, because of any difficulty moving or getting around?

(If yes, ask about specific activities, such as shopping, using public transportation, and so on).
- Are there any activities you would like to do, but do not do, because you are afraid of falling? (If yes, ask about specific activities, such as going up or down stairs, taking a bath or shower, and so on).

Observations Regarding Overall Musculoskeletal Performance

- Measure and record the person's present height and stated peak height.
- Observe the individual's walking and gait pattern.
- Observe the person rising from a chair.

Information From the Overall Assessment That Is Also Useful in Assessing Musculoskeletal Function

- Observe and document a functional assessment, as described in Chapter 11.
- How much exercise does the person get on a regular basis? In particular, how much weight-bearing exercise?
- Does the person smoke cigarettes?
- How much alcohol does the person consume?
- What is the person's usual daily intake of calcium and vitamin D?
- Does the person have any medical conditions that are associated with falls or osteoporosis (as summarized in Displays 18-1 and 18-2)?
- Is the person taking any medications that might create risks for falls (including over-the-counter medications)?
- Does the person have postural hypotension?
- Is the person moderately or seriously visually impaired?
- Does the person have any cognitive impairments or other psychosocial impairments that diminish his or her attention to the environment or interfere with the ability to respond to environmental stimuli?

Display 18-3 summarizes guidelines for assessing overall musculoskeletal performance in older adults.

Assessing Risk for Osteoporosis

Because some health promotion interventions for osteoporosis, such as adequate intake of calcium and vitamin D and participation in regular weight-bearing exercise, are universally applicable, nurses assess risks in all older adults. Nurses also identify modifiable risk factors, such as smoking and excessive amounts of alcohol, that can be alleviated through lifestyle interventions. If the nursing assessment identifies risk factors that cannot be modified (e.g., small bones), this information may be used to motivate the person to take action to eliminate the risks. Much of the information regarding risks for osteoporosis is obtained during an overall assessment or health history, and this information should be considered in relation to mobility and safety.

A diagnostic evaluation for osteoporosis is generally based on tests of BMD. Frequently used methods of measuring BMD include radiographic absorptiometry (RA), quantitative ultrasonography, dual photo absorptiometry (DPA), single photon absorptiometry (SPA), quantitative computed tomography (QCT), and dual-energy X-ray absorptiometry (DXA or DEXA). Sites that are evaluated include the hip, hand, wrist, heel, tibia, forearm, and lumbar spine. Because these tests have become widely available and community-based screening programs are becoming more common, nurses need to be knowledgeable about them so that they can provide health education to older adults about their value and the implications of their results. Universal screening is not recommended at this time, but guidelines emphasize that BMD measurement should be taken when the information will help the person and the health care practitioner make decisions about interventions or when monitoring of interventions is warranted (NIH, 2001). Medicare covers the cost of BMD testing every 2 years for the following five groups: people with vertebral abnormalities or primary hyperparathyroidism, women who are estrogen deficient or at clinical risk for osteoporosis, and patients taking long-term glucocorticoids therapy or being monitored for response to treatment with an FDA-approved osteoporosis medication.

With the increasing availability of safe and effective medical interventions, information provided by BMD tests has become more important, especially for people who have several risk factors for osteoporosis. Even people who are at lower risk for osteoporosis may find that information about BMD may assist in decisions about initiating medical treatment because some medical interventions involve risks (e.g., hormonal therapy) and can be quite expensive. For example, a woman with a BMD that is just slightly below normal may decide to forego prescription medications while she increases her weight-bearing activities and her intake of calcium and vitamin D. On the other hand, a woman whose BMD is 4 standard deviations below normal may feel that the risk and expense of prescription medications may be worthwhile. As new information evolves and new medical interventions are developed, guidelines for BMD tests are likely to expand, possibly to the point of universal screening for older men as well as women. Nurses should assess the older adult's awareness of BMD tests and ask whether the person has discussed them with his or her primary care practitioner. See Display 18-3 for assessment questions and considerations relating to osteoporosis.

Assessing Risk for Falls and Fear of Falling

Identifying fall risk is an essential part of health care for older adults because it is imperative to initiate preventive interventions for people at risk for falls. Standards for the management and prevention of falls in vulnerable older adults recommend that health care professionals ask an older person at least one screening question per year about the occurrence of falls (Rubenstein et al., 2001). This guideline is based on evidence that falls "are common, often preventable, frequently unreported, and often the cause of injury and unnecessary restriction of activity, which results in a reduction of overall health and quality of life. In addition, a recent history of falls is a strong predictor of future falls" (Rubenstein et al., 2001, p. 688). Guidelines also recommend further assessment for all older people who report even a single fall and for those who are observed to be unsteady (American Geriatrics Society et al., 2001).

Because prevention of falls and fall-related injuries is an important aspect of health promotion for older adults, all nurses working with older adults are responsible for assessing and documenting fall risk factors, particularly in institutional settings. Even in home and community settings where older adults are relatively independent, nurses can follow the guidelines of the American Geriatrics Society by observing for apparent risk factors and asking each person one question about the occurrence of falls annually. For any person with a history of falls or several other risk factors for falls, further fall risk assessment must be done and documented so that any modifiable factors can be addressed. In addition, nurses assess for factors that influence the risk for fall-related injury so that these can be addressed as well. See Display 18-3 for guidelines for assessment questions that are applicable to older adults who are independent or relatively independent.

Fall risk assessment is multidimensional and ideally includes observing the person in his or her usual environment. Although nurses in institutional settings focus their assessment on the person's immediate environment, they also must be concerned about the person's home environment as part of their discharge planning for people who are at risk for falls. Although the same assessment criteria are used for environmental safety, regardless of the setting, specific fall risks will vary according to the environment. For example, poor lighting and throw rugs are common fall risks in home environments, whereas assistive devices are common fall risks in institutional settings. The best assessment information is obtained by observing the person in the environment and paying particular attention to the person's awareness of and attention to the environment. Observations are especially helpful in identifying discrepancies between the person's perception of his or her abilities and his or her actual performance. Observations also provide information about adaptive behaviors that otherwise might not be acknowledged. For example, a person might state that he or she has no difficulty with stair climbing, but observations might reveal that the person performs this activity in a highly unsafe manner. Nurses in institutional settings generally do not have opportunities to observe home environments directly, but they can observe the person in the immediate environment and ask the person or their caregivers questions about the home setting and their ability to function safely in that setting. They can also consider referrals to home care agencies for home assessment as part of the discharge plan. The guidelines summarized in Display 18-4 can be used to assess the safety of any environment and can be applied to all older adults, particularly those who have intrinsic risk factors for falls.

In the past decades, many fall risk assessment tools have been developed and are now readily available for use in different settings. The purpose of these tools is to identify people who are at high risk for falls so that comprehensive assessment can be done and interventions can be planned. The two general types of fall risk assessment tools are functional assessment scales and nursing fall risk tools. Functional assessment scales, which focus on the person's mobility, are usually done by physical therapists or primary care practitioners. These tools specifically identify gait and balance problems that increase the risk for falls. Nurses can informally assess gait and balance by asking the person to sit in a firm straight-backed chair with armrests, stand up from the chair and walk a few steps, then turn around and return to the chair. Nurses also can observe the usual walking pattern of the person, paying particular attention to any gait or balance unsteadiness or unusual patterns. If any abnormalities are noted, nurses can suggest that further evaluation be done by a primary care provider. Nurses also can suggest that referrals be made to a physical therapist for further assessment and recommendations about a therapy program.

Nursing fall risk assessment tools are widely used in institutional settings as well as home and community-based settings. The Hartford Institute for Geriatric Nursing recommends the use of the Fall Assessment Tool (Figure 18-2) because it detects those people who are at high risk for falls, and a reassessment detects changes in risk factors (Farmer, 2000). Like many other nursing fall risk assessment tools, this tool assigns a numeric value to each factor, with a cumulative score that indicates degree of risk. Some assessment tools were developed specifically for one type of setting, and some studies have compared the use of various instruments. One study suggested that fall risk assessment for community-dwelling older adults focus simply and specifically on a combination of balance and mobility problems and a history of a fall during the previous year (Covinsky et al., 2001). A review of functional and nursing fall risk assessment tools concluded that functional assessment

tools are most appropriate for outpatient settings and that nursing assessment tools are more appropriate and efficient in acute care settings (Perell et al., 2001). This review also suggested that in extended care facilities, "where the majority of patients may be at high risk, applying universal precautions for falls may be more appropriate than relying on individual assessments, especially when nursing and rehabilitative interventions are already being utilized." (Perell et al., 2001, p. M765).

Fall risk assessment tools are useful in identifying people who are at high risk for falls, but they do not provide a base for comprehensive assessment of causative factors. If several risk factors are identified or if an older adult has already fallen, a more extensive assessment is required. Comprehensive fall assessments can be done by primary care practitioners, but they are often done in settings such as geriatric assessment or rehabilitation programs. Specialized fall assessment programs use a multidisciplinary approach to assess the following aspects of functioning: cognition, nutrition, medications, medical conditions, and gait and balance. Evaluation of previous falls and contributing factors also is included for people with a fall history. Gerontological nurses can encourage older adults who have fallen or who are at increased risk for falls to take advantage of these specialized programs, rather than accept falls as an inevitable consequence of aging.

Because fear of falling is now recognized as a serious functional consequence of falls that itself has negative functional consequences, at least one question about fear of falling should be asked in any assessment of falls and fall risk. Several tools are available to measure fear of falling in relation to specific activities. These tools can be used to assess fear of falling as well as avoidance of activities and self-confidence in performing activities that are often associated with falls (Tideiksaar, 1997). Assessment questions aimed at identifying fear of falling and related negative functional consequences are included in Display 18-3.

▶ Ms. M. is 75 years old and goes to the senior center three or four times weekly for lunch. You have been the wellness nurse at the center for 8 years and are quite familiar with Ms. M. because she frequently attends your weekly "Healthy Aging" classes. After your recent class on "Keeping Your Bones Healthy and Moving Well" she made an appointment to see you. She tells you she has significantly cut down on her exercise because she experienced pain in one knee about a month ago after she took a long walk in the park with her dog. She talked with her doctor about this and was told to start taking ibuprofen, but she has not started taking it

DISPLAY 18-4

Guidelines for Assessing the Safety of the Environment

Illumination and Color Contrast

- Is the lighting adequate but not glare producing?
- Are the light switches easy to reach and manipulate?
- Can lights be turned on before entering rooms?
- Are nightlights used in appropriate places?
- Is color contrast adequate between objects, such as a chair and the floor?

Hazards

- Are there highly polished floors, throw rugs, or other hazardous floor coverings?
- If area rugs are used, do they have a nonslip backing, and are the edges tacked to the floor?
- Are there cords, clutter, or other obstacles in pathways?
- Is there a pet that is likely to be running underfoot?

Furniture

- Are chairs the right height and depth for the person?
- Do the chairs have armrests? Are tables stable and of the appropriate height?
- Is small furniture placed well away from pathways?

Stairways

- Is lighting adequate?
- Are there light switches at the top and bottom of the stairs?
- Are there securely fastened handrails on both sides of the stairway?
- Are all the steps even?
- Are the treads nonskid?
- Should colored tape be used to mark the edges of the steps, particularly the top and bottom steps?

Bathroom

- Are grab bars placed appropriately for the tub and toilet?
- Does the tub have skid-proof strips or a rubber mat in the bottom?
- Has the person considered using a tub seat?
- Is the height of the toilet seat appropriate?
- Has the person considered using an elevated toilet seat?
- Does the color of the toilet seat contrast with surrounding colors?
- Is toilet paper within easy reach?

Bedroom

- Is the height of the bed appropriate?
- Is the mattress firm at the edges to provide enough support for sitting?
- If the bed has wheels, are they locked securely?
- Would full or partial side rails be a help or a hazard?
- When side rails are in the down position, are they completely out of the way?
- Is the pathway between the bedroom and bathroom clear of objects and adequately illuminated, particularly at night?
- Would a bedside commode be useful, especially at night?

- Is a light near the bed, and does the person have sufficient physical and cognitive ability to turn it on before getting out of bed?
- Is furniture positioned to allow safe use of assistive devices for ambulation?
- Is a telephone situated near the bed?

Kitchen

- Are storage areas used to the best advantage (e.g., are objects that are frequently used in the most accessible places)?
- Are appliance cords kept out of the way?
- Are nonslip mats used in front of the sink?
- Are the markings on stoves and other appliances clearly visible?
- Does the person know how to use the microwave safely?

Assistive Devices

- Is a call light available, and does the person know how to use it?
- What assistive devices are used?
- Would the person benefit from any assistive devices that are not being used?
- Are assistive devices being used safely and properly, or do they present additional hazards?

Temperature

- Is the temperature of the room(s) comfortable?
- Can the person read the markings on the thermostat and adjust it appropriately?
- During cold months, is the room temperature high enough to prevent hypothermia?
- During hot weather, is the room temperature cool enough to prevent hyperthermia?

Overall Safety

- How does the person obtain objects from hard-to-reach places?
- How does the person change overhead light bulbs?
- Are doorways wide enough to accommodate assistive devices?
- Do door thresholds create hazardous conditions?
- Are telephones accessible, especially for emergency calls? Would it be helpful to use a cordless portable phone?
- Would it be helpful to have some emergency call system available?
- Does the person wear sturdy shoes with nonskid soles?
- Does the person keep a list of emergency numbers by the phone?
- Does the person have an emergency exit plan in the event of fire?
- Are smoke alarms present and operational?
- Is there a carbon monoxide detector in an appropriate place (if the house has gas appliances, wood burning stoves, or another object that produces carbon monoxide)?

FALL RISK ASSESSMENT TOOL

Client Factors	Date	Initial Score	Date	Reassessed Score
History of falls		15		15
Confusion		5		5
Age (greater than 65 years)		5		5
Impaired judgement		5		5
Sensory deficit		5		5
Unable to ambulate independently		5		5
Decreased level of cooperation		5		5
Increased anxiety/emotional liability		5		5
Incontinence/urgency		5		5
Cardiovascular/respiratory disease affecting perfusion and oxygenation		5		5
Medications affecting blood pressure or level of consciousness		5		5
Postural hypotension with dizziness		5		5
Environmental Factors				
First week on unit (e.g., familiarity with facility, services)		5		5
Attached equipment (e.g., intravenous pole, chest tubes, appliances, oxygen, tubing)		5		5

Total points:_____

Implement fall precautions for a total score of 15 or greater.

FIGURE 18-2 A fall risk assessment tool is used to identify people who are at increased risk for falls. (Modified with permission from Hollinger, L., & Patterson, R. [1992]. A fall prevention program for the acute care setting. In S. G. Funk, E. M. Tomquist, M. T. Champagene, & R. A. Wiese [Eds.], *Key aspects of elder care: Managing falls, incontinence, and cognitive impairment*. New York: Springer.)

because she is not sure how much to take and her knee does not bother her except when she takes a long walk. She used to take her dog for daily walks but now ties him out so that she does not have to go out. Current prescription medications are enalapril, 5 mg twice daily, and hydrochlorothiazide, 25 mg daily. She also takes a multiple vitamin daily and acetaminophen, 1000 mg every 6 hours as needed. She continues to live in her one-floor house and is independent in doing all of her household chores. She also is responsible for all year-round outdoor maintenance activities, including mowing the lawn, raking leaves, and shoveling snow.

 THINKING POINTS

➤ What assessment questions from Display 18-3 would you ask Ms. M. at this time?

➤ Would you use any information from Displays 18-1, 18-2, or 18-4 at this time?

➤ What myths or misunderstandings might be influencing Ms. M. with regard to mobility and exercise?

➤ Would you take any steps to assess her home environment for fall risks?

NURSING DIAGNOSIS

Nurses working with older adults in any setting may identify risks for osteoporosis that can be addressed through health education. In community settings, postmenopausal women may express an interest in preventing osteoporosis because they are aware of the association between decreased estrogen and an increased likelihood of fractures. In these situations, Health-Seeking Behaviors may be an applicable nursing diagnosis, especially when there is a need for additional information about nutrition, exercise, and other interventions to prevent osteoporosis. This diagnosis is defined as "the state in which an individual in stable health actively seeks ways to alter personal health habits and/or the environment in order to move toward a higher level of wellness" (Carpenito, 2002, p. 466). In long-term care and rehabilitation settings, nurses frequently address the needs of older adults who have a diagnosis of osteoporosis or a history of fractures. In these situations, as well as in any situation in which someone has several risk factors for osteoporosis, the nurse may focus on secondary prevention by addressing modifiable risk factors. When this is a focus of care, a nursing diagnosis of Ineffective Health Maintenance may be appropriate. This is defined as "the state in which an individual or group experiences or is at risk of experiencing a disruption in health because of an unhealthy lifestyle or lack of knowledge to manage a condition" (Carpenito, 2002, p. 442).

Impaired Physical Mobility is a nursing diagnosis that is applicable when the assessment identifies limitations in mobility of an older adult, and is particularly applicable in rehabilitation settings. This diagnosis is defined as "a state in which the individual experiences or is at risk of experiencing limitation of physical movement but is not immobile" (Carpenito, 2002, p. 588). Related factors common in older adults include arthritis, depression, chronic pain, fractured hip, and neurologic disorders (e.g., dementia or Parkinson's disease). If the nursing assessment identifies a history of falls or any risks for falls, the nursing diagnosis of Risk for Falls would be applicable. This diagnosis is defined as "the state in which an individual has increased susceptibility to falling" (Carpenito, 2002, p. 551). Related factors common in older adults include all those factors listed in Display 18-2. When older adults express feelings associated with fallaphobia, the nurse may address this concern by applying a nursing diagnosis of Fear. Related factors would be postural instability, gait or balance disorders, or history of falls. This diagnosis is applicable when the nursing assessment reveals that the older adult limits his or her activities because of fallaphobia to the point that quality of life or level of functioning is affected.

OUTCOMES

Nursing care of older adults who are at risk for osteoporosis is directed toward preventing fractures and other serious consequences of osteoporosis. Because much of the focus is on primary and secondary prevention, pertinent nursing-sensitive outcomes for the nursing diagnosis of Ineffective Health Maintenance would include Health Promoting Behavior, Knowledge:

Health Behaviors, and Risk Control and Detection. Relevant indicators associated with Risk Control and Detection include the following: monitors environmental and personal behavioral risk factors, develops effective risk control strategies, modifies lifestyle to reduce risk, identifies potential health risks, and participates in screening at recommended intervals (Glick & Ressler, 2001). These outcomes are achieved primarily through health education interventions about osteoporosis, as discussed in the Interventions section.

Nursing goals for an older adult with a nursing diagnosis of Impaired Physical Mobility are to restore the person's functional abilities, to prevent further loss of function, and to prevent falls and other serious consequences of impaired mobility. Some nursing-sensitive outcomes that might be applicable to an older adult with a nursing diagnosis of Impaired Physical Mobility are Balance, Endurance, Mobility Level, Muscle Function, Pain Level, Comfort Level, and Active Joint Movement. Indicators related to these outcomes include the following: willingness to move; standing or walking balance; performance of usual routine; and muscle strength, tension, or movement (Maas & Specht, 2001).

Care of older adults with a nursing diagnosis of Risk for Falls focuses on preventing the occurrence of falls and fall-related injuries by implementing fall prevention programs. The following outcome labels can be used with regard to safety and fall prevention: Safety Behavior: Fall Prevention; Safety Behavior: Home Physical Environment; Safety Behavior: Personal; Safety Status: Physical Injury; and Safety Status: Falls Occurrence (Stolley et al., 2001). Examples of indicators for the nursing-sensitive outcomes associated with safety behavior include provision of lighting, elimination of clutter and glare, correct use of assistive devices, and adjustment of chair and toilet height as needed (Stolley et al., 2001). Risk control and detection outcomes and indicators also can be applied to prevention of falls and fall-related injuries. Maintaining quality of life is a nursing goal for older adults with fear of falling. Nursing-sensitive outcomes for the nursing diagnosis Fear include Coping, Fear Control, Anxiety Control, and Comfort Level (Moorhead & Brighton, 2001).

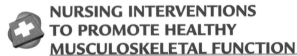

NURSING INTERVENTIONS TO PROMOTE HEALTHY MUSCULOSKELETAL FUNCTION

Healthy older adults will experience only a slight decline in overall musculoskeletal function, but they can compensate for these minor functional consequences by maintaining an active lifestyle. Various types of exercise are beneficial in promoting healthy musculoskeletal function, and older adults should try to incorporate several exercise strategies into their regular health behavior routines. Weight-bearing exercise is most helpful for osteoporosis, and resistance training has been found to increase muscle size, strength, and power in older adults. Flexibility exercises can improve range of motion, and balance training programs can improve safe mobility. Strength training exercise has several positive effects, including improved balance. Maintaining an active lifestyle can be enjoyable as well as physically beneficial. Walking, dancing, swimming, tai chi, and bicycle riding are a few examples of recreational and relaxation activities that can have very positive health benefits for musculoskeletal function. An excellent evidence-based nursing protocol for promoting exercise in older adults was recently developed by the Gerontological Nursing Interventions Research Center at the University of Iowa. The purpose of this protocol is to "help health care providers in all settings enhance or maintain exercise behavior, particularly walking, in older adults" (Jitramontree, 2001, p 7). Another excellent reference for developing care plans that address lifestyle interventions specifically for older adults is a recently published book entitled *Promoting Exercise and Behavior Change in Older Adults* (Burbank & Reibe, 2002).

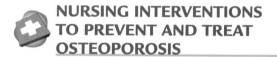

NURSING INTERVENTIONS TO PREVENT AND TREAT OSTEOPOROSIS

Goals of *Healthy People 2010* include reducing the proportion of adults with osteoporosis and reducing the proportion of adults who are hospitalized for vertebral fractures, which are the most common fracture due to osteoporosis (USDHHS, 2000). *Healthy People 2010* emphasizes that all older people, even those who have had a fracture, can benefit from treatment to prevent further bone loss or restore some lost bone to decrease the risk for further fractures. Osteoporosis is prevented and treated by using lifestyle, medical, and nutritional interventions. Lifestyle and nutritional interventions are applicable to all adults, and medical interventions are commonly used for people who have or are at risk for osteoporosis. Medical interventions are likely to be accompanied by at least a minimal risk for adverse effects, but for anyone with osteoporosis, the benefits and preventive effects are likely to far outweigh the risks. Because nutritional and lifestyle interventions have been found to be very safe as well as effective in both preventing and treating osteoporosis, there is much current emphasis on health education for all adults about them.

Although most studies on interventions for osteoporosis have focused on postmenopausal women,

there is growing attention to osteoporosis interventions for men and other groups of people at high risk, such as those taking long-term glucocorticoids and those living in long-term care facilities. In recent years, pharmaceutical companies have also started focusing their attention on developing medical interventions for osteoporosis in men and other high-risk groups. By 2010, it is likely that several medical interventions will be commonly used for osteoporosis in men. Recent attention also is focusing on osteoporosis in residents of long-term care facilities. This attention is warranted because it is estimated that up to 86% of white female nursing home residents meet the WHO criteria for osteoporosis (Lee, 2001). Interventions for osteoporosis should be viewed as an important part of fracture prevention programs in long-term care facilities.

Despite the sound medical evidence that osteoporosis interventions are effective, studies have found that many older adults with risk factors for osteoporosis are untreated or undertreated (Bellantonio et al., 2001; Cuddihy et al., 2002; Gallagher et al., 2002; Khan et al., 2001). Studies also have found that many patients receiving long-term glucocorticoid therapy are not adequately treated for osteoporosis (Yood et al., 2001). Gerontological nurses in any setting have numerous opportunities for educating older adults about lifestyle, nutritional, and medical interventions for osteoporosis.

Health Promotion Interventions

Because there is increasing attention to osteoporosis as a health concern that affects most older adults in the United States, nurses have almost limitless opportunities for educating older adults about preventing osteoporosis and fractures. Public awareness about osteoporosis in women is high, but awareness about osteoporosis in men is just beginning to develop. Thus, nurses have a particular responsibility for raising the level of awareness about osteoporosis in men and educating older men about risk factors for osteoporosis and fractures. Nurses also should focus health education efforts on older adults who already have had fractures and on people who have other risk factors because people who are more vulnerable to the serious consequences of osteoporosis may be more motivated to use preventive interventions.

Health education begins with providing information about risk factors for osteoporosis, as summarized in Display 18-1. Nurses can incorporate information about BMD tests in their health education about risk factors and advise older adults to discuss the appropriateness of this test with their primary care practitioner. Once risk factors are identified, nurses can help older adults develop a plan to address the modifiable risk factors. Nurses can encourage older adults with risk factors to discuss medical interventions with their primary care practitioner. Even in the absence of major risk factors, nutritional and lifestyle interventions should be encouraged for all older adults.

Nurses can teach older adults and their caregivers about the importance of adequate intake of calcium and vitamin D. A registered dietitian, if available, can be asked to evaluate a 3-day food history to determine the usual intake of calcium and vitamin D. If intake does not provide 1200 mg of calcium and 800 IU of vitamin D, then health education can focus either on increasing dietary intake to the recommended amount or taking a daily supplement. In long-term care facilities, a review of nutritional interventions for osteoporosis should be incorporated in care plans, especially in relation to prevention of fractures. Nurses can take the lead in initiating such a discussion and involving dietitians and primary care providers in developing and implementing appropriate preventive interventions. An article on management of osteoporosis in nursing homes stated that "unless there is clear contraindication, all residents should be taking recommended doses of calcium and vitamin D" (Lee, 2001, p. 34). Display 18-5 summarizes health promotion information that can be used as a guide for teaching older adults about osteoporosis.

Lifestyle Interventions

Lifestyle interventions aimed at preventing osteoporosis should be encouraged for all adults because of their many overall benefits. For example, quitting smoking, limiting alcohol intake, and engaging in regular weight-bearing exercise are health-promoting behaviors that are likely to reduce the risk for fractures and

---

DISPLAY 18-5
Health Promotion Teaching About Osteoporosis

Health Promotion Interventions for Early Detection and Treatment

- Review risk factors for osteoporosis as summarized in Display 18-1.
- Plan interventions for modifiable risk factors using Display 18-1 as a guide.
- Encourage discussion with primary care provider about bone mineral density (BMD) tests.
- Encourage discussion with primary care provider about medical interventions for osteoporosis if risk factors are present.
- Encourage discussion with primary care provider about prevention of fractures if osteoporosis is diagnosed.

Lifestyle Interventions

- Implement weight-bearing exercise regimen for 1/2 hour daily.
- Wear good support shoes.
- Discontinue cigarette smoking.
- Maintain ideal body weight.
- Avoid excessive alcohol intake.

Nutritional Interventions

- Calcium supplements often are recommended so that the total intake is 1500 mg per day (average daily calcium intake of older adults is less than 800 mg).
- Foods that are high in calcium include milk, cheese, yogurt, custard, ice cream, raisins, tofu, canned salmon or sardines, and broccoli and other dark green vegetables.
- Provide adequate dietary intake of vitamin D and use 400 to 800 IU of vitamin D supplement daily.

- Calcium carbonate, which is found in some antacids, is an effective and inexpensive source of elemental calcium.
- Limit consumption of beverages containing alcohol, caffeine, or phosphorus.
- Avoid phosphate food additives.
- Increase intake of foods high in plant estrogen (e.g., tofu, soy foods).
- Herbal sources of calcium include nettle, parsley, horsetail, and dandelion leaf.
- Sources of natural estrogen include sage, ginseng, licorice, motherwort, dong quai, black cohosh, and chaste tree.

Special Precautions

- Vitamin D in amounts greater than 400 to 600 IU per day, and vitamin A in amounts exceeding 5000 IU per day, can have detrimental effects.
- Calcium supplements are not recommended for people with poor kidney function or a predisposition for kidney stones.
- Because calcium may contribute to constipation, measures should be taken to promote bowel function (e.g., regular exercise and adequate fiber and fluid intake).
- Calcium supplements can interact with some medications (e.g., calcium decreases absorption of tetracycline).

Complementary and Alternative Care Practices

- Engage in activities such as yoga, swimming, massage, acupressure, tai chi, and chiropractic treatment.
- Acupuncture is helpful for arthritis and joint and muscle disorders.
- Homeopathic remedies include silica, calcarea phosphorica, and calcarea carbonica.

osteoporosis, as well as being highly beneficial for other aspects of health and function. Successful implementation of lifestyle interventions depends to a large degree on motivation, but motivation for change is based at least in part on knowledge about risk factors. Therefore, nurses have an important responsibility to provide health information not only about risk for osteoporosis and fractures but also about exercise and other lifestyle interventions that reduce this risk.

Nutritional Interventions

Adequate calcium is essential to maintaining musculoskeletal health, and there is widespread agreement that all adults aged 51 years or older should have a daily calcium intake of 1200 to 1500 mg. Because the average American adult diet provides only between 500 and 800 mg of calcium daily, calcium supplements are usually necessary. Two reviews of studies concluded that calcium supplementation reduces bone loss, increases BMD, lowers the fracture rate in older adults, and may be particularly helpful for postmenopausal women (Grossman & MacLean, 2001; Morgan, 2001). Calcium supplements, however, may have detrimental effects in older adults who take medications or in those who have physiologic disturbances such as renal impairments. They can interfere with absorption of zinc, iron, and other nutrients and medications such as atenolol, salicylates, propranolol, tetracyclines, and biphosphonates. Absorption of calcium supplements is optimal at doses of no more than 600 mg per dose (Morgan, 2001). The most common adverse effects of daily calcium supplements of 1500 mg or less are constipation, flatulence, and rebound gastric acidity.

An adequate intake of vitamin D also is essential for maintaining musculoskeletal health because it is necessary for the absorption of calcium. Most older adults do not have an adequate dietary intake of vitamin D. In addition, older adults who are not exposed to sunlight will not be able to synthesize vitamin D. Evidence supports the musculoskeletal benefits of 400 to 800 IU of vitamin D supplement daily. Caution should be used, however, because vitamin D is fat soluble, and excess amounts are not excreted. Adverse effects of vitamin D include hypercalcuria, hypercalcemia, and formation of kidney stones.

Medical Interventions

Effectiveness of medical interventions for osteoporosis is determined by their efficacy in both increasing BMD and reducing fracture risk. As new medications have become available, there has been more demand for randomized clinical trials that compare the effectiveness of various medical approaches for both treatment of osteoporosis and prevention of osteoporosis and fractures. Presently, major efforts are focused on developing medications that will reduce the occurrence of fractures, especially hip fractures. Medications that were initially approved only for treating osteoporosis may undergo further clinical trials and become approved for the additional indications of preventing osteoporosis or fractures. Because clinical trials have only recently started to address osteoporosis in men, recommendations about medical interventions for osteoporosis in men were limited in the early 2000s. Because this is a rapidly evolving area of medicine, it is important that nurses keep up to date with professional information about new developments so that they can provide health education about approved medical interventions. This section summarizes knowledge about and recommendations regarding medications for osteoporosis prevention and treatment in men and women in the early 2000s.

Since the early 1980s, studies have consistently found that oral or transdermal estrogen is effective in preventing bone loss and reducing the incidence of fractures in postmenopausal women. Thus, for 2 decades hormonal therapy has been the most well-established approach for osteoporosis treatment and prevention in postmenopausal women. Although estrogen is most effective when administered early in the postmenopausal period, it is also effective in preventing further bone loss even when treatment is begun at a late age. Many questions about the safety of estrogen replacement therapy arose during the 1970s, but at least some of the risk of the regimens initially prescribed has been reduced by using low doses and administering estrogen in combination with progesterone. In 2002, however, results of long-term studies identified additional serious risks from hormonal therapy, especially when it is used for more than a few years (see Chapter 22). Because of these findings, and because recent developments in pharmaceutical approaches to osteoporosis (discussed later in this section) have increased the number of medications available for prevention and treatment of osteoporosis, hormonal therapy is being used less commonly as a medical intervention for osteoporosis.

In 1984, calcitonin, a natural hormone that affects bone resorption, was approved by the FDA as the first nonestrogen medical intervention for treatment of osteoporosis. Initial limitations of calcitonin therapy included its high cost, the need for subcutaneous injections, and questions about its long-term effectiveness. In 1995, a nasal spray form of calcitonin was approved as an option for the treatment of low BMD. One therapeutic advantage of calcitonin over estrogen is that it has analgesic effects and can reduce the pain associated with vertebral fractures. A disadvantage is that it is not currently approved for prevention of osteoporosis, although it is under investigation for its effectiveness in preventing fractures.

The development of selective estrogen receptor modulators (SERMs) in the past decade created new hormonal treatment options for women with osteoporosis. SERMs, sometimes called designer estrogens, act like estrogen in some tissues but behave like estrogen blockers in others. The goal of these agents is to take advantage of the beneficial effects of estrogen on bone and to reduce or antagonize the detrimental effects on breast and endometrial tissue. Tamoxifen is a SERM that has been used since 1994 to treat breast cancer, and in recent years, there has been some evidence that it maintains bone mass and may prevent fractures. In late 1997, raloxifene became the first SERM to be approved for osteoporosis. The effectiveness of SERMs in preventing fractures is being investigated. Adverse effects of SERMs include hot flashes, leg cramps, and deep vein thrombosis.

In the mid-1990s, the biphosphonates became the first nonhormonal medications approved by the FDA for the prevention of fractures and bone loss. Biphosphonates are considered antiresorptive agents because they alter bone remodeling by reducing bone resorption. They are advantageous not only in preventing bone loss but also in increasing bone mass in women with postmenopausal osteoporosis. Studies have consistently found that they reduce the risk for vertebral fracture by 30% to 50% (NIH, 2001). Because of their effects on the gastrointestinal tract, biphosphonates need to be taken in the morning with a full glass of plain (not mineral) water at least 1/2 hour before any other food. In addition, the person must be in an upright position when taking this medication and avoid lying down for 1/2 hour after the dose. In 2001, a once-weekly dose of alendronate sodium was approved as therapeutically equivalent to the daily dose for treatment and prevention of postmenopausal osteoporosis. Adverse effects of biphosphonates include indigestion, diarrhea, flatulence, and abdominal pain.

All of the currently approved medical interventions can compensate for some bone loss and prevent further bone loss, but they do not have the ability to stimulate new bone growth. Pharmaceutical companies are now focusing much attention on developing anabolic agents that would cause bone formation to exceed resorption in bone remodeling. Sodium fluoride has been investigated since the 1980s as an anabolic agent for the treatment of osteoporosis, but results have been disappointing. Fluoride may be useful in stimulating new bone growth, but it does not reduce fracture risk, and, in fact, may increase risk for fractures because the quality of new bone is not good (Haguenauer et al., 2001). New drug development currently focuses on parathyroid hormone (PTH), an anabolic agent that has been found to be effective in stimulating new bone growth. A disadvantage of PTH is the need to administer it subcutaneously. Researchers are also investigating the length of treatment for PTH and whether it is more beneficial used in combination with other medical interventions or used intermittently in cycles with other types of agents. Although additional questions about safety and efficacy remain, this anabolic agent may evolve as another medical intervention for osteoporosis in the near future.

In summary, there is sound evidence for medically treating women with osteoporosis because medical intervention can improve BMD, reduce the rate of bone loss, and decrease the risk for fracture. The evidence about medical interventions for women who do not have osteoporosis but have risks for it is less clear, but medical interventions should be considered for all people who have risk factors for osteoporosis. As with other decisions about medical interventions, decisions about preventive medical interventions for people at risk for osteoporosis and fractures must be based on an appraisal of the relative risk and benefits of any particular intervention. Studies are just beginning to address the outcome of reducing the risk for fractures in women who have osteoporosis, a history of fractures, or risk factors for osteoporosis. It is likely that different medical interventions will be found to be effective for different aspects of prevention. In addition, nutritional and lifestyle interventions should be applied universally because these health behaviors are beneficial for all adults.

Because most clinical trials of medical interventions for osteoporosis have focused primarily on women, much less evidence is available about safe and effective medical treatments for men with the disease. Biphosphonates are the most widely studied medical interventions in men, and by 2002, the FDA had approved alendronate and risedronate for osteoporosis in men. It is likely that when additional biphosphonates are approved for treatment of osteoporosis, they will be approved for use in both men and women. Calcitonin is another medical intervention that can be used for men with osteoporosis, but its effectiveness in men is still being investigated. Testosterone therapy has been shown to improve BMD and may, in turn, decrease the risk for fracture in men, but it has only been shown to be effective in men with secondary osteoporosis associated with hypogonadism. One study of healthy older men with low serum testosterone levels found that transdermal testosterone prevented bone loss at the femoral neck, decreased body fat, and increased lean body mass (Kenny et al., 2001). Although it has not been found to be beneficial for older men who have normal testosterone levels, the administration of testosterone, alone or in combination with growth hormone, is under investigation for its effects in increasing BMD in men with primary osteoporosis (Christmas et al., 2002). Studies are addressing concerns about the long-term effects of testosterone therapy, and pharmaceutical companies are attempting to develop effective methods of delivering testosterone (Matsumoto, 2002). PTH and dehydroepiandrosterone (DHEA) are two additional hormonal treatments that are being investigated for osteoporosis in men, and vitamin D and calcium supplements are widely recommended as medical interventions.

> Recall that you are the nurse at the wellness program where Ms. M., who is 75 years old, regularly attends your health education programs. Based on additional assessment information, you know that Ms. M. does not take any calcium or vitamin D supplements because she drinks milk twice daily and believes that this should be sufficient. She stopped having menstrual periods when she was 50 years old and began hormonal therapy at that time. She stopped taking estrogen when she was 63 because she began "hearing too many bad things about estrogen." When she fractured her wrist 8 years ago, the orthopedic surgeon said that her x-rays showed that her "bones were pretty good for her age." She has not had any further x-rays or any BMD tests and says her doctor has never brought up the subject of osteoporosis because "I guess he's too worried about my heart problems to be concerned about my bones." Although she fell once when she was raking leaves last fall and tripped over a small tree stump, she has had no serious fall-related injuries since she fractured her wrist. She does not smoke and drinks alcohol only on major social occasions. When you assessed her blood pressure, you found her blood pressure while standing was 146/86 mm Hg and while lying was 128/78 mm Hg. Her record of self-monitored blood pressure readings indicates that her usual blood pressure is about 134/82 mm Hg. Her vision is adequate, but she has stopped driving at night and is being monitored by her ophthalmologist for progression of bilateral cataracts. Her eye doctor told her she is likely to need cataract surgery sometime during the next 2 to 3 years.

 THINKING POINTS

> What further assessment information would you want to have?

> What health promotion interventions would you advise for Ms. M.? Specifically, what health teaching would you do with regard to further assessment, lifestyle interventions, nutrition and nutritional supplements, and medical interventions?

> What educational materials would you use for Ms. M.?

> What follow-up health promotion would you consider for Ms. M.? Specifically, how would you work with Ms. M. to develop long-term health promotion interventions?

 MULTIDISCIPLINARY INTERVENTIONS TO PREVENT FALLS AND FALL-RELATED INJURIES

Gerontological nurses intervene to prevent falls and fall-related injuries, but because falls are multifaceted in their causes, prevention of falls and fall-related injuries is best done through efforts of multidisciplinary teams. Multidisciplinary interventions focus on actions that can be taken by nurses and other members of the health care team to eliminate and address all identified risk factors. Some of these interventions involve health education of older adults and their families. Formal fall prevention programs are now widely implemented in institutional as well as home care settings with the goals of preventing falls and fall-related injuries (e.g., Cumming, 2002; Jensen et al., 2002; Robertson et al., 2002; and Rose, 2002).

Implementing Fall Prevention Programs

Each fall prevention program addresses risk factors that are common in that particular setting and those factors that are unique to each at-risk person. Attention must be paid to intrinsic and extrinsic risk factors for falls, to factors that reduce the risk for falls, and to factors that reduce the risk for fall-related injuries. Key aspects of fall prevention programs are the identification of people who are at risk for falls and the consistent implementation of preventive actions by all staff. Thus, an important part of these programs is the education of all professional and nonprofessional staff members who have contact with the person who is at risk for falls. Education may involve strategies to heighten staff awareness of the importance of reducing the risks for falls. For example, posters and brochures may be used initially and periodically as reminders. Also, some form of patient/resident or chart identification can be used to draw attention to those people

DISPLAY 18-6
A Fall Prevention Program for Older Adults Being Cared for in Hospitals or Nursing Homes

Identification of Patients/Residents Who Are at Risk for Falling

- During the initial nursing or multidisciplinary assessment, identify any risks for falling and fall-related injuries (e.g., medications, osteoporosis, medical conditions, history of falls, impaired cognition, diminished alertness, impaired mobility, age 75 years or older).
- Document the risk factors on the designated fall assessment guide.
- Address any risk factors for falls, osteoporosis, or fall-related injuries that can be modified; this often requires a multidisciplinary approach.
- Reassess the risks for falls and fall-related injuries at predetermined times (e.g., every shift, every day, whenever there is a change in the patient's/resident's functional status).
- Use color-coded items (e.g., brightly colored stickers for the chart, a brightly colored identification band for the person's wrist, and signs near the person's bed and outside the room) to identify those who are included in the fall prevention program.

Education of the Staff, Patient/Resident, and Family

- Instruct the patient or resident and family about the fall prevention program using brochures that provide information about preventing falls and obtaining help if falls occur.
- Provide staff education about the fall prevention program and the risk factors for falls, especially those

factors that the staff influences (e.g., use of restraints, selection of footwear).

- Use posters and fliers to heighten staff awareness of the fall prevention program.

Interventions to Be Implemented for All High-Risk Patients/Residents

- Keep the call light within reach at all times.
- Offer assistance with activities of daily living (ADLs) and try to anticipate the person's needs before help is needed.
- Encourage the person to call for help when needed.
- Frequently check all people who cannot be relied on to call for help.
- Make sure the bed is in the lowest position possible and the wheels are locked.
- Carefully and frequently assess the environment for factors that increase the risk for either falls or fall-related injuries; address all modifiable risk factors.
- Consider the use of a movement detection device.
- Carefully evaluate the potential consequences of physical restraints, including bedrails.
- If restraints are used, reevaluate their use every shift.
- If appropriate, orient the person to person, place, and time every shift and as needed.
- Document fall prevention interventions on the person's chart.

who have an increased risk for falls. Display 18-6 describes a fall prevention program that could be adapted for use in institutional settings.

Addressing Intrinsic Risk Factors

Because any gait and balance impairment increases the risk for falls, any intervention that improves mobility is likely to be beneficial in preventing falls. Interventions for improving mobility are implemented primarily by therapists, nurses, and nursing staff, often through an interdisciplinary approach. Teaching about the proper use of mobility aids and other assistive devices is an important part of fall prevention programs (Figure 18-3). Nurses are responsible for raising questions about whether an older adult may benefit from the use of mobility aids or assistive devices and facilitating a referral to a physical therapist for evaluation and teaching regarding their use. In community settings, nurses may have to educate older adults and their caregivers about the availability of various mobility aids, transfer assistance devices, and other aids that might improve safety.

Nurses can suggest that older adults seek professional help with selecting appropriate mobility aids and assistive devices. Some suppliers of home health care equipment have therapists on staff who can provide advice and assist with processing of claims if the aids are covered by insurance. When mobility aids are prescribed, nurses are responsible for encouraging the use of such aids and making sure that they are accessible for the person's use. Nurses are responsible for facilitating referrals for reassessment if questions arise about the safety or effectiveness of mobility aids that are being used. Nurses also can advise older adults about wearing nonslip footwear whenever they are walking.

In recent years, fall prevention literature has emphasized the effectiveness of various exercise routines as an intervention for reducing fall risk. An important role for nurses is to identify those older adults who may benefit from gait and balance training programs and to facilitate referrals for physical therapy when appropriate. Nurses also are responsible for encouraging adequate and consistent follow-through with recommended exercise programs. In

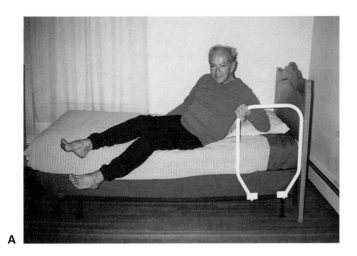

A

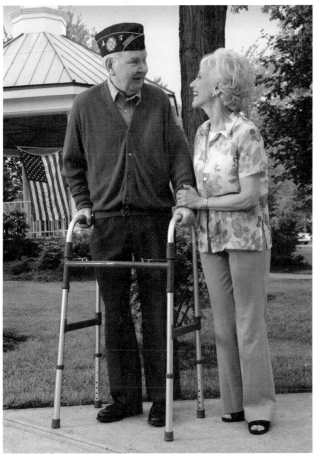

B

FIGURE 18-3 The use of assistive devices can help reduce the risk of falls. **(A)** Transfer assistive devices are used to facilitate safer transfer in and out of beds. **(B)** Walkers are available in various styles with wheels, brakes, baskets, seats, and other features to improve safety and mobility. (*Part A:* BED-BAR ® courtesy of Brown Engineering Corporation. *Part B:* Invacare ® Blue Release™ Walker. Photography © 2000 Invacare Corporation. Invacare is a registered trademark of Invacare Corporation.)

restorative nursing routines are essential aspects of fall prevention programs. Group exercise programs also are widely used as fall prevention interventions that are beneficial to all at-risk people. Many programs incorporate exercises that are aimed specifically at gait, balance, ankle strength, or other aspects of fall prevention. Tai chi, for example, is becoming more widely available in community and long-term care settings as a health promotion intervention for older adults. Studies have found that tai chi can reduce the risk for falls by improving balance, coordination, flexibility, and many other specific aspects of function that affect fall risk (McKenna, 2001). Nurses should incorporate information about the benefits of tai chi and other exercise routines into their health promotion education about fall prevention.

Most intrinsic risks cannot be reversed, but fall prevention programs generally include multidisciplinary interventions to address polypharmacy and medical conditions that increase the risk for falls. Nurses are responsible for knowing the common adverse effects of medications and raising questions about these effects, particularly in relation to fall risk. Medication regimens should be reviewed periodically, and nurses can take the lead in suggesting that pharmacists and prescribing practitioners evaluate medications in relation to fall risks. Another nursing responsibility with regard to medications is to assess for postural hypotension as a potential adverse medication effect and as a risk factor for falls.

Addressing Extrinsic Risk Factors

Many preventive interventions for extrinsic risk factors are applicable for older adults in any setting and often address environmental factors and the use of restraints. Educational interventions and assistance with modifications to reduce hazards based on a home hazard assessment have been found to be successful interventions in reducing fall hazards in homes (Stevens et al., 2001). Guidelines recommend that referrals be made for environmental home assessments when patients who are at risk for falls are discharged from hospitals (American Geriatrics Society et al., 2001). Display 18-4 can be used as a guide for planning interventions that may eliminate or reduce environmental risks. In addition, environmental modifications to improve a person's vision were discussed in Chapter 13 and are applicable to fall prevention.

Using Monitoring Devices

Monitoring devices can be very useful in alerting staff to potentially dangerous patient/resident activity, such as getting out of bed or a chair without assistance. Many types of devices are available, but they all have the ability to transmit a signal to a

long-term care settings, nurses generally oversee restorative nursing programs in which nursing assistants help residents with walking and other exercise regimens established by physical therapists. These remote location (e.g., a nursing station) when activated by certain levels of patient/resident movement. Some devices, such as a pad, are applied to the bed, whereas others are attached to the person's clothing. Other devices are programmed specifically for the person's movement in a confined environment such as their room. Most movement detection devices were originally designed for institutional use, but in recent years, simplified monitoring and signal systems have been developed for home use by family caregivers. In home settings, an auditory room-monitoring device may be useful when caregivers need to detect the sound of someone moving around in another room. These devices are widely available in stores where infant care supplies are sold. A major limitation of any movement detection device is that its effectiveness depends on the timely response of someone who is able to prevent the fall. These devices are not useful for people living alone or for people without responsible and responsive caregivers.

Preventing Fall-Related Injuries

When falls cannot be prevented, interventions are directed toward reducing the risk for fractures and other serious fall-related injuries. Because falls are the most common cause of injuries and trauma-related hospitalizations among older adults—with hip fractures being the most serious fall-related injury—one goal of *Healthy People 2010* is to reduce hip fractures in this population (USDHHS, 2000). Perhaps the most universally applicable intervention for prevention of fall-related injuries is to ensure that the measures for preventing and treating osteoporosis discussed earlier are taken. Environmental adaptations can also be considered universally as interventions to reduce the risk for fall-related injuries. For example, heavy furniture that is in a pathway where a fall is likely to occur can be moved out of the way, and sharp edges of furniture can be padded. Risk for injury from falling out of bed can be reduced by using a bed that can be adjusted to a low position. Soft pads can be placed near beds and in other locations where people are likely to fall, but caution must be used so that these pads do not become fall risks. External hip pads, designed as shock absorbers, have been available since the 1990s (Figure 18-4). Although studies have confirmed that wearing these protectors can significantly reduce the risk for hip fracture in people at risk for falls and fractures, compliance with wearing the pads may be problematic (Kannus et al., 2000). Information about hip protectors can be found on the Internet at http://www.hipprotector.com.

For people living alone, interventions also are directed toward providing assistance in a timely manner. A

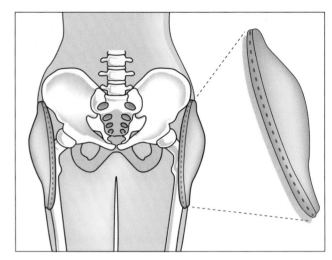

FIGURE 18-4 Hip protectors come in a variety of styles. This hip protector system consists of two padded shells that fit in undergarments with special inside pockets.

personal emergency response system (PERS) can be useful in summoning help in situations in which falls cannot be prevented. These devices involve the use of a small portable transmitter that is worn on the person's body or clothing. Examples of such devices are beeper-type devices worn on the belt or pendants worn as necklaces or bracelets. When the person falls, he or she can summon help by using the transmitter to signal a receiver unit that is attached to the phone. In turn, a call is automatically made to the PERS provider, who then checks in with the person and calls the local emergency response team or a contact person, such as a neighbor or family member. Some of these devices are set up so that a checkup call is made to the person during any 24-hour period in which the person does not push a reset button or otherwise notify the company that he or she is okay. The effectiveness of PERS depends on the ability of the fallen person to signal for help and on the availability of a helping person. A major limitation of such devices is that cognitively impaired people may not be able to learn to use them. Hospitals and home care agencies can provide information about local PERS programs, and information about national programs can be found on the Internet. Cordless phones, especially if preprogrammed for emergency help, may provide a practical alternative to such call systems for people who are able to use them.

Finally, use of bedrails and other types of restraints should be carefully evaluated, and decisions about restraints should take into consideration that restraints do not necessarily reduce the risk for falls and are associated with the occurrence of more serious fall-related injuries. Numerous nursing references can be found in professional journals, and organizations such as the American Nurses Association, the Health Care Financing Administration, and the Joint Commission on Accreditation of Healthcare Organizations have challenged the routine use of restraints (e.g., American Geriatrics Society et al., 2001; Hammond & Levine, 2000; Sullivan-Marx, 2001). Health care institutions have developed policies for restraint reduction or restraint-free care, and these policies emphasize the importance of developing individualized care plans for people at risk for falls. Restraint reduction policies also emphasize the importance of educating older adults, family members, and all caregiving staff members about the concept of restraint-free care as well as fall prevention measures. Nurses play an extremely important role in decisions about the use of restraints and in education about the risks associated with restraints.

Addressing Fear of Falling

Any interventions that reduce the risk for falls are likely also to reduce a person's fear of falling, but some people may need additional interventions to address this problem. Several models of group interventions have been published describing educational and psychosocial interventions to address fear of falling (Gentleman & Malozemoff, 2001; Tennstedt et al., 1998; Tennstedt et al., 2001). The "Falls and Feelings" discussion group is a nursing model that was designed to facilitate discussion of feelings related to falling experiences. The goal for the group members was "to enhance self-confidence and life satisfaction, resulting in empowerment of the individual to handle fear of falling" (Gentleman & Malozemoff, 2001, p. 36). Themes of the sessions included risks for falls, prevention of falls, falls and feelings, and fear as a consequence of falls (Gentleman & Malozemoff, 2001). Nurses can address fear of falling in the same way they address other fears: encourage the expression of feelings and provide education and reassurance about interventions that are being implemented as part of an individualized fall prevention care plan. Family members and caregivers should be included in nursing interventions and health education to address fear of falling. For people living alone, a PERS may be very reassuring and can at least alleviate the fear of not being helped if a fall occurs.

EVALUATING EFFECTIVENESS OF NURSING INTERVENTIONS

Nursing care for older adults with impaired musculoskeletal function is evaluated by the degree to which the person achieves and maintains the highest possible level of independence and safe mobility. Nursing care of older adults who are at high risk for osteoporosis is evaluated according to the degree to which the older adult incorporates preventive measures in his or her daily life. For example, older adults might begin a regimen of three 1/2-hour periods of weight-bearing exercise weekly. The nursing care of older adults who are at high risk for falls and fall-related injuries is evaluated according to the extent to which falls and serious injuries are prevented. Nurses cannot, of course, measure the number of falls that do not occur, but they can measure the risk factors that have been addressed in the care plan. Evaluation of these risk factors is facilitated by careful documentation of interventions, such as environmental modifications and fall prevention programs.

CHAPTER SUMMARY

Age-related changes in the musculoskeletal and central nervous systems affect the mobility and safety of older adults, increasing their susceptibility to falls and fall-related injuries. Osteoporosis is an age-related change that predisposes older adults to fractures. Although osteoporosis cannot totally be prevented in older adults, many risk factors can be addressed. Common risk factors for falls in older adults include medical problems, adverse medication effects, and environmental factors. Risk factors for fall-related injuries include restraints and osteoporosis. Functional consequences associated with age-related changes and risk factors include falls, fractures, and serious psychosocial effects.

Nursing assessment of overall musculoskeletal function focuses on identifying the risk factors for falls and osteoporosis as well as the functional consequences of age-related musculoskeletal changes. Particular emphasis is placed on identifying factors that can be alleviated through health education and other nursing interventions. Relevant nursing diagnoses include Impaired Physical Mobility and Risk for Injury. Health-Seeking Behaviors is a nursing diagnosis that would be applicable to older adults who are motivated to prevent osteoporosis and fractures. Nursing goals are directed toward alleviating or eliminating factors that increase the risk for falls and osteoporosis. Interventions to decrease the risk for falls and fall-related injuries are multidisciplinary and focus on environmental modifications and the implementation of fall prevention programs. Osteoporosis can largely be prevented through health promotion interventions. Nursing care is evaluated by documenting the use of fall prevention strategies and the implementation of interventions designed to prevent osteoporosis.

CONCLUDING CASE STUDY AND NURSING CARE PLAN

➤ Ms. M. is now 89 years old and has been admitted to the hospital for congestive heart failure. Additional medical problems include arthritis, osteoporosis, recurrent depression, early-stage dementia, and history of fractured hip. Current medications include furosemide, 40 mg twice daily; enalapril, 10 mg twice daily; digoxin, 0.125 mg daily; calcitonin nasal spray daily; OS-cal with D; and sertraline (Zoloft), 50 mg at bedtime. Ms. M. lives alone in an assisted-living facility, where she receives help with her medications and goes to the dining room for meals. You are the nurse on the acute care floor assigned to her care on the day of admission.

■ Nursing Assessment

During your initial nursing assessment, Ms. M. is quiet and withdrawn. When you ask about her living situation, she says she moved to the assisted-living facility 2 years ago, after she was hospitalized for treatment of a fractured hip. At the time of the injury, she had been living alone. She had fallen while making her way to the bathroom at night and remained lying on the floor until her daughter came to visit her the next morning. During the past year, Ms. M. reports that she has fallen twice in her room but that she has been able to call for help and has not had any serious injuries. You determine that Ms. M. will need help in ambulating to the bathroom and that she should be supervised whenever she gets out of bed.

Ms. M. confides that she is worried that she will have to move to the nursing home section of her facility if she falls again. She is very depressed about her lack of energy and her hospitalization for congestive heart failure. A mental status assessment indicates that Ms. M. is alert and oriented but that her short-term memory is impaired. She has a great deal of difficulty with abstract ideas, such as learning to use the call button. You check her vital signs, which are within normal range, with no evidence of postural hypotension.

■ Nursing Diagnosis

In addition to the nursing diagnoses related to Ms. M.'s medical condition, you identify a nursing diagnosis of Risk for Falls. Related factors include weakness, diuretic and cardiovascular medications, a history of falls, depression, and impaired cognition. You are concerned about preventing falls during her hospitalization.

■ Nursing Care Plan

The nursing care plan you develop for Ms. M. is presented in Display 18-7.

CRITICAL THINKING EXERCISES

1. Answer the following questions with regard to Ms. M. at 89 years old:
   - If you were the nurse on the acute care floor where Ms. M. was a patient, what concerns would you address in a discharge plan? Would you identify any additional nursing diagnoses related to safe mobility and musculoskeletal function? What additional nursing interventions would you plan to supplement the care plan described in this chapter?
   - If you were a nurse in the assisted-living facility where Ms. M. lives, what concerns would you have about her care? How would you address these concerns in a care plan?
2. Identify factors that increase or reduce the risk for osteoporosis.
3. Describe how each of the following age-related or risk factors might increase an older person's risk for falls and fractures: nocturia, osteoporosis, medications, altered gait, pathologic conditions, sensory impairments, cognitive impairments, functional impairments, slowed reaction time.
4. Describe the environmental factors that you would assess, in both home and institutional settings, to identify potential risks for falls.
5. Describe how you would design and implement a fall prevention program in a nursing home.
6. How would you deal with a daughter who demanded that restraints be used whenever her 84-year-old mother, who is a patient on your acute care floor, is sitting in a chair?
7. What information would you include in health education about osteoporosis?
8. Use the Internet to find information about fall prevention products that you might use in clinical practice.

DISPLAY 18-7 • NURSING CARE PLAN FOR MS. M.

EXPECTED OUTCOME	NURSING INTERVENTIONS	NURSING EVALUATION
Ms. M. will ambulate safely and avoid falls during her hospitalization.	• Identify Ms. M. as a participant in the fall prevention program by using an orange wrist bracelet, posting a Fall Alert sign near her bed, and placing an orange Fall Alert sticker on her chart. • Provide Ms. M. with a brochure that explains the fall prevention program. • Reassess fall risks every shift and document these on the Fall Assessment form included in Ms. M.'s chart. • Talk with Ms. M.'s physician about a referral for physical therapy. • Keep the call light button within her reach and review instructions for its use every shift. • Assess benefits and risks of using bed rails, and discuss with Ms. M. and her family. • Make sure that the bed is in the lowest possible position with the wheels locked. • Use a movement detection bed pad and explain to Ms. M. that the purpose of the pad is to ensure that the staff knows when she needs to get out of bed. • Every 2 hours, when Ms. M. is awake, the nursing staff will ask her if she needs to go to the bathroom.	• Ms. M. will receive assistance with ambulation every time she is out of bed. • Ms. M. will not fall during her hospitalization.

Future Directions for Healthier Aging: Focus on Mobility and Safety

THE FOLLOWING RESEARCH INITIATIVES OF THE NATIONAL INSTITUTE OF AGING ADDRESS MUSCULOSKELETAL FUNCTION:

• Identify underlying mechanisms of aging in bone, muscle, and joints with the goal of preventing disease and conserving or enhancing function.

• Develop effective prevention and intervention strategies for age-related musculoskeletal decline.

• Understand the underlying age-related changes that occur in the motor-control areas of the brain with the aim of developing therapeutic interventions.

• Identify factors that can predispose older people to fractures.

• Reduce the risk for falls through safety measures, improved therapies, environmental modifications, and health promotion and education (NIA, 2001).

EDUCATIONAL RESOURCES

American Menopause Foundation, Inc.
350 Fifth Avenue, Suite 2822, New York, NY 10118
(212) 714-2398
http://www.americanmenopause.org

Arthritis Foundation
P.O. Box 7669, Atlanta, GA 30357-0669
(800) 283-7800
http://www.arthritis.org

Joint Commission on Accreditation of Healthcare Organizations
601 13th Street, NW, Suite 1150N, Washington, DC 20005
(202) 783-6655
http://www.jcaho.org

National Arthritis and Musculoskeletal and Skin Diseases Information Clearinghouse
NAMSIC AMS Circle, National Institutes of Health,
1 AMS Circle, Bethesda, MD 20892-3675
(301) 495-4484
http://www.nih.gov/niams

National Center for Injury Prevention and Control
Mailstop K65, 4770 Buford Highway NE, Atlanta,
GA 30341-3742
(707) 488-1506
http://www.cdc.gov/ncipc

National Osteoporosis Foundation
Osteoporosis and Related Bone Diseases
  National Resource Center
1232 22nd Street N.W., Washington, DC 20037-1292
(202) 223-2226; (800) 624-2663
http://www.nof.org

North American Menopause Society
P.O. Box 94527, Cleveland, OH 44101
(440) 442-7550
http://www.menopause.org

Watch Your Step
Falls Prevention Initiative
http://www.chpna.ca/falls

REFERENCES

American Geriatrics Society, British Geriatrics Society, & American Academy of Orthopaedic Surgeons Panel on Falls Prevention. (2001). Guideline for the prevention of falls in older persons. *Journal of the American Geriatrics Society, 49,* 664–672.

American Nurses Association. (1999). *Testimony to Joint Commission on the Accreditation of Healthcare Organizations Behavioral Restraint Task Force.* Washington, DC: American Nurses Association.

Baldwin, R. L., Craven, R. F., & Dimond, M. (1996). Falls: Are rural elders at greater risk? *Journal of Gerontological Nursing, 22*(8), 14–21.

Baron, J. A., Farahmand, B. Y., Weiderpass, E., Michaëlsson, K., Alberts, A., Persson, I., & Ljunghall, S. (2001). Cigarette smoking, alcohol consumption, and risk of hip fracture in women. *Archives of Internal Medicine, 161,* 983–988.

Basante, J., Bentz, E., Heck-Hakley, J., Kenion, B., Young, D., & Holm, M. B. (2001). Fall risks among older adults in long-term care facilities: A focused literature review. *Physical and Occupational Therapy in Geriatrics, 19*(2) 63–85.

Bellantonio, S., Fortinsky, R., & Prestwood, K. (2001). How well are community-living women treated for osteoporosis after hip fracture? *Journal of the American Geriatrics Society, 49,* 1197–1204.

Brassington, G. S., King, A. C., & Bliwise, D. L. (2000). Sleep problems as a risk factor for falls in a sample of community-dwelling adults aged 64–99 years. *Journal of the American Geriatrics Society, 48,* 1234–1240.

Burbank, P. M., & Reibe, D. (Eds.) (2002). *Promoting exercise and behavior change in older adults.* New York: Springer.

Campbell, W. W., Trappe, T. A., Wolfe, R. R., & Evans. W. J. (2001). The recommended dietary allowance for protein may not be adequate for older people to maintain skeletal muscle. *Journal of Gerontology: Medical Sciences, 56A,* M373–M380.

Capezuti, E., Maislin, G., Strumpf, N., & Evans, L. K. (2002). Side rail use and bed-related falls outcomes among nursing home residents. *Journal of the American Geriatrics Society, 50,* 90–96.

Carpenito, L. J. (2002). *Nursing diagnosis: Application to clinical practice* (9th ed.). Philadelphia: Lippincott Williams & Wilkins.

Christmas, C., O'Connor, K. G., Harman, S. M., Tobin, J. D., Münzer, T., Bellantoni, M. F., St. Clair, C., Pabst, K. M., Sorkin, J. D., & Blackman, M. R. (2002). Growth hormone and sex steroid effects on bone metabolism and bone mineral density in healthy aged women and men. *Journal of Gerontology: Medical Sciences, 57A,* M12–M18.

Covinsky, K. E., Kahana, E., Kahana, B., Kercher, K., Schumacher, J. G., & Justice, A. C. (2001). History and mobility exam index to identify community-dwelling elderly persons at risk of falling. *Journal of Gerontology: Medical Sciences, 56A,* M253–M259.

Cuddihy, M. T., Gabriel, S. E., Crowson, C. S., Atkinson, E. J., Tabini, C., O'Fallon, W. M., & Melton III, L. J. (2002). Osteoporosis intervention following distal forearm fractures. *Archives of Internal Medicine, 162,* 421–426.

Cumming, R. G. (2002). Intervention strategies and risk-factor modification for falls prevention: A review of recent intervention studies. *Clinics in Geriatric Medicine, 18,* 175–189.

Cumming, R. G., Salkeld, G., Thomas, M., & Szonyi, G. (2000). Prospective study of the impact of fear of falling on activities of daily living, SF-36 scores, and nursing home admission. *Journal of Gerontology: Medical Sciences, 55A,* M299–M305.

Drozdick, L. W., & Edelstein, B. A. (2001). Correlates of fear of falling in older adults who have experienced a fall. *Journal of Clinical Geropsychology, 7*(1), 1–13.

Dunn, K. S. (2001). The effect of physical restraints on fall rates in older adults who are institutionalized. *Journal of Gerontological Nursing, 27*(10), 40–48.

Ellis, A. A., & Trent, R. B. (2001). Do the risks and consequences of hospitalized fall injuries among older adults in California vary by type of fall? *Journal of Gerontology: Medical Sciences, 56A,* M686–M692.

Espino, D. V., Palmer, R. F., Miles, T. P., Mouton, C. P., Wood, R. C., Bayne, N. S., & Markides, K. P. (2000). Prevalence, incidence, and risk factors associated with hip fractures in community-dwelling older Mexican Americans: Results of the Hispanic EPESE study. *Journal of the American Geriatrics Society, 48,* 1252–1260.

Evans, W. J. (2000). Exercise strategies should be designed to increase muscle power. *Journal of Gerontology: Medical Sciences, 55A,* M309–M310.

Farmer, B. C. (2000). Fall risk assessment. *Journal of Gerontological Nursing, 26*(7), 6–7.

Fransen, M., Woodward, M., Norton, R., Robinson, E., Butler, M., & Campbell, A. J. (2002). Excess mortality or institutionalization after hip fracture: Men are at greater risk than women. *Journal of Geriatrics Society, 50,* 685–690.

Gallagher, T. C., Geling, O., & Comite, F. (2002). Missed opportunities for prevention of osteoporotic fracture. *Archives of Internal Medicine, 162,* 450–456.

Gentleman, B., & Malozemoff, W. (2001). Falls and feelings: Description of a psychosocial group nursing intervention. *Journal of Gerontological Nursing, 27*(10), 35–39.

Gill, J., Allum, J. H. J., Carpenter, M. G., Held-Ziolkowska, M., Adkin, A. L., Honegger, F., & Pierchala, K. (2001). Trunk sway measures of postural stability during clinical balance tests: Effects of age. *Journal of Gerontology: Medical Sciences, 56A,* M438–M447.

Glick, O. J., & Ressler, C. (2001). Altered health maintenance. In M. L. Maas, K. C. Buckwalter, M. D. Hardy, T. Tripp-Reimer, M. G. Titler, & J. P. Specht (Eds.), *Nursing care of older adults: Diagnoses, outcomes, and interventions* (pp. 6–22). St. Louis: Mosby.

Grossman, J. M., & MacLean, C. H. (2001). Quality indicators for the management of osteoporosis in vulnerable elders. *Annals of Internal Medicine, 135,* 722–730.

Haguenauer, D., Welch, V., Shea, B., & Tugwell, P. (2001). Anabolic agents to treat osteoporosis in older people: Is there still a place for fluoride? *Journal of the American*

Geriatrics Society, 49, 1387–1389. (Reprinted: Cochrane review in: The Cochrane Library, 2000, issue 4, Oxford).

Hammond, M., & Levine, J. M. (2000). Bedrails: Choosing the best alternative. *Geriatric Nursing, 20,* 297–300.

Hanger, H. C., Ball, M. C., & Wood, L. A. (1999). An analysis of falls in the hospital: Can we do without bedrails? *Journal of the American Geriatrics Society, 47,* 529–531.

Harrison, B., Booth, D., & Algase, D. (2001). Studying fall risk factors among nursing home residents who fell. *Journal of Gerontological Nursing, 27*(10), 26–34.

Israel, E., Banerjee, T. R., Fitzmaurice, G. M., Kotlov, T. V., LaHive, K., & LeBoff, M. S. (2001). Effects of inhaled glucocorticoids on bone density in premenopausal women. *New England Journal of Medicine, 345,* 941–947.

Jensen, J., Lundin-Olsson, L., Nyberg, L., & Gustafson, Y. (2002). Falls and injury prevention in older people living in residential care facilities. *Annals of Internal Medicine, 136,* 733–741.

Jitramontree, N. (2001). Evidence-based protocol: Exercise promotion—encouraging older adults to walk. *Journal of Gerontological Nursing, 27*(10), 7–18.

Kannus, P., Parkkari, J., Niemi, S., Pasanen, M., Palvanen, M., Jarvinen, M., & Vuori, I. (2000). Prevention of hip fracture in elderly people with use of a hip protector. *New England Journal of Medicine, 343,* 1506–1513.

Kay, G. G. (2000). The effects of antihistamines on cognition and performance. *Journal of Allergy and Clinical Immunology, 105,* 622–627.

Kenny, A. M., & Prestwood, K. M. (2000). Osteoporosis: Pathogenesis, diagnosis, and treatment in older adults. *Rheumatic Diseases Clinics of North America, 26,* 569–591.

Kenny, A. M., Prestwood, K. M., Gruman, C. A., Marcello, K. M., & Raisz, L. G. (2001). Effects of transdermal testosterone on bone and muscle in older men with low bioavailable testosterone levels. *Journal of Gerontology: Medical Science, 56A,* M266–M272.

Khan, S. A., de Geus, C., Holroyd, B., & Russell, A. S. (2001). Osteoporosis follow-up after wrist fractures following minor trauma. *Archives of Internal Medicine, 161,* 1309–1312.

Lee, V. K. (2001). Management of osteoporosis in the nursing home setting. *Annals of Long-Term Care: Clinical Care and Aging, 9*(9), 32–42.

Loeser, R. F., Jr. (2000). Aging and the etiopathogenesis and treatment of osteoarthritis. *Rheumatic Diseases Clinics of North America, 26,* 547–567.

Lord, S. R., & Dayhew, J. (2001). Visual risk factors for falls in older people. *Journal of the American Geriatrics Society, 49,* 508–515.

Maas, M. L., & Specht, J. P. (2001). Impaired physical mobility. In M. L. Maas, K. C. Buckwalter, M. D. Hardy, T. Tripp-Reimer, M. G. Titler, & J. P. Specht (Eds.), *Nursing care of older adults: Diagnoses, outcomes, and interventions* (pp. 337–365). St. Louis: Mosby.

Magaziner, J., Hawkes, W., Hebel, J. R., Zimmerman, S. I., Fox, K. M., Dolan, M., Felsenthal, G., & Kenzora, J. (2000). Recovery from hip fracture in eight areas of function. *Journal of Gerontology: Medical Sciences, 55A,* M498–M507.

Maki, B. E. (1997). Gait changes in older adults: Predictors of falls or indicators of fears? *Journal of the American Geriatrics Society, 45,* 313–320.

Matsumoto, A. M. (2002). Andropause: Clinical implications of the decline in serum testosterone levels with aging in men. *Journal of Gerontology: Medical Science, 57A,* M76–M99.

McKenna, M. (2001). The application of tai chi chuan in rehabilitation and preventive care of the geriatric population. *Physical and Occupational Therapy in Geriatrics, 18*(4), 23–34.

Moorhead, S. A., & Brighton, V. A. (2001). Anxiety and fear. In M. L. Maas, K. C. Buckwalter, M. D. Hardy, T. Tripp-Reimer, M. G. Titler, & J. P. Specht (Eds.), *Nursing care of older adults: Diagnoses, outcomes, and interventions* (pp. 571–592). St. Louis: Mosby.

Morgan, S. L. (2001). Calcium and vitamin D in osteoporosis. *Rheumatic Diseases Clinics of North America, 27*(1), 101–130.

Morley, J. E. (2002). A fall is a major event in the life of an older person. *Journal of Gerontology: Medical Sciences, 57A,* M492–M495.

Murphy, J., & Isaacs, B. (1982). The post-fall syndrome. *Gerontology, 28,* 265–270.

Murphy, S. L., Williams, C. S., & Gill, T. M. (2002). Characteristics associated with fear of falling and activity restriction in community-living older persons. *Journal of American Geriatrics Society, 50,* 516–520.

National Institute on Aging (NIA). (2001). *Action plan for aging research: Strategic plan for fiscal years 2001–2005* (NIH Pub No. 01-4961). Washington, DC: U.S. Department of Health and Human Services.

National Institutes of Health (NIH). (2001). *National Institutes of Health consensus development conference statement* (March 27–29, 2000). Washington, DC: U.S. Department of Health and Human Services.

Ottenbacher, K. O., Ostir, G. V., Peek, M. K., Goodwin, J. S., & Markides, K. S. (2002). Diabetes mellitus as a risk factor for hip fracture in Mexican American older adults. *Journal of Gerontology, 57A*(10), M648–M653.

Patrick, L., & Blodgett, A. (2001). Selecting patients for falls-prevention protocols: An evidence-based approach on a geriatric rehabilitation unit. *Journal of Gerontological Nursing, 27*(10), 19–25.

Pavol, M. J., Owings, T. M., Foley, K. T., & Grabiner, M. D. (2001). Mechanisms leading to a fall from an induced trip in healthy older adults. *Journal of Gerontology: Medical Sciences, 56A,* M428–M437.

Perell, K. L., Nelson, A., Goldman, R. L., Luther, S. L., Prieto-Lewis, N., & Rubenstein, L. Z. (2001). Fall risk assessment measures: An analytic review. *Journal of Gerontology: Medical Sciences, 56A,* M761–M766.

Ray, W. A., Thapa, P. B., & Gideon, P. (2000). Benzodiazepines and the risk of falls in nursing home residents. *Journal of the American Geriatrics Society, 48,* 682–685.

Robertson, M. C., Campbell, A. J., Gardner, M. M., & Devlin, N. (2002). Preventing injuries in older people by preventing falls: A meta-analysis of individual-level data. *Journal of American Geriatrics Society, 50,* 905–911.

Rose, D. J. (2002). Promoting functional independence among "at risk" and physically frail older adults through community-based fall-risk-reduction programs. *Journal of Aging and Physical Activity, 10,* 207–225.

Rubenstein, L. Z., & Josephson, K. R. (2002). The epidemiology of falls and syncope. *Clinics in Geriatric Medicine, 18,* 141–158.

Rubenstein, L. Z., Powers, C. M., & MacLean, C. H. (2001). Quality indicators for the management and prevention of falls and mobility problems in vulnerable elders. *Annals of Internal Medicine, 135,* 686–693.

Sato, Y., Kondo, I., Ishida, S., Motooka, H., Takayama, K., Tomita, Y., Maeda, H., & Satoh, K. (2001). Decreased bone mass and increased bone turnover with valproate therapy in adults with epilepsy. *Neurology, 57,* 445–449.

Shaw, F. E. (2002). Falls in cognitive impairment and dementia. *Clinics in Geriatric Medicine, 18,* 159–173.

Sheldon, J. H. (1960). On the natural history of falls in old age. *British Medical Journal, 2,* 1685–1690.

Shorr, R. I., Guillen, M. K., Rosenblatt, L. C., Walker, K., Caudle, C. E., & Kritchevsky, S. B. (2002). Restraint use, restraint orders, and the risk of falls in hospitalized patients. *Journal of the American Geriatrics Society, 50,* 526–529.

Shreyasee, A., & Felson, D. T. (2001). Osteoporosis in men. *Rheumatic Diseases Clinics of North America, 27,* 19–47.

Si, M., Neufeld, R. R., & Dunbar, J. (1999). Removal of bedrails on a short-term nursing home rehabilitation unit. *Gerontologist, 39,* 611–614.

Stevens, M., Holman, C. D. J., & Bennett, N. (2001). Preventing falls in older people: Impact of an intervention to reduce environmental hazards in the home. *Journal of the American Geriatrics Society, 49,* 1442–1447.

Stolley, J. M., Lewis, A., Moore, L., & Harvey, P. (2001). Risk for injury: Falls. In M. L. Maas, K. C. Buckwalter, M. D. Hardy, T. Tripp-Reimer, M. G. Titler, & J. P. Specht (Eds.), *Nursing care of older adults: Diagnoses, outcomes, and interventions* (pp. 23–33). St. Louis: Mosby.

Sullivan-Marx, E. M. (2001). Achieving restraint-free care of acutely confused older adults. *Journal of Gerontological Nursing, 27*(4), 56–61.

Tennstedt, S., Howland, J., Lachman, M., Peterson, E., Kasten, L., & Jette, A. (1998). A randomized, controlled trial of a group intervention to reduce fear of falling and associated activity restriction in older adults. *Journal of Gerontology: Psychological Sciences, 53B,* P384–P392.

Tennstedt, S. L., Lawrence, R. H., & Kasten, L. (2001). An intervention to reduce fear of falling and enhance activity: Who is most likely to benefit? *Educational Gerontology, 27,* 227–240.

Tideiksaar, R. (1997). *Falling in old age: Prevention and management* (2nd ed.). New York: Springer.

Tideiksaar, R., & Kay, A. D. (1986) What causes falls? A logical diagnostic procedure. *Geriatrics, 41*(12), 32–50.

Twersky, J. I. (2001). Long-term care in geriatrics: Falls in the nursing home. *Clinics in Family Practice, 3,* 653–666.

U.S. Department of Health and Human Services (USDHHS). (2000). *Healthy people 2010* (2nd ed). Washington, DC: U.S. Government Printing Office.

Walker-Bone, K., Dennison, E., & Cooper, C. (2001). Epidemiology of osteoporosis. *Rheumatic Diseases Clinics of North America, 27,* 1–18.

Wang, P. S., Bohn, R. L., Glynn, R. J., Mogun, H., & Avorn, J. (2001). Zolpidem use and hip fractures in older people. *Journal of the American Geriatrics Society. 49,* 1685–1690.

Weintraub, D., & Spurlock, M. (2002). Change in the rate of restraint use and falls on psychogeriatric inpatient unit: Impact of the health care financing administration's new restraint and seclusions standards for hospitals. *Journal of Geriatric Psychiatry and Neurology, 15,* 91–94.

Westerterp, K. R., & Meijer, E. P. (2001). Physical activity and parameters of aging: A physiological perspective. *Journal of Gerontology: Series A, 56A*(Special Issue II), 7–12.

Woollacott, M. H. (2000). Systems contributing to balance disorders in older adults. *Journal of Gerontology: Medical Sciences, 55A,* M424–M438.

Wu, F., Mason, B., Horne, A., Ames, R., Clearwater, J., Liu, M., Evans, M. C., Gamble, G. D., & Reid, I. R. (2002). Fractures between the ages of 20 and 50 years increase women's risk of subsequent fractures. *Archives of Internal Medicine, 162,* 33–36.

Yardly, L., & Smith, H. (2002). A prospective study of the relationship between feared consequences of falling and avoidance of activity in community-living older people. *Gerontologist, 42,* 17–23.

Yood, R. A., Harrold, L. R., Fish, L., Cernieux, J., Emani, S., Conboy, E., & Gurwitz, J. (2001). Prevention of glucocorticoid-induced osteoporosis: Experience in a managed care setting. *Archives of Internal Medicine, 161,* 1322–1327.

Zamboni, M., Zoico, E., Tosoni, P., Zivelonghi, A., Bortolani, A., Maggi, S., DiFrancesco, V., & Bosello, O. (2002). Relation between vitamin D, Physical performance, and disability in elderly persons. *Journal of Gerontology: Medical Sciences, 57A,* M7–M11.

Skin

LEARNING OBJECTIVES

1. Delineate age-related changes that affect the skin and its appendages.
2. Describe risk factors that can affect the skin of older adults.
3. Discuss the functional consequences of age-related changes and risk factors that affect the skin and its appendages.
4. Describe interview questions, inspection techniques, and observations that apply to the assessment of skin and its appendages in older adults.
5. Identify interventions that address the following aspects of skin care: maintenance of healthy skin, prevention of xerosis, detection and treatment of harmful skin lesions, and prevention of pressure ulcers.

The skin, hair, and nails have many physiologic and social functions. The skin participates in the following physiologic processes: (1) thermoregulation; (2) excretion of metabolic wastes; (3) protection of underlying structures; (4) synthesis of vitamin D; (5) maintenance of fluid and electrolyte balance; and (6) sensation of pain, touch, pressure, temperature, and vibrations. The social functions of the skin include facilitating communication and serving as an indicator of race, gender, work status, and other personal characteristics. As an important visible indicator of age, skin appearance may more accurately reflect the combined effects of biologic aging, lifestyle, and environment, rather than simply the person's chronologic age.

Hair serves to protect underlying organs, primarily the skin, from injury and adverse temperatures. In addition, in social contexts, the length and style of one's hair can reflect certain characteristics, such as age, gender, and personality. Hair is one of the most visible manifestations of aging, and gray hair is an age-related characteristic that can easily be altered when it is viewed as an undesirable indicator of age. Like the skin and hair, nails also have both a physiologic and social capacity. Physiologically, nails protect the underlying tissue from injury. In social contexts, nails can reflect personal characteristics, such as grooming and occupational activities.

 ## AGE-RELATED CHANGES THAT AFFECT THE SKIN

The skin is the largest, as well as the most visible, body organ. Structurally, the skin is composed of three layers: the epidermis, the dermis, and the subcutaneous tissue. Hair, nails, and sweat glands are considered to be skin appendages. As with other changes that affect older adults, distinguishing between those changes in the skin and its appendages that are strictly attributable to aging and those that occur because of risk factors is difficult. Most likely, lifestyle and environmental factors have a greater impact on skin aging than chronologic age alone. Genetic factors also may have a strong influence, especially with regard to baldness and gray hair.

Epidermis

The epidermis is the relatively impermeable outer layer of skin that serves as a barrier, preventing both the loss of body fluids and the entry of substances from the environment. Density of the epidermis varies, depending on the part of the body it covers. The epidermis consists of layers of cells that undergo a continual cycle of regeneration, cornification, and shedding. Corneocytes and melanocytes, respectively, account for about 85% and 3% of epidermal cells; both develop in the innermost layer of the epidermis, called the basal layer, or stratum germinativum. Corneocytes continually migrate to the surface of the skin, where they are shed. With increasing age, corneocytes become larger and more variable in shape; these changes are more marked in sun-exposed skin than in sun-protected skin. In addition, the rate of epidermal turnover decreases about 30% to 50% between the third and eighth decades of life (Yaar & Gilchrest, 2001).

Papillae serve to give the skin its texture and connect the epidermis to the underlying dermis at the dermal–epidermal junction. With increased age, the papillae retract, causing a flattening of the dermal–epidermal junction and diminishing the surface area between the epidermis and dermis. This age-related change slows the transfer of nutrients

between the dermis and epidermis. In contrast to other epidermal changes that are more prominent on exposed skin surfaces, this change is found to some degree on all skin surfaces.

Melanocytes, located in the basal layer of the epidermis, give the skin its color and provide a protective barrier against ultraviolet radiation. The primary age-related factor affecting melanocytes is a decrease of 10% to 20% in the number of active cells each decade beginning at about the age of 25 years. Although this decline occurs in both sun-exposed and sun-protected skin, the density of melanocytes in exposed skin is double or triple that in unexposed skin. With increased age, the number of Langerhans cells, which serve as macrophages, decreases in both sun-exposed and sun-protected skin; the decrease ranges from 50% to 70% in sun-exposed skin. Another age-related change that has been identified is a decrease in the moisture content of the outer epidermal layer, also known as the stratum corneum. Objective measures of skin water content, however, have raised questions about this conclusion and suggest that skin dryness in older adults is associated with the decreased proliferation of the epidermal layer rather than with actual water loss in the stratum corneum (Leveque, 2001).

In women, skin changes in the epidermis occur sharply between the ages of 40 and 60 years, but in men, the rate of decline is more constant throughout adulthood (Yaar & Gilchrest, 2001).

Dermis

The primary functions of the dermis are provision of support for structures within and below this layer and nourishment of the epidermis, which has no blood supply of its own. In addition, the dermis has a role in skin coloration, sensory perception, and temperature regulation. Collagen, which constitutes 80% of the dermis, confers elasticity and tensile strength, which help to prevent tearing and overstretching of the skin. Elastin, which constitutes 5% of the dermis, maintains skin tension and allows for stretching in response to movement. The dermal ground substance, which has a water-binding capacity, determines skin turgor and elastic properties. Blood vessels in the deep plexus play a role in thermoregulation, and those in the superficial plexus supply nutrients to the epidermal layer. Cutaneous nerves in the dermis receive information from the environment regarding pain, pressure, temperature, and deep and light touch.

Beginning in early adulthood, dermal thickness gradually diminishes, with collagen thinning at a rate of 1% per year. Elastin increases in quantity and decreases in quality because of age-related and environmentally induced changes. The dermal vascular bed is decreased by about one third with increased age; this contributes to the atrophy and fibrosis of hair follicles and sweat and sebaceous glands. Additional age-related changes in the dermis include a decrease in the number of fibroblasts and mast cells.

Subcutaneous Tissue and Cutaneous Nerves

The subcutis is the inner layer of fat tissue that protects the underlying tissues from trauma. Additional functions include storage of calories, insulation of the body, and regulation of heat loss. With increased age, some areas of subcutaneous tissue atrophy, particularly in the plantar foot surface and in sun-exposed areas of the hands, face, and lower legs. Other areas of subcutaneous tissue hypertrophy, however, with the overall effect being a gradual increase in the proportion of body fat between the third and eighth decades. This increased body fat is more pronounced in women than in men and is most noticeable in the waists of men and the thighs of women. Age-related changes also affect the cutaneous nerves responsible for sensations of pressure, vibration, and light touch.

Sweat and Sebaceous Glands

Eccrine and apocrine sweat glands originate in the dermal layer. Eccrine glands open directly onto the skin surface and are most abundant on the palms, soles, and forehead. Apocrine glands are larger than eccrine glands and open into hair follicles, primarily in the axillae and genital area. Although eccrine glands are important in thermoregulation, apocrine glands function solely in the production of secretions that are decomposed by skin bacteria to create a distinctive body odor. Both eccrine and apocrine glands decrease in number and functional ability with increased age.

Sebaceous glands are present in the dermal skin layer over every part of the body except the palms of the hands and the soles of the feet. These glands continually secrete sebum, a substance that combines with sweat to form an emulsion. Functionally, sebum prevents the loss of water and serves as a mild retardant of bacterial and fungal growth. Beginning in the third decade, sebum secretion declines steadily, with women having a greater decline than men. In younger adults, sebum production is closely related to the size of the sebaceous glands. In older adults, however, while the size of the sebaceous glands increases, the amount of sebum produced decreases.

Nails

The rate of nail growth is influenced by many factors, including age, climate, state of health, circulation to and around the nails, and activity of the fingers and toes. Nail growth begins to slow in early adulthood, with a gradual decrease of 30% to 50% over the life span. Other age-related changes affecting the nails include the development of longitudinal striations and a decrease in lunula size and nail plate thickness. Because of these changes, the nails become increasingly soft, fragile, and brittle and are increasingly likely to split. In appearance, the older nail is dull, opaque, longitudinally striated, and yellow or gray in color.

Hair

Hair color and distribution are altered to some degree in all older adults, with the most noticeable changes being baldness and gray hair. By the age of 50 years, about 50% of people have graying hair, and about 60% of white men have a noticeable degree of baldness. Graying of the hair is caused by a decline in melanin production and the gradual replacement of pigmented hairs by nonpigmented ones. Hair distribution is also affected by age-related changes, with patches of coarse terminal hair developing over the upper lip and lower face in older women, and in the ears, nares, and eyebrows of older men. Most older adults experience an age-related, progressive loss of body hair, initially in the trunk, then in the pubic area and axillae. In addition, some men are genetically predisposed to baldness, which is attributable to a change in production from coarse terminal hair to fine vellus hair (Figure 19-1).

> Whites develop wrinkles and gray hair at an earlier age than do other ethnic groups in the United States. Gray hair usually first appear in the mid-30s in whites, in the early 40s in the Japanese population, and in the mid-40s in African Americans (Hordinsky et al., 2002).

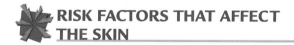 RISK FACTORS THAT AFFECT THE SKIN

The risk factors that influence the skin and appendages of older adults include heredity, pathologic conditions, adverse medication effects, and lifestyle

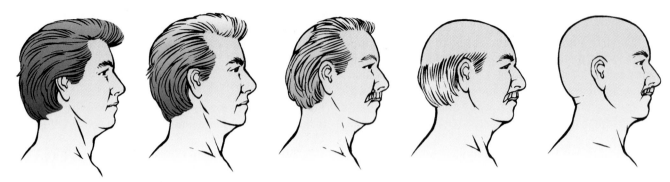

FIGURE 19-1 Typical age-related pattern of hair loss in men. (Reprinted with permission from Smeltzer, S. C., & Bare, B. G. [2000]. *Brunner and Suddarth's textbook of medical-surgical nursing* [9th ed., p. 1450]. Philadelphia: Lippincott Williams & Wilkins.)

and environmental factors. Genetic influences, which are irreversible, have only a small impact on the skin and its appendages, whereas lifestyle and environmental factors, which are the most amenable to interventions, have a significant impact. Thus, it is important to identify those risk factors, such as exposure to ultraviolet radiation, that can be alleviated through relatively simple interventions.

Genetic Influences

Heredity plays an important role in the development of pathologic and age-related skin and hair changes. People with fair skin, light hair, and light eyes are more sensitive to the effects of ultraviolet radiation than people with dark skin, as evidenced by the fact that skin cancers are common in light-skinned people of northern European ancestry but rare in African Americans.

Lifestyle and Environmental Influences

Lifestyle and environmental factors that can significantly affect skin aging include smoking, sun exposure, emotional stress, and substance or alcohol abuse (Antell & Taczanowski, 1999). Exposure to ultraviolet radiation is the most significant environmental factor, but adverse climate conditions also can cause negative functional consequences. For example, because the water content of the stratum corneum is influenced by relative humidity, xerosis (dry skin) is exacerbated when the relative humidity is below 30%.

The skin changes that occur as a result of exposure to ultraviolet radiation are referred to as *photoaging*. Some of the distinct characteristics of ultraviolet radiation–damaged skin are a thickened epidermis, enlarged sebaceous glands, a marked decrease in elasticity, dilated and tortuous blood vessels, decreased amounts of

mature collagen, large quantities of thickened and tangled elastic fibers, and the presence of pathologic lesions and seborrheic and actinic keratoses. Photoaged skin appears coarse, leathery, and ruddy or yellowed. In addition, it has many deep wrinkles, particularly on the face and neck. Exposure to ultraviolet radiation, even at levels that do not cause any detectable sunburn, can still damage skin collagen and lead to photoaging (Kang et al., 2001). Although these skin changes have been viewed as premature or accelerated aging, ultraviolet radiation–related skin changes are distinct from age-related changes. One reason for the common misconception that photoaging is an age-related change is that the cumulative effects of ultraviolet radiation may not be evident until later adulthood. Another reason for the difficulty in distinguishing between age-related and environmentally induced skin changes is that some skin changes, such as slowed wound healing, are thought to be accelerations or exacerbations of age-related processes.

Cigarette smoking is another factor that has been associated with detrimental skin changes as well as with hair changes, such as balding and gray hair (Antell & Taczanowski, 1999). The skin of people who smoke has been found to have more wrinkles and a grayish discoloration, and these changes are more pronounced in women. Cigarette smoking also diminishes the ability of the skin to protect against ultraviolet radiation damage and increases the risk for skin cancer. Epidemiologic studies suggest that the carcinogens in cigarettes directly affect epidermal and dermal cells (Yaar & Gilchrest, 2001).

Cultural factors, societal attitudes, and advertising trends influence hygiene and skin care practices. People in industrialized societies place a high value on frequent bathing and the use of commercial products for hygienic and cosmetic purposes. Although most of the personal practices arising from these values are desirable or harmless in younger adults, they may create risks for negative functional consequences in older adults. For example, frequent bathing with harsh deodorant soaps may cause or exacerbate dry skin problems in an older person.

> Hair loss patterns that commonly occur in older Hispanic and African American women (i.e., balding at the frontal and temporal hairline) may be associated with both biologic factors (e.g., fewer elastic fibers to anchor hair follicles) and cultural practices, such as tight braids and ponytails (Taylor, 2002).

Medication Effects

Common adverse medication effects involving the skin include pruritus, dermatoses, and photosensitivity reactions. Less common adverse medication effects on the skin and hair include alopecia and pigmentation changes of the skin or hair. Age-related skin changes also may be exacerbated by medications. For example, fluid loss from diuretics can exacerbate xerosis and cause further discomfort or skin problems for the older adult.

Dermatoses, or rashes, are the most frequently cited adverse medication effect, and they can be caused by virtually any medication. Medication-related skin eruptions vary widely in their manifestations and have no specific characteristics. In contrast to dermatoses arising from other causes, however, medication-related dermatoses tend to be redder in appearance, more abrupt in onset, and more widespread and symmetric in distribution. Although adverse dermatologic reactions frequently occur early in the course of treatment with a new medication, they can occur at any time during an initial or subsequent treatment course. Penicillin and penicillin-based medications are the medications most often associated with skin eruptions. Other medications that are commonly associated with dermatoses include sulfonamides, cephalosporins, barbiturates, and salicylates.

Photosensitivity is an adverse medication effect that causes an intensified response to ultraviolet radiation. The inflammatory reaction initially is distributed over sun-exposed areas but may spread to nonexposed areas and persist even after a medication is discontinued. Photosensitivity may begin during a seasonal exposure to bright sunlight or during a vacation in an unusually hot climate. Thiazides, phenothiazines, tetracyclines, amiodarone, and sulfonamides are the medications most often associated with photosensitivity reactions. Some herbal preparations also may increase the risk for photosensitivity (e.g., fennel, St. John's Wort).

Factors That Increase the Risk for Skin Breakdown

Although most older adults do not have mobility or activity limitations that are serious enough to increase the risk for skin breakdown, for the small percentage of older people who do, this risk is a major problem with far-reaching negative functional consequences. Because the primary contributing factor in the development of pressure ulcers is persistent pressure, people who lack the ability to move around independently are most vulnerable (Figure 19-2). Thus, the prevention of pressure ulcers is the focus of much of the nursing care for dependent older adults in any setting. Other risk factors that combine with activity limitations to cause pressure ulcers are moisture; friction; shearing force; poor hydration or nutrition (especially hypoproteinemia); and certain pathologic conditions (especially those that alter the person's level of consciousness). Age-related changes in the skin and pathologic conditions that occur more commonly in older adults also increase the risk for pressure ulcers and delay wound healing once pressure ulcers develop.

PATHOLOGIC CONDITIONS THAT CAN AFFECT SKIN

A nursing definition of pressure ulcers is "localized areas of cellular necrosis that occur over bony prominences exposed to pressure for a sufficient period of time to cause tissue ischemia" (Frantz, 2001). Although pressure ulcers are not a common problem for healthy older adults, they are a major problem for dependent older adults in any setting. A report from the National Pressure Ulcer Advisory Panel (NPUAP) found the following prevalence and incidence rates in various settings:

- Acute care: 10.1% to 17% prevalence, 0.4% to 38% incidence
- Long-term care: 2.3% to 28% prevalence, 2.2% to 23.9% incidence
- Home health care: 0% to 29% prevalence, 0% to 17% incidence (Cuddigan et al., 2001)

These figures are based on a review of more than 300 studies published between January 1, 1990 and December 31, 2000. Older adults account for about 70% of all patients with pressure ulcers (Thomas, 2001). In recent years, much attention has focused on the cost of prevention as well as treatment of pressure ulcers. Emphasis also has been placed on the presence or absence of pressure ulcers as an indicator of the quality of nursing care in institutional settings (Amlung et al., 2001; Berlowitz et al., 2000;

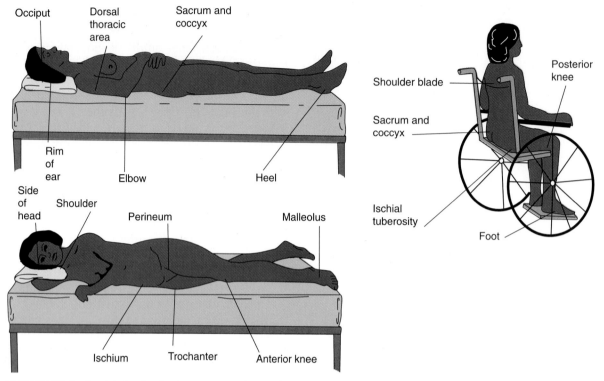

FIGURE 19-2 The risk for developing pressure ulcers is higher at these points. (Reprinted with permission from Craven, R. F., & Hirnle, C. J. [2003]. *Fundamentals of nursing: Human health and function* [4th ed., p. 988]. Philadelphia: Lippincott Williams & Wilkins.)

Meraviglia et al., 2002). *Healthy People 2010* added a goal of reducing the proportion of nursing home residents with a current diagnosis of pressure ulcers from a baseline of 16 diagnoses per 1000 nursing home residents in 1997 to a target of 8 diagnoses per 1000 residents (USDHHS, 2000).

FUNCTIONAL CONSEQUENCES ASSOCIATED WITH SKIN IN OLDER ADULTS

Age-related changes and risk factors negatively affect many functions of the skin, including thermoregulation, tactile sensitivity, and response to injury. Psychosocial consequences may occur when changes in the appearance of the skin and hair are associated with negative attitudes about visible indicators of aging.

The Impact of Skin Changes on Susceptibility to Injury

Under normal circumstances, age-related changes do not interfere with the protective function of the nails, and the primary consequences are generally cosmetic. Because the nails in older persons are fragile and

brittle, however, they are more likely to split. Moreover, if the nail has been injured, or if onychomycosis (a fungal infection of the nail) occurs, these age-related changes are likely to prolong the healing process.

Under most circumstances, age-related changes in the dermis and epidermis do not cause negative functional consequences. In the presence of any threat to skin integrity, however, age-related changes interfere with the protective function of the skin. Because of the flattened dermal–epidermal junction, older skin is less resistant to shearing forces than younger skin and is, therefore, more susceptible to bruises and shear-type injuries. Older skin is also more likely to develop blisters in response to disease processes. The age-related decrease in dermal thickness compounds the effects of the flattened dermal–epidermal junction, further increasing the susceptibility of older skin to injury and the effects of mechanical stress and ultraviolet radiation. Collagen changes also interfere with the tensile strength of the skin, causing it to be less resilient and more susceptible to damage from abrasive or tearing forces. Consequently, skin tears are common occurrences in older adults, especially those who have impaired mobility.

Regeneration of healthy skin takes twice as long for an 80-year-old person than for a 30-year-old person.

In perfectly intact skin, this slowed regeneration will not have any noticeable effects. When skin integrity is compromised, however, this age-related change contributes to delayed wound healing, even for superficial wounds. Consequences of age-related changes that affect the healing of deep wounds include an increased risk for postoperative wound disruption, decreased tensile strength of healing wounds, and increased risk for secondary infections.

The Impact of Skin Changes on Response to Ultraviolet Radiation

The age-related decrease in melanocytes causes older adults to tan less deeply and more slowly when exposed to ultraviolet radiation, and the increased variability in the melanocyte density in exposed and unexposed skin may cause a mottled and irregular appearance in the overall pigmentation. A positive functional consequence of age-related melanocyte changes is a decrease in the occurrence of moles beginning around the fourth decade. Aside from these cosmetic effects, a more serious functional consequence of the age-related decrease in melanocytes is the increased incidence of skin cancers in older adults. Other factors that increase the susceptibility of older adults to skin cancers are increased age, decreased number of Langerhans cells, and cumulative exposure to ultraviolet radiation.

The Impact of Skin Changes on Comfort and Sensation

Dry skin (xerosis) is one of the most universal complaints of older adults; indeed, it has been observed in up to 85% of noninstitutionalized older people. Age-related changes, such as diminished output of sebum and eccrine sweat, contribute to a decrease in the moisture content of the skin. Risk factors that may contribute to xerosis include stress, smoking, sun exposure, dry environments, excessive perspiration, adverse medication reactions, excessive use of soap, and certain medical conditions (e.g., hypothyroidism).

Tactile sensitivity begins to decline at about the age of 20 years, eventually causing older adults to have a diminished and less intense response to cutaneous sensations. This decline is attributable, at least in part, to age-related changes in pacinian and Meissner's corpuscles, which are the skin receptors that respond to vibration. Other contributing factors include lower body temperature and functional alterations in the central nervous system. A negative functional consequence of decreased tactile sensitivity is the increased susceptibility of older adults to

scald burns because of their diminished ability to feel dangerously hot water temperatures.

Thermoregulation is affected by age-related reductions in eccrine sweat, subcutaneous fat, and dermal blood supply. These age-related changes interfere with sweating, shivering, peripheral vasoconstriction and vasodilation, and insulation against adverse environmental temperatures. Thus, they increase the susceptibility of older adults to hypothermia and heat-related illnesses, as discussed in Chapter 21.

The Impact of Skin Changes on Quality of Life

The overall cosmetic effect of age-related skin changes is that the skin looks paler, thinner, and more translucent and is irregularly pigmented. Additional indicators of age-related skin changes include sagging, wrinkling, and various growths and lesions. Skin coloration changes are attributable to decreased melanocytes and dermal circulation. Wrinkling and sagging of the skin are caused by age-related changes in the epidermis and dermis, particularly those changes that affect the collagen fibers. The age-related decrease in subcutaneous tissue contributes to sagging of the skin, especially over the upper arms, by allowing the skin to be pulled downward by gravity.

Although these changes in appearance are gradual and do not interfere significantly with physiologic function, the psychosocial consequences of these changes can be significant because of the social value placed on personal appearance and negative attitudes that may be held about growing old. Regardless of age, one's physical appearance has been shown to be an important determinant of self-perception, and modern societies associate attractiveness with young-looking skin. Thus, age-related cosmetic changes will have psychosocial consequences in proportion to the prevalence of negative societal attitudes about aging and the extent to which the older adult adopts these attitudes.

Because of the high visibility of the face and neck, any signs of increased age that are prominent around the eyes and mouth may be especially bothersome to the person who wants to avoid visible indications of age. Characteristic signs of advanced age that are evident around the eyes include increased pigmentation, crow's-feet wrinkles, and fat and fluid accumulation in the upper lid and under the eye. Also, because of diminished skin elasticity and loss and shifting of subcutaneous fat, the neck skin sags, and a double chin may be evident.

Table 19-1 summarizes the age-related changes of the skin and its appendages as well as the associated functional consequences. Figure 19-3 illustrates

TABLE 19-1 ● Age-Related Changes Affecting Skin and Appendages

Change	Consequence
Decreased rate of epidermal proliferation	Delayed wound healing; increased susceptibility to infection
Flattened dermal–epidermal junction; thinning of dermis and collagen; increased quantity, but decreased quality, of elastin	Decreased resiliency; increased susceptibility to injury, bruising, mechanical stress, ultraviolet radiation, and blister formation
Reductions in dermal blood supply and the number of melanocytes and Langerhans' cells	Decreased intensity of tanning; irregular pigmentation; increased susceptibility to skin cancer; diminished dermal clearance, absorption, and immunologic response
Reductions in eccrine sweat, subcutaneous fat, and dermal blood supply	Decreased sweating and shivering; increased susceptibility to hypothermia or hyperthermia
Decreased moisture content	Dry skin; discomfort
Decreased number of Meissner's and pacinian corpuscles	Diminished tactile sensitivity; increased susceptibility to burns
Slowed nail growth	Increased susceptibility to cracking and injury; delayed healing
Changes in hair color, quantity, and distribution	Negative impact on self-esteem in proportion to negative attitudes

the age-related changes, risk factors, and negative functional consequences affecting the skin and its appendages.

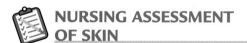

NURSING ASSESSMENT OF SKIN

Because the skin is the largest and most visible organ of the body, it is relatively easy to identify problems that affect functional aspects of the skin and its appendages. In addition, the skin may yield clues to other areas of physiologic and psychosocial function, such as nutrition, hydration, and personal care. Nurses collect information about the skin and its appendages during an assessment interview and through physical examination procedures. Opportunities for direct examination also arise during routine nursing care activities, such as assisting with personal care or listening to the lungs and apical heart rate. Information about other areas of function may be obtained by noting the characteristics of the skin and its appendages and using this information to validate or raise questions about other clinical impressions. For example, the observation that an older man has a beard of several days' growth, when combined with assessment information about his overall function, may support conclusions about possible depression or the need for assistance with personal care activities.

Identifying Opportunities for Health Promotion

Interview questions are aimed at identifying the person's perception of any problems, any risk factors that may contribute to skin problems, and the per-son's personal care behaviors that influence hair and skin status. Assessing these aspects of skin care can help identify opportunities for health education about risk factors and healthy skin care practices. Older adults often initiate a discussion about age spots or other noticeable skin changes, and they are usually very receptive to information about skin and hair care. Information about medications and other risk factors can be obtained as part of the overall assessment, and this information is incorporated into the skin assessment. Likewise, other pertinent information obtained during a comprehensive assessment, such as information about fluid intake, nutritional status, and mobility and safety, is applicable to the assessment of the skin and its appendages. Assessment questions about skin and its appendages are summarized in Display 19-1.

Observing Skin and Appendages

Close inspection of the skin and its appendages in a warm, private, and well-lit environment is an essential component of skin assessment. Examination of the skin is especially important in older adults because benign conditions, such as xerosis, may be the focus of complaints, whereas more serious conditions, such as skin cancer, may go unnoticed. The skin should be inspected for color, turgor, dryness, overall condition, and any growths or pathologic conditions. Cultural variations should be observed and documented. For example, older adults of Latin, Asian, or African ancestry may have faded Mongolian spots (i.e., irregular areas of blue coloration common on the buttocks and lower back, and, sometimes, on the arms, thighs, and abdomen) that might be mistaken for bruises. Also, when assessing for erythema or pressure areas, nurses should keep in mind that

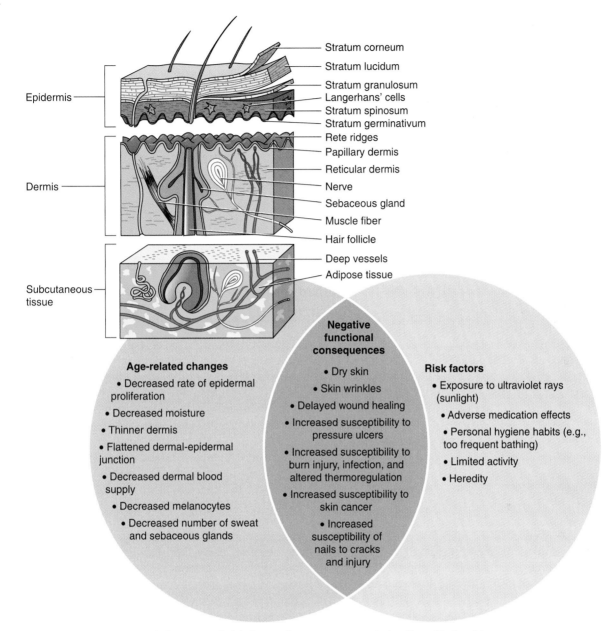

FIGURE 19-3 Age-related changes and risk factors intersect to negatively affect skin in older adults. (Inset of skin redrawn with permission from Skin care: Keeping the outside healthy. [1999]. *Nursing* 99 [Suppl.], December. Supported by Sage Products, Inc.)

early skin changes may be difficult to detect in people with darkly pigmented skin.

> Mongolian spots occur in 90% of African Americans, 80% of Asians and American Indians, and 9% of whites.

The common occurrence of various skin lesions complicates the assessment of skin in older adults. Although most of these changes are harmless, except in terms of their cosmetic consequences, some are cancerous or precancerous. An important aspect of health promotion is to reassure the older adult about the harmless changes and to encourage medical evaluation of the questionable ones. In general, a skin change with any of the following characteristics should be evaluated further: redness, swelling, dark pigmentation, moisture or drainage, pain or discomfort, and raised or irregular edges around a flat center. Also, any lesion that undergoes change, or any sore that does not heal within a reasonable period of time, should be evaluated further. Evaluation is also indicated when, because of its location, a mole or other

DISPLAY 19-1
Interview Questions for Assessing the Skin and Its Appendages

Questions to Assess Risk Factors and Skin Problems

- Do you have any concerns about or trouble with your skin?
- Do you have any sores that will not heal?
- Do you bruise easily?
- Have you ever been treated for skin cancer or any other skin problems?
- How much time do you spend in the sun?
- Do you spend time in tanning booths?
- Do you do anything to protect yourself from the effects of the sun?
- Do you have any problems with rashes, itching, swelling, or dry skin?

Questions to Assess Personal Care Practices

- How do you manage your bathing?
- How often do you take a bath or shower?
- What temperature water do you use?
- Do you use soap every time you bathe?
- What kind of soap do you use?
- Do you use any kind of skin lotion, creams, or ointments? What kind do you use and how frequently do you use it? Where do you apply it?
- Do you have any problems with your fingernails or toenails?
- Do you get or need any help with nail care?

skin lesion is subject to frequent rubbing or irritation. When a questionable skin lesion is observed, the following characteristics should be assessed and documented: size, shape, color, location, macular (flat) versus papular (raised), superficial versus penetrating, discrete versus diffuse borders, and the presence or absence of inflammation, redness, or discharge. Terminology related to various skin lesions in older adults is confusing, and many terms are used interchangeably for the same changes. Table 19-2 describes some of the terms used in conjunction with skin lesions that are common in older adults; some of these lesions are shown in Figure 19-4.

The skin and its appendages may provide clues to a broad spectrum of physiologic functional characteristics, particularly when nursing observations are combined with additional assessment information. For example, brown-stained fingertips are an indication of cigarette use, and feces under the fingernails and around the cuticle may be a clue to constipation. In some circumstances, toenails provide clues to mobility difficulties, especially when extremely long nails curl under the toes. Observations of the skin

may provide the only objective evidence of serious functional problems that the older person might not otherwise acknowledge. For example, multiple bruises, especially in various stages of healing, may be a significant clue to falls, alcoholism, self-neglect, or physical abuse. Observation and documentation of these signs are especially important when neglect or abuse is suspected but the older adult or caregiver denies any such problems.

In assessing the skin and its appendages for clues to broader aspects of function, it is important to understand that some of the usual manifestations may be altered in older adults. For example, nurses often assess skin turgor on the hands or arms as an indication of hydration status. Because of xerosis and decreased elasticity in the skin of older adults, however, skin turgor is not necessarily a reliable indicator of hydration status in this population. Although the hands or arms may be convenient and socially acceptable sites of inspection, the skin over protected areas, such as the sternum or abdomen, is a more accurate indicator of hydration status in older adults. In nonmedicated, older adults, the oral mucous membranes usually are reliable indicators of hydration. However, many medications, including over-the-counter preparations containing anticholinergic ingredients, cause dry mouth. Another age-related change that complicates assessment of the skin is delayed wound healing. This change makes it difficult to assess patterns of wound healing using the same standards that are applied to younger adults.

Observations of the hair, skin, and nails provide multiple clues to self-esteem and other aspects of psychosocial function. Physical limitations can interfere with personal grooming, as can psychosocial influences, such as lack of motivation or awareness. Thus, evidence of self-neglect in grooming may indicate depression, dementia, or social isolation. The use of hair coloring may reflect the person's attitudes about aging, and unusually deep hues of hair coloring or facial cosmetics may indicate impaired color perception. Display 19-2 summarizes observations that are made in the assessment of skin and its appendages.

> Ms. S. is an 84-year-old white woman who lives in her own home on the coast of Florida. She is quite active and healthy and enjoys golfing and "beach combing." She attends the local senior center, where you are the Wellness Nurse. The local chapter of the American Cancer Society is cosponsoring a "Skin Cancer Screening Day" at the senior center, and you have been asked to prepare a health education program entitled "Checking Your Skin for Serious Changes." You are also assisting the dermatologist with the screening examinations. Ms. S. attends the health

TABLE 19-2 • Common Skin Lesions in Older Adults

Common Term(s)	Description
Age spots, liver spots, senile lentigines, senile freckles	Pale to dark brown macules, occurring most frequently on exposed areas
Actinic keratosis, solar keratosis	Red, yellow, brown, or flesh-colored papules or plaques; gritty texture; surrounded by erythema; *premalignant*
Seborrheic keratosis	Brown or black papules or plaques with sharp edges and a waxy or wart-like texture; appearing most frequently on trunk and face
Sebaceous hyperplasia	Yellowish, doughnut-shaped elevations; common on face, especially in men
Senile angiomas, cherry or ruby angiomas, telangiectasia	Bright, ruby-red, pinpoint, superficial elevations of small blood vessels
Spider angiomas	Tiny, red papules with radiating arms; *may indicate a pathologic condition*
Venous stars	Bluish, irregular, sometimes spider-shaped lesions, appearing mainly on legs or chest
Venous lakes	Bluish papules with sharp borders, appearing mainly on lips or ears
Acrochordons, skin tags	Flesh-colored, pedunculated, or stalk-like lesions
Corns, calluses	Hard masses of keratin caused by repeated pressure or irritation
Xanthelasma	Fatty deposits, usually around the eyes; *may be related to a pathologic condition,* especially if large or numerous

education part of your program and says she's not sure if she can stay for the screening. She just has one "age spot," and she knows it's not serious because she's "had a couple skin cancers removed and this one looks different." You look at the questionable spot and you assess it as a brown, raised plaque with a gritty texture, about 1 cm in diameter.

 THINKING POINTS

➤ What additional assessment information would you want to obtain from Ms. S.?

➤ How would you use Table 19-2 and Displays 19-1 and 19-2 in your assessment?

➤ What advice would you give to Ms. S. about her skin?

Assessing Pressure Ulcers

Nurses are responsible for assessing risks for pressure ulcer development, the presence of pressure ulcers, and changes in the status of pressure ulcers. Several screening tools have been developed for assessing and rating risk factors for pressure ulcer development. In the United States, the Braden scale (Figure 19-5) is the most commonly used screening tool, and extensive testing supports its validity and reliability. The Hartford Institute for Geriatric Nursing recommends this tool as the best practice for identifying older adults who are at risk for developing pressure ulcers (Ayello, 1999). Although the Minimum Data Set-2 (MDS-2) includes risk assessment information about skin and is

widely used in long-term care facilities, the NPUAP has issued a report addressing several problems with the application of the MDS-2 as a screening tool for pressure ulcers (NPUAP, 1996). Rosenberg (2002) proposed a Checklist for Pressure Ulcer Prevention, which includes assessment of factors such as patient and caregiver knowledge about pressure ulcers. Nurses also need to consider a nutritional assessment as an essential component of pressure ulcer risk assessment (Schmidt, 2002).

> When using the Braden scale to evaluate pressure ulcer risk in African American and Latino people, a cutoff score of 17 or 18, rather than 16, is needed to prevent underprediction of risk in these populations (Ayello, 1999).

Recommended frequency of using a pressure ulcer screening tool varies and generally is based on the person's acuity and the frequency of change in his or her condition. Recommended frequency also depends on the clinical setting and length of time in that setting. For example, because most pressure ulcers develop within 3 weeks of admission to a long-term care facility, it would be important to use the screening tool frequently during that period. Recommended frequencies for using a screening tool in any setting are on admission and whenever the person's condition changes. Additional recommendations for specific settings are as follows: in acute care, reassess at least every 48 hours; in long-term care, reassess weekly for the first 4 weeks, then monthly to quarterly; in home health care, reassess with every nurse visit (Ayello & Braden, 2002).

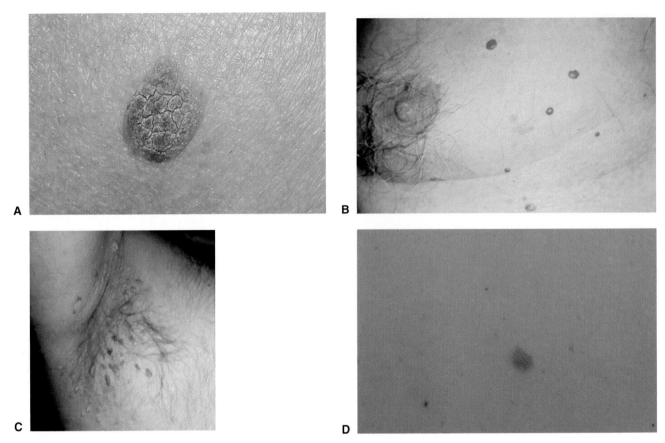

FIGURE 19-4 Common skin lesions in older adults. **(A)** Seborrheic keratosis. **(B)** Cherry angioma. **(C)** Skin tag. **(D)** Mole. (*Part A: Reprinted with permission from Goodheart, H. P. [1999]. A photo guide of common skin disorders: Diagnosis and management. Baltimore: Lippincott Williams & Wilkins, 1999. Parts B and D: Reprinted with permission from Weber, J., & Kelley, J. [2002]. Health Assessment in Nursing [2nd ed., pp. 131, 132]. Philadelphia: Lippincott Williams & Wilkins, 2002. Part C: Courtesy of Steifel Laboratories, Inc.*)

Assessment of pressure ulcers is important for developing appropriate interventions and for monitoring the effectiveness of interventions. One commentary emphasized that "the most common mistake that wound care novices make is inappropriate wound assessment" (Siegler & Ayello, 2001). Since the 1980s, pressure ulcers have been widely categorized by health care professionals according to stages I through IV (Table 19-3). This staging system was first published in 1975 by an orthopedic surgeon and has been modified and widely promulgated by the NPAUP (1995) in recent years. In 1998, the definition of stage I was revised to reflect more up-to-date information about assessment variations in lightly and darkly pigmented skin.

Appropriate assessment of pressure ulcers involves visual inspection and consideration of factors that can contribute to false conclusions. For example, darkly pigmented skin can mask stage I ulcers, and eschar can mimic hyperpigmented healthy skin. Lesions must be palpated to detect the softness of the tissue and differences in skin temperatures (Siegler & Ayello, 2001). The presence or absence of odors and the type of odor detected are additional factors that must be assessed and documented.

Once a pressure ulcer develops and is assessed according to the four stages, it must be assessed on an ongoing basis for changes. In the late 1980s, some nurses began documenting improvements in pressure ulcers by using a "reverse staging" method in which a stage IV pressure ulcer progressing through the healing sequence was documented as proceeding through stages III, II, and I. Since the mid-1990s, the NPAUP has advised against this practice and has stated that "pressure ulcer staging is only appropriate for defining the maximum anatomic depth of tissue damage" (NPUAP, 2000). The NPAUP further emphasizes that stage IV pressure ulcers can never become stage III, II, or I pressure ulcers because there is a permanent replacement of epidermis, dermis, subcutaneous, muscle, and bone tissue with granulation tissue. Therefore, there are significant structural

DISPLAY 19-2
Observations Regarding the Skin and Its Appendages

Examination of the Skin
- What is the color?
- Are there any areas of irregular pigmentation?
- Are there any areas of sunburn or tan?
- Are there areas that are discolored in any way?
- Are there any indications of poor circulation, especially in the extremities (e.g., varicosities, or areas of red, blue, or brown discoloration indicative of chronic stasis problems in the lower extremities)?
- What is the skin temperature?
- Is there a marked difference between the temperature of the extremities and that of the rest of the body?
- How does the skin feel in terms of moisture? Is it dry? Clammy? Oily?
- What is the skin's texture? Is it smooth or rough?
- Does the skin look tissue-paper thin?
- What is the turgor of the abdominal skin?
- Are scars present? (If so, describe their location and appearance.) Are there any signs of falling or physical abuse?
- Are any of the lesions described in Table 19-2 present?

Examination of the Hair and Nails
- What are the color, texture, and general condition of the hair?
- What is the distribution pattern of the hair?
- Is there any evidence of dandruff, scaling, or other problems with the hair?
- What are the color, length, cleanliness, and general condition of the toenails and fingernails?
- What are the color and general condition of the nail beds of the toes and fingers?

Personal Care Practices
- What is the person's overall appearance with regard to grooming and attention to personal attractiveness?
- If grooming is poor, does the person express concern about this or provide an explanation?
- Are there any psychosocial factors that influence personal care practices (e.g., is the person socially isolated or overburdened with caregiving responsibilities and, therefore, inattentive to personal care)?
- Are any of the following signs of neglect evident: presence of a body odor; unkempt, uncut, or matted hair; unusually long and unkempt fingernails or toenails; patches of brown crust on the skin; bruises; or any pathologic skin conditions?

and anatomic differences between a healed or healing stage IV pressure ulcer and any other pressure ulcer (NPUAP, 1995). Since 1996, the NPAUP has developed and validated a tool for assessing changes in pressure ulcers called the Pressure Ulcer Scale for Healing (PUSH) tool (Thomas et al., 1997; NPUAP, 2000). The PUSH tool scores pressure ulcers according to size, exudates, and tissue type, with changes in the PUSH score over time indicating the progression or regression of the pressure ulcer. Studies of the validity of the PUSH model found that it provides a simple, accurate, and clinically useful method of measuring progress toward wound healing (Stotts et al., 2001). This tool and instructions for its use are available from the NPUAP at http://www.npuap.org.

NURSING DIAGNOSIS

For functionally impaired older adults, the nursing diagnosis of Impaired Skin Integrity (or Risk for Impaired Skin Integrity) might be applicable. This is defined as a "state in which the individual experiences or is at risk for damage to the epidermal and dermal tissue" (Carpenito, 2002, p. 705). Some of the related factors that increase the risk for skin break-

down that are commonly found in functionally impaired older adults include incontinence, malnutrition, dehydration, limited mobility, prolonged bed rest, or a combination of these factors.

If the older adult has any suspicious-looking skin lesion, the nursing diagnosis of Ineffective Health Maintenance might be applicable. This is defined as "the state in which an individual or group experiences or is at risk of experiencing a disruption in health because of an unhealthy lifestyle or lack of knowledge to manage a condition" (Carpenito, 2002, p. 442). This diagnosis also would be applicable for people who are exposed to ultraviolet radiation (from sunlight or tanning booths) and who do not use protective measures.

OUTCOMES

Three nursing-sensitive outcomes associated with the nursing diagnosis of Impaired Skin Integrity are Comfort Level, Symptom Control, and Skin Tissue Integrity. Reported satisfaction with symptom control is an indicator of Comfort Level, and indicators for Symptom Control include recognition of symptom onset, variation, and persistence and use of relief and preventive measures. Indicators for Skin

Braden Scale
FOR PREDICTING PRESSURE SORE RISK

Patient's Name _____ Evaluator's Name _____ Date of Assessment

SENSORY PERCEPTION Ability to respond meaningfully to pressure-related discomfort	**1. Completely Limited:** Unresponsive (does not moan, flinch, or grasp) to painful stimuli, due to diminished level of consciousness or sedation. OR limited ability to feel pain over most of body surface.	**2. Very Limited:** Responds only to painful stimuli. Cannot communicate discomfort except by moaning or restlessness. OR has a sensory impairment which limits the ability to feel pain or discomfort over 1/2 of body	**3. Slightly Limited:** Responds to verbal commands, but cannot always communicate discomfort or need to be turned. OR has some sensory impairment which limits ability to feel pain or discomfort in 1 or 2 extremities.	**4. No Impairment:** Responds to verbal commands. Has no sensory deficit which would limit ability to feel or voice pain or discomfort.	
MOISTURE Degree to which skin is exposed to moisture	**1. Constantly Moist:** Skin is kept moist almost constantly by perspiration, urine, etc. Dampness is detected every time patient is moved or turned.	**2. Very Moist:** Skin is often, but not always moist. Linen must be changed at least once a shift.	**3. Occasionally Moist:** Skin is occasionally moist, requiring an extra linen change approximately once a day.	**4. Rarely Moist:** Skin is usually dry, linen only requires changing at routine intervals.	
ACTIVITY Degree of physical activity	**1. Bedfast:** Confined to bed	**2. Chairfast:** Ability to walk severely limited or non-existent. Cannot bear own weight and/or must be assisted into chair or wheelchair.	**3. Walks Occasionally:** Walks occasionally during day, but for very short distances, with or without assistance. Spends majority of each shift in bed or chair.	**4. Walks Frequently:** Walks outside the room at least twice a day and inside room at least once every 2 hours during waking hours.	
MOBILITY Ability to change and control body position	**1. Completely Immobile:** Does not make even slight changes in body or extremity position without assistance.	**2. Very Limited:** Makes occasional slight changes in body or extremity position but unable to make frequent or significant changes independently.	**3. Slightly Limited:** Makes frequent though slight changes in body or extremity position independently.	**4. No Limitations:** Makes major and frequent changes in position without assistance.	
NUTRITION Usual food intake pattern	**1. Very Poor:** Never eats a complete meal. Rarely eats more than 1/3 of any food offered. Eats 2 servings or less of protein (meat or dairy products) per day. Takes fluids poorly. Does not take a liquid dietary supplement. OR is NPO and/or maintained on clear liquids or IVs for more than 5 days.	**2. Probably Inadequate:** Rarely eats a complete meal and generally eats only about 1/2 of any food offered. Protein intake includes only 3 servings of meat or dairy products per day. Occasionally will take a dietary supplement. OR receives less than optimum amount of liquid diet or tube feeding.	**3. Adequate:** Eats over half of most meals. Eats a total of 4 servings of protein (meat, dairy products) each day. Occasionally will refuse a meal, but will usually take a supplement if offered. OR is on a tube feeding or TPN regimen which probably meets most of nutritional needs.	**4. Excellent:** Eats most of every meal. Never refuses a meal. Usually eats a total of 4 or more servings of meat and dairy products. Occasionally eats between meals. Does not require supplementation.	
FRICTION AND SHEAR	**1. Problem:** Requires moderate to maximum assistance in moving. Complete lifting without sliding against sheets is impossible. Frequently slides down in bed or chair, requiring frequent repositioning with maximum assistance. Spasticity, contractures or agitation leads to almost constant friction.	**2. Potential Problem:** Moves feebly or requires minimum assistance. During a move skin probably slides to some extent against sheets, chair, restraints, or other devices. Maintains relatively good position in chair or bed most of the time but occasionally slides down.	**3. No Apparent Problem:** Moves in bed and in chair independently and has sufficient muscle strength to lift up completely during move. Maintains good position in bed or chair at all times.		

Braden Scale Scores
   1=Highly Impaired
   3 or 4 = Moderate to Low Impairment
   Total Points Possible: 23
   Risk Predicting Score: 16 or Less

NPO: Nothing by Mouth

IV: Intravenously

TPN: Total parenteral nutrition

Total Score

FIGURE 19-5 The Braden Scale is a widely used screening tool to identify people at risk for pressure ulcers. (Courtesy of Barbara Braden and Nancy Bergstrom. Copyright, 1988. Reprinted with permission.)

TABLE 19-3 • Stages of Pressure Ulcer Development

Stage	Description
I	An observable pressure-related alteration of intact skin whose indicators, as compared with the adjacent or opposite area on the body, may include changes in one or more of the following: skin temperature (warmth or coolness), tissue consistency (firm or boggy feel), and sensation (pain, itching). The ulcer appears as a defined area of persistent redness in lightly pigmented skin, whereas in darker skin tones, the ulcer may appear with persistent red, blue, or purple hues.
II	Partial-thickness skin loss involving epidermis, dermis, or both. The ulcer is superficial and presents clinically as an abrasion, blister, or shallow crater.
III	Full-thickness skin loss involving damage to, or necrosis of, subcutaneous tissue that may extend down to, but not through, underlying fascia. The ulcer presents clinically as a deep crater with or without undermining of adjacent tissue.
IV	Full-thickness skin loss with extensive destruction, tissue necrosis, or damage to muscle, bone, or supporting structures (e.g., tendon, joint capsule). Undermining and sinus tracts also may be associated with stage IV pressure ulcers.

Source: National Pressure Ulcer Advisory Panel. (1995). Statement on reverse staging of pressure ulcers. *NPUAP Report, 4*(2).

Tissue Integrity include skin intactness and color in expected range (Hardy, 2001). Outcomes are achieved through interventions that promote healthy skin and prevent xerosis, as discussed in the Nursing Interventions section of this chapter. A nursing-sensitive outcome for Impaired Skin Integrity: Pressure Ulcer would be Wound Healing: Secondary Intention. Indicators of healing include granulation, epithelialization, decreased area, and resolution of wound (Frantz, 2001). This outcome is achieved through interventions that promote wound healing, as discussed in the Nursing Interventions section.

The nursing goal for older adults with risk factors for Impaired Skin Integrity is to prevent skin breakdown. Nurses who care for dependent older adults are directly responsible for providing skin care or for supervising caregivers who provide it. Interventions directed toward this goal are discussed in the following sections. For older adults with a nursing diagnosis of Altered Health Maintenance, outcomes might include Risk Control, Health Seeking Behaviors, and Knowledge: Health Behaviors (Glick & Ressler, 2001).

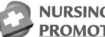

NURSING INTERVENTIONS TO PROMOTE HEALTHY SKIN

Maintaining Healthy Skin

Because the condition of the skin depends largely on the overall health of the person, the maintenance of optimal nutrition and hydration is an important

DISPLAY 19-3
Health Promotion Teaching About Skin Care for Older Adults

Maintaining Healthy Skin

- Include adequate amounts of fluid in the daily diet.
- Use humidifiers to maintain environmental humidity levels of 40% to 60%.
- Apply emollient lotions twice daily or more often.
- Use emollient lotions immediately after bathing, when the skin is still moist.
- Avoid massaging over bony prominences when applying lotions. Do not use rubbing alcohol.
- Avoid skin care products that contain perfumes or isopropyl alcohol.
- Avoid multiple-ingredient preparations because unnecessary additives may cause allergic responses.

Personal Care Practices

- When bathing or showering, use soap sparingly or use a mild, superfatted, nonperfumed soap (e.g., Castile, Dove, Tone, Basis).
- Maintain water temperatures for bathing at about 90°F to 100°F.
- Make sure skin is well rinsed after soap use. Whirlpool baths stimulate circulation, but moderate temperatures should be maintained.
- Apply emollient products after bathing, rather than using them in the bath water, to minimize the risk for falls on oily surfaces and to maximize the benefits of the emollient.
- Use emollient products containing petrolatum or mineral oil (e.g., Keri, Eucerin, Aquaphor).
- If you use bath oils, take extra safety precautions to prevent slipping.
- If emollient products are applied to the feet, don nonskid slippers or socks before walking.
- Make sure your skin is dried thoroughly, especially between your toes and in other areas where your skin rubs together.
- When drying your skin, use gentle, patting motions rather than harsh, rubbing motions.
- Obtain regular podiatric care.

Avoiding Sun Damage

- Wear wide-brimmed hats, sun visors, sunglasses, and long-sleeved garments when exposed to the sun.
- Wear clothing made of cotton, rather than polyester fabrics, because ultraviolet rays can penetrate polyester.
- Apply sunscreen lotions generously and frequently, beginning 1 hour before sun exposure.
- Use sunscreen lotions with an SPF of 15 or higher. Avoid exposure to the sun between 10:00 AM and 3:00 PM.
- Protect yourself from ultraviolet rays even on cloudy days and when you are in the water.
- Artificial tanning booths use ultraviolet type A rays, which are advertised as harmless, but which have been found to cause damage in high doses.

Preventing Injury From Abrasive Forces

- Do not use starch, bleach, or strong detergents when laundering clothing or linens.
- Use knit or percale bed linens.
- Use soft terry or cotton washcloths.
- If plastic-lined pads are necessary, make sure that an adequate amount of soft, absorbent material is placed over the plastic.

Nutritional Considerations

- Include adequate intake of zinc, magnesium, and vitamins A, B-complex, C, and E.

Complementary and Alternative Care Practices

- Herbs for topical use as emollients include aloe vera and calendula.
- Herbs for itching and inflammation include burdock, chickweed, marigold, chamomile, purslane, pineapple, marshmallow, peppermint oil, witch hazel, walnut leaves, and evening primrose oil.
- Bergamot, chamomile, lavender, and geranium can be used for aromatherapy.

---

intervention in the skin care of older adults. Because environmental conditions and personal care practices also influence the health of the skin, interventions are directed toward educating the older adult about these factors. Display 19-3 summarizes the teaching points that should be included in the education of older adults, or caregivers of dependent older adults, regarding skin health. Although much of the gerontological nursing literature advocates limiting the number of baths or showers to one to three times weekly, it is not clear that there is a cause-and-effect relationship between bathing or showering and dry skin. Factors such as smoking, dehydration, sun exposure, low environmental humidity, and the use of harsh cleansing products are more likely than frequency of bathing to contribute to dry skin in older adults (Sheppard & Brenner, 2000).

In recent years, nursing literature has addressed a variety of products and methods that are being introduced for bathing of older adults. Dawson and colleagues (2001) compared the cost and effectiveness of a no-rinse skin cleanser and regular bathing soap and found that cost was the only difference between the two products, with the no-rinse product being twice as expensive. Sheppard and Brenner (2000) investigated the use of the Bag Bath/Travel Bath and concluded that this prepackaged bed bath kit provided an easy, convenient, and effective method of bathing that improved skin quality for nursing home residents. Institutional settings are now making their own bag bath kits and finding that this is cost effective because of reduced use of staff time and other resources. These kits generally contain all the supplies needed for a bed bath, and the washcloths and towels often are warmed in a microwave before being used for a bath. Some of these kits use disposable materials to eliminate the need for laundering. Prepackaged bed bath kits also are available at drug stores for home use.

Preventing Skin Wrinkles

The best methods of preventing skin wrinkles are avoiding exposure to sunlight and using a sunscreen with a sun protection factor (SPF) of 15 or higher when exposure to the sun is unavoidable. Sunscreens also can prevent the occurrence of keratoses (Lawrence, 2000), and topical products containing α- or β-hydroxy acids may be beneficial in reversing wrinkles and promoting the regression of solar keratoses. Hormonal therapy may improve dryness, elasticity, fine wrinkling, collagen content, and wound healing in postmenopausal women (Phillips et al., 2001). Information about the harmful effects of sunlight should be included in health education about maintenance of healthy skin and prevention of undesirable cosmetic and pathologic skin changes. Also, nurses can encourage women who are concerned about wrinkles and dry skin to discuss medical interventions with their primary care provider.

Preventing Dry Skin

Dry skin discomfort may be alleviated with moisturizers, which can act either as occlusive agents that prevent evaporation of water from the skin or as humectant agents that attract water from the skin layers to the stratum corneum. Petrolatum is the most effective occlusive moisturizer, and silicones are the newest type of occlusive moisturizer. Lanolin is an effective occlusive moisturizer, but it is expensive and tends to cause allergic reactions. Honey, urea, and glycerin are examples of humectant moisturizers. Unless the environmental humidity is at least 70%, humectants alone are not effective in hydrating the skin because they draw moisture from the dermis to the epidermis (Draelos, 2000).

Emollients are skin care products that moisturize and lubricate the skin. Because the effectiveness of an emollient is based on its ability to prevent water evap-

oration, its beneficial effects will be enhanced when it is applied to skin that already has some degree of moisture. Thus, an emollient applied to moist skin immediately after bathing will trap moisture and be more effective than an emollient that is added to the bath water. See Display 19-3 for information on the use of emollients and other interventions designed to prevent or care for dry skin in older adults.

Detecting and Treating Harmful Skin Lesions

Early detection and treatment of cancerous or precancerous skin lesions are key factors in the prevention of negative functional consequences because the cure rate for most skin cancers approaches 100% with early excision. The role of the nurse is to detect any suspicious-looking lesions and to encourage or facilitate further evaluation. If the older adult or caregiver has avoided medical evaluation because of fears about cancer, the nurse can provide assurance about the high cure rate and the minimal chance of long-term problems if early treatment is sought. Older adults, and caregivers of dependent older adults, will often respond to a nurse's encouragement to obtain medical care for skin lesions, especially if any unreasonable fears are allayed.

Preventing and Managing Pressure Ulcers

Prevention of pressure ulcers is one of the most important responsibilities of any nurse caring for dependent older adults who have activity or mobility limitations. Because skin tissue breakdown is attributable to both impaired circulation and external pressure, the key intervention for preventing skin breakdown is to ensure adequate circulation and minimal external pressure. Thus, the nurse makes sure that older adults with mobility limitations change position at a minimum of 2-hour intervals and that pressure-relieving measures are instituted to relieve any external pressure areas. A review of studies found that pressure-reducing mattresses were superior to standard mattresses, with a 70% relative risk reduction, but there was no significant difference in the relative effectiveness of different devices, such as alternating air mattress and low-air-loss beds (Thomas, 2001). This review concluded that patients who are at risk for developing a pressure ulcer should be treated with a pressure-reducing device, with the choice based on cost, comfort, and availability. Gel, foam, and low-air-loss pressure-relieving overlays and cushions also are available and should be used for chairs.

In addition to preventing persistent pressure on the skin, it is important to avoid any friction or shearing forces and to ensure that the skin is free of excess moisture. The nurse also should promote good skin circulation by applying moisturizing agents at frequent intervals, avoiding massage over bony prominences. Good personal hygiene and the quick removal of irritants, such as urine, are important interventions, as are measures aimed at promoting optimal hydration and nutrition. Many of the interventions summarized in Display 19-3 are effective in preventing pressure ulcers as well.

Guidelines for the treatment of pressure ulcers have been developed by the Agency for Healthcare Research and Quality, and a wealth of up-to-date information is available from the NPUAP; both resources are listed in the Educational Resources at the end of this chapter. Bates-Jenson (2001) provides an excellent summary of supporting evidence for commonly used interventions for prevention and management of pressure ulcers. Numerous interventions are available for direct wound care, with much agreement on the benefit of maintaining a moist wound environment as compared with using dry or wet-to-dry dressings or exposing the wound to air. Choices of saline or occlusive dressings depend on wound location and characteristics such as exudate (Thomas, 2001). Medical interventions include débridement, treatment of infections, and surgical closure.

In addition to direct wound care interventions, treatment interventions focus on nutrition, with particular attention to protein intake. A reasonable protein intake for optimal healing of pressure ulcers is between 1.2 and 2 g/kg/day (Lewis, 2001; Thomas, 2001). Zinc or vitamin C supplements above the recommended daily allowance have not been found to improve pressure ulcer healing, and supplementation of more than 100 mg/day of zinc may be detrimental (Houston et al., 2001; Thomas, 2001). Similarly, the effectiveness of enteral feeding as an intervention for pressure ulcers has not been established (Thomas, 2001). Hormonal therapy is currently under investigation for pressure ulcer prevention, with one study finding a 32% reduction in the risk for developing pressure ulcers in older women taking hormonal therapy (Margolis, 2002).

▶ Recall that Ms. S. attends the senior center in Florida where you are responsible for presenting a health education program entitled "Maintaining Healthy Skin." You plan to emphasize the importance of self-care techniques, such as checking for skin changes. Ms. S. is very interested in attending the program and told you she will be bringing her 80-year-old sister, who also lives in Florida. Ms. S. worries about her sister because she uses a wheelchair and is very frail. You know that several of the participants at the senior program use wheelchairs, and you plan to include health education about prevention of pressure ulcers.

THINKING POINTS

➤ Outline your health education points for a 1/2-hour program, including specific points about prevention of pressure ulcers.

➤ How would you use Table 19-2 and Display 19-3 in your program?

➤ Find additional information that you would consider using as educational materials for this program.

EVALUATING EFFECTIVENESS OF NURSING INTERVENTIONS

Nursing care for older adults with dry or itching skin is evaluated by determining the degree to which the interventions alleviate the person's complaints. It may take several weeks for older adults to feel the full effects of skin care interventions because of an age-related delay in dermal response to external stimuli. Also, there is a great deal of individual variation among older adults in their response to interventions. Thus, it may be necessary to evaluate the effects of one type of soap or lotion for several weeks before trying a different brand if the problem does not resolve. Because environmental humidity affects skin comfort, the evaluation of interventions also may be influenced by environmental conditions.

Effectiveness of interventions for older adults at risk for skin breakdown is measured by the absence of pressure ulcers. Effectiveness of interventions for pressure ulcers that have developed is determined by rate of healing and prevention of complications, such as osteomyelitis. Because significant cost and quality-of-life issues are associated with pressure ulcers, the prevention of skin breakdown can have far-reaching positive consequences for older adults who are at risk for developing pressure ulcers.

CHAPTER SUMMARY

Gray hair and skin wrinkles are the most visible signs of aging. Less visible changes in the skin and its appendages include slowed nail growth, decreased moisture content, a slowed rate of epidermal proliferation, and reductions in sweat glands and subcutaneous fat tissue. Although some skin changes are inevitable consequences of aging, most are associated with heredity and the cumulative effects of exposure to ultraviolet radiation. Likewise, balding and graying hair are strongly associated with heredity. Functionally, the age-related changes that affect the skin and its appendages have few significant physiologic consequences for healthy older adults. Negative functional consequences include dry skin, delayed wound healing, and increased susceptibility to altered thermoregulation and shear-type injury. Because of negative stereotypes about old age, older adults with gray hair and skin wrinkles may experience negative psychosocial consequences, particularly if they have not challenged these stereotypes. Pressure ulcers are not a normal part of aging, but frail older adults are likely to have factors that increase the risk for skin breakdown. Risk factors for pressure ulcers include activity limitations, moisture, friction, poor hydration or nutrition, and altered level of consciousness.

Nursing assessment of the skin and its appendages focuses on identifying factors that increase the risk for negative functional consequences (e.g., increased susceptibility to injury or altered thermoregulation). In addition, the nursing assessment might identify factors that cause physical or psychosocial discomfort for the older adult (e.g., dry skin or embarrassment about skin wrinkles). Nurses assess any skin lesions to determine the need for medical evaluation of potentially harmful ones. Nurses also are responsible for assessing for risk factors for skin breakdown in vulnerable older adults. Relevant nursing diagnoses are Impaired Skin Integrity and Altered Comfort related to dry skin. Nursing care focuses on alleviating uncomfortable skin conditions, addressing risk factors that contribute to skin problems, and referring older adults with questionable skin lesions for further evaluation. The risk factors that are most amenable to interventions are exposure to ultraviolet radiation and personal care habits that contribute to dry skin. Nursing care is evaluated according to the degree to which the interventions alleviate risk factors or relieve the person's complaints.

CONCLUDING CASE STUDY AND NURSING CARE PLAN

➤ Ms. S. is now 92 years old and lives in an assisted-living facility in Florida. She ambulates with a walker and needs assistance with meals, medications, and personal care. Three months ago, her doctor prescribed hydrochlorothiazide, 25 mg, every morning for isolated systolic hypertension. She has a history of arthritis but does not take any medication for it. Ms. S. attends your monthly nursing clinic for health education and blood pressure monitoring. When she comes to see you in January, she complains of dry skin and discomfort.

■ Nursing Assessment

You interview Ms. S. about her personal care practices and find out that she soaks in the tub in lukewarm water three times weekly and enjoys using bath salts and perfumed skin lotions. She spends much of her leisure time outdoors on the patio or in the air-conditioned solarium. She does not use sunscreens because she thinks they are unnecessary and too oily. She states that she has not had a sunburn for several years and that she's built up a good tolerance to the sun. She does not wear sunglasses or sun hats. She reports that she has had three skin cancers removed in the past 10 years, one from her cheek, one from her arm, and one from her ear lobe. She says she does not worry about recurrent skin cancer because she no longer swims outside or sits by the swimming pool. Also, because she doesn't get sunburned, she believes she is not at risk for skin cancer.

Inspection of Ms. S.'s skin reveals dry, wrinkled skin on her face and arms and unevenly tanned skin on her face, neck, and extremities. She has many age spots over the exposed skin areas but no suspicious-looking lesions. Ms. S. has blue eyes and fair skin.

■ Nursing Diagnosis

Your nursing diagnosis is Ineffective Health Maintenance related to excessive sunlight exposure and insufficient knowledge of the effects of ultraviolet light. Evidence for this diagnosis comes from her misconceptions about risk factors for skin cancer and other skin problems. Also, you identify her lack of knowledge about the potential photosensitivity of hydrochlorothiazide as a factor that contributes to Ineffective Health Maintenance.

■ Nursing Care Plan

Your nursing care plan for Ms. S. is given in Display 19-4.

 CRITICAL THINKING EXERCISES

1. What would a healthy 85-year-old person notice with regard to his or her skin, hair, and nails?
2. Describe the questions you would ask and the observations you would make to assess the skin, hair, and nails of an 82-year-old person.
3. Describe at least eight skin lesions that are normal and three skin lesions that require further evaluation.
4. You are asked to give a 20-minute presentation on "Maintaining Healthy Skin" at a senior center.

DISPLAY 19-4 • NURSING CARE PLAN FOR MS. S.

EXPECTED OUTCOME	NURSING INTERVENTIONS	NURSING EVALUATION
Ms. S.'s discomfort from dry skin will be alleviated.	• Discuss and describe age-related skin changes. • Discuss risk factors that contribute to skin discomfort (e.g., bath salts, perfumed lotions, unprotected exposure to sunlight). • Use Display 19-3 to teach Ms. S. about skin care practices directed toward alleviating dry skin.	• Ms. S. will report that she no longer experiences skin discomfort and dryness.
Ms. S.'s knowledge about risk factors for skin cancer will be increased.	• Discuss the relationship between skin cancer and exposure to ultraviolet rays. • Explain that any exposure to ultraviolet rays is a risk factor for skin cancer. • Emphasize that a history of skin cancer increases the chance of recurrent skin cancer.	• Ms. S. will verbalize an awareness of the risk factors for skin cancer.
The factors that increase Ms. S.'s risk of skin problems and skin cancer will be eliminated.	• Inform Ms. S. that hydrochlorothiazide may increase the risk for photosensitivity, making protective measures increasingly important. • Use Display 19-3 as a guide for discussing measures to avoid sun damage. • Emphasize the importance of using sunscreens and wearing wide-brimmed hats when in the solarium or outside.	• Ms. S. will use measures to reduce the risk for skin cancer and sun damage.

Outline the content of your health education program.

5. What would you teach the family caregivers of a 74-year-old woman who is confined to a wheelchair with regard to the prevention of pressure sores?

Future Directions for Healthier Aging: Focus on Skin

• Studies are addressing various sequential treatment protocols for pressure ulcers. For example, a study found that sequential treatment with 4 weeks of calcium alginate followed by treatment with hydrocolloid dressing healed pressure ulcers faster than hydrocolloid dressing alone (Belmin et al., 2002).
• Studies are addressing the potential role for topical application of nerve growth factors (also called *cytokine therapy*) for the treatment of pressure ulcers, with particular emphasis on using different types of growth factors sequentially.

EDUCATIONAL RESOURCES

Agency for Health Care Policy and Research
U.S. Department of Health and Human Services
2101 Jefferson Street, Suite 501, Rockville, MD 20852
(301) 594-1364
http://www.ahcpr.gov

American Cancer Society
1599 Clifton Road, NE, Atlanta, GA 30329
(800) 227-2345
http://www.cancer.org

Canadian Cancer Society
10 Alcorn Avenue, Suite 200, Toronto,
    ON M4V 3B1
(416) 961-7223
http://www.cancer.ca

National Arthritis and Musculoskeletal and Skin Diseases Information Clearinghouse (NAMSIC)
National Institutes of Health, AMS Circle, Bethesda, MD 20892-3675
(877) 226-4267
http://www.nih.gov/niams

National Pressure Ulcer Advisory Panel (NPUAP)
12100 Sunset Hills Road, Suite 130, Reston,
    VA 20190-5202
(703) 464-4849
http://www.npuap.org

REFERENCES

Amlung, S. R., Miller, W. L., & Bosley, L. M. (2001). The 1999 national pressure ulcer prevalence survey: A benchmarking approach. *Advances in Skin and Wound Care, 14,* 297–301.

Antell, D. E., & Taczanowski, E. M. (1999). How environment and lifestyle choices influence the aging process. *Annals of Plastic Surgery, 43,* 585–588.

Ayello, E. A. (1999). Predicting pressure ulcer sore risk. *Journal of Gerontological Nursing, 25*(10), 7–9.

Ayello, E. A., & Braden, B. (2002). How and why to do pressure ulcer risk assessment. *Advances in Skin and Wound Care, 15,* 125–130.

Bates-Jensen, B. M. (2001). Quality indicators for prevention and management of pressure ulcers in vulnerable elders. *Annals of Internal Medicine, 135,* 744–751.

Belmin, J., Meaume, S., Rabus, M-T, & Bohbot, S. (2002). Sequential treatment with calcium alginate dressings and hydrocolloid dressings accelerates pressure ulcer healing in older subjects. *Journal of the American Geriatrics Society, 50,* 269–274.

Berlowitz, D. R., Bezerra, H. Q., Brandeis, G. H, Kader, B., & Anderson, J. J. (2000). Are we improving the quality of nursing home care? The case of pressure ulcers. *Journal of the American Geriatrics Society, 48,* 59–62.

Carpenito, L. J. (2002). *Nursing diagnosis: Application to clinical practice* (9th ed.). Philadelphia: Lippincott Williams & Wilkins.

Cuddigan, J., Berlowitz, D. R., & Ayello, E. A. (2001). Pressure ulcers in America: Prevalence, incidence, and implications for the future. *Advances in Skin and Wound Care, 14,* 208–215.

Dawson, M., Pilgrim, A., Moonsawmy, C., & Moreland, J. (2001). An evaluation of two bathing products in a chronic care setting. *Geriatric Nursing, 22,* 91.

Draelos, Z. D. (2000). Dermatologic aspects of cosmetics: Therapeutic moisturizers. *Dermatologic Clinics, 18,* 597–607.

Frantz, R. A. (2001). Impaired skin integrity: Pressure ulcer. In M. L. Maas, K. C. Buckwalter, M. D. Hardy, T. Tripp-Reimer, M. G. Titler, & J. P. Specht (Eds.), *Nursing care of older adults: Diagnoses, outcomes, and interventions* (pp. 121–136). St. Louis: Mosby.

Glick, O. J., & Ressler, C. (2001). Altered health maintenance. In M. L. Maas, K. C. Buckwalter, M. D. Hardy, T. Tripp-Reimer, M. G. Titler, & J. P. Specht (Eds.) *Nursing care of older adults: Diagnoses, outcomes, and interventions* (pp. 137–144). St. Louis: Mosby.

Hardy, M. D. (2001). Impaired skin integrity: Dry skin. In M. L. Maas, K. C. Buckwalter, M. D. Hardy, T. Tripp-Reimer, M. G. Titler, & J. P. Specht (Eds.), *Nursing care of older adults: Diagnoses, outcomes, and interventions* (pp. 137–144). St. Louis: Mosby.

Hordinsky, M., Sawaya, M., & Roberts, J. L. (2002). Hair loss and hirsutism in the elderly. *Clinics in Geriatric Medicine, 18,* 121–133.

Houston, S., Haggard, J., Williford, J., Meserve, L., & Shewokis, P. (2001). Adverse effects of large-dose zinc supplementation in an institutionalized older population with pressure ulcers. *Journal of the American Geriatrics Society, 49,* 1130–1131.

Kang, S., Fisher, G. J., & Voorhees, J. J. (2001). Photoaging: Pathogenesis, prevention, and treatment. *Clinics in Geriatric Medicine, 17,* 643–660.

Lawrence, N. (2000). New and emerging treatments for photoaging. *Dermatologic Clinics, 18,* 99–112.

Leveque, J. L. (2001). Quantitative assessment of skin aging. *Clinics in Geriatric Medicine, 17,* 673–690.

Lewis, M. M. (2001). Nutrition in long-term care. *Clinics in Family Practice, 3,* 627–651.

Margolis, D. J. (2002). Hormone replacement therapy and prevention of pressure ulcers and venous leg ulcers. *Lancet, 359,* 675–677.

Meraviglia, M., Becker, H., Grobe, S. J., & King, M. (2002). Maintenance of skin integrity as a clinical indicator of nursing care. *Advances in Skin and Wound Care, 15,* 24–29.

National Pressure Ulcer Advisory Panel. (1995). Statement on reverse staging of pressure ulcers. *NPUAP Report, 4*(2).

National Pressure Ulcer Advisory Panel. (1996). Minimum Data Set-2 (MDS-2) and skin ulcer assessment. *NPUAP Report, 4*(3).

National Pressure Ulcer Advisory Panel. (2000). The facts about reverse staging in 2000: The NPUAP position statement. *NPUAP Report, 4*(2).

Phillips, T. J., Demircay, Z., & Sahu, M. (2001). Hormonal effects on skin aging. *Clinics in Geriatric Medicine, 17,* 661–672.

Rosenberg, C. J. (2002). New checklist for pressure ulcer prevention. *Journal of Gerontological Nursing, 28*(8), 7–12.

Schmidt, T. (2002). Pressure ulcers: Nutrition strategies that make a difference. *Caring, June,* 18–24.

Sheppard, C. M., & Brenner, P. S. (2000). The effects of bathing and skin care practices on skin quality and satisfaction with an innovative product. *Journal of Gerontological Nursing, 26*(10), 36–45.

Siegler, E. L., & Ayello, E. A. (2001). Pressure ulcer prevention and treatment. In M. D. Mezey (Ed.), *The encyclopedia of elder care* (pp. 521–523). New York: Springer.

Stotts, N. A., Rodeheaver, G. T., Thomas, D. R., Frantz, R. A., Bartolucci, A. A., Sussman, C., Ferrell, B. A. (2001). An instrument to measure healing in pressure ulcers: Development and validation of the Pressure Ulcer Scale for Healing (PUSH). *Journal of Gerontology: Medical Sciences, 12,* M795–M799.

Taylor, S. C. (2002). Understanding of skin color. *Journal of the American Academy of Dermatology, 46*(2 Suppl), S41–S62.

Thomas, D. R. (2001). Issues and dilemmas in the prevention and treatment of pressure ulcers: A review. *Journal of Gerontology: Medical Science, 12*(56A), M328–M340.

Thomas, D. R., Rodeheaver, G. T., Bartolucci, A. A., Franz, R. A., Sussman, C., Ferrell, B. A., et al. (1997). Pressure ulcer scale for healing: Derivation and validation of the PUSH tool. *Advances in Wound Care, 10*(5), 96–101.

U.S. Department of Health and Human Services (USDHHS). (2000). *Healthy people 2010* (2nd ed). Washington, DC: U.S. Government Printing Office.

Yaar, M., & Gilchrest, B. A. (2001). Skin aging: Postulated mechanisms and consequent changes in structure and function. *Clinics in Geriatric Medicine, 17,* 617–630.

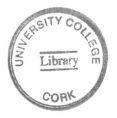

Sleep and Rest

LEARNING OBJECTIVES

1. Delineate age-related changes that affect sleep and rest patterns in older adults.
2. Describe psychosocial, environmental, and physiologic risk factors that influence sleep and rest in older adults.
3. Discuss sleep changes and problems common in older adults.
4. Identify assessment techniques that are useful in identifying opportunities for health promotion and planning interventions to improve sleep in older adults.
5. Identify interventions that can be implemented to promote optimal sleep and to address risks that interfere with sleep in older adults.

About one third of a person's lifetime is spent in sleep and rest activities, yet little attention is paid to the essential physiologic and psychosocial functions accomplished through these activities. During periods of sleep and rest, many metabolic processes decelerate, production of growth hormone increases, and tissue repair and protein synthesis accelerate. During the deeper stages of sleep, cognitive and emotional information is stored, filtered, and organized. Thus, physiologic function and psychosocial well-being both are affected by the quality and quantity of sleep.

Before the 1930s, research on sleep was nonexistent, and nocturnal sleep was viewed as the absence of daytime activity rather than as an activity in its own right. In the 1950s, the identification of sleep cycles through the use of polygraphic measurements greatly improved our understanding of sleep. By the 1960s, rapid eye movement (REM), non–rapid eye movement (NREM), and waking stages were recognized as three distinct states of consciousness. In the 1970s, sleep disorder centers were established to conduct research on sleep and to offer comprehensive evaluation and treatment programs for persons suffering from sleep disorders. By the late 1990s, the American Sleep Disorders Association, a professional organization of primary care providers involved in the diagnosis and treatment of sleep disorders, had more than 2000 members. In the early 2000s, print and broadcast media focused public attention on the detrimental effects of sleep deprivation and the large numbers of people in developed countries affected by inadequate sleep. Numerous Internet sites sprang up, and sleep apnea syndromes became part of the common language. Because older adults are as likely as younger adults to benefit from newer information and technology, it is important to understand the specific sleep problems of older adults so that they too can benefit from the most recent approaches to addressing this quality-of-life concern.

 ## AGE-RELATED CHANGES THAT AFFECT SLEEP AND REST PATTERNS

Sleep research initially focused on identifying the characteristics of each phase of the sleep cycle across the life span, with some attention directed to the unique aspects of the sleep structure and patterns of older adults. Although age-related changes in the sleep cycle are now fairly well understood, many questions remain to be answered about sleep-related phenomena, such as apnea and circadian rhythms, that often affect older adults. A sleep cycle is characterized according to the quantity of time spent in bed while awake or asleep, and the depth and quality of sleep. Age-related changes have little impact on the overall quantity of sleep of older adults, but they do have a significant impact on the quality of sleep and the quantity of rest. Complaints about sleep disturbances rank high among the problems for which older adults medicate themselves or seek medical care (Giron et al., 2002). Although some complaints about the quality of sleep may be attributable to age-related changes, most sleep disturbances are the result of risk factors and external influences. Sleep patterns and disturbances are affected by a wide range of physiologic, environmental, and psychosocial factors that interact, and these interrelationships become even more complex with increasing age.

Time in Bed and Total Sleep Time

Researchers agree that older adults spend increasing amounts of time in bed, not always attempting to sleep, with a decreasing proportion of time in actual sleep. They disagree, however, about changes in total sleep time. There is some agreement that healthy older adults are likely to experience the same duration of sleep as younger adults, but older adults spend more time in bed. One meta-analysis of 41 published studies on age-related sleep changes concluded that polysomnography results show diminished nighttime sleep in older adults, but self-reports did not reflect the same age-related changes (Floyd et al., 2000).

Both older and younger adults spend an average of 6.5 to 7.5 hours sleeping during a 24-hour period, but older adults spend an additional 3 to 4 hours resting in order to attain the same amount of sleep attained by younger adults. Compared with younger adults, older adults spend more time napping and are likely to nap earlier in the afternoon (i.e., between noon and 3:00 PM). The major reasons why older adults nap are to relieve excessive daytime sleepiness and to obtain other benefits, such as improved alertness (Tamaki et al., 2000).

Sleep Efficiency and Number of Arousals

Sleep efficiency, or the percentage of time asleep during time in bed, influences perceived quality of sleep. Sleep efficiency ranges from 80% to 95% for younger people and is about 70% for older people. This diminished sleep efficiency is attributed both to prolonged sleep latency, which is the time required to fall asleep, and to an increased number of awakenings during the night. Beginning in the fourth decade, the number of awakenings during the night gradually increases to the point that, by later adulthood, as much as one fifth of the night may be spent in periods of wakefulness.

As with many other changes that commonly occur in older adults, there is much controversy about whether the changes are attributable to pathologic conditions or to nonpathologic, age-related phenomena. The increased number of awakenings in older adults may be the result of any of the following factors: sleep apnea, physical discomfort, dementia or depression, pathologic processes, lower auditory arousal threshold, or increased levels of plasma norepinephrine. Whether these conditions are age-related or pathologic, they occur with increased frequency in older adults and must be considered as risk factors for disturbed sleep.

Sleep Stages

Normal Sleep Stages

Nocturnal sleep patterns are described in terms of sleep cycles and sleep stages. Each sleep cycle, which lasts between 70 and 120 minutes, is a combination of sleep stages. Sleep stages are classified according the presence or absence of REM. A typical cycle consists of four NREM stages (also called *slow-wave stages*) and one REM stage (also called the *dream stage*). At the beginning of each cycle, the NREM stages occur sequentially from stage I (lightest sleep) through stage IV (deepest sleep). These stages then occur in reverse order until stage I is reached again and is followed by REM sleep. The cycle repeats during the night, with the length of REM increasing and the length of stages III and IV gradually diminishing (i.e., more time is spent in dream stage and less time in deeper NREM stages as the night progresses). During the NREM stages, muscles gradually relax, body systems function at low levels, and heart and respiratory rates are slower and more regular than during REM or waking periods. Stages III and IV are the deepest stages, and essential restorative functions and the release of hormones take place during the fourth stage.

Although some dreaming takes place in NREM stages, most active and vivid dreaming takes place during REM sleep. In addition to rapid eye movement, REM sleep is characterized by the following physiologic changes:

- Flaccid muscles
- Fluctuating blood pressure
- Diminished thermoregulatory functions
- Increased gastric acid secretions
- Production of more highly concentrated urine by the kidneys
- About 40% increase in cerebral blood flow
- Irregular and increased rate and rhythm of pulse and respirations
- Clitoral engorgement and increased vaginal blood flow (in women)
- Penile tumescence (in men)

The physiologic alterations that occur during REM may exacerbate some medical problems. For example, increased gastric acid secretion during REM sleep may precipitate gastrointestinal pain for people with peptic ulcer disease. Likewise, people with chronic obstructive pulmonary disease (COPD) may experience dyspnea or even a respiratory crisis because of decreased oxygen saturation during REM periods.

Age-Related Changes in Sleep Stages

Throughout adulthood, the duration of stage I sleep increases gradually, from 5% of a younger adult's sleep to about 20% of an older adult's sleep. In the early part of the night, older adults experience longer periods of drowsiness without actual sleep in comparison to younger adults. During the night, older adults have more frequent shifts in and out of stage I sleep than do younger adults, but the length of stage II does not differ in older and younger adults. Stage III sleep shows a greater degree of variability in older adults as compared with younger adults, and many older adults have little or no stage III sleep. Similarly, stage IV sleep decreases to the point that it is absent in many older adults. Roth and Roehrs (2000) studied sleep stages in adults aged 30 to 59 years and found that the subjects in the fourth-decade group spent 10% of the night in stages III and IV and the subjects in the sixth-decade group spent 6% in these stages. In both younger and older adults, stage IV sleep increases significantly during the night after sleep loss. The same number of episodes of REM sleep tend to occur in both younger and older adults, but each episode is shorter in older adults. In early childhood, more than 40% of sleep time is spent in dream stages, but this decreases to about 25% by the age of 70 years (Blazer, 1998). Also, in older adults, REM sleep occurs more uniformly throughout the night, rather than occurring more predominantly during the second half of the night, as occurs in young adults. Table 20-1 summarizes the usual adult

TABLE 20-1 • Age-Related Changes in Sleep

Sleep Stage	Young Adults	Older Adults
NREM: slow eye movements, normal muscle tension		Increased number of shifts into NREM
Stage I	5% TST	Steady increase to 10%–20%
Stage II	50% TST	Generally unchanged
Stage III	10% TST	Little or no change
Stage IV	10% TST	Very short or absent, especially in men
REM: rapid eye movements, weak muscle tension, vivid dreams	25% TST	Shorter, less intense, more evenly distributed
OVERALL CHANGES		Longer time required to fall asleep More frequent arousals Different quality of sleep, with less time in deep sleep More time in bed Same quantity of sleep during a 24-hour period

NREM, nonrapid eye movement; REM, rapid eye movement; TST, total sleep time.

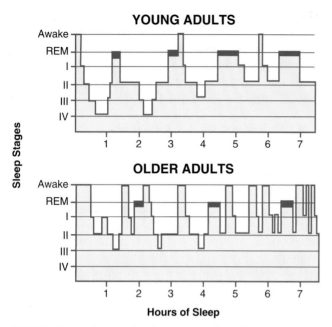

FIGURE 20-1 Changes in the sleep cycle with aging. Older adults typically take longer to fall asleep and experience more frequent arousals. Older adults also usually spend less time in deep sleep.

sleep cycle and typical age-related changes in sleep patterns. Typical sleep cycles for younger and older adults are illustrated in Figure 20-1.

Circadian Rhythm

Sleep patterns are determined, in part, by an individual's circadian rhythm, also known as a *biologic clock*. Body functions that have a circadian pattern include thermoregulation, sleep–wake cycles, and secretion of many hormones, including cortisol and melatonin. The sleep–wake circadian rhythm generally causes adults to become sleepy between 10:00 PM and midnight and to wake feeling rested between 6:00 AM and 8:00 AM. With increasing age, the circadian rhythm advances, causing older adults to become sleepy earlier in the evening and to awaken earlier in the morning. Alterations in circadian rhythm may also account for difficulties maintaining sleep as well as difficulty returning to sleep after awakening during the night. This phenomenon is sometimes called *advanced sleep phase*. Sleep disturbances associated with altered circadian rhythm are not necessarily caused by age-related changes alone and are likely to be exacerbated by lack of exposure to bright light (Klerman et al., 2001). Also, older adults may be predisposed to irregular sleep–wake patterns and circadian rhythm disorders because they do not have external demands to go to bed or get up at specific times (Blazer, 2002).

Gender-Related Differences in Sleep Patterns

Beginning at puberty, sleep patterns of men and women differ, with men having a relatively higher percentage of stage I sleep and more awakenings during the night. The gender differences in stage I sleep remain consistent throughout adulthood, but by the eighth decade, there are no gender differences in the number of awakenings during the night. Also, older men have shorter but more frequent REM episodes and decreased amounts of both total sleep time and stages III and IV sleep compared with women. In all age categories, however, women consistently report more sleep complaints than men.

Recent research has focused on the potential influence of hormones and sleep, with separate studies being done on men and women. Shaver and Zenk (2000) concluded that insomnia is associated with hot flashes, night sweats, and other factors (e.g., stress) in menopausal women. In men, age-related changes in REM and slow-wave sleep may be associated with hormonal alterations, such as decreased production of growth hormone (Van Cauter et al., 2000).

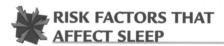

RISK FACTORS THAT AFFECT SLEEP

The common complaint of sleep problems among older adults is associated not only with age-related changes that occur even in healthy older adults but also with the many psychosocial or physiologic risk factors that frequently affect older adults. In addition, environmental conditions, particularly in institutional settings, can significantly affect the sleep patterns of older adults.

Psychosocial Factors

Beliefs and attitudes about sleep can have a powerful impact on sleep, with many beliefs having a detrimental, anxiety-producing effect. For example, older adults who believe that arousals during the night are abnormal and unhealthy may think they have insomnia and seek treatment with medications. Rigid beliefs about the amount of sleep required during the night, or the need for the same amount of sleep every night, may also lead to false definitions of insomnia and inappropriate treatment. Likewise, worrying, negative thoughts, and anxious thoughts about awakening may add to distress about insomnia for older adults (Libman et al., 1997). Maggi and colleagues (1998) found that thoughts, memories, anxiety, and other psychological factors account for most reported difficulties falling asleep.

Anxiety, dementia, depression, and sensory impairments are psychosocial disorders associated with disrupted sleep. Anxiety and dementia are likely to be manifested by difficulty falling asleep and may also lead to frequent arousals during the night, after which it may be difficult to return to sleep. People with dementia have been found to have the following sleep alterations: no stage IV sleep, disrupted sleep–wake cycle, very little REM or stage III sleep, and frequent nighttime arousals and daytime napping. Compared with people unaffected by depression, people who are depressed typically take longer to fall asleep, have less deep sleep and more light sleep, awaken more frequently during the night and earlier in the morning, and feel less rested in the morning. In addition, the presence of dementia, depression, or sensory impairments may interfere with the person's ability to respond to time cues and environmental stimuli, thereby disrupting the overall sleep–wake pattern. For example, the association between visual impairments and sleep complaints may be due to an inability to regulate light stimuli (Zizi et al., 2002).

Daytime boredom and lack of social demands or environmental stimulation can also interfere with sleep habits. Older adults with little or no structured activities, work responsibilities, or social responsibilities may find it particularly difficult to establish healthy sleeping patterns. A study of more than 13,000 adults in several European countries concluded that aging per se was not associated with insomnia, but inactivity and dissatisfaction with social life were two of the strongest predictors of insomnia (Ohayon et al., 2001). These researchers concluded that being active and satisfied with one's social life protects against insomnia at any age. Older adults with dementia or depression who are living alone are particularly susceptible to disturbed sleep patterns because of the tendency to stay in bed during the day out of boredom, lack of motivation, an inability to concentrate on stimulating activities, or a desire to withdraw from stressful situations.

Environmental Factors

Perhaps more than any other factor, environmental circumstances can significantly influence sleep patterns. For people who do not live alone, the actions and demands of other people in the home or institutional setting, especially those sharing the same sleeping area, influence sleep patterns. For adults at any age, a change in the sleeping environment usually requires a period of adjustment before optimal sleep patterns are established. Thus, older adults may have a particularly difficult time sleeping in institutional settings, especially during the first few nights in a new environment.

In institutional settings, lack of quiet and privacy, conflicting needs of various people, and sleeping in close proximity to others are all factors that can interfere with sleep. Older adults who are accustomed to sleeping alone or with family members may feel their privacy is being violated in institutional settings where they are required to wear nightclothes, remove their dentures, and share a room with people from outside their family. Difficulty falling asleep also may arise if environmental circumstances do not allow the performance of usual pre-bedtime activities, such as listening to music or reading a book. Schedules of caregivers also may interfere with the sleeping habits of the older adult. For example, in institutional settings, the time for awakening patients/residents is often based on the most efficient use of nursing and dietary time, and patients/residents are expected to adjust their sleep routines accordingly. Likewise, in home settings, dependent older adults may have to adjust their sleep routines to the schedule of their caregivers, who may have work and other responsibilities.

Noise, uncomfortable temperature, and lighting are environmental factors that interfere with sleep and often can be modified, especially in institutional settings. Beginning at about the age of 40 years, people become more sensitive to noise when they are sleeping and can be awakened by less intense auditory stimuli. Cruise and colleagues (1998) found a strong association between sleep disruption and noise and incontinence care practices in nursing homes. Uncomfortably low or high temperatures, perhaps caused by inadequate heating or cooling systems, also contribute to decreased sleep efficiency. Lighting is a potent influence on circadian rhythms and can affect sleep patterns in several ways. Excessive light in rooms and hallways as well as intermittent use of bedside or overhead lighting during nighttime care routines may disrupt sleep. Poor environmental lighting also disrupts the sleep–wake cycle, and the effect of environmental lighting on sleep patterns has been the focus of recent research. For example, Mishima and colleagues (2001) found that the older participants who were exposed to lower levels of environmental lighting had significantly diminished nocturnal melatonin secretions and experienced more sleep difficulties. Another study of older nursing home residents (mean age, 86 years) found an association between higher light levels during the day and fewer nighttime awakenings (Shochat et al., 2000).

Environmental factors can interfere with the sleep of older adults in home settings as well. For example, older adults who are caregivers may have their sleep interrupted by dependent family members who demand attention during the night. Conditions such as fear, loneliness, and neighborhood noise are environmental factors that can interfere with sleep in home settings. In any of these situations, a move to an institution may provide the supports and security needed for more peaceful sleeping. Finally, in any setting, if an older adult spends all of his or her time in the same room, the lack of differentiation between space for waking and sleeping activities may interfere with sleep patterns.

Physiologic Factors

Pathologic processes, physical pain or discomfort, and adverse effects of chemicals and medications are physiologic factors that can interfere with sleep. As with many other risk factors, although they are not unique to older adults, they are increasingly likely to occur in older adults and are more detrimental in the presence of age-related changes and other risk factors.

Pathologic Processes

Disease processes and physical discomfort interfere with sleep patterns in many ways, with some pathologic conditions being exacerbated during sleep, particularly during REM sleep stages. Specific disease conditions that may be exacerbated during sleep, especially REM stages, include angina, hypertension, duodenal ulcers, coronary artery disease, and COPD. Acute and chronic pain and discomfort are significant factors contributing to sleep disturbances. Cramps in the calf or foot muscles are a nighttime problem for some older adults and may interrupt sleep patterns. Table 20-2 lists specific processes and

their effects on sleep, including some processes that are not pathologic.

Sleep Apnea and Neuromuscular Disorders

Although medical literature in the late 1880s referred to syndromes in which sleep disorders were associated with brief interruptions in respirations, this phenomenon received little attention until the mid-1970s. Sleep apnea syndromes have received widespread attention in the literature, largely because of research in sleep disorder centers, where they currently are a dominant focus. In 1988, the U.S. Congress established the National Commission on Sleep Disorders Research to promote prevention, diagnosis, and treatment of obstructive sleep apnea (OSA) and other sleep disorders. OSA is the involuntary cessation of airflow for 10 seconds or longer; the occurrence of more than five to eight of these episodes per hour is considered pathologic. This condition occurs because the muscles responsible for holding the throat open relax during sleep, narrowing the throat opening and blocking the passage of air. Symptoms of OSA include daytime fatigue, morning headaches, diminished mental acuity, and loud snoring punctuated by brief periods of silence. OSA is not exclusively a condition of older adults, but it is generally agreed that between one third and two thirds of adults aged 60 years or older experience five or more brief sleep interruptions per hour because of apnea episodes. The prevalence of apnea increases with advancing age, beginning around the fifth decade, and is higher in men than in women. In addition to being associated with increased age, sleep apnea is associated with obesity, dementia, depression, hypertension, hypothyroidism, kyphoscoliosis, deformities of the jaw or nasal structures, and the

TABLE 20-2 • Physiologic Factors Affecting Sleep

Risk Factor	Sleep Alteration
Arthritis	Chronic pain and discomfort that interfere with sleep
COPD	Awakening as a result of apnea and respiratory distress
Diabetes mellitus	Awakening secondary to nocturia or poorly controlled blood glucose levels
Gastrointestinal disorders, ulcers	Nocturnal pain secondary to increased gastric secretions during REM sleep
Hypertension	Early morning awakening
Hyperthyroidism	Increased difficulty falling asleep
Nocturnal angina	Awakening without perception of pain, especially during REM sleep
PLMS, RLS	Awakening caused by periodic, involuntary leg movements
Altered circadian rhythm	Earlier sleep time; earlier awakening in the morning; difficulty returning to sleep after arousals
Parkinsonism	Increased time awake; decreased amount of sleep

COPD, chronic obstructive pulmonary disease; PLMS, periodic limb movements in sleep; REM, rapid eye movement; RLS, restless leg syndrome.

use of nicotine, alcohol, and medications that depress the respiratory center.

Two neuromuscular disorders, restless leg syndrome (RLS) and periodic limb movements in sleep (PLMS), also have been a topic of interest and research in sleep disorder centers since the mid-1970s. RLS is the experience of an almost irresistible urge to move the legs, usually accompanied by unpleasant leg sensations. RLS may interfere both with initiating and maintaining sleep. Getting up and walking may provide relief. Phillips and colleagues (2000) found a prevalence of 10% in adults between the ages of 30 and 79 years and 19% in adults aged 80 years and older. In addition to being associated with increased age in this study population, RLS was associated with smoking, diabetes, poor health, lower income, lack of exercise, and higher body mass index (BMI) (Phillips et al., 2000). Other factors that increase the risk for RLS include neuropathy, anemia, uremia, rheumatoid arthritis, and Parkinson's disease. Medications that may worsen the symptoms of RLS include phenytoin, antidepressants, tranquilizers, dopamine blockers, and cold and allergy agents.

PLMS, also known as *nocturnal myoclonus*, is the occurrence of brief muscle contractions, spaced at intervals of about 30 seconds, that cause leg jerks or rhythmic movements of muscles in the foot or leg. They may occur several times to a couple hundred times nightly, and their prevalence increases with increasing age. There may be an association between sleep apnea and PLMS, but the exact relationship is not known at this time. PLMS may contribute to complaints of insomnia, frequent arousals, and increased daytime sleepiness. Risk factors for PLMS include caffeine, alcohol, increased age, and certain medications (e.g., benzodiazepines and antidepressants).

Chemical Effects and Adverse Medication Effects

Adverse effects of medications and chemicals, such as caffeine, alcohol, and nicotine, can interfere with sleep in a number of ways. Caffeine is a central nervous system stimulant that lengthens the sleep latency period and causes awakening during the night. Although low doses of nicotine can have relaxing and sedative effects, higher doses interfere with sleep because of nicotine's stimulant effect as well as its effects on respiration. Alcohol may induce drowsiness as an initial effect, but it suppresses REM sleep and increases the number of awakenings, especially during the latter half of the sleep period. The end result of alcohol consumption is a decrease in total sleep time and an increase in daytime sleepiness. Moreover, people who have consumed alcohol over many years may experience alcohol-related insomnia for a few years after withdrawing from it. If OSA is

an underlying causative factor of insomnia, the use of alcohol, hypnotics, or other central nervous system depressants may exacerbate the sleep disorder and lead to increased doses of medication and further detrimental effects. These chemical effects are not unique to older adults; however, adverse effects of medication are more likely to occur in older adults (discussed in Chapter 23).

Contrary to their primary purpose, hypnotic medications often cause or contribute to sleep disturbances in the following ways:

1. Although the initial response to hypnotics may be good, tolerance to these medications usually develops, sometimes within several days.
2. Because of central nervous system depression and the increased sensitivity of older adults to these medications, adverse effects are likely to occur, especially if the dose is increased to compensate for tolerance.
3. Hypnotics tend to have paradoxical effects, including nightmares and agitation.
4. Hypnotics interfere with REM and deep sleep stages.
5. Rebound insomnia and nightmares occur after the withdrawal of many hypnotics.
6. Some hypnotic medications, particularly those that have been in use for many years, tend to have very long half-lives, interfering with nighttime sleep by causing daytime drowsiness. For example, flurazepam is broken down to an active metabolite with an average half-life of 47 to 100 hours. When used nightly for 1 week, the blood level of flurazepam reaches a level 5 to 6 times that of the initial dose.

Other medications that have been associated with disturbed sleep include steroids, antidepressants, aminophylline preparations, thyroid extracts, antiarrhythmic medications, and centrally acting antihypertensives. Table 20-3 summarizes the effects of various medications and chemicals on sleep in older adults.

> Studies have found that women are twice as likely as men, and whites are almost three times as likely as African Americans, to be taking sedative-hypnotic medications (Blazer et al., 2000; Maggi et al., 1998).

FUNCTIONAL CONSEQUENCES ASSOCIATED WITH SLEEP CHANGES IN OLDER ADULTS

The functional consequences of age-related sleep changes can be summarized as follows: in comparison with younger adults, older adults have more

TABLE 20-3 • The Effect of Various Medications and Chemicals on Sleep

Medication or Chemical	Sleep Alteration
Alcohol	Suppression of REM sleep; early morning awakening
Alcohol or hypnotic withdrawal	Sleep disturbances; nightmares
Anticholinergics	Hyperreflexia; overactivity; muscle twitching
Barbiturates	Suppression of REM sleep; nightmares; hallucinations; paradoxical responses
Benzodiazepines	Awakening secondary to apnea
β-Blockers	Nightmares
Corticosteroids	Restlessness; sleep disturbances
Diuretics	Awakening for nocturia; sleep apnea secondary to alkalosis
Theophylline, levodopa, isoproterenol, phenytoin	Interference with sleep onset and sleep stages
Antidepressants	PLMS; suppression of REM sleep

PLMS, periodic limb movements in sleep; REM, rapid eye movement.

difficulty falling asleep, awaken more readily and more frequently, and spend more time in the drowsiness stage and less time in deep sleep. Functionally, these changes alone have little impact on the daily life of the older adult, especially because the total amount of sleep time is not significantly changed. However, the prevalence of risk factors that make the older adult more vulnerable to sleep disorders often gives rise to complaints of insomnia and feelings of excessive daytime sleepiness. In comparison with adults younger than 65 years, older adults are 1.5 times more likely to have sleep difficulties (Umlauf & Weaver, 2001). Factors that are associated with the increased likelihood of sleep complaints in older adults include angina, depression, white race, female gender, cognitive impairment, anxiety and worries, low educational level, poor self-rated health, and the presence of chronic health conditions. Older adults in nursing homes and other institutional settings experience significantly more sleep difficulties. For example, sleep–wake intervals for nursing home residents may be 1 hour or less.

> Older women report more difficulty than older men in falling asleep.

At least one third of older adults complain of some type of sleep disturbance, usually involving symptoms of daytime sleepiness, difficulty falling asleep, and frequent arousals during the night. In the late 1970s, sleep disorders were classified systematically, and standards were established to diagnose these disorders. *Insomnia* is classified as a disorder of initiating and maintaining sleep and is one of the most common sleep disorders of older adults. Excessive daytime sleepiness is classified as *hypersomnia* and

can be measured objectively with the Multiple Sleep Latency Test (MSLT). This test is based on polygraphic recordings of the speed of falling asleep at periodic intervals during a 24-hour period. Excessive daytime sleepiness, defined as the inability to maintain alertness, differs from fatigue, which manifests as difficulty sustaining a high level of performance (Umlauf & Weaver, 2001).

Although sleep deprivation is not a normal consequence of age-related changes, it may arise from a combination of age-related changes and risk factors in older adults. Psychosocial consequences of short-term sleep loss include confusion, irritability, excessive daytime sleepiness, an inability to concentrate, and poor performance on psychometric tests. Studies have found that sleep disturbances and complaints are associated with declines in cognitive abilities in both middle-aged and older adults (Jelicic et al., 2002). Manifestations of prolonged sleep deprivation include fatigue, irritability, disorientation, persecutory feelings, attention deficits, perceptual disturbances, and transient neurologic symptoms, such as hand tremors. When manifestations such as these (e.g., disorientation, attention deficits, and persecutory feelings) occur in older adults, they may mistakenly be attributed to dementia or other pathologic conditions rather than being recognized as effects of sleep deprivation. Figure 20-2 illustrates the age-related changes, risk factors, and negative functional consequences that affect sleep and rest in older adults.

> A 3-year study of more than 6000 older adults found that cognitive decline was associated with chronic insomnia in men, but in women, the cognitive decline was found only in those subjects who had both chronic insomnia and a high level of depression (Cricco et al., 2001).

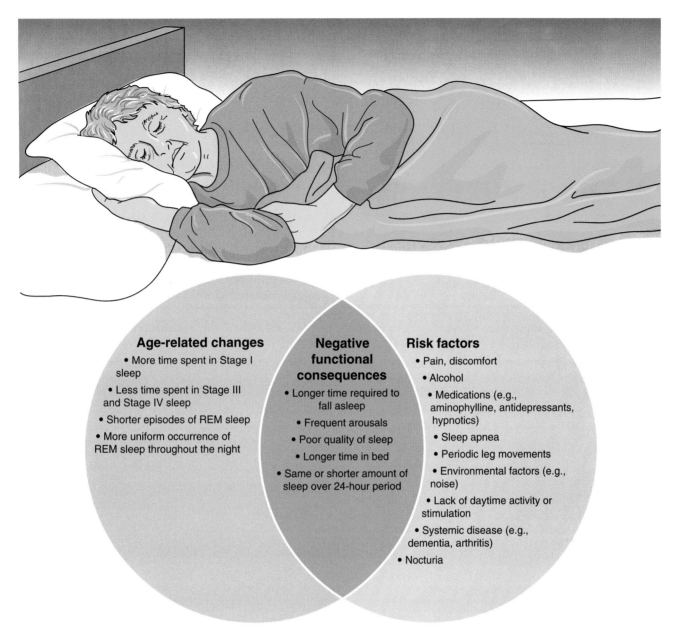

Age-related changes
- More time spent in Stage I sleep
- Less time spent in Stage III and Stage IV sleep
- Shorter episodes of REM sleep
- More uniform occurrence of REM sleep throughout the night

Negative functional consequences
- Longer time required to fall asleep
- Frequent arousals
- Poor quality of sleep
- Longer time in bed
- Same or shorter amount of sleep over 24-hour period

Risk factors
- Pain, discomfort
- Alcohol
- Medications (e.g., aminophylline, antidepressants, hypnotics)
- Sleep apnea
- Periodic leg movements
- Environmental factors (e.g., noise)
- Lack of daytime activity or stimulation
- Systemic disease (e.g., dementia, arthritis)
- Nocturia

FIGURE 20-2 Age-related changes and risk factors intersect to negatively affect sleep in older adults.

NURSING ASSESSMENT OF SLEEP PATTERNS

Identifying Opportunities for Health Promotion

The nurse assesses a person's sleep patterns to determine the adequacy of the person's usual sleep and rest pattern and to identify factors that may contribute to or interfere with the quality and quantity of sleep. During the assessment, the nurse listens for any indications of misinformation or a lack of knowledge that might contribute to sleep disorders. It is especially important to identify any detrimental behaviors, such as the prolonged use of hypnotics, that may be based on myths or misinformation. Identification of these factors will lay the groundwork for health promotion interventions. Display 20-1 provides guidelines for interviewing independent older adults and caregivers of dependent older adults about sleep and rest patterns.

In addition to obtaining subjective information from the older adult and from caregivers of the dependent older adult, the nurse observes behavioral cues of nighttime and daytime rest and activities. This is especially important when objective

DISPLAY 20-1
Guidelines for Assessing Sleep and Rest

Questions to Assess the Perception of Quality and Adequacy of Sleep

- On a scale of 1 to 10, with 10 as the highest, how would you rate your sleep?
- When you awaken in the morning, do you feel like you are rested?
- Do you feel drowsy or sleepy during the day or early evening?
- Does fatigue interfere with your desired daytime activity level?

Questions to Identify Opportunities for Education About Health Promotion

- Describe your usual activities during the evening hours before you fall asleep.
- What is your usual time for getting into bed?
- What are the factors that help you fall asleep (e.g., food or drink, relaxation strategies, environmental influences)?
- Do you take any medicines to help you sleep?
- Do you take medicines to help you stay awake during the day?

- Do you drink alcoholic or caffeinated beverages, or take medicines that contain alcohol or caffeine during the late afternoon or evening? (If yes, how much and what kind?)
- What kind of activities do you engage in during the day and evening?

Questions to Assess Nighttime Sleep Pattern

- Where do you sleep at night (e.g., bed, couch, recliner chair)?
- How long does it usually take to fall asleep after you get into bed?
- Do you think you lie awake too long before falling asleep?
- After you fall asleep, do you wake up during the night? (If so, how many times?)
- What kinds of things disturb your sleep during the night (e.g., getting up to urinate; activities of roommates or other people in the setting; environmental factors, like noise or lighting)?
- If changes in living arrangements have occurred in the past few months: Has your sleep pattern changed since . . . (e.g., since you came to this nursing home; since your spouse passed away)?

observations are contrary to subjective complaints. For example, older adults may complain of not sleeping at all, but when observed by caregivers, they may appear to be sleeping during the entire night. By contrast, older adults who deny any problems sleeping may nap frequently and readily fall asleep during daytime activities.

Using Sleep Assessment Tools

Nurses can perform a sleep history or ask older adults to keep a sleep–wake diary to help identify problem areas and plan appropriate interventions, as discussed and reviewed in nursing literature (e.g., Beck-Little & Weinrich, 1998; Schoenfelder & Culp, 2001). The Hartford Institute for Geriatric Nursing has identified the Pittsburgh Sleep Quality Index (PSQI) (Figure 20-3) as an effective instrument for initial and ongoing assessment of sleep quality and patterns in older adults in a variety of health care settings (Smyth, 1999).

> Mrs. Z. is 66 years old and recently retired from her job as office manager for a law firm. She considers herself to be in good health, although she has had hypertension for 20 years and osteoarthritis for the past several years. She self-monitors her blood pressure and takes atenolol,

100 mg daily. She occasionally takes an over-the-counter analgesic medication when her arthritis pain bothers her. She just started going to the local senior center once a week for lunch and social and educational activities. During one of your weekly Senior Wellness Clinics, Mrs. Z. comes to talk with you about her difficulty sleeping. She reports that since she has retired, she often wakes up several times during the night and has difficulty returning to sleep. She used to sleep an average of 7 to 8 hours nightly and could easily return to sleep if she woke up during the night. Now she is lucky if she gets 6 hours of sleep because she lays in bed for several hours. She used to go to bed between 10:00 PM and 11:00 PM and get up promptly between 6:30 AM and 7:00 AM. Now that she is retired, she goes to bed at about 11:00 PM but stays in bed until 10:00 AM if she wakes up during the night and does not get a full night's sleep.

THINKING POINTS

> What age-related changes may be contributing to Mrs. Z.'s dissatisfaction with her sleep?

> What risk factors might be contributing to Mrs. Z.'s dissatisfaction with her sleep?

> What further assessment information would you need to obtain and how would you obtain it?

PITTSBURGH SLEEP QUALITY INDEX

Instructions: The following questions relate to your usual sleep habits during the past month only. Your answers should indicate the most accurate reply for the majority of days and nights in the past month. Please answer all questions.

During the past month,
1. When have you usually gone to bed?_____
2. How long (in minutes) has it taken you to fall asleep each night?_____
3. When have you usually gotten up in the moring?_____
4. How many hours of actual sleep did you get that night? (This may be different than the number of hours you spend in bed)._____

5. During the past month, how often have you had trouble sleeping because you...	Not during the past month (0)	Less than once a week (1)	Once or twice a week (2)	Three or more times a week (3)
a. Cannot get to sleep within 30 minutes.				
b. Wake up in the middle of the night or early moring.				
c. Have to get up to use the bathroom.				
d. Cannot breathe comfortably.				
e. Cough or snore loudly.				
f. Feel cold.				
g. Feel too hot.				
h. Have bad dreams.				
i. Have pain.				
j. Other reason(s). Please describe, including how often you have had trouble sleeping because of this reason(s):				
6. During the past month, how often have you taken medicine (prescribed or over the counter) to help you sleep?				
7. During the past month, how often have you had trouble staying awake while driving, eating meals, or engaging in social activity?				
8. During the past month, how much of a problem has it been for you to keep up enthusiasm to get things done?				
	Very good (0)	Fairly good (1)	Fairly bad (2)	Very bad (3)
9. During the past month, how would you rate your sleep quality overall?				

Component 1 #9 Score.   C1_____
Component 2 #2 score (≤15 minutes = 0; 16 to 30 minutes=1; 31 to 60 minutes = 2; > 60 minutes = 3)
      + #5a Score (if sum is equal 0 = 0; 1 to 2 = 1; 3 to 4 = 2; 5 to 6 = 3)   C2_____
Component 3 #4 Score (>7 = 0; 6 to 7 = 1; 5 to 6 = 2; < 5 = 3)   C3_____
Component 4 (total number of hours asleep)/ (total number of hours in bed) x 100
      (>85% = 0; 75% to 84% = 1; 65% to 74% = 2; < 65% = 3)   C4_____
Component 5 Number sum or scores #5b to #5j (0 = 0; 1 to 9 = 1;10 to 18 = 2; 19 to 27 = 3)   C5_____
Component 6 #6 Score   C6_____
Component 7 #7 Score + #8 Score (0 = 0; 1 to 2 = 1; 3 to 4 = 2; 5 to 6 = 3)   C7_____
      Add the seven component scores together _____   **Global PSQI Score** _____

FIGURE 20-3 The Pittsburgh Sleep Quality Index (PSQI) is a tool that can be used to assess sleep habits and sleep quality. (Adapted from Buysse, D. J., Reynolds III, C. F., Monk, T. H., Berman, S. R., & Kupfer, D. J. [1989]. The Pittsburgh Sleep Quality Index: A new instrument for psychiatric practice and research. *Psychiatric Research, 28* (2), 193–213. Reprinted with permission from Elsevier Science.)

NURSING DIAGNOSIS

When older adults report dissatisfaction with their sleep or when nursing staff find that patients or residents have difficulty initiating or maintaining sleep, a nursing diagnosis of Disturbed Sleep Pattern is applicable. This is defined as the "state in which the individual experiences or is at risk of experiencing a change in the quantity or quality of his rest pattern that causes discomfort or interferes with desired lifestyle" (Carpenito, 2002, p. 872). Related factors common in older adults include pain, anxiety, depression, nocturia, incontinence, medication effects, menopausal hormonal changes, environmental changes or conditions, and pathologic conditions, such as dementia.

OUTCOMES

Indicators for the Nursing Outcomes Classification (NOC) of Sleep include sleep quality, pattern, efficiency, and routine; feelings of rejuvenation after sleep; napping appropriate for age and wakeful at appropriate times (Schoenfelder & Culp, 2001). Indicators are measured by directly observing older adults and by questioning them or their caregivers about their perceptions of sleep.

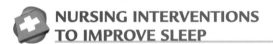

NURSING INTERVENTIONS TO IMPROVE SLEEP

Nursing interventions to promote healthy sleep include health education and direct interventions, such as environmental modifications and comfort and relaxation strategies. As with other aspects of nursing care for older adults, it is essential that care be individualized for each person's identified needs. Nurses in community and long-term care settings have numerous opportunities to teach older adults and their caregivers about interventions that can improve sleep and quality of life. In hospital settings, the nursing focus is primarily on acute medical problems, but quality-of-life concerns, such as sleep disturbances, should not be overlooked. The Hartford Foundation's Nurses Improving Care of the Hospitalized Elderly (NICHE) Project developed a standard of nursing practice to improve the quality of care and decrease the poorer outcomes of care associated with sleep disturbances of hospitalized older adults (Foreman & Wykle, 1995).

When older adults have sleep disturbances that do not respond to interventions and interfere with their quality of life, referrals for further evaluation and treatment should be suggested. One goal of *Healthy*

People 2010 is to increase the proportion of people with symptoms of OSA who seek medical evaluation and receive medical care for long-term management of their condition. *Healthy People 2010* emphasizes the need for health education about OSA, and gerontological nurses can play an important role in educating older adults about the importance of having any sleep disorder evaluated by a knowledgeable professional (USDHHS, 2000). Many behavioral, mechanical, and surgical interventions are available for the treatment of OSA, and obtaining a comprehensive evaluation and treatment at a sleep disorders clinic should be considered. A list of accredited sleep disorder centers can be obtained from the American Academy of Sleep Medicine (listed in the Educational Resources section at the end of this chapter).

Promoting Healthy Sleep Patterns

Health promotion interventions begin with educating independent older adults and caregivers of dependent older adults about age-related sleep changes that affect sleep (Figure 20-4). As discussed earlier, these changes can be summarized as follows: older adults may need more time to fall asleep, may awaken more readily and more often during the night, and may have greater difficulty falling back to sleep after awakening. A good understanding of the age-related changes in sleep patterns may alleviate anxiety about sleep problems. Also, nurses can emphasize the importance of establishing good sleep habits, even in older adults who do not report sleep problems. Older adults without sleep problems who participated in a year-long program of sleep-hygiene education and modest bed-restriction time reported an improved sense of well-being on awakening and improvements in sleep depth and continuity (Hoch et al., 2001). Health education about sleep is particularly important in community and long-term care settings, where nurses have more opportunities to focus on quality-of-life issues. Display 20-2 summarizes some measures that can be taken by older adults to promote healthy sleep as well as complementary and alternative care practices that may be used to promote sleep and rest.

Nursing actions are directed toward eliminating risk factors and promoting sleep when risk factors cannot be eliminated. Nurses who work evening or night shifts in institutional or home care settings have many opportunities to engage in activities that promote good nighttime sleep. For dependent older adults, nursing responsibilities include assisting with positioning in bed and ensuring the most comfortable environment possible. If dementia or depression interferes with sleep onset, the nurse may simply

ZZZZ'S ALERT: ONE OUT OF EVERY TWO SENIORS IS SLEEP-DEPRIVED.

Sleep Tips for Sleepy Seniors

Keep Regular Hours.
Try to go to bed at the same time each night and wake up at the same time each morning.

Go For A Walk. Natural sunlight and outdoor activity are mood-boosters — and sleep inducers.

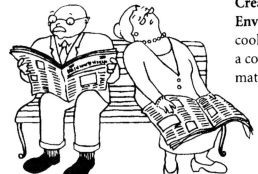

Create A Good Sleep Environment. Sleep in a cool, quiet, dark room on a comfortable, supportive mattress.

FIGURE 20-4 A flier that can be used for health education about sleep. (Courtesy of the Better Sleep Council. Statistic source: National Commission on Sleep Disorders Research. [1992]. *Wake up America: A national sleep alert*. Washington, D.C.: Author.)

stay with the older person to provide reassurance until the person is able to fall asleep. In addition, relief of pain and anxiety are nursing responsibilities that directly influence the sleep of older adults. Older adults who are cognitively impaired may not request analgesics but may give nonverbal cues that pain is interfering with sleep. Nurses should be alert to this possibility and assess for chronic or acute pain. An analgesic taken 30 minutes before bedtime may help induce sleep in people with chronic pain or discomfort.

Soft music and dim lighting also may be helpful as measures to promote sleep. Comfort and relaxation measures, such as backrubs, afternoon baths, and the use of therapeutic touch, are particularly helpful when emotional stress or physical pain interfere with sleep. Older adults who participated in four weekly 1-hour educational sessions that focused on relaxation techniques, sleep hygiene practices, and stimulus control measures experienced significant improvements in sleep efficiency and sleep quality (Lichstein et al., 2000). Stress management and other behavioral techniques are effective alternatives to medication for sleep problems in older adults who are caregivers (McCurry et al., 1998). Older adults and caregivers of dependent older adults can be taught to use relaxation techniques as an effective method of inducing sleep without any adverse effects. Cassette tape recorders with automatic shutoffs can be used to play soothing music or instructions for deep breathing, guided imagery, or relaxation exercises. These tapes are growing in popularity and can be purchased in many book and music stores or through the Internet. Display 20-3

summarizes simple instructions for relaxation and mental techniques designed to promote sleep.

Modifying the Environment to Promote Sleep

Environmental modifications are among the simplest and most effective interventions to improve sleep, especially in institutional settings. Activities such as closing bedroom doors and adjusting bedroom lighting may be quite effective in promoting adequate sleep for older adults. In long-term care settings, preferences for bedtime routines and measures that promote sleep can be documented on each resident's care plan and carried out by nursing staff. Elimination of unnecessary staff-initiated noise, especially conversations at the nursing station, is a helpful intervention for patients/residents located near the center of nursing activity. In long-term care settings, decisions about room assignments should be based partially on an assessment of sleep requirements and compatibility of individual needs. Once room assignments have been made, roommate behaviors that interfere with sleep may be addressed by a room change, if necessary.

If a noisy environment contributes to sleeping difficulties and the noise cannot be controlled or eliminated, the older person may wish to use earplugs. Any person who lives alone, however, should be cautioned about the danger of blocking out protective noises, such as that of a smoke detector. Environmental noise that cannot be eliminated can be masked by white noise (e.g., using a fan, air

DISPLAY 20-2
Health Promotion Teaching About Sleep

Actions To Take

- Establish a bedtime ritual that is effective for you, and try to follow it every night.
- Maintain the same daily schedule for waking, resting, and sleeping.
- Take a warm, relaxing bath in the afternoon or early evening.
- After 1:00 PM, avoid foods, beverages, and medications that contain caffeine, including tea, cocoa, coffee, chocolate candy, hot chocolate, and some over-the-counter pain relievers and cold preparations. In addition, avoid alcohol, sugar, refined carbohydrates, and food additives and preservatives.
- Pre-bedtime foods that promote sleep include milk (warm), chamomile tea, and a light snack of complex carbohydrates (e.g., whole grains).
- Use one or more of the following relaxation methods: imagery, meditation, deep breathing, progressive relaxation, passive exercise, soothing music, body or foot massage, rocking in a chair, reading nonstimulating materials, or watching nonstimulating television.
- Perform daily moderate aerobic exercise, preferably before the late afternoon, but avoid vigorous exercise in the evening.

Actions To Avoid

- Do not drink alcohol before bedtime because it may cause early morning awakening. If you use alcohol, use only in small amounts.
- Do not smoke cigarettes in the evening because nicotine is a stimulant.
- If your bedtime is temporarily changed, try to keep your waking time as close to the usual time as possible, and avoid staying in bed beyond your usual waking time.

- Do not use your bed for reading or other activities not associated with sleeping.
- If you awaken during the night and cannot return to sleep, get out of bed after 30 minutes and engage in a nonstimulating activity, such as reading, in another room.
- Arise at your usual time, even if you have not slept well.

Nutritional Considerations

- Provide adequate intake of zinc, calcium, magnesium, manganese, and vitamins B-complex and C.
- Vitamin E and folic acid may be helpful for restless leg syndrome.

Complementary and Alternative Care Practices

- Yoga, meditation, acupuncture, imagery, hypnotherapy, light therapy, progressive relaxation, and a warm bath or warm footbath may be effective in promoting sleep.
- Chamomile, coriander, lavender, and marjoram can be used as aromatherapy to promote sleep.
- Herbs commonly used for sleep problems include hops, ginseng, catnip, skullcap, lavender, chamomile, valerian, rose hips, lemon balm, passion flower, and St. John's wort.
- Homeopathic remedies include oat, arnica, aconite, coffea, arsenicum, chamomile, pulsatilla, rhus tox, nux vomica.

Special Precautions

- Although widely promoted as sleep aids, tryptophan and melatonin should be used with caution in older adults because of their possible adverse effects, and only under the supervision of a qualified health care provider.

conditioner, soft music, tape recordings of such sounds as waves or rain, or white noise machines). If outside neighborhood noise is bothersome, heavy draperies can be installed over windows to filter it out. In addition to addressing noise in the environment, interventions address temperature in the sleeping area. The nighttime room temperature should be comfortable and is usually slightly lower than during the day. In cooler environments, the older adult should wear a nightcap to prevent loss of heat through the head.

If the effects of lighting interfere with sleep, environmental modifications should be made to address these factors. Institutionalized older adults with dementia who were exposed to higher light levels during the day had less disturbed nighttime sleep (Shochat et al., 2000). Another study suggests that scheduled bright light exposure can be used to treat circadian phase disturbances in older adults (Klerman

et al., 2001). Efforts can be made to expose older adults to bright lights during daytime hours and to eliminate bright lights during nighttime hours.

Individualizing Care in Institutional Settings

Individualized care plans for older adults in residential settings focus on promoting better sleep for people with disturbed sleep patterns. Because they influence sleep patterns, daytime activities should be incorporated in plans to improve sleep of older adults in residential settings. One study of cognitively impaired older adults demonstrated that timing activities in relation to peak napping times and prescribing activities that held the attention of the residents improved their nocturnal sleep and reduced their daytime napping (Richards et al., 2001). Another study showed that participation in light physical

DISPLAY 20-3
Relaxation and Mental Imagery Techniques That Promote Sleep

Deep Breathing

- Focus your attention on your breathing; extend your belly and draw in a deep breath as you count.
- Hold your breath for 3 or 4 counts.
- Exhale completely.
- Repeat this pattern, focusing your total attention on breathing.
- Phrases, such as "I am sleepy," or counting may be repeated during each exhalation to help keep your attention focused on breathing.

Progressive Relaxation

- Start by focusing your attention on the muscles in your toes.
- Flex or tense these muscles, and then relax them.
- Repeat 2 or 3 times.
- Focus your attention on the muscles in your foot.
- Flex or tense, then relax these muscles, 2 or 3 times.
- Repeat this process, progressively focusing on different muscle groups and proceeding from your feet to your head.

Mental Imagery

- Begin with deep breathing exercises to relax yourself.
- Focus your attention on a serene and peaceful scene, visualize the setting, and imagine the sounds (e.g., a beach with waves gently washing ashore).
- Imagine yourself in the setting, lying relaxed, enjoying the environment.
- Keep your attention focused on the scene.
- Imagine repetitive motions, such as waves on the beach or sheep jumping over a fence.

activity and structured social activity resulted in improved slow-wave sleep in older adults living in an assisted-living facility (Naylor et al., 2000). Nighttime routines also need to be individualized to meet the needs of each resident. In one study, the usual nighttime nursing care regimens at predetermined times were replaced with nondisruptive care routines, which included hourly flashlight checks of residents and provision of care only when the resident was awake. The nondisruptive routine resulted in increased total and consecutive sleep times and did not compromise skin condition in the participants (O'Rourke et al., 2001). Nurses in residential care facilities are encouraged to individualize nighttime care practices to meet the needs of each resident. An individualized care plan is based on a comprehensive assessment of the various needs of the older adult and weighs the risks and benefits of addressing needs

that may conflict, including the need for a good night's sleep. Thus, for some older adults, the need for an uninterrupted night's sleep may outweigh the potential benefits of being awakened for nighttime care tasks. In many situations, the needs can be addressed during the person's usual waking time, rather than performing the tasks on a rigid schedule designed for the convenience of staff.

Educating Older Adults About Medications and Sleep

Hypnotics may be effective for short-term management of sleep disorders, especially in temporary circumstances, such as in acute care settings. In any community or long-term care setting, however, the adverse effects of hypnotics usually outweigh their advantages. A National Institute of Aging Consensus Statement on the treatment of sleep disorders in older people advises that hypnotic medications should not be the primary mode of management for most people with disturbed sleep (NIH, 1990). The statement also reports that there are no studies demonstrating the long-term effectiveness of hypnotic medications. The recommendation to avoid the use of hypnotics in older adults has been reaffirmed by guidelines for the use of psychopharmacologic medications in nursing homes (Ruby & Kennedy, 2001). Holbrook and colleagues (2001) analyzed studies of benzodiazepines as a treatment for insomnia and concluded that behavioral therapies, rather than benzodiazepines, should be the mainstay of insomnia treatment in older adults, because of adverse effects of benzodiazepines and the long-term efficacy of behavior therapies. These researchers suggested that behavioral therapies include health education to improve sleep habits and correct misperceptions about sleep.

If a hypnotic agent is used for older adults, special attention should be paid to its half-life. There is a great variability in half-life among the benzodiazepines, and some have an extremely long half-life in older adults. Benzodiazepines with longer half-lives are associated with a higher risk for adverse effects, including risks for falls. Table 20-4 provides information about the half-life of hypnotics in younger and older adults. Nurses can educate older adults and their caregivers about the effects of alcohol, medications, and certain chemicals on sleep. Display 20-4 summarizes the pertinent teaching points for older adults.

In addition to educating older adults about medications, nurses may need to address the use of other physiologically active substances (e.g., L-tryptophan and melatonin) because older adults are likely to be using these substances or asking questions about their

	Half-Life in Average Adult (hr)	Half-Life in Older Adult (hr)
TABLE 20-4 Half-Life of Benzodiazepines		
Medication		
Flurazepam (Dalmane)	47–100	120–160
Diazepam (Valium)	20–50	36–98
Estazolam (ProSom)	10–24	10–24*
Lorazepam (Ativan)	10–20	10–20*
Chlordiazepoxide (Librium)	5–20	15–30
Temazepam (Restoril)	9–13	8–20
Oxazepam (Serax)	5–20	5–20*
Alprazolam (Xanax)	6–20	6–20*
Triazolam (Halcion)	2–5	2–6

*Insufficient data available to determine a difference in younger and older adults.

use as sleep aids. L-Tryptophan is an amino acid essential to the synthesis of serotonin in the brain. About 0.5 to 2 g are consumed daily in the typical adult diet, primarily in protein and dairy products. L-Tryptophan has natural sedative qualities, especially in its effect on sleep latency and slow-wave sleep.

DISPLAY 20-4

Health Promotion Teaching About Medications and Sleep

- Hypnotic medications are not effective for long-term use because of increasing tolerance, which often develops within the first week and inevitably develops after a month of regular use.
- Hypnotics should not be used for more than 3 nights in a row.
- Sleeping medications, even over-the-counter ones, are likely to have adverse effects that interfere with daytime function and with the quality of nighttime sleep.
- Older adults are more susceptible than younger adults to the adverse effects of sleeping medications.
- Most hypnotics interfere with REM sleep. When hypnotics are discontinued, a rebound effect, characterized by nightmares and excessive dreaming, may occur.
- Over-the-counter sleeping preparations generally contain antihistamines and can have adverse effects, such as confusion, constipation, or blurred vision, either alone or in combination with other medications.
- Alcohol, in any amount, is likely to have detrimental effects on sleep, such as nightmares and awakenings during the latter part of the night.
- Medications that can interfere with sleep include steroids, diuretics, theophylline, anticonvulsants, decongestants, and thyroid hormone.
- Combining a sleeping medication with any other medication can be harmful and even fatal.
- L-Tryptophan probably has some hypnotic effects; it occurs naturally in milk, eggs, meat, fish, poultry, beans, peanuts, and green leafy vegetables.

L-Tryptophan, in doses of 1 g or less, shortens the sleep latency period for people who have difficulty falling asleep but has no impact on the number of awakenings during the night. Although doses of 1 g or less were thought to be harmless in humans, the Food and Drug Administration (FDA) declared a recall of synthetic L-tryptophan in late 1989, based on reports of an association between L-tryptophan and a rare, but potentially fatal, blood disorder. There is no contraindication to taking L-tryptophan in its natural form.

Melatonin is a hormone that is synthesized by the pineal gland as a byproduct of tryptophan. Serum levels of melatonin follow a circadian rhythm, with very low levels occurring during the day and peak levels occurring between 2:00 AM and 4:00 AM. Melatonin levels diminish with increased age, but the clinical significance of this, if any, has not been identified. Melatonin has been found to be effective for the treatment of jet lag and circadian rhythm disruptions associated with blindness, but its effectiveness as a treatment for insomnia is not clear. Zhdanova and colleagues (2001) used polysomnography to investigate the effects of three doses of melatonin on people aged 50 years and older who complained of insomnia. These researchers found that lower doses (0.1 mg and 0.3 mg) of melatonin were effective in restoring sleep efficiency without adverse effects, but the pharmacologic dose of 3.0 mg induced hypothermia and caused plasma melatonin levels to remain abnormally elevated in the daylight hours (Zhdanova et al., 2001). Adverse effects of melatonin include drowsiness, hypothermia, and loss of libido.

▶ Mrs. Z. returns for further discussion of her sleep problem after filling out a sleep log for 5 days. You review the log with her and find out that when she is home, she spends most of her time reading or doing crossword puzzles. She attends the senior center weekly, plays bridge 2 evenings a week, and goes to lunch with friends a few times every week. She enjoys gardening during the summer but has no other interest in physical activities. She avoids exercise because she is afraid that physical activity "will get the old arthritis all stirred up." On further questioning, she estimates that when she worked she walked about one-half mile daily. She drinks about "a pot" of coffee daily and has coffee and cookies at bridge games. She enjoys a glass of wine in the evenings. When she wakes up during the night, she usually gets up and goes to the bathroom, then returns to bed and lays there "thinking" until she returns to sleep. Her log reflects that she often stays awake for a couple of hours before returning to sleep. She says she's heard that melatonin is good for insomnia and asks your opinion about trying it.

 ## THINKING POINTS

> What myths and misunderstandings about sleep would you address?

> What risk factors might be addressed through health education?

> Since you can see Mrs. Z. weekly at the Wellness Clinic, you can develop a long-term teaching plan. How would you establish priorities for immediate and long-term goals?

> What information from Displays 20-2, 20-3, and 20-4 would you use for health education with Mrs. Z.?

EVALUATING EFFECTIVENESS OF NURSING INTERVENTIONS

The effectiveness of interventions for the nursing diagnosis of Disturbed Sleep Pattern can be measured subjectively or objectively. A subjective measurement would be that the older adult reports that he or she feels rested and refreshed upon awakening in the morning. If a sleep assessment tool is used during the initial assessment, it can be used again for a reassessment after interventions have been implemented. An example of an objective measurement would be that the older adult is able to sleep for 6 to 8 hours at night with only brief interruptions, and that the person looks and acts rested during the day.

CHAPTER SUMMARY

Healthy older adults may experience the following changes in their sleep patterns as compared with their earlier sleep patterns: it may take longer to fall asleep, they may awaken more frequently, and they may spend a longer time in bed but sleep for the same amount of time. Also, because they tend to awaken frequently and spend less time in the deep stages of sleep, they may feel that the quality of their sleep is unsatisfactory. Risk factors that may interfere with sleep patterns of older adults include OSA; PLMS; adverse effects of hypnotics and other medications; physical pain, illness, or discomfort; and psychosocial disturbances, such as anxiety, dementia, or depression.

Nursing assessment of sleep focuses on identifying the older adult's perception of his or her sleep and rest pattern and on identifying the risk factors that interfere with the quality and quantity of sleep. Nursing assessment of sleep is likely to identify many opportunities for health promotion education. A pertinent nursing diagnosis is Disturbed Sleep Pattern. Nursing care is directed toward improving the quantity and quality of sleep. Interventions focus on eliminating risk factors and establishing routines that promote good sleep. Interventions include health education about sleep and nursing actions directed toward individualized care in institutional settings. Nursing care is evaluated by the extent to which the older adult feels rested when he or she awakens in the morning.

CONCLUDING CASE STUDY AND NURSING CARE PLAN

> Mrs. Z. is now 79 years old and is being admitted to a nursing home for skilled care after a total hip replacement. Her diagnoses include osteoarthritis and osteoporosis. After a few weeks in the nursing home, she plans to return to her ranch-style home where she lives with her husband. Before surgery, she was independent in her activities of daily living (ADLs), and she expects to regain her independence and walk with a walker. The hospital transfer form has orders for nabumetone, 750 mg every morning, and temazepam, 15 mg at bedtime as needed.

■ Nursing Assessment

During the admission interview, you ask Mrs. Z. about her sleep patterns. She states that for the past few years, she has been awakened frequently at night by her hip pain and other arthritic discomforts. Also, she reports that she would usually get up three or four times during the night to go to the bathroom. When questioned further, she explains that the pain and discomfort would wake her, and she would go to the bathroom because she wanted to move around, not because she felt an urge to urinate that often. Although her doctor had advised her to take ibuprofen four times daily, she tried not to take this medication more than two times a day because the pills upset her stomach. She avoided taking any medications at night because she thought she shouldn't take the medications on an empty stomach. During her 1-week hospitalization, she had taken a sleeping pill several times. She had also taken Darvocet-N, 100 mg every 4 hours while she was in the hospital, but said that her doctor wanted her to start taking a nonsteroidal antiinflammatory drug (NSAID) on a regular basis for her arthritis and hip pain. She said he had prescribed a new drug that would not upset her stomach, but she had not yet begun to take it. Mrs. Z. expresses anxiety about sleeping in the nursing home because she says that the noise in the hospital was very disruptive to her sleep. She reports that she feels rested in the morning if she gets at least 6 hours of sleep during the 8 hours she spends in bed. During her hospitalization, she never felt rested in the morning and was unable to sleep for 6 hours except when she took sleeping pills. Mrs. Z. says that listening to relaxing music helps her to fall asleep.

■ Nursing Diagnosis

In addition to nursing diagnoses related to Mrs. Z.'s osteoarthritis and hip surgery, you identify a nursing diagnosis of Disturbed Sleep Pattern. Related factors are pain, age-related changes, and environmental conditions. You decide that you will not list nocturia as an associated factor because Mrs. Z. does not feel an urge to void during the night. Rather, she wakes up with pain and then goes to the bathroom. You decide to list age-related changes as a related factor because it is important for Mrs. Z. to understand that, even though she may not awaken with pain, she may awaken because of age-related changes.

■ Nursing Care Plan

The nursing care plan you develop for Mrs. Z. is presented in Display 20-5.

 CRITICAL THINKING EXERCISES

1. Answer the following questions in relation to Mrs. Z. at 79 years old:
   - What additional assessment information pertinent to Mrs. Z.'s sleep patterns would you like to have and how would you obtain this information?
   - What additional nursing interventions would you include in the care plan to address Mrs. Z.'s disturbed sleep pattern? Would you use any of the information in Display 20-2 or give her a copy of it?

DISPLAY 20-5 • NURSING CARE PLAN FOR MRS. Z.

EXPECTED OUTCOME	NURSING INTERVENTIONS	NURSING EVALUATION
Mrs. Z. will identify factors that influence her sleep pattern.	• Describe age-related changes in sleep patterns. • Discuss the important role of pain-relieving measures in promoting good sleep.	• Mrs. Z. will be able to describe the age-related changes and other conditions that affect her sleeping pattern.
Mrs. Z. will consistently obtain 6 hours of sleep nightly without the aid of sleeping medications.	• Administer nabumetone as ordered and evaluate its effectiveness in controlling Mrs. Z.'s pain. • Explain that sleeping medications should be avoided, except for periodic use in short-term situations. • Assign Mrs. Z. to a room that is not close to the nursing station. • Make sure Mrs. Z.'s door is closed at night. • Encourage Mrs. Z. to use her tape recorder to play quiet music at bedtime. • Give Mrs. Z. a copy of Displays 20-3 and 20-4 and discuss additional nonpharmacologic methods for promoting sleep.	• Mrs. Z. will report that she is not awakened by pain. • Mrs. Z. will report that she feels rested upon awakening in the morning.

- What concerns specifically related to sleep would you have about Mrs. Z. after she is discharged from the skilled nursing facility to her own home? How would you address these concerns in your health promotion interventions?

2. What is an older adult likely to experience with regard to sleep and rest patterns? How would you explain these changes to an older adult?

3. Identify three specific factors in each of the following categories that might interfere with sleep: environmental influences, physiologic disturbances, and psychosocial factors.

4. How would you assess an 82-year-old person who comes to the nursing clinic at the senior Wellness Center complaining of feeling tired all the time and not getting enough sleep?

5. What would you include in a half-hour presentation on Tips for Good Sleep for participants in a senior wellness program at a community-based center?

6. What information about sleep and rest would you include in an in-service program for evening and night-shift nursing assistants employed at a nursing home?

Future Directions for Healthier Aging: Focus on Sleep

A goal of the National Institute on Aging is to reduce the burden of sleep disturbances through further research on the following:

- Mechanisms underlying sleep–wake cycles
- Biorhythms of the aging nervous system
- Interactions between diseases and sleep in older adults

Source: National Institute on Aging, 2001.

EDUCATIONAL RESOURCES

American Academy of Sleep Medicine
One Westbrook Corporate Center, Suite 920, Westchester, IL 60154
(708) 492-0930
fax (708) 492-0943
http://www.aasmnet.org

American Sleep Apnea Association
1424 K Street N.W, Suite 302, Washington, DC 20005
(202) 293-3650
http://www.sleepapnea.org

Better Sleep Council
P.O. Box 19534, Alexandria, VA 22320-0534
http://www.bettersleep.org

Canadian Sleep Society
School of Psychology, Laval University
Ste-Foy, Quebec G1K 7P4
http://www.css.to

National Center on Sleep Disorders
NHLBI Information Center, Two Rockledge Center, Suite 10038
6701 Rockledge Drive, Bethesda, MD 20892-7920
(301) 251-1222
http://www.nhlbi.nih.gov/about/ncsdr/index.htm

National Sleep Foundation
1522 K Street NW, Suite 500, Washington, DC 20005
(202) 347-3471
http://www.sleepfoundation.org

REFERENCES

Ancoli-Israel, S., Martin, J. L., Kripke, D. F., Marler, M., & Klauber, M. R. (2002). Effect of light treatment on sleep and circadian rhythms in demented nursing home patients. *Journal of the American Geriatrics Society, 50,* 282–289.

Beck-Little, R., & Weinrich, S. P. (1998). Assessment and management of sleep disorders in the elderly. *Journal of Gerontological Nursing, 24*(2), 21–29.

Blazer, D. G. (1998). *Emotional problems in later life: Intervention strategies for professional caregivers* (2nd ed.). New York: Springer.

Blazer, D. G. (2002). *Depression in late life* (3rd ed.). New York: Springer.

Blazer, D., Hybels, C., Simonsick, E., & Hanlon, J. T. (2000). Sedative, hypnotic, and antianxiety medication use in an aging cohort over ten years: A racial comparison. *Journal of the American Geriatrics Society, 48,* 1073–1079.

Buysse, D. J., Reynolds, C. F., Monk, T. H., Berman, S. R., & Kupfer, D. J. (1989). The Pittsburgh Sleep Quality Index: A new instrument for psychiatric practice and research. *Psychiatry Research, 28,* 193–213.

Carpenito, L. J. (2002). *Nursing diagnosis: Application to clinical practice* (9th ed.). Philadelphia: Lippincott Williams & Wilkins.

Cricco, M., Simonsick, E. M., & Foley, D. J. (2001). The impact of insomnia on cognitive functioning in older adults. *Journal of the American Geriatrics Society, 49,* 1185–1189.

Cruise, P. A., Schnelle, J. F., Alessi, C. A., Simmons, S. F., & Ouslander, J. G. (1998). The nighttime environment and incontinence care practices in nursing homes. *Journal of the American Geriatrics Society, 46,* 181–186.

Floyd, J. A., Medler, S. M., Ager, J. W., & Janisse, J. J. (2000). Age-related changes in initiation and maintenance of sleep: A meta-analysis. *Research in Nursing and Health, 23*(2), 106–117.

Foreman, M. D., & Wykle, M. (1995). Nursing standard-of-practice protocol: Sleep disturbances in elderly patients. *Geriatric Nursing, 16,* 238–243.

Giron, M. S. T., Forsell, Y., Bersten, C., Thorslund, M., Winblad, B., & Fastbom, J. (2002). Sleep problems in a very old population: Drug use and clinical correlates. *Journal of Gerontology: Medical Sciences, 57A,* M236–M240.

Hoch, C. C., Reynolds, C. F. III, Buysse, D. J., Monk, T. H., Nowell, P., Begley, A. E., Hall, F., & Dew, M. A. (2001). Protecting sleep quality in later life: A pilot study of bed restriction and sleep hygiene. *Journal of Gerontology: Psychological Sciences, 56B*(1), P52–P59.

Holbrook, A. M., Crowther, R., Lotter, A., et al. (2001). The role of benzodiazepines in the treatment of insomnia. *Journal of the American Geriatrics Society, 49,* 824–926.

Jelicic, M., Bosma, H., Ponds, R. W., Van Boxtel, M. P., Houx, P. J., & Jolles, J. (2002). Subjective sleep problems in later life as predictors of cognitive decline. *International Journal of Geriatric Psychiatry, 17,* 73–77.

Klerman, E. B., Dijk, D. J., & Czeisler, C. A. (2001). Circadian phase resetting in older people by ocular bright light exposure. *Journal of Investigative Medicine, 49*(1), 30–40.

Libman, E., Creti, L., Amsel, R., Brender, W., & Fichten, C. S. (1997). What do older good and poor sleepers do during periods of nocturnal wakefulness? The Sleep Behaviors Scale: 60 + . *Psychology and Aging, 12*(1), 170–182.

Lichstein, K. L., Wilson, N. M., & Johnson, C. T. (2000). Psychological treatment of secondary insomnia. *Psychology and Aging, 15*(2), 232–240.

Maggi, S., Langlois, J. A., Minicuci, N., Grigoletto, F., Pavan, M., Foley, D. J., & Enzi, G. (1998). Sleep complaints in community-dwelling older persons: Prevalence, associated factors, and reported causes. *Journal of the American Geriatrics Society, 46,* 161–168.

McCurry, S. M., Logsdon, R. G., Vitiello, M. V., & Teri, L. (1998). Successful behavioral treatment for reported sleep problems in elderly caregivers of dementia patients: A controlled study. *Journal of Gerontology: Psychological Sciences , 53B,* P122–P129.

Mishima, K., Okawa, M., Shimizu, T., & Hishikawa, Y. (2001). Diminished melatonin secretion in the elderly caused by insufficient environmental illumination. *Journal of Clinical Endocrinology and Metabolism, 86*(1), 129–133.

National Institute on Aging (NIA). (2001). *Action plan for aging research: Strategic plan for fiscal years 2001–2005.* Washington, DC: U.S. Department of Health and Human Services. HIH Publication No. 01-4961.

National Institutes of Health Consensus Development Conference (NIH). (1990, March 26–28). *Treatment of sleep disorders of older people.* NIH Consensus Statement, 8(3). Washington, DC: NIH.

Naylor, E., Penev, P. D., Orbeta, L., Janssen, I., Ortiz, R., Colecchia, E. F., Keng, M., Finkel, S., & Zee, P. C. (2000). Daily social and physical activity increases slow-wave sleep and daytime neuropsychological performance in the elderly. *Sleep, 23*(1), 87–95.

Ohayon, M. M., Zulley, J., Guilleminault, C., Smirne, S., & Priest, R. G. (2001). How age and daytime activities are related to insomnia in the general population: Consequences for older people. *Journal of the American Geriatrics Society, 49,* 360–366.

O'Rourke, D. J., Klaasen, K. S., & Sloan, J. A. (2001). Redesigning nighttime care for personal care residents. *Journal of Gerontological Nursing, 27*(7), 30–37.

Phillips, B., Young, T., Finn, L., Asher, K., Hening, W. A., & Purvis, C. (2000). Epidemiology of restless legs symptoms in adults. *Archives of Internal Medicine, 160,* 2137–2141.

Richards, K. C., Sullivan, S. C., Phillips, R. L., Beck, C. K., & Overton-McCoy, A. L. (2001). The effects of individualized activities on the sleep of nursing home residents who are cognitively impaired. *Journal of Gerontological Nursing, 27*(9), 30–37.

Roth, T., & Roehrs, T. (2000). Sleep organization and regulation. *Neurology, 54*(5 Suppl. 1), 2–7.

Ruby, C. M., & Kennedy, D. H. (2001). Psychopharmacologic medication use in nursing-home care: Indicators for surveyor assessment of the performance of drug-regimen reviews, recommendations for monitoring, and nonpharmacologic alternatives. *Clinics in Family Practice, 3,* 577–598.

Schoenfelder, D. P., & Culp, K. R. (2001). Sleep pattern disturbance. In M. L. Maas, K. C. Buckwalter, M. D. Hardy, T. Tripp-Reimer, M. G. Titler, & J. P. Specht (Eds.), *Nursing care of older adults: Diagnoses, outcomes, and interventions* (pp. 401–413). St. Louis: Mosby.

Shaver, J. L., & Zenk, S. N. (2000). Sleep disturbance in menopause. *Journal of Women's Health & Gender-Based Medicine, 9*(2), 109–118.

Shochat, T., Martin, J., Marler, M., & Ancoli-Israel, S. (2000). Illumination levels in nursing home patients: Effects on sleep and activity rhythms. *Journal of Sleep Research, 9,* 373–379.

Smyth, C. (1999). The Pittsburgh Sleep Quality Index (PSQI). *Journal of Gerontological Nursing, 25,* 10–11.

Tamaki, M., Shirota, A., Hayashi, M., & Hori, T. (2000). Restorative effects of a short afternoon nap (> 30 min) in the elderly on subjective mood, performance and EEG activity. *Sleep Research Online, 3*(3), 131–139. Retrieved from http://www.sro.org/2000/_Tamaki/131/.

Umlauf, M. G., & Weaver, T. E. (2001). Daytime sleepiness. In M. D. Mezey (Ed.), *The encyclopedia of elder care* (pp. 182–184). New York: Springer.

U.S. Department of Health and Human Services (USDHHS). (2000). *Healthy people 2010* (2nd ed). Washington, DC: U.S. Government Printing Office.

Van Cauter, E., Leproult, R., & Plat, L. (2000). Age-related changes in slow wave sleep and REM sleep and relationship with growth hormone and cortisol levels in healthy men. *Journal of the American Medical Association, 284,* 861–868.

Wallace-Guy, G. M., Kripke, D. F., Hean-Louis, G., Langer, R. D., Elliott, J. A., & Tuunainen, A. (2002). Evening light exposure: Implications for sleep and depression. *Journal of the American Geriatrics Society, 50,* 738–739.

Zhdanova, I. V., Wurtman, R. J., Regan, M. M., Taylor, J. A., Shi, J. P., & Leclair, O. U. (2001). Endocrine care: Of special interest to the practice of endocrinology. *Journal of Clinical Endocrinology and Metabolism, 86,* 4727–4730.

Zizi, F., Jean-Louis, G., Magai, C., Greenidge, K. C., Wolintz, A. H., & Health-Phillip, O. (2002). Sleep complaints and visual impairment among older Americans: A community-based study. *Journal of Gerontology: Medical Sciences, 57A,* M691–M694.

Thermoregulation

AGE-RELATED CHANGES THAT AFFECT THERMOREGULATION

The primary function of thermoregulation is to maintain a stable core body temperature in a wide range of environmental temperatures. In the presence of infections, thermoregulation also assists in maintaining homeostasis. With increased age, subtle alterations in thermoregulation occur, and these become important considerations in caring for healthy, as well as frail, older adults. Under normal circumstances, the core body temperature is maintained at 97°F (36.1°C) to 99°F (37.2°C) through complex physiologic mechanisms governing heat production and dissipation. Nervous system control over thermoregulation is centered in the hypothalamus and is affected by both internal and external influences. The following internal factors affect temperature regulation: metabolism rate; disease processes; muscle activity; peripheral blood flow; amount of subcutaneous fat; function of the cutaneous nerves; ingestion of fluid, nutrients, and medications; and temperature of the blood flowing through the hypothalamus. External factors that influence thermoregulation include the environmental temperature, humidity level, and airflow as well as the type and amount of clothing and covering used.

Response to Cold Temperatures

In cold environmental temperatures, physiologic mechanisms are initiated to prevent loss of body heat and increase heat production. At the same time, protective behaviors are initiated, in response to central nervous system mechanisms, to warm the body and protect the person from adversely cold temperatures. Shivering, muscle contraction, increased heart rate, peripheral vasoconstriction, dilation of the blood vessels in the muscles, insulation of deeper tissues by subcutaneous fat, and the release of thyroxine and corticosteroid by the pituitary gland are all physiologic mechanisms that prevent heat loss and increase heat production. Actions that can be initiated to protect a person in cold temperatures include seeking of shelter, ingestion of warm fluids, use of warm clothing or covering, and an increase in activity to stimulate circulation.

The age-related changes that interfere with an older person's ability to respond to cold temperatures include inefficient vasoconstriction, decreased cardiac output, decreased muscle mass, diminished peripheral circulation, decreased subcutaneous tissue, and delayed and diminished shivering. Age-related changes affecting the response to cold usually begin during the fifth decade, but their impact is not felt until the seventh or eighth decade. The overall effect of these changes is a dulled perception of cold and a concomitant lack of stimulus to initiate protective actions, such as adding more clothing or raising the environmental temperature.

Response to Hot Temperatures

In hot environmental temperatures, or when metabolic heat production is high, the normal mechanisms for heat dissipation are the production of sweat to facilitate evaporation and the dilation of peripheral blood vessels to facilitate heat radiation. When exposed to hot climates or engaged in strenuous activity over a period of several days or weeks, healthy adults are able to acclimatize, or gradually increase their metabolic efficiency. The older person's response to heat is altered primarily by age-related dermal changes affecting sweating and vasoconstriction. Older adults have an increased threshold for the onset of sweating, a diminished response when sweating occurs, and a dulled sensation of warm environments. For example, the sweat response to exercise in healthy adults in their mid-60s is about half of that in adults in their mid-20s. Impaired sweating mechanisms and decreased cardiac output can interfere with the older person's ability to acclimatize. Consequently, older adults are more susceptible to heat stress, and their core body temperature may rise higher than that of younger adults (Young, 2001).

Normal Body Temperature and Febrile Response to Illness

Normal human body temperature is maintained at 98.6°F (37.0°C), plus or minus 1°F, with diurnal variations of 2°F. An elevated temperature, or fever, is the body's protective response to pathologic conditions such as cancer, infection, dehydration, or connective tissue disease. Normal body temperature decreases with increased age, particularly in people older than 75 years. Mean body temperatures in older adults range from 96.9°F (36.1°C) to 98.3°F (36.8°C) orally and 98°F (36.7°C) to 99°F (37.2°C) rectally.

Questions have been raised about the accuracy of oral and axillary temperatures as a measurement of core temperature in older adults because the difference between their core and skin temperatures is greater and more variable than in younger people. Although rectal temperature has long been viewed as the established standard for measuring body temperature, obtaining it is difficult and very invasive. In recent years, ear thermometry has become the method of choice because it is the least invasive and quickest way of obtaining temperatures, especially in acutely ill patients. Studies suggest that ear temperatures provide accurate estimates of core body temperature in older adults because they are the same as or less than one half degree celsius lower than rectal temperatures (Smitz et al., 2000). Fever threshold for older adults is 98.6°F (37°C) for oral and axillary, 99°F (37.2°C) for auditory, and 99.5°F (37.5°C) for rectal. It is important to keep in mind that there is wide individual variation in normal body temperature; thus, fevers need to be evaluated in relation to an individual's baseline temperature.

RISK FACTORS THAT AFFECT THERMOREGULATION

Age alone predisposes people to both hypothermia and hyperthermia. Whereas hypothermia develops in healthy young adults only when they are exposed to adversely cold temperatures, older adults can become hypothermic even in moderately cool environments, especially in the presence of additional risk factors. Likewise, healthy young adults can tolerate hot environmental temperatures without adverse effects, whereas heat-related illnesses may develop in older adults even in moderately hot temperatures. Any combination of environmental and other risk factors in the older adult is likely to lead to serious problems or even death because of impaired thermoregulatory mechanisms that increase the older adult's vulnerability to hypothermia and hyperthermia.

Environmental and Socioeconomic Influences

Environmental temperatures have a significant effect on the susceptibility of older adults to hypothermia or hyperthermia as is evident from the following statistics: heat waves can raise the number of heat-related deaths from an average 200 per year to thousands; and, average mortality rates from hypothermia are nearly 12 times greater in people aged 75 years and older compared with people aged 15 to 34 years (Hirsch, 1998). Although the weather cannot be controlled, many environmental factors that directly affect thermoregulation are amenable to disease prevention interventions.

Heat waves are especially hazardous for older adults living in environments with poor ventilation. The detrimental effects of heat waves are compounded when high temperatures are combined with high humidity levels and air pollutants. For older adults living in urban areas with high crime rates, ventilation may be restricted when windows are kept closed because of safety considerations. In Great Britain, the term "urban hypothermia" has been used to refer to older adults living alone in poorly heated dwellings. Likewise, the term "urban hyperthermia" could be applied to older adults living in poorly ventilated houses and apartments, particularly public housing, in cities where heat waves and air pollution are common.

In addition to the obvious environmental influence of cold or hot temperatures, substandard living conditions and diets deficient in protein and calories also have been associated with hypothermia and hyperthermia. Because hypothermia and hyperthermia usually are not self-reported disorders, social isolation and living alone are additional risk factors. Thus, during periods of extremely hot or cold weather, lack of daily contact with other people increases the risk for an older adult's progressive hypothermia or hyperthermia not being identified.

> The annual death rate from hypothermia in older people of African American and other races is much higher than that in whites; this may be associated with socioeconomic determinants that increase the risk for hypothermia (Hanania & Zimmerman, 1999).

Behaviors Based on Myths and Misunderstandings

Lack of knowledge about age-related vulnerability to hypothermia and hyperthermia may create risks secondary to inadequate protective measures. For example, when the use of heating or air conditioning is curtailed as a cost-saving measure, younger adults may be able to adjust to the moderately hot or cool temperature, whereas an older adult might become hyperthermic or hypothermic under the same circumstances. If older adults and their caregivers are not aware of the age-related decrease in the perception of environmental temperatures, appropriate measures to counteract hot or cold environments, such as removing or adding clothing, may not be taken.

In the presence of infection, lack of knowledge about age-related thermoregulatory changes may result in undetected illnesses. For example, if caregivers of older adults believe that an infectious disease is always accompanied by an elevated temperature, they may assume that no infection is present if there is no fever. Similarly, if they believe that the baseline temperature for all adults is 98.6°F (37.0°C), they may not recognize an elevated temperature in someone whose baseline temperature is lower than this. Lack of knowledge about diurnal temperature variations, the age-related decrease in body temperature, and the age-related increase in the difference between core and skin temperature also may contribute to false expectations and undetected illness. For example, if body temperatures are recorded only in the morning, when they are normally lower, a slight or modest temperature elevation may not be detected.

Chemical Effects and Adverse Medication Effects

Chemical effects and adverse medication effects alter thermoregulation by predisposing people to hypothermia and hyperthermia and by interfering

TABLE 21-1 • Risk Factors for Altered Thermoregulation

Risk Factor	Hypothermia	Hyperthermia
Age of 75 years or older	X	X
Slightly uncomfortable environmental temperatures	X	X
Dehydration	X	X
Electrolyte imbalances	X	X
Infections	X	X
Cardiovascular and cerebrovascular diseases	X	X
Peripheral vascular disease		X
Postural hypotension	X	
Diabetes	X	X
Hypoglycemia	X	
Hypothyroidism	X	
Hyperthyroidism		X
Parkinsonism	X	
Inactivity/immobility	X	
Hypertension		X
Obesity		X
Alcohol consumption	X	X
Phenothiazines	X	X
Anticholinergics		X
Barbiturates	X	X
Diuretics	X	X
Antidepressants	X	
Benzodiazepines	X	
Reserpine	X	
Cardiovascular drugs (e.g., sympatholytics, β-blockers, calcium channel blockers)		X

with the fever response in the presence of an illness. Antipsychotics, acetaminophen, steroid medications, and nonsteroidal anti-inflammatory agents, for example, may mask a fever. In usual doses, salicylates can predispose people to hypothermia and interfere with fever responses, and salicylate intoxication can induce hyperthermia by causing metabolic acidosis. Medications may predispose a person to hypothermia through mechanisms that suppress shivering and increase vasodilation. Medications may predispose a person to hyperthermia by inducing diuresis, increasing heat production, and interfering with sweating. Some medications, such as diuretics and phenothiazines, affect thermoregulation through several mechanisms, increasing the risk for both hypothermia and hyperthermia.

Alcohol ingestion increases the risk of hyperthermia by inducing diuresis, and it increases the risk of hypothermia by inducing vasodilation and interfering with shivering. When excessive alcohol is consumed, the risks are increased even further because sensory perception is dulled and the person is less able to initiate protective behaviors. Table 21-1, which summarizes some of the risk factors for altered

thermoregulation, includes some of the medications that may predispose a person to hypothermia or hyperthermia. If combinations of these medications are taken, or if any medication is taken in combination with alcohol, the risk for altered thermoregulation is greatly increased.

Physiologic Disturbances

Thermoregulation can be compromised by any condition that interferes with cardiac output or peripheral circulation. Cerebrovascular and cardiovascular diseases increase the risk for both hypothermia and hyperthermia. Fluid and electrolyte imbalances, especially dehydration and hypernatremia or hyponatremia, increase one's susceptibility to both hyperthermia and hypothermia. Also, diminished renal function may interfere with the febrile response of older adults. Half of patients undergoing surgery experience unintentional hypothermia, and this occurs more commonly in older patients and those who receive general anesthesia (Hirsch, 1998).

Endocrine dysfunctions commonly associated with hypothermia in older adults include hypoglycemia, hypothyroidism, and hypopituitarism. Thyrotoxicosis and diabetic ketoacidosis also may cause or contribute to hyperthermia in older adults. Infections, particularly pneumonia and sepsis, are common causes of elevated body temperature in younger adults; however, in older adults, these conditions may predispose the person to hypothermia. Neurologic impairment secondary to parkinsonism or any type of dementia also can cause or contribute to hypothermia.

Inactivity secondary to chronic physical illness or psychosocial factors, such as depression or isolation, can increase the risk for hypothermia. Likewise, fatigue and hypoxia can increase the risk for hypothermia by suppressing shivering. An inability to rise after falling may precipitate hypothermia in cool environmental temperatures, and this risk is increased for people living alone. Postural hypotension also may cause or contribute to hypothermia. In acute care settings, older surgical patients are particularly prone to developing hypothermia owing to a combination of conditions, such as immobility, body exposure, low environmental temperatures, age-related changes, and anesthesia and other medication effects.

In older adults, heat-related illness may be precipitated by moderate exercise in hot weather, especially if fluid intake is not sufficient to replace fluid loss. If older adults rely solely on their sensation of thirst to signal the need for fluid intake, they may become underhydrated or dehydrated because the thirst mechanism becomes less efficient with advancing age. Additional risks for dehydration and heat-related illnesses arise from the diminished efficiency of the older adult's kidneys in concentrating urine. Risks are compounded if the older adult who may have mobility problems restricts fluid intake to avoid inconvenient trips to the bathroom. If adequate rehydration is not provided between periods of exercise or during prolonged exposure to a hot climate, a heat-related illness is likely to develop in the older adult.

FUNCTIONAL CONSEQUENCES ASSOCIATED WITH THERMOREGULATION IN OLDER ADULTS

A healthy older adult in a comfortable environment will experience few, if any, functional consequences of altered thermoregulation. In the presence of any risk factor, however, hypothermia or hyperthermia may develop in an older adult. Even moderately adverse environmental temperatures may precipitate hypothermia or hyperthermia in an older adult, especially in the presence of additional predisposing factors, such as certain medications or pathologic conditions. Older adults with impaired thermoregulation may develop hypothermia after prolonged exposure to environmental temperatures lower than 95°F (35°C), even though most people would be comfortable or hot at these temperatures (Hirsch, 1998). In the United States, hypothermia and hyperthermia usually are seasonal hazards that occur during heat waves and cold spells, and these weather-related problems most often affect older adults who live in climates with extremes of weather. Older adults who live in climates where either hot or cold weather is the norm have been acclimatized to these conditions and usually live in housing environments that are suitable to the climate.

For older adults in whom hypothermia or hyperthermia develops, the risk for subsequent morbidity or mortality from this condition is greater than that for their younger counterparts. One study of deaths among elderly people from excessive heat and excessive cold found that three fifths of the preventable deaths were due to excessive cold (Macey & Schneider, 1993). It also found that minority and rural elderly adults were disproportionately likely to suffer deaths from temperature-related causes.

Altered Response to Cold Environments

Increased age is associated with an increased vulnerability to hypothermia because most older adults are less aware of a low core body temperature, less efficient in their physiologic response to cold, less perceptive of cold environments, and less apt to take corrective actions in them. One study of the response of younger and older adults to environmental temperatures suggested that older adults are at greater risk for altered thermoregulation because they may require a more intense thermal stimulus before taking appropriate actions (Taylor et al., 1995). Physiologic alterations, as well as behavioral factors, contribute to the increased risk for hypothermia in older adults.

Hypothermia is defined as a core body temperature of 95°F (35°C) or lower. A low environmental temperature usually contributes to hypothermia, and the term *accidental hypothermia* is used when it is the primary cause of the condition. Even in normal environmental temperatures, however, the condition can result from serious alterations in homeostasis, such as endocrine or neurologic diseases. Accidental hypothermia can occur in older adults as a consequence of exposure to moderately cool temperatures and is thought to affect as many as 10% of older adults living in winter climates, such as Great Britain, Canada, and parts of the United States.

In the early stages of hypothermia, the older adult probably will not shiver or complain of feeling cold. In the absence of any protective measures, hypothermia will progress, clouding mental function. The effects of impaired thermoregulation are cumulative, and hypothermia progresses rapidly after the core body temperature falls to 93.2°F (34.0°C). The age-related diminished ability of the kidney to conserve water and the common occurrence of inadequate fluid intake in older adults exacerbate the effects of hypothermia. If the process is not reversed, death from hypothermia will result from the myocardial effects of seriously impaired thermoregulation.

Altered Response to Hot Environments

The functional consequences of age-related changes in the older adult's ability to respond to hot environments include delayed and diminished sweating and inaccurate perception of environmental temperatures. Because of these functional consequences, the older adult is more likely to have heat-related illnesses, including heat stroke and heat exhaustion. Although "hyperthermia" is the term often used to refer to heat-related illnesses in older people, this term more accurately refers to any condition in which the body temperature is elevated above normal. In addition to being caused by impaired thermoregulation and environmental factors, hyperthermia can be caused by pyrogens and other pathologic conditions.

Heat exhaustion is a condition that develops gradually from depletion of fluid, sodium, or both. It can occur in active or immobilized older people who are dehydrated or underhydrated and exposed to hot environments. Heat stroke is an even more serious condition that is likely to occur in active older adults because of a combination of age-related thermoregulatory changes and risk factors, such as overexertion and warm environments. Heat stroke can also occur in immobilized older adults in hot environments, either as a progression of untreated heat exhaustion or as a result of a combination of risk factors, such as diabetes and certain medications. The underlying mechanism in heat stroke is an inability to balance the rates of heat production and dissipation. This balance depends primarily on sweating and cardiac output.

In hot environments, the effects of altered thermoregulation are cumulative, and heat-related illnesses progress rapidly after the body temperature reaches 105.8°F (40.6°C). If fluid volume is not adequate to meet the requirements for effective sweating, then hyperthermia will progress even more rapidly. The age-related decrease in thirst sensation may contribute to inadequate fluid intake and diminished thermoregulation. If hyperthermia is not reversed, death will result from respiratory depression.

> A study of heat- and cold-related deaths in elderly people found that older men were more likely to die from excessive cold, whereas older women were more likely to die from excessive heat (Macey & Schneider, 1993).

Altered Thermoregulatory Response to Illness

A diminished febrile response to illness and infections, such as bacteremia, occurs in many older adults as a consequence of age-related changes in the thermoregulatory centers of the hypothalamus. Thus, older adults are likely to have undetected infections, and these infections are often found upon admission to a hospital for a functional decline, a change in mental status, or other vague manifestations of illness. A common finding in older adults with infections is a normal or even lower than normal temperature, but when their temperature is compared with their baseline temperature, at least a slight elevation is evident. Thus, elevated temperature in older adults can be detected only in relation to their normal baseline temperature.

Altered Perception of Environmental Temperatures

A very common observation of nurses is that older adults frequently report feeling cool or cold, even in very warm environments. Also, older adults generally prefer environmental temperatures that are at least 75°F (23.9°C). Misperceptions of environmental temperatures are not necessarily caused by age-related changes but are probably associated with pathophysiologic conditions, such as dementia, thyroid disorders, or cardiovascular inefficiency.

Psychosocial Consequences of Altered Thermoregulation

Psychosocial consequences do not arise from age-related thermoregulatory changes alone; however, they can be caused by hypothermia, hyperthermia, or diminished fever response. If hypothermia or hyperthermia is overlooked, or if interventions are not initiated at an early stage, the condition may progress to the point of impairing cognitive function. Likewise, if a diminished or delayed febrile response to an infection is not recognized, a treatable condition may be overlooked, and treatment may unintentionally be delayed or denied. Unrecognized infections are likely to progress in severity and, in older adults, may manifest primarily as a functional decline, such as in cognitive function. Figure 21-1 illustrates the age-related changes, risk factors, and negative functional consequences affecting thermoregulation.

> Mrs. T. is 76 years old and lives alone in a large farmhouse in a rural county in central Ohio. She has lived on this 20-acre farm for 49 years and has been a widow for 2 years. She has four children and eight grandchildren, but they all live in other states. Mrs. T. has been able to manage her farm with a part-time farmhand who comes a couple times a week to help feed the several dozen chickens and collect eggs. When her farmhand doesn't come, she manages the chores by herself. She has hypertension and type II diabetes, and she manages pretty well medically. She adheres to her diabetic diet and takes her medications daily. She sends her farmhand to the city about once weekly for groceries and drives to the nearby church on Sundays. Once a month she attends the county senior center, where you are the nurse. It is the middle of July, and summer in Ohio this year has been unusually hot and humid. A drought and heat wave are predicted for central Ohio, and you are planning to present a health education program called "Hot Tips for Surviving the Summer." You are particularly concerned about Mrs. T. and several other

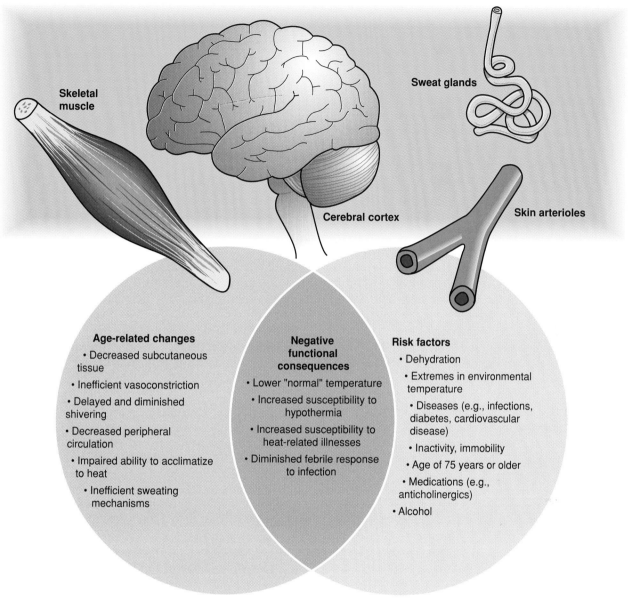

FIGURE 21-1 Age-related changes and risk factors intersect to negatively affect temperature regulation in older adults.

participants who live in isolated area and have little contact with others.

 THINKING POINTS

➤ What factors increase the risk for Mrs. T. developing a heat-related illness? Which ones would you discuss in your health education program?

➤ In your health education program, how would you explain heat-related illnesses and the associated signs and symptoms?

 NURSING ASSESSMENT OF THERMOREGULATION

Nursing assessment of thermoregulation is aimed at identifying the person's baseline body temperature, any risk factors for altered thermoregulation, manifestations of hypothermia or hyperthermia, and the older adult's febrile response to illness. Much of this information will be used as the basis for planning health education interventions to prevent hypothermia and hyperthermia. Information will also be used to detect hypothermia or heat-related illnesses as quickly as possible so that appropriate interventions can be initiated before serious or irreversible effects occur. Assessment information also is important in detecting infections at an early stage. Although much of the pertinent information about risk factors is collected as part of the overall assessment, specific information about thermoregulation is obtained by observing the environment, measuring the person's body temperature, and interviewing the older adult and the caregivers of dependent older adults.

Assessing Baseline Temperature

Body temperature measurements show a diurnal fluctuation of 1° to 2°F (0.6°–1.1°C), with a greater variation occurring during periods of fever-inducing illness. The highest temperature occurs in the evening, usually between 6:00 PM and 8:00 PM, and the lowest temperature occurs between 2:00 AM and 3:00 AM. Because older adults normally have a lower body temperature and may have a diminished febrile response to infection, it is especially important to determine the person's usual temperature as well as to characterize the usual pattern of diurnal variation. Older adults in home settings should be encouraged to determine their usual temperature by recording their oral temperature at different times of the day for several days when they are feeling well. If this is done seasonally by people who live in fluctuating climates and annually by those who live in stable climates, there will be a good basis for comparison when symptoms of illness or functional decline occur. The same procedure can be followed in long-term care settings, with the results recorded as baseline data on the person's chart. Display 21-1 summarizes the principles underlying nursing assessment of thermoregulation in older adults.

Identifying Risk Factors for Altered Thermoregulation

Anyone older than 75 years of age should be considered at risk for altered thermoregulation, as should any older adult who has one or more of the risk factors listed in Table 21-1. Because so many of the risk factors for altered thermoregulation are modifiable, it is important to identify those that can be addressed through health promotion interventions. Risk factors involving medications and physiologic disturbances usually are identified during the overall assessment, but they may be overlooked unless special attention is paid to their role in predisposing the person to hypothermia or hyperthermia. In addition to assessing for risks for hypothermia or heat-related illnesses, nurses must consider a low baseline body temperature as a risk for undetected fever. If a person's baseline temperature is below 98°F (36.7°C), it is important to document the usual baseline and note that this should be used as the base of comparison when assessing for an elevated temperature.

Although most nurses do not have the opportunity to assess the older adult's environment directly, nurses can ask pertinent questions and listen for clues to detect environmental risk factors. For example, older adults who live alone and express concern about paying utility bills or keeping the house warm in winter should be considered at risk for hypothermia. Likewise, older adults who live in poor housing conditions, or with family members who keep the house at low temperatures during winter months, should be considered at risk for hypothermia. Older adults in urban environments who express fears about keeping windows open in houses that are not air-conditioned or who live in poorly ventilated rooms should be considered to be at risk for hyperthermia during heat waves. Interview questions aimed at identifying risk factors for altered thermoregulation are listed in Display 21-1.

Assessing for Hypothermia

Hypothermia is best detected by measuring core body temperature with a thermometer that registers below 95°F (35°C). Cool skin in unexposed areas, such as the abdomen and buttocks, is a distinguishing characteristic of hypothermia. The environmental temperature may be only moderately cool, and the older person will not necessarily shiver or complain of feeling cold. Even in environmental temperatures of 68°F (20°C) or 69°F (20.6°C), an older person may become hypothermic, especially if other risk factors, such as immobility or hypothermia-inducing medications, are present. Early signs of hypothermia are subtle, and the most objective assessment tool is a comparison of the person's body temperature with his usual baseline temperature. As untreated hypothermia progresses, additional signs may include lethargy, slurred speech, mental changes, impaired gait, puffiness of the face, slowed or irregular pulse, low blood pressure, slowed tendon reflexes, and slow, shallow respirations. Severe stages of hypothermia are characterized by muscular rigidity, diminished urinary function, and a progression of all other manifestations to the point of stupor and coma. The skin will feel very cool, and, contrary to what might be expected, the color of the skin will be pink. Also contrary to what might be expected, a hypothermic person may not shiver, particularly if the body temperature is below 90°F (32.2°C).

DISPLAY 21-1
Guidelines for Assessing Thermoregulation

Principles of Temperature Assessment

- Document the person's baseline body temperature and its diurnal and seasonal variations.
- Assume that even a small elevation above the baseline temperature is a clue to the presence of a pathologic process.
- Document actual temperature and deviations from the baseline, rather than using such terminology as "afebrile."
- Carefully follow all the standard procedures for accurate temperature measurement. Use a thermometer that registers temperatures lower than 95°F (35°C).
- Consider the influence of temperature-altering medications when evaluating a temperature reading (e.g., medications that mask a fever).
- Do not assume that an infection will necessarily be accompanied by an elevated temperature.
- Remember that, in the presence of an infection, a decline in function or change in mental status may be an earlier and more accurate indicator of illness than an alteration in temperature.
- Do not assume that an older adult will initiate compensatory behaviors or complain of discomfort when exposed to adverse environmental temperatures.

Questions to Assess Risk Factors for Hypothermia or Hyperthermia

- Do you have any particular health problems that occur in hot or cold weather?
- Are you able to keep your house or room at a comfortable temperature in both summer and winter months?
- What do you do to cope with hot temperatures in the summer?
- Do you have any difficulty paying your utility bills?
- What forms of protection against the cold do you use in the winter months (e.g., electric blanket, supplemental sources of heat)?
- Have you ever received medical care for exposure to heat or cold?
- Have you ever fallen and not been able to get up or get help?

Observations to Assess Risk Factors for Hypothermia or Hyperthermia

- Does the older person live in a house where the temperature is kept below 70°F (21.1°C) during the winter?
- Does the person drink alcohol or take temperature-altering medications (see Table 21-1)?
- Does the person live alone? If so, what is the frequency of outside contacts?
- Does the person have any pathologic conditions that predispose him or her to hypothermia (e.g., endocrine, neurologic, or cardiovascular disorders)?
- Is the person's fluid and nutritional intake adequate?
- Does the person have postural hypotension? (See Table 16-2 and Displays 16-1 and 16-2 for assessment criteria relating to postural hypotension.)
- Is the person immobilized or sedentary? Is the person's judgment impaired because of dementia, depression, or other psychosocial disorders?
- Does the person live in a poorly ventilated dwelling without air conditioning?
- Are atmospheric conditions very hot, humid, or polluted?
- Does the person engage in active exercise during hot weather?
- Does the person have chronic illnesses, such as diabetes or cardiovascular disorders, that predispose him or her to hyperthermia?
- Is the person at risk for hyponatremia or hypokalemia because of medications or chronic illnesses?

Assessing for Hyperthermia

Manifestations of heat-related illnesses range from mild headache to life-threatening respiratory and cardiovascular disturbances. In the early stages of heat-related illness, the person will feel weak and lethargic and may complain of headache, nausea, and loss of appetite. The skin will be warm and dry, and the sweating response may be absent, especially if the person's fluid intake is low. As the heat-related condition progresses, these manifestations will be exacerbated, and the following signs will become evident: dizziness, dyspnea, tachycardia, vomiting, diarrhea, muscle cramps, chest pain, mental impairment, and a wide pulse pressure.

Assessing the Older Adult's Febrile Response to Illness

Because the manifestations of delayed or diminished febrile response to infections are likely to be very subtle, nurses assess for any temperature changes from the person's baseline, and they also observe for additional signs of illness, such as a decline in function. Nurses also should examine assumptions about temperature regulation that may apply to younger adults but not to older adults. For example, the expectation that pneumonia is accompanied by a temperature greater than 98.6°F (37.0°C) is not necessarily applicable to older adults. Hofland and Mort (1994) found that confusion was the only common sign of infection in nursing home residents that was identified by health care providers. Pals and colleagues (1995) also studied fevers in nursing home residents and found that 85% of the clinical manifestations were detected by staff rather than reported by residents. Thus, nurses in long-term care facilities need to be particularly vigilant about subtle temperature changes and other manifestations of fever. A more reliable indicator of elevated temperature in older adults would be an increase of 2°F (1°C) above the person's baseline. See Display 21-1 for a summary of some of these considerations.

NURSING DIAGNOSIS

If the nursing assessment identifies risks for impaired thermoregulation in an older adult, the nursing diagnoses of Risk for Imbalanced Body Temperature, Hypothermia, or Hyperthermia may be applicable. Hypothermia, as a nursing diagnosis, is defined as "the state in which an individual has or is at risk of having a sustained reduction of body temperature of below 35.5°C (96°F) rectally because of increased vulnerability to external factors" (Carpenito, 2002, p. 140). The definition of the nursing diagnosis Hyperthermia is "the state in which an individual has or is at risk of having a sustained elevation of body temperature of greater than 37.8°C (100°F) orally or 38.8°C (101°F) rectally due to external factors" (Carpenito, 2002, p. 137).

If several factors are identified that place the older person at risk for both hypothermia and hyperthermia, then the nursing diagnosis of Risk for Imbalanced Body Temperature may be appropriate. For example, an 83-year-old woman with diabetes, dementia, and hypertension who is taking a diuretic, haloperidol, and an oral hypoglycemic would have many risk factors for both hypothermia and hyperthermia. Related factors that are common in older adults include immobility, advanced age, medication effects, adverse environmental conditions, and acute and chronic illnesses. For older adults living alone, social isolation may be a related factor that increases the risk for experiencing more serious consequences if hypothermia or hyperthermia occurs.

OUTCOMES

Nursing care for an older adult with a diagnosis of Risk for Hypothermia or Hyperthermia is directed toward eliminating the risk factors and maintaining the person's normal body temperature. Related nursing-sensitive outcomes include Risk Control and Thermal Stability. Risk control outcomes are aimed at reducing the likelihood of hypothermia by increasing either patient awareness or caregiver surveillance and by monitoring for the need for assistance in the event of exposure to cold. Thermal stability is aimed at successfully maintaining the body temperature within safe thermal ranges, and the outcome indicator would be thermal comfort (Holtzclaw, 2001).

Outcomes vary depending on the setting. In acute care settings, nurses are more likely to focus on nursing-sensitive outcomes such as Thermoregulation, Risk Control, Fluid Balance, and Vital Signs: Body Temperature. In home and other community settings, nurses might be able to provide group or individual health education for older adults who are at risk for developing hypothermia or heat-related illness, especially during times of extreme weather conditions. In these situations, outcomes might include Risk Control, Risk Detection, Health Promoting Behavior, Knowledge: Health Behavior, and Safety Behavior: Home Physical Environment. In long-term care settings, nurses would address Risk Detection and Risk Control outcomes as well as Thermoregulation, and Vital Signs: Body Temperature.

 ## NURSING INTERVENTIONS TO PROMOTE HEALTHY THERMOREGULATION

Health promotion interventions to address altered thermoregulation can be directed toward primary prevention of hypothermia and heat-related illness. Many risk factors for altered thermoregulation can be eliminated through health education or direct interventions that reduce the vulnerability of older adults to hypothermia or heat-related illnesses. Health promotion interventions also address early detection of altered thermoregulation and prompt initiation of interventions to restore thermal balance and to prevent detrimental effects. Comfort interventions are initiated to promote well-being in older adults.

Addressing Risk Factors

Maintenance of an environmental temperature of about 75°F (23.9°C) is the single most important intervention to prevent hypothermia or hyperthermia. In addition, relative humidity can be altered to minimize the discomfort and detrimental effects associated with extremely warm or cool environments.

With comfortable indoor temperatures, the ideal humidity is between 40% and 50%, whereas an acceptable range is between 20% and 70%. Older adults can be encouraged to humidify the air in their homes during the dry winter months by using humidifiers, either alone or in conjunction with their heating systems. Simpler measures, such as keeping wet towels near heating vents or using a vaporizer near the bed at night, may be appropriate if a humidifier is unavailable. Older adults living in hot, humid climates may need assistance in applying to elder care community programs that provide window air conditioners, fans, and assistance with summer electric bills.

Interventions for the socially isolated older adult include establishing a system of social contact, such as a friendly phone call program, that ensures daily contact during periods of adversely hot or cold weather. In many areas of the United States and Canada in which cold winters are the norm, financial assistance for heating bills may be available through government-sponsored programs, such as the Low Income Home Energy Assistance Program's (LIHEAP) Fuel Assistance Program. Other government-sponsored programs provide financial assistance, such as low-interest loans, for home winterization and modernization measures to protect against adverse weather conditions. Older people and their family caregivers should be encouraged to take advantage of these programs, applications for which can be obtained from the LIHEAP contact listed in the Educational Resources at the end of this chapter.

Promoting Healthy Thermoregulation

In cool environmental temperatures, hypothermia can be prevented through the use of proper clothing and covering and the avoidance of risk factors. Older adults should be encouraged to wear several layers of warm clothing during the daytime and caps and warm socks while sleeping. Electric blankets used during the night are a relatively inexpensive form of protection in cool environments, but proper safety precautions must be taken. Space heaters often are used to provide intense heat in a small area, but they can create serious fire and safety hazards. In addition to environmental considerations, special attention must be directed toward ensuring adequate nutrition, including fluid intake, and toward the treatment of any pathologic conditions.

During heat waves, hyperthermia can affect older adults living in their own homes or in long-term care settings that are not air-conditioned. Nurses in long-term care facilities without air conditioning must

ensure that adequate fluids are provided. They must also observe for early signs of hyperthermia, especially in residents who are immobile or who have medical problems, such as endocrine or circulatory disorders, that predispose older adults to hyperthermia. If only parts of the facility are air-conditioned, nurses can encourage residents to spend time in those areas and can provide assistance for residents who have mobility limitations.

Older adults living in community settings can be instructed about measures to cool the environment, such as those summarized in Display 21-2. Older adults may be reluctant to use fans or air conditioners because of a desire to save money on utility bills. If they understand the health risks associated with hyperthermia, however, they may be prompted to use these appliances judiciously. If the home setting cannot be cooled adequately during heat waves, older adults can be encouraged to spend time in air-conditioned public places. Older adults who have difficulty getting to these places can take advantage of transportation programs that are available through senior centers. Additional interventions to prevent hyperthermia during heat waves include the provision of adequate fluids and the avoidance of heavy meals and strenuous exercise. Display 21-2, which summarizes interventions for the prevention of hyperthermia, can be used as an educational tool for older adults.

Promoting Comfort

Nurses have many opportunities to improve the comfort of older adults who live in environments where they frequently feel cold. Interventions directed toward warming the hands, feet, and head are particularly effective because these areas of the body have the heaviest concentration of nerve endings that are sensitive to heat loss. Nurses can encourage older adults to wear caps, thermal socks, and leg warmers. These interventions are likely to increase the older adult's comfort level and perception of warmth, even if they do not increase the core body temperature (Holtzclaw, 2001). Additional measures that can be used to increase comfort are summarized in Display 21-2, along with nutritional considerations and complementary and alternative care practices that also may improve quality of life with regard to preventing infections.

> Recall that Mrs. T. is 76 years old and a participant at the county senior center where you will be presenting a health education program.

DISPLAY 21-2
Health Promotion Teaching About Hypothermia and Heat-Related Illness

Environmental and Personal Protection Considerations for Preventing Hypothermia

- Maintain a constant room temperature as close to 75°F (23.9°C) as possible, with a minimum temperature of 70°F (21.1°C).
- Use a reliable, clearly marked thermometer to measure room temperature.
- Wear close-knit, but not tight, undergarments to prevent heat loss; wear several layers of clothing.
- Wear a hat and gloves when outdoors; wear a nightcap and socks for sleeping.
- Wear extra clothing in the early morning when your body metabolism is at its lowest point.
- Use flannel bed sheets or sheet blankets.
- Use an electric blanket set on a low temperature.
- Take advantage of programs that offer assistance with utility bills and home weatherization.

Environmental and Personal Protection Action to Prevent Heat-Related Illnesses

- Maintain room temperatures at below 85°F (29.4°C).
- If your residence is not air-conditioned, use fans to circulate the air and cool the environment.
- During hot weather, spend time in public air-conditioned settings, such as libraries or shopping malls.
- Drink extra noncaffeinated, nonalcoholic liquids, even if you don't feel thirsty.
- Wear loose-fitting, lightweight, light-colored, cotton clothing.
- Wear a hat or use an umbrella to protect yourself against sun and heat when you are outside.
- Avoid outdoor activities during the hottest time of the day (i.e., between 10:00 AM and 2:00 PM); perform them during the cooler hours of the morning or evening.
- Place an ice pack or cold, wet towels on your body, especially on the head, the groin area, and armpits. Take cool (about 75°F [23.9°C]) baths or showers several times daily during heat waves, but do not use soap every time.

Health Promotion Actions for Maintaining Optimal Body Temperature

- Maintain adequate fluid intake by drinking 8 to 10 glasses of noncaffeinated, nonalcoholic liquid daily.
- Do not rely on your thirst sensation as an indicator of the need for fluid.
- Eat small, frequent meals rather than heavy meals.
- Avoid drinking caffeinated beverages, such as cola and coffee.
- Avoid drinking alcohol.
- In cold weather, engage in moderate physical exercise and indoor activities to increase circulation and heat production.

Nutritional Considerations

- Maintain good nutrition, especially zinc, selenium, and vitamins A, C, and E.

Complementary and Alternative Care Practices

- Herbs for preventing infections include garlic, ginger, thyme, sage, rosemary, echinacea, goldenseal, licorice, and ginseng.

Preventive Measures and Additional Approaches

- Know your normal temperature in the morning, when you get up and in the mid-evening.
- Know the difference in your temperature in the winter and the summer.
- Obtain pneumonia and influenza immunizations (as discussed in Chapter 17).
- Obtain tetanus and diphtheria vaccinations every 10 years.
- Be aware that melatonin and other bioactive substances (see Table 21-1) might alter temperature regulation; use these substances only under the advice of a health care professional.
- Engage in exercise, massage, imagery, and meditation.

 THINKING POINTS

➤ How would you incorporate assessment information into your health education program?

➤ How would you use information from Display 21-2 to teach about preventing heat-related illnesses?

➤ What specific suggestions would you make about early detection of heat-related illnesses to the participants at this rural senior center?

➤ How would you find health education materials to use for your program?

EVALUATING EFFECTIVENESS OF NURSING INTERVENTIONS

Nursing care of older adults who are diagnosed as being at Risk for Hypothermia/Hyperthermia or Imbalanced Body Temperature is evaluated according to the extent to which the goals have been achieved. A common nursing goal is the elimination of risk factors. For example, housing and financial factors that increase the risk for hypothermia and heat-related illnesses might be addressed by referring an older adult to LIHEAP. When the goal is to educate older adults and their caregivers about the prevention of hypothermia and heat-related illnesses, the nurse can use the information in Display 21-2 as a teaching tool. Evaluation of this intervention would be based on the person's ability to describe ways of decreasing the risk factors for hypothermia or heat-related illnesses.

CHAPTER SUMMARY

Thermoregulation in older adults is altered by age-related changes that interfere with their ability to adapt effectively to environmental temperatures. Because of these changes, older adults are more likely to experience hypothermia or heat-related illnesses. In addition, older adults may have a lower normal body temperature and a delayed or diminished febrile response to illness. Risk factors that can further impair the thermoregulatory response of older adults include diseases, immobility, medication effects, and adverse environmental temperatures.

Nursing assessment of thermoregulation focuses on ascertaining the person's baseline body temperature and identifying any risk factors for hypothermia or heat-related illnesses. Other aspects of the nursing assessment address the detection of illnesses in the absence of temperature elevations in the usual febrile range. Applicable nursing diagnoses include Risk for Hypothermia, Risk for Hyperthermia, and Risk for Imbalanced Body Temperature. Nursing goals are directed toward eliminating risk factors, maintaining the person's normal body temperature, and improving the comfort of older adults who frequently feel cold.

Nursing interventions focus on modifying environments, addressing socioeconomic factors, implementing measures to maintain normal body temperature, and educating older adults and their caregivers about the prevention of hypothermia and heat-related illnesses. Nursing care is evaluated according to the degree to which risk factors are eliminated. Another measure of nursing care is the absence of complaints about feeling cold.

CONCLUDING CASE STUDY AND NURSING CARE PLAN

➤ Mrs. T. is now 87 years old and continues to live alone in her own home in a rural area of central Ohio. She has a history of hypertension and diabetic retinopathy and was recently hospitalized for uncontrolled diabetes. Upon discharge from the hospital in November, she was referred to the Visiting Nurses Association for teaching about insulin administration and monitoring of her diabetic care.

■ Nursing Assessment

During your initial visit, you observe that Mrs. T.'s house is poorly maintained and has no insulation or other weatherization. Mrs. T. tells you that she has lived in this house for 60 years and that, in recent years, she has had difficulty keeping up with its maintenance because of her poor eyesight and limited income. She has few social contacts, but her daughter visits her every other week and a neighbor visits weekly and brings her groceries. About once a month, friends pick her up and take her to church. Your assessment reveals that although Mrs. T. has difficulty preparing meals because of her poor eyesight, she is independent in all other activities of daily living.

During your initial visit, you identify several risk factors for hypothermia, so during subsequent visits, you follow up with further assessment. You learn that Mrs. T. was taken to the emergency room in January 2 years ago to be treated for hypothermia. She recalls that her daughter had come for her usual visit and had found her in a very weak and confused state. Her description of the situation is that "they just warmed me up at the hospital and sent me home again. I could have done that myself if my daughter would have just let me be." It is apparent that she did not consider her condition to be of particular concern. In the winter, she keeps her utility bills low by using a small, portable heater in the living room during the day and moving it into the bedroom at night. Mrs. T. keeps her thermostat at 65°F (18.3°C) during the day and 60°F (15.6°C) at night. A neighbor told her that the county office on aging had a program to assist with utility bills, but she is embarrassed to ask her daughter to drive her to the county office to apply for this "welfare help."

■ Nursing Diagnosis

In addition to addressing the nursing diagnoses related to Mrs. T.'s diabetes, you identify a nursing diagnosis of Risk for Imbalanced Body Temperature, Hypothermia. Related factors include advanced age, diabetes, social isolation, poor housing conditions, low environmental temperatures, and a history of hypothermia.

■ Nursing Care Plan

The nursing care plan you develop for Mrs. T. is presented in Display 21-3.

DISPLAY 21-3 • NURSING CARE PLAN FOR MRS. T.

EXPECTED OUTCOME	NURSING INTERVENTIONS	NURSING EVALUATION
Mrs. T.'s knowledge about risk factors for hypothermia will be increased.	• Discuss and describe risk factors for hypothermia, with emphasis on Mrs. T.'s diabetes, social isolation, environmental conditions, and history of hypothermia.	• Mrs. T. will be able to state at least four factors that place her at risk for hypothermia.
Mrs. T.'s knowledge about ways of preventing hypothermia will be increased.	• Use Display 21-2 to discuss interventions to prevent hypothermia and to explore ways of applying these interventions to Mrs. T.'s situation.	• Mrs. T. will implement strategies aimed at reducing her risk for hypothermia.
The risk factor of low temperatures in Mrs. T.'s house will be eliminated.	• Inform Mrs. T. that she is eligible for the Low Income Home Energy Assistance Program (LIHEAP) and can qualify for assistance with utility bills as well as help with weatherization. • Emphasize that LIHEAP is an important health-related program aimed at preventing hypothermia in older adults. • Ask Mrs. T.'s permission to arrange for a home assessment by a LIHEAP staff person.	• Mrs. T. will accept assistance from the LIHEAP program. • Mrs. T. will have her house weatherized. • Mrs. T. will keep her thermostat at 70°F (21.1°C) during the winter.
The risk factor of social isolation will be eliminated.	• Suggest home-delivered meals to Mrs. T. as a means of providing prepared meals and daily contact. • Emphasize that one of the purposes of such programs is to ensure that socially isolated older adults have daily contact with someone who can monitor their well-being. • Ask Mrs. T. for permission to contact her daughter to suggest that she call her mother daily during cold spells to make sure she is okay.	• Mrs. T. will accept home-delivered meals. • Mrs. T.'s daughter will phone daily during cold spells.

CRITICAL THINKING EXERCISES

1. Answer the following questions in relation to Mrs. T.:
   • How would you address Mrs. T.'s perception that hypothermia does not have serious health-related implications?
   • What additional interventions might you consider to address Mrs. T.'s risk for hypothermia?
2. Describe four major functional consequences that an older adult is likely to experience with regard to thermoregulation. How would you explain these changes to an older adult?
3. Explain how each of the following factors might affect an older person's thermoregulation: medications, pathologic conditions, environmental conditions, socioeconomic factors, and myths and misunderstanding.
4. What would you include in an assessment of thermoregulation in an older adult?
5. What would you teach older adults about hypothermia and its prevention?
6. What would you teach older adults about heat-related illnesses and their prevention?
7. Find appropriate health education materials on the Internet to use in teaching older adults about hypothermia and heat-related illnesses.

EDUCATIONAL RESOURCES

Administration on Aging
One Massachusetts Ave., Washington, DC 20201
(202) 619-0724
http://www.aoa.dhhs.gov/

American Academy of Family Physicians
11400 Tomahawk Parkway, Leawood, KS 66211
(800) 274-2237
http://www.aafp.org

Canadian Safety Council
http://www.safety-council.org/

National Institute on Aging (NIA)
Age Pages NIA Information Center
P.O. Box 8057, Gaithersburg, MD 20898-8057
(800) 222-2225
http://www.nia.nih.gov/health

REFERENCES

Carpenito, L. J. (2002). *Nursing diagnosis: Application to clinical practice* (9th ed.). Philadelphia: Lippincott Williams & Wilkins.

Hanania, N. A., & Zimmerman, J. L. (1999). Accidental hypothermia. *Critical Care Clinics, 15,* 235–249.

Hirsch, C. H. (1998). Hypothermia and hyperthermia. In E. Duthie (Ed.), *Practice of geriatrics* (3rd ed., pp. 244–255). Philadelphia: WB Saunders.

Hofland, S. L., & Mort, J. (1994). Infections in long-term care facilities: Issues for practice. *Geriatric Nursing, 15,* 260–264.

Holtzclaw, B. J. (2001). Risk for altered body temperature. In M. L. Maas, K. C. Buckwalter, M. D. Hardy, T. Tripp-Reimer, M. G. Titler, & J. P. Specht (Eds.), *Nursing care of older adults: Diagnoses, outcomes, and interventions* (pp. 201–216). St. Louis: Mosby.

Macey, S. M., & Schneider, D. F. (1993). Deaths from excessive heat and excessive cold among the elderly. *Gerontologist, 33,* 497–500.

Pals, J. K., Weinberg, A. D., Beal, L. F., Levesque, P. G., Cunningham, T. J., & Minaker, K. L. (1995). Clinical triggers for detection of fever and dehydration: Implications for long-term care nursing. *Journal of Gerontological Nursing, 21*(4), 13–19.

Prentice, D., & Moreland, J. (1999). A comparison of infrared ear thermometry with electronic predictive thermometry in a geriatric setting. *Geriatric Nursing, 20,* 314–317.

Smitz, S., Giagoultsis, T., Dewé, W., & Albert, A. (2000). Comparison of rectal and infrared ear temperatures in older hospital inpatients. *Journal of the American Geriatrics Society, 48,* 63–66.

Taylor, N. A. S., Allsopp, N. K., & Parkes, D. G. (1995). Preferred room temperature of young vs. aged males: The influence of thermal sensation, thermal comfort, and affect. *Journal of Gerontology: Medical Sciences, 50A,* M216–M221.

Young, J. B. (2001). Effects of aging on the sympathoadrenal system. (2001). In E. J. Masoro & S. N. Austad (Eds.), *Handbook of the biology of aging* (5th ed., pp. 269–296). San Diego: Academic Press.

Sexual Function

LEARNING OBJECTIVES

1. List age-related changes that affect sexual function in men and women.

2. Examine the risk factors that influence older adults' interest in, opportunities for, and performance of sexual activities.

3. Discuss the functional consequences of age-related changes and risk factors that affect reproduction, interest in sexual activity, and response to sexual stimulation.

4. Explain the reasons for, and the components of, an assessment of nurses' attitudes about sexual function in older adults.

5. Define the goals of assessment of sexual function in older adults.

6. Describe guidelines for interviewing older adults about sexual function.

7. Identify appropriate nursing interventions to address risk factors that influence sexual function in older adults.

Because sexual function in older adults encompasses many physiologic and psychosocial aspects of sexuality and intimate relationships, this chapter's perspective is broad. Although sexual function is not a dominant focus of gerontological nursing care in most situations, it is a very important component of quality of life for many older adults. Thus, in situations in which quality of life is a focus of care (especially long-term care settings), nurses need to be prepared to assess sexual function and provide health education interventions related to concerns about sexual function.

 ## AGE-RELATED CHANGES THAT AFFECT SEXUAL FUNCTION

A loss of reproductive ability at the onset of menopause in women is the age-related change in sexual function that is most easily delineated. Erectile dysfunction in older men, often addressed as an age-related change, is more strongly associated with risk factors than with age-related changes and is discussed in the risk factors and pathologic conditions sections. Other more subtle age-related changes in sexual function include diminished reproductive abilities in older men and alterations in both male and female responses to sexual stimulation. In the absence of risk factors, these changes have little impact because older adults generally do not desire high levels of reproductive ability and can readily compensate for any altered physiologic response to sexual stimulation. In the presence of risk factors, however, the sexual function of older adults may be severely compromised. This is because the risk factors, not the age-related changes, are the strongest determinants of sexual function in older adults.

Changes Affecting Female Reproductive Function

Female reproductive function is governed by hormonally regulated cycles, called menses. With the onset of menses during adolescence, the cyclic release of ova marks the beginning of female reproductive abilities. Reproductive abilities decline around the fifth decade, when the frequency of ovulation diminishes and the menstrual cycle becomes shorter and more irregular. Menopause (the cessation of menses), which typically occurs at about 49 to 51 years of age, is a clear indicator that reproduction is no longer possible.

In addition to affecting reproductive ability, menopause influences other aspects of sexual function, predominantly because of the accompanying decline in endogenous estrogen levels. Before menopause, the primary source of estrogen is the production of estradiol by the ovaries. After menopause, the primary source of estrogen is the conversion of androstenedione to estrone in skin and fat tissue. Endogenous estrogen levels decline in all postmenopausal women, but the extent and manifestations of estrogen deficiency vary.

Factors that may influence postmenopausal levels of endogenous estrogen include the interval since the onset of menopause; the production of hormones by the adrenal cortex; changes in the clearance rates of androgens and estrogens; and body weight, with higher body fat being positively correlated with higher levels of estrogen.

Diminished estrogen levels cause the following changes, which may affect sexual function:

- The cervix, uterus, and fallopian tubes atrophy.
- The vaginal wall and mucosa become thinner.
- The length and width of the vagina are reduced.
- Bartholin's glands atrophy and secrete less fluid.
- The amount of vaginal lubrication during periods of sexual excitement is diminished.
- The labia lose their fullness owing to diminished subcutaneous fat.
- The amount of pubic hair diminishes.

Decreased estrogen levels also affect the breasts of older women, causing a gradual replacement of mammary gland tissue with fat tissue. In addition to this estrogen-related effect on the breasts, age-related connective tissue changes cause the breasts of older women to become less firm and more pendulous.

Changes Affecting Male Reproductive Function

Male reproductive function depends on the secretion of hormones, the production and release of sperm, and the motility of sperm through the penile urethra. Luteinizing hormone and follicle-stimulating hormone are the two gonadotropins that regulate the production of testosterone and sperm in men. For many decades, researchers and gerontologists have debated the extent to which diminished testosterone in older men is due to age-related changes or risk factors. Recent research reviews conclude that when risk factors, such as medications and pathologic conditions, are controlled for, serum levels of testosterone decrease at a rate of 1% to 2% per year beginning around the age of 30 years (Anderson et al., 2002). Currently, researchers agree that diminished testosterone levels—which occur in about 20% of men older than 60 years and 50% of men older than 80 years—are caused by a combination of age-related changes and risk factors (Anderson et al., 2002; Matsumoto, 2002; Vermeulen, 2001).

The testes, paired oval-shaped organs in the scrotal sac, contain hundreds of seminiferous tubules in which sperm is produced and testosterone is secreted. The seminiferous tubules undergo the following age-related changes: increased fibrosis; thinning of the epithelium; thickening of the basement membrane;

and narrowing of the lumen, eventually to the point of obliteration of some of the tubules. Beginning in the sixth decade, the number of viable sperm gradually diminishes, but questions have been raised about the degree to which this is caused by age-related changes or risk factors, such as pathologic conditions. Gerontologists also raised questions about the universality and extent of this decline in viable sperm because some men never lose their reproductive abilities.

The seminal vesicles, prostate gland, and Cowper's (or bulbourethral) glands are accessory structures that produce semen, a mixture of sperm cells and secretions whose primary function is to nourish and transport sperm and facilitate reproductive functions. The following degenerative changes affect the seminal vesicles: the mucosa becomes smoother, the epithelium becomes thinner, connective tissue replaces the muscle tissue, and the fluid-retaining capacity is reduced. The degenerative changes that affect the prostate gland include diminished secretions, atrophy of the gland cells, the formation of hard masses around the prostatic urethra, replacement of muscle tissue by connective tissue, and a change in the shape of epithelial cells from columnar to cuboidal and irregular. Age-related changes in Cowper's glands have not been documented.

Beginning around the fourth decade, the penis also undergoes age-related changes, but these degenerative changes do not affect reproductive function. These changes may, however, affect sexual pleasure and contribute to erectile dysfunction (discussed in the section on Functional Consequences). The primary age-related penile changes are venous and arterial sclerosis and fibroelastosis of the corpus spongiosum. The weight and volume of the testes may decrease, but this is associated with pathological conditions rather than age-related changes.

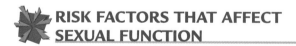

RISK FACTORS THAT AFFECT SEXUAL FUNCTION

Attitudes and Stereotypes of Older Adults

Personal attitudes about sexuality, which are shaped in part by societal influences, can affect sexual behaviors and enjoyment of sexual activity. Thus, it is important to consider the societal context and historical perspective of attitudes about aging and sexuality. As long ago as the Middle Ages, Western cultural beliefs "have held that sexual drive disappears with old age, that sex is perverse in old age, and that those elderly who attempt it practice self-deception. In addition, traditional concepts related to sexuality, such as beauty,

attractiveness, sexual potency, and female orgasm, did not refer to elderly people, but excluded them" (Covey, 1989, p. 93). In the early 20th century, strict Victorian standards of morality in Europe and North America strongly influenced the attitudes and behaviors of people who currently are older adults. According to Victorian standards, masturbation, homosexual activity, public displays of affection, and sex with anyone except a marital partner were totally taboo. Moreover, masturbation was considered to be more detrimental than sex outside of marriage, as evidenced by the Victorian norm of tolerating prostitution for the purpose of obviating the need for men to practice masturbation (Brecher, 1984). Currently, people in Western societies associate sexual attractiveness with physical attractiveness in very gender-specific and stereotypic ways. For example, male sexuality is associated with the image of a tanned, muscular, and youthful man, whereas female sexuality is associated with the image of a thin, but adequately endowed, young woman. Because these images contrast sharply with typical portrayals of older adults as physically unattractive, they foster a stereotype of "sexless seniors."

A serious negative consequence of these many societal influences is the false perception that older adults are no longer interested in, or capable of engaging in, sexual activity. This can become a self-fulfilling prophecy if older adults believe this stereotype. If older adults do not believe these stereotypes and societal perceptions, they may be embarrassed to acknowledge their sexual desires and activities for fear of being ridiculed or considered abnormal.

Attitudes and Stereotypes of Families and Caregivers

Adult children of older people often find it difficult to deal with the sexuality of their parents because they are influenced by the common stereotype that older adults are asexual. In addition, children of older adults who are widowed may discourage intimate relationships because of concern about their inheritance (Cooney & Dunne, 2001). If the adult child can successfully deny the existence of his or her older parent's sexual needs, then the possibility of threatening relationships also can be ignored.

In institutional settings, attitudes of staff can significantly affect the way in which residents express or repress their sexual needs. Researchers have consistently found that nursing home staff hold negative or patronizing attitudes about sexual expression among older adults and that these attitudes are based largely on insufficient knowledge about sexuality and aging (Walker & Harrington, 2002). Although staff in nursing homes are gradually becoming more accepting and permissive in their attitudes about sexual expressions, and their attitudes may in fact be more positive and tolerant than those of the residents and spouses of the residents (Gibson et al., 1999), most often, caregivers ignore the sexual needs of dependent older adults, and when they acknowledge sexual needs, it is usually because they judge the sexual behaviors as inappropriate.

The sexual needs of residents usually are ignored by staff members unless a resident is discovered engaging in a sexual activity. If staff members do acknowledge sexual activities, they often judge these activities as inappropriate and may punish the sexually active resident. Typically, the only expression of sexual needs by residents of long-term facilities that is considered appropriate and socially acceptable is a private, medically approved visit by a spouse. Any sexual activities in which a solitary resident or two unmarried people engage usually are not tolerated, even if done in private. When the staff of long-term care facilities become aware of sexual activities that are not considered to be acceptable, family members often are asked to intervene, even when the resident is a competent adult. Decisions regarding sexual activity, even between spouses, usually are dealt with as strictly medical matters. In addition to the prerequisite of medical approval for sexual activity, the permission of family members often is sought as part of the staff decision to allow or tolerate sexual activity.

Social Circumstances

Sexual activity at any age is influenced by such social circumstances as the response and availability of an acceptable and desirable partner. For older adults, particularly older women, social circumstances often are the strongest determinants of sexual activity because the level of sexual activity for older women is directly related to their marital status, whereas the level of sexual activity for older men is not as closely associated with marital status. Men at all ages report a higher frequency of extramarital sexual relationships, and older widowers have the advantage of a higher likelihood of remarriage in comparison with older widows. Statistics on the ratio of women to men provide one logical explanation for the gender differences in availability of sexual partners. With increasing age, the ratio of men to women gradually changes, from a ratio of 82 men per 100 women in the age group of 65 to 74 years to a ratio of 41 men per 100 women in the age

group of 85 years and older (Hetzel & Smith, 2001). The frequency and enjoyment of sexual activities during older adulthood is strongly associated with the importance assigned to sexual activity in the past. As a group, never-married women have the lowest rate of sexual activity compared with other categories of older adults. Although women of all ages are less sexually active than men in their cohort, the difference in their levels of sexual activity widens with increasing age.

Homosexuality is another social circumstance that significantly influences one's sexual activity and relationships because prejudiced attitudes toward lesbians and gay men can seriously interfere with their freedom to cultivate and express satisfying sexual relationships. This may be particularly problematic for lesbians and gay men who live in institutional settings because nursing home staff are likely to be intolerant or condemning of homosexuality among residents (Cahill, 2002). Because lesbians and gay men have become increasingly visible and more accepted in American society only recently, older adults who have experienced decades of feeling stigmatized may find it particularly difficult to meet partners and enjoy satisfying sexual activities and relationships. Despite their experience of long-term prejudice, however, older lesbians and gay men report levels of emotional well-being similar to those of older heterosexual people. Similarly, the social support they receive is comparable to that of heterosexual people, but the sources of support differ in that older lesbians and gay men are likely to receive assistance from friends, selected relatives, and current or former lovers (Cooney & Dunne, 2001).

Constraints in Long-Term Care Settings

Privacy is generally considered a requisite for sexual activity, and adults who live in their own homes are usually able to arrange for this. However, older adults who live in institutions, group settings, or family homes may find it difficult or impossible to arrange for privacy, especially if their sexual needs are ignored or considered abnormal by their caregivers or those with whom they live. Although privacy is a basic right of nursing home residents, "privacy in nursing homes is virtually nonexistent" because of physical environments and staff attitudes (Bauer, 1999, p. 40). Even if privacy is provided in institutional settings, additional environmental constraints include the inability to lock doors and ensure total privacy and the unavailability of anything larger than a single bed. Confidentiality of information is another constraint in nursing homes because sharing information about day-to-day activities of residents "is accepted and taken for granted as part of the caregiving role" and nursing home staff frequently share intimate information about residents lives (Bauer, 1999, p. 39).

Adverse Effects of Medications, Alcohol, and Nicotine

Before the 1980s, the role of medication as a cause of disorders of sexual function was largely ignored, but in recent years, adverse medication effects have received increased attention, primarily because of sexual dysfunction in younger men due to antidepressants and cardiovascular medications. This problem was first brought to the public's attention in 1983 in a *New York Times* article that cited medications as the single largest cause of erectile dysfunction in men and listed more than 50 medications with potentially adverse sexual effects (Brody, 1983). Brody cited a study that had been published in the *Journal of the American Medical Association* (Slag et al., 1983) of 1180 male patients in a medical clinic. Thirty-four percent of these subjects were impotent, and 25% of the 188 subjects who subsequently underwent further evaluation were found to have medication-induced erectile dysfunction.

Research on medication-related sexual dysfunction has grown because of the increased attention to adverse medication effects that affect quality of life. Until recently, most scientific literature on medication-induced sexual dysfunction focused on men, particularly middle-aged or younger men. The lack of attention to medication-induced sexual dysfunction in women and older adults is not the result of an absence of such problems in these groups. Rather, it is because investigators usually select younger men as their subjects because of cultural biases and the relative ease with which male sexual response is measured compared with female sexual response. Although researchers are only beginning to address adverse medication effects on sexual function in women, it is likely that such medications as antidepressants, antipsychotics, and spironolactone can cause female sexual dysfunction (Giraldi & Victor, 2002).

Medications adversely affect sexual function through a variety of mechanisms, including their influence on the release of hormones and their actions on the autonomic and central nervous systems. For example, with the exception of trazodone and bupropion, all antidepressants are likely to cause erectile dysfunction (Thomas et al., 2003). Specific adverse medication effects that interfere with sexual function in men include a decreased or absent libido; difficulty obtaining or maintaining an erection; dry, premature, or retrograde ejaculation; and inability to achieve orgasm. A less common adverse medication effect is priapism, an erection that persists beyond or is unrelated to sexual stimulation, which can lead to permanent erectile dysfunction (Berger, 2001). Medications that can cause this condition include antipsychotics, antidepressants, anticoagulants, antihypertensives, and medications used for the treatment of erectile dysfunction (Thomas et al., 2003). Women may experience the following medication-induced limitations in sexual function: diminished vaginal lubrication, decreased or absent libido, and inability to achieve orgasm. Display 22-1 lists some of the medications that are commonly associated with sexual dysfunction. These effects usually disappear when the medication is discontinued; occasionally, the effects will disappear with a mere decrease in the dose.

DISPLAY 22-1
Medications That Can Interfere With Sexual Function

Antihypertensives and Cardiovascular Agents
α-Adrenergic blockers
β-blockers
Calcium channel blockers
Digoxin
Hydralazine
Spironolactone
Thiazide diuretics
Cyclic antidepressants
Lithium
Monoamine oxidase inhibitors (MAOIs)
Selective serotonin reuptake inhibitors (SSRIs)

Agents That Act on the Central Nervous System
Benzodiazepines
Phenothiazines
Antihistamines
Chlorpheniramine
Diphenhydramine

Antiparkinson Agents
Benztropine
Trihexyphenidyl

Gastrointestinal Agents
Anticholinergics
Histamine H_2 antagonists (e.g., cimetidine)

Miscellaneous Medications
Alcohol
Allopurinol
Colchicine
Cytotoxic agents

Because alcohol is a central nervous system depressant, it can interfere with sexual function. In men, chronic alcohol use affects testosterone and gonadotropin production and can cause impotence and reduced libido (Nudell et al., 2002). Although in social settings, alcohol can decrease inhibitions and heighten sensual and sexual interest, in excessive amounts, the central nervous system depressant effect of alcohol usually counteracts any beneficial effects and interferes with sexual performance. Moderate amounts of alcohol normally do not interfere with sexual performance; however, in combination with other risk factors, such as medications or pathologic conditions, even small amounts of alcohol may be detrimental to the sexual performance of older adults.

Researchers first reported that cigarette smoking was a risk factor for erectile dysfunction in the mid-1980s (Virag et al., 1985), and in recent years, researchers have identified cigarette smoking as both an independent risk factor and a factor that exacerbates the risk associated with medications and pathologic conditions (Lewis, 2001; Nudell et al., 2002; Solomon et al., 2003). Nicotine has a detrimental effect on sexual function because it interferes with circulation to the sexual organs and accentuates the effects of other risk factors, such as hypertension and vascular disease. Recently, the importance of smoking cessation as an intervention to improve sexual function has been emphasized.

Functional Impairments and Pathologic Conditions

Functional impairments and pathologic conditions can interfere with sexual functioning by interfering with enjoyment of sexual activity. For example, people with chronic obstructive pulmonary disease may experience hypoxia and severe shortness of breath in response to the high physiologic demands of sexual activity. Similarly, people with arthritis or other musculoskeletal disorders may be reluctant to engage in sexual activity because of pain, stiffness, muscle spasms, and limited flexibility (Nusbaum et al., 2003). Some functional impairments, such as urinary incontinence or the effects of strokes, can interfere with satisfying sexual relationships in people of any age, but are more likely to affect older adults and interact with other risk factors.

Functional impairments may indirectly affect sexual function because of cultural biases that lead to the conclusion that disabled people are asexual. This perception, along with other effects of disabilities on self-image, may have a negative impact on sexual function. This may be more problematic for men because society tends to associate male sexual

performance with physical vigor. Although these effects are not unique to older adults, functional limitations increase with advancing age and are likely to combine with other risk factors to interfere with sexual function. Because sensory stimulation is an important part of sexual pleasure and intimate communication, sensory impairments can interfere with sexual pleasure. An older adult whose hearing ability is seriously impaired may find it difficult or impossible to carry on the intimate conversations that are often a part of sexual stimulation with a partner. Hearing impairments may also interfere with professional efforts to assess and counsel the older adult on this sensitive topic. Likewise, impairments affecting vision, smell, or touch can interfere with some of the usual sensual stimulation associated with sexual activities.

In recent years, gerontologists and clinicians have focused attention on sexual function and intimate relationships in people with dementia. Although the majority of people with dementia are indifferent about sex by the later stages of the disease, issues related to sexual function and intimate relationships commonly need to be addressed during early and middle stages (Kuhn, 2002; Mace & Rabins, 1999). Loss of sexual desire is the most common effect of dementia on sexual function, but some people with dementia develop hypersexuality and demand frequent sexual intercourse, especially men and especially during the middle stages. Hypersexuality in people with dementia may be caused by neuropathologic changes, particularly those that affect the temporal and frontal lobes of the brain (Robinson, 2003). Between 7% and 17% of nursing home residents with dementia exhibit behaviors that are considered sexually inappropriate; however, some of these behaviors, such as removing clothing or getting into bed with someone, are caused by cognitive impairments rather than sexual impulses (Velez & Peggs, 2001).

The negative impact of certain chronic illnesses on erectile dysfunction has been well documented. Specifically, the pathologic conditions that most often cause erectile dysfunction in older men include vascular, neurologic, and endocrine disorders. The conditions most commonly associated with sexual dysfunction are diabetes mellitus and ischemic heart disease. Because nurses care for many older adults with these conditions, the effects of each of these conditions on the sexual function of older adults are discussed in detail below. Other pathologic conditions that may cause erectile dysfunction include hypertension, hyperlipidemia, atherosclerosis, hormonal insufficiencies, and injury from trauma, irradiation, or surgery (e.g., prostate surgery).

Diabetes mellitus is a common cause of penile neuropathy in diabetic men at any age and has been identified as the chronic disease most strongly associated with erectile dysfunction (Bacon et al., 2002; Lewis, 2001; Solomon et al., 2003). Prevalence rates of erectile dysfunction in men with diabetes range from 35% to 75% (Sasaki et al., 2003); Bacon and colleagues (2002) found that the prevalence of erectile dysfunction in men with and without diabetes was 46% and 24%, respectively. Increased rates are strongly associated with older age, longer duration of diabetes, and the presence of concurrent conditions such as heart disease or hypertension. Erectile dysfunction may be an early manifestation of uncontrolled diabetes, and the degree of sexual dysfunction may vary in accordance with the degree of diabetic control. The ability to ejaculate is not lost, but it may be retrograde. Libido and orgasm are not affected to the same degree that erection is. Although very little research has been done on the sexual function of diabetic women, one research review concluded that the prevalence of sexual problems in diabetic women was similar to that of men with diabetes (Buvat, 2001). The most common sexual dysfunction in women with diabetes is delayed and greatly diminished vaginal lubrication.

Cardiovascular disease is associated with many aspects of sexual dysfunction, including decreased libido, impaired performance and pleasure, and decreased frequency of sexual activities. For example, people who have had myocardial infarctions may avoid sexual activities, even when no physiologic basis exists for abstaining from sexual intercourse with a regular partner. Researchers generally agree that sexual activity with a marital partner can be resumed when the affected person can perform moderate exercise—such as climbing two flights of steps—without experiencing harmful cardiac effects (Nusbaum et al., 2003). The risk that sexual activity will trigger a heart attack, even in people with cardiovascular disease, is very small and can be reduced with regular exercise (Bernardo, 2001). Thus, a major barrier to sexual function following a heart attack is the influence of psychological factors, such as fatigue, depression, partner's decision, lack of information, fears and anxiety, and diminished sexual desire. Cardiovascular disease is a risk factor for erectile dysfunction because atherosclerosis is the most significant cause of penile arterial insufficiency (Milbank & Goldfarb, 2003). In addition, people with hypertension and other cardiovascular disease commonly take medications that affect sexual function (see Display 22-1).

Factors That Affect the Level of Sexual Activity of Older Adults

Researchers have tried to identify factors that affect the level of sexual activity of older adults and have identified relative influences that differ for men and women. For older men, a decline in sexual activity is primarily related to dissatisfaction with their health and to factors that contribute to erectile dysfunction such as medications and medical conditions (Avis, 2000; Beutel, 2002). For older women, however, health is a less important factor: the most important variable is having a functioning and sexually interested partner (Avis, 2000; Weismiller, 2002). A study of married men between the ages of 50 and 80 years found that declines in sexual activity were most closely related to the wife's desire for intercourse and the man's ability to maintain an erection (Mazur, 2002). Factors that interfere with sexual activity for nursing home residents include having poor health, feeling unattractive, lacking privacy, and not having a partner (Lichtenberg, 1997).

PATHOLOGIC CONDITIONS ASSOCIATED WITH SEXUAL FUNCTION IN OLDER ADULTS

Because of age-related changes and risk factors, older adults are more susceptible to gender-specific pathologic conditions associated with sexual function. Prostatic hyperplasia is a pathologic condition that affects 50% of 50-year-old men and 90% of 90-year-old men that is caused, at least in part, by age-related hormonal changes. This condition is a common cause of urinary incontinence, which can interfere with enjoyment of sexual activities. Another condition that commonly affects older men is diminished frequency and rigidity of nocturnal penile tumescence, which is a reflex erection that occurs during sleep. A condition that commonly affects sexual function in older women is increased susceptibility to urethritis and vaginitis because of the thinning of the vaginal tissue and the decreased acidity and quantity of vaginal secretions. After intercourse, older women may experience urinary urgency and burning that persists for several days. Fibroid cysts also are more likely to develop in older women than in younger women.

Since the 1990s, knowledge about erectile dysfunction has been growing at a rapid pace, and much of the information that was thought to be accurate has been disproved. For example, erectile dysfunction is no longer viewed as an inevitable consequence of aging, and physiologic, rather than psychological, factors are recognized as the most common cause. In the early 1990s, the National Institutes of Health proposed that the term "impotence" be replaced by "erectile dysfunction," defined as the inability to achieve or maintain an erection sufficient for satisfactory sexual function (National Institutes of Health, 1992). More than half of men over the age of 40 years have some degree of erectile dysfunction, and the incidence rate doubles during each decade after 40 years of age (Johannes et al., 2000). Erectile dysfunction is strongly associated with increasing age, but it is caused by risk factors that occur more commonly in older men rather than by age-related changes alone. It is currently viewed as a complex disease that is associated with several interacting factors, the most common physiologic causes being adverse medication effects and pathologic conditions, as discussed in the section on risk factors (Heaton & Morales, 2003). Although the primary cause of erectile dysfunction most often is physiologic, psychological factors such as anxiety, depression, self-esteem, relationship issues, fear of failure, and childhood sexual trauma need to be considered as factors that contribute to or are consequences of erectile dysfunction in almost all situations (Chun & Carson, 2001; Rosen, 2001). As Masters and Johnson reported many decades ago, "Fears [of failure to perform] were expressed, under interrogation, by every male subject beyond forty years of age, irrespective of reported levels of formal education" (1966, p. 202). They concluded that "the fallacy that secondary impotence is to be expected as the male ages is probably more firmly entrenched in our culture than any other misapprehension" (1966, p. 202). Much progress has been made in understanding and addressing erectile dysfunction since the Masters and Johnson reports, but researchers estimate that more than 70% of men with erectile dysfunction are not diagnosed because of reluctance to discuss it with health care professionals (Chun & Carson, 2001). The recent trend in promoting medications for treatment of erectile dysfunction is likely to prompt more men and health care practitioners to discuss this topic and identify causes and treatments.

In recent years, health care practitioners and pharmaceutical companies have starting addressing female sexual dysfunction, similar to the way in which erectile dysfunction has been addressed since the early 1990s. Female sexual dysfunction is defined as a "multicausal and multidimensional medical problem that has biologic and psychosocial components. It is age related, progressive, and highly prevalent, affecting 30% to 50% of American women" (Berman & Goldstein, 2001, p. 405). This condition causes significant personal distress and negatively affects interpersonal relationships and quality of life (Munarriz et al., 2002). Any of the four phases of sexual function—libido, arousal, orgasm, and satisfaction—can be affected. Many of the same physiologic risk factors that are associated with erectile dysfunction also are associated with female sexual dysfunction: hypertension, hypercholesterolemia, cigarette smoking, pelvic surgeries, and adverse medication effects. In addition, diminished estrogen level in menopausal women who are not taking hormonal therapy is a major contributing factor. Urinary incontinence, disorders of the pelvic floor (cystocele, vaginal prolapse), and any type of pelvic surgery (e.g., hysterectomy or procedures for urinary incontinence) increase the risk for female sexual dysfunction (Pauls & Berman, 2002). Depression and a history of sexual trauma are two psychological factors that may cause female sexual dysfunction (Kaplan, 2002).

FUNCTIONAL CONSEQUENCES ASSOCIATED WITH SEXUAL FUNCTION IN OLDER ADULTS

Sexual function involves reproduction, response to sexual stimulation, and interest and participation in sexual activity. Whereas reproduction is directly affected by age-related changes, the other two aspects of sexual function are affected more directly by risk factors. In addition, andropause and menopause are considered in the context of functional consequences associated with sexual function in older adults.

The Impact of Sexual Function Changes on Reproductive Ability

Loss of reproductive ability is a functional consequence of menopause, caused by the cessation of ova production within 1 year of the last menstrual cycle. Another functional consequence affecting reproduction in women is the increased risk that a fetus will be defective if ova are fertilized during the premenopausal years. The reproductive ability of men, by contrast, gradually declines but does not cease completely.

The Impact of Sexual Function Changes on the Response to Sexual Stimulation

The Kinsey reports (1948, 1953) are recognized as landmark studies of human sexual behaviors, whereas the Masters and Johnson investigation

(1966) is recognized as the landmark study of human physiologic response to sexual stimulation. The Masters and Johnson study of 694 adults in a laboratory setting identified four phases of physiologic response to sexual stimulation in men and women. An analysis of data on older subjects led to the conclusion that the ability of older adults to respond to sexual stimulation is maintained, but their response is slower and less intense. Masters and Johnson also concluded that older adults who regularly engage in sexual activity experience fewer changes in their response to sexual stimulation than those who are sexually inactive. Any additional changes in an individual's response to sexual stimulation or ability to be sexually stimulated are thought to be associated with the many risk factors that commonly occur in older adults. Although older adults were greatly underrepresented in this study, the findings of Masters and Johnson have been widely accepted as the knowledge base about age-related changes in physiologic response to sexual stimulation. Normal male and female responses to sexual stimulation and the associated age-related changes are discussed in the following sections and summarized in Table 22-1.

Response of Women to Sexual Stimulation

During the initial excitement phase of sexual stimulation, the following physiologic changes occur in women: the breasts enlarge and the nipples become erect; the skin over the upper chest becomes flushed; voluntary muscles become tense; the heart rate and blood pressure increase; the labia and clitoris enlarge and become vasocongested; the vaginal barrel expands, distends, and becomes lubricated and vasocongested; and the uterus elevates slightly. Older women are likely to experience some changes in the intensity of these responses. For instance, the breasts enlarge to a smaller degree; the sexual flush is absent or less noticeable; the length and width of vaginal expansion are diminished; vaginal lubrication is decreased and takes longer to occur; the elevation of the uterus is delayed and less marked; and the labia are less vasocongested.

During phase two—the plateau phase—the following responses normally occur: the breasts enlarge to a greater degree, and the areola become engorged; the sexual flush spreads over the body and becomes more intense; the voluntary muscles become more tense; the rectal sphincter is voluntarily contracted; the blood pressure, heart rate, and respiratory rate increase; the clitoral shaft and glans withdraw; the vaginal barrel increases further in width and depth; the uterus elevates fully, and the cervix elevates; the labia become more vasocongested; and Bartholin's glands secrete mucoid material. Because of age-related changes, older women experience these responses to a lesser degree, as summarized in Table 22-1.

TABLE 22-1 • Age-Related Changes in Response to Sexual Stimulation

	Female Response	Male Response
Excitement Phase	Breasts not as fully engorged Sexual flush absent or diminished Delayed or diminished vaginal lubrication Decreased expansion of vaginal wall Decreased vasocongestion of labia	Longer time required to attain erection Less firm erection Longer maintenance of erection before ejaculation Increased difficulty regaining an erection if lost Reduced or absent scrotal and testicular vasocongestion
Plateau Phase	Decreased areolar engorgement Less intense sexual flush Less intense myotonia Decreased degree of deepening of labial color Decreased vasocongestion of labia Reduced Bartholin's gland secretions Slower/less marked uterine elevation	Diminished or absent nipple turgidity and sexual flush Less intense muscle tension Slower penile erectile response No color change in glans penis Delayed and diminished testicular elevation
Orgasmic Phase	Decreased frequency of rectal sphincter contractions Decreased number and intensity of orgasmic contractions	Decreased frequency of rectal sphincter contractions Diminution of ejaculatory expulsion force by about 50% Absent or diminished sense of ejaculatory inevitability Fewer and less intense ejaculatory contractions
Resolution Phase	Slower loss of nipple erection Quicker return to pre-excitement stage	Slower loss of nipple erection Longer refractory period Very rapid penile detumescence Very rapid testicular descent

The orgasmic phase of female sexual response is characterized by the following: sexual flush increases in intensity, parallel to the intensity of orgasm; muscle groups contract involuntarily; the rectal sphincter contracts involuntarily; pulse, blood pressure, and respirations increase further; the orgasmic platform contracts at intervals, with gradual lengthening of the intervals and weakening of the contractions; and the uterus contracts with an intensity parallel to that of the orgasm. As with other phases of sexual excitement, all the responses of the orgasmic phase are less intense in older women. In addition, the involuntary rectal sphincter contractions occur only with high tension levels, and the number of orgasmic contractions decreases by about 50%. Because postmenopausal women are no longer concerned about the reproductive consequences of sexual intercourse, however, their anxieties might be decreased, and their capacity for orgasm may actually be increased. Some women experience orgasm or multiple orgasms for the first time during their postmenopausal years.

The resolution phase involves a gradual return to the pre-excitement state, beginning with a loss of deep vasocongestion. The breasts return to their normal appearance, the sexual flush disappears, muscle tone returns to a normal state within 5 minutes, vital signs return to normal, and all pelvic organs resume their pre-excitement characteristics. With the exception of a slower loss of nipple erection, the resolution phase occurs more rapidly in older women.

Response of Men to Sexual Stimulation

During the excitement phase of sexual stimulation, men experience the following physiologic changes: nipples may become erect; voluntary muscles become more tense; heart rate and blood pressure increase; the penis becomes erect; the scrotal sac flattens and elevates; and the testes become partially elevated. The most noticeable age-related change in this phase is a delay in attaining erection because of the need for longer or more intense stimulation. In addition, the erection may be less firm, but it can be maintained longer before ejaculation. If the erection subsides before ejaculation, however, a refractory period occurs, and older men may have greater difficulty than younger men regaining a full erection. Scrotal and testicular vasocongestion is markedly reduced in older men, as is testicular elevation. In general, all responses of the excitement phase are less intense and are influenced more by arousal conditions than by autonomic nervous system responses.

During the plateau phase, men experience the following: the nipples become erect and turgid; the skin over the head and trunk becomes flushed; voluntary and involuntary muscle tone increases; the rectal sphincter is voluntarily contracted; the pulse, respirations, and blood pressure are increased; penile circumference increases at the coronal ridge; the testes elevate and enlarge by 50%; and Cowper's glands emit pre-ejaculatory fluid. Age-related changes in these responses include an absence of or great diminution in sexual flush, nipple erection, and muscle tension. Full penile erection often occurs later in this stage, just before ejaculation, and testicular elevation is delayed or diminished because of less intense vasocongestion.

The orgasmic phase is characterized by the following changes: the skin flush is well developed and parallels the intensity of excitement; there is a loss of voluntary control of muscles, and the rectal sphincter and some muscle groups involuntarily contract; heart rate, blood pressure, and respirations increase above normal; the penis contracts at intervals and with an expulsive force; and a sensation of ejaculatory inevitability is experienced and the ejaculatory process initiated. Masters and Johnson (1966) identified the following changes in the orgasmic phase in older men: ejaculation is less powerful; seminal fluid emerges under less pressure; penile contractions are fewer and less intense; rectal sphincter contractions occur less frequently; and intercontractile intervals lengthen rapidly after the second expulsive contraction. Older men also reported a decreased sense of ejaculatory inevitability.

During the resolution phase, the manifestations of sexual excitement gradually disappear, and all physiologic responses return to the pre-excitement state. A refractory period occurs, during which the man is unable to redevelop an erection that is accompanied by ejaculation. With the exception of a slower loss of nipple erection, if present, all other responses to sexual stimulation return to their pre-excitement state more rapidly in older men as compared with younger men. In older men, the refractory period may last for a day or two, but erection without ejaculation may be able to be achieved during this time.

The Impact of Sexual Function Changes on Quality of Life

Diminished estrogen levels that occur during menopause affect sexual function and many other aspects of functioning. One of the most noticeable effects of estrogen deficiency in menopausal women is the occurrence of hot flashes, described as "the sudden, transient sensation of heat spreading over the upper body, usually starting in the neck and face, then extending to the chest, back, and arms, the hot flash may also bring on flushing and sweating, and then a sensation of chilling" (Taylor, 2002, p. 559). They are commonly accompanied by nausea, anxiety, palpitation, air hunger, and head stuffiness or fullness. Additional functional consequences include embarrassment, discomfort, and interruptions in activities, including sexual activities. Hot flashes affect up to 85% of all menopausal women, with as many as 57% reporting persistent but less severe hot flashes for 10 years after their last menstrual period (Taylor, 2002). Factors that increase the intensity and frequency of hot flashes during menopause include obesity and cigarette smoking (Whiteman, 2003). For some women, hot flashes may occur frequently throughout the day and night and last for as long as half an hour. About 25% of women characterize their hot flashes and sweats as severe and disruptive of their quality of life (Taylor, 2002). Another effect of diminished estrogen is significantly diminished vaginal secretions, which can affect sexual intercourse unless compensatory interventions, such as using lubricant, are used.

Andropause is a term that is used to describe the age-related decline in testosterone in men that is analogous to the age-related decline in estrogen in women (Anderson et al., 2002; Matsumoto, 2002). Manifestations of andropause that affect sexual function and quality of life include fatigue, depression, and diminished sexual desire and erectile capacity (Matsumoto, 2002; Wespes, 2002). Researchers currently are investigating the use of testosterone therapy, as discussed in the section on Interventions.

The Impact of Sexual Function Changes on Sexual Interest and Activity

The first large-scale surveys of human sexual behavior, conducted by Kinsey and associates, were published in 1948 (*Sexual Behavior in the Human Male*) and 1953 (*Sexual Behavior in the Human Female*). These surveys of the sexual behaviors of more than 20,000 adults in the United States brought information about sexual behavior of older adults to public attention. The Kinsey report challenged many myths about sexual activity and generated further interest in and research on this previously taboo topic. Although fewer than 300 participants in the Kinsey report were aged 61 years or older, many of its conclusions about sexual activity of older adults have been confirmed by subsequent studies. For example, the Kinsey report's conclusions about the occurrence of a gradual decline in sexual activity were confirmed

by a 1978 to 1979 Consumers Union survey of more than 4000 people between the ages of 50 and 93 years (Brecher, 1984). Because 61% of the participants in the Kinsey report and 73% of those participating in the Consumers Union survey were born between 1905 and 1924 (Brecher, 1984), these two reports provide an overview of sexual interest and activity in people who currently are aged 80 years and older.

Since the 1980s, studies of sexuality and aging have included more older subjects and have focused on broader aspects of sexual function, such as affection, friendships, and intimacy. For older adults, these aspects of sexual function may become more important as the number of acceptable opportunities for direct sexual activities diminishes. For example, in one of the first studies addressing sexual behaviors other than intercourse and masturbation, Bretschneider and McCoy (1988) found that the most common sexual activities in a sample of 202 adults aged 80 to 102 years were touching and caressing without sexual intercourse. Similarly, Johnson (1996) found that older adults (mean age, 66 years) reported that the sexual activities of kissing, hugging, and hearing loving words were more important than masturbation, oral sex, or sexual conversation. In this study, older women ascribed greater importance to sexual activities of sitting and talking, making oneself more attractive, and saying loving words than did men. By contrast, older men reported greater interest in sexual activities, such as erotic movies and readings, sexual daydreams, and physically intimate activities. Studies of nursing home residents suggest that it would be more appropriate to view intimacy and sexual function as a continuum, ranging from social intimacy to sexual-physical intimacy (Lichtenberg, 1997). In light of these findings, conclusions drawn from studies considering only the frequency of masturbation or sexual intercourse as indicators of sexual activity may be quite limited in their applicability to older adults because other expressions of physical intimacy (e.g., hugging, kissing, and holding hands) may be more meaningful.

Although the frequency of sexual activity gradually declines with increasing age, the level of sexual interest and the sexual competence of older adults do not necessarily decline. Sexual interest, attitudes, activity, and satisfaction are a continuation of lifelong patterns, and they remain stable in older adulthood unless risk factors interfere with sexual function. Risk factors that commonly affect sexual interest and activity in older adults include social circumstances, pathologic conditions, adverse medication effects, and influences of family and caregivers. The social circumstances that most frequently lead to decreased sexual activity are spousal death or illness and lack of an available partner. The sexual needs and interest of older adults, including residents of long-term care facilities, do not necessarily decrease, but their opportunities for sexual activity are often limited.

In summary, older adults do not lose their interest in or capacity for sexual activity because of age-related changes, but risk factors such as misinformation, social circumstances, pathologic conditions,

environmental constraints, and adverse medication effects do commonly interfere with sexual function. Because of age-related changes, however, the response of older men and women to sexual stimulation is slower, less intense, and of shorter duration. As one 79-year-old man confided to this author, "It's like sparklers, not fireworks." Figure 22-1 illustrates the age-related changes, risk factors, and negative functional consequences that affect sexual function.

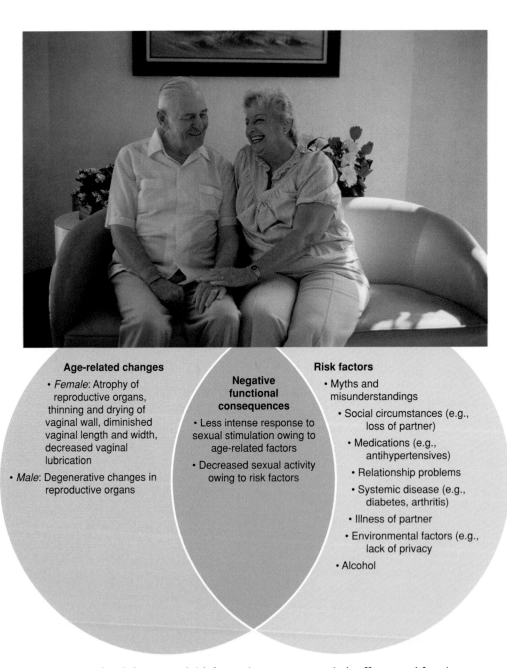

FIGURE 22-1 Age-related changes and risk factors intersect to negatively affect sexual function in older adults.

➤ You are the "wellness nurse" at the senior center where Mr. and Mrs. S. come for the meal program and socialization. Mr. S. is 73 years old and has hypertension and a history of a heart attack. He takes atenolol, 100 mg daily; hydrochlorothiazide, 25 mg daily; and digoxin, 0.125 mg daily. Mrs. S., who is 71 years old, describes herself as generally healthy, but with a history of depression and some arthritis. She takes ibuprofen, 400 mg four times daily, and sertraline, 50 mg daily. During your nursing clinics, Mr. S. and several other men have asked you about the new drug that is advertised on television for men who have trouble satisfying their partners. The senior center director also has noticed an increased interest in this topic and has asked that you plan a group health information session about "Sexuality and Aging."

THINKING POINTS

➤ Develop a teaching plan for discussing normal age-related changes in sexual function in older adults.

➤ What risk factors would you discuss in relation to sexuality and aging?

➤ What educational materials would you use?

➤ What teaching would you do about interventions?

NURSING ASSESSMENT OF SEXUAL FUNCTION

Sexual function is not necessarily included in every nursing assessment, but it should be included in any comprehensive assessment that addresses quality-of-life issues that affect the person's day-to-day function. It is, however, often neglected in an assessment of older adults. Thus, assessment of sexual function is especially important in home care and long-term care settings (e.g., nursing homes, group homes, and assisted-living facilities). Major reasons that sexual function is neglected in nursing assessments include the high degree of privacy associated with sexual function and the stereotype of the "sexless senior" that is prevalent in our society. In addition, gender or generational differences between the health professional and the older person may interfere with an assessment of sexual function. Although all of these factors may explain why sexual function in older adults is so often overlooked, they do not justify its exclusion. Rather, the potential detrimental consequences of ignoring the sexual needs of older adults and the relatively simple and effective educational interventions that can

be initiated to address them make assessment of the sexual function of older adults an essential component of gerontological nursing care.

Self-Assessment of Attitudes About Sexual Function in Older Adults

Because of the private nature of sexual function and its associated emotional responses and cultural factors, nurses are often uncomfortable discussing it. Additional discomfort occurs because many nurses do not learn about sexual function and assessment, especially regarding older adults, in their professional education. Thus, an assessment of personal attitudes about sexuality and aging is a prerequisite for the gerontological nurse addressing the sexual function of older adults. The goal of this self-assessment is to increase the nurse's level of comfort with, openness to, and sensitivity about issues of sexual function. Display 22-2 lists some of the questions nurses can use to examine their attitudes toward the sexual function of older adults. The self-assessment includes questions specific to attitudes of nursing staff in long-term care facilities because of the importance of addressing sexual function as a quality-of-life issue and because of the dominant role that nurses play in addressing this issue in long-term care facilities. Kuhn (2002) developed a self-assessment tool, called the Staff Attitudes About Intimacy and Dementia (SAID), that can be used by nursing home staff to identify personal attitudes about aging, intimacy, sexuality, and dementia.

Significant cultural differences between the nurse and the older adult may increase the difficulty of discussing sexual function. Culture Box 22-1 summarizes some cultural aspects of sexual function that may be applicable to nursing assessment. Nurses also may be uncomfortable discussing sexual function with older adults who are involved in same-sex or other nontraditional relationships. Thus, an important aspect of self-assessment is to identify attitudes toward nontraditional sexual activities because these attitudes can influence the assessment and care of people who do not conform to the nurse's expectations. When assessing sexual function of older gays and lesbians, it is important that nurses are nonjudgmental, have an awareness of gay and lesbian culture, and understand the importance of relationships for older lesbians and of sexual activity for older gay men (Pope, 1997). In addition, it is important to use gender-neutral pronouns when asking questions about significant relationships. For example, ask if the person has anyone who is a confidant or is very important, rather than asking if the person is married.

DISPLAY 22-2
Assessing Personal Attitudes Toward Sexuality and Aging

What do I believe about sexuality and aging?

- Do I believe that older people, especially unmarried ones, are no longer interested in or capable of sexual activities?
- Do I believe the subtle messages associating sexual activities with youth and attractiveness?
- Do I hold age-specific standards regarding sexual activity and romantic relationships? (For example, do I think it is okay for young adults to kiss or hold hands, but inappropriate or "cute" for older people to do this?)

What do I believe about the nurse's role with regard to the sexual function of older adults?

- Do I believe that sexual function is strictly a private matter that should not be addressed by health professionals?
- Do I view sexual function as an activity of daily living that should be included in a comprehensive assessment of long-term care needs of older adults?
- Do I feel more comfortable discussing sexual function with people who are of the same gender and age range as myself, but very uncomfortable in discussing this matter with people who are old enough to be my parents or grandparents?
- Do I avoid discussion of sexual function with older adults because I believe they are not interested in sexual activity or are uncomfortable discussing this topic?
- Do I avoid discussing sexual function with older adults who are not in traditional marital relationships?

- Do I hold different beliefs about the assessment of sexual function based on the age of the person? For example, do I think sexual function should be assessed in sexually active teenagers who are at risk for unwanted pregnancy, but not older people?

What is my attitude about various expressions of sexual activity?

- How do I view sexual activity and romantic relationships between unmarried people, or between people of the same gender?
- How do I view masturbation?
- Do my views about masturbation or sexual activity between unmarried or same-gender people influence my assessment of and interventions for people who engage in these activities?
- Am I tolerant and nonjudgmental toward people whose views and practices are nontraditional or different from mine?

For nurses in settings where long-term needs are addressed:

- How do I feel about the rights of residents to engage in sexual activity in private, either with themselves or people of their own choosing?
- Do I try to ensure privacy for those residents who desire it?
- If I am aware of the sexual activities of a resident, do I think that I should inform the administrator, a family member, or another "responsible adult"?

CULTURE BOX 22-1   **Cultural Aspects of Sexual Function**

Expressions of Sexuality and Intimacy

- In some cultures, direct eye contact, especially between a man and woman, is interpreted as an expression of intimacy.
- In some cultures, it is taboo for a man to be alone with a woman other than his wife.
- Touching another person (particularly of the opposite sex) is considered taboo in many cultures.
- In some cultures, heterosexual men and women commonly hold hands with another person of the same gender.
- Only a few cultures value sexual equality between men and women.
- Homosexuality is accepted in some cultures but is considered taboo or is kept secret among family members in others.

Assessment Considerations

- In some cultures, it is considered taboo for post-menopausal women to have their breasts or vagina examined, even by a health care provider.
- Menopausal manifestations may vary in different cultural groups (e.g., most Japanese women do not experience hot flashes).

Assessing Sexual Function in Older Adults

The goals of assessment of sexual function in older adults are (1) to provide an opportunity for the older adult to address any issues related to sexual function that are important or relevant; and (2) to identify risk factors, particularly attitudinal influences and lack of information, that interfere with the older person's sexual function and quality of life. Although the extent of the assessment will vary according to individual circumstances, it should include, at a minimum, questions about the gynecologic aspects of female sexual function and the genitourinary aspects of male sexual function. These questions are easily incorporated into a routine assessment of overall function. If these questions are followed by an open-ended question about sexual interest and activities, the nurse can then respond to the individual needs of the older adult. If problems or risk factors are identified, the nurse is not expected to conduct an in-depth assessment of all aspects of sexual function, but should obtain enough information to suggest appropriate resources for further evaluation. Display 22-3 summarizes guidelines for assessing sexual function in

DISPLAY 22-3
Guidelines for Assessing Sexual Function in Older Adults

Interview Atmosphere and Communication Techniques

- Ensure both privacy and comfort.
- Be nonjudgmental and matter-of-fact in verbal and nonverbal communication.
- If feasible, sit face-to-face in chairs, rather than conducting the interview while the person being interviewed is in bed.
- If feasible, allow the person being interviewed to wear usual daytime clothing, rather than a hospital gown.

Initiation and Discussion of the Topic

- Begin by acknowledging feelings of discomfort and by stating the reason for discussing this topic. (For example, "I know that sexuality is a private matter and people are often uncomfortable discussing this topic. However, as a nurse, I consider sexuality to be an aspect of health and well-being, and it may have a significant bearing on your overall care.")
- Include statements that address stereotypes and require a response from the older adult. (For example, "Our society tends to view old people as being uninterested in sex, but for most older people, this is not true. Many older people are less sexually active than when they were younger, but this is not because of age-related changes. Have you experienced any changes in your sexual activities in the past few years?")
- Initiate the topic near the end of a comprehensive assessment interview, and begin with questions about the physiologic aspects of male or female function, such as those that follow.

Interview Questions to Assess Male Sexual Function

- Have you ever had prostate problems or related surgery? Have you ever been told that you have or had an enlarged prostate?
- How often do you undergo a complete medical examination? When was your last complete physical?
- Do you ever experience dribbling of urine or have problems holding your water?
- Do you have any trouble initiating the stream of urine?
- After you have urinated (passed water), do you still feel like you haven't emptied your bladder completely?
- Do you have to get up during the night to empty your bladder? If so, how many times?
- Have you ever noticed any blood in your urine?
- Do you ever have any discharge from your penis?
- Do you have any sores, lumps, ulcers, irritations, or areas of inflammation on your penis or scrotum?
- Do you have any trouble with erection or ejaculation?

Interview Questions to Assess Female Sexual Function

- How many children, if any, have you had? How many pregnancies?
- At what ages did your menstrual periods begin and end?
- Have you ever had a Pap (Papanicolaou) test? When was your most recent Pap test and gynecologic examination?
- Have you ever had a mammogram? When was the most recent one?
- Have you ever been taught to examine your breasts for lumps?
- Do you examine your breasts for lumps? How often?
- Have you noticed any changes in your breasts? Do you ever have any discharge from your nipples?
- Do you have any burning, itching, or irritation in the vaginal area?
- Do you ever have any vaginal discharge or bleeding?
- Do you have any difficulties with sexual intercourse?

Principles for Assessing Sexual Interest and Activities

- If the older adult makes a clear statement that this topic is irrelevant, do not insist on further questions. If the older adult responds to questions, however, do not discontinue the interview because of your own discomfort.
- Do not assume that an assessment of sexual function is irrelevant to unmarried people.
- For both married and unmarried older adults, use open-ended questions to elicit information about intimate relationships (e.g., "Is there anything you would like to ask or discuss about intimate relationships?").
- For a married person, open-ended questions may be asked about the partner's influence on sexual activities (e.g., "Has your husband experienced any changes in his health that have affected your sexual activities?").
- Listen for statements that reflect myths, a negative self-image, or self-fulfilling prophecies, such as "Of course, I stopped being interested in sex after menopause," or "I can't have an erection because I have prostate trouble."
- If risk factors, such as certain medications or pathologic conditions, have been identified earlier in the interview, ask additional questions, such as "Have you had any difficulties with sexual activities since your heart attack?" or "Do you have any questions about the possible effects of diabetes on sexual activity?"
- Emphasize the clinical reason for the questions. ("Sometimes certain illnesses or medications interfere with sexual function, and we want to identify any problems you might be having in this area.")
- Use open-ended questions that allow for either closure of the topic or a further discussion of issues. ("Is there anything you would like to discuss with regard to your sexual relationships?")

older adults. The Hartford Institute for Geriatric Nursing recommends that nurses use the PLISSIT assessment model as a routine nursing assessment for older adults (Wallace, 2001). The four components of this model are as follows:

- Obtaining **P**ermission from the client to initiate sexual discussion
- Providing **L**imited **I**nformation about sexual function
- Giving **S**pecific **S**uggestions for the individual to proceed with sexual relations
- Providing **I**ntensive **T**herapy surrounding the issues of sexuality for the client

NURSING DIAGNOSIS

When the nursing assessment identifies risks that interfere with sexual function, or when older adults express an interest in discussing their sexual function, the appropriate nursing diagnosis is Ineffective Sexuality Patterns. This is defined as "the state in which an individual experiences or is at risk of experiencing a change in sexual behaviors or sexual health" (Carpenito, 2002, p. 852). Related factors commonly identified in older adults include medication effects (e.g., from antihypertensive medications); endocrine diseases (e.g., diabetes); cardiovascular diseases (e.g., congestive heart failure); genitourinary conditions (e.g., vaginitis, prostatitis, incontinence); functional impairments secondary to chronic conditions (e.g., limited range of motion as a result of arthritis); psychosocial circumstances (e.g., lack of a partner); and myths and misunderstandings about age-related changes. The case example at the end of this chapter addresses this nursing diagnosis.

OUTCOMES

Because problems with sexual function in older adults often are caused by lack of information about age-related changes and risk factors, providing accurate information about sexual function is the primary intervention, and increased knowledge about sexual functioning is an expected outcome. In nursing home settings, an appropriate outcome might be increased knowledge of staff about aging and sexuality. Additional nursing-sensitive outcomes most commonly identified for Ineffective Sexuality Patterns include control of menopausal symptoms, acceptance of aging body image, improved communication skills about sexual functioning, and improved ability to

obtain desired levels of sexual intimacy (Wright, 2001).

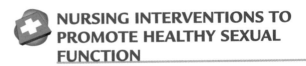

NURSING INTERVENTIONS TO PROMOTE HEALTHY SEXUAL FUNCTION

Role of the Nurse in Education About Sexual Function

The role of the nurse in educating older people about sexual function differs from that of a primary health care provider or sex therapist because the nurse is not expected to provide direct interventions (other than educational interventions) or sex counseling. Major goals of nursing interventions are to change attitudes of caregivers and older adults by providing information and to facilitate appropriate referrals for further evaluation and treatment of identified problems. Gerontological nurses are not expected to know all the answers about sexual function, but they are expected to provide accurate information about normal sexual function, age-related changes, risk factors that cause or contribute to problems with sexual function, and resources for dealing with identified problems and risk factors.

Providing Health Education About Sexual Function

Older adults, as well as their caregivers, may need to be educated about age-related changes that affect sexual function. This is not always easily accomplished, however, because of the perception that this topic is strictly private. Therefore, excellent communication skills are required for providing health education about sexual function in older adults. A survey of older adults found that they prefer that health care professionals use open, respectful, nonjudgmental, and plain English communication when discussing sexuality (Johnson, 1997). Group sex education programs for older adults can be effective in achieving positive attitudinal changes and improving knowledge, confidence, and sensitivity of participants (Wiley & Bortz, 1996). Tunstull and Henry (1996) describe a nursing model of a group education program, called the Intimacy Group, that can be used for nursing home residents.

Written materials are helpful in providing a basis for education and discussion. Many excellent resources that can be used by professionals and lay people alike are available in bookstores and on the Internet. Display 22-4 is a sample of a teaching tool that is written in nontechnical terms so that it can be used for older adults and caregivers as a basis of

Health Education About Sexual Activity for Older People

- Older people remain fully capable of enjoying orgasm, but their response to sexual stimulation usually is slower, less intense, and of shorter duration. Increasing the amount and diversity of sexual stimulation and experimenting with different positions can compensate for these changes and increase sexual enjoyment.
- The "use it or lose it" principle applies to sexual activity.
- Sexual problems in older people occur for the same reasons they occur in younger people. That is, they may be related to illness or disability, medications or alcohol, or psychological and relationship factors. The only cause of sexual problems that is unique to older people is the self-fulfilling prophecy of the "sexless senior" stereotype.
- The following habits enhance sexual enjoyment: exercising regularly, avoiding or limiting consumption of alcohol, maintaining optimal health and nutrition, using hearing aids and corrective lenses as needed, and engaging in sexual activities when you are relaxed and your energy level is at its peak.
- If you experience problems with sexual function, seek advice from a professional who is skilled in working with older people. Medical help can be obtained from a urologist, gynecologist, or other medical specialist. If there is no medical basis for the problem, a sex therapist or marriage counselor might be helpful.

Facts Specific to Older Men
- Periodic difficulties with erection and ejaculation do not necessarily indicate that you are impotent.

- After you've reached orgasm, it may be 1 or 2 days before you are able to reach full orgasm again.
- Many new treatment options are available for treating erectile dysfunction (impotence). If your health care provider cannot provide up-to-date information about these options, ask for a referral for an appropriate evaluation and discussion of various options.

Facts Specific to Older Women
- Using a water-soluble lubricant will compensate for decreased vaginal lubrication. Do *not* use petroleum jelly because it is not a very effective lubricant for this purpose and can predispose you to infection.
- Estrogen is beneficial in preventing some problems with sexual function, but the relative risks and benefits of such therapy should be considered and discussed thoroughly with your primary care provider.
- You may have vaginal irritation or urinary tract infections, especially after sexual intercourse, because of age-related thinning of the vaginal wall. Such problems may be avoided by the following interventions:
  1. Drink plenty of fluids.
  2. Use an estrogen cream or vaginal lubricant.
  3. Maintain good hygiene in the vaginal area.
  4. If you have a male partner, have him thrust his penis downward, toward the back of your vagina.
  5. Empty your bladder before and after intercourse.

discussion about sexual function. Table 22-1 may be used as a basis for a more detailed discussion of age-related changes that affect sexual function in older adults. An additional teaching point for older women is that sildenafil and other medications are currently being investigated for female sexual dysfunction (Modelska & Cummings, 2003). An additional teaching point for older men is that many interventions are now available for erectile dysfunction (as discussed in this chapter) and that additional ones are being investigated. Thus, older adults should seek further advice about these conditions from their primary care provider or other appropriate health care professional.

Providing Health Education About Medication Effects and Pathologic Conditions

If an older adult has acknowledged a problem with sexual function and also has a pathologic condition, takes a medication, or uses a chemical substance that might be a contributing factor, the nurse can educate the older adult about the potential influence of these

risk factors on sexual function. This is especially important when the nurse has identified pertinent risk factors, but the older adult attributes sexual dysfunction to old age. For example, an older man may attribute a problem with attaining an erection to age-related changes, when, in fact, he has diabetes and takes an antihypertensive medication that is associated with erectile dysfunction. Nurses can use Display 22-1 to identify some of the medications and chemicals that can interfere with sexual function. If a potential relationship exists between risk factors and problems with sexual function, an appropriate nursing intervention is to suggest that the older adult seek appropriate professional consultations for assessment and treatment. A complete medical evaluation by a primary care provider who is knowledgeable about the sexual problems of older adults is usually the best starting point. After any medical problems have been satisfactorily addressed, the older adult may be referred to a mental health professional for counseling if problems with sexual function persist. If medications are causing or contributing to sexual dysfunction, the primary care provider should consider prescribing different medications or reduced doses if medically feasible. For example, people with hypertension are less likely to have sexual dysfunction when treated with calcium channel blockers, angiotensin-converting enzyme inhibitors, or peripheral α-adrenergic receptor blockers.

Arthritis is one of the most common pathologic conditions affecting older adults, and it is often self-managed with little or no medical supervision. Often, the symptoms are not severe enough to motivate the older adult to seek medical evaluation and treatment, but they may be severe enough to interfere with sexual activities. In such cases, the nurse may be the health professional most likely to address the sexual problems that may be caused by the pain, fatigue, and joint limitations associated with arthritis. Nurses can provide health education about simple interventions that may be effective in improving the quality of sexual activities for the older adult with arthritis. Pamphlets about arthritis and sexual activity are available from local chapters of the Arthritis Foundation. Display 22-5 can be used for health education about sexual activity for people with arthritis.

Another pathologic condition often associated with sexual dysfunction is coronary artery disease, especially in those who have had myocardial infarctions or

DISPLAY 22-6
Health Education About Sexual Activity for People With Cardiovascular Disease

- Participation in a medically supervised exercise program can reduce oxygen requirements during sexual activity and improve the quality of your sex life.
- The typical energy expenditure for sexual intercourse is equivalent to that used for climbing two flights of steps.
- Do not engage in sexual activity in extremely hot and humid environments.
- Wait 3 hours after consuming alcohol or a large meal before initiating sexual activity.
- Engage in sexual activity when your energy is at its peak and you are feeling rested and relaxed.
- Avoid sexual activity during times of intense emotional stress.
- Avoid engaging in sexual activity with a partner with whom you are uncomfortable (e.g., an extramarital partner).
- Experiment with different positions to find one that is least demanding of your energy.
- Consider using nitroglycerin, if ordered by your primary care provider, as needed before sexual activity.
- Consult your primary care provider if you experience chest pain during or after sexual activity, or breathlessness or heart palpitations persisting for 15 minutes after orgasm.

DISPLAY 22-5
Health Education About Sexual Activity for People With Arthritis

The pain, fatigue, and joint limitations of arthritis may interfere with, but do not have to curtail, your enjoyment of sexual activity. In fact, sexual activity can be beneficial to you because it stimulates the release of cortisone, adrenalin, and other chemicals that are natural pain relievers. The following actions may enhance your sexual enjoyment and minimize the effects of arthritis:

- Engage in sexual activity when you feel least fatigued and most relaxed.
- Use analgesic medications and other methods of pain relief before engaging in sexual activity.
- Use relaxation techniques before engaging in sexual activity. Relaxation techniques that may be helpful for arthritis include warm baths or showers and the application of hot packs to the affected joints.
- Maintain optimal health through good nutrition and a proper balance of rest and activity.
- Experiment with different sexual positions and use pillows for comfort and support.
- Increase the time spent in foreplay.
- Use a vibrator if your ability to massage is limited by arthritis.
- Use a water-soluble jelly for vaginal lubrication.

who have undergone coronary artery bypass surgery. Although educational and rehabilitation programs for patients with cardiac disease usually provide information about sexual function, older adults are likely to need additional information to address specific concerns about sexual function. Nurses can encourage older adults to discuss these concerns with their primary care practitioner and provide health education using the general guidelines outlined in Display 22-6.

NURSING INTERVENTIONS TO PROVIDE SEXUAL HEALTH EDUCATION TO WOMEN

Since the 1940s when estrogen was first prescribed for treatment of menopausal symptoms, the relative risks and benefits of hormonal therapy have been hotly debated. Researchers and health care practitioners agree that estrogen is an effective intervention for alleviating hot flashes, vaginal atrophy, and other manifestations of menopause that interfere with comfort, sexual function, and quality of life. However, there have been mounting concerns about risks and increasing controversy about any additional potential benefits. Questions about the safety of estrogen therapy were first raised during the 1970s when studies began showing an association between estrogen therapy and increased rates of breast cancer and endometrial cancer and hyperplasia. Although initial studies raised questions about the risk-to-benefit ratio of estrogen, later studies suggested that the administration of a combination of estrogen and progestin could reduce or eliminate such risks for most women. Around the same time, studies found that estrogen was effective in preventing osteoporosis and fractures in postmenopausal women. By the 1980s, studies indicated that hormonal therapy had far-reaching benefits and might even reduce mortality, prevent skin aging, and decrease the incidence of dementia, depression, and cardiovascular disease. By the late 1990s, hormonal therapy was widely recommended not only for menopausal symptoms but also for preventing osteoporosis, fractures, and heart disease. By the early 2000s, however, findings from two major long-term studies—the Women's Health Initiative and the Heart and Estrogen/Progestin Replacement Study—contradicted many of the findings of earlier studies.

In July 2002, a major part of the Women's Health Initiative study was suddenly halted, and study participants were advised to discontinue using the same hormonal therapy regimen that millions of women worldwide had been using for many decades. Results of this study, which "caused a leap in knowledge" and its premature discontinuation, had enormous implications for women and health care practitioners, who began to ask, "How could we have been so wrong?" (Laine, 2002, p. 290). Nurses need to be familiar with results of recent studies on hormonal therapy and explanations of why these results differed so significantly from previous studies so that they can provide health education about hormonal therapy and other aspects of menopause and sexual function in older women. Nurses also need to be familiar with recommendations about nonhormonal interventions for menopausal symptoms.

Recent Conclusions and Recommendations About Hormonal Therapy

The Women's Health Initiative and Heart and Estrogen/Progestin Replacement Study concluded that the most commonly prescribed hormonal therapy regimen, called continuous-combined estrogen-progestin (i.e., daily administration of 0.625 mg of conjugated equine estrogens plus 2.5 mg of medroxyprogesterone acetate), increased the risk for all of the following: heart disease, blood clots, stroke, breast cancer, and symptomatic

gallbladder disease (Grady et al., 2002; Hulley et al., 2002; Women's Health Initiative Investigators, 2002). Positive effects of hormonal therapy identified in these studies included a decreased risk for colorectal cancer, improved bone mineral density, and decreased rates of fractures. After weighing both risks and benefits, the researchers concluded that the risks exceeded the benefits, even though the risk for developing an adverse event was relatively small. For example, based on the findings of the Women's Health Initiative study, 100 women would have to take hormonal therapy for 5 years to develop one additional adverse effect (Sherman, 2002). Because of these studies, organizations such as the U.S. Preventive Services Task Force updated their guidelines and cautioned against the long-term use of hormonal therapy (U.S. Preventive Services Task Force, 2003).

In January 2003, the U.S. Food and Drug Administration (FDA) mandated that the label on all medications containing estrogen must warn about the increased risk for heart disease, heart attacks, stroke, and breast cancer. Labels on hormonal therapy products also should do the following:

- Suggest that topical vaginal products be used for treatment of vulvar or vaginal atrophy
- Suggest that nonestrogen treatments be considered for prevention of postmenopausal osteoporosis
- Encourage practitioners to prescribe the lowest dose for shortest duration of time
- Emphasize that decisions about hormonal therapy be individualized, based on an evaluation of potential risks and benefits
- Suggest that menopausal women may still want to rely on these products for relief of severe vasomotor symptoms

In summary, hormonal therapy is no longer recommended for prevention of any chronic condition (including osteoporosis and cardiovascular disease). It continues to have a place in the treatment of menopausal symptoms such as hot flashes, but its use should be limited to the lowest dose for the shortest duration.

Explanation of Differences Between Recent and Earlier Study Conclusions

Many questions have been raised about how these recent studies could so blatantly contradict earlier findings and lead to major reversals of recommendations made by highly respected health care organizations. It is important to recognize that conclusions were based on different types of studies. Until the early 2000s, conclusions about hormonal therapy were based on observational studies (e.g., the Nurses' Health Study) that found that women taking hormonal therapy had lower rates of cardiovascular disease than women who were not taking estrogen. Observational studies also found that women taking hormonal therapy had decreased serum levels of low-density lipoproteins and increased serum levels of high-density lipoproteins, two factors that reduce the risk for cardiovascular disease (Gupta & Aronow, 2002). By the early 2000s, "a large body of observational data" suggested that hormonal therapy caused a "sizable reduction in the risk for coronary events" in postmenopausal women (Humphrey et al., 2002; Laine, 2002). Researchers then speculated that there was a possible cause–and-effect relationship between the use of hormonal therapy and improved cardiovascular health; therefore, they designed longitudinal and well-controlled prospective studies (e.g., the Women's Health Initiative and Heart and Estrogen/Progestin Replacement Study) to shed additional light on these issues. Contrary to what was expected, however, the well-controlled studies did not support findings from observational studies and, in fact, contradicted many conclusions of earlier studies. An explanation for this contradiction is that the Nurses' Health Study did not control for the fact that women taking hormonal therapy were more likely to be better educated, have better access to medical care, and lead healthier lifestyles. This so-called "healthy woman effect" accounted for the decreased rate of cardiovascular disease in subjects who took hormonal therapy. In summary, the observational data were misleading because they did not adequately account for socioeconomic status: rather than hormonal therapy keeping women healthy, healthy women were taking hormonal therapy (Laine, 2002).

Current Recommendations About Interventions for Menopausal Symptoms

Currently, an advisory panel of the Women's Health Initiative is investigating the following questions:

- Do lower doses of estrogen plus progestin reduce the risk for adverse events?
- Is the risk for adverse effects changed with the use of transdermal estrogen and progestin?
- What is the best way of discontinuing hormonal therapy?
- Which risks are associated with estrogen and which are associated with progestin?

Until these questions are answered, women who have taken hormonal therapy for more than 3 to 5 years are advised to talk with their primary care practitioner about discontinuing the medication and seeking other treatments for the menopausal symptoms

that need to be addressed. Although some women have no major adverse effects from abruptly discontinuing hormonal therapy, many find that a process of gradual tapering is more comfortable and allows their body to adjust better to the changes. Some women who discontinue hormonal therapy find that the benefits outweigh the risks and choose to resume hormonal therapy because they cannot find other effective ways of managing menopausal symptoms. Women need to understand that decisions about hormonal therapy are highly individualized and should be made only after careful consideration by the woman and her health care practitioner.

Researchers and health care practitioners are trying to identify interventions (e.g., medications, herbal and botanical products) that are both safe and effective for managing menopausal symptoms, but most studies to date are inconclusive or not well designed. Because information about the use of hormonal therapy and other interventions for menopausal symptoms is rapidly evolving, nurses need to keep up to date about these issues so that they can provide accurate, complete, and objective information. The Women's Health Initiative is investigating many of these issues, and ongoing findings and recommendations can be found on their website: http://www.whi.org. The website of the North American Menopause Society (http://www.menopause.org) is another excellent source of up-to-date information about interventions for menopausal symptoms. Display 22-7 can be used for educating older women about menopause and hormonal therapy.

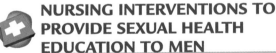

NURSING INTERVENTIONS TO PROVIDE SEXUAL HEALTH EDUCATION TO MEN

Until recently, attention to men's sexual health issues focused primarily on erectile dysfunction, and even that attention was limited because erectile dysfunction was viewed as a relatively inevitable and untreatable condition of older adulthood. However, the recent development of oral agents that are easy to use and relatively safe and effective for erectile dysfunction has significantly increased the interest of researchers, clinicians, and pharmaceutical companies in men's sexual health. Another change that is occurring in issues related to sexual health of older men is the interest in testosterone therapy for treating symptoms of andropause. Nurses need to be familiar enough with both of these emerging issues so that they can provide health education to older men and facilitate appropriate referrals.

DISPLAY 22-7
Health Education About Interventions for Menopause

Health promotion interventions to reduce the frequency or intensity of hot flashes:

- Engage in regular exercise (especially aerobic exercise).
- Avoid caffeine, alcohol, hot beverages, spicy foods.
- Perform relaxation techniques (e.g., slow, deep breathing) several times daily and at the onset of a hot flash.
- Wear layers of lightweight clothing.
- Keep environmental temperatures cool.

Over-the-counter products that may be effective in reducing the frequency or intensity of hot flashes:

- Black cohosh
- Isoflavones (e.g., soy protein)
- Progesterone cream

Prescription medications that may be effective in reducing the frequency or intensity of hot flashes:

- Progesterone and progestational agents (e.g., megestrol, 20–40 mg daily).
- Antidepressants (e.g., venlafaxine, 75 mg daily; fluoxetine, 20 mg daily; paroxetine, 12.5–25 mg daily; sertraline, 50–100 mg daily).
- Clonidine, 0.1 mg daily.
- Gabapentin, 100–900 mg daily.

Clinical trials have *not* supported the use of any of the following interventions for hot flashes:

- Vitamin E.
- Herbal products: sage, ginseng, licorice, sarsaparilla, dong quai, fish oil, wild yam, flaxseed oil, gotu kola, ginkgo biloba, valerian root, evening primrose oil.

Interventions that need further investigation of their potential effectiveness for hot flashes:

- Chasteberry.
- Hypnosis.
- Acupuncture.
- Biofeedback.

Health promotion interventions for other symptoms of menopause:

- Engage in regular weight-bearing exercises for prevention of osteoporosis.
- Provide daily intake of 1,500 mg calcium and 600 IU vitamin D for prevention of osteoporosis.
- Talk with your primary care practitioner about assessment of and interventions for osteoporosis.
- Perform pelvic muscle exercises for prevention of urinary incontinence.
- Use lubricants for vaginal dryness.

Testosterone Therapy

In recent years, researchers and practitioners have attempted to address questions about the role of testosterone therapy for treatment of andropausal symptoms and erectile dysfunction, but many questions remain about its safety and efficacy. Testosterone therapy in healthy older men may have beneficial effects on libido, muscle strength, cognitive function, cardiovascular function, body composition, bone mineral density, and general well-being (Kenny et al., 2002; Matsumoto, 2002). These effects may be greater in younger rather than older men and are most significant in men who have low serum levels of testosterone because there is a "threshold effect" (i.e., a level at which no further benefits are seen) (Vermeulen, 2001). Because detrimental effects of testosterone therapy, including prostatic hyperplasia and increased risk for prostate cancer, may outweigh the benefits, it is not widely recommended for management of andropause or sexual dysfunction and is contraindicated in men with breast cancer or prostate cancer. A recent research summary concluded that "the most prudent course of action is to treat only older men with repeatedly low serum T levels and symptoms and signs consistent with androgen deficiency in whom the potential benefits of therapy clearly outweigh the potential risks, and to carefully monitor treated men for adverse effects" (Matsumoto, 2002). Currently approved methods of administering testosterone therapy in the United States include gels, patches, and intramuscular injections; a buccal preparation is under investigation. Testosterone pills are available outside the United States, but they are not recommended because they are less effective and are associated with potentially serious adverse effects (e.g., hepatotoxicity and cardiovascular disease). Information about testosterone therapy is rapidly evolving, but some of the information is disseminated by companies whose primary goal is to sell testosterone products; hence, there is a great need for well-controlled studies of testosterone therapy.

Treatments for Erectile Dysfunction

Since the 1990s, erectile dysfunction has been recognized as a very common and treatable condition that should be addressed by health care professionals.

TABLE 22-2 • Interventions for Erectile Dysfunction

Intervention	Mode of Action	Comment
Oral medications (e.g., sildenafil, vardenafil)	Causes penile engorgement by increasing the blood flow and relaxing the smooth muscles	Cannot be used by men taking nitrate medications. Adverse effects include headache, indigestion, and facial flushing
Sublingual apomorphine	Acts on the dopamine receptors in the brain to stimulate erection	Can be used by men taking nitrate medications. Adverse effects include nausea, sweating, dizziness, and somnolence
Testosterone therapy (oral, sublingual, or injectable preparations)	Increases serum testosterone in the small number (1% to 5%) of men who have testosterone deficiency	May worsen prostate problems and increase the risk for prostate cancer
Vacuum pumps and constriction devices	Stimulates an erection by using an airtight plastic cylinder to create a vacuum; a constriction band is then placed around the base of the penis to retain the erection, and the cylinder is removed	Requires a high degree of manual dexterity; is intrusive and cumbersome; may cause ejaculatory discomfort
Intracavernosal injection of vasoactive drug (e.g., alprostadil)	Injects medication directly into the erectile tissue to cause vasodilation and relaxation of the smooth muscles of the penis	Adverse effects include priapism, bruising, and local pain
Transurethral alprostadil suppository	Aids erection by causing vasodilation and relaxation of smooth muscle tissue after the active agent is absorbed from the urethral tissue	Adverse effects include hypotension, syncope, and transient burning sensation in the urethra
Topical medications (e.g., herbal combinations, vasodilators)	Enhance erections by increasing blood flow	Not approved by the Food and Drug Administration; vasodilators should not be used by men with cardiovascular disease
Yohimbine (alone or in combination with L-arginine or trazodone)	Stimulates receptors in the brain associated with libido and erections	Low success rate (not proven effective in clinical trials); adverse effects include nausea, insomnia, nervousness, dizziness, and hypertension
Penile prostheses (require a surgical procedure)	Facilitates erection by improving penile rigidity without affecting urination, ejaculation, or orgasm	High rate of success, is the only intervention that is permanent

Many surgical and medical interventions are now available for erectile dysfunction, ranging from surgical procedures (e.g., penile prostheses) to oral medications (Table 22-2). In 1998, the FDA approved the first oral medication for erectile dysfunction, sildenafil, which simplified the treatment of this disorder and stimulated much public debate and attention. Sildenafil is currently the first-line treatment for erectile dysfunction, and men prefer it to other interventions even though its efficacy rate—between 42% and 66%—is lower than that of other methods (Fink et al., 2002; Padma-Nathan & Giuliano, 2001).

Interventions also are directed toward addressing risk factors, in addition to improving sexual function. For example, smoking cessation and optimal management of diabetes can improve erectile dysfunction in men with these contributing factors. If blood flow is blocked, vascular surgery to restore normal circulation to the penis may be an appropriate intervention. Psychotherapy and behavioral therapy may be used as primary or adjunctive treatment options to address the psychosocial issues that may be contributing to erectile dysfunction. Pelvic muscle exercises, commonly performed as a treatment for urinary incontinence, may also be useful in the treatment of erectile dysfunction. The technique for performing these exercises is described in Chapter 15. Decisions about appropriate treatment options must be based on a comprehensive evaluation by a urologist or by a primary care provider who is knowledgeable about erectile dysfunction. The primary responsibility of the gerontological nurse is to keep up to date on the types of interventions that are available and to educate older men about the importance of seeking help for erectile dysfunction.

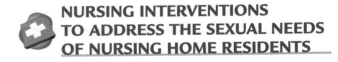

NURSING INTERVENTIONS TO ADDRESS THE SEXUAL NEEDS OF NURSING HOME RESIDENTS

In addressing the sexual needs of older adults, the responsibilities of nurses in long-term care facilities differ from those of nurses in acute care or home settings in the following ways:

- Because of the intense medical needs of patients in acute care settings, sexual needs are often irrelevant or have a very low priority.
- Because of the short duration of stay in acute care settings, it is not necessary to address the long-term sexual needs of patients.
- Because people in their own homes have a high degree of privacy and autonomy in meeting their personal needs, a nurse who provides home care does not routinely have to be concerned about sexual needs.

Residents of long-term care facilities, however, generally are not acutely ill, are planning to stay in the facility for a long time, and do depend on the nursing staff to ensure the privacy necessary to meet their personal needs. Thus, the nurses in long-term care facilities must address the sexual needs of residents as an integral part of the overall care plan.

Because many of the barriers to meeting the sexual needs of older adults in long-term care facilities are based on myths and attitudes of the staff, education of the staff is the most effective starting point for addressing these issues (Kuhn, 2002; Walker & Harrington, 2002). Education of staff members in long-term care facilities can be accomplished through in-service programs that address issues related to various aspects of sexual function, including the lifelong interest in and need for sexual activity and intimate relationships. Audiovisual materials can be used to stimulate discussion about the unique aspects of meeting sexual needs in institutional settings and about the responsibilities and limitations of staff. When staff express concerns about the ability of a cognitively impaired resident to give informed consent, a model for assessing competence to participate in an intimate relationship may be used. An example of such a model is discussed by Lichtenberg (1997) and can be used by an interdisciplinary team. Emphasis should be placed on the rights of residents, as defined by the federal government in the Residents' Rights Bill (Health Care Financing Administration, 1980). Specific rights pertaining to the sexual needs of residents of long-term care facilities include (1) the right to private visits with a spouse and the right to share a room with a spouse unless medically contraindicated, and (2) the right to associate, communicate, and meet privately with people of their choice, unless this infringes on the rights of another resident. The effectiveness of in-service programs may be enhanced if social service and administrative staff members are included as planners and participants. Presenters and discussion leaders should use a nonjudgmental and matter-of-fact approach to provide the

staff with an appropriate role model for addressing this sensitive topic.

In addition to educating staff members about the sexual needs and rights of residents, nurses are responsible for taking measures to ensure privacy for those residents who desire it. If a resident does not have a private room, efforts must be made to provide privacy, while still respecting the rights of any roommates. Sometimes, the role of the nurse will be that of a negotiator, assisting residents in reaching mutually acceptable agreements about privacy and shared space.

EVALUATING EFFECTIVENESS OF NURSING INTERVENTIONS

Nursing care for older adults with the diagnosis of Ineffective Sexuality Patterns is evaluated by the degree to which risk factors are eliminated, particularly through the provision of accurate information. For example, older adults may verbalize an improved understanding of the age-related changes that affect response to sexual stimulation. In turn, this information can alleviate anxiety about sexual performance and may improve the older adult's quality of life. Interventions to alleviate risk factors, such as medical conditions or adverse medication or chemical effects, would be judged to be successful if the older adult follows through with a referral to an appropriate resource. One measure of successful intervention in nursing home settings would be that staff members increase their understanding of the sexual needs of older adults and are more comfortable allowing appropriate means of sexual expression by the residents.

CHAPTER SUMMARY

Age-related changes do not significantly interfere with the ability of older adults to pursue and maintain satisfying sexual activities and relationships, but risk factors commonly interfere with sexual expression. Myths and lack of knowledge about age-related changes and risk factors that influence sexual function are important risk factors that can be alleviated through educational interventions. Risk factors that cannot be alleviated, such as medical conditions or social circumstances, may be addressed through referrals for further evaluation or counseling. Nursing assessment is directed toward identifying the concerns that older adults have about their sexual function. Nursing assessment also aims to identify any risk factors that interfere with an older adult's sexual function and quality of life. Assessment of sexual function is particularly important in home and long-term care settings, where nursing care focuses on quality-of-life issues that affect the older adult's daily life. Because nurses usually are not well prepared to assess sexual function, a self-assessment of their personal attitudes toward sexual function in older adults increases their comfort with this aspect of nursing care. Ineffective Sexuality Patterns is an appropriate nursing diagnosis for older adults who express concerns about, or have risk factors that interfere with, their sexual function. Nursing interventions are directed toward alleviating risk factors and improving or maintaining the older adult's quality of life. Specific nursing interventions include health education and referrals for counseling or further evaluation. Nursing care is evaluated according to the degree to which the older adult increases his or her knowledge about age-related changes and risk factors that influence sexual function. Another measure of successful interventions would be that the older adult expresses improved satisfaction with sexual activities and relationships.

CONCLUDING CASE STUDY AND NURSING CARE PLAN

➤ Mr. and Mrs. S. are now 75 and 73 years old, respectively, and they have moved to an assisted-living facility where you are the nurse. Their health conditions have not changed significantly in the past 2 years, with the exception of Mrs. S. having more difficulty walking because of her arthritis. Mr. and Mrs. S. recently moved to the facility because they needed help with transportation and wanted to live in a place where they had fewer responsibilities and more time to enjoy life. During one of their appointments, Mrs. S. becomes tearful and says she has been disappointed in their move from their own home. She says, "Now we have the time to enjoy our life together, but we seem to be in each other's way all the time. When we lived in our own home we were so busy with the yard and the housekeeping and all the daily chores, we never had time to think about what we enjoy together. Now I don't have to cook meals and worry about getting to the grocery store, but we aren't enjoying the time we have together."

■ Nursing Assessment

On further discussion, Mrs. S. acknowledges that she has talked with her husband about having more "intimate time and resuming sexual activities that have petered out in the past few years because we were always so tired and never seemed to have much time." In reply, Mr. S. has stated that "We're probably too old to do those things, and old people shouldn't expect to have the fun we used to have." Mrs. S. says she used to believe that, but recently

she's been talking with some of the other women in the assisted-living facility who seem to be enjoying sexual activities. Mr. and Mrs. S. relate that they had a good sexual relationship until Mr. S.'s heart attack 5 years ago. After that, he lost interest in sexual activities, even though he was told he could resume all his usual activities except for very strenuous activity, such as shoveling snow. Mrs. S. says she masturbates occasionally, but she doesn't find that very satisfying. Mrs. S. expresses concern about being comfortable in the sexual position they used previously because her arthritis has gotten worse in the past few years.

■ Nursing Diagnosis

You address Ineffective Sexuality Patterns as your nursing diagnosis for Mr. and Mrs. S. Related factors include myths and lack of information about the age-related changes and risk factors that influence sexual function. Potential risk factors that you identify are Mr. S.'s medications and his lack of information about sexual function after a heart attack.

■ Nursing Care Plan

The care plan you develop for Mr. and Mrs. S. is given in Display 22-8.

 CRITICAL THINKING EXERCISES

1. Address the following questions in relation to Mr. and Mrs. S, the subjects of the case study.
   - What risk factors are likely to influence Mrs. S.'s enjoyment of sexual activity?
   - What risk factors are likely to affect Mr. S.'s enjoyment of sexual activity?
   - What health education would you provide for Mrs. S. and what would you use for patient teaching tools?
   - What health education would you provide for Mr. S. and what would you use for patient teaching tools?
2. Describe the attitudinal risk factors, on the parts of society, older adults, and health care providers, that can interfere with healthy sexual function in older adults.
3. Summarize the functional consequences that are likely to affect sexual function in healthy older men and women.
4. What are the responsibilities of nurses in each of the following settings relating to assessment of sexual function in older adults: community setting, acute care facility, and long-term care facility?

DISPLAY 22-8 • NURSING CARE PLAN FOR MR. AND MRS. S.

EXPECTED OUTCOME	NURSING INTERVENTIONS	NURSING EVALUATION
Mr. and Mrs. S.'s knowledge about age-related changes and risk factors that affect sexual function will be increased.	• Use Display 22-4 as a basis for discussion of sexual function in later adulthood.	• Mr. and Mrs. S. will verbalize correct information about sexual function in older adulthood.
The risk factors associated with Mr. S.'s heart attack and medication regimen will be addressed.	• Explain that many medications for heart problems and high blood pressure are associated with problems with sexual function. • Use Display 22-6 as a basis for discussing sexual activity as it relates to people with heart problems. • Encourage Mr. S. to talk with his primary care provider about his medication regimen and about his heart condition. Suggest that he inquire whether a different medication would effectively treat his high blood pressure without interfering with sexual function.	• Mr. S. will agree to talk with his primary care provider about the potential relationship between his medications and heart condition and his lack of sexual activity.
The risk factors associated with Mrs. S.'s arthritis will be addressed.	• Use Display 22-5 to discuss sexual activity as it relates to people with arthritis.	• Mrs. S. will identify ways to increase her comfort during sexual activities.

5. Describe the assessment and health education approaches you might use for a 73-year-old married man who confides that he has difficulty making his wife "happy in bed."
6. Spend a few minutes answering all the questions included in Display 22-2, Assessing Personal Attitudes Toward Sexuality and Aging. What did you learn about yourself?

EDUCATIONAL RESOURCES

American Association of Sex Educators, Counselors and Therapists
P.O. Box 5488, Richmond, VA 23220-0488
http://www.aasect.org

American Menopause Foundation, Inc.
350 Fifth Avenue, Suite 2822, New York, NY 10118
(212) 714-2398
http://www.americanmenopause.org

North American Menopause Society
P.O. Box 94527, Cleveland, OH 44101
(800) 774-7680
http://www.menopause.org

Pride Senior Network
22 West 23rd Street, 5th Floor, New York, NY 10010
(212) 675-1936
http://www.pridesenior.org
A nonprofit organization for aging gays and lesbians

Senior Action in a Gay Environment (SAGE)
305 Seventh Avenue, 16th Floor, New York, NY 10001
(212) 741-2247
http://www.sageusa.org

Sexuality Information and Education Council of the United States
130 West 42nd Street, Suite 350, New York, NY 10036-7802
(212) 819-9770
http://www.siecus.org

REFERENCES

Anderson, J. K., Faulkner, S., Cranor, C., Briley, J., Gevirtz, F., & Roberts, S. (2002). Andropause: Knowledge and perceptions among general public and health care professionals. *Journal of Gerontology: Medical Sciences, 57A*, M793–M796.

Avis, N. E. (2000). Sexual functioning and aging in men and women: Community and population-based studies. *Journal of Gender-Specific Medicine, 3*(2), 37–41.

Bacon, C. G., Giobanucci, E., Glasser, D. B., Mittleman, M. A., & Rimm, E. B. (2002). Association of type and duration of diabetes with erectile dysfunction in a large cohort of men. *Diabetes Care, 25*, 1458–1463.

Bauer, M. (1999). Their only privacy is between their sheets: Privacy and sexuality of elderly nursing home residents. *Journal of Gerontological Nursing, 25*(8), 37–41.

Berger, R. (2001). Report of the American Foundation for Urologic Disease Thought Leader Panel for evaluation and treatment of priapism. *International Journal of Impotence Research, 13*(Suppl 5), S39–S43.

Berman, J. R., & Goldstein, I. (2001). Female sexual dysfunction. *Urologic Clinics of North America, 28*(2), 405–416.

Bernardo, A. (2001). Sexuality in patients with coronary disease and heart failure. *Herz, 26*(5), 353–359.

Beutel, M. E. (2002). Sexual activity, sexual and partnership satisfaction in ageing men—results from a German representative community study. *Andrologia, 34*(1), 22–28.

Brecher, E. M. (1984). *Love, sex, and aging: A Consumers Union Report.* Boston: Little, Brown & Company.

Bretschneider, J. G., & McCoy, N. L. (1988). Sexual interest and behavior in healthy 80- to 102-year-olds. *Archives of Sexual Behavior, 17,* 109–129.

Brody, J. E. (1983, September 28). Drugs can be bad medicine for lover. *New York Times,* p III, 1:1.

Buvat, J. (2001). [Sexuality of the diabetic woman.] *Diabetes and Metabolism, 27*(4 Pt 2), S67–S75.

Cahill, S. (2002). Long term care issues affecting gay, lesbian, bisexual and transgender elders. *Geriatric Care Management Journal, 12*(3), 4–8.

Carpenito, L. J. (2002). *Nursing diagnosis: Application to clinical practice* (9th ed.). Philadelphia: Lippincott Williams & Wilkins.

Chun, J., & Carson, C. C. (2001). Physician-patient dialogue and clinical evaluation of erectile dysfunction. *Urologic Clinics of North America, 28*(2), 249–258.

Cooney, T. M., & Dunne, K. (2001). Intimate relationships in later life. *Journal of Family Issues, 22,* 838–858.

Covey, H. C. (1989). Perceptions and attitudes toward sexuality of the elderly during the middle ages. *Gerontologist, 29*(1), 91–103.

Fink, H. A., MacDonald, R., Rutks, I. R., Nelson, D. B., & Wilt, T. J. (2002). Sildenafil for male erectile dysfunction: A systemic review and meta-analysis. *Archives of Internal Medicine, 162,* 1349–1360.

Gibson, M. C., Bol, N., Woodury, M. G., Beaton, C., & Janke, C. (1999). Comparison of caregivers', residents', and community-dwelling spouses' opinions about expressing sexuality in an institutional setting. *Journal of Gerontological Nursing, 25*(4), 30–39.

Giraldi, A. G., & Victor, J. (2002). Female sexual dysfunction as an adverse effect of pharmacological treatment. *Ugeskrift for Laeger, 164,* 4757–4760.

Grady, D., Herrington, D., Bittner, V., Blumenthal, R., Davidson, M., Hlatky, M., et al. (2002). Cardiovascular disease outcomes during 6.8 years of hormone therapy: Heart and Estrogen/Progestin Replacement Study follow-up (HERS II). *Journal of the American Medical Association, 288*(1), 49–57.

Gupta, G., & Aronow, W. S. (2002). Hormone replacement therapy: An analysis of efficacy based on evidence. *Geriatrics, 57*(8), 18–24.

Health Care Financing Administration. (1980, July 1). Rule 5101:3-3-08. *Residents' rights in long-term care facilities.* Washington, DC: U.S. Government Printing Office.

Heaton, J. P. W., & Morales, A. (2003). Endocrine causes of impotence (nondiabetes). *Urologic Clinics of North America, 30*(1), 73.

Hetzel, L., & Smith, A. (2001). *Census Brief. The 65 years and over population: 2000.* Washington, DC: U.S. Census Bureau.

Hulley, S., Furberg, C., Barrett-Connor, E., Cauley, J., Grady, D., Haskell, W., et al. (2002). Noncardiovascular disease outcomes during 6.8 years of hormone therapy. Heart and Estrogen/Progestin Replacement Study follow-up (HERS II). *Journal of the American Medical Association, 288*(1), 58–66.

Humphrey, L. L., Chan, B. K. S., & Sox, H. C. (2002). Postmenopausal hormone replacement therapy and the primary prevention of cardiovascular disease. *Annals of Internal Medicine, 137,* 273–284.

Johannes, C. B., Araujo, A. B., Feldman, H. A., Derby, C. A., Kleinman, K. P., & McKinlay, J. B. (2000). Incidence of erectile dysfunction in men ages 40–69: Longitudinal results form the Massachusetts male aging study. *Journal of Urology, 163*(2), 460–463.

Johnson, B. (1997). Older adults' suggestions for health care providers regarding discussions of sex. *Geriatric Nursing, 18*(2), 65–66.

Johnson, B. K. (1996). Older adults and sexuality: A multidimensional perspective. *Journal of Gerontological Nursing, 22*(2), 6–15.

Kaplan, M. J. (2002). Approaching sexual issues in primary care. *Primary Care: Clinics in Office Practice, 29*(1), 113–124.

Kenny, A. M., Bellantonio, S., Gruman, C. A., Acosta, R. D., & Prestwood, K. M. (2002). Effects of transdermal testosterone on cognitive function and health perception in older men with low bioavailable testosterone levels. *Journal of Gerontology, Series A, Biological Sciences and Medical Sciences, 57*(5), M321–M325.

Kinsey, A. C., Pomeroy, W. B., & Martin, C. E. (1948). *Sexual behavior in the human male.* Philadelphia: W. B. Saunders.

Kinsey, A. C., Pomeroy, W. B., & Martin, C. E. (1953). *Sexual behavior in the human female.* Philadelphia: W. B. Saunders.

Kuhn, D. (2002). Intimacy, sexuality, and residents with dementia. *Alzheimer's Care Quarterly, 3*(2), 165–176, Appendix A.

Laine, C. (2002). Postmenopausal hormone replacement therapy: How could we have been so wrong? *Annals of Internal Medicine, 137,* 290.

Lewis, R. W. (2001). Epidemiology of erectile dysfunction. *Urologic Clinics of North America, 28*(2), 209–216.

Lichtenberg, P. A. (1997). Clinical perspectives on sexual issues in nursing homes. *Topics in Geriatric Rehabilitation, 12*(4), 1–10.

Mace, N. L., & Rabins, P. V. (1999). *The 36-hour day* (3rd ed.) Baltimore: The Johns Hopkins University Press.

Masters, W. H., & Johnson, V. E. (1966). *Human sexual response.* Boston: Little, Brown & Company.

Matsumoto, A. M. (2002). Andropause: Clinical implications of the decline in serum testosterone levels with aging in men. *Journal of Gerontology: Medical Sciences, 57A,* M76–M99.

Mazur, A. (2002). Causes of sexual decline in aging married men: Germany and America. *International Journal of Impotence Research, 14*(2), 101–106.

Milbank, A. J., & Goldfarb, D. A. (2003). Urologic manifestations of vascular disease. *Urologic Clinics of North America, 30*(1), 13.

Modelska, K., & Cummings, S. (2003). Female sexual dysfunction in postmenopausal women: Systematic review of placebo-controlled trials. *American Journal of Obstetrics and Gynecology, 188*(1), 286–293.

Munarriz, R., Kim, N. M., Goldstein, I., & Traish, A. M. (2002). Biology of female sexual function. *Urologic Clinics of North America, 29*(3), 685–693.

National Institutes of Health. (1992, December 7–9). *Consensus statement: Impotence.* Washington, DC: Author.

Nudell, D. M., Monoski, M. M. & Lipshultz, L. I. (2002). Common medications and drugs: How they affect male fertility. *Urologic Clinics of North America, 29*(4), 347–354.

Nusbaum, M. R., Hamilton, C., & Lenahan, P. (2003). Chronic illness and sexual functioning. *American Family Physicians, 67*(2), 347–354.

Padma-Nathan, H., & Giuliano, F. (2001). Oral drug therapy for erectile dysfunction. *Urologic Clinics of North America, 28*(2), 321–334.

Pauls, R. N., & Berman, J. R. (2002). Impact of pelvic floor disorders and prolapse on female sexual function and response. *Urologic Clinics of North America, 29*(3), 677–683.

Pope, M. (1997). Sexual issues for older lesbians and gays. *Topics in Geriatric Rehabilitation, 12*(4), 53–60.

Robinson, K. M. (2003). Understanding hypersexuality: A behavioral disorder of dementia. *Home Healthcare Nurse, 21*(1), 43–47.

Rosen, R. C. (2001). Psychogenic erectile dysfunction. *Urologic Clinics of North America, 23*(2), 269–278.

Sasaki, K., Yoshimura, N., & Chancellor, M. B. (2003). Implications of diabetes mellitus in urology. *Urologic Clinics of North America, 30*(1), 1–12.

Sherman, F. T. (2002). Hormone replacement therapy: The sudden half of a clinical trial shakes long held beliefs. *Geriatrics, 57*(8), 7–8.

Slag, M., Morley, J. E., Elson, M. K., Trence, D. L., Nelson, C. J., Nelson, A. E., Kinlaw, W. B., Beyer, H. S., Nuttall, F. Q., & Shafer, R. B. (1983). Impotence in medical clinic patients. *Journal of the American Medical Association, 249,* 1736–1740.

Solomon, H., Man, J. W., Wierzbicki, A. S., & Jackson, G. (2003). Relation of erectile dysfunction to angiographic coronary artery disease. *American Journal of Cardiology, 91*(2), 230–231.

Taylor, M. (2002). Alternative medicine and the perimenopause: An evidence-based review. *Obstetrics and Gynecology Clinics, 29*(3), 555–573.

Thomas, A., Woodard, C., Rovner, E. S., & Wein, A. J. (2003). Urologic complications of nonurologic medications. *Urology Clinics of North America, 30*(1), 123–131.

Tunstull, P., & Henry, M. E. (1996). Approaches to resident sexuality. *Journal of Gerontological Nursing, 22*(6), 37–42.

U.S. Preventive Services Task Force. (2003). Postmenopausal hormone replacement therapy for the primary prevention of chronic conditions: Recommendations and rationale. *American Family Physician, 67*(2), 358–364.

Velez, L., & Peggs, J. (2001). Managing behavioral problems in long-term care. *Clinics in Family Practice, 3*(3), 561–576.

Vermeulen, A. (2001). Special articles: Hormones and reproductive health. *Journal of Clinical Endocrinology and Metabolism, 86,* 2380–2390.

Virag, R., Bouilly, P., & Frydman, D. (1985). Is impotence an arterial disorder? *Lancet, 1,* 181–184.

Walker, B. L., & Harrington, D. (2002). Effects of staff knowledge and attitudes about sexuality. *Educational Gerontology, 38,* 639–654.

Wallace, M. (2001). Sexuality. *Journal of Gerontological Nursing, 7*(2), 10–11.

Weismiller, D. G. (2002). The perimenopause and menopause experience. *Clinics in Family Practice, 4*(1), 1–12.

Wespes, E. (2002). Male andropause: Myth, reality, and treatment. *International Journal of Impotence Research, 14*(Suppl 1), S93–S98.

Whiteman, M. K., Staropoli, C. A., Langenberg, P. W., McCarter, R. J., Kjerulff, K. H., and Flaws, J. A. (2003). Smoking, body mass, and hot flashes in midlife women. *Obstetrics and Gynecology, 101,* 264–272.

Wiley, D., & Bortz, W. M. (1996). Sexuality and aging: Usual and successful. *Journals of Gerontology: Medical Sciences, 51A,* M142–M146.

Women's Health Initiative Investigators. (2002). Risks and benefits of estrogen plus progestin in healthy postmenopausal women: Principal results from the Women's Health Initiative randomized controlled trial. *Journal of the American Medical Association, 288*(3), 321–333.

Wright, L. K. (2001). Altered sexuality patterns. In M. L. Maas, K. C. Buckwalter, M. D. Hardy, T. Tripp-Reimer, M. G. Titler, & J. P. Specht (Eds.), *Nursing care of older adults: Diagnoses, outcomes, and interventions* (pp. 750–761). St. Louis: Mosby.

5

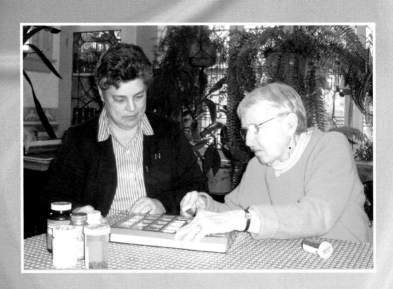

MEDICATION
MANAGEMENT

Medications and the Older Adult

LEARNING OBJECTIVES

1. Delineate age-related changes that affect the action of medications in the body and skills involved with taking medications.

2. Examine risk factors that affect medication action and patterns of medication use in older adults.

3. Describe interactions that can occur between medications and any of the following substances: other medications, nutrients, alcohol, caffeine, nicotine, and herbs.

4. Identify the adverse effects that are likely to occur in older adults because of age-related changes and risk factors.

5. Describe the purposes of medication assessment and the relationship between the medication assessment and the overall assessment of older adults.

6. Describe observations and interview questions that are used for a comprehensive medication assessment.

7. Identify interventions directed toward enhancing the therapeutic effectiveness of medications, reducing the risks for adverse effects, and minimizing the negative functional consequences of adverse effects.

Although the topic of medications and the older adult is not a distinct category of function in the same sense as physiologic and psychosocial aspects of function (e.g., vision and cognition), it is an extremely important consideration and can be addressed from the same perspective as other aspects of function. Thus, this chapter addresses age-related changes, risk factors, and functional consequences in relation to medication effects and patterns of medication use by older adults.

AGE-RELATED CHANGES THAT AFFECT MEDICATIONS IN OLDER ADULTS

Age-related changes that affect medications in older adults are discussed in relation to those that affect the action of medications in the body and those that affect the skills involved with taking medications correctly. The factors that have the most significant impact on medication effectiveness in older adults are not age-related changes, but risk factors, and are considered in the section on Risk Factors.

Changes That Affect the Action of Medications in the Body

• Effects of medications in the body are usually considered in relation to *pharmacokinetics* (i.e., how the drug is absorbed, distributed, metabolized, and excreted) and *pharmacodynamics* (i.e., how the body is affected by the drug at the cellular level and in relation to the target organ). Age-related changes in renal function, liver function, and body composition affect the distribution, metabolism, and excretion of drugs and alter the *elimination half-time* (also called the *serum half-life*). Age-related changes in receptor sensitivity and homeostatic mechanisms affect pharmacodynamics. •

Absorption refers to the passage of a medication from its site of introduction, usually the gastrointestinal tract, into the general circulation. Absorption of oral medications can be affected by diminished gastric acid, increased gastric pH, delayed gastric emptying, and the presence of other substances (e.g., food, nutrients, inert ingredients of medications). Because most oral medications are absorbed by passive diffusion across the small intestine—a process that is not pH-dependent—they are not usually affected by any alterations in gastric acidity. The unique chemical properties of each medication determine the degree to which it is susceptible to any gastrointestinal changes, regardless of age. For example, pH-sensitive medications, such as penicillin and ferrous sulfate, are more likely to be affected by altered gastric acid levels or by prolonged exposure to these acids because of delayed emptying. Although some gerontological references suggest that absorption of oral medications is influenced by age-related gastric acid changes, researchers have not identified any clinically significant effect of gastrointestinal changes in healthy older adults (Cusack & Vestal, 2000; Beyth & Shorr, 2002). If absorption of medications is affected, it is likely to be associated with risk factors (e.g., drug interactions and pathologic conditions) rather than with age-related changes.

An age-related decline in glomerular filtration rate, which begins in early adulthood and progresses at an annual rate of 1% to 2%, may affect drug concentrations in the body. As with other aspects of pharmacokinetics, however, the specific chemical characteristics of each medication determine the degree to which age-related changes affect excretion. For example, medications that are dependent on glomerular filtration (e.g., gentamicin) or tubular secretion (e.g., penicillin) for elimination will be more directly influenced by diminished renal function than those that are metabolized more extensively in the liver before excretion. Likewise, the effect of diminished renal function will be greater on medications that have a narrow therapeutic index, like digoxin, than on medications with a wide therapeutic index. Display 23-1 lists some medications that are likely to be affected by age-related renal changes.

Hepatic blood flow declines by 35% between the ages of 40 and 65 years. This age-related change may influence the serum concentration and volume of distribution of some medications (Display 23-2). For example, the effect of medications that are rapidly metabolized and, therefore, greatly influenced by the speed of delivery to the liver may be affected by diminished hepatic blood flow. The specific impact of these age-related liver changes on medication metabolism is unclear, however, because other factors (e.g., diet, disease, smoking, and genetic variations) are likely to affect drug metabolism simultaneously and to exert a stronger influence than any age-related factors.

Two measures of the efficiency of metabolism and elimination are elimination half-time and clearance rate. Elimination half-time is the time required to decrease the drug concentration by one half of its original value. It takes five half-times to reach

---

DISPLAY 23-1

Medications Likely to be Affected by Age-Related Renal Changes

Amantadine
Amikacin
Chlorpropamide
Ciprofloxacin
Digoxin
Enalapril
Furosemide
Hydrochlorothiazide
Nitrofurantoin
Quinapril
Ranitidine
Streptomycin

<table>
<tr><td>

DISPLAY 23-2

Medications Likely to be Affected by Age-Related Changes in Hepatic Blood Flow

Chlordiazepoxide
Diazepam
Ibuprofen
Imipramine
Meperidine
Morphine
Naproxen
Nortriptyline
Propranolol
Quinidine
Theophylline
Trazodone
Verapamil

</td><td>

DISPLAY 23-3

Medications Likely to be Affected by Age-Related Changes in Body Composition

Medications That May Become More Concentrated in Older Adults

Cimetidine
Digoxin
Ethanol (alcohol)
Gentamicin
Morphine
Quinine

Medications That May Become Less Concentrated in Older Adults

Chlordiazepoxide
Phenobarbital
Prozosin
Thiopental
Tolbutamide

</td></tr>
</table>

steady-state concentrations after a drug is initiated or to eliminate a medication completely from the body after a drug is discontinued. The clearance rate measures the volume of blood from which the medication is eliminated per unit of time. An increase in serum half-life or a decrease in clearance rate may result in accumulation of the medication. The result is that the therapeutic effect is likely to be altered, and the risk for adverse effects is likely to be increased.

An age-related decrease in total body water and an increase in the proportion of body fat to lean body mass can alter medication action in older adults. Between the ages of about 20 and 80 years, the following changes in body composition occur: body fat gradually increases by 15% to 20%, lean tissue decreases by about 20%, and total body water is reduced by 10% to 15%. Loss of lean body mass accelerates after the age of 80 years, even in healthy older adults (Kyle et al., 2001). Because these age-related changes in body composition will affect medications according to their degree of fat or water solubility, drugs that are distributed primarily in body water or lean body mass may reach higher serum concentrations in older adults, and their effects may be more intense. Similarly, the serum concentration of highly fat-soluble medications, which are distributed and stored in fat tissue, may be lowered, and these medications have an increased tendency to accumulate in adipose tissue. Consequently, fat-soluble medications may have a prolonged duration of action, be more erratic in their effects, and have less intense immediate effects. Display 23-3 identifies the effects of age-related changes in body composition on some medications.

As medications are distributed and metabolized in the body, some molecules are bound to serum albu-

min and other proteins so that the bound portion becomes inactive, whereas the unbound molecules remain active. Because the unbound portion is the amount available for metabolism, tissue perfusion, and renal excretion, the protein-binding capacity of a drug is an important determinant of its potential for both therapeutic and adverse effects. The degree of protein binding of each medication varies, with some medications, such as warfarin, having a protein-binding capacity of 99%. The binding capacity of protein-bound medications can be influenced by diminished serum albumin levels in older adults. Additional factors that affect the degree of protein binding for any medication include the strength of the binding and the number of chemicals competing for the binding sites.

Although researchers disagree about the extent and cause of decreased serum albumin levels in older adults, it is generally agreed that the serum albumin level diminishes by as much as 20% in the later decades of life. Diminished serum albumin levels are associated with a combination of factors, including nutrition, disease processes, decreased mobility, and age-related liver changes. Regardless of the cause, a decrease in serum albumin level will lead to an increased amount of the active portion of protein-bound medications. Highly protein-bound medications, which are commonly taken by older adults, are especially likely to be affected. Examples of medications that are likely to be altered by low serum albumin levels and decreased binding opportunities are digoxin, furosemide, phenylbutazone, phenytoin, salicylic acid, theophylline, warfarin, and thyroid hormone.

DISPLAY 23-4
Some Medications That Compete at Protein-Binding Sites

Salicylates and oral hypoglycemics
Sulfonamides and oral hypoglycemics
Warfarin and chloral hydrate
Warfarin and clofibrate
Warfarin and nalidixic acid
Warfarin and phenylbutazone
Warfarin and sertraline

DISPLAY 23-5
Medications With Increased or Decreased Receptor Sensitivity in Older Adults

Increased Sensitivity (increased potency)
Angiotensin-converting enzyme (ACE) inhibitors
Diazepam
Digoxin
Diltiazem
Enalapril
Felodipine
Levodopa
Lithium
Midazolam
Morphine
Temazepam
Verapamil
Warfarin

Decreased Sensitivity (may have delayed signs of toxicity)
β-Blockers
Bemetamide
Dopamine
Furosemide
Isoproterenol
Propranolol
Tolbutamide

When more than one protein-bound medication is consumed, the influence of decreased albumin level is intensified. Even in the presence of adequate serum albumin levels, highly protein-bound medications compete for the same sites. Thus, if the serum albumin level is low, the competition will be increased, as will the potential for altered effects. Display 23-4 identifies some medication combinations that are competitive by virtue of their protein-binding capabilities and that, therefore, are likely to be affected by diminished serum albumin levels.

Independent of any changes that affect pharmacokinetics of medications, age-related changes in receptor sensitivity can influence pharmacodynamics and cause older adults to be more or less sensitive to particular medications. For example, an increased sensitivity of the older brain to centrally acting psychotropic medications may potentiate both the therapeutic and adverse effects of these medications. This is particularly true for benzodiazepines, which have stronger sedative effects in older adults. Display 23-5 lists examples of drugs that have increased or decreased sensitivity in older adults. Another age-related change that can affect pharmacodynamics is diminished efficiency of homeostatic mechanisms, such as thermoregulation, fluid regulation, and baroreceptor control over blood pressure. For example, inefficient fluid regulation may alter the action of medications, such as lithium, that are particularly sensitive to fluid and electrolyte balance.

Changes That Affect the Skills Involved With Taking Medications

For any adult, the appropriate consumption of medications is significantly influenced by the following factors:

- Motivation
- Some level of understanding about the purpose of the medication

- An ability to obtain the correct amount of medication, an ability to distinguish the correct container, and an ability to read directions
- An ability to hear and remember verbal instructions
- An ability to understand the correct timing for medication administration and to follow the correct dosage regimen
- Fine motor movement and coordination to remove the medication from the container and administer it

When the medication is to be taken orally, the person must also possess the ability to swallow it. Additional skills related to coordination, manual dexterity, and visual acuity may be required when medications are administered nasally, transdermally, subcutaneously, or by other methods. Age-related changes in hearing or vision can interfere with a person's ability to understand instructions and read directions, especially labels on medicine bottles. Any limitations in fine motor movement of the hands may interfere with the ability to remove lids from medication containers, especially when the lids are tamper resistant. Although the skills related to taking medications are sometimes influenced by age-related changes, more often they are influenced by risk factors that commonly occur in older adults.

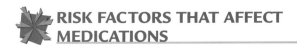

RISK FACTORS THAT AFFECT MEDICATIONS

The effects of medication in the body and the medication-taking behaviors of older adults are affected to a small degree by age-related changes and to a much larger degree by risk factors that are common in older adults. The consumption of more than one medication greatly increases the potential for adverse effects and altered therapeutic effect. Because older adults take a disproportionately greater number of medications than do younger people, they have an increased susceptibility to adverse or altered medication effects. Additional risks arise from myths and misunderstandings that affect the medication consumption patterns of older adults. Finally, certain factors that are unrelated to age, such as weight, gender, and smoking habits, combine with age-related changes and risk factors to increase further the risk for adverse and altered effects.

Weight and Gender

Because body size affects volume of distribution of medications, it also affects both the therapeutic and adverse effects of medications. Thus, older adults who are small or have lost or are losing weight may be particularly at risk for adverse medication effects. Despite the close association between body size and volume of distribution, body weight is not always considered when determining adult medication doses.

Women are at higher risk than men for altered therapeutic effects and increased adverse medication effects. Although little is known about causal relationships, altered medication effects may be associated with any of the following factors that affect women to a greater degree than men: smaller size, hormonal influences, and a higher proportion of body fat to lean body tissue. An additional factor is that women use more drugs than men, particularly psychoactive and antiarthritic agents (Cusack & Vestal, 2000).

Pathologic Processes and Functional Impairments

Because the purpose of any medication is to relieve or control symptoms of pathologic conditions, it can be assumed that people who take medications have at least one disease-related symptom. Disease processes may influence not only the action of medications in the body, but also the skills related to medication consumption, especially if functional limitations

accompany the disease process. Medication–disease interactions may manifest themselves in any of the following ways:

1. Disease processes tend to exacerbate age-related changes that would otherwise have little or no impact on the medication. (For example, malnutrition further decreases serum albumin, thereby increasing both the therapeutic and adverse effects of medications with a high protein-binding capacity.)
2. Disease processes potentiate the therapeutic and adverse effects of medications. (For instance, congestive heart failure decreases both the metabolism and the excretion of most medications.)
3. Adverse medication effects alter disease processes. (For example, anticholinergics may exacerbate prostatic hyperplasia, causing acute urinary retention.)

Any condition that affects the skills involved with taking medications correctly can interfere with the person's ability to comply with medication regimens. For example, hearing and vision impairments can significantly affect the older adult's ability to understand directions and read labels and instructions. Cognitive impairment interferes with the ability to self-manage medication regimens (Akishita et al., 2002). Dysphagia or any condition that affects chewing and swallowing can interfere with the ability to take medications orally.

Behaviors Based on Myths and Misunderstandings

Myths and misunderstandings influence attitudes about medication consumption held by older adults as well as their caregivers. An attitude that can be potentially harmful for older adults is that medications, particularly over-the-counter products, provide a "quick fix" for any uncomfortable symptom. For example, messages promoting constipation remedies reinforce false beliefs about bowel function and lead to laxative abuse. Adults of any age can be influenced by these attitudes, but older adults are more likely than their younger counterparts to have negative consequences because they are more vulnerable to adverse effects and drug interactions when they take medications.

Another potentially harmful attitude is that over-the-counter remedies are always safe, even in extra-strength doses. Although over-the-counter preparations may be relatively safe for healthy younger adults, they often create problems for older adults, particularly in the presence of pathologic conditions and in combination with other medications. For example, many over-the-counter preparations, like remedies for colds and insomnia, contain anticholinergic ingredients that have adverse effects in older adults. In these situations, the addition of a seemingly harmless over-the-counter product to an already complex regimen of prescription medications can be the factor that tips the scale of safety and causes a serious adverse effect, such as delirium.

Attitudes and expectations about medications as quick-fix remedies also can influence the prescribing patterns of primary care practitioners. For example, when over-the-counter remedies are ineffective, people expect their health care practitioners to provide an otherwise unobtainable remedy, through a prescription, for their discomfort. Sometimes, a nonmedication remedy is safer than, and just as effective as, a prescription medication, but these remedies usually demand more of the practitioner's time and some degree of patient motivation. Another factor contributing to the reluctance of practitioners to suggest nonmedication remedies is that there are more controlled clinical trials supporting the use of medications and many of the nonmedication remedies are not as well studied. Sleep and anxiety complaints are examples of conditions that respond to nonmedication treatments but that are often addressed by prescription medications because of attitudes of the patient or primary care practitioner.

Communication Barriers

Another factor that may contribute to increased use of prescriptions by older adults is the older adult's reluctance to challenge or question the primary care practitioner because he or she perceives the primary care practitioner as all knowing. Although the image of the infallible physician is subsiding, older adults are still inclined to accept advice from prescribing practitioners without question.

Communication barriers and lack of confidence in one's communication skills may further inhibit someone from discussing prescriptions and other treatments with a health care practitioner. Because medical knowledge has been expanding at a tremendous pace in recent years, decisions about medical conditions are becoming increasingly more complex. Consequently, older adults and other health care consumers may hesitate to ask questions about medical decisions out of fear of appearing ignorant. Hearing impairments and other sensory impairments that are common in older adults also may interfere with patient-directed discussions of a medication plan. Other communication barriers, such as an attitude of impatience on the part of the health care practitioner, also may thwart discussion. In addition, poor command of the English language, on the part of either the older adult or the health care practitioner, can interfere with a discussion of health issues and lead to misunderstandings.

Lack of Information

Despite the fact that older adults are the primary consumers of prescription and over-the-counter medications, our knowledge about medication effects in older adults is insufficient and still in an early phase. Before the 1980s, research on the influence of age on the action of specific medications was virtually nonexistent, and pharmaceutical companies determined normal adult doses based on clinical trials of healthy adult men with an average weight of about 150 pounds (70 kg). In addition, the few studies of age-related influences on medications were cross-sectional rather than longitudinal and identified age differences rather than age-related changes. Moreover, older adults who are included in clinical trials tend to be healthier and young-old rather than medically frail or old-old (Beyth & Shorr, 2002).

Information about medication–medication interactions also is lacking, especially for newly approved medications. Because the U.S. Food and Drug Administration (FDA) does not require the testing of a medication as it interacts with other medications, medication–medication interactions may not be identified until after the medication has been marketed. Thus, any recently approved medication should be used cautiously in older adults who are taking more than one medication because of the increased risk for unpredictable drug interactions. Cimetidine is an example of a medication that is relatively safe when taken alone but that is likely to interact with other medications, potentially causing serious adverse effects, such as mental changes, especially in older people. Examples of other medications that are likely to cause serious adverse effects when consumed with another medication include alcohol, phenytoin, digoxin, analgesics, theophylline, anticoagulants, and psychotropic agents.

In 1982, the U.S. Pharmacopoeia, which sets the official standards for medications in the United States, established a geriatrics advisory panel to examine age-related influences on medication action. By the late 1980s, two trends emerged in the pharmaceutical industry that may benefit older adults: (1) pharmaceutical companies began testing medications on older adults, and (2) they began focusing on adverse medication effects, including medication interactions. Although pharmaceutical companies do not routinely recommend geriatric doses, some progress has been made, and geriatric dosage adjustments are sometimes recommended when new medications are released. Pharmaceutical companies also are providing information about drug interactions when new drugs are released and on an ongoing basis when drug interactions are discovered after a drug has been on the market. In addition, because of the emphasis on adverse reactions, new medications are developed and promoted not only for their therapeutic effectiveness but also for their lack of unwanted effects.

Inappropriate Prescribing Practices

During the late 1980s, geriatricians began to address medication-related problems of older adults because of widespread concerns about the large numbers as well as the types of drugs prescribed for older adults (Giron et al., 2001). The term *inappropriate medications* was used to describe drugs that were not appropriate for use with older adults (Sloane et al., 2002). In 1991, an international panel of experts in geriatrics and pharmacology developed and published explicit criteria for identifying inappropriate medication use in nursing home residents (Beers et al., 1991). Drugs were judged inappropriate by the expert panel if better drugs were available or if they were ineffective or had poor safety profiles (Dhalla et al., 2002). For example, diazepam was deemed inappropriate because it increases the risk for falls and fractures, and therapeutic effectiveness can be achieved with shorter-acting benzodiazepines that are safer. These criteria were later updated and expanded to include potentially inappropriate medication use for any person 65 years of age or older (Beers, 1997).

These "Beers criteria" have been widely used by clinicians, researchers, and drug utilization reviewers, and the Health Care Financing Administration has been using a modified version of the criteria since 1999 in nursing home surveys (Gurwitz & Rochon, 2002; Sloane et al., 2002). Studies published during the 1990s concluded that inappropriate prescribing practices for older adults, particularly in relation to psychotropic medications, were common in nursing homes, community settings, outpatient departments, and board and care homes (Hanlon et al., 2002; Mort & Aparasu, 2000; Pitkala et al., 2002; Sloane et al., 2002). Several studies using these criteria found that the number of drugs prescribed was the most significant predictor of inappropriate prescribing and that amitriptyline, long-acting benzodiazepines, and nonsteroidal antiinflammatory drugs were the most common classes of inappropriate drug use (Dhalla et al.,

2002; Hanlon et al., 2000). Although inappropriate prescribing practices are still common, more recent studies suggest "that there have been meaningful improvements in the quality of medication use in elderly patients since 1987" (Gurwitz & Rochon, 2002, p. 1670). Studies also suggest that the 1987 Nursing Home Reform Act, which mandated that the Health Care Financing Administration address the overuse of psychotropic drugs in nursing facilities, has resulted in more appropriate use of antipsychotics and antianxiety agents for nursing home residents (Hughes et al., 2000).

Much of the attention during the 1990s was on the inappropriate prescribing of medications that should not be used in older adults because of the risk for serious adverse effects. By the early 2000s, however, some geriatricians viewed this "good drug–bad drug" approach as inappropriately narrow because it did not address the more important issue of underuse of beneficial therapies in older adults (Gurwitz & Rochon, 2002). Researchers and clinicians began raising concerns about the underuse of medications for both treatment and prevention of conditions and symptoms such as pain, stroke, osteoporosis, hypertension, depression, hyperlipidemia, and cardiovascular disease (Knight & Avorn, 2001; Rochon & Gurwitz, 1999). Currently, geriatricians are advising that underutilization of necessary medications receive the same level of attention that recently has been given to problems of overuse and misuse of drug therapies in older adults (Gurwitz & Rochon, 2002; Knight & Avorn, 2001). One recent summary emphasized, "Finding the right balance between too few and too many drugs will ensure increased longevity, improved overall health, and enhanced functioning and quality of life for the aging population" (Williams, 2002, p. 1917).

Polypharmacy and Inadequate Monitoring of Medications

Polypharmacy refers to the use of multiple medications, often from multiple sources. A typical older adult in the United States takes four to five prescription and two over-the-counter drugs at a time and fills 12 to 17 prescriptions per year (Cusack & Vestal, 2000). This level of medication use is primarily associated with the increased prevalence of chronic illness among older adults, and it is usually appropriate and therapeutic; however, polypharmacy is also associated with a significant increase in drug interactions and adverse medication effects. As the number and sources of medications increase, the need for monitoring becomes more important, from the time of the initial prescription until the termination of treatment. The following risk factors are likely to interfere with medication monitoring in older adults:

- Patient consultations with multiple health care providers, who usually do not communicate about the patient's care
- Health care practitioners' lack of information about medications obtained from a variety of sources (i.e., prescription medications offered by friends and relatives, or nonprescription products, such as herbs, nutritional supplements, and over-the-counter products)
- Health care practitioners' lack of information about a patient's nonadherence to a treatment regimen
- A patient's fear of disclosing information about folk remedies or about medications obtained from sources other than the prescribing health care practitioner
- A patient's fear about disclosing information about self-directed changes in the medication regimen
- An assumption by the patient or health care practitioner that, once most medications are started, they should be continued indefinitely
- An assumption by the patient or health care practitioner that, once an appropriate medication dosage is established, it will not need to be changed
- An assumption by the patient or health care practitioner that a lack of adverse effects early in the course of treatment indicates that adverse effects will never occur
- Changes in the patient's weight, especially weight loss, which may affect pharmacokinetics
- Changes in the patient's daily habits, which may affect pharmacokinetics (e.g., smoking, activity level, or nutrient and fluid intake)
- Changes in the patient's mental-emotional status, which may affect medication consumption patterns
- Changes in the patient's health status, which may affect medication actions, increasing the potential for adverse effects

Medication Nonadherence and Financial Factors

Medication nonadherence (also called noncompliance) refers to medication-taking patterns that differ from the prescribed pattern, including missed doses, not filling prescriptions, or taking medications too frequently or at inappropriate times. Nonadherence occurs to some degree in about half of all adults for whom long-term medication regimens have been prescribed. Although health care practitioners often view nonadherence as a problem more strongly associated with older than younger adults, this perspective is not necessarily accurate. Studies have found that a busy lifestyle influences medication adherence, which may be better in older adults than in middle-aged adults (Park et al., 1999; Renteln-Kruse, 2000). Other factors that contribute to nonadherence include living alone, financial considerations, type of disease, adverse medication effects, complex medication regimens, increased frequency of dosing, cognitive and sensory impairments, poor understanding of the medication regimen, and the relationship between the patient and the primary care practitioner.

In recent years, there is increasing attention to the rapidly increasing cost of medications and the lack of health insurance coverage for prescriptions. More than one third of Medicare beneficiaries do not have any prescription drug coverage, and nearly half of those who do have coverage have limited or intermittent benefits (Stuart & Shea, 2001). Moreover, the cost of prescription drugs is increasing rapidly and significantly. A report by Families USA (2002) found that between January 2001 and January 2002, the prices of the brand-name drugs most commonly used by older people increased 8.1%, which is three times the rate of inflation. Older adults are affected disproportionately by increasing drug prices because they consume more than one third of all prescriptions and account for more than 42% of total drug expenditures (Families USA, 2002). Both the high cost of medications and the lack of prescription drug insurance contribute to nonadherence because these factors cause older adults to avoid filling prescriptions, save medications for future use, take less than the prescribed dose, and take medications that are prescribed for another person (Mitchell et al., 2001).

Insufficient Recognition of Adverse Medication Effects

In older adults, manifestations of adverse effects often are misinterpreted or not recognized as such because of their similarity to age-related changes or commonly occurring pathologic conditions in older adults. Studies have found that nurses and physicians in acute care settings detect only 5% to 15% of ongoing adverse medication effects (Hohl et al., 2001). When an older adult experiences an adverse medication reaction, two or three potential causes, other than the medication, usually can be identified. For example, when an older adult becomes depressed, a psychosocial factor, such as widowhood, may be identified as the source of the depression. Even if the person is taking a medication that is known to cause depression (e.g., benzodiazepines, propranolol), the depression may be viewed as a primary problem. As two noted geriatricians recently stated, "Another important aspect of medication use in vulnerable elders is that the patient, caregivers, or even physician often mistake side effects for the onset of new illness, or worse, for aging itself" (Knight & Avorn, 2001, p. 703). This mistake may lead to treatment with additional medications, rather than the direct and more appropriate approach of dealing with the adverse effect. Although adverse effects are not unique to older adults, they occur more commonly with increasing age and are more likely to be attributed erroneously to pathologic conditions or age-related changes and circumstances. Table 23-1 summarizes adverse medication effects that are likely to remain unrecognized in older adults because of their similarity to age-related changes.

MEDICATION INTERACTIONS WITH OTHER SUBSTANCES

Medications can interact with almost any other substance, including herbs, caffeine, nutrients, alcohol, nicotine, and other medications. These interactions occur not only with prescription medications but also with over-the-counter products (e.g., analgesics, antihistamines). Outcomes of medication interactions with other substances include altered or erratic therapeutic effect, increased potential for adverse effects, and, in rare cases, a decreased potential for adverse effects.

Medication–Medication Interactions

The risk for adverse effects from interactions between two or more medications increases exponentially according to the number of medications being consumed. Because older adults are more likely than younger people to take two or more medications

TABLE 23-1 • Some Adverse Medication Effects That May Remain Unrecognized in Older Adults

Manifestation	Medication Type	Specific Examples
Cognitive impairment	Antidepressants; antipsychotics; antianxiety agents; anticholinergics; hypoglycemics; OTC cold, cough, and sleeping preparations	Perphenazine, amitriptyline, chlorpromazine, diazepam, chlordiazepoxide, benztropine, trihexyphenidyl, cimetidine, digoxin, barbiturates, tolazamide, tolbutamide, chlorpheniramine, diphenhydramine
Depression	Antihypertensives, antiarthritics, antianxiety agents, antipsychotics	Reserpine, clonidine, propranolol, indomethacin, haloperidol, barbiturates
Urinary incontinence	Diuretics, anticholinergics	Furosemide, doxepin, thioridazine, lorazepam
Constipation	Narcotics, antacids, antipsychotics, antidepressants	Codeine, chlorpromazine, calcium carbonate, aluminum hydroxide, amoxapine
Vision impairment	Digitalis, antiarthritics, phenothiazines	Digoxin, indomethacin, ibuprofen, chlorpromazine
Hearing impairment	Mycin antibiotics, salicylates, loop diuretics	Gentamicin, aspirin, furosemide, bumetanide
Postural hypotension	Antihypertensives, diuretics, antipsychotics, antidepressants	Guanethidine, furosemide, propranolol, chlorpromazine, imipramine, clonidine
Hypothermia	Antipsychotics, alcohol, salicylates	Haloperidol, aspirin, alcohol, fluphenazine
Sexual dysfunction	Antihypertensives, antipsychotics, antidepressants, alcohol, antihypertensives	Timolol, clonidine, thiazides, haloperidol, amitriptyline, alcohol, cimetidine, propranolol, methyldopa
Mobility problems	Sedatives, antianxiety agents, antipsychotics, ototoxic medications	Chloral hydrate, diazepam, furosemide, gentamicin
Dry mouth	Anticholinergics, corticosteroids, bronchodilators, antihypertensives	Chlorpromazine, haloperidol, prednisone, furosemide, sertraline, theophylline
Anorexia	Digitalis, bronchodilators, antihistamines	Digoxin, theophylline, diphenhydramine
Drowsiness	Antidepressants, antipsychotics, OTC cold preparations, alcohol, barbiturates	Amitriptyline, haloperidol, chlorpheniramine, secobarbital
Edema	Antiarthritics, corticosteroids, antihypertensives	Ibuprofen, indomethacin, prednisone, reserpine, methyldopa
Tremors	Antipsychotics	Haloperidol, chlorpromazine, thioridazine

OTC, over-the-counter.

concurrently, they are at increased risk for medication–medication interactions. Medication–medication interactions are often caused by the competitive action of chemicals, but they may be caused by any mechanism that influences the absorption, distribution, metabolism, or elimination of any of the medications. Effects of medication–medication interactions include increased or decreased serum levels of either one or both of the medications, with subsequent altered therapeutic effects and increased risk for adverse or toxic effects. Table 23-2 summarizes specific mechanisms of medication–medication interactions and examples of each type that are most likely to occur in older adults.

Medication–Nutrient Interactions

Interactions between a medication and a nutrient or dietary supplement can affect either the nutrient or the medication. Because the influence of medications on nutrients was addressed in Chapter 14, this chapter focuses on the effects of nutrients and dietary supplements on medications. In the context of medication–nutrient interactions, the term *nutrient* includes foods, beverages, and enteral formulas. Commonly consumed foods that can affect medications include cocoa, coffee, fiber, alcohol, protein, cabbage, caffeinated tea, and brussels sprouts. In addition, food preparation methods, such as charcoal

broiling, can affect certain medications. As with other interactions, medication–nutrient interactions are not unique to older adults, but they are likely to have more serious consequences in older adults. Nutrients can affect medication by altering absorption of oral medications in the stomach through any of the following mechanisms:

- Delayed transit time or slowed gastric emptying
- Competitive binding of molecules
- Diminished stomach secretions

In many situations, the effect of the nutrient is to diminish the absorption of the medication, causing the serum levels to be lower than expected. In other situations, however, the effect on the medication is delayed absorption, which increases the time required to reach peak serum levels but does not necessarily affect the total amount absorbed. In some situations, delayed gastric emptying increases the amount of medication that is absorbed before it passes into the small intestine. Table 23-3 summarizes common medication–nutrient interactions.

Medication–Alcohol Interactions

Alcohol interacts with medications in the same way as other central nervous system depressants, but because of societal attitudes about alcohol consumption, medication–alcohol interactions often are not

TABLE 23-2 • Types and Examples of Medication–Medication Interactions

Type of Interaction	Example	
	Interaction	*Effect*
Binding effect (e.g., an oral drug diminishes the absorption of another drug in the stomach)	Magnesium- or aluminum-containing antacids may bind with tetracycline in the stomach	Decreased effects of tetracycline
Metabolism interference effect (e.g., one drug interferes with liver metabolism of another drug)	Ciprofloxacin and anticonvulsants inhibit metabolism of warfarin	Increased effects of warfarin
Metabolism enhancing effect (e.g., one drug activates the drug-metabolizing enzymes in the liver)	Phenobarbital increases metabolism of warfarin	Decreased effects of warfarin
Elimination interference effect (e.g., one drug interferes with the renal elimination of another drug)	Furosemide can interfere with elimination of salicylates	Increased effects of salicylates
Elimination enhancement effect (e.g., renal reabsorption is blocked because of altered urinary pH)	Sodium bicarbonate can enhance excretion of lithium, tetracyclines, and salicylates	Decreased effects of lithium, tetracycline, or salicylate
Competitive or displacement effect (e.g., two drugs compete at receptor sites)	Diphenhydramine may interfere with effect of cholinergic agents (e.g., tacrine, donepezil)	Decreased effects of tacrine or donepezil
Potentiating effect (e.g., two drugs produce greater effects when taken together even though they have different actions)	Acetaminophen taken with codeine has a greater analgesic effect than either medication taken alone	Increased analgesic effect
Additive effect (e.g., two drugs produce greater effect because they have similar action)	Verapamil or diltiazem may have additive effect when taken with a β-blocker	Increased effect on blood pressure

TABLE 23-3 • Medication–Nutrient Interactions	
Effect on Medication	**Example of Interaction Effect**
Delayed absorption rate, no effect on amount absorbed	Ingestion of food may delay absorption of cimetidine, digoxin, and ibuprofen.
Reduced rate and amount of absorption	Calcium decreases absorption of tetracycline. A high-protein or high-fiber meal decreases absorption of levodopa.
Reduced absorption because of nonnutrient components	Caffeinated tea and fiber intake interfere with iron absorption.
Increased absorption	High-fat foods increase serum levels of griseofulvin.
Decreased therapeutic effect	Vitamin K decreases the effectiveness of warfarin. Charcoal broiling of foods diminishes the effectiveness of aminophylline or theophylline.
Increased rate of metabolism	A high-protein diet increases the metabolism of theophylline.

TABLE 23-4 • Medication–Alcohol Interactions	
Type of Interaction	**Example of Interaction Effect**
Altered metabolism of benzodiazepines when combined with alcohol	Increased psychomotor impairment and adverse effects
Altered metabolism of barbiturates and meprobamate when combined with alcohol	Central nervous system depression
Competition between alcohol and chloral hydrate at metabolic sites	Increased serum levels of alcohol and chloral hydrate
Altered metabolism of alcohol when combined with chlorpromazine	Increased serum levels of alcohol and acetylhyde; increased psychomotor impairment
Enhanced vasodilation as a result of a combination of alcohol and nitrates	Severe hypotension and headache, enhanced absorption of nitroglycerin
Altered hepatic gluconeogenesis, which influences the action of oral hypoglycemics, as a result of alcohol	Potentiation of oral hypoglycemics by alcohol

addressed. Health care practitioners may not inquire about a patient's use of alcohol, and even when people are asked, they may not accurately acknowledge the amount of alcohol used. Alcohol is consumed not only in beverages, but also in over-the-counter preparations, some of which are composed of up to 40% alcohol. Categories of over-the-counter preparations that are most likely to contain alcohol include mouthwashes, vitamin and mineral tonics, and liquid cough and cold preparations. When taken in combination with medications, alcohol can alter the therapeutic action of the medication and increase the potential for adverse effects. Older adults may be more susceptible to developing medication–alcohol interactions because age-related changes in body composition cause higher serum levels of alcohol, as compared with those achieved when a younger person consumes an equivalent amount of alcohol. In addition, an age-related decrease in the stomach enzymes that metabolize alcohol can cause a concomitant increase in serum level of alcohol (Fingerhood, 2000). As with other types of medication–medication interactions, medication–alcohol interactions can alter either the alcohol or the medication. Table 23-4 lists some of the medication–alcohol interactions that are most likely to occur in older adults.

Physiologically, women are more vulnerable to the toxic effects of alcohol compared with men of the same stature (Ludwick et al., 2000).

Medication–Caffeine and Medication–Nicotine Interactions

Medication–caffeine and medication–nicotine interactions have received little attention despite the widespread use of caffeine and nicotine and the fact that interactions between these substances and medications can be as harmful as medication–medication interactions. Caffeine is found not only in food and beverages but also in many over-the-counter analgesics and cold preparations. Most medication–caffeine interactions affect the action of the medication rather than that of the caffeine; however, a few medications alter caffeine metabolism and increase its serum half-life. Table 23-5 lists examples of medication–caffeine interactions.

Medication–nicotine interactions arise from cigarette smoking and are affected by fluctuations in smoking habits. Nicotine can affect medications through the following actions:

- Vasoconstriction
- Stimulation of the central nervous system
- Increased gastric acid secretions
- Altered metabolism of liver enzymes

Most often, the medication–nicotine interaction interferes with the therapeutic action of the medication, and smokers may require higher doses of a medication than nonsmokers to achieve the same therapeutic effects. For example, smokers may require increased doses of insulin, anticoagulants, antihypertensives, and pain relievers (Lee & D'Alonzo, 1993).

TABLE 23-5 • Medication–Caffeine Interactions

Type of Interaction	Example of Interaction Effect
Caffeine-induced increase in gastric acid secretion	Decreased absorption of iron
Caffeine-induced gastrointestinal irritation	Decreased effectiveness of cimetidine; increased gastrointestinal irritation from corticosteroids, alcohol, and analgesics
Altered caffeine metabolism	Prolonged effect of caffeine when combined with ciprofloxacin, estrogen, or cimetidine
Caffeine-induced cardiac arrhythmic effect	Decreased effectiveness of antiarrhythmic medications
Caffeine-induced hypokalemia	Exacerbated hypokalemic effect of diuretics
Caffeine-induced stimulation of the central nervous system	Increased stimulation effects from amantadine, decongestants, fluoxetine, and theophylline
Caffeine-induced increase in excretion of lithium	Decreased effectiveness of lithium

Table 23-6 lists common medication–nicotine interactions.

Medication–Herb Interactions

With the recent dramatic increase in the use of herbs by people in the United States, it is becoming increasingly important to address potential interactions between herbs and other bioactive agents, such as

TABLE 23-6 • Medication–Nicotine Interactions

Type of Interaction	Example of Interaction Effect
Nicotine-induced alteration in metabolism	Decreased efficacy of analgesics, lorazepam, theophylline, aminophylline, β-blockers, and calcium channel blockers
Nicotine-induced vasoconstriction	Increased peripheral ischemic effect of β-blockers
Nicotine-induced central nervous system stimulation	Decreased drowsiness from benzodiazepines and phenothiazines
Nicotine-induced stimulation of antidiuretic hormone secretion	Fluid retention, decreased effectiveness of diuretics
Nicotine-induced increase in platelet activity	Decreased anticoagulant effectiveness (heparin, warfarin); increased risk of thrombosis with estrogen use
Nicotine-induced increase in gastric acid	Decreased or negated effects of H_2 antagonists (cimetidine, famotidine, nizatidine, ranitidine)

TABLE 23-7 • Medications and Herbs with Similar Bioactivity

Medication	Herb
Aspirin	Birch bark Willow bark Wintergreen Meadowsweet
Anticoagulants	Feverfew Garlic Ginkgo biloba
Caffeine	Guarana Kola nut
Ephedrine	Ephedra
Estrogen	Black cohosh Fennel Red clover Stinging nettle
Lithium	Thyme Purslane
Monoamine oxidase inhibitors	Ginseng St. John's wort Yohimbe
Nicotine	Lobelia
Calcium channel blockers	Angelica

medications. Herbs that are similar in bioactivity to over-the-counter or prescription medications can potentiate the effects of the medication and increase the risk for adverse effects and drug interactions. Table 23-7 lists some herbs and medications that have similar bioactivity. In addition, many medication–herb interactions have been identified in recent years because of increased use of herbs and increased attention to interactions, and medication–herb interactions are now commonly listed in pharmacology references. Table 23-8 lists some of the medication–herb interactions that are likely to occur in older adults.

FUNCTIONAL CONSEQUENCES ASSOCIATED WITH MEDICATIONS IN OLDER ADULTS

The major functional consequence of age-related changes that affect medication effectiveness and use, even in healthy older adults, is an increased potential for both altered therapeutic action and adverse medication effects. Polypharmacy and other risk factors further increase the potential for these negative functional consequences and can cause additional functional consequences, such as medication interactions with other substances. Age-related changes and risk factors also affect medication consumption patterns, increasing the possibility of nonadherence and the potential for adverse and altered therapeutic effects.

deserves special attention with regard to older adults for the following reasons:

- Older adults are more likely than younger adults to experience tardive dyskinesia.
- Advanced age correlates with both an earlier onset and increased severity of tardive dyskinesia.
- The chance of reversing tardive dyskinesia decreases with increasing age.
- When combined with age-related changes and risk factors, tardive dyskinesia can seriously impair the ability of the older adult to perform activities of daily living (ADLs).
- When combined with psychosocial influences, the negative impact of tardive dyskinesia on self-esteem can be especially detrimental.
- Tardive dyskinesia is associated with the long-term use of antipsychotic medications, which are sometimes used inappropriately in older adults for behaviors that could be managed with nonmedication interventions.

Factors that can increase the risk for tardive dyskinesia include dementia, depression, age-related neurochemical changes, and early extrapyramidal reactions to medications. The reversibility of tardive dyskinesia depends on early detection of the signs and discontinuation of the causative medication. Vitamins B_6 and E have been used effectively to reverse tardive dyskinesia in some patients.

Increased Potential for Altered Mental Status

Although medications can cause mental changes (e.g., delirium, depression) in anyone, older adults are at increased risk for medication-induced altered mental status because of age-related changes and risk factors. In addition, when older adults experience a change in their mental status, these changes are likely to be attributed to dementia or another pathologic condition, rather than being recognized as adverse medication effects. Nurses need to be alert to the possibility that even a simple over-the-counter product, such as diphenhydramine, is a common cause of mental changes in older adults.

Delirium is an acute confusional state that can be precipitated by any medication or by medication interactions. Older adults are particularly susceptible to medication-induced delirium because of altered neurochemical activity in the brain. Moreover, their risk for medication-induced delirium is increased by some pathologic conditions, such as dementia, dehydration, malnutrition, head injury, or central nervous system infection. Even at nontoxic serum levels, or at doses considered normal, medications can cause mental changes in older adults.

Older adults are particularly susceptible to mental changes and other adverse effects from medications with anticholinergic effects (e.g., many psychotropic agents and over-the-counter preparations for coughs, colds, and insomnia). In recent years, geriatricians are emphasizing the importance of assessing the "total anticholinergic burden," described as the cumulative effect of medications that have anticholinergic effects, even though they are not specifically designated as anticholinergic agents (Knight & Avorn, 2001). Some drugs commonly used by older adults that have strongly anticholinergic effects, despite not being categorized primarily as anticholinergic agents, include digoxin, cimetidine, ranitidine, nifedipine, prednisolone, theophylline, warfarin, and isosorbide mononitrate (Tune, 2001). An anticholinergic burden score can be calculated to determine the combined effect of all anticholinergic agents that are taken by someone during 1 day (Aizenberg et al., 2002). Table 23-10 lists medications that have detectable anticholinergic effects and can cause mental changes, even in healthy older adults.

Older adults with dementia are doubly jeopardized by anticholinergic drugs because dementia is associated with decreased levels of acetylcholine in the brain. Older adults with dementia have been found to be even more likely than healthy older adults to develop medication-induced cognitive impairment, particularly from anticholinergic drugs (Roe et al., 2002). In addition, the therapeutic effectiveness of the cholinesterase inhibitors for people with dementia is associated with the ability of these drugs to increase available acetylcholine in the brain. Thus, if a cholinesterase inhibitor is being used to treat dementia, an anticholinergic agent may counteract the effects of the antidementia drug and negate any therapeutic effectiveness. This is an important consideration for people with dementia who are taking antidepressants, antipsychotics, antispasmodics, or antiparkinsonian agents. Even over-the-counter antihistamines, such as diphenhydramine, can interfere with the therapeutic effectiveness of the cholinesterase inhibitors. Some medications that are likely to cause mental changes in older adults, as well as the mechanisms underlying these adverse actions, are listed in Table 23-11.

Psychosocial Consequences of Adverse Effects

Older adults experience serious psychosocial consequences when adverse medication effects precipitate mental changes, especially if the cause of the mental change is not recognized. Depression, delirium, and dementia are common adverse medication effects that interfere with one's functional abilities and quality of

TABLE 23-10 • Medications With Anticholinergic Effects

Drug Category	Examples of Medications With Potent Anticholinergic Effects
Antidepressants	Amitriptyline Doxepine Nefazodone Trazodone
Antihistamines	Chlorpheniramine Cyproheptadine Dexchlorpheniramine Diphenhydramine Hydroxyzine Meclizine Promethazine Tyripelennamine
Antipsychotics	Chlorpromazine Clozapine Fluphenazine Prochlorperazine Promethazine Thioridazine Triflupromazine
Gastrointestinal agents	Belladonna Cimetidine Clinidium Dicyclomine Diphenoxylate Hyoscyamine Ranitidine
Urinary antispasmodics	Oxybutynin
Antiparkinson agents	Benztropine Trihexyphenidyl
Cardiovascular agents	Digoxin Disopyramide Isosorbide dinitrate Lanoxin Nifedipine
Miscellaneous agents	Furosemide Prednisolone Theophylline Warfarin

TABLE 23-11 • Mechanisms of Action for Mental Changes Caused by Adverse Medication Effects

Mechanism of Action	Examples
Anticholinergic effects	Atropine, scopolamine, antihistamines, antipsychotics, antidepressants, antispasmodics, antiparkinsonian agents
Decreased cerebral blood flow	Antihypertensives, antipsychotics
Depression of respiratory center	Central nervous system depressants
Fluid and electrolyte alterations	Diuretics, alcohol, laxatives
Altered thermoregulation	Alcohol, psychotropics, narcotics
Acidosis	Diuretics, alcohol, nicotinic acid
Hypoglycemia	Hypoglycemics, alcohol, propranolol
Hormonal disturbances	Thyroid extract, corticosteroids
Depression-inducing action	Reserpine, methyldopa, indomethacin, barbiturates, fluphenazine, haloperidol, corticosteroids

NURSING ASSESSMENT OF MEDICATION USE AND EFFECTS

The nurse assesses the older adult's use of medications, and the effects of the medications being used, to accomplish the following:

- Determine the effectiveness of the medication regimen
- Identify any factors that interfere with the correct regimen
- Ascertain risks for adverse effects or altered therapeutic actions (with particular attention to older adults at increased risk)
- Detect adverse medication effects
- Identify opportunities for health education

During a medication assessment, the nurse clarifies the prescribed medication regimen as well as the person's actual medication-taking behavior, which may differ from the prescribed regimen. Assessment information is obtained by interviewing the older adult and his or her caregivers and by observing patterns of medication use by the older adult.

Using Communication Techniques to Obtain Accurate Information

Obtaining accurate information about medications and medication-taking behaviors is difficult for a variety of reasons. Time limitations and lack of a

life and, if not reversed, may have long-term or permanent detrimental effects. It is important to keep in mind that medication-induced mental changes do not always subside immediately after the offending medication is discontinued. In some cases, it may take several weeks after the medication is decreased or discontinued for mental function to return to the pre-medication level.

Other adverse medication effects can cause serious and long-term detrimental psychosocial consequences through their effects on functional abilities. For example, medication-induced postural hypotension has been identified as a contributing factor in falls and fractured hips.

Figure 23-1 summarizes age-related changes, risk factors, and functional consequences as they relate to medications and the older adult.

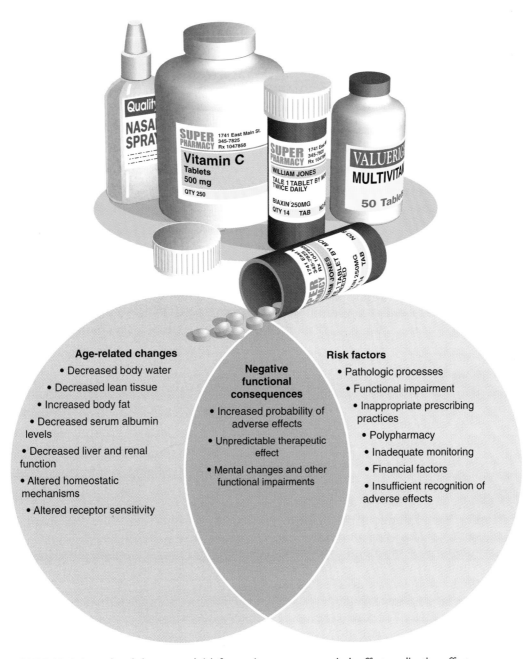

FIGURE 23-1 Age-related changes and risk factors intersect to negatively affect medication effects and compliance in older adults.

trusting relationship may present barriers to obtaining an accurate medication assessment. Because medication assessments often are very time consuming, and because the older adult may not think of all the information during the first interview or may initially be reluctant to reveal accurate information, it may be necessary to conduct the medication assessment over the course of two or more visits.

Another barrier to an effective medication assessment may be a reluctance on the part of the

older adult to share information. Older adults may hesitate to answer questions about their medications because they perceive this information, including information about the use of alcohol, as being very private. Many older adults have received care from primary care practitioners who have communicated an attitude of secrecy about prescription medications, blood pressure readings, and other aspects of medical care. Although this attitude of secrecy is no longer common among health care providers, many older adults have learned not to ask questions, and they may believe that they are not entitled to information about medical aspects of their care. Also, they may be unsure of what questions to ask. Many older adults welcome the opportunity to discuss medications with a nurse, but initially they may hesitate to ask questions or share information. Once the nurse has established a trusting relationship and has initiated a medication interview, the assessment often provides an excellent basis for uncovering and discussing questions about medications. In addition, it often helps the nurse identify many opportunities for health education about medications.

Another barrier to obtaining accurate medication information is the older adult's fear of judgment, especially if the prescribed regimen is not being followed exactly, or if home remedies, alternative therapies, or over-the-counter medications are being used. Because people are reluctant to admit that they do not follow the health care practitioner's orders exactly as expected, they are likely to recite the prescribed regimen, rather than describe what they actually do. People also may be reluctant to discuss the reasons they do not follow a medication regimen, and this can create additional barriers. For example, older adults who cannot afford medications may be embarrassed to discuss their limited finances.

Nurses can use open-ended questions and convey a nonjudgmental attitude during the medication interview to address these barriers to obtaining accurate information. For example, if the question "Are you taking anyone else's medications?" is asked in a matter-of-fact way, an honest response may be elicited. Similarly, asking the question "What do you do when you miss a dose of medicine?" in a matter-of-fact way may elicit a more honest response than asking, "Do you ever miss a dose of medication?" with a judgmental tone of voice. People are more likely to be honest if they view the nurse as a problem solver, rather than as an authority figure who judges or criticizes their health habits. Information about the use of home remedies and over-the-counter preparations is more likely to be elicited by posing open-ended questions than by asking specific questions about medications used for particular problems. For example, the question "What do you do to help you sleep?" is more open-ended than the question "Do you take any medications for sleep?" because the latter may be interpreted only in relation to prescription medications.

In addition to using open-ended questions, nurses can use leading questions to identify risk factors that interfere with the older person's ability to take medications accurately. These questions are based on the nurse's knowledge about factors that commonly interfere with obtaining medications. For example, because the high cost of medications and lack of insurance coverage for medications is a commonly acknowledged problem, the nurse can ask a leading question such as "I know that some of these medications that are prescribed for you can be quite expensive; do you have any problems with getting them?" Similarly, asking a question such as "I know you don't drive—are you able to have your medications delivered, or do you have someone who helps you get them from the pharmacy?" may elicit information about transportation barriers.

The nursing assessment also includes questions about the person's ability to take his or her medications as prescribed, based on the nurse's observations. For example, if the nurse observes that a prescribed medication is very large or difficult to take, a question such as, "Do you have any trouble swallowing these capsules?" might be appropriate. Similarly, if the nurse knows that the older adult has limited hand strength, an appropriate assessment question would be "Do you have any difficulty getting the caps off your medication bottles?"

Information obtained from an interview with the older adult can be supplemented by information derived from caregivers and direct observations of the older person. A nonthreatening technique that may elicit more accurate information than direct questions is to ask about the person's method of organizing medications. For example, people taking medications often have a method of organizing their regimen by using divided medication boxes or written charts or schedules. They usually are willing to show this organizational system to the nurse and, in fact, may be proud to discuss their method with the nurse during the medication assessment.

Observing Patterns of Medication Use

In addition to obtaining medication assessment information through questions and discussions, nurses obtain essential assessment information by reviewing the person's array of medications. When nurses conduct the medication assessment in the home setting, they can ask to see all the medications that the older person uses. In settings other than the home, the nurse can ask the older adult ahead of time to bring in all of his or her medications. In community settings, such as senior meal programs, nurses might sponsor a "brown bag" medication review session. Program participants are asked to bring all their medications with them to an educational session, during which the nurse provides group education and individual assessment and counseling regarding the medications. Because older people often are very comfortable discussing medications with their peers, this method is both non-threatening and quite effective.

Direct observation of medication containers provides useful information, such as the actual prescription instructions and the dates of prescription refills. Nurses must use this information cautiously, however, because the contents of the medication containers may not be the original medications. Inconsistencies between the prescription label and the contents of the container may be used as a basis for further questioning. For example, if the label indicates that the original prescription was for 30 pills and the prescription has not been refilled for 1 year, the nurse might inquire about the reason for this. The patient may explain that the prescription is so expensive that he or she takes it only occasionally. Often the nurse will find that the original container is not being used because it has a childproof cap that the person cannot manipulate. The pills may then be stored in an incorrectly labeled container, which increases the risk for medication errors.

Another reason for direct examination of medication containers is to discover information about sources of care and duplication of medications. People who are seeing more than one health care practitioner may not acknowledge multiple sources of prescriptions, but this information can be discovered by reading prescription labels. Nurses also may discover that the same or similar medications are being prescribed by more than one health care practitioner, or under more than one brand name. Because of the use of generic medications and the increasing number of brand names and similar medications, people can inadvertently be taking duplicate medications. The person taking the duplicate medication usually is unaware of this because the medications are dispensed with different names on the labels.

Dates on labels also reveal important information that can lead to additional questions. For example, if there are three types of antihypertensive medications, each prescribed at a different time, the nurse can inquire whether the second or third medication was supposed to replace or supplement the original medication. Finally, checking the prescription container can provide valuable clues to adherence. By looking at the date on the label, the amount of the last refill, and the contents of the prescription container, nurses can make a rough estimate of the consumption pattern.

Performing a Comprehensive Medication Assessment

In the 1960s, Doris Schwartz, a nurse-researcher who was among the first to investigate problems of medication use in elderly people, advocated the use of a 24-hour drug history, similar to a nutrition history, to gather information (Schwartz et al., 1962). Such a history may be obtained by asking the older person about a typical day: "When you first get up in the morning, what medicine do you take?" "What medicine is next?" and so on, continuing through the day and night in this way. This approach is more likely to elicit accurate information than simply asking the person to recite the prescribed regimen.

During the medication interview, the nurse inquires about prescription and over-the-counter medications, home remedies, vitamins and minerals, and herbal and homeopathic remedies as well as alcohol, caffeine, and nicotine. In addition to inquiring about pills and liquid medications, nurses ask about remedies and medications administered by any other route (e.g., nasal, aural, topical, optical, injection, dermal patch). Nurses must be alert to the increasing use of alternative products and should include open-ended questions about any products that might be considered nontraditional in Western cultures. Most herbs, home remedies, and alternative products contain relatively safe doses of active ingredients; however, some have the potential for interactions and adverse effects, as already discussed. A discussion of home remedies and alternative health care practices may be valuable in identifying health beliefs and in obtaining information about medication-taking behaviors. Also, it is important to elicit information about medications that are used only sporadically or as needed because these can contribute to medication interactions, erratic medication effects, and adverse effects when they are taken. Information about doses of vitamins and minerals is important because megavitamins or high doses of some preparations may be harmful. For example, pyridoxine (vitamin B_6) can interfere with coordination or cause peripheral neuropathy at doses greater than the recommended dietary allowance. Moreover, even low doses of iron or calcium carbonate can be constipating.

Information about the brand names of over-the-counter medications is important in identifying additives that may be causing problems or increasing the risk for altered medication action. Examples of additives that may cause difficulties are caffeine in some analgesics, lactose in some antacids, or highly allergenic sulfites in some bronchodilators. Reading the labels on over-the-counter medications is a reliable way of finding out about some additives, such as caffeine, if the nurse is not familiar with ingredients in specific brand names. Keep in mind, however, that the FDA does not require the listing of so-called inert ingredients, such as sulfites, other preservatives, or dissolving agents.

One of the most important aspects of the medication interview is assessing the person's understanding of the purpose of medications. This information reflects not only the person's understanding of the medication regimen, but also the person's understanding of overall health problems. Misinformation or a lack of information can provide clues about the communication patterns between the patient and the primary care practitioner as well as about the person's interest in and understanding of his or her own health status. As with other parts of the medication assessment, it is essential to phrase questions in as open-ended and nonjudgmental a manner as possible. Asking "What do you take this pill for?" with a tone of curiosity will likely elicit more information than asking questions such as, "What do you take for your heart?" or "Why do you take digoxin?" Nurses cannot assume that the person has been told the reason for a particular medication or that the person fully understood the explanation that was provided. The person's explanations for taking or not taking medications can lay the groundwork for many hours of health teaching!

Another aspect of the nursing assessment is obtaining and documenting information about the person's perception of and preferences for various forms of medications (Culture Box 23-1). This information may be important in decisions about medication interventions, especially when there are several options that may be equally effective. Similarly, nurses should assess the older adult for any cultural factors that might influence adherence to the regimen or the person's understanding of the purpose of the medication. For example, Chinese people are likely to perceive illness as an imbalance of hot and cold forces. If the illness makes the body hot, then the remedy should make it cooler. Teaching about medications should be framed accordingly. Practical information about illness and health beliefs from many cultural perspectives is described in an excellent pocket guide, written by nurses, entitled *Culture and Nursing Care* (Lipson et al., 1996).

Obtaining information about allergies and adverse reactions is essential because anyone with a

---

CULTURE BOX 23-1	**Cultural Considerations With Regard to Medication Assessment and Interventions**

- Medications that are not readily available or that are prescription medications in the United States may be available over the counter in other countries, such as Mexico, Canada, and Latin American countries.
- Older Hispanics may view wine and other forms of alcohol as a food staple, not a social drug, because they may be used as a healthy alternative to potentially contaminated water in their home country.
- People of Vietnamese and other cultural groups may view injections as being more effective than pills, and pills as being more effective than drops.
- Some Chinese and other Asian people may have the following preferences:
  - Balms and ointments rather than pills for local pain
  - Teas and soups rather than antacids for indigestion
  - Herbs rather than prescription drugs
- Teaching about medications should be done in the context of culturally based beliefs about health, illness, and remedies.

---

history of medication-related problems will need to be closely monitored, especially if the medications being administered are similar to those that caused the reaction. Sometimes people state that they are allergic to a medication, but when they are asked about the symptoms, they describe an adverse effect, rather than an allergic reaction. Therefore, rather than simply documenting that the person is allergic to a certain medication, the nurse should document the specific reaction that occurred if the person can describe it. Nurses can organize the data about medication regimens in a list or chart that is revised and updated as additional information is obtained and changes are made in the regimen. Older adults in community settings can be taught and encouraged to keep their own medication charts.

Another component of a comprehensive medication assessment is obtaining information about various sources of health care. This is particularly important when someone receives care from more than one health care practitioner, as is often the case with older adults who have more than one medical condition. Nurses also can ask specifically about whether the person receives care from non-Western health care practitioners, such as herbalists, spiritual healers, naturopathic practitioners, or Ayurvedic doctors. Questions about alternative and complementary remedies must be phrased in nonjudgmental terms. Culture Box 23-2 summarizes some culturally specific sources of health care and treatment modalities that older adults might use.

CULTURE BOX 23-2	Culturally Specific Health Care Sources and Practices		

Cultural Group	*Sources of Care**	*Common Practices**
African Americans	Home remedies, faith healers, "church nurses"	Folk remedies (e.g., teas, herbs); magic or voodoo (especially in rural areas)
American Indians	Native practitioners	Roots, herbs, physical modalities (e.g., purification rituals)
Cambodians (Khmer)	Vietnamese or Cambodian practitioners	Herbs, medicated strips of adhesive tape, and physical modalities
Chinese Americans	Herbalists, acupuncturists	Herbs, food, beverages, and other remedies to balance yin and yang
Japanese Americans	Herbalists	Herbs, self-care practices
Mexican Americans	Traditional healers, pharmacists	Herbs, teas, soups, rituals, physical modalities (massage, manipulation)
Puerto Ricans	Pharmacists	Tea, herbs, folk remedies
Russians	Folk remedies	Herbal teas, sweet liquor, physical modalities (oils, ointments, enemas, mud baths)
South Asians (Indo-Americans)	Homeopathic or Ayurvedic doctors, spiritual healers	Yoga, diet, fasting, prayer, rituals

*In the United States, Western practitioners and medicine often are used in conjunction with these sources of care and common practices.
Source: Lipson, J. G., Dibble, S. L., & Minarik, P. A. (1996). *Culture and nursing care*: A pocket guide. San Francisco: UCSF Nursing Press.

Display 23-7 summarizes the information that is included in a medication assessment.

Linking the Medication Assessment to the Overall Assessment

The nurse uses information from the medication interview in conjunction with the overall health assessment in several ways. First, information about past and present medication behaviors may provide clues to identified problems or complaints. For example, if the person complains of nervousness or difficulty sleeping, the nurse can inquire about the use of caffeine-containing medications because these may be a contributing factor. Information about recent medication-taking behaviors can also shed light on current problems, such as the recurrence of symptoms that once were controlled by medications. For example, if someone has stopped taking an antiarrhythmic medication, symptoms of dizziness might be related to this. Recent medication-taking behaviors also may account for health problems that are residual or latent adverse medication effects. Examples of residual adverse effects include arthritic changes after a vaccination, blood dyscrasia after a course of chloramphenicol, diarrhea occurring after a course of antibiotics, and gastrointestinal symptoms arising from the administration of antiinflammatory medications.

Second, the overall health assessment provides the basis for evaluating the effectiveness of a medication regimen. Nurses are responsible for determining the expected and actual outcomes and usual dosage of medications. The expected outcomes of medications usually are evaluated through subjective and objective assessment information. For example, analgesic effectiveness is measured by the person's report of pain relief, and the effectiveness of antihypertensive medications is judged according to lowered blood pressure readings.

Third, the overall health assessment will help answer the question, Can the person, or caregivers, safely and effectively administer medications? This is a complex question that addresses all of the following functional areas: cognitive ability to understand the regimen and remember to perform medication-related tasks; motivation to perform the tasks; and physical skills to obtain and administer the medication. Some physical skills that may be required include visual acuity, manual dexterity, and an ability to swallow. The environment also should be assessed in relation to certain conditions, such as accessibility of water and the availability of a refrigerator (if this is necessary for medication storage), that can affect medication-taking behaviors. The overall assessment also might provide information about financial limitations or mobility or transportation problems that interfere with obtaining medications.

DISPLAY 23-7
Guidelines for Medication Assessment

Information About the Therapeutic Agents

- Prescription pills, liquids, injections, eye drops, ear drops, nasal sprays, transdermal patches, and topical preparations
- Over-the-counter preparations (identified by brand names) that are used regularly or occasionally
- Vitamins, minerals, and nutritional supplements
- Pattern of alcohol, caffeine, or tobacco use
- Herbs and herbal preparations
- Homeopathic remedies
- Home remedies
- Sources of health care

Interview Questions to Assess Medication-Taking Behaviors

- How would you describe your usual daily routine for taking medications and remedies, beginning when you get up in the morning?
- Is there anything else you do or use to treat illness or to maintain your health, such as using herbs, ointments, home remedies, or nutritional supplements?
- Are you taking anyone else's medications?
- What do you do when you miss a dose of medication?
- What do you take for constipation? What do you do to help you sleep (or to alleviate any other identified problem)?
- How do you get your prescriptions filled? (Where do you get your remedies?)
- Do you have any difficulty taking your pills?
- What method do you use to keep track of your medications and remedies?
- Is there anything you do to help you remember to take your medicines or remedies at the appropriate time?

Interview Questions to Assess the Person's Understanding of the Purpose of Medications and Other Remedies

- What is this medication (or herb, etc.) for?
- For medications (or remedies) that are used as needed (PRN): How do you decide when to take this pill (or remedy)?
- What did your health care practitioner tell you about this medication (or herb, etc.)?
- What problems were you having when the health care practitioner prescribed this medication (or suggested that you use this remedy)?

Interview Questions to Elicit Additional Information

- Are there any medications or remedies you were taking at one time but are no longer taking?
- Have you ever had an allergic reaction, or any other bad reaction, to a medication or remedy? (If yes, describe what happened.)
- Where do you store your medications and remedies?

Questions and Observations Based on Reading of Prescription Labels

- Who is the prescribing health care practitioner?
- If there is more than one health care practitioner, does each practitioner know all the medications that are being used?
- Are any medications the same or similar and prescribed by different health care practitioners?
- If the dates on various prescriptions are different, were the later medications supposed to be added to the medication regimen, or were they intended to replace previously prescribed medications?
- Are the date of the last refill and the number of pills in the bottle consistent with the prescribed regimen?

Fourth, if the home environment can be observed as part of the overall assessment, important clues to health problems and medication-taking behaviors may be disclosed. For example, observing that nitroglycerin is stored on a windowsill may explain why the medication is not effective in relieving angina. An assessment of the home environment also may lead to additional pertinent information, as when the nurse notices over-the-counter preparations and home remedies on a kitchen counter and asks about these items.

Finally, the overall health assessment serves as the basis for identifying the many factors that can increase the risk for nonadherence, altered therapeutic effects, and adverse medication effects. For example, the nursing assessment of the older adult's cognitive abilities and abilities to perform daily activities provides valuable information about factors than can significantly influence medication-taking behaviors. Similarly, the nursing assessment of depression and other psychosocial aspects of functioning can provide important information about motivational and behavioral factors that can influence medication-taking behaviors.

Identifying Adverse Medication Effects

The first, and sometimes most difficult, step in alleviating adverse medication effects is to recognize their existence. Because many adverse effects are subtle and superimposed on one or more symptoms of illness, they often are attributed to pathologic conditions rather than to the treatment of the condition. Nurses often are the first to recognize adverse medication effects because they generally spend more time with patients than do primary care practitioners. Nurses also are more attentive to long-term monitoring of changes in day-to-day function, in contrast to the medical practitioner's focus on acute illness. Especially in long-term care and home settings, the nurse is the health professional most likely to notice subtle changes in function that may be attributable to adverse medication effects. In community settings, older adults often view the nurse as the health care professional who is most accessible for a discussion of medications and their potential adverse effects.

Health care practitioners may hesitate to discuss adverse medication effects with patients for any of the following reasons: (1) they may be uncertain about the potential adverse effects of a prescribed drug, especially when newer medications are prescribed; (2) they may assume that the power of suggesting possible adverse effects will become a self-fulfilling prophecy; or (3) they may fear that the patient will choose not to take the medication. The nurse can serve as an interpreter between the prescribing practitioner and the patient by emphasizing the medication's benefits as well as pointing out the problems that are most likely to arise. The nurse also can provide health education about ways to avoid adverse effects. For example, if a medication is likely to cause stomach irritation, this adverse effect may be avoided by taking the medication after meals or with milk. The nurse does not automatically initiate a discussion of all the potential adverse effects of a medication, but when a change in the person's health status may be related to adverse medication effects, the nurse can raise that possibility.

Changes in mental status are a potentially devastating adverse medication effect that is often overlooked as such, especially when superimposed on an existing dementia. Any medication-related change in mental status, such as confusion, lethargy, depression, or agitation, can be sudden and obvious or subtle and gradual. Mental status changes, such as delirium or hallucinations, usually are very obvious, but they may be attributed mistakenly to pathologic processes, rather than to medication effects. Whenever an older person experiences changes in mental status, medication intake must be assessed carefully. Over-the-counter medications and alcohol consumption must be considered, especially in relation to medication interactions. Questions that must be asked include the following:

- Can any medications be eliminated?
- Can any doses be lowered?
- Is the mental change interfering with consumption patterns and causing additional problems? (For example, if the person's memory is impaired because of adverse medication effects, is the person taking too much medication and experiencing further mental changes?)

When assessing mental changes that may be associated with medications, it is important to recognize that adverse medication effects are not always alleviated immediately after discontinuation of the medication or a dosage adjustment, and it may take a few days or several weeks before mental function returns to the premedication level. The resolution time depends on the particular medication involved, the length of time it was consumed, and the person's general health status.

NURSING DIAGNOSIS

When the nursing assessment identifies factors that interfere with safe and accurate medication self-administration (e.g., lack of knowledge or functional impairments affecting memory, vision, or hearing), an applicable nursing diagnosis is Instrumental Self-Care Deficit. This is defined as "a state in which the individual experiences an impaired ability to perform certain activities or access certain services essential for managing a household" (Carpenito, 2002, p. 789).

The nursing diagnosis of Noncompliance is defined as "the state in which an individual or group desires to comply but factors are present that deter adherence to health-related advice given by health professionals" (Carpenito, 2002, p. 602). Related factors that might be identified include complex medication regimens, inadequate social supports, adverse effects of medications, lack of money or transportation, and lack of understanding of instructions.

If the nursing assessment identifies adverse effects of medications, particularly those that affect one's safety or quality of life, the nurse might address these through a nursing diagnosis that is specific to the adverse effect. Examples of nursing diagnoses that might be related to adverse medication effects include Constipation, Urinary Incontinence, Imbalanced Nutrition, Impaired Memory, Ineffective Thermoregulation, Sexual Dysfunction, Disturbed Sleep Pattern Impaired Physical Mobility, and Risk for Injury because of medication-related falls and postural hypotension. These nursing diagnoses are discussed in other chapters of this text.

OUTCOMES

Nursing interventions for older adults who are taking medications are directed toward enhancing the therapeutic effectiveness of medications, reducing the risk for adverse effects, and minimizing the negative functional consequences of adverse effects. An outcome criterion for the nursing diagnosis of Instrumental Self-Care Deficit is that the person describes a method to ensure adherence to the medication schedule. An outcome criterion for the nursing diagnosis of Noncompliance is that the person will verbalize a desire to change or initiate change, as indicated by the person stating reasons for the suggested regimen and identifying barriers to adhering to the regimen (Carpenito, 2002).

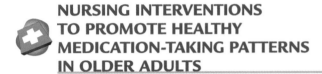

NURSING INTERVENTIONS TO PROMOTE HEALTHY MEDICATION-TAKING PATTERNS IN OLDER ADULTS

Providing Health Education About Medications

Medications are most therapeutic and least risky when they are taken as prescribed and when the medication regimen is periodically reevaluated for maximum effectiveness and minimal risk for adverse reactions. Most community-living older adults take medications with little advice or supervision from health care practitioners; therefore, health education about medications—including self-medication with over-the-counter products—can be an important and effective intervention to promote responsible medication-taking behaviors (Neafsey & Shellman, 2002; Neafsey et al., 2001).

An easy and nonthreatening way to initiate health education about medications is to have the person write a list of all medications taken, including over-the-counter preparations, and to list specifically any medication allergies. The nurse emphasizes that this list is a convenient way of helping health care practitioners keep track of the person's medications, and it should be available to health care practitioners at all times. If the person seeks the care of more than one health care practitioner, this list is especially important. The nurse explains that a medication list facilitates communication and reminds the health care practitioner to reevaluate the medication regimen periodically. The nurse can discuss each medication on the list and provide appropriate information based on an assessment of the person's knowledge and understanding. The person might ask additional questions, and the nurse usually will have ample opportunities for medication education while the list is being written.

Some older adults are uncertain about what information they are entitled to know about their med-

ications, and they may hesitate to question their health care practitioners. Therefore, in any discussion of medications, the nurse suggests pertinent questions that older persons might ask their primary health care provider. In addition, nurses educate older adults and their caregivers about obtaining medication-related information from knowledgeable sources, such as pharmacists. People need to understand that prescribing practitioners are skilled in diagnosing illnesses and deciding the most appropriate interventions, and that pharmacists are the health care practitioners who are most knowledgeable about the specific actions and interactions of medications. Nurses can explain which medication questions are best answered by prescribing practitioners and which are best addressed by pharmacists. Display 23-8 can be used to educate older adults about medications.

Nurses also can educate older adults and caregivers about using consumer references for information about herbs, homeopathy, medications, and alternative therapies. Particularly in community settings, the nurse might use such a book with the older adult and demonstrate how to obtain pertinent information. People taking medications may be interested in purchasing a reference, obtaining one from the library, or using the Internet for information. The nurse can indicate that some good references have been published in recent years, but that some of the references are biased and some information should be used cautiously because it is published primarily for promoting a particular product. Although older adults may find valuable information in these references, they should be advised that it is best to discuss specific remedies and medications with a health professional who can interpret the information in relation to the person's unique situation.

When older adults have trouble adhering to their medication regimen, nurses can provide health education about methods of improving adherence. This is particularly important for older adults who have memory impairments or who manage complex regimens. For example, "unit-dose" medication systems, which have been widely used in institutional settings, are becoming more available for use in home settings and may be helpful in improving medication adherence, especially when medication regimens are complex. A variety of simple "pill organizers" (i.e., containers with separate compartments designated for each day of the week and with one to four compartments for each day) are widely available in stores. In addition, more sophisticated devices to enhance independence and improve adherence are available and may be particularly helpful for people with cognitive

DISPLAY 23-8
Tips on Safe and Effective Medication Use

- Carry an up-to-date list of all your medications, including herbs and over-the-counter preparations, and show the list to your health care practitioner(s).
- When your health care practitioner suggests a medication, ask if there is any way to take care of the problem without medication.
- Ask your health care practitioner the following questions about each new, regularly scheduled medication:
  - What is the reason for taking the medication?
  - How will I know if it's doing what it's meant to do?
  - How soon can I expect to feel the beneficial effects?
  - What will happen if I don't take it?
  - How often am I supposed to take it?
  - How long should I continue taking it?
  - What should I do if I miss a dose?
  - When will you want to see me again, and what will you want me to tell you so that you can determine whether the medication is effective?
- Ask your health care practitioner the following questions at follow-up visits:
  - Do I still need to take this medication?
  - Can the dosage be reduced?
- Ask your health care practitioner the following questions about each medication that is prescribed on an "as-needed" (PRN) basis:

- What is the reason for taking the medication, and how should I determine whether I need the medication?
- How often can I take it? Is there a range of frequency?
- What is the maximum dose I can take within 24 hours?
- What should I do if the medication does not relieve the symptoms (e.g., if chest pain continues after taking several nitroglycerin tablets)?
- Ask your pharmacist the following questions:
  - What are the generic and brand names for this medication?
  - Is it likely to interact with the other medications I'm taking?
  - Is it likely to interact with herbs, cigarettes, alcohol, or any nutrient?
  - What is the best time of day to take it?
  - Does it matter if I take it before or after meals?
  - Are there any side effects I should watch for?
  - Is there anything I can do to minimize the risk of side effects (e.g., taking the medication with milk or meals to reduce stomach irritation)?
  - Is there anything I should avoid while I'm taking this medication (e.g., milk, certain foods, driving)?
  - Are there any special instructions for storing this medication?

or functional impairments. For example, human voice recordings, telephone-computer services, and beeping watches or key chains can be used to remind the person to take medications at designated times. Medication-dispensing systems, which can be filled monthly and programmed to dispense medications at specific times, also are available. Internet sites that provide information about these more technologically advanced systems include http://www.epill.com, http://www.ontimerx.com, and http://www.med-prompt.com. Nurses can encourage older adults and their caregivers to investigate different types of devices and systems (Figure 23-2) that can be used to improve medication adherence.

Addressing Financial Barriers to Medication Adherence

Older adults and people with chronic conditions, such as diabetes and hypertension, are particularly affected by the high cost of medications, which currently average more than $1000 per year for each prescription (Families USA, 2002). Thus, health education interventions need to address financial barriers

that affect the older adult's adherence to medication regimens because even a person who has an adequate income may decide that a medication is not worth the high cost, especially on an ongoing basis. Nurses can encourage older adults to be candid with their health care practitioners in discussing the high cost of medications and to inquire whether a less costly medication might be just as effective as the more expensive one. Many of the newer, but more costly, medications are developed because they are safer or more effective than older medications; thus, it is important that questions about both the cost and effectiveness of newer but more expensive medications be addressed.

Health education about medications can address questions about the use of generic medications. The FDA authorizes the manufacture of generic drugs when a patent on a brand name drug expires, and they require these drugs to be bioequivalent (i.e., identical) to their brand name counterparts in dosage form, safety, strength, quality, intended use, performance characteristics, and route of administration. When generic drugs initially become available, they typically cost 20% to 25% less than the identical brand name drug; however, as competition among

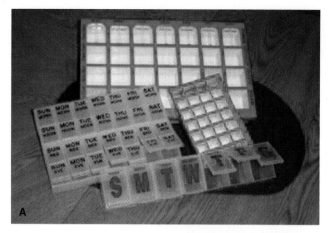

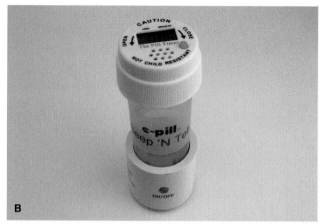

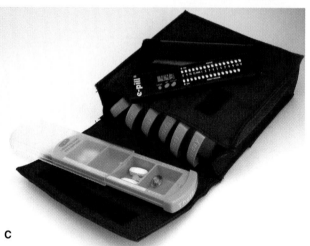

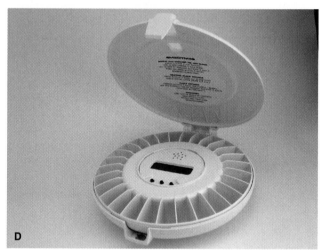

FIGURE 23-2 A sampling of the many devices and systems that are available to improve medication adherence. **(A)** Many simple pill organizers are available in drug stores. **(B)** The Beep 'N Tell pill bottle can be programmed to sound a beeping alarm or play a recorded message. **(C)** The 7-Day Organizer & Reminder has daily pill containers with four large compartments and a multi-alarm electronic reminder system. **(D)** The Automatic Medication Dispenser can be filled with 28 doses of pills and programmed to move the compartments for opening at a predetermined time. It also has a lock and audible alarm with three different sounds. (*Part A:* Courtesy of Tracey Moulton. *Parts B, C, and D:* Courtesy of www.e-pill.com, 70 Walnut Street, Wellesley, MA 02481, 800-549-0095.)

manufacturers increases, the cost of generic drugs gradually decreases to 80% of the brand name (Mohler & Nolan, 2002). About half of the drugs manufactured today are available in generic form. With the exception of drugs that have a very narrow therapeutic range, the use of generic drugs is a safe and effective way of reducing the cost of drugs. Examples of drugs that should not be used in generic form are digoxin, lithium, phenytoin, warfarin, quinidine, theophylline, carbamazepine, and valproic acid.

In April 2002, the American Association for Retired People (AARP) launched a major educational campaign, called "Check Up on Your Prescriptions," with the goal of helping consumers talk with their health care providers and make good decisions about generic drugs. Organizations such as the American Geriatrics Society, United Health Group, and American Medical Women's Association have joined AARP in this major educational initiative. Nurses play key roles in educating older adults and their caregivers about generic drugs. For example, if a patient cannot afford to purchase a medication, the nurse can suggest that the patient ask the prescribing practitioner if a drug that is available generically could be used just as effectively. Nurses can find up-to-date information about generic drugs on the Internet at http://www.fda.gov, and educational information about the AARP campaign is available at http://www.aarp.org/wiseuse.

In addition to educating older adults about generic medications, nurses can educate older adults about economical ways of purchasing prescriptions. For example, when most people begin a new medication regimen, they automatically have the entire prescription filled because this is more convenient and economical than purchasing smaller quantities. Nurses can suggest that patients explain to the pharmacist that they have a new prescription and that they want only a few days' supply of the drug so that they can determine its effectiveness. Many pharmacists will fill the smaller quantity at the same proportionate cost as the larger quantity if the customer intends to purchase the entire prescription after the trial doses. This method saves money if the medication is not effective. In addition, this method deters the person from finishing the prescribed medication, even if it is not effective, or from saving the unused portion just because it has been purchased.

Additional methods of decreasing the cost of medications include obtaining free samples of medications from primary care practitioners and enrolling in medication assistance programs. A medication assistance program provides a particular brand of medication at little or no cost to people who meet certain financial criteria and do not have prescription drug insurance coverage. Pharmaceutical companies have sponsored medication assistance programs for several decades, but traditionally, information about these programs has not been widely disseminated. In recent years, the rapidly rising costs of drugs and the increasing availability of information on the Internet have brought more attention to these programs. These programs have gradually expanded, and by 1999, about 53% of the top 200 prescribed medications were offered through assistance programs to patients who qualified financially (Chisolm & DiPiro, 2002). Financial eligibility varies widely, but usually it is based on being at or within a certain percentage of the federal poverty limits. For example, one program might designate the annual income criterion as less than twice the federal poverty level, and another program might designate income criterion as less than $25,000. Programs require some physician involvement in the application process, but many programs allow nurses and other health care providers to act as advocates to initiate referrals, facilitate the process, and assist with the application.

Nurses can take an active role in educating older adults and their caregivers about the availability of medication assistance programs. In addition, they can provide information about such programs and facilitate referrals. Because these programs are particularly important for older adults with limited financial resources who need to take a brand name drug, nurses need to be familiar with some of these programs and to suggest that older adults and their caregivers ask their prescribing practitioners about these programs. Nurses might also ask their employing institutions to purchase a directory of medication assistance programs for handy reference for use with their patients. Several Internet sites provide helpful information, and some sites assist with enrollment for a processing fee, which usually ranges between $5 and $25. Some of the most useful Internet sites are http://www.medshelp4u.com, http://www.needymeds.com, http://www.helpingpatients.org, http://www.rxassist.org, and http://www.themedicineprogram.com. Printed directories of medication assistance programs are available from several of these sites.

Educating Older Adults About Communicating With Health Care Providers

Because good communication skills are essential to obtaining answers to the questions listed in Display 23-8, it may be necessary for the nurse to suggest ways of communicating effectively with pharmacists and other health care practitioners. For example, before visits for health or medical care, the person can prepare a list of questions to discuss with the health care practitioner. The nurse can help write this list and suggest which questions are most important for each medication. With regard to communicating with pharmacists, nurses can suggest that older adults call the pharmacist at a time of day, such as late morning, that is less likely to be as busy as a peak time. Again, it is helpful to prepare a list of questions that the pharmacist can answer about each medication. In home settings, nurses might call the health care practitioner to discuss medications in the presence of the older adult or caregiver. By demonstrating good communication skills, the nurse will serve as a role model. If older adults or their caregivers can hear the nurse discussing medications using plain English, rather than medical terminology, they may acquire confidence about their own ability to communicate with health care practitioners.

Decreasing the Number of Medications

Because the chance of adverse medication effects increases in proportion to the number of medications consumed, a key intervention is to decrease the number of medications to as few as possible. This is accomplished by coordinating the efforts of the prescribers to discontinue duplicate medications or medications that are no longer appropriate, and by educating the older person about the judicious use of medications that are not medically necessary. In home settings and long-term care facilities, nurses have a great deal of autonomy regarding medications, and in any setting, nurses have many opportunities to raise questions about medication regimens and to communicate with prescribing practitioners about medications. Meredith and colleagues (2002) developed a program to improve medication use in home care settings by using the home care nurses to identify and address unnecessary therapeutic duplication (which affects 4% of home care patients) and the use of medications that have high potential for adverse effects. This intervention can be implemented with minimal use of outside resources and within the context of routinely provided care.

When an older adult is admitted to an acute care facility, he or she may receive care from a primary care practitioner who has not cared for the person before or who has not prescribed many of the person's medications. The nurse usually is the health professional who obtains the medication history on admission, and the prescribing practitioner may automatically order the medications that are listed on the nursing assessment. Careful questioning of the older adult, or the caregivers of dependent older adults, by the nurse may help identify some medications that are either unnecessary or duplicative. The nurse may even discover that medications or medication interactions contribute to or directly cause the problem for which the patient is hospitalized. The nurse is responsible for raising questions about preadmission medication regimens, rather than assuming that the regimen is safe, effective, and warranted. The hospital admission is usually an ideal time to reevaluate the medication regimen, and the medication history obtained by the nurse on admission provides a good basis for this evaluation.

When medications are prescribed for behavioral reasons rather than for a medical condition, the nurse is responsible for educating the older adult and his or her caregivers about these medications and potential nonmedication alternatives. For example, older adults may request antianxiety medications because they perceive medications as a simple and safe solution to nervousness. Nursing staff in institutional settings or caregivers of dependent older adults in home settings may request medications for management of undesirable behaviors. After these medications are prescribed, they often are given or taken over long periods of time without reevaluation, even though the situation may have changed. It is especially important, therefore, to educate older adults and their caregivers about medications, such as alco-

hol, hypnotics, and antianxiety agents, that are used for symptoms that might respond to nonmedication remedies. If the older person has symptoms serious enough to warrant the long-term use of antipsychotic or antidepressant medications, consultation with a mental health professional may be warranted and helpful.

In community settings, it is important to educate older adults and caregivers about criteria for using medications that are used *as needed* (i.e., PRN) because caregivers may not understand the purpose of a particular medication and nonmedication interventions may be equally effective and safer. For example, a caregiver of someone with dementia may be instructed to give a behavior-modifying medication as needed when the person becomes agitated. Although the episodes of agitation may be precipitated by environmental factors (e.g., noise or overstimulation), the caregiver might think the agitation is an inherent part of the illness and use medications unnecessarily rather than modifying the environmental factors to achieve the same outcome. In contrast to this situation, a caregiver may withhold medications that could improve the quality of life for the older person and the caregiver because of misunderstandings or lack of information about the appropriate use of medications. Nurses can educate caregivers about nonmedication interventions as well as the appropriate use of medications for behavior management, particularly for people with dementia (discussed in Chapter 24).

In institutional settings, nurses must establish clear criteria for administering medications for behavior management. These criteria must be based primarily on the patient's needs, rather than primarily on the staff's needs. In home settings, different criteria for behavioral medication might be justified, and the needs of the caregivers may take precedence over the needs of the dependent older adult. For example, if nighttime wakening of a dependent older person interferes with the caregiver's sleep, medication intervention might be warranted. In an institutional setting, however, the nursing staff who are paid to provide around-the-clock care might try nonmedication interventions or allow the person to be awake at night, rather than immediately turning to the use of medications.

Behavioral problems are one example of the types of symptoms that can be managed medically but might be managed just as well, and with fewer risks, through nonmedication interventions. Other types of problems that can be managed without pharmacologic agents are those that are related to comfort, anxiety, and chronic illnesses. The nurse is the health professional who is best able to encourage the use of nonmedication interventions, such as complementary and alternative medicine practices, for certain health problems.

Providing Information About Herbal and Homeopathic Remedies

Homeopathy, herbal medicine, and folk remedies are nontraditional approaches to preventing and treating illness, despite the fact that these approaches have a long tradition in many non-Western cultures. In recent years, there has been a growing trend in the United States toward the use of alternative healing products that have not traditionally been a part of Western medicine. Thousands of alternative healing products are widely available and are being used increasingly by older adults. Even the National Institutes of Health have established the National Center for Complementary and Alternative Medicine and have funded clinical trials of herbs, such as ginkgo biloba and St. John's wort.

Nurses, primary care providers, and other health care practitioners need to be knowledgeable about a variety of therapies so that health care consumers can be advised about their use and effectiveness and so

that some of these therapies can be used judiciously in clinical practice. The challenge for health care practitioners is to be able to educate health care consumers about these remedies, just as people are educated about medications. Throughout this text, information is provided about some of the alternative remedies that are being used more commonly in the United States for particular conditions. This information should be considered in the broader context of the precautions and information discussed in the following sections. This chapter provides information about herbal and homeopathic products because these two alternative and complementary interventions are commonly used as alternatives or supplements to medications. Display 23-9 can be used to teach older adults about the use of herbal and homeopathic remedies, and additional information about alternative and complementary medicine is provided throughout this text in relation to particular aspects of function.

Herbal Remedies

Herbs were perhaps the original "over-the-counter" products used by people who found the remedies they needed in their natural environment. In fact, before the last half of the 20th century, the natural

---

DISPLAY 23-9
Tips on Use of Herbs and Homeopathic Remedies

- Before treating any symptom with a nonprescription product, make sure you are not overlooking a condition that requires medical attention.
- Discuss the use of any nonprescription product with your primary health care provider(s).
- Be cautious about substituting herbal or homeopathic products for prescribed medications.
- Seek information from objective sources and check any warnings on the label or package.
- Observe for beneficial and harmful effects.
- Report any possible side effects to your primary health care provider for evaluation.
- Keep in mind that some products are not required to meet FDA standards for safety and efficacy.
- Introduce only one new substance at a time.
- Start with a low dose and increase the dose gradually.
- Doses may need to be lowered when combining two or more herbs or an herb and a medication.
- Some herbs and homeopathic remedies are for short-term use only.
- Some herbs need to be taken for 1 to 3 months before effects are noticed (e.g., ginkgo biloba, St. John's wort).

- Herbs can interact with all of the following: other herbs, food, beverages, caffeine, nutrients, prescription medications, and over-the-counter medications.
- Some herbs are contraindicated in people with the following conditions: stroke, glaucoma, diabetes, hypertension, heart disease, thyroid disorder, and any bleeding disorder or condition requiring anticoagulation.
- Some herbs are most effective when taken on an empty stomach.
- Many herbs can cause gastrointestinal effects (e.g., anorexia, nausea, diarrhea).
- Some herbs, especially those that are applied externally, can cause skin rashes.
- Herbs can cause allergic reactions.
- Some herbs are extremely toxic, or fatal, if ingested.
- A few herbs, or ingredients in herbs, can be toxic when taken in large doses or for a long time. (For example, Oregon grape, used for prostatitis, may cause heart failure.)
- A few herbs are thought to be carcinogenic.
- Herbs that are used for anxiety or insomnia should not be taken before driving a car.
- Be skeptical about exaggerated claims; if it sounds too good to be true, it probably is!

FDA, U.S. Food and Drug Administration.

environment was the primary source for all healing agents. Most herbs are safe, but some have serious adverse effects, and some can interact with medications, as discussed previously. Because herbs have been used for centuries in European and non-Western cultures, a wealth of information is available. There is much concern about the increasing popularity of herbal remedies in the United States, however, because there has been very little testing that meets the standards established by the FDA for medications. Because herbs are considered to be dietary supplements, they are not required to be tested for safety or efficacy, and little or no reliable information is available about herbal supplements' additional ingredients, potential harmful effects, quantity of active ingredients, or suitability of form for use by the human body. Health care consumers, therefore, need to seek information from sources that do not have a vested interest in selling a particular product. When the decision is made to use an herbal product, the product should be obtained from a reputable source.

Homeopathic Remedies

Three concepts are key to understanding homeopathy as a German physician, Samuel Hahnemann, initially proposed it two centuries ago. First, there is the law of similars, or "like cures like." According to this concept, homeopathy treats an illness by stimulating the body's self-healing abilities through the use of a small amount of a substance similar to the substance that caused the illness. For example, quinine can produce symptoms of malaria in a healthy person, and it can cure malaria when administered in minute doses. The second key concept is that the more a substance is diluted, the more potent it becomes. Based on this concept, homeopathic remedies are diluted repeatedly, and each dilution is vigorously shaken to increase its potency. The third concept is that illnesses are highly individualized, and therefore, the treatment must be individualized. Based on this principle, homeopathic practitioners focus on treating the person, not the disease, and they spend a lot of time interviewing and assessing patients before prescribing a homeopathic remedy. Homeopathy is widely used in India, Russia, Mexico, and European countries, and it is gaining acceptance in the United States as a safe alternative to conventional medicine.

Although most homeopathic remedies are now available for self-treatment, a few are available only through health care practitioners. Unlike herbs, homeopathic remedies are regulated by the FDA as over-the-counter products. Remedies come in a variety of single-substance or combination forms, including powders, wafers, small tablets, and alcohol-based liquids. Over-the-counter homeopathic products are too weak to cause adverse effects, and there are very few precautions, interactions, or contraindications that apply to these products. People who are taking homeopathic remedies are advised to limit the amount taken and the length of time they are taken. Other precautions include avoiding food, caffeine, beverages, toothpaste, and mouthwashes for 15 to 60 minutes before and after taking the substance. Also, oils of camphor, eucalyptus, and peppermint should be avoided during homeopathic treatments. Information about homeopathic remedies and homeopathic practitioners can be obtained from the National Center for Complementary and Alternative Medicine (see the listing in the Educational Resources section).

EVALUATING EFFECTIVENESS OF NURSING INTERVENTIONS

Nursing care of older adults with medication-related nursing diagnoses is evaluated according to the degree to which the older adult follows a safe and effective medication regimen. This involves an evaluation of medication-taking behaviors as well as an evaluation of the therapeutic effects of the medication. Another evaluation criterion is the extent to which negative functional consequences, such as side effects and medication interactions, are avoided, alleviated, or controlled. Nurses in home settings have the ideal opportunity to evaluate the effectiveness of their health education about medication regimens through observations of the medication-taking patterns of the older adult. In any setting, nurses can evaluate the knowledge of the older adult and his or her caregivers about safe and effective medication management.

CHAPTER SUMMARY

Age-related changes in many physiologic mechanisms affect medication action, potentially altering the therapeutic effect and increasing the likelihood of adverse effects. The impact of these age-related changes on any particular medication is determined by the chemical characteristics of the medication, the extent of the age-related changes, and the presence of risk factors. The risk factors that most significantly influence medication action in older adults include polypharmacy, lack of information, inappropriate prescribing practices, pathologic processes and functional impairments, and insufficient recognition of adverse medication effects. In addition, medications can interact with many other substances (e.g., herbs, nutrients, and other medications). The primary functional consequence of these age-related changes, risk factors, and interactions is that older adults are likely to experience altered therapeutic effects and an increased chance of adverse effects of medications. Additional and serious consequences occur when adverse medication effects are not recognized as such in older adults.

The purpose of the nursing assessment is to determine the effectiveness of the medication regimen and to identify the factors that influence medication-taking behaviors. The assessment focuses on detecting adverse effects, identifying the factors that increase the risk for adverse effects or altered therapeutic effects, and identifying cultural factors that influence medication-taking behaviors. Instrumental Self-Care Deficit and Noncompliance are two nursing diagnoses that may be applicable for older adults with medication-related problems. Nursing interventions include educating older adults and their caregivers, facilitating communication between older adults and health care providers, decreasing the number of medications, and providing information about herbs and homeopathy. Nursing care is evaluated by the degree to which the older adult adheres to a safe and effective medication regimen and avoids adverse effects.

CONCLUDING CASE STUDY AND NURSING CARE PLAN

➤ Mrs. M., who is 76 years old, is being discharged to her home after a stay in a nursing home for rehabilitation following a stroke. Residual problems from the stroke include left-sided weakness and visual-perceptual difficulties. In addition to the stroke, Mrs. M.'s medical problems include glaucoma, depression, and congestive heart failure. Her medications include the following: Centrum Silver, 1 tablet daily; furosemide, 20 mg, 2 tablets twice a day; Lanoxicaps, 0.1 mg daily except Mondays and Thursdays; Ecotrin, 81 mg, 1 tablet daily; Transderm-Nitro, 0.2 mg/hr daily; Zoloft, 50 mg daily; Cardizem, 60 mg three times a day; and Timoptic, 0.25% twice daily. The nursing home regimen for administering the medications is as follows:

7:30 AM: Lanoxicaps (except Mondays and Thursdays)
          Cardizem, 60 mg
          Furosemide, 20 mg, 2 tablets
          Timoptic, 0.25% in each eye

9:00 AM: Transderm-Nitro, 0.2 mg/hr
1:00 PM: Centrum Silver, 1 tablet
          Ecotrin, 81 mg, 1 tablet
          Cardizem, 60 mg
3:30 PM: Furosemide, 20 mg, 2 tablets
7:30 PM: Timoptic, 0.25% in each eye
          Cardizem, 60 mg
9:00 PM: Zoloft, 50 mg

■ Nursing Assessment

Your assessment reveals that, before her hospitalization and nursing home stay, Mrs. M. administered her medications independently, but the only medications she took were the eye drops, furosemide (20 mg once daily), and Lanoxicaps. The functional assessment indicates that Mrs. M. has weakness and limited use of her left arm and hand, causing difficulty performing tasks that require fine motor movements. She has full use of her right upper extremity, and she is right-hand dominant. She ambulates independently, but slowly, with a walker. A mental status assessment reveals that Mrs. M. is alert, oriented, and has no memory deficits; however, her abstract thinking and time perception have been impaired by the stroke. She has some expressive aphasia, but she seems to understand instructions, especially if ideas are reinforced by using concrete examples and demonstrations.

Mrs. M. expresses motivation to take her medications, but she admits to being overwhelmed by the complexity of the regimen, stating that, at the nursing home, they administered her medications at six different times. She is also concerned about self-administering her eye drops because she used to use her left hand to hold her eyelids open. With regard to furosemide, she says she does not like taking it twice a day because it makes her go to the bathroom too much. While at the nursing home, she has not had any trouble with incontinence, but she worries about what she'll do at home because there is no bathroom on the first floor. She asks whether she can take the entire dose of furosemide at nighttime so that she will only have to get up during the night to go to the bathroom, which is located near the bedroom.

In response to your questions about medication management routines before her stroke, Mrs. M. reports using a compartmentalized medication container and taking her two medications and the eye drops after breakfast, around 9:30 AM. She would administer the second dose of eye drops around

DISPLAY 23-10 • NURSING CARE PLAN FOR MRS. M.

EXPECTED OUTCOME	NURSING INTERVENTIONS	NURSING EVALUATION

Mrs. M.'s medication routine will be simplified.	• Work with the pharmacist and the prescribing practitioner to simplify the medication regimen.
	  • Discuss with Mrs. M.'s prescribing practitioner the problem of the complexity of the regimen and the cost of medications. Ask Mrs. M.'s prescribing practitioner if she can take Cardizem CD, 180 mg daily, rather than Cardizem, 60 mg three times a day. (This will be less expensive and will eliminate two doses of medication daily.)
	  • Ask the pharmacist about combining medications to allow twice-daily administration.
	• Assist Mrs. M. in establishing a routine for self-administering medications that will fit in with her usual activities.
	• At least 3 days before discharge from the nursing home, arrange for Mrs. M. to assume responsibility for her own medication management, using pill containers that she herself fills.
		• Mrs. M. will be able to follow a twice-daily medication dosing schedule.

Mrs. M.'s concerns about furosemide will be addressed.	• Explain the importance of taking furosemide, as ordered, to control congestive heart failure effectively. • Suggest that Mrs. M. obtain a portable commode for use downstairs during the day.	• Mrs. M. will take furosemide as ordered and will not experience difficulty with urinary incontinence.
Mrs. M.'s concerns about the cost of medications will be addressed.	• Encourage Mrs. M. to talk with her primary care practitioner about her concerns over the cost of the prescribed medications. • Suggest that Mrs. M. consider using the pharmacy services provided by the American Association of Retired Persons (AARP) to obtain her prescriptions.	• Mrs. M. will be able to afford her prescribed medications.
A system for self-administering eye drops will be identified.	• Ask an occupational therapist to evaluate Mrs. M.'s ability to self-administer her eye drops and to identify any assistive devices that may increase her independence and reliability in performing this task. • Have Mrs. M. practice self-administering her eye drops before she is discharged from the nursing home, with staff providing whatever assistance is necessary. • Talk with Mrs. M. about the possibility of her husband assisting with the eye drop procedure if she is unable to do this independently. • Ask Mrs. M.'s ophthalmologist whether the eye drop regimen can be simplified to once-daily dosing by prescribing an extended-action eye drop formula.	• Mrs. M. will self-administer her eye drops or will receive the assistance she needs for eye drop administration from her husband.

9:30 PM, before getting ready for bed. She had no difficulty remembering the medications because she kept the pill container and one bottle of eye drops near the toaster, and she kept a second bottle of eye drops on her nightstand. Now, though, she expresses concern about the number of times she must take medications if the regimen remains the same as in the nursing home, and she thinks that she will need six pill containers, but is not sure where she should put all of them. She also worries about the cost of all the medications.

Mrs. M. lives with her husband, who is physically healthy but has early-stage Alzheimer's disease. Their daughter lives nearby and visits two or three times weekly to assist with grocery shopping, laundry, and household chores. She also provides transportation to stores and appointments.

■ Nursing Diagnosis

You decide on a nursing diagnosis of Noncompliance because Mrs. M. expresses a desire to take her medications, but several factors deter adherence to the current regimen. Related factors include functional impairments, complex medication regimens, negative side effects of furosemide, and concern about the cost of medications.

■ Nursing Care Plan

The care plan you develop for Mrs. M. is shown in Display 23-10.

 CRITICAL THINKING EXERCISES

1. As the nurse working with Mrs. M. in the skilled nursing facility, address each of the following questions:
   - What are the factors that influence Mrs. M.'s ability to manage her medications independently?
   - What additional assessment information would be helpful in establishing a plan for Mrs. M. to manage her medications independently?
   - What health education would you provide to address Mrs. M.'s concerns about the cost of her medications?
   - What steps would you take to ensure that expected outcomes are achieved after Mrs. M. is back in her own home?
2. You are asked to give a half-hour presentation on "Medications and Aging" to a local senior citizens group. Describe the following:
   - What points would you cover about age-related changes?

   - How would you address the risk factors that affect medication action and medication-taking behaviors?
   - What tips would you give about taking medications?
   - What educational materials would you use?
   - How would you involve the group participants in the discussion?
3. Carefully read the interview questions in Display 23-7 and decide which questions you would use and how you would phrase the questions in your own words for each of the following situations:
   - You are doing an admission interview for a 78-year-old man who lives alone and has been admitted to the hospital for the third time in 18 months for congestive heart failure.
   - You are working in a Senior Wellness program in an urban setting with a large number of older adults who were born in Mexico. You are preparing for 15-minute interviews with older adults who have agreed to participate in an educational session to which they must bring all their pills in a bag and ask the nurse about them.
4. Carefully read the information in Displays 23-8 and 23-9 and describe what information you would be likely to use in each of the following situations:
   - Discharge planning for the 78-year-old man described in Exercise 3, bullet 1
   - Health education for the people described in the Senior Wellness program in Exercise 3, bullet 2

EDUCATIONAL RESOURCES

American Association of Retired Persons (AARP)
601 E Street, NW, Washington, DC 20049
(800) 424-3410
http://www.aarp.org

National Center for Complementary and Alternative Medicine
P.O. Box 7923, Gaithersburg, MD 20898
(888) 644-6226
http://nccam.nih.gov

National Council on Patient Information and Education
4915 Saint Elmo Avenue, Suite 505, Bethesda, MD 20814-6082
(301) 656-8565
http://www.talkaboutrx.org

The Peter Lamy Center for Drug Therapy and Aging
University of Maryland School of Pharmacy
515 West Lombard Street, 1st Floor, Baltimore, MD 21201
(877) 706-2434
http://www.pharmacy.umaryland.edu/lamy

Therapeutic Products Directorate
Holland Cross, Tower B, 6th Floor
Address Locator 3106B, 1600 Scott Street, Ottawa, Ontario K1A 0K9, Canada
http://www.hc-sc.gc.ca

U.S. Food and Drug Administration
5600 Fishers Lane, HFE-88, Rockville, MD 20857
(888) 463-6332
http://www.fda.gov

REFERENCES

Aizenberg, D., Sigler, M., Weizman, A., & Barak, Y. (2002). Anticholinergic burden and the risk of falls among elderly psychiatric inpatients: A 4-year case-control study. *International Psychogeriatrics, 14,* 307–310.

Akishita, M., Toba, K., Nagano, K., & Ouchi, Y. (2002). Adverse drug reactions in older people with dementia. *Journal of the American Geriatrics Society, 50,* 400–401.

Avorn, J., & Gurwitz, J. H. (1997). Principles of pharmacology. In C. K. Cassel, E. B. Larson, D. E. Meier, N. M. Resnick, L. Z. Rebenstein, & L. B. Sorenson (Eds.), *Geriatric medicine* (3rd ed., pp. 55–70). New York: Springer.

Beers, M. H. (1997). Explicit criteria for determining potentially inappropriate medication use by the elderly: An update. *Archives of Internal Medicine, 157,* 1531–1536.

Beers, M. H., Oslander, J. G., Rollingher, J., Brooks, J., Reuben, D., & Beck, J. C. (1991). Explicit criteria for determining potentially inappropriate medication use by the elderly. *Archives of Internal Medicine, 151,* 1825–1832.

Beyth, R. J., & Shorr, R. I. (2002). Principles of drug therapy in older patients: Rational drug prescribing [Review]. *Clinics in Geriatric Medicine, 18*(3), 577–592.

Birkett, D. P., Dumanuing, N., & Singh, K. (2001). Neuroleptic sensitivity in the elderly. *Clinical Gerontologist, 23* (1/2), 145–151.

Carpenito, L. J. (2002). *Nursing diagnosis: Application to clinical practice* (9th ed.). Philadelphia: Lippincott Williams & Wilkins.

Chisolm, M. A., & DiPiro, J. T. (2002). Pharmaceutical manufacturer assistance programs. *Archives of Internal Medicine, 162,* 780–784.

Cusack, B. J., & Vestal, R. E. (2000). Clinical pharmacology. In M. H. Beers & R. Berkow. *The Merck manual of geriatrics,* pp. 54–74. Whitehouse Station, NJ: Merck Research Laboratories.

Dhalla, I. A., Anderson, G. M., Mamdani, M. M., Bronskill, S. E., Sykora, K., & Rochon, P. A. (2002). Inappropriate prescribing before and after nursing home admission. *Journal of the American Geriatrics Society, 50,* 995–1000.

Families USA. (2002). *Bitter pill: The rising prices of prescription drugs for older Americans.* Washington, DC: Families USA.

Field, T. S., Gurwitz, J. H., Avorn, J., McCormich, D., Jain, S., Eckler, M., et al. (2001). Risk factors for adverse drug events among nursing home residents. *Archives of Internal Medicine, 161,* 1629–1634.

Fingerhood, M. (2000). Substance abuse in older people. *Journal of the American Geriatrics Society, 48,* 985–995.

Giron, M. S., Wang, H-X., Bernsten, C., Thorslund, M., Winblad, B., & Fastbom, J. (2001). The appropriateness of drug use in an older nondemented and demented population. *Journal of the American Geriatrics Society, 49,* 277–283.

Glazer, W. M. (2000). Extrapyramidal side effects, tardive dyskinesia, and the concept of atypicality. *Journal of Clinical Psychiatry, 61*(Suppl 3), 16–21.

Goldberg, J. F. (2000). New drugs in psychiatry. *Emergency Medicine Clinics of North America, 18*(2), 211–231.

Gurwitz, J. H., Field, T. S., Harrold, L. R., Rothschild, J., Debellis, K., Seger, A. C., et al. (2003). Incidence and preventability of adverse drug events among older persons in the ambulatory setting. *Journal of the American Medical Association, 289*(9), 1107–1116.

Gurwitz, J. H., & Rochon, P. (2002). Improving the quality of medication use in elderly patients: A not-so-simple prescription. *Archives of Internal Medicine, 162,* 1670–1672.

Hanlon, J. T., Fillenbaum, G. G., & Schmader, K. E. (2000). Inappropriate drug use among community-dwelling elderly. *Pharmacotherapy, 20,* 575–582.

Hanlon, J. T., Schmader, K. E., Boult, C., Artz, M. B., Gross, C. R., Fillenbaum, G. G., et al. (2002). Use of inappropriate prescription drugs by older people. *Journal of the American Geriatrics Society, 50,* 26–34.

Hohl, C., Dankoff, J., Colacone, A., & Afilalo, M. (2001). Polypharmacy, adverse drug-related events, and potential adverse drug interactions in elderly patients present to an emergency department. *Annals of Emergency Medicine, 36*(6), 666–671.

Hughes, C. M., Lapane, K. L., Mor, V., Ikegami, N., Jonsson, P. V., Ljunggren, G., & Sgadari, A. (2000). The impact of legislation on psychotropic drug use in nursing homes: A cross-national perspective. *Journal of the American Geriatrics Society 48*(8), 931–937.

Jeste, D. V., Rockwell, E., Harris, J. B., & Larco, J. (1999). Conventional vs. newer antipsychotics in elderly patients. *American Journal of Geriatric Psychiatry, 7*(1), 70–76.

Knight, E. L., & Avorn, J. (2001). Quality indicators for appropriate medication use in vulnerable elders. *Archives of Internal Medicine, 135,* 703–710.

Kyle, U. G., Genton, L., Hans, D., Karsegard, V. L., Michel, J-P., Slosman, D. O., et al. (2001). Total body mass, fat mass, fat-free mass, and skeletal muscle in older people: Cross-sectional differences in 60-year-old persons. *Journal of the American Geriatrics Society, 49,* 1633–1640.

Lantz, M. S. (2001). Serotonin syndrome: A common but often unrecognized psychiatric condition. *Geriatrics, 56*(1), 52–53.

Lee, E. W., & D'Alonzo, G. E. (1993). Cigarette smoking, nicotine addiction, and its pharmacological treatment. *Archives of Internal Medicine, 153,* 34–48.

Lipson, J. G., Dibble, S. L., & Minarik, P. A. (1996). *Culture & nursing care: A pocket guide.* San Francisco: UCSF Nursing Press.

Ludwick, R. E., Sedlak, C. A., Doheny, M. O., & Martsolf, D. S. (2000). Alcohol use in elderly women: Nursing considerations in community settings. *Journal of Gerontological Nursing, 26*(2), 44–49.

Mamo, D. C., Sweet, R. A., Mulsant, B. H., Pollock, B. G., Miller, M. D., Stack, J. A., et al. (2000). Effect of nortriptyline and paroxetine on extrapyramidal signs and symptoms: A prospective double-blind study in depressed elderly patients. *American Journal of Geriatric Psychiatry, 8*(3), 226–231.

Meredith, S., Feldman, P., Grey, D., Giammaro, L., Hall, K., Arnold, K., et al. (2002). Improving medication use in newly admitted home healthcare patients: A randomized controlled trial. *Journal of the American Geriatrics Society, 50,* 1584–1941.

Mitchell, J., Mathews, H. F., Hunt, L. M., Cobb, K. H., & Wataon, R. W. (2001). Mismanaging prescription medications among rural elders: The effects of socioeconomic status, health status, and medication profile indicators. *Gerontologist, 41,* 348–356.

Mohler, P., & Nolan, S. (2002). What every physician should know about generic drugs: Are generic drugs second-class medicine or prudent prescribing? *Family Practice Management, 9*(3), 45–46.

Mort, J. R., & Aparasu, R. R. (2000). Prescribing potentially inappropriate psychotropic medications to the ambulatory elderly. *Archives of Internal Medicine, 160,* 2825–2831.

Neafsey, P. J., & Shellman, J. (2002). Interactions of prescription medicines. *Journal of Gerontological Nursing, 28*(9), 30–39.

Neafsey, P. J., Strickler, Z., Shellman, J., & Padula, A. T. (2001). Delivering health information about self-medication to older adults. *Journal of Gerontological Nursing, 27*(11), 19–27.

Park, D. C., Hertzog, C., Leventhal, H., Morrell, R. W., Leventhal, E., Birchmore, D., et al. (1999). Medication adherence in rheumatoid arthritis patients: Older is wiser. *Journal of the American Geriatrics Society, 47,* 172–183.

Pitkala, K. H., Strandberg, T. E., & Tilvis, R. S. (2002). Inappropriate drug prescribing in home-dwelling, elderly patients. *Archives of Internal Medicine, 162,* 1707–1712.

Renteln-Kruse, W. V. (2000). Medication adherence: Is and why is older wiser? *Journal of the American Geriatrics Society, 48,* 457–458.

Rochon, P. A., & Gurwitz, J. H. (1999). Prescribing for seniors: Neither too much nor too little. *Journal of the American Medical Society, 282,* 113–115.

Roe, C. M., Anderson, M. J., & Spivack, B. (2002). Use of anticholinergic medications by older adults with dementia. *Journal of the American Geriatrics Society, 50,* 835–842.

Schwartz, D., Wang, M., Zeitz, L., & Goss, M. (1962). Medication errors made by elderly, chronically ill patients. *American Journal of Public Health, 52,* 2018–2029.

Sloane, P. D., Zimmerman, S., Brown, L. C., Ives, T. J., & Walsh, J. F. (2002). Inappropriate medication prescribing in residential care/assisted living facilities. *Journal of the American Geriatrics Society, 50,* 1001–1011.

Stuart, B., & Shea, D. (2001). Dynamics in drug coverage of Medicare beneficiaries: Finders, losers, switchers. *Health Affairs (Millwood), 20,* 86–99.

Tune, L. E. (2001). Anticholinergic effects of medication in elderly patients. *Journal of Clinical Psychiatry, 62*(Suppl 21) 11–14.

Williams, C. M. (2002). Using medications appropriately in older adults. *American Family Physician, 66*(10), 1917–1924.

6

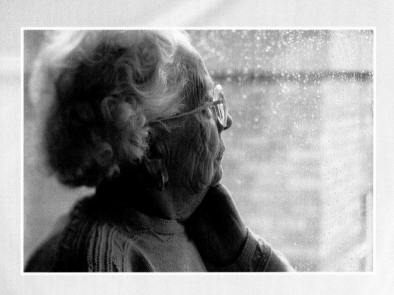

IMPAIRED PSYCHOSOCIAL FUNCTION IN OLDER ADULTS

Impaired Cognitive Function: Delirium and Dementia

LEARNING OBJECTIVES

1. State the characteristics of delirium.
2. Define and differentiate between the various terms used to describe impaired cognitive function in older adults.
3. Discuss theories about Alzheimer's disease.
4. Describe vascular dementia, frontotemporal dementia, and dementia with Lewy bodies.
5. List the factors that increase the risk for dementia.
6. Discuss the functional consequences of impaired cognitive function in older adults and the impact of these consequences on caregivers.
7. Describe guidelines for assessing cognitively impaired older adults.
8. Identify environmental modifications and communication techniques as interventions for people with dementia.
9. Discuss the cholinergic medications currently used for treating dementia.

Healthy older adults experience only minor changes in cognitive abilities (as described in Chapter 7), but as people age, they are increasingly more likely to develop pathologic conditions that have a major impact on cognitive function. When impaired cognitive functioning causes a progressive loss of abilities that affects all aspects of functioning, it is one of the most devastating losses that older adults and their caregivers must confront. Nurses in all settings frequently care for older adults who have dementia or delirium—the two main causes of significant cognitive impairment in older adults. Nurses are responsible for differentiating between delirium and dementia and for identifying causes of impaired cognitive functioning in older adults. In addition, nurses and the other people who care for people with dementia must meet the challenge of preserving as much of the person's dignity and quality of life as possible, despite the serious and progressive losses the person with dementia experiences. Although this chapter differs from most others in its focus on pathologic conditions, it addresses impaired cognitive function from the perspective of the role of the nurse in promoting wellness for people with dementia and their caregivers. Because knowledge about dementia is progressing at a rapid pace, nurses and all gerontological health care providers are encouraged to use the Internet to supplement information in this chapter by obtaining up-to-date information from the many excellent sites listed in the Educational Resources section.

DELIRIUM

Researchers and practitioners are increasingly recognizing delirium as a major and treatable cause of cognitive impairment in older adults. *Delirium* is a medical diagnosis characterized by the following:

- Altered levels of consciousness with reduced ability to focus, sustain, or shift attention
- Mental status changes (e.g., disorientation, altered perception, deficits in thinking or memory)
- Unsafe or disruptive behaviors (e.g., loud vocalizations, hitting caregivers, attempts to remove clothing or medical equipment)

Hypoactive delirium, which occurs less commonly, is characterized by inactivity and withdrawn and sluggish behavior. Manifestations of either form of delirium develop over a short period of time (hours or days), fluctuate over the course of the day (usually affecting the sleep–wake cycle), and are not directly caused by a dementia or depression. Nurses commonly use the term *acute confusion* (or *acute confusional state*) to describe the medical syndrome of delirium, and most health care professionals use these terms interchangeably (Rapp et al., 2001).

Researchers and practitioners cite delirium as the most frequent complication of hospitalization for older adults (Inouye et al., 2001), and health care providers are currently focusing a great deal of attention on this as a major problem for older adults. Current research is particularly focusing on the common occurrence of delirium in people with dementia and in people who are recovering from hip fracture surgery (Fick et al., 2002; Millisen et al., 2002). Recent studies indicate that delirium occurs in the following:

- 22% to 89% of all people aged 65 years and older who have dementia (Fick et al., 2002)

- 14% to 80% of all elderly patients hospitalized for acute physical illness (Foreman et al., 2001)
- 40% to 60% of nursing home residents (Rapp et al., 2001)
- 13% to 61% of patients with hip fractures (Morrison et al., 2003)

Researchers and practitioners also are trying to determine the most common time frame for the onset and duration of delirium symptoms. For older adults, the onset is likely to occur during the first 2 days of hospitalization; it occurs only occasionally after the sixth day (Rapp et al., 2001). The duration is likely to be prolonged in older adults and may last for up to 6 months after discharge from an acute care setting (Marcantonio et al., 2003). Marcantonio and colleagues (2003) found that 23% of people discharged from acute care had symptoms of delirium on admission to rehabilitation or skilled nursing facilities; 64% of that group had the same number or more symptoms 1 week later, and an additional 4% of the newly admitted group had developed symptoms. These researchers concluded "in patients newly admitted to post-acute care facilities from acute care hospitals, delirium symptoms are prevalent, persistent, and associated with poor functional recovery" (Marcantonio et al., 2003, p. 4).

Although delirium occurs in people of any age, it is more likely to affect older adults because they have more risk factors for delirium. Dementia is the factor most consistently identified as a risk factor for delirium, and researchers have identified all of the following additional risk factors:

- Age 80 years and older
- Concurrent medical conditions (Display 24-1)
- Poor hydration and nutrition
- Medical or chemical restraints
- Medications (e.g., benzodiazepines, anticholinergics, cardiovascular agents; see Chapter 23, Table 23-11)
- Undertreated pain
- Immobility
- Vision or hearing impairment, sensory deprivation
- Depression
- General anesthesia
- Social isolation or sensory overload (Foreman et al., 2001; Han et al., 2001; Inouye et al., 2001; McCusker et al., 2001; Morrison et al., 2003; Zeleznik, 2001)

Particular problems arise when delirium occurs in older adults who have dementia because the acute changes are likely to be superimposed on already existing cognitive deficits, and families and health

DISPLAY 24-1
Some Medical Conditions That Can Cause Delirium

- Fluid and electrolyte disturbances (e.g., dehydration, volume depletion, acidosis, alkalosis, hypercalcemia, hypokalemia, hyponatremia or hypernatremia, hypoglycemia or hyperglycemia, hypomagnesemia)
- Cardiovascular disturbances (e.g., atrial fibrillation, myocardial infarction, congestive heart failure)
- Infections (e.g., pneumonia, septicemia, meningitis, encephalitis, urinary tract infection)
- Metabolic and endocrine disorders (hypothyroidism or hyperthyroidism, hypopituitarism or hyperpituitarism, parathyroid disorders, hypoadrenocorticism or hyperadrenocorticism)
- Trauma (e.g., fractures, head injury)
- Respiratory disorders (e.g., tuberculosis, pulmonary embolism)
- Collagen and rheumatoid disease (e.g., temporal arteritis)
- Bowel impaction
- Acute abdominal disorder
- Malignant disease
- Malnutrition
- Heavy metal or carbon monoxide intoxication
- Alcoholism
- Hypothermia or hyperthermia
- Hepatic or renal failure
- Seizures and postconvulsive states

care professionals are likely to attribute the recent changes to the dementia. Researchers and clinicians also are focusing on the very common occurrence of physicians and nurses failing to recognize delirium, especially when it is superimposed on dementia. Nursing studies have concluded that all of the following factors contribute to failure to recognize delirium: not assessing mental status, failing to recognize the hypoactive form, the absence of standardized assessment protocols, and a lack of knowledge about differentiating between dementia and delirium (Fick et al., 2002; Fick & Foreman, 2000; Foreman et al., 2001).

Delirium causes serious functional consequences in older adults, including the following:

- Longer hospital stays
- Increased mortality
- Increased nursing care
- Immediate and long-term functional impairment
- Higher rates of institutionalization (Fick & Foreman, 2000; McCusker et al., 2001: Morrison et al., 2003)

In addition, people with both delirium and dementia are more likely to be readmitted to the hospital within 1 month of discharge, as compared with people with delirium alone or those with neither delirium nor dementia (Fick & Foreman, 2000).

In recent years, nursing and medical journals increasingly emphasize the importance of detecting delirium in acute and long-term care settings and of using standardized assessment instruments (Inouye et al., 2001). The Mini-Mental State Examination (MMSE; discussed in Chapter 10) is a commonly used screening tool to identify a person's level of cognitive function, but it is not specific for identifying delirium. Moreover, its usefulness for identifying changes in mental status depends on administering it more than once; thus, it is more effective for evaluating the progression of mental status changes than the onset of changes. Although health care professionals often focus on orientation as a key indicator of mental status, this is one of the least sensitive indicators of delirium (Fick & Foreman, 2000). Thus, identification of delirium requires the assessment of all the following factors: mental status, risk factors, and specific indicators of delirium. Since the 1990s, nurses have developed several models for assessing delirium, as described in Table 24-1.

The nursing diagnosis of Acute Confusion is applicable when the onset of mental changes is abrupt or caused by risk factors such as medical conditions and adverse medication effects. Nursing goals for people with delirium focus on alleviating the contributing factors, improving mental status, and preventing injury. Nursing-sensitive outcomes related to these goals include Memory, Thinking, and Perception (Wakefield et al., 2001).

Nurses and other health care professionals have important roles in preventing and managing delirium by developing care plans that address the individual needs of patients. Some interventions, such as providing aids to orientation (e.g., clock, watch, calendar) and aids to improve sensory function (e.g., eyeglasses, hearing aids) are relatively simple. Additional interventions that are effective in preventing or managing delirium are as follows:

- Environmental modification (e.g., noise reduction, familiar objects)
- Psychological support (e.g., cognitive and social stimulation)
- Identification and management of adverse medication effects
- Physiologic stability (e.g., low-dose oxygenation, maintenance of fluid and electrolyte balance)
- Adequate pain management

TABLE 24-1 • Models for Nursing Assessment of Delirium

Assessment Model	Description	Recent References
Confusion Assessment Method (CAM)	Easy-to-use standardized instrument used to screen for overall cognitive impairment and assess the four aspects of cognitive function that are most indicative of delirium: acute onset and fluctuating course, inattention, disorganized thought, and altered level of consciousness	Inouye et al., 2001; Laplante & Cole, 2001; Wakefield et al., 2001; Waszynski, 2002
NEECHAM Confusion Scale	Nine-item interactive observational scale with three subscales: processing, behavior, and physiologic	Wakefield et al., 2001
Acute Confusion/Delirium Protocol	Recommends combination of MMSE, CAM and NEECHAM and provides algorithm for interventions	Cacchione, 2002; Rapp et al., 2001

MMSE, Mini-Mental State Examination.

- Physical activity (e.g., ambulation, physical therapy)

OVERVIEW OF DEMENTIA

Terminology to Describe Dementia

An understanding of impaired cognitive function is complicated by the many terms that have been used interchangeably—and often inaccurately—to describe dementia. Although the recent and rapid expansion of knowledge about impaired cognitive function has led to improved ability to distinguish different types of dementia, it has also led to the use of more terms to describe dementia. Perhaps more than any other terms used in reference to older adults, those associated with cognitive impairments are the most misused, misunderstood, and emotionally charged. For example, the term *senility* is usually associated with the false belief that the behaviors are normal accompaniments of old age, whereas the term *demented* is commonly associated with bizarre, socially inappropriate, or even criminal behaviors. Different terms are more or less acceptable to different people—including health care professionals—in the same way that various terms associated with cancer are more or less acceptable to different people. The following are some of the terms that health care professionals use in reference to cognitive impairment in older adults: confusion, dementia, senility, Alzheimer's disease, small strokes, memory problems, "old timer's disease," organic brain syndrome, and "hardening of the arteries." The selection of a term sometimes is based on emotional preferences and sometimes on a lack of understanding. Because cognitive impairment is an emotionally charged subject, nurses must understand the correct terminology and

then choose the most appropriate term based on an understanding of the underlying causes for the impairment and an assessment of what term is most acceptable to the older adult and his or her caregivers.

Senility was the first term applied to cognitive impairment in older adults. By definition, senility means old age, or pertaining to old age, and originally, it was a neutral term. Only in the past two centuries has the term referred to a state of being mentally and physically infirm as a result of old age, and only in the last century has it consistently been associated with disease conditions and feeblemindedness. Unfortunately, the use of this term to describe cognitively impaired older adults implies that the impairments are a necessary consequence of being old. As recently as the 1970s, senility was the explanation given for any condition associated with "aging" that was viewed as needing no further investigation or treatment. Almost two decades ago, a commentary on terms that nurses should never use in reference to older adults made the following point:

> *The word senile is an archaic, negative, prejudicial term which usually refers to general mental decline in the elderly. . . . But the word senile is not a professional term and should never be used to describe an older person.* (Hogstel, 1988, p. 7).

In the early 1900s, the phrase *hardening of the arteries* became a popular diagnostic label for cognitive impairment in older adults. This label was an improvement over the senility label because it referred to a causative factor; however, the causative factor still was viewed as an inevitable, albeit pathologic, consequence of aging. This label, therefore, did nothing to challenge the myth that cognitive impairments were an integral part of aging. Like senility, this term is now considered outdated and is not used in reference to cognitive impairments.

By the 1950s, the term *organic brain syndrome* (OBS) had become the popular medical label for cognitive impairment in older adults. This label described a constellation of manifestations that could be attributed to the neurologic effects of underlying pathologic conditions. Along with the use of the term OBS, there came a distinction between acute and chronic conditions. Acute OBS, also called delirium, was viewed as a manifestation of a pathologic process that would resolve after the underlying cause was treated. By contrast, *chronic organic brain syndrome* (COBS) was viewed as the manifestation of irreversible brain damage, and it was thought to be closely associated with underlying vascular pathology. The use of the terms OBS and COBS was a step in the right direction in that cognitive impairments no longer were considered to be an inevitable result of old age. The step was not a very big step, however, because, the cause of cognitive impairments in older adults still was attributed to untreatable vascular disease.

In the 1960s, autopsy examination of brain specimens provided the first scientific evidence about the underlying causes of cognitive impairments. Based on these findings, researchers and practitioners began to realize that many of the changes previously attributed to COBS or untreatable vascular diseases actually were manifestations of treatable conditions. By the early 1980s, much of the geriatric literature was reporting that as many as 25% of older adults had been misdiagnosed as having COBS when they actually had treatable conditions.

During the 1970s, geriatricians began using the term *pseudodementia*—which had originally been applied to psychiatric disorders that resembled dementia but did not cause irreversible cognitive impairment—in reference to cognitive impairments caused by physiologic conditions. In recent years, this term is applied primarily to cognitive impairment associated with depression (discussed in Chapter 25). Since the 1990s, geriatricians have debated the merits of continuing to use this term and currently are discouraging its use and emphasizing the increasing capability of identifying specific underlying causes of dementia (Reifler, 2000).

Dementia is the term that most accurately describes progressive declines in cognitive function. Dementia is "a syndrome of impaired cognition caused by brain dysfunction" and characterized by multiple cognitive deficits, such as memory impairment, aphasia, apraxia, agnosia, or impaired executive functions (Morris, 2000, p. 774). In addition,

noncognitive manifestations, such as changes in personality and behavior, are manifestations of dementia. Unfortunately, this medical term is also associated with the lay term *demented*, which has a long history of pejorative use in popular language and which may be viewed as even more derogatory than the word senile. Thus, nurses can use phrases such as "a person with dementia" or a "person with a dementing illness" to refer accurately to the medical syndrome of impaired cognitive function while avoiding pejorative connotations.

An additional point must be emphasized with regard to the term *dementia*. Because dementia is not a single disease but a syndrome, the term refers to a unique combination of manifestations that calls for the identification of an underlying cause. Because Alzheimer's disease is the most common type of dementia, accounting for one half to two thirds of the cases of dementia, health care professionals and lay people frequently use the terms *Alzheimer's disease* and *dementia* interchangeably, even though this may not be accurate. Alzheimer's disease is the type of dementia that was first identified and is most widely studied. However, researchers and geriatricians are increasingly recognizing and addressing vascular dementia, frontotemporal dementia, and dementia with Lewy bodies as commonly occurring types of dementia in older adults.

Another evolving trend is to use distinct terminology for different stages of progressive cognitive impairment. For example, researchers and practitioners use the term *mild cognitive impairment* in reference to a predementia stage. People with mild cognitive impairment do not meet the criteria for dementia; although they have some cognitive impairment that is not normal for their age, the impairment does not interfere significantly with everyday functioning. Specifically, they are likely to have short-term memory impairment, executive function impairment, and difficulty with written arithmetic (Griffith et al., 2003). A similar approach to terminology is applied to early stages of other types of dementia. For example, *vascular cognitive impairment* has been proposed to describe people who have cognitive difficulties that arise from vascular causes that are noticeable but not serious enough to be called *vascular dementia* (Wentzel et al., 2001).

An important consideration regarding terminology is that there are significant overlaps in manifestations of different types of dementia and that two (or more) types of dementia can coexist in the same person. Thus, the term *mixed dementia* has been used since the 1960s in reference to the co-occurrence of two or more conditions that cause dementia, with Alzheimer's disease and vascular dementia being the combination that occurs most frequently (Zekry et al., 2002b). Researchers are focusing on the probability that the presence of vascular dementia intensifies the manifestations of Alzheimer's (Snowden, 1997; Zekry et al., 2002a). The term *modifiable dementia* is similar to mixed dementia, in that it refers to a combination of a dementia and a medical condition that will cause progressive cognitive impairment if left untreated (e.g., thyroid disorder, vitamin B_{12} deficiency) (Massoud et al., 2000).

Theories to Explain Dementia

The major changes in terminology used to describe impaired cognitive function reflect the significant developments in our understanding of this phenomenon during the past century. Major progress has been made in identifying pathologic changes and behavioral manifestations that characterize different types of dementia, and some progress has been made in identifying various causes of dementia. However, despite more than 100 years of research on causes of impaired cognitive function in older adults, theories to explain dementia are inconclusive and still evolving.

During the 1800s, European physicians discovered neuritic plaques in the brains of older adults and identified these changes as the cause of senility, or senile dementia. Around that same time, medical scientists discovered that arteries throughout the body lose their elasticity and become hardened during later adulthood, and they theorized that this was the underlying cause of the brain changes in older adults. In 1906, Alois Alzheimer, a German physician, discovered neuritic plaques in the autopsied brain specimens from a woman who was 55 years old when she died and had initially manifested cognitive and behavior changes around the age of 50 years. Alzheimer concluded that these pathologic brain changes caused a relatively rare disease called *presenile dementia* (or *Alzheimer's disease*), and he published these findings in a psychiatric journal (Alzheimer, 1907). Deductions of Alzheimer and other physicians and researchers at the time lead to the following conclusions:

- Neuritic plaques caused presenile dementia.
- Hardening of the arteries caused senile dementia.
- Alzheimer's disease and senile dementia were distinct diseases differentiated by age at onset.

Simply stated, if the onset of the cognitive impairment occurred before the age of 65 years, it was called Alzheimer's disease, whereas if the onset took place after the age of 65 years, it was called senility or hardening of the arteries.

The chronologic distinction between senile and presenile dementia was not challenged until the 1960s, when questions were raised on the basis of autopsy studies in which no association was found between the degree of arteriosclerotic brain changes and the clinical manifestations of dementia during the person's lifetime. Landmark studies by Tomlinson and colleagues (1968, 1970) led to the theory that the neuropathologic changes of Alzheimer's disease represent a single disease process, regardless of the age at onset. Furthermore, studies of autopsy brain specimens from subjects with and without dementia revealed that Alzheimer's disease was the underlying cause of progressive dementia in most cases. Based on these and other studies, the causes of irreversible dementia were delineated as follows: 50% of the cases were attributable to Alzheimer's disease; 15% were the result of multiinfarct dementia; an additional 25% were attributable to a combination of Alzheimer's disease and multiinfarct dementia; and the remaining 10% were the result of less common causes, such as Pick's disease.

In 1974, Hachinski and colleagues published a landmark paper asserting that cerebral atherosclerosis was the cause of cognitive impairments in older adults and was also the most common medical misdiagnosis. Moreover, these scientists denounced the use of the phrase "hardening of the arteries" and suggested that the term *multiinfarct dementia* be used to describe dementias of cerebrovascular origin. Their rationale was that dementia was not caused by atherosclerosis or chronic ischemia, but by the occurrence of multiple cerebral infarcts. Another major contribution of this publication was that Hachinski and colleagues (1974) supported the findings of Tomlinson and associates (1968, 1970), emphasizing that Alzheimer's disease was the most common cause of progressive dementia. By the late 1980s, the term *multiinfarct dementia* was viewed as too narrow because it referred only to completed infarcts, and the term *vascular dementia* was used instead. The original Hachinski criteria for multiinfarct dementia are still being used, but several other clinical criteria have been proposed in recent years with the intent of more accurately reflecting the broad dimensions of ischemic brain injury (Chui, 2000; Ikeda et al., 2001).

As knowledge about vascular dementia and Alzheimer's disease increased, researchers discovered that some brain changes and patterns of behavior and cognitive impairment did not fit in existing diagnostic classifications. Much of this information has evolved since the 1990s, when brain imaging techniques were developed to provide information about different aspect of brain function. For example, computed tomography (CT) and magnetic resonance imaging (MRI) provide information about structural brain changes and lesions that can cause cognitive impairment. Single photon emission computed tomography (SPECT) and positron emission tomography (PET) scans provide specific information about metabolism rates for glucose and oxygen in the brain. Researchers currently use information from imaging techniques to supplement information from autopsies, clinical records, mental status tests, and other sources. In addition, many longitudinal studies provide valuable information about lifestyle patterns and cognitive function during adulthood, and some studies are designed to evaluate this information in relation to autopsy findings. Many of the current theories focus on the role of specific proteins as causative factors, and some researchers suggest that dementias be classified according to the type of protein abnormality. According to these theories, Alzheimer's disease, dementia with Lewy bodies, and frontotemporal dementia are associated with abnormalities of specific proteins, such as tau or amyloid precursor protein (Rogan & Lippa, 2002).

TYPES OF DEMENTIA

This chapter reviews current information about all types of dementia, but more emphasis is placed on Alzheimer's disease because that is the type of dementia that is most common and most widely studied. It is important to recognize that as dementia progresses, it becomes more difficult to distinguish one type of dementia from another. Thus, information about the different types of dementia is more relevant to making an accurate diagnosis and addressing the unique manifestations of the disease during the early and middle stages. As medications and other treatments are developed for each type of dementia, it will become more important to diagnose accurately specific types of dementia.

Alzheimer's Disease

Various figures on the prevalence of Alzheimer's disease have been quoted, with many estimates indicating that 50% of people aged 85 years or older and up to 80% of nursing home residents have Alzheimer's disease. Although studies about the rates of Alzheimer's disease at specific ages vary, gerontologists agree that the chance of having Alzheimer's disease increases with increasing age. Current consensus on prevalence rates—that is, the number of people who have Alzheimer's disease at a particular age—indicates the following rates: 1% to 3% of people aged 65 to 74 years, 6% to 11% of people aged 75 to 84 years, and 30% of people aged 85 years and older. Some recent studies have challenged the notion that the prevalence of Alzheimer's disease increases exponentially with increasing age. These studies suggest that a leveling-off effect occurs around the age of 85 to 90 years and that a decline in incidence begins at age 93 years for men and 97 years for women (Miech et al., 2002). However, studies of centenarians have found prevalence rates of between 51% and 64% for mild to severe dementia (Andersen-Ranberg et al., 2001; Silver et al., 2001).

Pathologic Changes Associated With Alzheimer's Disease

The presence of neuritic plaques and neurofibrillary tangles—first described by Alzheimer in 1907—are the hallmark pathologic criteria for Alzheimer's disease, as confirmed by numerous autopsy studies done since the 1960s (Figure 24-1). Although these pathologic alterations also occur in normal aging and other neurodegenerative diseases, the combination of a higher density in specific regions (e.g., the neocortex) and a clinical history consistent with Alzheimer's disease confirms the diagnosis of Alzheimer's disease (Tsuang & Bird, 2002). Loss or degeneration of neurons and synapses, particularly in the neocortex and hippocampus, is another central feature of the brain changes associated with Alzheimer's disease (Figure 24-2). In addition, Alzheimer's disease is associated with a marked reduction in brain weight.

Alzheimer first described beta-amyloid as a "peculiar substance" in 1907, but this substance was not named or defined until 1984. By the early 1990s, scientists had identified the presence of beta-amyloid in the plaques and blood vessels as another pathologic hallmark of Alzheimer's disease. The discovery that beta-amyloid was a normal substance produced by many cells in the body laid the groundwork for much of the current research on the role of beta-amyloid and its precursor protein. Scientists now know that beta-amyloid is a tiny, insoluble protein fragment of a much larger protein called the *amyloid precursor protein*. The exact functions of the amyloid precursor protein have not been identified, but researchers recognize that this protein has multiple essential roles in cells throughout the body. It is not known how beta-amyloid is released from the amyloid precursor protein. In some cases, a genetic mutation is thought to be an underlying factor, as discussed in the next section. What is known is that excessive amounts of beta-amyloid are found in the neuritic plaques and the walls of the blood vessels in the brains of people

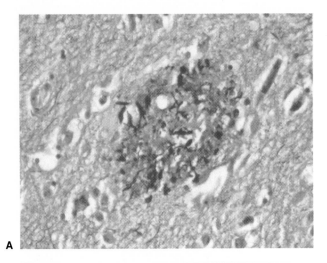

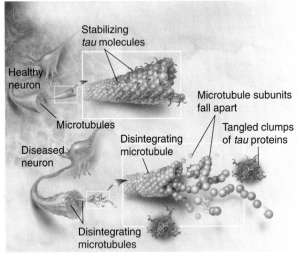

FIGURE 24-1 The hallmark neuropathologic findings in Alzheimer's disease. (A) Amyloid plaque. (B) Neurofibrillary tangle. (Images courtesy of the Alzheimer's Disease Education and Referral Center, a service of the National Institute on Aging.)

with Alzheimer's disease and Down's syndrome. These deposits cause damage by triggering a reaction in nearby healthy neurons that leads to their degeneration, and eventually, to cell death (Conway et al., 2003).

Currently, beta-amyloid plaques are the most widely studied neuropathologic change associated with Alzheimer's disease. Researchers are exploring whether the abnormal accumulation of beta-amyloid results from excessive production or insufficient removal and whether it is the cause or effect of pathologic processes. In addition, researchers are trying to find enzymes to reduce beta-amyloid, perhaps through drugs that stop its production. They also are trying to find ways of reducing the toxicity of beta-amyloid and reducing the associated inflammation of the brain. Researchers developed an Alzheimer's disease vaccine with the expectation

that it would stimulate the immune system to destroy beta-amyloid; however, clinical trials were halted in the early 2000s because of serious adverse events in the subjects who were vaccinated. Pharmaceutical companies are testing secretase drugs that are designed to inhibit the enzymes that divide the amyloid precursor protein.

Pathologic brain changes of Alzheimer's disease trigger degeneration in the neurotransmitters, and these changes may cause both cognitive and behavioral symptoms. Changes in neurotransmitters that are associated with Alzheimer's disease include the following:

- A loss of serotonin receptors and reduced serotonin uptake into platelets
- A 50% or greater reduction in the production of acetylcholine in the areas of the brain that contain plaques and tangles
- A reduction in the amount of acetylcholinesterase, which serves to break down acetylcholine after it has been secreted
- A reduction in the amount of choline acetyltransferase, with the greatest reduction in the areas most affected by plaques and tangles

Based on these findings, pharmaceutical companies have focused on developing drugs that affect neurotransmitter pathways. Initial drug interventions were directed toward increasing the brain's supply of choline and choline precursors by the use of such substances as choline and lecithin. Because this approach was not successful, the focus shifted to finding ways of preventing or slowing the breakdown of acetylcholine through cholinesterase inhibitors (e.g., tacrine, donepezil, rivastigmine, and galantamine). Recent and current approaches to drug development are discussed in the section on Nursing Interventions.

Theories About the Causes of Alzheimer's Disease

Researchers first raised questions about genetic factors as a cause of Alzheimer's disease in the mid-1930s, but it was not until the late 1970s that the term *familial Alzheimer's disease* appeared in the literature. Current studies suggest that an identifiable genetic mutation is found in 5% to 10% of cases of Alzheimer's disease (Rogan & Lippa, 2002). In familial Alzheimer's disease, the children of an affected parent have a 25% to 50% chance of having Alzheimer's disease if they live to be old enough for the disease to manifest itself. The risk is higher if the disease occurs in more than one generation and when the onset of the disease is before the age of 65 years (Tsuang & Bird, 2002). Abnormalities on chromosomes 1, 14, and 21 are associated with early-onset, or

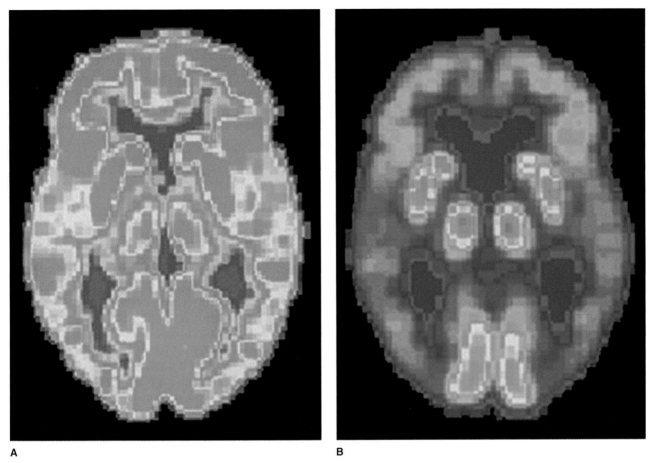

A   B

FIGURE 24-2 **(A)** A positron emission tomography (PET) scan of a brain of a healthy person. **(B)** A PET scan of a brain of a person with Alzheimer's disease. The blue areas indicate reduced brain activity. (Images courtesy of the Alzheimer's Disease Education and Referral Center, a service of the National Institute on Aging.)

familial, Alzheimer's disease, but researchers have yet to identify one fourth to one half of the genes for this disease (Kukull & Bowen, 2002). Recent discoveries related to beta-amyloid, chromosomal mutations, and the amyloid precursor protein form the basis for much genetics research. For example, people with Down's syndrome have an extra chromosome 21, where the amyloid precursor protein gene is located, and they inevitably show Alzheimer's disease–like brain changes at about 40 years of age. In addition, there is an increased risk for Down's syndrome in the families of individuals with Alzheimer's disease.

Researchers are particularly interested in genetic factors associated with the nonfamilial type of Alzheimer's disease, which constitutes between 90% and 95% of the cases. To this end, intensive efforts are being directed toward elucidating the role of apolipoprotein E (APOE). A relationship between the APOE genotype on chromosome 19 and Alzheimer's disease was discovered in the 1990s in conjunction with research on triglyceride metabolism

and cholesterol levels in cardiovascular disease (Roses, 1995). There are three variants of the *APOE* gene, designated as *APOE-$_E$2*, *APOE-$_E$3*, and *APOE-$_E$4*. Each person inherits one *APOE* gene from each parent, so there are six possible combinations (2/2, 2/3, 2/4, 3/3, 3/4, and 4/4). The inherited combination may be at least partially predictive of the risk for Alzheimer's disease as well as the age at onset. For example, an increased risk for Alzheimer's disease and a younger age at onset of Alzheimer's disease are associated with *APOE-$_E$4*, particularly in women (Choi et al., 2003; Tsuang & Bird, 2002). By contrast, *APOE-$_E$2* is associated with both a decreased risk for Alzheimer's disease and a later age at onset if the disease does develop. Current research is focusing on the practical implications of the role of *APOE* in causing or preventing Alzheimer's disease.

In addition to studying genetic factors, researchers are investigating numerous other factors thought to be associated with Alzheimer's disease. Researchers are particularly interested in the mechanisms involved with inflammatory processes that affect brain function because studies indicate that long-term use of nonsteroidal antiinflammatory drugs (NSAIDs) may reduce the risk for Alzheimer's disease (Landi et al., 2003; Zandi et al., 2002). The role of nerve growth factors (i.e., proteins that regulate nerve cell maturation) is another major focus of research and drug development. Researchers also are investigating potential roles of estrogen, antihypertensives, statin medications, and antioxidants (e.g., vitamins C and E) in preserving cognitive function and preventing or treating Alzheimer's disease (Crisby et al., 2002; Forette et al., 2002; Hajjar et al., 2002; Masaki et al., 2000; Murray et al., 2002). Similarly, researchers are investigating the role of nutritional deficits, hypertension, and elevated serum cholesterol as potential risk factors (Kivipelto et al., 2002). Other causative factors currently under investigation are head trauma, environmental toxins, the flow of calcium in and out of brain cells, and the possibility that Alzheimer's disease is a systemic metabolic disorder with some specificity for brain tissue.

Some theories have been studied for many decades and are inconclusive but still being investigated. For example, the discovery in 1920 of the virus that caused Creutzfeldt-Jakob disease generated theories about a viral cause of dementia, and these theories are still being investigated in relation to subtypes of Alzheimer's disease. Theories about aluminum as a cause of Alzheimer's disease have been widely publicized since the 1960s, based on findings that the brains of people with Alzheimer's disease contained abnormally high levels of aluminum. Some, but not all, subsequent studies confirmed this finding, and no study has determined whether increased aluminum levels were a cause or an effect of Alzheimer's disease. Based on current studies, there is no reason to believe that increased aluminum levels are related to the amount of aluminum ingested through the diet. Nor is there adequate evidence that high levels of aluminum are a causative factor in Alzheimer's disease.

Scientists are also studying other minerals as potential contributing factors in Alzheimer's disease, either alone or in combination with aluminum. For example, some studies have suggested that high fluoride levels in drinking water may have a preventive role in Alzheimer's disease, perhaps because fluoride can block absorption of aluminum in the intestinal tract. Another factor that is being investigated is the relationship between calcium and aluminum in the brain. Finally, zinc levels are known to be relatively low in people with Alzheimer's disease, but, as with aluminum and Alzheimer's disease, no cause-and-effect relationship has been established.

Despite the long history of intense research on Alzheimer's disease, no one theory has yet emerged to explain the causes of Alzheimer's disease. Many gerontologists are concluding that Alzheimer's disease, like dementia in general, is a syndrome of heterogeneous diseases caused by multiple interacting factors (e.g., aging, environmental influences, genetic mutations) (Kukull & Bowen, 2002). Perhaps in the near future, gerontologists will be able to identify several subtypes of Alzheimer's disease as well as effective preventive and treatment modalities.

Theories About the Stages of Alzheimer's Disease

In recent years, researchers have described the progression of Alzheimer's disease through stages of increasing involvement of the brain, and they currently are endeavoring to correlate pathologic brain changes with cognitive impairments and behavior changes (Perl, 2000) (Figure 24-3). Gerontologists are particularly interested in results of longitudinal studies that address questions about whether Alzheimer's disease and normal aging are distinct entities or part of a continuum. Similarly, some gerontologists suggest that Alzheimer's disease is a process of accelerated aging in which neurons are lost at a more rapid rate than normal (Chan, 2002). Because some longitudinal studies suggest that pathologic changes in the brain may begin years before the onset of clinical disease manifestations, the concept of preclinical Alzheimer's disease has emerged recently.

Gerontologists are now proposing that people can be classified in three distinct groups according to the degree of brain changes and the level of cognitive function. The first group is composed of people who do not have degenerative brain changes but exhibit the cognitive changes that are commonly called *age-associated memory impairment* (also called *benign senescent forgetfulness* or *age-associated cognitive decline*, as described in Chapter 7). The second group is composed of minimally cognitively impaired people who are in the predementia stage called *mild cognitive impairment*. Mild cognitive impairment is considered an early or incipient stage of Alzheimer's disease (Boeve et al., 2003; Ritchie et al., 2001; Storandt et al., 2002). People with mild cognitive impairment have higher death rates and are at increased risk for developing Alzheimer's disease, as compared with those in cognitively unimpaired control groups (Bennett et al., 2002; Morris, 2000). About half of people with mild cognitive impairment develop Alzheimer's disease within 4 years (Brandt, 2001). The third group in this categorization is comprised of people who have Alzheimer's disease.

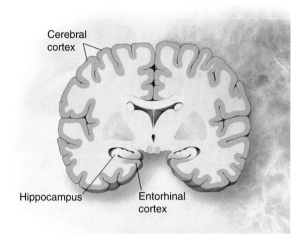

A

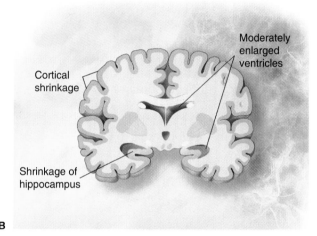

B

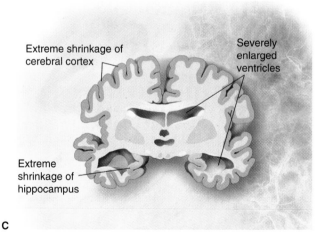

C

FIGURE 24-3 **(A)** Preclinical Alzheimer's disease. Subtle degenerative changes begin to occur in the cortex, and the person develops mild cognitive impairment. **(B)** Mild Alzheimer's disease. Degenerative changes affect the areas of the brain that control memory, language, and reasoning. **(C)** Severe Alzheimer's disease. Degenerative brain changes have caused significant atrophy in many areas. (Images courtesy of the Alzheimer's Disease Education and Referral Center, a service of the National Institute on Aging.)

Vascular Dementia

Much progress has been made in our understanding of vascular dementia since it was first described several decades ago. In contrast to the early belief that dementia was caused directly by arteriosclerosis or atherosclerosis, the current understanding is that vascular dementia is caused by the death of nerve cells in the regions nourished by the diseased vessels. Most commonly, vascular dementia is caused by a single major stroke or multiple small strokes (also called *transient ischemic attacks*). In these cases, the *terms poststroke dementia* and *multiinfarct dementia*, respectively, are applicable. Factors that increase the risk for vascular dementia after a stroke—which occurs in one fourth to one third of patients within 3 months of the first stroke—include older age, diabetes mellitus, recurrent strokes, fewer years of education, and involvement of the left hemisphere (Chui, 2000; Desmond et al., 2000; Roman, 2002).

The concept of ischemic brain injury encompasses a broader perspective and addresses all factors that can cause acute or chronic ischemia, which is the predominant pathophysiologic mechanism responsible for vascular dementia (Chui, 2000). Gerontologists now understand that vascular dementia is caused by ischemic processes, which in turn can be caused by conditions such as the following:

- Single or multiple emboli or atherosclerotic occlusions of large blood vessels
- Microinfarcts (lacunar strokes of the small arteries)
- Diffuse lesions involving the white matter (e.g., Binswanger's disease)
- Hemorrhage of large or small blood vessels
- Hypoxic lesions
- Hypoperfusion secondary to global brain ischemia following cardiac arrest or profound hypotension
- Hypoperfusion from chronic conditions such as orthostatic hypotension, cardiac arrhythmias, or congestive heart failure
- Narrowing of the lumen associated with diabetes, hypertension, or arteriosclerosis

Clinical manifestations of vascular dementia vary according to the area of the brain that is affected by the ischemia. Common manifestations include cognitive impairments (e.g., aphasia, memory impairment), behavior changes (e.g., apathy, depression, emotional lability), and sensory-motor deficits (hemiparesis, gait disturbances, hemisensory loss, urinary incontinence).

Many references state that the main features distinguishing vascular dementia from Alzheimer's disease are its tendency to have an abrupt onset and a stepwise progression; however, when vascular dementia is caused by numerous small infarcts, it may have a gradual onset and a linear progression. Recent studies suggest that the clinically silent presentations are more common and that the classic presentation of sudden onset with stepwise deterioration occurs less than half the time (Ross & Bowen, 2002). In addition, diagnostic procedures usually can trace the pathologic processes to damage in particular areas of the brain. A distinguishing characteristic of vascular dementia is that it is likely to be associated with identifiable risk factors, such as smoking, diabetes, hypertension, hyperlipidemia, previous strokes, cardiovascular pathology, and a sedentary lifestyle, all of which can be addressed through preventive and treatment measures.

Frontotemporal Dementia

Since the early 1990s, gerontologists have been investigating frontotemporal dementia (e.g., Pick's disease) as a distinct and common type of early-onset dementia (Ratnavalli et al., 2002). Neuronal atrophy, rather than plaques and tangles, affect primarily the frontal and anterior temporal lobes of the brain in this type of dementia. A distinguishing pathologic characteristic of frontotemporal dementia is the accumulation of abnormal forms of the tau protein (comparable to the accumulation of beta-amyloid protein in Alzheimer's disease). Other distinguishing features include a family history of a similar disorder and an onset before the age of 65 years.

Clinical manifestations of frontotemporal dementia differ significantly from those of other types of dementia during early stages; but as the disease progresses, they are similar to other dementias. Initially, behavioral disturbances, rather than memory impairments, are prominent, and many of the characteristic manifestations are associated with executive functions (e.g., abstraction, planning, self-regulation of behavior). If memory impairment occurs during early stages, it is usually due to difficulty concentrating or lack of concern or effort. Common behavioral characteristics of early-stage frontotemporal dementia include the following:

- Apathy or hyperactivity
- Impulsivity
- Distractibility
- Emotional lability
- Urinary incontinence
- Personality changes
- Withdrawal from social contact
- Lack of insight into appropriate social behavior
- Disinhibition (e.g., inappropriate jocularity, sexually provocative behavior)

- Loss of personal awareness (e.g., neglect of personal care)
- Language impairment (e.g., incorrect use of words, echoing what others say)
- Hyperorality (e.g., excessive or compulsive eating or drinking)
- Perseverative activity (e.g., repetitive clapping, humming, or singing)

Recent research suggests that another characteristic of frontotemporal dementia is increased sensitivity to extrapyramidal effects of neuroleptic medications, similar to that which occurs in dementia with Lewy bodies (Pijnenburg et al., 2003).

Because the onset of frontotemporal dementia often occurs before the age of 65 years and the manifestations can mimic behaviors associated with psychiatric disorders, this type of dementia is commonly misdiagnosed. In 2001, well-known dementia disease researchers and clinicians developed criteria for frontotemporal dementia and emphasized the importance of recognizing this condition as a dementia rather than a psychiatric disorder (McKhann et al., 2001). This will become increasingly important as new medications are developed for specific types of dementia.

Dementia With Lewy Bodies

Another type of dementia that currently is under intense investigation is dementia with Lewy bodies (i.e., spherical, intraneuronal inclusions that are formed by a protein in the neuron). Some gerontologists consider this condition a subtype of Alzheimer's disease because about 20% to 30% of autopsied brains of people with dementia have significant numbers of Lewy bodies in the neocortex and brainstem (Lopez et al., 2000). Other gerontologists consider this condition a form of Parkinson's disease because these conditions share many clinical and pathologic characteristics (McKeith et al., 2003). Still others consider it a separate type of dementia. Currently, there is much debate among researchers and dementia experts about the criteria for, and classification of, this type of dementia.

Although guidelines for diagnosing dementia with Lewy bodies have been developed, gerontologists and clinicians have questioned the criteria in recent years because all the so-called hallmark symptoms of dementia with Lewy bodies—parkinsonism, visual hallucinations, and fluctuations in cognitive skills—also occur commonly in other dementias and in Parkinson's disease. In particular, many questions pertain to whether the clinical manifestations are caused by the disease itself or are adverse effects of medications commonly used in people with this condition (Serby & Samuels, 2001). This is especially relevant because a characteristic of dementia with Lewy bodies that is widely recognized is that it causes hypersensitivity to many medications that act on the central nervous system. Thus, people who have dementia with Lewy bodies commonly experience serious adverse medication effects that are similar to the manifestations of dementia. For example, visual hallucinations and cognitive fluctuations may be secondary to the medications that are commonly used for people with dementia (Serby & Samuels, 2001). Similarly, researchers are trying to identify how (or if) the pattern of cognitive fluctuation of dementia with Lewy bodies differs from that of other dementias (Walker et al., 2000).

Increased neuroleptic sensitivity is a characteristic of dementia with Lewy bodies that has important clinical implications because people with this type of dementia are likely to have extreme, sometimes fatal, reactions to cholinergic-type medications, such as antipsychotics. Gerontological nurses and other health care practitioners need to be alert to the possibility that someone with dementia with Lewy bodies is likely to have idiosyncratic reactions or have extreme responses even to low doses of neuroleptic medications. For example, sedatives may cause extreme agitation, somnolence, or sleeplessness. Likewise, antipsychotic medications or medications for Parkinson's disease may cause or exacerbate delusions and visual hallucinations. Another clinically important characteristic is that people with dementia with Lewy bodies are medically frail and may decompensate rapidly and significantly when they have a medical condition (e.g., minor infection) or when their environment is changed (Rogan & Lippa, 2002). Because of the serious clinical implications of this type of dementia and because it is difficult to diagnose, nurses need to be alert to the possibility that someone may have undiagnosed dementia with Lewy bodies.

RISK FACTORS ASSOCIATED WITH DEMENTIA

Factors That Increase the Risk for Developing Dementia

Epidemiologic studies of people who are cognitively impaired are flourishing, and researchers are trying to identify conditions that increase the risk for developing dementia. Some studies focus on dementia in general, whereas others focus on a particular type of dementia (e.g., Alzheimer's disease, vascular dementia). Still others focus on preclinical dementia (e.g., mild cognitive impairment). Thus, conclusions about risk factors are clouded by differing scopes of studies

and overlapping and poorly defined terminology. The previous section on the four most common types of dementia discussed current findings about risk factors for each of these dementias. Researchers have identified the following risk factors for nonspecific dementia:

- Nonrheumatic atrial fibrillation (Sabatini et al., 2000)
- Hypertension (Birkenhager et al., 2001; Wu et al., 2003)
- Folate or vitamin B_{12} deficiency (Reynish et al., 2001; Whyte et al., 2002)
- Diabetes mellitus (Gregg et al., 2000)

As gerontologists discover more information about different types of dementia, it is very likely that they will be able to relate some of these risk factors to specific types of dementia.

Factors That Interfere With Assessment of and Interventions for Dementia

Attitudes, myths, and lack of information are risk factors that interfere with appropriate assessment of, and interventions for, dementia. In recent years, gerontologists have made tremendous progress in understanding and identifying causes of impaired cognitive function; hence, health care providers are increasingly less likely to attribute serious cognitive impairments to "normal aging." However, many older adults and their families and caregivers still falsely believe that "senility" is an expected and normal concomitant of aging. When this happens, treatable conditions are likely to be overlooked, and older adults are denied the appropriate interventions to treat or manage their conditions. Although there currently is no cure for dementia, treatment options are becoming more widely available. Even in the absence of curative treatments, many interventions are effective in delaying the progression of the condition, managing symptoms, and assisting with long-term planning. Nurses are not primarily responsible for diagnosing dementia, but they are responsible for educating older adults and their caregivers about normal age-related changes in cognitive function and encouraging assessment of any cognitive impairment that is beyond the range of normal. Therefore, nurses must challenge any attitudes that reflect the "what-do-you-expect-you're-old" syndrome and encourage appropriate assessment of cognitive impairment.

Attitudes about dementia are highly influenced by cultural factors, such as perceptions of aging and illness. For example, some cultural groups accept dementia as a normal process in old age, whereas other cultural groups view dementia-related behaviors as shameful. It is imperative that all health care providers demonstrate sensitivity toward various cultural interpretations of aging, illness, and dementia-related behaviors. Many such cultural interpretations create barriers to treatment and support services.

FUNCTIONAL CONSEQUENCES ASSOCIATED WITH DEMENTIA IN OLDER ADULTS

The functional consequences of impaired cognition focus more on those associated with Alzheimer's disease, rather than on those associated with other types of dementia, because researchers and clinicians have described functional consequences of Alzheimer's disease since the 1950s, making this the most widely studied type of dementia. Less is known about functional consequences associated with other types of dementia because researchers are just beginning to identify unique manifestations of different dementias. Because many of the functional consequences are common to all of the dementias, much of what is known about functional consequences of Alzheimer's disease is applicable to other types of dementia. Moreover, by the later stages of dementia, the functional consequences are similar in all types of dementia. However, during all stages and in all types, functional

consequences vary tremendously among individuals because of unique personality characteristics, coexisting conditions (e.g., depression, functional impairments), and other influencing factors.

Fifty years ago, Sjögren, a Scandinavian psychiatrist, described stages of Alzheimer's disease as: (1) memory loss; (2) impairment of language, motor ability, and object recognition; and (3) the terminal stage, which is marked by loss of continence, ambulation, and all language skills. This three-stage classification was widely used until the 1980s when an American psychiatrist, Reisberg, proposed a more detailed approach based on seven specific stages of Alzheimer's disease. Reisberg subdivided the last two stages (6 and 7) to reflect the loss of functional abilities in reverse order from that in which they were acquired during development—a process he refers to as *retrogenesis* (Reisberg, 1986; 2002). Reisberg's staging schema, which has been updated and refined, is referred to as the Global Deterioration Scale/Functional Assessment Staging, or GDS/FAST (Auer & Reisberg, 1997). This staging system is widely used and has been found to be valid and reliable for staging Alzheimer's disease in diverse settings. Table 24-2 summarizes the functional consequences associated with each of the seven stages of the GDS/FAST. It should be noted that the diagnosis of Alzheimer's disease is made retrospectively because it is based on a progression of manifestations.

TABLE 24-2 • Global Deterioration Scale/Functional Assessment Staging (GDS/FAST) of Alzheimer's Disease

Stage	Effects on Functioning
1: Normal adult	No deficits or complaints
2: Age-associated memory impairment	Deficits consistent with normal aging (i.e., no objective findings, difficulty with word finding, forgets location of objects)
3: Mild cognitive impairment	Some deficits in performing complex tasks, especially in demanding social and employment settings; diminished organizational skills; deficits noted by others for the first time
4: Mild dementia	Diminished ability to perform complex tasks (e.g., meal planning, financial management); decreased knowledge of current and recent events; flattened affect and withdrawal from challenging situations
5: Moderate dementia	Obvious cognitive deficits; unable to manage complex daily tasks without some supervision or assistance; difficulty remembering names of familiar people
6: Moderately severe dementia	Increasingly obvious cognitive deficits (e.g., disorientation, significant short-term memory impairment); personality and emotional changes (e.g., anxiety, delusions). Loss of abilities in the following order: (a) Difficulty putting clothing on properly without assistance (b) Unable to bathe independently (c) Unable to handle all aspects of toileting (e.g., does not wipe properly) (d) Occasional or frequent urinary incontinence (e) Occasional or frequent fecal incontinence
7: Severe dementia	Progressive loss of all verbal and psychomotor abilities: (a) Verbal abilities limited to six or fewer different words (b) Verbal abilities limited to a single intelligible word (c) Unable to walk without assistance (d) Unable to sit without assistance (e) Unable to smile (f) Unable to hold up head independently

Reisberg, B. [1986]. Dementia: A systematic approach to identifying reversible causes. *Geriatrics, 41*[4], 30–46.

Although the GDS/FAST schema has become widely accepted, researchers and practitioners recognize that people with Alzheimer's disease show a great deal of variability in the manifestations of the progressive decline from onset until death. For example, all people with Alzheimer's disease lose cognitive skills progressively through their remaining lifetime, but the changes differ significantly in the rates of decline and the precise skills that are affected. Thus, researchers are trying to identify cause-and-effect relationships between functional consequences and variables such as emotional response, concurrent conditions, caregiver supports, and environmental factors. Researchers also are trying to identify functional consequences that may be predictive of Alzheimer's disease but occur before the disease can be diagnosed (e.g., in stage 2 of the GDS/FAST schema). For example, Gates and colleagues (2002) found that decreased ability to process speech occurs in the preclinical stage and may be caused by pathologic changes that affect the auditory pathway or the frontotemporal lobes.

In recent years, gerontologists and health care practitioners are increasingly recognizing that death is the ultimate functional consequence of Alzheimer's disease, which is one of the 10 leading causes of death among older adults (Foley et al., 2003). The life expectancy of people with dementia is one half to one third that of people the same age without dementia; and the usual time from diagnosis until death is 10 years, with the end stage occurring during the last 2 to 3 years (Shuster, 2000). Currently, health care practitioners consider dementia a terminal illness and advocate for referrals for hospice care when a person has reached stage 7 on the GDS/FAST scale (Shuster, 2000).

Researchers, clinicians, people with dementia, and families and caregivers are intensely interested in identifying factors that influence survival time and rate of progression. The most consistently identified predictor of shorter survival time is poor functional status (Aguero-Torres et al., 2002). Other factors that may be associated with a faster rate of cognitive and functional decline include younger age at time of onset, fewer years of education, longer duration of illness, family history of dementia, and history of alcohol use (Santillan et al., 2003). Cerebrovascular disease (e.g., stroke) and other concurrent diseases and the presence of extrapyramidal symptoms are additional factors associated with faster progression and shorter survival (Carlson et al., 2001; Knopman et al., 2003; Santillan et al., 2003).

Impact of Dementia on the Person

One of the myths associated with dementia is that people with dementia deny their symptoms or have no awareness of their deficits. Unfortunately, this fallacy has led to serious misunderstandings on the part of some health care professionals, as exemplified by statements such as, "If they can ask if they have Alzheimer's disease, then they don't have it." In recent years, this perception of a high prevalence of so-called denial in people with dementia is diminishing, and gerontologists are researching *anosognosia* (i.e., the lack of awareness of cognitive deficit) and insight in people with dementia. Early studies suggested that insight and awareness are determined largely by neuropathologic factors, with damage to the frontal lobes and right hemisphere being more closely associated with anosognosia. However, recent studies emphasize that awareness is influenced by the interaction between cognitive impairment and psychosocial processes, such as coping skills and personality characteristics (Clare, 2002a). Gerontologists also thought that insight and awareness progressively diminish as the disease progresses; however, this conclusion has been challenged recently. For example, Arkin and Mahendra (2001) found that insight fluctuates during the course of the disease and does not necessarily diminish, but the ability to verbalize it diminishes with progression of the disease. Similarly, nurse-researchers found that subjects with MMSE scores of 7 or less "communicated either verbally or nonverbally their awareness that they had some impairment with remembering or being able to say what they wanted to say" (Mayhew et al., 2001, p. 109). Awareness of cognitive deficits varies among people at all stages of dementia and is on a continuum: whereas some people with dementia have full awareness of their deficits, others have no insight or awareness.

Common emotions and behaviors of people with dementia during the early stages include fear, shame, anger, anxiety, frustration, loneliness, depression, uselessness, self-blame, diminished affect, and withdrawal from challenging activities. Very commonly, people with dementia try to cover up their deficits to protect themselves and their families. These behaviors are not necessarily associated with denial, unawareness, or lack of insight; rather, they may reflect acceptance and positive coping (Clare, 2002a).

During the early stages, only the people who live, work, or have close contact with a person with dementia will notice the initial changes, such as impaired judgment and short-term memory. When the changes are noticed, numerous explanations may be applicable, and the deficits may be attributed to such factors as depression or the occurrence of a major life event (e.g., retirement, widowhood). People in the early stages of dementia may withdraw from complex tasks as a way of protecting themselves from the effects of diminishing cognitive abilities. For example, employed people may retire without acknowledging cognitive impairments as the reason. People who do not have to perform complex intellectual or psychomotor tasks may be able to conceal or compensate for the cognitive losses until the deficits seriously interfere with activities of daily living (ADLs). As the disease progresses, however, the person with dementia will be less able to cover up the changes, and people with less intimate contact will begin to question the underlying cause of the deficits.

Clare (2002b) interviewed people in the early stages of Alzheimer's disease and their partners to identify coping mechanisms they used to adjust to the onset of this disease. The most commonly identified coping mechanisms can be categorized as follows:

- Holding on (e.g., trying harder, taking medications, sticking to routine)
- Compensating (e.g., using memory aids, relying on partner)
- Developing a fighting spirit (e.g., obtaining information, talking about it, finding new roles, fighting it as long as possible)
- Coming to terms (e.g., finding a balance between hope and despair, accepting losses)

A common objective of all coping mechanisms was achieving a positive outcome for the self.

Cohen and associates (1984) described six phases of emotional response through the course of Alzheimer's disease. According to this model, phase 1 occurs before diagnosis and is characterized by a recognition and concern that something is seriously wrong. Phase 2, which begins when the diagnosis of Alzheimer's disease is made, is characterized by denial. After the diagnosis, during phase 3, people with Alzheimer's disease and their family members experience and must resolve the following feelings: shock, guilt, anger, depression, confusion, and questioning. Phase 4 is the coping stage, during which the person and family plan for present and future problems. Phases 5 and 6 occur if the person lives long enough after the onset of the disease. Phase 5, called maturation, is characterized both by an acceptance of the necessary losses and a striving to maintain functional abilities. Phase 6, a stage that "no patient has ever been able to express," is the point at which people can react to certain environmental stimuli but do not have the ability to respond actively (Cohen et al., 1984, p. 14).

Nurses must keep in mind that there is significant individual variation in the emotional responses of people with dementia, but there is always some emotional response. Feelings of fear, shame, anger, anxiety, and frustration may occur at any stage or last throughout the course of the disease, but they will vary in their manifestations.

Even in the later stages of dementia, when cognitive abilities are severely impaired, emotional response may be blunted or altered, but it is never absent. As dementia progresses, the person is likely to express emotions nonverbally and behaviorally. Thus, two important responsibilities of caregivers are to encourage and interpret nonverbal communication, which becomes the primary mode of communication during later stages of dementia (Hubbard et al., 2002).

People with dementia exhibit a wide range of behaviors—often referred to as *noncognitive symptoms*—that are superimposed on the cognitive impairments. The most commonly occurring noncognitive symptom is apathy, which occurs in up to 92% of people with Alzheimer's disease (Landes et al., 2001). *Apathy* is defined as a loss of motivation that is accompanied by behaviors such as indifference, diminished initiation, poor persistence, lack of interest, lack of insight, low social engagement, and blunted emotional response (Landes et al., 2001). Additional noncognitive behaviors associated with dementia include the following:

- Delusions
- Hallucinations
- Personality changes
- Agitation (physical or verbal)
- Inappropriate social and sexual actions
- Mood disturbances (depression, euphoria, emotional lability)
- Aberrant motor movements (pacing, rummaging, wandering)
- Neurovegetative changes (appetite changes, sleep disturbances)

Researchers have investigated many facets of these behaviors and have concluded that these behaviors:

- Occur in at least 90% of people with dementia at some time during the course of the disease
- Are extremely variable
- May herald the onset of the disease
- Show patterns of recurrence and fluctuation
- Are associated with more impaired functioning and a more rapid decline
- Increase in frequency as the disease progresses
- Often lead to institutionalization
- Are probably caused by neuropathologic changes
- May improve with treatment (e.g., cholinergic therapy, psychotropic agents) (Chung & Cummings, 2000)

Not all behavioral changes are problematic for caregivers, but the geriatric literature tends to focus on those behaviors that cause management problems. This is unfortunate because it reinforces fears and anxieties about the functional consequences of dementia that may never occur. This author has heard such remarks as, "I know he doesn't have Alzheimer's disease because he doesn't hallucinate," or "I know she doesn't have Alzheimer's disease because she's not violent." These comments reflect a false belief that certain difficult behaviors are an inevitable consequence of dementia. Another caregiver recently asked, "Can you tell me if my mother will be the 'nice kind' or the 'mean kind' as her Alzheimer's gets worse?" This question at least acknowledges that not all people with dementia are difficult, but it reflects another negative and false belief about categorical types of behaviors in people with dementia. Environmental influences and perceptions of caregivers determine whether behaviors are viewed as problematic. For example, in a locked institutional unit, wandering behaviors might not be problematic, whereas in a home setting, wandering may be both unsafe and otherwise problematic. Likewise, nighttime restlessness creates more problems for a spouse who is the sole caregiver than for nursing staff who are paid to provide 24-hour care.

The term *agitation* is applied to a wide variety of dementia-related behaviors: anxiety, wandering, irritability, sleep disturbances, restless walking, repetitive motor activity, nonaggressive or repetitive vocalizations, or verbally and physically aggressive behavior. In addition to being a dementia-related behavior, agitation can be a manifestation of certain types of depression, or it can arise from physiologic disturbances or adverse medication effects. Therefore, agitation cannot automatically be attributed to a dementing illness just because it occurs in someone with dementia. In fact, agitation in a person with dementia often is an early and prominent sign of a change in physical condition, such as an infection.

The term *catastrophic reaction* is commonly used in reference to behaviors associated with dementia. The term is applied to a wide range of behaviors that occur in people with brain damage and that are disproportionate to the reactions that would normally be expected in a situation (Mace & Rabins, 1999). These behaviors involve a sudden and exaggerated response to a situation that the person with dementia perceives as threatening. The onset of a catastrophic reaction may be signaled by a sudden change in mood, increased restlessness, stubbornness, or wandering. In addition, any of the following behaviors may be a component of the catastrophic reaction: anger, crying, shouting, anxiety, irritability,

combativeness, and physical or verbal aggression. Caregivers may interpret the overreaction as intentional and think the person is being obstinate, critical, or overemotional. Caregivers sometimes can identify specific precipitants of these episodes. For example, a catastrophic reaction may be precipitated by the caregiver assisting with essential ADLs, such as bathing or incontinence care, because the person with dementia may perceive this as embarrassing or threatening. At other times, caregivers may be unable to identify any precipitating factor. Catastrophic reactions resolve when the perceived threat is removed or when the person with dementia again feels safe and secure.

Gerontologists also are focusing on the meaning of behaviors for the person with dementia. For example, Johansson and colleagues (2002) found that caregivers interpreted "picking behavior" in people with dementia as a means of diminishing anxiety and striving for control, normalization, and a sense of staying in contact with others. Because of the growing recognition that behaviors are a primary mode of nonverbal communication for people with dementia, researchers and practitioners are emphasizing the importance of using neutral terms that more accurately reflect the meaning of behaviors (Cohen-Mansfield, 2000a; Richards et al., 2000). For example, references to behaviors as "disruptive," "problematic," or "disturbing," focus on the caregiver's response rather than on the perspective of the person with dementia (Talerico & Evans, 2000). Similarly, the term *aggressive* is commonly used to describe behaviors that are "among the most distressing of behavioral symptoms to caregivers, often resulting in institutionalization and significant caregiver injury" (Talerico & Evans, 2000, p. 77). In recent years, researchers and practitioners have increasingly recognized that people with dementia communicate their needs and feelings through behaviors that may be perceived as problematic (Talerico et al., 2002). Thus, the term *aggressive-protective* is more appropriate for describing behaviors that are rooted in a need for self-protection (Talerico & Evans, 2000).

Impact of Dementia on the Caregivers

Since the 1980s, gerontological references have addressed issues related to caregivers of older adults, with particular emphasis on those who care for relatives who have dementia. Focus on this topic has increased in recent years, as indicated by numerous articles in gerontological literature as well as countless books on caregiving that are widely available in bookstores. This attention is warranted because family and friends, despite the proliferation and availability of formal services for older adults in the United States, provide 80% to 90% of the care given to dependent older adults in the community.

The term *caregiver burden* is commonly used to describe the financial, physical, and psychosocial problems that are experienced by family members caring for impaired older adults. Most studies of caregiver burden focus on stresses related to caring for people in home settings, but recent studies suggest that moving the dependent person to a nursing home does not alleviate or even diminish the stress (Larrimore, 2003; Pearson, 2001). Researchers have identified the following specific functional consequences of caregiving (Acton, 2002; Larrimore, 2003; Narayan et al., 2001):

- Depression
- Disturbed sleep
- Social isolation
- Family discord
- Career interruptions
- Financial difficulties
- Lack of time for self
- Poor physical health
- Impaired immune function
- Mental, physical, and emotional strain
- Feelings of anger, guilt, grief, anxiety, hopelessness, helplessness, and chronic fatigue

Although most attention has been focused on the burdens of caregiving, there is increasing recognition that caregivers experience positive as well as negative consequences. For example, Narayan and colleagues (2001) found that spouse caregivers of people with dementia experienced their caregiving role as self-fulfilling and affirming while at the same time experiencing the losses and hardships of their role. The caregiving experience can cause anger, ambivalence, and emotional fragility; however, it can also be a source of strength and personal growth (Acton, 2002). Gerontologists currently emphasize the need to assess the caregiving experience in the context of the caregiver's whole life and to identify burdensome as well as beneficial aspects (Suwa, 2002). Nurses can use the Caregiver Strain Index, which is a reliable and valid assessment tool, to identify families with potential caregiving concerns (Sullivan, 2002).

NURSING ASSESSMENT OF DEMENTIA IN OLDER ADULTS

Despite the tremendous evolution of information about dementia, many questions remain unanswered. There is consensus among researchers and clinicians that dementia is a most complex syndrome that frequently involves several overlapping and coexisting conditions. Gerontologists also agree that different types of dementia have common pathologic features as well as some distinct features. The diagnosis of dementia is currently viewed as a two-step process. The first step is to determine that the person has dementia; the second step is to determine the type of dementia. Despite many recent advances in diagnostic modalities, the specific type of dementia still cannot be determined definitively until autopsy findings are considered in conjunction with information about the person's functional level during the course of the illness. Comprehensive geriatric assessment programs and research settings have significantly improved the ability to diagnose dementia, differentiate between the types of dementia, and identify other conditions that cause the cognitive impairment. For example, Massoud and colleagues (2000) found that between 8% and 9.3% of people diagnosed with dementia have a partially reversible condition and that less than 3% have a fully reversible condition. It is important to keep in mind that many people with dementia will have more than one disease condition that may be causing the cognitive impairment, behavior changes, and other clinical manifestations. Advances in knowledge are bringing us closer to the day when we will be able to diagnose accurately, treat successfully, and perhaps prevent dementia.

Initial Assessment

With the exception of delirium and poststroke dementia, impaired cognitive function is a slowly progressive process that requires assessment but does not usually require immediate attention. Often, the changes slowly occur over a period of years, and an assessment is delayed until the changes significantly interfere with normal functioning. The assessment process usually takes place over weeks or months and involves the compilation of information about both medical and psychosocial functioning. Because progressive cognitive impairment is a very complex phenomenon, it is quite difficult for a single health care professional to obtain and evaluate all the information necessary to determine the causes accurately. Thus, the assessment process generally is multidisciplinary, requiring input from primary care providers, psychiatrists, nurses, social workers, and rehabilitation therapists. Members of the assessment team must work with the family and other caregivers to obtain information and determine the appropriate level of involvement of the cognitively impaired person with regard to discussing assessment results and planning care. The major nursing focus is to

General Principles

- Assessment of impaired cognitive function usually takes place during several visits, and it might include a home assessment.
- Recognize that the person with impaired cognitive function may not be a reliable reporter and that health care professionals may need to check the accuracy of information.
- Health care professionals must respect the person's rights and ask permission before obtaining information from others, including family members.
- Do not assume that the family has drawn accurate conclusions about events of the past (e.g., family members may state that the person retired and then showed cognitive deficits when, in reality, the person retired because of an inability to cope with job demands).

Focus of the Assessment

- The primary purpose of the assessment is to identify causes of the cognitive impairment.
- An assessment of a person with impaired cognitive function is multidisciplinary and includes the following components: complete medical history and physical examination, including a review of all medications; a functional assessment; a comprehensive psychosocial and formal mental status assessment; and an assessment of environmental and caregiver influences, with particular emphasis on those factors that affect functional abilities.

- The assessment includes an interview with caregivers, family members, and other people who can describe the progression of the manifestations of impairment.
- Information about lifelong patterns of personality, coping, and performance characteristics is considered in relation to the person's current functional level.
- It may be necessary to ask probing questions to help family members recognize clues to cognitive deficits retrospectively.

Considerations in Assessing Risk Factors That Contribute to Impaired Cognitive Function

- Never assume that all cognitive impairments and behavioral manifestations stem from a dementing illness.
- Because risk factors can either cause the initial cognitive impairments or develop later, causing additional impairments, they must be reassessed periodically.
- The following categories of risk factors must be assessed, both initially and on an ongoing basis: depression, physiologic alterations, functional impairments, adverse medication effects, and environmental and psychosocial influences.
- Early in the assessment, ensure that vision and hearing impairments are compensated for as much as possible and that the environment does not interfere with the person's performance (e.g., make sure the person is using eyeglasses and a hearing aid if needed, and make sure the lighting is optimal).
- A priority is to identify and treat those factors that are reversible before deciding on a long-term management plan.

determine the person's level of function, to identify the factors that affect the person's level of function, and to identify the person's response to the illness. Frequently, the nurse serves as the team leader and is responsible for coordinating information and facilitating communication among team members and with the older adult and his or her family or other caregivers. Display 24-2 provides guidelines for assessing progressive cognitive impairment in older adults.

Ongoing Assessment

Because dementia is a progressive condition that commonly coexists with other conditions, all people with dementia require ongoing assessment of the following:

- Changes in cognitive and psychosocial function related to the dementia (e.g., a decline in cognitive abilities, the onset of anxiety or depression)

- Changes in mental status related to concurrent conditions (e.g., delirium due to a medical condition or adverse medication effects)
- Changes in functional abilities
- Causes of behavioral changes related to treatable conditions (e.g., anxiety, physical discomfort, environmental factors)

A major goal of ongoing assessment is to identify factors that interfere with the person's level of functioning or quality of life so that interventions can be initiated to alleviate these contributing factors. It is important to recognize that even though dementia is a progressive condition that gradually affects all levels of functioning, not all changes are caused by the dementia—many problems are caused by concurrent conditions and other variables that affect the level of functioning. Thus, ongoing assessment to identify all factors that affect level of functioning is essential. Another goal of ongoing assessment is to identify both strengths and limitations in the person's abilities so that individualized interventions can be

TABLE 24-3 ● Models for Nursing Assessment of Dementia

Assessment Model	Description	Recent References
Functional Assessment Staging Tool-Action Checklist	Assessment tool based on seven stages of dementia as defined in the FAST model (Table 24-2) with corresponding health education interventions identified	Gerdner & Hall, 2001; Connolly et al., 2000
Progressively Lowered Stress Threshold (PLST)	Assesses stressors that commonly trigger dysfunctional behaviors and excess disability: fatigue; change of routine, environment, or caregiver; demands that exceed functional capacity; inappropriate stimuli; affective response to loss (e.g., anger, depression); and physical stressors (e.g., illness, adverse medication effects)	Gerdner & Hall, 2001; Stolley et al., 2002
Dementia Care Mapping	Assesses 24 domains of quality of life ("well-being" and "ill-being") based on 6 hours of observations in a care setting and "maps" behaviors with emphasis on the viewpoint of the person with dementia (person-centered approach)	Kuhn et al., 2000
Cognitive Performance Evaluation	Uses functional tasks to assess an individual's level of information processing; emphasizes the person's abilities, encourages as much independence as possible, and identifies level of assistance that is necessary	Sevier & Gorek, 2000

planned to improve the person's functioning and quality of life. Because of the progressive and fluctuating nature of impaired cognitive function, the person's strengths and limitations will change periodically; thus, care plans must be updated frequently. Table 24-3 describes several models for ongoing assessment of people with dementia.

NURSING DIAGNOSIS

A nursing diagnosis most often applied to older adults who have dementia is Chronic Confusion, defined as "a state in which an individual experiences an irreversible, long-standing, and/or progressive deterioration of intellect and personality" (Carpenito, 2002, p. 237). Additional nursing diagnoses that are applicable to functional consequences associated with psychosocial responses to dementia include Fear, Anxiety, Hopelessness, Impaired Memory, Social Isolation, Self-Esteem Disturbance, and Ineffective Individual Coping. During the later stages when dementia affects the person's functional abilities, applicable nursing diagnoses include Wandering, Imbalanced Nutrition, Urinary Incontinence, Self-Care Deficit, Impaired Verbal Communication, Risk for Falls, Risk for Injury, Disturbed Sensory Perception, and Disturbed Sleep Pattern. If cognitive deficits interfere with the person's ability to take medications accurately, the nurse might apply the diagnosis of Ineffective Therapeutic Regimen Management.

Nursing diagnoses also may be used to address the needs of caregivers because much of the care of people with dementia focuses on helping the family and other caregivers address the day-to-day needs and issues of the person with dementia. Nursing diagnoses that might be used to address caregiver needs include Family Coping and Caregiver Role Strain (or Risk for Caregiver Role Strain). During the later stages of dementia, the nursing diagnosis Anticipatory Grieving may be appropriate, particularly for spousal caregivers.

OUTCOMES

The primary nursing goal for older adults in any stage of dementia is to promote function at the highest level of independence possible, while providing the supports that are necessary for the highest quality of life. Additional goals for nursing care of people with dementia include alleviating anxiety, maintaining reality orientation, promoting cognitive function, and facilitating optimum communication. Nursing Outcomes Classifications applicable to people with dementia include the following:

- Safety Behavior: Home Physical Environment
- Nutritional Status: Food and Fluid Intake
- Sleep
- Comfort Level
- Communication Ability
- Social Interaction Skills
- Coping
- Symptom Control
- Mood Equilibrium
- Leisure Participation
- Self-Care: Activities of Daily Living
- Quality of Life (Gerdner & Hall, 2001)

When the person with dementia is cared for by friends, family members, or paid caregivers, nursing goals address the needs of the caregivers. In the early stages of dementia, the caregiver's foremost need might be for information about the disease and about resources that address the changing needs of the person with dementia and the caregiver's own needs. As the dementia progresses, caregivers are likely to need emotional support and practical assistance. Nursing-sensitive outcomes for caregivers of people with dementia include: Caregiver Well-Being, Caregiver Emotional Health, Grief Resolution, and Quality of Life (Gerdner & Hall, 2001).

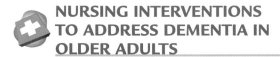

NURSING INTERVENTIONS TO ADDRESS DEMENTIA IN OLDER ADULTS

Information about interventions to address dementia is evolving at a rapid pace, and findings from recent studies are shedding light on appropriate interventions for treating the disease and managing the functional consequences. Most of the research on interventions has focused on Alzheimer's disease, but studies are expanding to address other types of dementia. For example, all the initial research on drug development focused on Alzheimer's disease, but recent studies address the use of these drugs for other types of dementia, such as vascular dementia and dementia with Lewy bodies. Regardless of underlying causes, however, many interventions are applicable to all people with dementia and are individualized according to specific manifestations (e.g., reassurance for anxiety and confusion, redirection for unsafe or inappropriate behaviors). Similarly, health promotion interventions (e.g., exercise and nutrition) are applicable for primary and secondary prevention for all types of dementia.

The approach to diagnosing and treating dementia can be likened to the approach taken when diagnosing and treating an infection. An infection is a generic diagnosis indicating the presence of a constellation of signs and symptoms (e.g., malaise, elevated temperature), but it does not indicate the causative factor. As additional information is collected, the specific type of infection is identified (e.g., pneumonia, urinary tract infection), and sometimes more than one infection is discovered. Until the specific causative agent is identified, generic measures are taken (e.g., antipyretics, broad-spectrum antibiotics). After the specific causative agent is identified (e.g., through culture and sensitivity tests), the infection is treated with very specific antimicrobial agents. At all stages, comfort measures are used.

Analogously, dementia is a generic diagnosis indicating the presence of a constellation of signs and

symptoms (e.g., memory impairment, personality changes), but initially little or no information is available about the cause. Because there are no clear indicators during early stages of most types of dementia, the cause is difficult to identify until the condition progresses. As further information evolves (e.g., patterns of cognitive and behavioral changes emerge, or the person has strokes or transient ischemic attacks) and clues are considered (e.g., the person's mother and father both had Alzheimer's disease), one or more causative factors are likely to be identified. As these factors are recognized, specific interventions can be used (e.g., cholinesterase inhibitors for Alzheimer's disease). Unfortunately, there are no "culture and sensitivity" tests for dementia, and sophisticated diagnostic procedures are not widely available; therefore, it is difficult to distinguish between different types of dementia until the condition progresses or unless specific risk factors are identified. Similarly, there currently are no pharmaceutical agents to cure dementia, although some drugs can delay the progression of the disease. Continuing the analogy, scientific developments for treating dementia are still in the "preantibiotic" phase. At any phase of dementia, and regardless of the cause, numerous interventions can be used to address comfort, functioning, and quality of life.

As anyone who has cared for a person with dementia knows, interventions must be highly individualized and frequently modified. An intervention that works for one person may not work for others, and interventions that are effective one day will not necessarily be effective the next day. Currently, a dominant theme of both research and practice is the implementation of person-centered interventions that are based on a comprehensive and ongoing assessment of the person's unique and changing needs. Thus, caring for people with dementia is a creative process and a most challenging aspect of gerontological nursing.

A comprehensive discussion of interventions for specific behaviors associated with dementia is beyond the scope of this chapter, but there are many practical references available on the management of dementia, and Table 24-4 lists some of the recent nursing studies of interventions for various dementia-related behaviors. In addition to professional nursing references, numerous books have been written by highly qualified and experienced caregivers and are excellent references for any nurse caring for people with dementia. The Alzheimer's Association and other resources listed at the end of this chapter provide health education materials and additional reliable information about interventions for people with dementia and their caregivers. This text

TABLE 24-4 • Studies of Interventions for Dementia-Related Behaviors

Reference	Intervention	Dementia-Related Behavior Addressed
Brush et al., 2002	Enhanced lighting in the dining room	Poor nutritional intake
DeYoung et al., 2002	Music therapy and management strategies such as encouraging independence, using time-outs, providing consistency in routines, and knowing the residents as unique individuals	Aggressive, agitated, disruptive behaviors
Dunn et al., 2002	Modified bed bath (thermal bath)	Agitation during bathing
Futrell & Melillo, 2002; Peatfield et al., 2002	Environmental modification; devices for safety, physical, and psychosocial interventions; support and education of caregivers	Wandering
Kolanowski et al., 2002	Diversional activities (e.g., games, sing-alongs, objects for tactile and visual stimulation)	Physical aggression, disruptive vocalization, non-aggressive physical behavior
Kovach & Wells, 2002	Pacing of sensory stimulation and sensory calming activity	Agitation
Lim, 2003	Systematic prompting and social reinforcement, using a series of one-step commands	Grooming behaviors
Lucero, 2002	Participation in structured recreational group activity and engagement in purposeful work-related activities	Wandering
Mickus et al., 2002	Privacy, Reassurance, Information, Distraction, and Evaluation (PRIDE)	Agitation during bathing
Miller et al., 2001	Audio presence intervention	Agitation
Moss et al., 2002	Reminiscence group activities	Impaired communication
Rader & Barrick, 2000	Person-centered, rather than task-centered, focus	Agitation during bathing
Roberts & Durnbaugh, 2002	Modifications of dining room milieu	Poor nutritional intake

will provide an overview of the theoretical frameworks that form a basis for common nursing interventions and explain how interventions may vary depending on the setting where the person is receiving care. Commonly employed nursing interventions will then be discussed.

Theoretical Frameworks for Nursing Interventions

Hall and Buckwalter (1987) first proposed a theoretical framework for nursing interventions for people with dementia, called the Progressively Lowered Stress Threshold (PLST) model. Briefly stated, this model posits that dysfunctional behaviors indicate a progressive lowering of the stress threshold, which, in turn, interferes with the person's function and ability to interact with the environment. The goal of nursing care, then, is to maximize the person's function by relieving stressors that cause excess disability. The choice of interventions is based on an ongoing assessment of anxiety "as a barometer to determine how much activity and stimuli the anxious person can tolerate at any point during their illness. As anxious behaviors occur, activities and environmental stimuli are modified and simplified until the anxiety disappears" (Hall & Buckwalter, 1987, p. 403). This approach is highly individualized, and from a nursing perspective, it is analogous to adjusting insulin doses

according to serum glucose levels. Display 24-3 summarizes the principles of this approach.

In recent years, researchers have developed many additional theoretical frameworks to explain behavioral problems in people with dementia. These theoretical frameworks, which are not mutually exclusive, focus on the following causes of dementia-related behaviors:

- Neuropathologic changes inherent in the disease
- Unmet needs of the person with dementia
- Behavioral patterns that are controlled by antecedents and consequences
- Environmental effects (Cohen-Mansfield, 2000b)

Nurses and other health care professionals are using these models to develop interventions that address the underlying problems, rather than simply addressing the behaviors. Many recent nursing models focus on unmet needs. These models propose that problematic behaviors in people with dementia reflect an attempt to communicate needs that the person may not consciously recognize and cannot express verbally. For example, the Need-Driven, Dementia-Compromised Behavior (NDB) model has been used to identify interventions for numerous behaviors that occur in people with dementia (e.g., Cohen-Mansfield, 2001; Colling & Buettner, 2002; Richards et al., 2000; Whall, 2002). The NDB model is used "to assess strengths that can be improved, weaknesses that can be circumvented, and adaptation patterns that can be

DISPLAY 24-3

Nursing Interventions for People With Dementia Based on the Progressively Lowered Stress Threshold Model (PLST)

- Maximize safety by modifying the environment to compensate for cognitive losses.
- Control any factors that increase stress, such as fatigue; physical stressors; competing or overwhelming stimuli; changes in routine, caregiver, or environment; and activities or demands that exceed the person's functional ability.
- Plan and maintain a consistent routine.
- Implement regular rest periods to compensate for fatigue and loss of reserve energy.
- Provide unconditional positive regard.
- Remain nonjudgmental about the appropriateness of all behaviors except those that present threats to safety.
- Recognize individual expressions of fatigue, anxiety, and increasing stress, and intervene to reduce stressors as soon as possible.
- Modify reality orientation and other therapeutic interventions to incorporate only that information needed for safe function.
- Use reassuring forms of therapy, such as music and reminiscence.

(Hall, G. R., & Buckwalter, K. C. [1987]. Progressively lowered stress threshold: A conceptual model for care of adults with Alzheimer's disease. *Archives of Psychiatric Nursing, 1*, 399–406.)

supported" (Buettner & Kolanowski, 2003, p. 22). Similarly, Cohen-Mansfield (2000a) applies the Treatment Routes for Exploring Agitation (TREA) unmet needs model to verbal agitation and other types of aggression in people with dementia.

General Principles of Nursing Interventions in Different Settings

Long-Term Care Settings

In recent years, there has been increasing implementation of multifaceted interventions for people with dementia in nursing home settings. For example, dementia care programs based on the principles incorporated in the Eden Alternative (discussed in Chapter 5) are becoming more widely implemented in many nursing home settings. This attention is warranted because almost 90% of nursing home residents are cognitively impaired, and about half are severely cognitively impaired (Teresi et al., 2000).

Another recent trend is the development of specially designed special care units (SCUs) for people with dementia. Essential features of these nursing home units for cognitively impaired residents include environmental modifications, family involvement, individualized care plans, dementia-specific activity programs, and specially trained and selected staff. Many positive outcomes of SCUs have been identified for the staff, the residents with dementia, and the families of these residents. For example, less resident depression and agitation and improved social interaction and friendships among residents are positive effects of smaller units (i.e., fewer than 30 residents) (Calkins, 2001). Many of the positive outcomes that area associated with SCUs can be achieved in nursing care units that address the individualized needs of the residents, even if these units are not specifically designated as SCUs. Currently, these programs are viewed as a stimulus to "raise the general standard of care" for people with dementia (Maslow & Ory, 2001). Many assisted-living facilities also have special dementia care units and programs. These units and programs are similar to those in nursing homes, but are not always able to provide care for people in later stages of dementia.

Acute Care Settings

Although an older adult may be hospitalized for an initial evaluation of dementia, especially if there are primary or secondary physiologic causes, the more common scenario is that a person with dementia is hospitalized for evaluation and treatment of an acute medical problem that is superimposed on the dementia. Consequently, nurses in hospital settings usually deal not only with the acute illness, but also with the dementia-related behaviors, which are exacerbated by the medical problem, the hospital environment, the unfamiliar caregivers, and the change in routines. Thus, nurses in acute care settings face a tremendous challenge in caring for people with dementia.

One of the most important initial interventions is to involve at least one of the older adult's usual caregivers in planning and implementing nursing care for the cognitively impaired person. Although the person with dementia is likely to exhibit different behaviors in the hospital than at home, nurses must begin by identifying any interventions that were effective in the home environment. During the admission process, nurses may save a lot of time and frustration by interviewing the caregivers about specific methods that help or hinder care. For example, knowing that the person eats only sandwiches or needs to be assisted to the toilet at specific times may facilitate the planning of effective interventions. It is important to remember that people with dementia may not express their needs directly or verbally. Usually, family caregivers have a good understanding of the needs of the person and the expressions of those needs, but if this information is not obtained at the time of admission, the person's needs may not be addressed.

In addition to obtaining information from one of the usual caregivers, nurses may consider involving the caregiver in the person's care or asking him or her to provide a familiar presence during the hospitalization. Although family members and other caregivers deserve a respite from caregiving responsibilities, they may be willing to assist at some level with the care of the patient. This may be particularly helpful during the first few days of hospitalization, and with patients who are especially difficult to manage. Often, the family will be relieved to be able to participate in the care, especially if they have never had any outside assistance.

Community Settings

In community settings, professional nurses usually work with family members or paid caregivers, rather than directly implementing the interventions for the person with dementia. Thus, their primary responsibilities are to serve as role models and to educate caregivers about interventions that will promote the highest level of function for the person with dementia and the least burden for the caregivers. An intervention that might be most effective, as well as efficient, is to encourage caregivers to participate in educational or support groups. Caregiver support groups are widely available and have been found to be successful in diminishing caregiver stress and helping caregivers cope with challenging situations (Hebert et al., 2003). The number of groups addressing the needs of caregivers is increasing rapidly, and information about these groups is available from the Alzheimer's Association or local hospitals. Nurses also can encourage caregivers to purchase one of the many caregiver guides that are available in bookstores or through the Internet and to contact the Alzheimer's Association and other resources for information. Connolly and colleagues (2000) developed an excellent guide to providing health education to caregivers and people with dementia through the stages of dementia.

In addition to educating caregivers about specific management problems, nurses in community settings must be ready to discuss resources for medical care, home services, and other community-based services for people with dementia and their caregivers. As the number and range of services increase, it is becoming more and more difficult to keep up to date on the resources in one's own community. Although nurses cannot be expected to know all the details about all available community services, they should know about the general types of services available. In addi-

tion, they must be able to suggest at least one information and referral resource from which caregivers can obtain specific information. A good rule of thumb is to suggest that caregivers call the local area agency on aging because this type of organization serves every part of the United States. Additionally, local chapters of the Alzheimer's Association provide information about resources for care, and many chapters provide direct services. Information about these services can be obtained from the national Alzheimer's Association and the Eldercare Locator, listed in the Educational Resources section at the end of this chapter. In addition, various types of services that may be helpful to people with dementia and their caregivers are discussed in Chapter 26.

Improving Safety and Function Through Environmental Adaptations

Environmental modifications are important interventions for people with dementia because environmental factors profoundly affect their functioning, particularly in the middle and later stages of the disease. Environmental interventions are particularly important for ensuring safety, fostering independence in ADLs, and preventing and addressing problematic behaviors (e.g., wandering). Examples of environmental factors that significantly affect the safety, functioning, and well-being of people with dementia are as follows:

- Noise
- Floor surfaces
- Colors and color contrast
- Lighting (e.g., glare, shadows, brightness)
- Design and placement of exits and bathrooms
- Presence of living things (e.g., plants, birds, fish, pets)
- Furniture (seating, placement, heights of tables and chairs)
- Use of safety devices (e.g., rails, grab bars)
- Provisions for privacy and social interaction
- Presence of items that improve comfort and home-likeness (e.g., decorative items, textured items, meaningful personal belongings)
- Absence of potentially harmful items (e.g., clutter, obstacles, sharp knives, cleaning solutions and other potentially toxic products)

Display 24-4 summarizes environmental interventions and techniques to address safety and independence in ADLs.

During the 1960s, gerontologists emphasized the role of environmental modifications in providing stimulation, and they suggested that reality orientation programs be widely implemented, particularly in

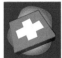

DISPLAY 24-4

Environmental Adaptations and Techniques for Improving Safety and Functioning in People With Dementia

General Environmental Modifications

- Modify the environment to compensate as much as possible for sensory deficits and other functional impairments. (Refer to interventions in Chapters 12 through 15 and 18.)
- Use clocks, calendars, daily newspapers, and simple written cues for orientation (e.g., day, date, names, place, and events).
- Use simple pictures, written cues, or color codes for identifying items and places (e.g., toilet, bedroom).
- Use simple written cues to clarify directions for operating radios, televisions, appliances, and thermostats (e.g., on, off, directional arrows).
- Place pictures of familiar people in highly visible places, but use nonglossy pictures and nonglare glass in picture frames.
- Turn lights on as soon as or before it begins to get dark.
- Use nightlights, or leave dim lights on during the night.
- Provide adequate environmental stimuli while avoiding overstimulation.

Techniques to Ensure Safety

- Make sure the person carries some form of identification, along with the phone number of someone to call.
- Adapt the environment for safety (e.g., use alarm devices for doors to prevent wandering).
- Keep the environment uncluttered.

- Keep medications, cleaning solutions, and any poisonous chemicals in inaccessible places.
- Enroll the person in a protective program, such as the Safe Return program sponsored by the Alzheimer's Association.

Techniques to Facilitate Independent Performance of Activities of Daily Living (ADLs)

- Keep all activities as simple and routine as possible.
- Establish routines that allow for maximum independence and the least amount of frustration.
- While keeping the routines as consistent as possible, recognize that they will have to be changed as the person's level of function changes.
- Lay out one set of clothing in the order in which the items are to be donned.
- If the person needs assistance with hygiene, use matter-of-fact statements, such as "It's time for your bath."
- Arrange personal care items, such as grooming and hygiene aids, in a visible and uncluttered place, in the order in which the items are to be used.
- Leave a toothbrush on the bathroom sink with toothpaste already on it.
- Establish an individualized toileting plan that allows for maximum independence but minimal risk for incontinence episodes.
- Offer finger foods and nutritious snacks if the person will not sit at the table to eat a meal.

nursing homes and other residential care settings. Reality orientation involves the repeated use of verbal and nonverbal indicators of time, place, and person in the context of the individual, group, and environment. For example, nurses and nursing assistants give verbal information about the time of day, and "reality orientation boards" display large-print information about the day, date, and weather. The goals are to improve the person's self-esteem and sense of control and to reduce his or her confusion, anxiety, and disorientation. Reality orientation may be effective for some people with dementia, especially when combined with other strategies, but it should not necessarily be applied to all people with dementia, and it must be tailored to individual needs.

Currently, gerontologists are emphasizing the important role of the total physical environment as "a therapeutic resource to promote well-being and functionality among people with dementia" (Day et al., 2000). Researchers are emphasizing that, to be therapeutic, environmental modifications must be individualized and adapted to meet the needs of people at different stages of dementia (Teresi et al., 2000).

Lighting and sensory stimulation are two specific aspects of environmental interventions that researchers have addressed recently. For example, Ancoli-Israel and colleagues (2003) found that morning exposure to bright light (from sun or artificial sources) improved sleep patterns and diminished agitation in people with dementia, and this effect may be particularly beneficial during the mild or moderate stages. A comprehensive nursing review of studies on the use of multisensory stimulation for people with dementia—achieved by using aromatherapy, soft music, favorite foods, and colored lighting effects—concluded that this type of intervention "may be one effective intervention with a positive view and an intent to provide pleasure. As nurses, we should use it" (Chitsey, et al., 2002, p. 48).

Communicating With Older Adults With Dementia

Communication techniques, particularly nonverbal methods (e.g., touch, facial expression), are extremely important nursing interventions for people with dementia throughout the entire course of the disease (Hendryx-Bedalov, 2000). Currently, both researchers and practitioners are emphasizing the importance of maintaining two-way communication through all stages of dementia, despite the person's declining ability to communicate verbally. There is much agreement that people with dementia communicate through their behaviors at all stages of the disease, even though they gradually lose the ability to communicate verbally (Hubbard et al., 2002). Although people with dementia are often labeled as "confused" because they cannot use words accurately to communicate their thoughts, it may be more appropriate to identify the listener as confused because he or she is unable to interpret accurately the verbal expressions of the person with dementia (Mayhew et al., 2001). Thus, a major challenge of communicating with people who have dementia is interpreting verbal and nonverbal communication.

Gerontologists are emphasizing the importance of sensory stimulation strategies to improve communication by enhancing the memory processes that are involved with communication. Bourgeois (2002) described the following examples of such strategies:

- Printed materials using highlighting, bright colors, enlarged type, high contrast, and color coding
- Labels, nametags, calendars, post-it notes, message boards
- Devices to enhance auditory communication (e.g., alarms, times, hearing aids, assistive listening devices)
- Memory aids: watches, cue cards, notebooks, tape recorded messages
- Verbal communication: smile, establish visual contact
- Auditory communication: calm and positive speech, frequent use of proper names
- Tactile communication: touch, familiar objects

Touch, including gentle massage, is a method of sensory stimulation that is well received by nursing home residents and is within the scope of nursing (Sansone & Schmitt, 2000). Display 24-5 summarizes techniques for facilitating communication with people with dementia.

Providing Health Education About Medications

Because they are the health care professionals who most often counsel older adults who have dementia and their families about interventions for dementia,

nurses play an important role in providing health education about medications for dementia. Medications are becoming increasingly more important in treating dementia because recent studies and guidelines support and encourage the use of cholinesterase inhibitors during the early and middle stages of dementia. In addition, other types of medications are being investigated for treatment of dementia, and many over-the-counter products are being promoted for prevention and treatment of dementia. Nurses also are frequently involved with decisions about medications for managing dementia-related symptoms.

Drugs for Slowing the Progression of Dementia

Since 1993, when the first drug was approved for the treatment of Alzheimer's disease, much progress has been made in our knowledge about pharmaceutical treatment and prevention strategies for Alzheimer's disease as well as other types of dementia. By 2001, the U.S. Food and Drug Administration (FDA) had approved four cholinesterase inhibitors for the treatment of Alzheimer's disease. Tacrine (Cognex), the first drug approved, is still available, but the other three drugs—donepezil (Aricept), rivastigmine (Exelon), and galantamine (Reminyl)—are much more widely used because they have fewer adverse effects. Despite these advances in knowledge, however, 2002 was the first year since 1999 in which no new drugs were approved for the treatment of dementia.

Cholinesterase inhibitors currently are the standard of medical therapy for dementia. Researchers have consistently found that these drugs exert modest positive effects in improving or delaying the progression of functional decline and cognitive and behavioral symptoms (Bonner & Peskind, 2002; Cummings, 2003; Purandare et al., 2002; Trinh et al., 2003). In the early 2000s, researchers began publishing studies of the effects of cholinesterase inhibitors on types of dementia other than Alzheimer's disease. There is increasing evidence that these drugs are effective for vascular dementia and dementia with Lewy bodies, but as of 2003, the FDA had not approved of these drugs for any dementia other than Alzheimer's disease. Nurses can use Display 24-6, which summarizes current information about cholinesterase inhibitors, for health education of older adults and their families.

As of 2003, no medication had been determined to be effective in reversing or permanently improving the symptoms of dementia, but many drugs were being investigated. Particular emphasis is on antioxidants (e.g., ginkgo biloba), NSAIDs, memantine, and drugs with neuroprotective effects. Vitamin E, taken

DISPLAY 24-5

Facilitating Communication With People Who Have Dementia

Verbal Communication

- Adapt your level of communication to the abilities of the person with dementia.
- Use very simple sentences.
- Present only one idea at a time.
- Allow enough time for processing.
- Avoid infantilization (e.g., do not talk baby talk or use a demeaning or condescending tone of voice).
- Assist with word finding (e.g., supply missing words, repeat the person's sentence with the correct word).
- Avoid shaming the person (e.g., do not emphasize deficits).
- Paraphrase what the person says and ask for clarification about the meaning.
- If the person does not understand a statement, repeat the statement using the same words, or simplify the wording.
- Do not argue with the person, unless it is a matter of safety.
- Avoid complex or sarcastic humor.
- Use positive statements (i.e., avoid using statements containing the word "don't" or other negative commands).
- Involve the person with decisions to the best of his or her ability by offering simple and concrete choices (e.g., "Do you want chicken or steak?" rather than "What do you want to eat?").
- Do not ask questions that you know the person cannot answer correctly.

- Do not test the person's memory unnecessarily.
- Listen to the feelings the person is trying to express and respond to the feelings, rather than the statement.
- When discussing activities of daily living (ADLs), avoid statements such as "You need a bath now," which may be interpreted as judgmental.

Nonverbal Communication

- Attract and maintain the person's attention (e.g., through eye contact, pleasant facial expressions).
- Use a relaxed and smiling approach.
- Reinforce verbal communication with appropriate nonverbal communication (e.g., demonstrate what you are asking the person to do).
- Use simple pictures rather than written cues.
- Use appropriate touch for communication (e.g., to gain the person's attention or reinforce feelings of concern), unless the person responds negatively to touch.
- Be aware of your own nonverbal communication.
- Keep in mind that your nonverbal cues will probably communicate more than your spoken words and will not necessarily be interpreted correctly.
- Closely observe all nonverbal cues exhibited by the person, especially those that express feelings.
- Assume that all nonverbal expressions of the person with dementia are attempts to communicate needs or feelings.

alone or in combination with selegiline (a drug prescribed for the management of Parkinson's disease), can delay the progression of Alzheimer's disease. The effects of the drugs are thought to be attributable to their antioxidant properties, which may improve overall health and function. Current recommendations are that people with dementia take vitamin E (starting with 400 IU daily and increasing gradually to 1000 IU twice daily) to slow disease progression (Bonner & Peskind, 2002). Display 24-7 summarizes findings from recent studies published about medications for dementia.

Drugs for Managing Dementia-Related Symptoms

Behavior-modifying medications may be an effective and essential intervention for the safety and comfort of people with dementia as well as their caregivers, but decisions about the use of these medications are very complex for several reasons. First, because difficult behaviors are often precipitated by factors such as medical conditions, environmental influences, and adverse medication effects (e.g., anticholinergic medications), efforts should be made to identify and address any treatable causes before initiating behavior-modifying medications. For example, in some situations, the most effective intervention is to discontinue a medication rather than begin a medication. Second, there is always a risk that medications will further interfere with function and perhaps even cause serious harm. A third consideration is whether the behaviors justify the risks associated with medications. Bothersome or socially inappropriate behaviors might better be ignored or tolerated than treated with medications. However, if the behavior is unsafe, uncomfortable, or interferes with the function of the person with dementia, then pharmaceutical intervention is probably justified if other interventions are not successful. Moreover, if the behavior interferes with the rights of the caregivers or other people in the environment, then consideration might be given to medication management. In any situation, health care professionals

Cholinesterase Inhibitors Available in the United States in 2003

- Tacrine (Cognex)
- Donepezil (Aricept)
- Rivastigmine (Exelon)
- Galantamine (Reminyl)

Effectiveness of Cholinesterase Inhibitors for Dementia

- There is increasing support for starting a cholinesterase inhibitor early in the course of Alzheimer's disease and continuing the treatment during the early and middle stages.
- Cholinesterase inhibitors stabilize cognitive function and delay the progression of dementia symptoms; they noticeably improve cognitive function in about one third of people with dementia.
- Cholinesterase inhibitors stabilize or improve all the following: memory, language skills, functional abilities (e.g., activities of daily living), and behaviors such as pacing, delusions, and uncooperativeness.
- Cholinesterase inhibitors may have similar positive effects in people with vascular dementia or dementia with Lewy bodies, but these drugs are currently approved only for Alzheimer's disease.

- Because the effectiveness of a cholinesterase inhibitor is significantly diminished if it is stopped and then restarted, it is important to ensure regular administration of this type of drug.
- All cholinesterase inhibitors are equally effective for Alzheimer's disease, but tacrine is no longer initiated because the newer drugs have fewer adverse effects and a more convenient dosing schedule.

Dosing and Adverse Effects

- The usual dosing schedule for the commonly used drugs is once daily for donepezil and twice daily for rivastigmine and galantamine.
- Nausea, vomiting, diarrhea, and loss of appetite are common adverse effects, but these effects can be prevented or reduced by starting with a low dose and gradually increasing to the maximum dose.
- Less common adverse effects include sleep disturbances, extrapyramidal symptoms, and cardiorespiratory events.
- Rivastigmine may be more likely than donepezil or galantamine to cause gastrointestinal adverse effects but less likely interact with other medications.

Cholinesterase Inhibitors

- Rivastigmine is less likely to interact with other drugs (particularly those that are metabolized in the liver) and therefore may be safer and better tolerated in people with concomitant illnesses (Inglis, 2002).
- Rivastigmine is more likely than donepezil or galantamine to cause gastrointestinal adverse effects, but these effects can be avoided by starting with a low dose and increasing it gradually and by administering the medication with food (Inglis, 2002).
- Rivastigmine may be effective for at least 2 years in improving behavioral and cognitive symptoms in people with Alzheimer's disease, vascular dementia, and dementia with Lewy bodies (Farlow, 2002; Robert, 2002; Rosler, 2002; Wesnes, 2002).
- Galantamine is effective in cognitive and behavioral symptoms in both Alzheimer's disease and vascular dementia; in mild stages, the improvement is primarily cognitive, and in later stages, the improvement is primarily in behavioral symptoms (Erkinjuntti, 2002).
- Donepezil is effective in improving cognitive function in people with vascular dementia (Meyer, 2002).

Other Medications

- Long-term use of nonsteroidal antiinflammatory drugs (NSAIDs) may reduce the risk for Alzheimer's disease if people begin using it well before the onset of dementia (Zandi et al., 2002).
- Statins are effective in reducing the prevalence of dementia and arresting the progression of cognitive impairment (Hajjar et al., 2002)
- Nimodipine (Nimotop), a calcium channel blocker used since 1988 for cardiovascular disease, is prescribed for dementia in European countries and may be of some benefit (Lopez-Arrieta, 2002).
- People with Alzheimer's disease showed significant cognitive improvement after 2 months of treatment with Cerebrolysin (Cere), a neurotropic (Panisset et al., 2002).
- Memantine, which has been used for more than a decade in European countries, is effective for the treatment of Alzheimer's disease and vascular dementia, and is sometimes used in combination with a cholinesterase inhibitor (Hartmann & Mobius, 2003; Orogozo et al., 2002).

DISPLAY 24-8
Guidelines for Decisions About Behavior-Modifying Medications for People With Dementia

Considerations Regarding Behavior-Modifying Medications

- Assess whether any of the following factors cause or contribute to the difficult behaviors: environmental conditions; psychosocial factors, such as anxiety or depression; or physiologic factors, such as pain, discomfort, or medical disorders. If any of these factors are implicated, interventions should be directed at the causative factor.

- Are the behaviors caused by adverse medication effects? In this case, the appropriate intervention might be to reduce the dose of or discontinue a medication, rather than begin a new medication.

- Treatment with medication should be implemented for behavior problems only after a trial of nonmedication interventions.

- Do the behaviors truly justify the use of medications, or are the caregivers requesting medications for their own comfort and convenience?

Considerations Regarding the Choice and Dose of Medications

- The specific goals of and expectations for the medication interventions should be clear to all caregivers.

- If the person is depressed, antidepressants may be effective in treating the depression, and some functional improvement may occur, as the depression is alleviated.

- Caregivers should not assume that, just because medications are necessary and appropriate during one

stage of dementia, they will be necessary and appropriate on an ongoing basis.

- Medication regimens should be reevaluated as the dementia progresses or as other conditions, such as medical disorders, affect the person's functional level.

- People with dementia exhibit a wide range of responses to various medications, and the selection of a particular medication should be based on current manifestations as well as prior experiences with medications.

- Some people with dementia, especially those with dementia with Lewy bodies, are highly sensitive to even minute doses of psychotropic medications.

- Any behavior-modifying medication is likely to interfere with cognitive function.

- The type of behavior-modifying medication should be appropriate for the type of behavioral manifestations (e.g., antipsychotics for delusions and hallucination, antianxiety agents for anxiety).

- The initial dose should be one half to one third the normal adult dose.

- Dosage should be increased gradually until therapeutic effects are achieved, all the while observing the person for adverse effects.

- Medications with long half-lives (e.g., flurazepam, diazepam, chlordiazepoxide) should be avoided.

- The half-life of a medication should be considered in determining the frequency of doses.

---

should view behavior-modifying medications as one component of a comprehensive management plan that addresses the complex nature of dementia-related behaviors. Display 24-8 summarizes guidelines for decisions about behavior-modifying medications for people with dementia.

Several types of medications are effective for treating behavioral problems that commonly occur in people with dementia. The so-called atypical antipsychotics (i.e., more recently developed antipsychotics that have fewer adverse effects than older drugs such as haloperidol) are the most commonly used medications for behavioral disturbances in people with dementia. Olanzapine (Zyprexa), quetiapine (Seroquel), and risperidone (Risperdal), are effective for managing dementia-related behaviors such as agitation, delusions, hallucinations, and physical aggression. Antidepressants and mood stabilizers (e.g., valproate, carbamazepine) may be effective for people with dementia who also have mood disturbances. Melatonin (6 mg daily) may improve sleep and reduce evening agitation in people with Alzheimer's disease (Cardinali et al., 2002).

Providing Health Education About Complementary and Alternative Care Practices

Nutrition, exercise, and general mental, physical, and spiritual health practices have long been considered essential components of maintaining optimal cognitive function in people with and without dementia. Recently, however, attention has been focused on a quest for remedies, such as "brain boosters," that can enhance cognitive performance for people of all ages. Currently, there is widespread interest in products that are promoted for their ability to improve cognitive function (e.g., herbs, antioxidants, ginkgo biloba). The physiologic effects of some of these products are similar to those of medications that currently are used or under investigation for dementia. For example, willow bark has antiinflammatory effects; ginkgo biloba has antioxidant effects; and sage and rosemary affect acetylcholine levels. The National Institutes of Health (NIH), many medical institutions, and Alzheimer's research centers in the United States are studying these herbs and other alternative care

DISPLAY 24-9
Health Education About Complementary and Alternative Care Practices for People With Dementia

Nutritional Supplements

- Vitamin E, 1000 IU twice daily (start with 400 IU daily, and add 400 IU daily each week until the maximum dose is reached), but do not take high doses if you are taking an anticoagulant (e.g., warfarin sodium [Coumadin])
- Beta-carotene, 5000 IU
- Selenium, 100 μg twice daily
- Magnesium, 250 mg

Herbal Therapies

- Ginkgo biloba, 120–160 mg daily in two or three doses, increases blood supply to the brain and may improve cognitive function (especially memory and attention) to a small degree in some people with dementia. Ginkgo

biloba may cause serious bleeding if taken with anticoagulants or nonsteroidal antiinflammatory drugs (NSAIDs; e.g., ibuprofen).

Additional Therapies That May be Effective for Managing Symptoms

- Bright light therapy, ½ hour daily to reduce agitation and improve sleep
- Aromatherapy (inhaled or applied to the skin): rosemary for mental stimulation, lavender oil or lemon balm for calming effects
- Relaxation therapies: music, massage, touch therapy, deep breathing
- Acupuncture for anxiety and depression in people with dementia

---

practices that are widely used in other countries. Nurses can use Display 24-9 for health education about complementary and alternative approaches to management of dementia.

Facilitating Decisions About the Care of People With Dementia

Nurses are frequently asked to facilitate decisions about care of people with dementia because families face complex decisions and assume uncomfortable levels of responsibility for people who once were able to make their own decisions. Although some families take on too much decision-making power, most are reluctant to make decisions about dependent older adults. Decision making is especially difficult when the older adult is physically healthy but mentally impaired, or when the person voices strong opinions about unwise or unsafe actions. For example, families of people with dementia often deal with decisions about the person driving a car. Decisions about specific behaviors, like driving, may be relatively easy compared with decisions about long-term care or end-of-life care, decisions that most families of people with progressively declining conditions must confront. In addition to basic safety and medical concerns, these decisions involve complex emotional and financial issues. Because several people are involved in these decisions, differing opinions and interests may complicate the process.

The role of the nurse in facilitating decision making varies in different settings. For example, if decisions about long-term care are made during a

hospitalization, much of the decision-making responsibility may be assumed by or relegated to the primary care provider and the decision may be based primarily on medical concerns. When the person is being cared for at home, however, the decision-making process is more nebulous, and the responsibility rests primarily with families. When the dependent person primarily needs social activities or supervision of daily care, the decision is more psychosocial than medical. In many situations, especially in home or residential settings, nurses are the only health care professionals who maintain close and ongoing relationships with dependent older adults and their caregivers. Thus, the nurse often becomes a support person or a care manager. Nurses can use the following six-step decision-making model as a guide to assisting families with this challenging process. Specific questions and considerations for each of the six steps are listed in Display 24-10. It is important to keep in mind that the identification of caregivers and decision makers should be done with a high degree of cultural sensitivity because decision-making and caregiver patterns are strongly influenced by cultural factors.

Step I: Assessing the Decision-Making Situation

To facilitate decisions about long-term care for cognitively impaired older adults, nurses begin by assessing all of the following: (1) physical and psychosocial function of the dependent person, (2) resources that can be used to meet identified needs, and (3) factors that influence the decision on the part of the caregivers and the dependent person. This assessment

DISPLAY 24-10
Model for Facilitating Decisions About the Care of People With Dementia

Step I: Assess the decision-making situation.
- What are the typical decision-making patterns in the family?
- Who influences the decision making, either directly or indirectly?
- How do family relationships help or hinder the decision-making process?
- Are there patterns of passive nondecisions, as well as active decisions?
- What is each person's perception of the situation?
- How objective are the perceptions of the various decision makers?
- What does each person in the decision-making process have to gain or lose based on various decisions?

Step II: Obtain consensus about problems and needs.
- Have the most involved caregivers describe the problems first.
- After those who are most involved voice their opinions, those who are less involved can be asked to describe the problems.
- Provide objective information to ensure that the various needs of the dependent person are recognized.
- Address the needs of the caregivers as well as the needs of the person with dementia.
- Summarize the identified needs of the older adult and the caregivers.

Step III: Discuss the potential resources.
- Ask caregivers to suggest potential solutions and resources.
- Identify resources for the caregivers' needs as well as for those of the person with dementia.
- Supplement the family's knowledge about resources and potential solutions.
- Discuss the positive and negative consequences of each option for the person with dementia and for the caregivers.

- As the family members discuss solutions, assess their attitudes about using various services and spending family resources to purchase services.
- Provide information about the long-range benefits that the caregivers might not perceive.
- Summarize important points on paper or a blackboard for all participants to review.

Step IV: Agree on a plan of action.
- Eliminate the least acceptable options.
- Agree on the two or three most acceptable alternatives.
- Emphasize the fact that any plan of action will be given a trial period and should not be viewed as a permanent decision.
- Suggest a time frame and criteria for evaluating the plan of action.
- Identify one or two people who will evaluate the plan and make appropriate changes.

Step V: Involve the person with dementia.
- Discuss the ability of the person with dementia to understand the decision.
- Identify the most realistic level of involvement for the person with dementia.
- Identify the best approach to take in involving the person with dementia.
- Identify the roles of caregivers and professionals in assisting the person with dementia to understand the decision.

Step VI: Summarize the plan and clarify roles.
- Review and summarize the plan of action.
- Have the caregivers state their roles in very specific terms.
- Clarify the role of the nurse and other professionals.
- Assure caregivers that you will be available for further discussion and problem solving, or provide the name of someone who can assume this role.

usually is very complex and time-consuming. If this step is done well, however, the nurse will save time in the end, and the plan is increasingly likely to succeed.

Step II: Obtaining Consensus About Problems and Needs

After obtaining as much assessment information as possible, it usually is effective and efficient to gather all the decision makers together. Once the decision makers are gathered together, the nurse leads the conference to obtain consensus about problems and needs. When caregivers do not have a broad perspective on the dependent person's needs, the nurse may provide additional input about the person's needs.

For example, the nurse might point out that social activities and interactions with others are important ways of meeting psychosocial needs and helping cognitively impaired people maintain the highest level of function. Although group activities cannot be provided in home settings, they are available in residential facilities or community-based programs, like adult day care centers.

Step III: Discussing Potential Resources

After summarizing the older person's needs, the nurse then initiates and guides a discussion about potential resources for addressing the problems. Attention is focused on the needs of the caregivers as well as the needs of the dependent older person. Often, the needs of caregivers may be addressed through support groups or individual counseling. Many families are not aware of the range of housing options and community-based services that are available. Nurses who are not familiar with these resources should arrange for a social worker to participate in the conference. As resources are identified, advantages and disadvantages are discussed from various perspectives. The nurse can begin with a statement such as "As we identify different options, let's look at the good points and bad points of each. We need to look at the financial costs and emotional costs that affect each of you, as well as the person for whom we are planning the care." Because the financial aspects are the most objective, they often are a good starting point. Financial decisions, however, can involve many repercussions for spouses and for anyone who might inherit money from the dependent older adult. Sometimes, some of the decision makers may be more concerned about protecting their own financial interests than implementing a plan that is in the best interests of the dependent elder. Another pertinent question that may be asked regarding the advantages and disadvantages of various options is, "What is the cost of not providing this service?" This approach is especially effective in broadening the caregivers' perspective when their viewpoint is very narrow. For example, the nurse may be able to use professional knowledge and experience to convince a family that the long-term benefits of a particular plan may far outweigh the immediate cost of services.

Step IV: Agreeing on a Plan of Action

After reviewing the options, the nurse then summarizes the information and eliminates those options that are least acceptable. The nurse then tries to identify two options that are the best (or only) alternatives. There are always at least two final choices: to do nothing or to make a change. If caregivers are reluctant to accept any of the options identified, the nurse might review the consequences associated with doing nothing as well as the consequences of implementing one or two of the possible action steps. When neither alternative is deemed acceptable initially, it may be helpful to say, "I realize that neither of these choices may seem desirable, but there are no other options." Families sometimes need to hear this kind of conclusion, and they may accept it more readily when it is based on professional experience and knowledge. Once the choices are defined, the decision makers must agree on what action to take. At this point, it is helpful to emphasize that no decision is permanent

and to set a specific timeframe for evaluating the decision after a trial period. If the caregivers understand that the decision can be altered after a fair trial period, they usually are more comfortable with a particular action. Because this decision-making process can be very time-consuming, it is important to identify ways of streamlining the process as much as possible. Therefore, when many people are involved in the conference, one or two key people should be designated as the ones responsible for follow-up. Unless there is a major change in the situation, effective communication networks can eliminate the need for additional conferences with all the decision makers. The evaluation plan may even be carried out through phone contact, rather than in-person contact.

Step V: Involving the Person With Dementia

When the older adult cannot participate in the decision-making conference, the participants must determine the best way of involving that person in the decision. The decision-making process just described applies primarily to situations in which the dependent older person is not able to make decisions on his or her own behalf. In any situation, it is crucial to address the rights and wishes of the dependent older person at every step. In situations in which the person has serious cognitive impairments, the decision makers may simply need to identify the best way to gain acceptance and cooperation. In situations in which the person has some problem-solving abilities, the caregivers may identify the person who is best able to discuss the decision. When spouses are involved in the decision making, they usually assume the role of communicating the decision to the dependent older person. At times, the nurse, physician, or other professional person may assume the role of an authority figure to assist in explaining the decision to the dependent older adult.

Step VI: Summarizing the Plan and Clarifying Roles

The final step is to clarify the roles of various people. The nurse and other professionals who are part of the decision-making process should inform the caregivers about their ongoing roles. If several caregivers are involved with the plan, each person should state his or her understanding of his or her role.

EVALUATING THE EFFECTIVENESS OF NURSING INTERVENTIONS

Care of a person with dementia is evaluated according to the extent to which the person receives needed supports and maintains his or her dignity and quality of life. Because a decline in function is an inherent part of dementia, nursing care must be evaluated on an ongoing basis as the person's condition changes. Nurses evaluate the degree to which quality of life is maintained by obtaining feedback about life satisfaction, which people in the early and middle stages of dementia usually can express verbally or nonverbally. For example, nurses can evaluate the extent to which the person enjoys or participates in meaningful activities and interactions. As the dementia progresses, it becomes more difficult to obtain this kind of information and nurses rely more on feedback from caregivers and their own judgment about the person's quality of life. During the later stages of dementia, measures of quality of life focus more on comfort and basic physical needs. Throughout the course of dementia, care can be evaluated by the extent to which the person is free from pain, fear, and anxiety.

Another consideration in evaluating care for a person with dementia is the extent to which the needs of the caregiver are met. An evaluation criterion is whether caregivers express satisfaction with their own quality of life, despite the demands of the situation. Other evaluation criteria may be a caregiver's attendance at support groups and the use of resources to assist with or guide care.

CHAPTER SUMMARY

Dementia is a syndrome characterized by a progressive loss of cognitive abilities that has significant functional consequences for older adults and their families and caregivers. Alzheimer's disease is the most common type of dementia, but in recent years, gerontologists have developed criteria for other types, including vascular dementia, frontotemporal dementia, and dementia with Lewy bodies. Delirium, or acute confusional state, is a common and reversible cause of impaired cognitive function in older adults. Different types of dementia can occur concurrently, as can dementia and delirium. Although much progress has been made in identifying causes of dementia in recent years, there currently is no one theory to explain dementia. Dementia is viewed as a heterogeneous disorder, and many underlying, probably interacting, factors are being studied. Risk factors for dementia include genetic factors, medical conditions, and environmental influences. Functional consequences of dementia begin with mild cognitive impairments in the early stages and progress to global cognitive and functional impairments in the last stage. Throughout the course of the disease, the person with dementia

experiences a wide range of emotional and psychosocial consequences (e.g., anxiety, depression). The final functional consequence is death. In addition, dementia significantly affects the physical and mental health and quality of life of caregivers and families of people with dementia.

Nursing assessment of people with impaired cognitive function is multidisciplinary and must consider a number of factors. Additional important nursing responsibilities are recognizing delirium as a cause of cognitive impairment and providing ongoing assessment of people with dementia. Chronic Confusion and Acute Confusion are nursing diagnoses that are applied to older adults with dementia and delirium, respectively. Additional nursing diagnoses address problems associated with functional impairments, the emotional needs of the person with dementia, and the needs of caregivers. Nursing interventions, which include communication techniques and environmental modifications, must be highly individualized and frequently evaluated and modified. Nursing care is evaluated by the extent to which quality of life is maintained for both the older adult with dementia and his or her caregivers.

CONCLUDING CASE STUDY AND NURSING CARE PLAN

➤ Mrs. D. is 85 years old and lives with her 86-year-old husband in a high-rise apartment for the elderly. Two years ago, Mrs. D. was diagnosed as having Alzheimer's disease but she was able to participate in her usual activities until the past year. Now she is neglecting her personal care and is unsafe in meal preparation.

When she wakes up several times nightly to go to the bathroom, she sometimes goes to the apartment door rather than returning to the bedroom. Mr. D. worries that she will leave in the middle of the night, and his sleep is disrupted because he maintains a state of constant vigilance. Mr. D. has called a home care agency requesting home health aide assistance, and you are the nurse responsible for the initial assessment and for working with the home health aides.

■ Nursing Assessment

During your initial assessment, you find that Mrs. D. is pleasant and receptive, but has little insight into her need for help. She acknowledges that her doctor has told her she has "a memory problem." Mrs. D. reports that this problem doesn't affect her daily life, except that her husband has to remind her about things like turning the stove off after cooking meals.

She acknowledges being lonely and says she misses being able to read books and talk to people. Mrs. D. takes Aricept and vitamin E, and is otherwise physically healthy.

With regard to her ADLs, Mrs. D. has not taken a bath or shower in several months, and she gets very angry if Mr. D. suggests that she take one. She gets confused about her clothing and sometimes wears her underwear over her regular clothes, or wears a skirt and slacks at the same time. She insists on doing the meal preparation, but she is unsafe using the stove and gets confused about ingredients in recipes (e.g., she may use salt instead of sugar). Mrs. D. always has done the laundry and housekeeping, but in the past months, she has "made a lot of mistakes," such as using powdered milk for laundry detergent.

Mr. D. reports feeling very stressed about the full-time responsibilities of caring for his wife, and this stress has escalated in the past month because he no longer feels he can leave her alone. Mrs. D. "shadows" him and feels very insecure if he is out of her sight for more than a few minutes. Mr. D. has taken her everywhere with him for the past year, but in the last few months, this has become increasingly more difficult. For example, when they are in the grocery store, Mrs. D. gets very impatient and pushes the cart into other people. Also, while they are waiting in the checkout line, she insists on taking one of each of the tabloids and magazines near the counter, and she creates a big scene if he doesn't buy them for her.

Mr. D. confides that he expected to be able to care for his wife at home "until the end," but now he has doubts about his ability to keep her at home. He perceives her as being "senile" and feels he should be able to meet her needs. There are no nearby family members who can help with her care, but his son and daughter have offered to help pay for some services. Mr. D. is aware of support groups offered by the Alzheimer's Association, but he has not attended any because he cannot leave his wife alone. When asked about his health, Mr. D. says, "I see the doctor for my arthritis and heart problems, but I get along OK, except that I'm supposed to have cataract surgery and I don't know how I'll manage to get that done."

■ Nursing Diagnosis

Your nursing diagnosis for Mrs. D. is Altered Thought Processes related to the effects of dementia. You use the nursing diagnosis of Caregiver Role Strain for Mr. D. because you recognize the need to address Mr. D.'s problems. Your immediate goal is to arrange for supportive services and assistance with Mrs. D.'s care because this will improve the quality of life for both Mr. and Mrs. D., and it will alleviate some of the caregiver stress for Mr. D. A long-term goal is to arrange for respite services so Mr. D. can undergo cataract surgery. You also recognize the need for educational and support services for Mr. D.

■ Nursing Care Plan

The care plan you develop for Mr. and Mrs. D. is shown in Display 24-11.

 CRITICAL THINKING EXERCISES

1. Apply the following to the concluding case study and care plan:
   - Use the FAST/GDS in Table 24-2 to assess Mrs. D.'s stage of dementia.
   - What would you identify as Mr. D.'s needs as a caregiver?
   - What health education information would you plan for Mr. D.?
   - What approaches would you suggest for Mr. D. and home care workers for communicating with Mrs. D.?
   - What challenges would you anticipate having to address as you provide ongoing supervision of the home health aide and continue to work with Mr. and Mrs. D.?

2. Define each of the following terms and describe the relevance of each term according to our current understanding of impaired cognitive function: senility, organic brain syndrome, hardening of the arteries, pseudodementia, delirium, dementia, and Alzheimer's disease.

3. Describe the characteristics of early and middle stages of each of the following types of dementia: Alzheimer's disease, vascular dementia, frontotemporal dementia, and dementia with Lewy bodies.

4. You are working in a nursing clinic at a senior center. How would you respond to the following questions, posed by a 74-year-old woman: "I've been having memory problems lately, but I know it's not Alzheimer's because I haven't done anything really stupid. What do you think I should do? My friend says ginkgo helps her a lot, and I was thinking of trying that. Do you know how much of it I should take?"

5. You are planning an in-service program to nursing home staff about medications used in the treatment of dementia and the management of dementia-related behaviors. What information would you present?

DISPLAY 24-11 • NURSING CARE PLAN FOR MR. AND MRS. D.

EXPECTED OUTCOME	NURSING INTERVENTIONS	NURSING EVALUATION
Mrs. D. will function at her highest level of independence.	• Work with Mr. D. to identify ways to improve Mrs. D.'s ability to function safely and independently in performing her ADLs. (For instance, Mr. D. can involve Mrs. D. in selecting an outfit to wear and can set out the clothing in the order in which it should be donned.) • Arrange for an HHA to work with Mrs. D. and assist her with complex tasks, such as laundry, housekeeping, and meal preparation. • Teach the HHA to assume an "assistant" and "friend" role by providing only subtle supervision and minimal direct help with activities such as laundry.	• Mrs. D. will perform ADLs and IADLs with minimal assistance.
Mrs. D.'s quality of life will be maintained.	• Work with Mr. D. and the HHA to identify activities that are interesting, satisfying, and intellectually stimulating (e.g., "word find" games). • Explore the possibility of Mrs. D.'s attending an adult day care program for group activities. • Support Mrs. D. in carrying out familiar roles and meaningful activities.	• Mrs. D. will continue to engage in activities that are satisfying.
Mr. D. will use sources of support to alleviate caregiver-related stress.	• Arrange the HHA's schedule to enable Mr. D. to attend caregiver support groups and educational programs. • Help Mr. D. in identifying one activity per week that he could do to promote his own well-being (e.g., going to lunch with a friend). • Provide HHA assistance for 4-hour periods to allow Mr. D. time for grocery shopping and pursuing his own interests. • Provide Mr. D. with information about the "Caregiver Connection Hot Line" at the Alzheimer's Association, and suggest that he join this telephone support network.	• Mr. D. will verbalize feelings of being able to cope effectively with caregiver responsibilities. • Mr. D. will participate in one activity per week that is focused on his own needs and interests.

ADLs, activities of daily living; IADLs, instrumental activities of daily living; HHA, home health aide.

Future Directions for Healthier Aging: Focus on Treatment of Dementia

Researchers and pharmaceutical companies are focusing on the following promising developments in the treatment of dementia:

• Clinical trials of statins for treatment of Alzheimer's disease
• The use of stem cell therapies
• Development of vaccination with beta-amyloid fragments
• Development of β- and γ-secretase inhibitors

EDUCATIONAL RESOURCES

Alzheimer's Association
225 North Michigan Avenue, Suite 1700, Chicago, IL 60601
(800) 272-3900
http://www.alz.org

Alzheimer's Disease Education and Referral (ADEAR) Center
P.O. Box 8250, Silver Spring, MD 20907-8250
(800) 438-4380
http://www.alzheimers.org

Alzheimer's Society of Canada
20 Eglington Avenue West, Suite 1200, Toronto, ON M4R 1K8
(416) 488-8772
(800) 488-3778 (valid only in Canada)
http://www.alzheimer.ca

Eldercare Locator
U.S. Administration on Aging
(800) 677–1116
http://www.eldercare.gov/

Family Caregiver Alliance
690 Market Street, Suite 600, San Francisco, CA 94104
(800) 445-8106
http://www.caregiver.org

National Institute of Neurological Disorders and Stroke
P.O. Box 5801, Bethesda, MD 20824
(800) 352-9424
http://www.ninds.nih.gov

National Institute on Aging (NIA)
National Institutes of Health
Bldg. 31, Rm. 5C27, Bethesda, MD 20892-2292
(800) 222-2225
http://www.nih.gov/nia

U.S. Agency for Healthcare Research and Quality
2101 East Jefferson Street, Suite 501, Rockville, MD 20852
(800) 358-9295
http://www.ahcpr.gov

REFERENCES

Acton, G. J. (2002). Self-transcendent views and behaviors: Exploring growth in caregivers of adults with dementia. *Journal of Gerontological Nursing, 28*(12), 22–30.

Aguero-Torres, H., Qiu, C., Winblad, B., & Fratiglioni, L. (2002). Dementing disorders in the elderly: Evolution of disease severity over 7 years. *Alzheimer Disease and Associated Disorders, 16,* 221–227.

Alzheimer, A. (1907). Uber eine eigenartige Erkrankung der Hirnrinde. *Assgemeine Zeitschrift Fur Psychiatrie und Psychisch-GerichtlicheMedicin, 64,* 146–148.

Ancoli-Israel, S., Martin, J. L., Gehrman, P., Sochat, T., Corey-Bloom, J., Marler, M., et al. (2003). Effect of light on agitation in institutionalized patients with severe Alzheimer disease. *American Journal of Geriatric Psychiatry, 11,* 194–203.

Andersen-Ranberg, K., Vasegaard, L., & Jeune, B., (2001). Dementia is not inevitable: A population-based study of Danish centenarians. *Journal of Gerontology: Psychological Science, 56B,* P152–P159.

Arkin, S., & Mahendra, N. (2001). Insights in Alzheimer's patients: Results of a longitudinal study using three assessments methods. *American Journal of Alzheimer's Disease and Other Dementias, 16,* 211–224.

Auer, S., & Reisberg, B. (1997). The GDS/FAST Staging System. *International Psychogeriatrics, 9*(Suppl. 1), 167–171.

Bennett, D. A., Wilson, R. S., Schneider, J. A., Evans, D. A., Beckett, L. A., Aggarwal, N. T., et al. (2002). Natural history of mild cognitive impairment in older adults. *Neurology, 59,* 198–295.

Birkenhager, W. H., Forette, F., Seux, M. L., Wang, J. G., Staessen, J. A. (2001). Blood pressure, cognitive functions, and prevention of dementias in older patients with hypertension. *Archives of Internal Medicine, 161,* 152–156.

Boeve, B., McCormick, J., Smith, G., Ferman, T., Rummans, T., Carpenter, T., et al. (2003). Mild cognitive impairment in the oldest old. *Neurology, 60,* 477–480.

Bonner, L. T., & Peskind, E. R. (2002). Pharmaceutical treatments of dementia. *Medical Clinics of North America, 86,* 657–674.

Bourgeois, M. S. (2002). The challenge of communicating with persons with dementia. *Alzheimer's Care Quarterly, 3*(2), 132–144.

Brandt, J. (2001). Mild cognitive impairments in the elderly. *American Family Physician, 63,* 625–626.

Brush, J. A., Meehan, R. A., & Calkins, M. P. (2002). Using the environment to improve intake for people with dementia. *Alzheimer's Care Quarterly, 3,* 330–338.

Buettner, L., & Kolanowski, A. (2003). Practice guidelines for recreation therapy in the care of people with dementia. *Geriatric Nursing, 24,* 18–23.

Cacchione, P. Z. (2002). Four acute confusion assessment instruments: Reliability and validity for use in long-term care facilities. *Journal of Gerontological Nursing, 28*(1), 12–19.

Calkins, M. P. (2001). Special care units and the environment: Advances of the past decade. *Alzheimer's Care Quarterly, 2*(3), 41–48.

Cardinali, D. P., Brusco, L. I., Liberczuk, C., & Furio, A. M. (2002). The use of melatonin in Alzheimer's disease. *Neuroendocrinology Letters, 23*(Suppl 1), 20–23.

Carlson, M. C., Brandt, J., Steele, C., Baker, A., Stern, Y., & Lyketsos, C. G. (2001). Predictor index of mortality in dementia patients upon entry into long-term care. *Journal of Gerontology: Medical Sciences, 56A,* M567–M570.

Carpenito, L. J. (2002). *Nursing diagnosis: Application to clinical practice* (9th ed.). Philadelphia: Lippincott Williams & Wilkins.

Chan, D. K. Y. (2002). A new hypothesis (concept) of diagnosing Alzheimer's disease. *Journal of Gerontology: Medical Sciences, 57A,* M645–M647.

Chitsey, A. M., Haight, B. K., & Jones, M. M. (2002). A multisensory intervention. *Journal of Gerontological Nursing, 28*(3), 41–49.

Choi, Y-H., Kim, J-H., Kim, D. K., Kim, J-W., Kim, D-K., Lee, M. S., et al. (2003). Distributions of ACE and APOE Polymorphisms and their relations with dementia status in Korean centenarians. *Journal of Gerontology: Medical Sciences, 58A,* 227–231.

Chui, H. (2000). Vascular dementia, a new beginning: Shifting focus from clinical phenotype to ischemic brain injury. *Neurologic Clinics, 18,* 951–978

Chung, J. A., & Cummings, J. L. (2000). Neurobehavioral and neuropsychiatric symptoms in Alzheimer's Disease. *Neurologic Clinics, 18,* 829–846.

Clare, L. (2002a). Developing awareness about awareness in early-stage dementia. *Dementia, 1,* 295–312.

Clare, L. (2002b). We'll fight it as long as we can: Coping with the onset of Alzheimer's disease. *Aging & Mental Health, 6*(2), 139–148.

Cohen, D., Kennedy, G., & Eisdorfer, C. (1984). Phases of change in the patient with Alzheimer's dementia. *Journal of the American Geriatrics Society, 32*(1), 11–15.

Cohen-Mansfield, J. (2000a). Nonpharmacologic management of behavioral problems in persons with dementia: A TREA model. *Alzheimer's Care Quarterly, 1*(4), 22–34.

Cohen-Mansfield, J. (2000b). Theoretical frameworks for behavioral problems in dementia. *Alzheimer's Care Quarterly, 1*(4), 8–21.

Cohen-Mansfield, J. (2001). Nonpharmacologic interventions for inappropriate behaviors in dementia: A review, summary, and critique. *American Journal of Geriatric Psychiatry, 9,* 361–381.

Colling, K. B., & Buettner, L. L. (2002). Simple pleasures. *Journal of Gerontological Nursing, 28*(10), 16–20.

Connolly, D. M., MacKnight, C., Lewis, C., & Fisher, J. (2000). Guidelines for stage-based supports in Alzheimer's care: The FAST-ACT. *Journal of Gerontological Nursing, 26*(11), 34–45.

Conway, K. A., Baxter, E. W., Felsenstein, K. M., & Reitz, A. B. (2003). Emerging beta-amyloid therapies for the treatment of Alzheimer's disease. *Current Pharmaceutical Design, 9,* 427–447.

Crisby, M., Carlson, L. A., & Winblad, B. (2002). Statins in the prevention and treatment of Alzheimer disease. *Alzheimer Disease and Associated Disorders, 16,* 131–136.

Cummings, J. L. (2003). Use of cholinesterase inhibitors in clinical practice: Evidence-based recommendations. *American Journal of Geriatric Psychiatry, 11,* 131–145.

Day, K., Carreon, D., & Stump, C. (2000). The therapeutic design of environments for people with dementia: A review of the empirical research. *Gerontologist, 40,* 397–416.

Desmond, D. W., Moroney, J. T., Paik, M. C., Sano, M., Mohr, J. P., Aboumatar, S., Tseng, C-L., et al. (2000). Frequency and clinical determinants of dementia after ischemic stroke. *Neurology, 54,* 1124–1131.

DeYoung, S., Just, G., & Harrison, R. (2002). Decreasing aggressive, agitated, or disruptive behavior. *Journal of Gerontological Nursing, 28*(6), 22–31.

Dunn, J. C., Thiru-Chelvam, B., & Beck, C. H. M. (2002). Bathing: Pleasure or pain? *Journal of Gerontological Nursing, 28*(11), 6–12.

Erkinjuntti, T., Kurz, A., Gauthier, S., Bullock, R., Lilienfield, S., & Damaraju, C. V. (2002). Efficacy of galantamine in probable vascular dementia and Alzheimer's disease combined with cerebrovascular disease: A randomized trial. *Lancet, 359*(9314), 1283–1290.

Farlow, M. R. (2002). Do cholinesterase inhibitors slow progression of Alzheimer's disease? *International Journal of Clinical Practice, Supplement, 127,* 37–44.

Fick, D. M., Agostini, J. V., & Inouye, S. K. (2002). Delirium superimposed on dementia: A systematic review. *Journal of the American Geriatrics Society, 50,* 1723–1732.

Fick, D., & Foreman, M. (2000). Delirium superimposed on dementia. *Journal of Gerontological Nursing, 26*(1), 30–40.

Foley, D. J., Brock, D. B., & Lanska, D. J. (2003). Trends in dementia mortality from two National Mortality Followback Surveys. *Neurology, 60*(4), 709–711.

Foreman, M. D., Wakefield, B., Culp, K., & Milisen, K. (2001). Delirium in elderly patients. *Journal of Gerontological Nursing, 27*(4), 12–20.

Forette, F., Seux, M. L., Staessen, J. A., Thijs, L., Babarskiene, M. R., Babeanu, S., et al. (2002). The prevention of dementia with antihypertensive treatment. *Archives of Internal Medicine, 162,* 2046–2052.

Futrell, M., & Melillo, K. D. (2002). Evidence-based protocol: Wandering. *Journal of Gerontological Nursing, 28*(11), 14–22.

Gates, G. A., Beiser, A. Rees, T. S., D'Agostino, R. B., & Wolf, P. A. (2002). Central auditory dysfunction may precede the onset of clinical dementia in people with probable Alzheimer's disease. *Journal of the American Geriatrics Society, 50,* 482–488.

Gerdner, L. A., & Hall, G. R. (2001). Chronic confusion. In M. L. Maas, K. C. Buckwalter, M. D. Hardy, T. Tripp-Reimer, M. G. Titler, & J. P. Specht (Eds.), *Nursing care of older adults: Diagnoses, outcomes, and interventions* (pp. 421–441). St. Louis: Mosby.

Gregg, E. W., Yaffe, K., Cauley, J. A., Rolka, D. B., Blackwell, T. L., Narayan, K. M. V., et al. (2000). Is diabetes associated with cognitive impairment and cognitive decline among older women? *Archives of Internal Medicine, 160,* 174–180.

Griffith, H. R., Belue, K., Sicola, A., Krzywanski, S., Zamrini, E., Harrell, L., & Marson, D. C. (2003). Impaired financial abilities in mild cognitive impairment. *Neurology, 60,* 449–457.

Hachinski, V. C., Lassen, N. A., & Marshall, J. (1974). Multi-infarct dementia: A cause of mental deterioration in the elderly. *Lancet, 2,* 207–209.

Hajjar, I., Schumpert, J., Hirth, V., Wieland, D., & Eleazer, G. P. (2002). The impact of the use of statins on the prevalence of dementia and the progression of cognitive impairment. *Journal of Gerontology: Medical Science, 57A,* M414–M418.

Hall, G. R., & Buckwalter, K. C. (1987). Progressively lowered stress threshold: A conceptual model for care of adults with Alzheimer's disease. *Archives of Psychiatric Nursing, 1,* 399–406.

Han, L., McCusker, J., Cole. M., Abrahamowicz, M., Primeau, F., Flie, M., et al. (2001). Use of medications with anticholinergic effect predicts clinical severity of delirium symptoms in older medical inpatients. *Archives of Internal Medicine, 161,* 1099–1105.

Hartmann, S., & Mobius, H. J. (2003). Tolerability of memantine in combination with cholinesterase inhibitors in dementia therapy. *International Clinical Psychopharmacology, 18,* 81–85.

Hebert, R., Levesque, L., Vezina, J., Lavoie, J. P., Ducharme, F., Gendron, C., et al. (2003). Efficacy of a psychoeducative group program for caregivers of demented persons living at home: A randomized controlled trial. *Journal of Gerontology: Social Science, 3,* S58–S57.

Hendryx-Bedalov, P. M. (2000). Alzheimer's dementia. *Journal of Gerontological Nursing, 26*(8), 20–24.

Hogstel, M. O. (1988). Forget these three words. *Journal of Gerontological Nursing, 14*(12), 7.

Hubbard, G., Cook, A., Tester, S., & Downs, M. (2002). Beyond words older people with dementia using and interpreting nonverbal behaviour. *Journal of Aging Studies, 16,* 155–167.

Ikeda, M., Hokoishi, K., Maki, N., Nebu, A., Tachibana, N., Komori, K., et al. (2001). Increased prevalence of vascular dementia in Japan. A community-based epidemiological study. *Neurology, 57,* 839–844.

Inglis, F. (2002). The tolerability and safety of cholinesterase inhibitors in the treatment of dementia. *International Journal of Clinical Practice, 127*(Suppl), 45–63.

Inouye, S. K., Foreman, M. D., Mion, L. C., Katz, K. H., & Cooney, L. M. (2001). Nurses' recognition of delirium and its symptoms: Comparison of nurse and researcher ratings. *Archives of Internal Medicine, 161,* 2467–2473.

Johansson, K., Norberg, A., & Lundman, B. (2002). Family members' and care providers interpretations of picking behavior. *Geriatric Nursing, 23,* 258–261.

Kivipelto, M., Helkala, E. L., Laakso, M. P., Hanninen, T., Hallikinen, M., Alhinen, K., et al. (2002). Apolipoprotein E 4 allele, elevated midlife total cholesterol level, and high midlife systolic blood pressure are independent risk factors for late-life Alzheimer disease. *Annals of Internal Medicine, 137,* 149–155.

Knopman, D. S., Rocca, W. A., Cha, R. H., Edland, S. D., & Kokmen, E. (2003). Survival study of vascular dementia in Rochester, Minnesota. *Archives of Neurology, 60,* 85–90.

Kolanowski, A. M., Richards, K. C., & Sullivan, S. C. (2002). Activity preferences of persons with dementia. *Journal of Gerontological Nursing, 28*(10), 12–15.

Kovach, C. R., & Wells, T. (2002). Pacing of activity as predictor of agitation. *Journal of Gerontological Nursing, 28*(1), 28–35.

Kuhn, D., Ortigra, A., & Kasayka, R. (2000). Dementia care mapping: An innovative tool to measure person-centered care. *Alzheimer's Care Quarterly, 1*(3), 7–15.

Kukull, W. A., & Bowen, J. D. (2002). Dementia epidemiology. *Medical Clinics of North America, 86,* 573–590.

Landes, A. M., Sperry, S. D., Strauss, M. E., & Geldmacher, D. S. (2001). Apathy in Alzheimer's disease. *Journal of the American Geriatric Society, 49,* 1700–1707.

Landi, F., Cesari, M., Onder, G., Russo, A., Torre, S., & Bernabei, R. (2003). Non-steroidal anti-inflammatory drugs (NSAID) use and Alzheimer Disease in community-dwelling elderly patients. *American Journal of Geriatric Psychiatry, 11,* 179–185.

Laplante, J., & Cole, M. G. (2001). Detection of delirium using the Confusion Assessment Method. *Journal of Gerontological Nursing, 27*(9), 16–23.

Larrimore, K. L. (2003). Alzheimer disease support group characteristics: A comparison of caregivers. *Geriatric Nursing, 24,* 32–35, 49.

Lim, Y. M. (2003). Nursing intervention for grooming of elders with mild cognitive impairments in Korea. *Geriatric Nursing, 24,* 11–15.

Lopez, O. L., Hamilton, R. L., Becker, J. T., Wisniewski, S., Kaufer, D. I., DeKosky, S. T., et al. (2000). Severity of cognitive impairment and the clinical diagnosis of AD with Lewy bodies. *Neurology, 54,* 1780–1787.

Lopez-Arrieta, J. M. (2002). Nimodipine for primary degenerative, mixed and vascular dementia. *Cochrane Database Systems Review, 3,* CD000147.

Lucero, M. (2002). Intervention strategies for exit-seeking wandering behavior in dementia residents. *American Journal of Alzheimer's Disease and Other Dementias, 5,* 277–280.

Mace, N. L., & Rabins, P. V., (1999). *The 36-hour day.* (3rd ed.). Baltimore: The Johns Hopkins University Press.

Marcantonio, E. R., Simon, S. E., Bergmann, M. A., Jones, R. N., Murphy, K. M., Morris, J. N., et al. (2003). Delirium symptoms in post acute care: Prevalent, persistent, and associated with poor functional recovery. *Journal of the American Geriatrics Society, 51,* 4–9.

Masaki, K. H., Losonczy, K. G., Izmirlian, G., Foley, D. J., Ross, G. W., Petrovitch, H., et al. (2000). Association of vitamin E and C supplement use with cognitive function and dementia in elderly men. *Neurology, 54,* 1265–1272.

Maslow, K., & Ory, M. (2001). Review of a decade of dementia special care unit research: Lessons learned and future directions. *Alzheimer's Care Quarterly, 2*(3), 10–16.

Massoud, F., Devi, G., Moroney, J. T., Stern, Y., Lawton, A., Bell, K., et al. (2000). The role of routine laboratory studies and neuroimaging in the diagnosis of dementia: A clinicopathological study. *Journal of the American Geriatrics Society, 48,* 1204–1210.

Mayhew, P. A., Acton, G. J., Yauk, S., & Hopkins, B. A. (2001). Communication from individuals with advanced DAT: Can it provide clues to their sense of self-awareness and well-being? *Geriatric Nursing, 22,* 106–110.

McCusker, J., Cole, M., Abrahammowicz, M., Han, L., Podoba, J. E., Ramman-Haddad, L., et al. (2001). Environmental risk factors for delirium in hospitalized older people. *Journal of the American Geriatrics Society, 49,* 1327–1334.

McKeith, I. G., Burn, D. J., Ballard, C. G., Collerton, D., Jaros, E., Morris, C. M., et al. (2003). Dementia with Lewy bodies. *Seminars in Clinical Neuropsychiatry, 8,* 46–57.

McKhann, G. M., Albert, M. S., Grossman, M., Miller, B., Dickson, D., Trojanowski, J. Q., & Work Group on Frontotemporal Dementia and Pick's Disease. (2001). Clinical and pathological diagnosis of frontotemporal dementia: Report of the Work Group on Frontotemporal Dementia and Pick's Disease. *Archives of Neurology, 58*(11), 1803–1809.

Meyer, J. S. (2002). Donepezil treatment of vascular dementia. *Annals of the New York Academy of Sciences, 977,* 482–486.

Mickus, M. A., Wagenaar, D. B., Averill, M., Colenda, C. C., Gardiner, J., & Luo, Z. (2002). Developing effective bathing strategies for reducing problematic behavior for residents with dementia: The PRIDE approach. *Journal of Mental Health and Aging, 8*(1), 37–43.

Miech, R. A., Breitner, J. C., Zandi, P. P., Khachaturian, A. S., Anthony, J. C., Mayer, L., et al. (2002). Incidence of AD may decline in the early 90s for men, later for women: The Cache County study. *Neurology, 58,* 209–218.

Miller, S., Vermeersch, P. E. H., Bohan, K., Renbarger, K., Kruep, A., Sacre, S., et al. (2001). Audio presence intervention for decreasing agitation in people with dementia. *Geriatric Nursing, 22,* 66–70.

Millisen, K., Foreman, M. D., Wouters, B., Driesen, R., Godderis, J., Abraham, I. L., & Broos, P. L. O. (2002). Documentation of delirium in elderly patients with hip fracture. *Journal of Gerontological Nursing, 28*(11), 23–29.

Morris, J. C. (2000). The nosology of dementia. *Neurologic Clinics, 18,* 773–788.

Morrison, R. S., Magaziner, J., Gilbert, M., Koval, K. J., MaLaughlin, M. A., Orosz, G., et al. (2003). Relationship between pain and opioid analgesics on the development of delirium following hip fracture. *Journal of Gerontology: Medical Science, 58A,* 76–81.

Moss, S. E., Polignano, E., White, C. L., Minichiello, C. L., & Sunderland, T. (2002). Interaction in Alzheimer's disease. *Journal of Gerontological Nursing, 28*(8), 36–44.

Murray, M. D., Lane, K. A., Gao, S., Evans, R. M., Unverzagt, F. W., Hall, K. S., et al. (2002). Preservation of cognitive function with antihypertensive medications. *Archives of Internal Medicine, 162,* 2090–2096.

Narayan, S., Lewis, M., Tornatore, J., Hepburn, K., & Corcoron-Perry, S. (2001). Subjective responses to caregiving for a spouse with dementia. *Journal of Gerontological Nursing, 27*(2), 19–28.

Orogozo, J. M., Rigaud, A. S., Stoffler, A., Mobius, H. J., & Forette, F. (2002). Efficacy and safety of memantine in patients with mild to moderate vascular dementia: A randomized, placebo-controlled trial. *Stroke, 33,* 1834–1839.

Panisset, M. Gauthier, S., Moessler, H., Windisch, M., & The Cerebrolysin Study Group. (2002). Cerebrolysin in Alzheimer's disease: A randomized, double-blind, placebo-controlled trial with a neurotropic agent. *Journal of Neural Transmission, 109,* 1089–1104.

Pearson, A. (2001). Nursing home admission. In M. D. Mezey (Ed.), *The encyclopedia of elder care* (pp. 450–452). New York: Springer.

Peatfield, J. G., Futrell, M., & Cox, C. L. (2002). Wandering. *Journal of Gerontological Nursing, 28*(4), 44–50.

Perl, D. P. (2000). Neuropathology of Alzheimer's disease and related disorders. *Neurologic Clinics, 18,* 847–864.

Pijnenburg, Y. A., Sampson, E. L., Harvey, R. J., Foc, N. C., & Rossor, M. N. (2003). Vulnerability to neuroleptic side effects in frontotemporal lobar degeneration. *International Journal of Geriatric Psychiatry, 18,* 67–72.

Purandare, N., Bloom, C., Page, S., Morris, J., & Burns, A. (2002). The effects of anticholinesterases on personality changes in Alzheimer's disease. *Aging & Mental Health, 6*(4), 350–354.

Rader, J., & Barrick, A. L. (2000). Ways that work: Bathing without a battle. *Alzheimer's Care Quarterly, 1*(4), 35–49.

Rapp, C. G., & Iowa Veterans Affairs Nursing Research Consortium. (2001). Acute confusion/delirium protocol. *Journal of Gerontological Nursing, 27*(4), 21–33.

Ratnavalli, E., Brayne, C., Dawson, K., & Hodges, J. R. (2002). The prevalence of frontotemporal dementia. *Neurology, 58,* 1615–1621.

Reifler, B. V. (2000). A case of mistaken identity: Pseudodementia is really predementia. *Journal of the American Geriatrics Society, 48,* 593–594.

Reisberg, B. (1986). Dementia: A systematic approach to identifying reversible causes. *Geriatrics, 41*(4), 30–46.

Reisberg, B., Franssed, E. H., Souren, L. E., Auer, S. R., Akram, I., & Kenowsky, S. (2002). Evidence and mechanisms of retrogenesis in Alzheimer's and other dementias: Management and treatment import. *American Journal of Alzheimer's Disease and Other Dementias, 17,* 169–174.

Reynish, W., Andrieu, S., Nourhashemi, F., & Vellas, B. (2001). Nutritional factors and Alzheimer's disease. *Journal of Gerontology: Medical Sciences, 56A,* M675–M680.

Richards, K., Lambert, C., & Beck, C. (2000). Deriving interventions for challenging behaviors from the need driven, dementia-compromised behavior model. *Alzheimer's Care Quarterly, 1*(4), 62–76.

Ritchie, K., Artero, S., & Touchon, J. (2001). Classification criteria for mild cognitive impairment a population-based validation study. *Neurology, 56,* 37–42.

Robert, P. (2002). Understanding and managing behavioural symptoms in Alzheimer's disease and related dementias: Focus on rivastigmine. *Current Medical Research and Opinion, 18,* 156–171.

Roberts, S., & Durnbaugh, T. (2002). Enhancing nutrition and eating skills in long-term care. *Alzheimer's Care Quarterly, 3*(4), 316–329.

Rogan, S., & Lippa, C. F. (2002). Alzheimer's disease and other dementias: A review. *American Journal of Alzheimer's Disease and Other Dementias, 17,* 11–17.

Roman, G. C. (2002). Vascular dementia revisited: Diagnosis, pathogenesis, treatment, and prevention. *Medical Clinics of North America, 86,* 477–499.

Roses, A. D. (1995). Apolipoprotein E and Alzheimer's disease. *Science and Medicine, 2*(5), 16–25.

Rosler, M. (2002). The efficacy of cholinesterase inhibitors in treating the behavioral symptoms of dementia. *International Journal of Clinical Practice, 127*(Suppl), 20–36.

Ross, G. W., & Bowen, J. D. (2002). The diagnosis and differential diagnosis of dementia. *Medical Clinics of North America, 86,* 455–476.

Sabatini, T., Frisoni, G., Barbisoni, P., Bellelli, G., Rozzini, R., & Trabucchi, M. (2000). Atrial fibrillation and cognitive disorders in older people. *Journal of the American Geriatrics Society, 48,* 387–390.

Sansone, P., & Schmitt, L. (2000). Providing tender touch massage to elderly nursing home residents: A demonstration project. *Geriatric Nursing, 21,* 303–308.

Santillan, C. E., Fritsch, T., & Geldmacher, D. S. (2003). Development of a scale to predict decline in patients with mild Alzheimer's disease. *Journal of the American Geriatrics Society, 51,* 91–95.

Serby, M., & Samuels, S. C. (2001). Diagnostic criteria for dementia with Lewy bodies reconsidered. *American Journal of Geriatric Psychiatry, 9,* 212–216.

Sevier, S., & Gorek, B. (2000). Cognitive evaluation in care planning for people with Alzheimer disease and related dementias. *Geriatric Nursing, 21,* 92–97.

Shuster, J. L. (2000). Palliative care for advanced dementia. *Clinics in Geriatric Medicine, 16,* 373–386.

Silver, M. H., Jilinskaia, E., & Perls, T. T. (2001). Cognitive functional status of age-confirmed centenarians in a population-based study. *Journal of Gerontology: Psychological Science, 56B,* P134–P140.

Snowden, D. A. (1997). Aging and Alzheimer's disease: Lessons for the Nun Study. *Gerontologist, 37,* 150–156.

Stolley, J. M., Reed, D., & Buckwalter, K. C. (2002). Caregiving appraisal and interventions based on the progressively lowered stress threshold model. *American Journal of Alzheimer's Disease and Other Dementias, 17,* 110–120.

Storandt, M., Grant, E. A., Miller, J. P., & Morris, J. C. (2002). Rates of progression in mild cognitive impairment and early Alzheimer's disease. *Neurology, 59,* 1034–1041.

Sullivan, M. T. (2002). Caregiver Strain Index (CSI). *Journal of Gerontological Nursing, 28*(8), 4–5.

Suwa, S. (2002). Assessment scale for caregiver experience with dementia. *Journal of Gerontological Nursing, 28*(12), 2–12.

Talerico, K. A., Evans, L. K., & Strumpf, N. E. (2002). Mental health correlates of aggression in nursing home residents with dementia. *Gerontologist, 42,* 169–177.

Talerico, K. A., & Evans, L. K. (2000). Making sense of aggressive/protective behaviors in person with dementia. *Alzheimer's Care Quarterly, 1*(4), 77–88.

Teresi, J. A., Holmes, D., & Ory, M. G. (2000). The therapeutic design of environments for people with dementia: Further reflections and recent finding from the National Institute on Aging Collaborative Studies of Dementia Special Care Units. *Gerontologist, 40,* 417–421.

Tomlinson, B. E., Blessed, G., & Roth, M. (1968). Observations on the brains of non-demented old people. *Journal of Neurological Science, 7,* 331–356.

Tomlinson, B. E., Blessed, G., & Roth, M. (1970). Observation on the brains of demented old people. *Journal of Neurological Science, 11,* 205–242.

Trinh, N. H., Hoblyn, J., Mohanty, S., & Yaffe, K. (2003). Efficacy of cholinesterase inhibitors in the treatment of neuropsychiatric symptoms and functional impairment in Alzheimer disease: A meta-analysis. *Journal of the American Medical Society, 289,* 210–216.

Tsuang, D. W., & Bird, T. D. (2002). Genetics of dementia. *Medical Clinics of North America, 86*(3), 591–614.

Wakefield, B., & Johnson, J. A. (2001). Acute confusion in terminally ill hospitalized patients. *Journal of Gerontological Nursing, 27*(4), 49–55.

Wakefield, B., Mentes, J. Mobily, P., Tripp-Reimer, T., Culp, K. R., Rapp, C. G., et al. (2001). Acute confusion. In M. L. Maas, K. C. Buckwalter, M. D. Hardy, T. Tripp-Reimer, M. G. Titler, & J. P. Specht (Eds.), *Nursing care of older adults: Diagnoses, outcomes, and interventions* (pp. 442–454). St. Louis: Mosby.

Walker, M. P., Ayre, G. A., Cummings, J. L., Wesnes, K., McKeith, I. G., O'Brien, J. T., et al. (2000). Quantifying fluctuation in dementia with Lewy bodies, Alzheimer's disease, and vascular dementia. *Neurology, 54,* 1616–1625.

Waszynski, C. M. (2002). Confusion Assessment Method (CAM). *Journal of Gerontological Nursing, 28*(4), 4–5

Wentzel, C., Rockwood, K., MacKnight, C., Hachinski, V., Hogan, D. B., Feldman, H., et al. (2001). Progression of impairment in patients with vascular cognitive impairment without dementia. *Neurology, 57,* 414–416.

Wesnes, K. A. (2002). Effects of rivastigmine on cognitive function in dementia with Lewy bodies: A randomized placebo-controlled international study using the cognitive drug research computerized assessment system. *Dementia and Geriatric Cognitive Disorders, 13,* 183–192.

Whall, A. L. (2002). Natural environment and implicit memories. *Journal of Gerontological Nursing, 28*(10), 21–23.

Whyte, E. M., Mulsant, B. H., Butters, M. A., Qayyum, M., Towers, A., Sweet, R. A., et al. (2002). Cognitive and behavioral correlates of low vitamin B_{12} levels in elderly patients with progressive dementia. *American Journal of Geriatric Psychiatry, 10,* 321–327.

Wu, C., Zhou, D., Wen, C., Zhang, L., Como, P., Qiao, Y. (2003). Relationship between blood pressure and Alzheimer's disease in Linxian County, China. *Life Sciences, 72,* 1125–1133.

Zandi, P. P., Anthony, J. C., Hayden, K. M., Mehta, K., Mayer, L., & Breitner, J. C. S. (2002). Reduced incidence of AD with NSAID not H_2 receptor antagonists. *Neurology, 59,* 880–886.

Zekry, D., Duyckaerts, C., Moulias, R., Belmin, J., Geoffre, C., Herrmann, F., & Hauw, J. J. (2002a). Degenerative and vascular lesions of the brain have synergistic effects in dementia of the elderly. *Acta Neuropathologica, 103,* 481–487.

Zekry, D., Hauw, J. J., & Gold, G. (2002b). Mixed dementia: Epidemiology, diagnosis and treatment. *Journal of the American Geriatrics Society, 50,* 1431–1438.

Zeleznik, J. (2001). Delirium: Still searching for risk factors and effective preventive measures. *Journal of the American Geriatrics Society, 49,* 1729–1732.

Impaired Affective Function: Depression

LEARNING OBJECTIVES

1. Delineate theories to explain late-life depression.
2. Examine risk factors that cause or contribute to depression in older adults.
3. Discuss the functional consequences of late-life depression.
4. Describe the following aspects of assessment of late-life depression: manifestations of depression that differ in younger and older adults, cultural variations in the expression of depression, distinguishing features of dementia and depressive pseudodementia, and potential for suicide.
5. Identify interventions for alleviating risk factors for late-life depression, treating depression in older adults, and preventing suicide.

Depression is the most common impairment of psychosocial function in older adulthood, yet it has the unfortunate distinction of being the most undetected and untreated of the treatable mental disorders in older adults. The term *depression* is difficult to define because it is considered a mood, a complaint, a syndrome, and a disease; however, gerontological references commonly use the term *depressive symptoms* to describe a constellation of symptoms that profoundly affect the quality of life of a significant number of older adults. Gerontologists have developed theories to explain depression in older adults, which is often called *late-life depression*, and health care practitioners have developed assessment tools to identify depression in older adults. Nurses have important roles in addressing depression because there is a range of nursing interventions that can have a significant positive impact on the quality of life of older adults.

THEORIES ABOUT LATE-LIFE DEPRESSION

Although theories attempt to identify specific causative factors for late-life depression, most discussions of late-life depression emphasize the complex relationships among multiple interacting influences. MacMahon and Pugh (1970) used the term *web of causation* to describe the complex relations among all the factors that interact to cause depression. Blazer (1993) used this concept to illustrate some components in the etiology of late-life depression (Figure 25-1). Some of the more common psychosocial, cognitive, and biologic theories

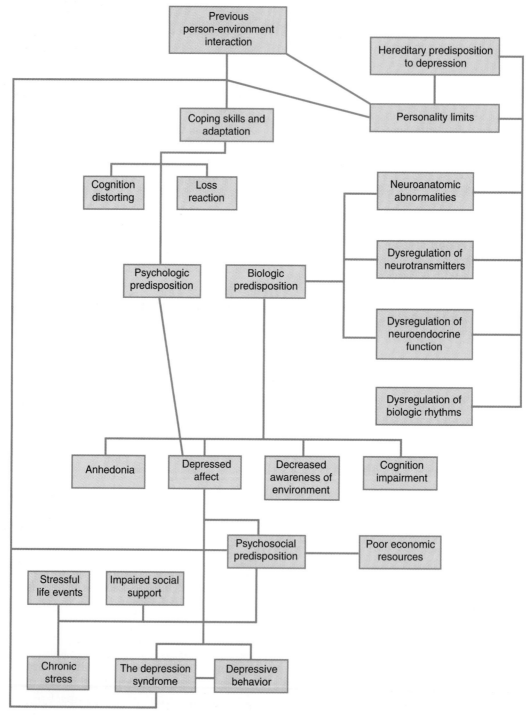

FIGURE 25-1 Possible etiologic factors contributing to depression in late life. (From Blazer, D. G. [1993]. *Depression in late life* [2nd ed.]. St. Louis: Mosby. Used with permission.)

about late-life depression (which are discussed in the following sections) can be used to explain causative factors from various perspectives. A major focus of recent research is the relationship between dementia and depression, and studies are just beginning to address questions about the very common co-occurrence of these two conditions.

Psychosocial Theories

Psychosocial theories hypothesize "that late-life depression arises from the loss of self-esteem, loss of meaningful roles, loss of significant others, and diminished social contacts" (Reker, 1997, p. 709). Many psychosocial theories emphasize the interrelationship among variables, especially the buffering effects of social supports and the social network in protecting against depression. Blazer (2002a) reviewed psychosocial theories related to late-life depression and identified the following potential contributing factors:

- Ageism, loss of social roles, and lower socioeconomic status
- Early experiences, including impoverishment and childhood trauma
- Recent social stressors, including stressful life events
- Inadequate social network (e.g., no spouse, few friends, small family network)
- Diminished social interaction
- Poor social integration (e.g., unstable environment, lack of strong religious affiliation)
- Combination of above factors

The learned helplessness theory also has been used to explain late-life depression. A cognitively oriented formulation of this theory describes depression as a deficit in the following four areas: cognitive, motivational, self-esteem, and affective-somatic (Seligman, 1981). According to this theory, depression occurs when people expect bad things to happen, believe they can do nothing to prevent them, and perceive that the events result from internal, stable, and global factors (Seligman, 1981). Thus, late-life depression occurs because older adults are more likely than younger adults to be placed in situations in which their own behavior has little effect on the behavior of others (Blazer, 2002b). In addition to being used to explain why older people become depressed, the learned helplessness theory has been used to identify factors that can protect older adults from depression. For example, Reker (1997) found that the freedom to choose and be responsible for those choices protected community-living older people from depression; whereas having a purpose, a

sense of order, a reason for existence, and an optimistic outlook protected institutionalized elderly from depression. Similarly, Blazer (2002b) suggested that strategies to strengthen self-efficacy in older adults could prevent depression.

Cognitive Triad Theory

Beck proposed the cognitive triad theory as a way of explaining depression in general and late-life depression in particular (Beck, 1967; Beck et al., 1979). According to this theory, people appraise themselves by the "cognitive triad" of their self-image, their environment or experiences, and their future. Depressed people judge these three realms as lacking some features that are necessary for happiness. Examples of negative appraisals are feelings of worthlessness, interpretations of neutral events as bad, and unrealistic feelings of hopelessness. Beck postulates that depression is caused not by adverse events, but by distorted perceptions, which impair one's ability to appraise oneself and the event in a constructive manner. The second element of Beck's theory involves schemas, or consistent cognitive patterns. Schemas are assumptions, or unarticulated rules, that influence thoughts, feelings, and behaviors. Depressed people typically hold negative assumptions that lead to faulty conclusions. For instance, a depressed person might believe, "I must not be important because the nurse didn't stop to see me." The third component of Beck's theory is the existence of certain logical errors, such as personalization, minimization, magnification, and overgeneralization. This theory is supported by studies that have found a relationship between late-life depression and cognitive distortions or negative cognitions (Blazer, 2002a).

Biologic Theories

Biologic theories about late-life depression investigate the relationship among aging, depression, and changes in the brain, nervous system, and neuroendocrine system. Many theories have addressed the role of neurotransmitters, with particular emphasis on serotonin, dopamine, acetylcholine, and norepinephrine as causative or contributing factors. In addition, the following changes in the neuroendocrine system are associated with depression: elevated plasma cortisol levels, altered growth hormone secretion, altered response of thyroid hormones, and increased activity in the hypothalamic-pituitary-adrenal axis. Other biologic theories address genetic predisposition, neuroanatomic brain changes (e.g., lesions in white or deep gray matter), neurophysiologic brain changes (e.g., decreased cerebral blood flow), and disruption of circadian rhythms (e.g., sleep patterns). Researchers also are trying to identify neuroendocrine changes, such as diminished serotonin, that may contribute to the increased risk for suicide (Mann, 2002).

A major focus of investigation is the relationship between the age-related changes and the biologic changes associated with depression. Because many of these changes are similar, the risk for developing a depressive disorder that is associated with biologic changes increases with increasing age (Blazer, 2002a). Researchers have not been able to draw clear conclusions about cause-and-effect relationships among aging, depression, and biologic changes; however, there is undisputed evidence that "the more severe depressive disorders are strongly influenced by psychobiologic changes" (Blazer, 2002a, p. 117).

Theories About Depression and Dementia

Gerontologists recognize a high correlation between depression and dementia, with many studies finding that depression occurs in 30% to 50% of people with Alzheimer's disease and in 30% to 60% of people with vascular dementia (Blazer, 2002a; Olin et al., 2002a). Similarly, memory deficits and other types of cognitive impairment are more characteristic of depression in older people than in younger people. Both dementia and depression share common characteristics of apathy, loss of interest, diminished cognitive function, and psychomotor agitation or retardation (Moretti et al., 2002). Researchers have identified common neuropathologic changes for dementia and depression, but they have not identified a specific cause-and-effect relationship, nor do they know which condition precedes the other (Blazer, 2002a). Current theories are addressing questions about depression as a causative factor for dementia and vice versa and the implications of these relationships.

Depressive pseudodementia refers to a condition that appears to be a cognitive impairment—and may be labeled as a dementia—but whose underlying cause is depression. A similar concept, called *reversible dementia*, refers to a condition in which the remission of the depression causes a resolution of the cognitive deficits (Olin et al., 2002a). Long-term studies suggest that the type of depression that is accompanied by more severe cognitive deficits increases the risk for developing dementia in the future (Blazer, 2002a). Thus, from this perspective, depression is a risk factor for dementia.

In the mid-1990s, researchers started investigating the possible relationship between late-life depression and atrophy of brain cells, with particular attention on the relationship between vascular dementia and depression. Theories about vascular depression (also called *poststroke depression*) propose that major or minor depression can arise in late life from cerebrovascular damage and that this type of depression has a distinct etiology and a different clinical presentation, which is described at the end of the following section (Miller et al., 2002; Simpson et al., 2000; Tateno et al., 2002).

TYPES OF DEPRESSION

Three of the mood disorders defined in the *Diagnostic and Statistical Manual of Mental Disorders (DSM-IV)* are bipolar disorders, major depressive disorder, and dysthymic disorder (American Psychiatric Association, 1994). In addition, the *DSM-IV* lists criteria for bereavement and adjustment disorder with depressed mood, which are closely associated with late-life depression. The majority of older adults who are admitted to hospitals for mood disorders are diagnosed with major depressive disorder, but dysthymic disorder and bereavement are much more common in community settings (Blazer, 2002a).

Because most early studies of mood disorders of later life focused primarily on major depression, which affects less than 3% of older adults, gerontologists have identified the need to broaden the scope of studies to address the depressive symptoms that occur more commonly in older adults. Judd and Akiskal (2002) suggested that the narrow definitions of major depressive disorder could account for significant underdiagnosis and undertreatment of depression, and they advised both clinicians and researchers to take any level of severity of depressive disorders very seriously. Consequently, terms such as *minor, subthreshold, subclinical,* and *subsyndromal depression* are currently used to reflect more accurately depressive symptoms in older adults (Blazer, 2003; Flint, 2002). This more recent conceptualization places late-life depression on a continuum, ranging from no depression to major depression, and emphasizes that all types of late-life depression "can be associated with significant functional impairment and disability, impaired quality of life, and increased use of health services and medications" (Flint, 2002, p. 230). This reconceptualization is based on studies suggesting that minor and major depressions are not distinct disorders but rather are distinguished by severity of symptoms (Hybels et al., 2001; Lavretsky & Kumar, 2002; Oxman & Sengupta, 2002). Characteristics that most commonly occur, with varying degrees of severity, in any type of depression in older adults are discussed in the section on Functional Consequences.

Another recent trend in classifying depression in older adults is to identify the unique characteristics of depression with vascular dementia or Alzheimer's disease. In 2002, a group of researchers and clinicians with extensive experience related to both late-life depression and Alzheimer's disease proposed diagnostic criteria for depression of Alzheimer's disease (Olin et al., 2002a). Criteria for depression of Alzheimer's disease include the manifestations of depression listed in Display 25-1, all the criteria for the diagnosis of dementia of the Alzheimer's type (discussed in Chapter 24), and additional criteria such as "the symptoms cause clinically significant distress or disruption in functioning" (Olin et al., 2002a, p. 136). Specific diagnostic criteria have not

---

DISPLAY 25-1
Functional Consequences of Late-Life Depression

Impact on Physical Function

- Loss of appetite
- Weight loss
- Digestive system complaints, especially dysphagia, flatulence, constipation, stomach distress, or early satiety
- Insomnia, hypersomnia, frequent awakening, early-morning awakening, and other sleep disturbances
- Fatigue, loss of energy
- Pain, discomfort, dyspnea, general malaise
- Slowed or increased psychomotor activities
- Loss of libido and/or other problems with sexual function

Impact on Psychosocial Function

- Affect: sad, low, "blue," worried, unhappy, "down in the dumps"
- Absence of feelings; feeling numb or empty
- Diminished life satisfaction
- Low self-esteem
- Loss of interest or pleasure
- Passivity, lack of motivation to do things
- Inattention to personal appearance
- Feelings of guilt, hopelessness, self-blame, unworthiness, uselessness, helplessness
- Anxiety, worry, irritability
- Slowed thinking, poor memory, inability to concentrate, poor attention span, inability to make decisions, exaggeration of any mental deficits
- Rumination about past and present problems and failures

---

been proposed for vascular depression, but studies have identified some unique characteristics of this type of depression (Miller et al., 2002; Tateno et al., 2002). Compared with other types of depression, vascular depression is characterized by poor insight, less agitation, increased disability, more cognitive impairment, more psychomotor retardation, and less depressive ideation (e.g., feelings of guilt).

 RISK FACTORS FOR DEPRESSION IN OLDER ADULTS

Risk factors that are likely to cause or contribute to depression in older adults include demographic factors and psychosocial influences, medical conditions and functional impairments, and effects of medications and alcohol. Although these factors can increase the risk for depression in people of any age, older adults are more likely than younger people to have one or more of these variables. In the following sections, each category of risk is discussed in relation to older adults. In addition, cognitive impairments and dementia can be considered risk factors for depression, as discussed in other sections of this chapter.

Demographic Factors and Psychosocial Influences

Demographic factors and personal characteristics that are associated with depression include female gender; low income; low educational level; personal or family history of depression; and divorced, widowed, or separated marital status. When race and ethnic differences have been identified as risk factors for depression, the differences are explained socioeconomically, and these differences have been shown to diminish with the increasing age of the individual (Blazer, 2002a).

The major psychosocial influences associated with increased risk for depression include loneliness, chronic stress, recent social stressors, a stressful social environment, loss of meaningful social interaction, and the lack of social supports, particularly regarding significant roles and intimate relationships. For example, Ugarriza (2002) found that poor health, loss of roles, and death of loved ones are causative factors for depression in older women. Similarly, older adults who are immigrants to the United States or Canada may have higher rates of depression because of the many losses and stresses associated with the move from their homeland (e.g., loss of social status, stress of acculturation, change in living situation) (McKenna, 2003). Additional psychosocial influences that are associated with depression in older adults are current or previous experiences of abuse or neglect and being a caregiver (including assuming primary care of a grandchild). Although losses and stress can be risk factors for depression, the presence of social supports (e.g., having at least one close relationship) and the use of effective coping mechanisms can protect older adults from depression. Thus, the stressors alone are not the primary risk factor for depression; rather, it is the combination of the presence of stressors and the absence of social supports that increases the risk for depression.

Medical Conditions and Functional Impairments

The relationship between depression and the presence of a functional impairment or medical condition is complex and interactive. Minicuci and colleagues (2002) examined the interrelationship and concluded that medical conditions increase the risk for depression only when they interfere with the person's level of functioning. Urinary incontinence is an example of a functional impairment that significantly increases the risk for depression (Nygaard et al., 2003). Moreover, the relationship can be synergistic or cyclic, with depression contributing to medical illness and disability, and medical illness and disability contributing to depression (Lenze et al., 2001; Mehta et al., 2002; Oslin et al., 2002). For example, depression is common in people who have had a myocardial infarction, and it is an independent risk factor for higher morbidity and mortality in the first 4 months after a myocardial infarction (Bush et al., 2001; Romanelli et al., 2002). Researchers have found a synergistic relationship for positive effects of interventions because treatment of depression can improve disability and rehabilitation can improve depression (Lenze et al., 2001). Examples of the interrelationship between depression and medical conditions or functional impairments include the following:

- Depression is strongly associated with numerous medical conditions (Display 25-2); it may cause the medical condition or be an effect of the medical condition.
- Depression in medically ill older adults is associated with increased mortality, longer hospitalizations, and extended recovery time.
- Depression in medically ill older adults can lead to other health problems, such as hip fracture and increased susceptibility to infection.

- Chronic pain is a common cause of depression, and it is sometimes a symptom of depression.
- Depression worsens pain and pain worsens depression.
- Functional impairment is associated with depression as both a contributing factor and a consequence.
- Depression is a common cause of nutritional deficits in older adults.

Explanations for inclusion of functional impairment as a risk factor for depression generally empha-

DISPLAY 25-2
Medical Conditions That Can Cause Depression

Central Nervous System Disorders
Parkinson's disease
Dementia
Strokes
Hemorrhage or hematoma
Tumors
Neurosyphilis
Normal-pressure hydrocephalus

Nutritional Deficiencies
Folate or vitamin B_{12} deficiency
Pernicious anemia
Iron deficiency

Cardiovascular Disturbances
Myocardial infarction
Congestive heart failure
Subacute bacterial endocarditis

Miscellaneous
Rheumatoid arthritis
Cancer, particularly of the pancreas or intestinal tract
Tuberculosis
Tertiary syphilis

Metabolic and Endocrine Disorders
Diabetes
Hypothyroidism/hyperthyroidism
Hypoglycemia/hyperglycemia
Parathyroid disorders
Adrenal diseases
Hepatic or renal disease

Fluid and Electrolyte Disturbances
Hypercalcemia
Hypokalemia
Hyponatremia

Infections
Meningitis
Viral pneumonia
Hepatitis
Urinary tract infections

size the role of disability as a major stressor. Researchers have found that physical disability is associated with all of the following psychosocial risk factors for depression: social isolation, low self-esteem, restricted social activity, strained interpersonal relationships, loss of perceived control, and increased negative life events (Lenze et al., 2001). In addition, chronic illnesses create daily hassles (i.e., chronic stressors) and continually or frequently place demands on coping energy. Acute medical illnesses can threaten survival, independence, self-concept, role functions, economic resources, and sense of well-being.

Another risk factor is that depression often goes unrecognized as a concomitant condition in older adults with medical conditions (Goldstein, 2002). Researchers have found that health care providers overlook depression in 43% to 86% of nursing home residents (McCurren, 2002). Although this is not a risk factor for causing depression, it is a risk factor for the progression of depression when it is untreated. Untreated depression leads to increased functional decline and increased morbidity and mortality (Fabacher et al., 2002).

Effects of Alcohol and Medications

People of any age may experience depression as an adverse medication effect, but older adults are more likely than younger adults to be taking medications. Medications as risk factors for depression can be described as follows:

- Adverse medication effects can cause a depressive syndrome that improves or disappears when the medication is stopped.
- Adverse medication effects can induce a depression that does not remit when the medications are stopped.
- Adverse medication effects can simulate a depressive syndrome by causing lethargy, insomnia, and irritability.
- A depressive syndrome can result from the withdrawal of certain medications, such as psychostimulants.

Depression as an adverse effect of medications is usually related to the use of prescription medications for medical conditions; however, benzodiazepines—the type of medication that is most frequently abused by older adults—also present a risk factor for depression. Table 25-1 lists some medications that may cause depression as an adverse effect.

Alcohol is the drug that is most commonly used by older people for its central nervous system effects as a sedative and antianxiety agent (Blazer, 2002a). Moreover, although people of any age may experience

TABLE 25-1 • Medications That Can Cause Depression	
Types of Medications	**Examples**
Analgesics	Ibuprofen, indomethacin, narcotics, propoxyphene
Antihypertensives	Clonidine, guanethidine, hydralazine, methyldopa, propranolol, reserpine
Antiparkinsonian agents	Levodopa
Cardiovascular agents	Digoxin, digitalis
Central nervous system agents	Alcohol, barbiturates, benzodiazepines, fluphenazine, haloperidol, meprobamate
Histamine blockers	Cimetidine
Steroids	Corticosteroids, estrogen, progesterone

adverse effects from alcohol, older people are more sensitive to these adverse effects because of age-related changes. Alcohol and depression have a cyclic and synergistic relationship: alcohol causes depression, and depression leads to alcohol abuse, which exacerbates the depression. For example, depression is associated with higher alcohol intake, an increased risk for suicide, more frequent relapses in drinking, and a more severe course of alcoholism (Blow & Barry, 2000).

FUNCTIONAL CONSEQUENCES ASSOCIATED WITH DEPRESSION IN OLDER ADULTS

Depression has serious functional consequences for people of any age, but for frail and seriously depressed older adults, the effects can be life-threatening. Functional consequences range from a small negative impact on well-being and quality of life to the most serious consequence, which is suicide. In addition to focusing on specific functional consequences of depression, this section discusses types of depression that commonly affect older adults and terminology associated with depression in older adults.

Impact of Depression on Physical Health and Functioning

A decline in physical functioning is one of the most consistently identified functional consequences of depression in older adults (e.g., Blazer, 2002a; Mehta et al., 2002). Depression is more likely to interfere with daily functioning when the older person also is cognitively impaired (Kiosses et al., 2001). Moreover, older adults with major depression have higher mortality rates than their counterparts without depression (Blazer et al., 2001; Meyers, 2002; Rozzini et al., 2002; Unutzer et al., 2002). Additional functional consequences that affect physical health and functioning are a high number of physical complaints and worse self-reported health (Han, 2002; Oxman et al., 2000; Xavier et al., 2002). Display 25-1 lists ways in which depression affects physical health and functioning.

Appetite disturbances, especially anorexia, are among the most common physical complaints of depressed older adults. Sometimes, the depressed person does not complain of anorexia and may even deny the problem, but a caregiver or family member may note that the person is not interested in food and is losing weight. Other gastrointestinal complaints that may be functional consequences of depression include flatulence, constipation, early satiety, and attention to bowels. Any of these disturbances may be attributed to or actually caused by other factors, such as medical conditions or adverse medication effects, but depression must be considered as a possible underlying factor. Like weight loss and diminished appetite, sleep changes commonly occur in older adults, and they may or may not be caused by depression. Waking up more during the night and early-morning awakening are two changes in sleep patterns that are characteristic of depression. Chronic fatigue and diminished energy are additional functional consequences of late-life depression that are likely to be attributed to or caused by other conditions.

Older adults, like seriously depressed people of any age, are likely to experience psychomotor agitation or retardation. Psychomotor retardation is manifested as slowed body movements and slowed verbal responses, sometimes to the point of muteness. A monotonous or whispering tone of voice might also be an indicator of psychomotor retardation. Affected people often complain of feeling extremely fatigued and having little or no energy. In contrast to people with psychomotor retardation, people with psychomotor agitation present an atypical picture of depression. These people manifest high levels of activity, such as pacing and hand wringing. They may be unable to sit still and may have verbal outbursts, such as shouting. Another activity associated with psychomotor agitation is compulsive behavior, such as frequent toileting or hand washing.

Older depressed women have more appetite disturbances, and older depressed men have more agitation (Kockler & Heun, 2002).

Impact of Depression on Psychosocial Function and Quality of Life

Depression is inherently characterized by a depressed mood or sad affect, but older adults may not perceive or acknowledge these mood disturbances in themselves. Rather than acknowledging that they are depressed, older adults are more likely to talk about being "blue" or "down in the dumps." Depressed older people may feel like crying but may not be able to. They may have difficulty identifying an underlying reason for their sadness. Depressed older adults frequently express feelings of diminished life satisfaction.

Cultural factors may influence the expression of depression, and nurses must consider these in assessing depression. Culture Box 25-1 identifies some of

CULTURE BOX 25-1 Cultural Variations in Expressions of Depression

Cultural Group	Expressions of Depression
African Americans	Fatigue and somatic complaints. "I sure have a lot of troubles;" "I know God won't give me more than I can handle."
Native Americans	Heart problems, being out of harmony
Chinese Americans	Shameful to discuss; may be called "neurasthenia" (i.e., symptoms produced by social stressors)
Cubans	Attribute symptoms to "nerves," anxiety, or extreme stress
Filipinos	Shameful to discuss; may refer to *Lungknot* (i.e., sadness)
Japanese Americans	Shameful to discuss
Koreans	Nonverbal expressions; *Chim-ool haumnida*
Mexican Americans	Sign of weakness, shameful to discuss, common response to stress
Puerto Ricans	References to *Ataque de nervios*
South Asians	References to *Dil uddas hona*, associated with spiritual unhappiness
People from countries with a recent history of war, violence, or political upheaval	May be associated with posttraumatic stress disorder; feelings of helplessness; memories of war-related brutalities

(Lipson, J. G., Dibble, S. L., & Minarik, P. A. [1996]. *Culture and nursing care: A pocket guide.* San Francisco: UCSF Nursing Press; and Andrews, M. M., & Boyle, J. S. [2003]. *Transcultural concepts in nursing care* [4th ed.] Philadelphia: Lippincott Williams & Wilkins.)

the cultural variations that are characteristic of depressed older adults.

Anxiety, irritability, diminished self-esteem, and negative feelings about self are some of the more generalized affective consequences of depression. The absence of feelings, or a feeling of emptiness, also can be a functional consequence of depression. A loss of interest in social activities may be the depression-related psychosocial change that is most obvious to others. Similarly, other people are likely to observe that the depressed older person has little or no concern about personal appearance. In addition, the depressed person may be overly or unrealistically worried about illnesses, financial affairs, and family issues.

Cognitive impairments can occur because of depression, and in older adults, these deficits are likely to be viewed as a primary problem rather than as a consequence of another problem. Depressed older adults may, in fact, exaggerate cognitive deficits and make statements about global deficits, such as "I can't remember anything at all." In particular, they may emphasize memory deficits and attribute these to normal aging, when the underlying problem is actually a depression-related difficulty in concentrating. See Display 25-1 for a list of functional consequences of depression that affect psychosocial function.

Depression has a major negative impact on quality of life. For example, depressed older adults report unsatisfactory social functioning, lower levels of life satisfaction, and poor perceptions of physical and mental health. (Doraiswamy et al., 2002; Meyers, 2002; Xavier et al., 2002). In addition, many of the symptoms of depression (e.g., worry, fatigue, sad affect, sleep disturbances, loss of interest) directly interfere with well-being and quality of life. Moreover, a sense of meaninglessness, which is a common symptom in late-life depression, can have a significant negative effect on quality of life because this causes the older adult to "view the structure and purpose of his or her life in negative ways" (Blazer, 2002a, p. 179).

Suicide

Despite the fact that suicide is the most serious functional consequence of late-life depression, nurses and other health care workers tend to overlook this risk. This tendency is partially attributable to the fact that old age is associated with passivity and nonviolence, whereas suicide is associated with aggressiveness and violence. In 1999, people aged 65 years and older constituted 12.7% of the population in the United States, but they committed 18.8% of all suicides (Conwell &

Pearson, 2002). These rates do not reflect the "drastic underreporting" of suicides in older adults that occurs for reasons such as family efforts to conceal evidence and difficulty determining the actual cause of death in medically ill people (Roff, 2001). Nor do these rates reflect the unrecognized suicidal acts that older adults indirectly or subtly use to take their own lives, such as refusal to eat, failure to take medically necessary medications, and other means of self-neglect. In addition to having the highest rate of suicide, older people have the highest rate of completed suicides in proportion to unsuccessful attempts.

In most countries, men have a higher rate of completed suicide, whereas women have a higher rate of attempted suicide (Mann, 2002).

Suicide rates among older adults in the United States vary significantly by gender and ethnicity, as illustrated in Table 25-2. Across cultures, there is a general trend for a higher rate of suicide among elderly people as compared with young people, and among elderly men as compared with elderly women (Corin, 1996). Worldwide, the suicide rate increased by approximately 35% in men and 10% in women between 1950 and 1995 (Mann, 2002). Researchers have addressed cross-cultural differences in suicide among elderly persons and are attempting to identify the potential impact of culture on suicide rates (Corin, 1996). This is important because studies of suicide rates among various immigrant groups indicate that the factors that influence suicide rates in a country of origin continue to influence suicide rates

TABLE 25-2 • Differences in Suicide Rates for People 65 Years and Older in the United States According to Race and Gender (2000)

Race and Gender	Suicide Deaths per 100,000
White male	34.5
Hispanic male	17.4
Asian or Pacific Islander male	13.9
African American male	12.0
Asian or Pacific Islander female	6.5
White female	4.6
Hispanic female	2.2
African American female	1.5

(National Center for Health Statistics. [2002]. *Health, United States, 2001* [Table 47]. Hyattsville, MD: U.S. Department of Health and Human Services.)

among immigrants in their new country (Burvill, 1996).

> The suicide rate in men is more than four times that in women. In women, suicide rates remain relatively stable throughout adulthood; but in men, suicide rates increase substantially and gradually beginning in their mid-70s (Mann, 2002).

NURSING ASSESSMENT OF DEPRESSION IN OLDER ADULTS

Because Chapter 10 addresses all aspects of psychosocial assessment, this section is limited to the following specific aspects of late-life depression: identifying the unique manifestations of depression in older adults, differentiating between dementia and depressive pseudodementia, using screening tools to identify late-life depression, and assessing suicide risk in older adults. The assessment information in Chapter 10, particularly Display 10-6, can be used with the information in the following sections as a guide for assessing depression in older adults.

Identifying the Unique Manifestations of Depression in Older Adults

Assessment of late-life depression is complicated by a wide array of possible manifestations, as reviewed in the section on Functional Consequences. Moreover, manifestations of depression in older adults differ from those in younger adults. Although it is difficult to generalize about manifestations of

TABLE 25-3 • Comparison of Depression in Younger and Older Adults	
Depressed Younger Adults	**Depressed Older Adults**
More likely to report emotional symptoms	Report more cognitive and physical symptoms
Sense of hopelessness, uselessness, and helplessness	Apathy; exaggeration of personal helplessness
Negative feelings toward self	Sense of emptiness, loss of interest, withdrawal from social activities
Insomnia	Hypersomnia; early morning awakening
Eating disorders	Anorexia, weight loss
More verbal expressions of suicidal ideation than successful attempts; more passive means of suicide	Less talk about suicide, but more successful attempts and more violent means of suicide

depression according to age categories, some conclusions about the differences in younger and older adults are summarized in Table 25-3.

In assessing depression in any cognitively impaired older adult, the most problematic area is distinguishing between manifestations of depression and dementia. Table 25-4, which identifies specific features that are most likely to be associated with either dementia or depression, can be used as a guide for nursing assessment to differentiate between these two conditions. It is important to keep in mind that older adults frequently have conditions that contribute to both depression and cognitive impairment; hence, manifestations will not always be clearly distinguished.

Using Screening Tools to Assess for Depression in Older Adults

Concerns about depression being overlooked and underdiagnosed in older people have stimulated the development of very brief, two- or three-item screening tools that health care professionals can use in a variety of settings (e.g., Fabacher et al., 2002; National Institute of Mental Health, 2001; Thobaben, 2002). For example, the U.S. Preventive Services Task Force recently emphasized that there is sufficient research evidence to suggest that primary care practitioners should routinely screen for depression in all adults (Agency for Healthcare Research and Quality, 2002). The Task Force recommends that use of the following two questions may be as effective as using longer screening instruments (Agency for Healthcare Research and Quality, 2002):

1. During the past 2 weeks, have you felt down, depressed, or hopeless?
2. During the past 2 weeks, have you felt little interest or pleasure in doing things?

A positive response to either of these two questions warrants further assessment with a depression scale.

The Geriatric Depression Scale (GDS) is a 30-question screening tool that has been widely used across health care settings for older adults who are healthy, medically ill, or mild to moderately cognitively impaired. The Hartford Institute for Geriatric Nursing recommends the use of this screening tool—which is reliable, sensitive, and takes an average of 12 minutes to administer—to facilitate assessment of depression in older adults (Kurlowicz, 1999). Shorter forms of the GDS, consisting of 12 or 15 items (Figure 25-2), have been developed for use with residents in long-term care settings

TABLE 25-4 • Distinguishing Features of Dementia and Depression

Parameter	Dementia	Depression
Onset of symptoms	Gradual onset, recognized only by hindsight	Abrupt onset, possibly involving a triggering event
Presentation of symptoms	Unawareness of symptoms, or attribution to nonpathologic causes	Exaggeration of memory problems and other cognitive deficits
Memory and attention	Impaired memory, especially for recent events; poor attention; strong attempts to perform well	Memory and attention deficits attributable to lack of motivation and inability to concentrate
Emotions	Labile affect that changes in response to suggestions; possible apathy owing to cognitive impairments	Consistent feelings of sadness and being "down in the dumps"; unresponsive to suggestions
Response to questions	Evasive, angry, sarcastic; use of humor, confabulation, or social skills to cover up deficits	Slowed, apathetic, frequent response of "I don't know," with no effort expended
Personal appearance	Inappropriate dress and actions owing to impaired perceptions and thought processes	Little or no concern about appearance because of lack of motivation or diminished self-esteem
Physical complaints	Vague fatigue and weakness; complaints are inconsistent and easily forgotten	Anorexia, weight loss, constipation, insomnia, decreased energy
Neurologic features	Aphasia, agnosia, agraphia, apraxia, perseveration	Complaints of dysphagia without any physical basis
Contact with reality	Denial of reality; illusions more predominant than hallucinations; if present, delusions are aimed at explaining deficits	Exaggerated sense of gloom; possible auditory hallucinations or self-derogatory delusions

(McCurren, 2002; Sutcliffe et al., 2000). Because of the high correlation between depression and medical illness, Piven (2001) developed a protocol to improve detection of depression in medically compromised but cognitively intact older adults in health care facilities. This protocol advises the weekly use of the Folstein Mini-Mental State Examination (MMSE) and the short-form GDS to detect depression. The protocol includes a form to monitor detection of depression.

A brief screening tool, which takes about 2 minutes to administer, is available for identifying Puerto Rican older adults who need further evaluation of depression (Robison et al., 2002).

Geriatric Depression Scale (Short Form)

1. Are you basically satisfied with your life?	Yes	No
2. Have you dropped many of your activities and interests?	Yes	No
3. Do you feel that your life is empty?	Yes	No
4. Do you often get bored?	Yes	No
5. Are you in good spririts most of the time?	Yes	No
6. Are you afraid that something bad is going to happen to you?	Yes	No
7. Do you feel happy most of the time?	Yes	No
8. Do you often feel helpless?	Yes	No
9. Do you prefer to stay at home rather than go out and do new things?	Yes	No
10. Do you feel you have more problems with memory than most?	Yes	No
11. Do you think it is wonderful to be alive now?	Yes	No
12. Do you feel pretty worthless the way you are now?	Yes	No
13. Do you feel full of energy?	Yes	No
14. Do you feel that your situation is hopeless?	Yes	No
15. Do you think that most people are better off than you are?	Yes	No

Score:___/15   One point for "No" to questions 1, 5, 7, 11, 13
One point for "Yes" to other questions

Normal	3 ± 2
Mildly depressed	7 ± 3
Very depressed	12 ± 2

FIGURE 25-2 Geriatric Depression Scale (short form). (From Yesavage, J. A., Brink, T. L., Rose, T. L., et al. [1983]. Development and validation of a geriatric depression screening scale: A preliminary report. *Journal of Psychiatric Research, 17,* 37–49. Used with permission.)

Assessing the Risk for Suicide in Older Adults

Nursing assessment of suicide risk is especially important because older people usually give clues, sometimes to many people, about potential suicide. Up to 90% of older adults who commit suicide have a knowledgeable informant (Younger et al., 1990). These clues, however, may be subtle, and the person who hears them may not associate them with suicide risk, particularly in older adults. Although 70% of older people who commit suicide visit their primary care provider within 1 month before the act, fewer than 5% of depressed older adults directly express suicidal ideation to their primary care practitioner (Bartels et al., 2002). Even when older adults express suicidal ideation to primary care practitioners, they are less likely than younger adults to be viewed as having a serious and treatable condition (Uncapher & Arean, 2000). Thus, the nursing assessment of suicide risk must be based primarily on identification of potential risk factors for suicide in older adults, such as the following:

- Limited social support
- Poor impulse control
- Poor sleep quality
- Recent stressful life event (e.g., widowhood)
- Strong sense of hopelessness
- Lack of a reason for living
- Nonadherence to medical treatment
- Immediate access to a lethal method
- Serious medical illness (e.g., cancer, neurologic disorders)
- Moderate to severe functional impairment (e.g., visual impairment)
- Moderate to severe depression, often co-occurring with anxiety disorder (Bartels et al., 2002; Turvey et al., 2002; Waern et al., 2002)

Because depression is the factor most consistently identified across studies as a risk factor for suicide, it is important to assess for suicidal ideation in any depressed older adult. In addition to these factors that alert the nurse to risk for suicide, the factors that are most strongly predictive of actual suicide are a history of previous attempts and current suicide ideation that includes a plan or evidence of preparation of a plan (Mann, 2002). Display 25-3 summarizes risk factors for suicide in older adults, verbal and nonverbal clues to suicide intent, and specific questions to assess immediate suicide risk.

When risk factors or clues to potential suicide have been identified, an assessment of the immediate potential for a suicide attempt must be done. This assessment is multilevel, with each level of questions depending on the response to the previous level. The assessment begins with questions to determine the presence or absence of suicidal thoughts. Health care professionals may be reluctant to initiate questions about suicide because they fear that this line of questioning may "put ideas in the person's head." This fear is unfounded. People who do not have suicidal thoughts usually respect the necessity of the questions but do not begin thinking about suicide just because the topic was broached. Rather than asking a person "Do you ever think about committing suicide?" the nurse can phrase the question in such a way that the person will give clues to his or her intent if it exists, but will not be offended by the question if it does not.

If suicidal thoughts are suspected or identified at level 1, additional questions must be asked. Although level 1 questions are indirect, level 2 questions must be more direct and are aimed at determining the presence or absence of thoughts about self-harm. If the answer to any of these questions is positive, level 3 questions are asked to determine whether the person has a realistic suicide plan. Questions at this level must be very direct and specific because this information is crucial to assessing the immediate risk for suicide. If the person describes a detailed plan and has access to all the necessary implements, the potential for suicide is close to 100%. By contrast, if the person has a plan that is vague or that cannot possibly be carried out, the immediate potential for suicide is lower. For example, if the plan involves a gun, but the person does not have a gun and cannot get out of the house, then the chance of a successful suicide is low. By contrast, if the person threatens to consume the bottle of barbiturates that is readily available in the medicine cabinet, then the chance of a successful suicide is quite high. Level 4 questions are asked to assess further the immediacy of the risk when the person has described a plan. When answers to level 3 or 4 questions are positive, the nurse must plan immediate interventions to deal with the suicide risk.

NURSING DIAGNOSIS

Nurses currently are advocating for the development of a nursing diagnosis of Depression, but in the absence of this specific nursing diagnosis, applicable nursing diagnoses include Powerlessness, Hopelessness, and Chronic Low Self-Esteem (Piven & Buckwalter, 2001).

DISPLAY 25-3
Guidelines for Assessing Suicide Risk

Risk Factors for Suicide in Older Adults

- Demographic factors: white race, male gender, divorced or widowed, low socioeconomic status
- Depression, especially when accompanied by insomnia, agitation, and self-neglect
- Chronic illness with increasing dependence and helplessness; diagnosis of cancer or a terminal illness
- Poor social supports; social isolation, especially recent isolation
- History of psychiatric illness, especially major depression
- Onset of major depression within the past year
- Family history of suicide; personal or family history of suicide attempts
- Patterns of impulsive behavior
- Alcohol abuse
- Poor communication skills

Verbal Clues to Suicide Intent

- "Pretty soon you won't have to worry about me."
- "I would be better off dead."
- "I don't want to be a burden to others."
- Expressions of hopelessness
- Remarks about life being unbearable
- Reflections on the worthlessness of life

Nonverbal Clues to Suicide Intent

- Making a will; giving belongings away; preparing for own funeral
- Serious self-neglect, especially in people who have no cognitive impairments
- Frequent visits to primary care provider(s)
- Excessive use of medications or alcohol
- Accumulation of prescription medications
- Unusual preoccupation with self and withdrawal from others

Interview Questions to Assess the Immediate Risk of Suicide

Level 1
- "Do you ever think life is not worth living?"
- "Do you ever think about escaping from your problems?"

Level 2
- "Do you ever think about harming yourself?"
- "Do you ever think of taking your own life?"

Level 3
- "Do you have a plan?"
- "What would you do to take your life?"

Level 4
- "Have you ever started to act on a plan to harm yourself?"
- "Under what circumstances would you act on that plan?"

Another appropriate nursing diagnosis is Ineffective Individual Coping, defined as "a state in which the individual experiences, or is at risk to experience, an inability to manage internal or environmental stressors adequately due to inadequate resources (physical, psychological, behavioral and/or cognitive)" (Carpenito, 2002, p. 257). Related factors commonly found in older adults are relocation, ageist attitudes, financial concerns, social isolation, caregiving responsibilities, multiple social stressors, loss of significant roles or relationships, functional impairments (including cognitive deficits), and increased dependence (e.g., owing to the loss of the ability to drive).

If the nursing assessment identifies risk factors for suicide, an applicable nursing diagnosis would be Risk for Suicide, defined as "a state in which an individual is at risk for killing himself or herself" (Carpenito, 2002, p. 837). Related factors would include any risk factors and verbal and nonverbal clues to suicide. An example is an 85-year-old widower who says his life is no longer worthwhile and who makes frequent visits to his doctor for complaints of weight loss and sleep disturbance.

OUTCOMES

Nursing-sensitive outcomes and related indicators that pertain to depressed older adults, as outlined by Piven and Buckwalter (2001), include the following:

- Hope, as indicated by the person expressing inner peace, will to live, belief in self, and positive future orientation
- Coping, as indicated by the person identifying effective and ineffective coping patterns and verbalizing sense of control or acceptance of situation
- Mood equilibrium, as indicated by the person exhibiting concentration, impulse control, appropriate affect, nonlabile mood, and absence of suicidal ideation
- Suicide self-restraint, as indicated by the person expressing feelings, maintaining connectedness in relationships, seeking help when feeling self-destructive, and refraining from gathering the means for suicide

The following nursing-sensitive outcomes are applicable for the nursing diagnosis of Ineffective

Individual Coping: appropriate morale, good somatic health, satisfying social functioning, and healthy religiosity and spirituality (Stolley, 2001).

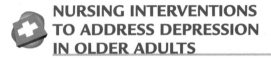

NURSING INTERVENTIONS TO ADDRESS DEPRESSION IN OLDER ADULTS

Gerontological nurses in any setting are responsible for addressing depression in older adults. Particularly in long-term care settings, nurses are the health care providers most likely to identify manifestations of depression and to request further evaluation and treatment. In recent years, primary care physicians and nurse practitioners have been the health care professionals who are evaluating and managing depression, and referrals to psychiatrists and other mental health professionals for depression have become less common. This trend is due to the emphasis on cost-effectiveness and the availability of safer and more effective antidepressant medications. Nursing protocols for depression in elderly patients emphasize the important responsibility of nurses in reducing the negative consequences of depression through early recognition, intervention, and referral of patients with depression (Kurlowicz & NICHE Faculty, 1997; Piven, 2001). The next sections review the role of the gerontological nurse in planning and implementing interventions for late-life depression.

Promoting Health by Alleviating Risk Factors

Health promotion interventions for depressed older adults address the risk factors that can cause depression in older adults and can be alleviated through nursing interventions. Some of the risk factors that are most amenable to nursing intervention include functional impairments, adverse medication effects, and excess alcohol use. The role of nurses in addressing these risk factors is discussed in this section. In addition, nurses have dominant roles in addressing medical conditions, but these interventions are beyond the scope of this text and are addressed in medical-surgical texts.

Because functional impairment is a common contributing factor for depression, nursing interventions that are directed toward improved level of functioning also are interventions for alleviating or preventing depression. For example, sensory impairments, urinary incontinence, mobility impairments, and dementia are examples of conditions that might contribute to depression and improve with the

implementation of nursing interventions discussed in the corresponding chapters of this text (Chapters 12, 13, 15, 18, and 24). As discussed throughout this text, many functional impairments are unnecessary consequences of myths, misinformation, or lack of information. In these situations, the nurse is the professional person most able to provide information and facilitate referrals for a thorough assessment and appropriate interventions.

If adverse medication effects cause or contribute to depression, nurses can educate the person about this potential relationship and identify problem-solving strategies regarding adverse effects of medications. One such strategy is to educate the older adult about ways of communicating with the prescribing health care provider (as discussed in Chapter 23) because most older adults are unaccustomed to questioning their primary care provider about medications. For example, if the older person understands that there is a wide array of antihypertensive medications, and that not all of them will cause depression, the person can use this information in discussing the problem with his or her primary care provider. Nurses also can assure the older adult that it is acceptable to initiate this kind of problem-solving discussion with health care practitioners. When the nurse, rather than the patient, is the one who communicates with the primary care provider, appropriate questions can be raised about depression as an adverse medication effect. This problem-solving approach is especially important when the primary care provider is considering adding an antidepressant medication to a regimen that includes a depression-inducing medication. In these situations, the solution may be to change medications, rather than to add another medication and increase the risk for adverse effects.

If excess alcohol use is a risk factor for depression, individual and group interventions can be effective, particularly when the alcohol abuse is a reaction to recent losses. Alcoholics Anonymous (AA) is the most widely used group program for alcoholics of any age, and in some areas, age-homogeneous groups have been established, including some for older adults. Nurses can encourage older adults to initiate contact with AA, or they might directly facilitate the referral if the person agrees to this. Individual and family counseling also may be effective, and nurses can suggest or facilitate referrals for these mental health services.

Promoting Health by Improving Psychosocial Function

In addition to alleviating the risk factors for depression, health promotion interventions can improve psychosocial health and prevent depression from occurring or progressing. Blazer (2002b) emphasized the importance of primary prevention of late-life depression through interventions that enhance self-efficacy and alleviate sadness and loneliness. In addition to health promotion interventions for psychosocial health (discussed in Chapter 8), nurses can identify interventions to strengthen social supports and foster meaningful roles.

Because social supports significantly affect the mental health of older adults, any intervention that strengthens social supports may prevent or alleviate depression. Nurses can encourage older adults to participate in group meal or social programs. Most communities in the United States have some social programs for older adults, and many provide transportation. Many churches and religious organizations also have programs designed to meet the social needs of isolated older adults. Volunteer visitor or phone call programs, for example, are sometimes available to address the needs of people who have difficulty getting out of the house. Other programs, such as pet therapy or "Adopt a Grandparent," are available in some home, community-based, and long-term care settings, and they can be helpful in alleviating loneliness and depression.

Involvement in volunteer activities can enhance self-esteem and provide a meaningful role for older adults who are mildly depressed. Nurses can suggest that older adults explore opportunities for volunteer activities through organizations such as the National Senior Service Corps (previously called the Retired Senior Volunteer Program), which is one of the many programs in the United States that assists older adults in becoming involved in volunteer activities (see the Educational Resources at the end of this chapter).

Promoting Health Through Exercise and Nutrition Interventions

The beneficial effects of exercise with regard to anxiety, depression, self-esteem, and other components of mental health are widely acknowledged. Researchers have identified the effects of physical exercise in both alleviating and preventing depression in older adults (e.g., Blazer 2002b; Penninx et al., 2002; Singh et al., 2001; Strawbridge et al., 2002). Older adults, however, may not view exercise as important, or they may be reluctant to participate in exercise programs because of chronic illnesses, such as arthritis. If older adults understand the benefits of exercise for both their physical and mental health, and an individually tailored program is developed for them, they may be more willing to become involved in exercise programs. In community and long-term care settings, nurses can facilitate the establishment of group exercise programs and encourage depressed older adults to participate in them.

Nutrition is an important consideration as an intervention for depression for three reasons. First, nutritional status often is negatively affected by depression, and this can cause additional negative consequences. Second, good nutrition has a positive effect on mental health and cognitive function. Third, constipation is both a consequence of depression and an adverse effect of some antidepressant medications, and it usually can be alleviated through nutritional interventions. During phases of serious depression, malnutrition can lead to medical problems, which may progress to the point of being life-threatening. Nutritional supplements, hyperalimentation, or tube feedings may be necessary interventions when depression seriously interferes with eating. When depression is severe enough to lead to malnutrition, the older person must be evaluated for psychiatric care. Interventions for less severely depressed older people are aimed at maintaining adequate hydration and nutrition and preventing or managing constipation. The interventions discussed in Chapter 14 can be applied to the care of the depressed older adult.

Providing Counseling

Many types of individual and group psychosocial therapies are effective for late-life depression. For example, when multiple stressors challenge the person's coping abilities and contribute to depression, individual or group therapy can be an important intervention for improving the person's psychosocial health and alleviating depression. Nurses provide counseling and emotional support for depressed older adults, and in some situations, they participate in providing specific psychosocial therapies.

Counseling, which is defined as "the use of an interactive helping process focusing on the needs, problems, or feelings of the patient and significant others to enhance or support coping, problem-solving, and interpersonal relationships" (Iowa Intervention Project, 2000, p. 238), can be effective in alleviating depression. Some of the activities listed under this intervention that are most applicable for depressed older adults include the following:

- Establish a therapeutic relationship.
- Encourage expression of feelings.
- Demonstrate empathy, warmth, and genuineness.
- Encourage new skill development, as appropriate.
- Provide factual information, as necessary and appropriate.

- Assist patient to identify strengths and reinforce these (Piven & Buckwalter, 2001).

Another nursing intervention that can be universally applied to care of depressed older adults is Emotional Support, defined as "provision of reassurance, acceptance, and encouragement during times of stress" (Iowa Intervention Project, 2000, p. 300).

Nurses need to be at least minimally familiar with some of the individual therapies that have been found acceptable to and effective for depressed older adults so that they can encourage or facilitate referrals for these interventions. Therapies that are identified as effective and acceptable for depressed older adults include the following:

- Behavior therapy (e.g., problem solving, practicing assertiveness, setting up a daily schedule)
- Cognitive therapy (e.g., conscious restructuring of negative thought processes)
- Interpersonal therapy (e.g., modification of relationships or expectations about relationships)
- Supportive therapy (e.g., evaluating the person's strengths and weaknesses and facilitating choices that improve coping abilities)
- Dynamic psychotherapy (e.g., resolution of intrapsychic conflicts)
- Bibliotherapy (e.g., readings and exercises to assist the person in identifying and reducing dysfunctional thought processes) (Blazer 2002a; Landreville, et al., 2001; Piven & Buckwalter; 2001)

In recent years, group therapies have been recognized as an effective and efficient intervention for depressed older adults. Group therapy is effective for depressed older adults because it imparts information, improves self-esteem, enhances social interaction, encourages attitudinal changes, and facilitates personal development (Blazer, 2002a). Support and self-help groups are commonly used interventions to improve psychosocial function and alleviate depression in older adults who are coping with life events, such as caregiving, widowhood, or grief reactions, and nurses can educate older adults about the availability of such groups. Numerous studies have found that support groups are particularly effective for caregivers of people with dementia.

Nurses generally do not lead psychotherapy groups as a routine responsibility, but they are increasingly assuming group leadership roles, particularly in community and long-term care settings. Other group models used as interventions for late-life depression include reminiscence, relaxation, art therapy, focused imagery, creative movement, and cognitive-behavioral strategies. In addition to groups specifically targeted for depression, groups such as the Healthy Aging Class (described in Chapter 8), which are directed toward developing coping skills, may be effective in alleviating depression.

Although adult day care programs are not primarily a group therapy for depressed older adults, they are a commonly available resource for providing structured social and therapeutic activities. Similarly, many community-based senior programs provide opportunities for group meals, exercise, and social interaction, and these can be quite effective in alleviating mild to moderate depression in older adults. Information about these and other group programs for older adults can be obtained from local offices on aging, and nurses can encourage older adults or their caregivers to seek out such information and take advantage of these programs.

Facilitating Referrals for Psychosocial Therapies

Older adults who are seriously depressed must be referred to appropriate mental health professionals and psychiatric services. Nurses frequently facilitate referrals for appropriate psychosocial therapies. Hospital-based geropsychiatric programs, which are becoming increasingly available, can provide assessment and treatment of the unique aspects of late-life depression. Some community mental health centers also are beginning to address the mental health needs of older adults, and they may provide special programs for depressed older adults. Nurses can either suggest or directly facilitate referrals to these programs. Older adults or their caregivers may perceive depression as an untreatable problem, but they may follow through on suggestions for help if they understand that the condition can be resolved. Often, the primary role of the nurse is to convince the older person that depression is not a necessary consequence of old age and that help is available.

Educating Older Adults About Antidepressant Medications

Types of Antidepressant Medications

Biochemical theories of depression have guided the development of various antidepressant medications. For example, the observation that depression was a common adverse effect of drugs that deplete the brain of catecholamine led to the development of tricyclic and other cyclic antidepressants, which block the reuptake of chemical messengers at neuronal synapses in the brain. As scientists have discovered more information about brain function and neurotransmitters, pharmaceutical companies have made major advances in developing safe and effective antidepressants.

Monoamine oxidase inhibitors (MAOIs) were the first medications used as antidepressants. After their use became widespread in the 1960s, it was discovered that this category of medication could cause dangerous and even fatal adverse effects (e.g., hypertensive crisis) when they interacted with many other medications and with some types of food. Another disadvantage of using MAOIs is the common occurrence of confusion, restlessness, agitation, and paranoid ideation in older adults who are cognitively impaired (Blazer, 2002a). Because there are so many contraindications to the use of MAOIs in older adults, they are used with extreme caution and only when other therapies have been found to be ineffective. Thus, older adults who are taking an MAOI are usually very closely supervised and evaluated by a psychiatrist or other primary care practitioner. Examples of MAOIs are phenelzine, isocarboxide, and tranylcypromine.

Cyclic antidepressants, used widely since the late 1950s, are thought to be particularly effective in alleviating the following depression-related symptoms: loss of libido, sleep and appetite disturbances, and loss of interest and pleasure in activities. Cyclic antidepressants are usually categorized as tricyclic antidepressants (which were the first ones developed) and second-generation agents (which have been widely used since the mid-1980s). Cyclic antidepressants differ more in their potential for adverse effects than in their therapeutic effects. Because cyclic antidepressants affect several neurotransmitters, they are associated with a variety of anticholinergic and other detrimental effects. Two particular areas of concern in geriatric care are the potential for adverse cardiovascular and anticholinergic effects. The most likely cardiovascular effects are orthostatic hypotension and altered cardiac rate and rhythm. The most serious anticholinergic effects are blurred vision, urinary retention, and cognitive impairments. Additional common side effects are sedation, constipation, dry mouth, and weight gain. Because of these side effects, people with glaucoma, prostatic hyperplasia, or cardiac conduction abnormalities should not take cyclic antidepressants. In addition, cyclic antidepressants should be avoided in people with dementia or Parkinson's disease because of the potential adverse effect of cognitive impairment. Anticholinergic potency varies among the tricyclic antidepressants, with amitriptyline having the strongest anticholinergic

effects and desipramine having the weakest. As a rule of thumb, cyclic agents with weaker anticholinergic effects should be prescribed over those with stronger anticholinergic effects.

During the late 1980s, pharmaceutical companies developed a class of antidepressant drugs that were more selective in their action than the cyclic antidepressants. Called selective serotonin reuptake inhibitors (SSRIs), these drugs are chemically unrelated to cyclic or other types of antidepressants. The therapeutic effectiveness of SSRIs is similar to that of cyclic antidepressants, but they have minimal cholinergic, histaminic, dopaminergic, and noradrenergic effects. SSRIs currently are considered the first-line medications for depression because they are effective for most people, and their adverse effects are more tolerable and less dangerous (Blazer, 2002a; Snow et al., 2000; Williams et al., 2000). For example, an important consideration for older adults is that SSRIs are less likely than cyclics to cause orthostatic hypotension and anticholinergic effects. This is particularly important for mentally frail elderly people who are susceptible to confusion and for physically frail elderly people who are at high risk for falls.

Although SSRIs are safer than other types of antidepressants, nurses need to be aware of important adverse effects and drug interactions. For example, SSRIs are metabolized in the liver, and some of them are highly bound to plasma protein; thus, they may be affected by interactions with other drugs that are metabolized in the liver or are highly protein bound. In addition, when an SSRI is prescribed, special attention should be paid to potential interactions with nicotine, alcohol, and other medications (including some over-the-counter products). Drug interactions may occur even after an SSRI with a long half-life (e.g., fluoxetine) has been discontinued. Common adverse effects of SSRIs include nausea, vomiting, diarrhea, headache, nervousness, insomnia, tremor, dry mouth, and sexual dysfunction. A recent study found that SSRIs significantly increased the risk for gastrointestinal bleeding, and this risk was increased with concurrent use of nonsteroidal antiinflammatory drugs or low-dose aspirin (Dalton et al., 2003). Withdrawal effects of SSRIs include nausea, tremor, anxiety, dizziness, palpitations, and paresthesias. Fluoxetine, the first available drug in this category, may cause agitation in as many as 20% to 30% of the patients taking it. Also, because of its long half-life, it may take 2 to 4 weeks to reach a steady state in older adults, and side effects may not resolve until 7 to 10 days after the drug is discontinued. Sertraline and paroxetine differ from fluoxetine in that they have shorter half-lives and no

TABLE 25-5 • Antidepressants Commonly Used for Older Adults

Category	Examples	Trade Names
Selective serotonin reuptake inhibitors (SSRIs)	Citalopram Fluoxetine Fluvoxamine Paroxetine Sertraline	Celexa Prozac Luvox Paxil Zoloft
Serotonin and norepinephrine reuptake inhibitors	Mirtazapine Venlafaxine	Remeron Effexor
Serotonin modulators	Nefazodone Trazodone	Serzone Desyrel
Dopamine reuptake inhibitors	Buproprion	Wellbutrin
Cyclic antidepressants	Amoxapine Desipramine Imipramine	Asendin Norpramin Tofranil

depression and dementia, antidepressant medications may improve the affective symptoms so that overall abilities are improved and the person is able to function more effectively and independently.

Nursing responsibilities regarding antidepressant medication therapy include observing for both adverse and therapeutic effects and educating the older adult about the unique aspects of these medication therapies. Another important responsibility is educating older adults about the ongoing need for continued evaluation and treatment of depression, including the monitoring of antidepressant medication use. Older adults who have been diagnosed with major depressive disorder are at high risk for recurrence, and this risk is increased if antidepressant medications are not maintained for at least 6 months (Geddes et al., 2003; Glick et al., 2001; Meyers et al., 2001). Older adults often want to discontinue medications when their depressive symptoms resolve, and nurses need to teach them about the importance of ongoing antidepressant therapy and periodic reevaluations after medications are discontinued. This is especially important in nursing home settings because there is a very high rate of underdiagnosis and undertreatment of depression among nursing home residents (Brown et al., 2002). Display 25-4 summarizes guidelines for the nursing responsibilities regarding antidepressant medications.

anticholinergic effects. Fluvoxamine, like fluoxetine, may have mild anticholinergic effects.

In addition to the cyclic antidepressants, MAOIs, and SSRIs, several other types of antidepressants are used for older adults, as listed in Table 25-5. Special considerations in the use of these other types of antidepressants are as follows: venlafaxine may cause an increase in blood pressure; trazodone and nefazodone are very sedating and may be useful in the treatment of depression with sleep disturbances; and buproprion has a stimulating effect, which sometimes can be therapeutic, but is contraindicated in people with a seizure disorder. Lithium is sometimes used to augment the effects of another antidepressant, particularly for people with bipolar disorders. Psychomotor stimulants (e.g., methylphenidate) have been used for decades for certain types of depression, but these drugs are not antidepressants, and they are not widely used, especially in older adults. Some antidepressants are available in liquid or long-acting formulations to increase compliance and ease of administration.

Nursing Responsibilities Regarding Antidepressants

An important nursing responsibility regarding antidepressants is to educate older adults about the primary purpose of these medications, which is to alleviate depressive symptoms so that the person is able to respond to additional interventions, such as psychosocial therapy. For older adults who have both

Educating Older Adults About Electroconvulsive Therapy

Electroconvulsive therapy (ECT) is increasingly being used as a low-risk treatment that has an efficacy rate of at least 80% for older depressed people, including patients as old as 102 years (Kelly & Zisselman, 2000; Manly et al., 2000). Researchers have found that ECT is at least as effective as, and perhaps more effective than, medications for older depressed patients, and it can be life saving for seriously depressed older adults (Kujala et al., 2002). Although ECT is usually recommended only after the person fails to respond adequately to a course of antidepressant medications, the American Psychiatric Association states that it should be considered a first-line treatment when a rapid and definitive response is needed for a severely depressed person (Kelly & Zisselman, 2000).

Prevalent negative attitudes about ECT are attributable, in part, to the alleged inhumane use of this procedure when it was first developed a half-century ago. In recent years, however, the technique for administering ECT has been refined, and the risks, discomfort, and side effects are now quite minimal.

DISPLAY 25-4

Health Education About Antidepressant Medications

Information to Be Shared with the Older Adult

- Immediate improvement will not be evident, but a fair trial must be given to the medication as long as serious adverse effects are not noticed.
- The fair trial may take as long as 12 weeks, but some positive effects should be noticed within 2 to 4 weeks.
- If one type of antidepressant is not effective, another type may be effective.
- Antidepressants cannot be used on an "as needed" basis.
- Antidepressants should be viewed as part of a comprehensive approach to treating depression, and psychosocial therapies should be considered along with antidepressants.
- Antidepressants can interact with alcohol, nicotine, and other medications, including over-the-counter medications, possibly altering the effects of the medication or increasing the potential for adverse effects.
- The prescribing health care practitioner should be asked about potential adverse effects and drug–drug or food–drug interactions.
- The prescribing health care practitioner should be consulted before discontinuing an antidepressant.
- If postural hypotension occurs, the effects can be minimized through such interventions as changing position slowly and maintaining adequate fluid intake.

- If monoamine oxidase inhibitors (MAOIs) are prescribed, certain medications must be avoided, and a low-tyramine diet must be followed (i.e., avoidance of beer, yogurt, red wine, fermented cheese, and pickled foods, as well as excessive amounts of caffeine and chocolate).

Principles Regarding Dosage and Length of Treatment

- Older adults should be started at one half to one third the normal adult dose.
- Dosages can be increased gradually until maximal therapeutic levels are reached, while observing for adverse effects.
- Age-related changes may increase the time needed for medication to reach maximal effectiveness.
- A once-daily regimen usually is effective.
- Bedtime administration of an antidepressant may facilitate sleep as a result of the drug's hypnotic effects, but some antidepressants (e.g., fluoxetine) may be better taken in the morning because of side effects, such as agitation.
- The length of treatment is usually 6 months for a first-time depression, 1 to 2 years for people with a history of a prior depressive episode, and lifetime maintenance for people with a history of three or more depressive episodes.

Most adverse effects—such as headache, nausea, bradycardia, memory impairment, and muscle pain—are transient, and there is no evidence that ECT causes any long-term structural brain changes (Blazer, 2002a). Except in psychiatric settings, nurses will not be involved with the care of people who are undergoing ECT. Nurses caring for depressed people in any setting, however, need to maintain an open mind about this therapy. In addition, gerontological nurses may be in the position of encouraging older adults or their caregivers to seek advice about ECT from knowledgeable professionals.

Educating Older Adults About Alternative Health Care Practices

In recent years, there has been increasing interest in herbs and other natural remedies for depression. St. John's wort (also called *hypericum extract*) has been widely used in Europe as an alternative to prescription antidepressants, and it has been found to be equally effective for many people. Since 1998, the National Center for Complementary and Alternative Medicine has sponsored randomized, controlled, double-blind studies in the United States to compare

placebo effect, St. John's wort, and prescription antidepressants. Currently, studies suggest that St. John's wort is "probably more effective than placebo in the treatment of mild to moderate depression" (Gaster & Holroyd, 2000). St. John's wort is widely available and relatively inexpensive, but products are not standardized or regulated for quality. Although St. John's wort is not likely to cause any serious adverse reactions, precautions that apply to herbal products (discussed in Chapter 23) should be heeded.

Bright-light therapy has been used to improve sleep in people with disturbed circadian rhythm, and it is an established therapy for treatment of seasonal affective disorder (Remick, 2002). Sumaya and colleagues (2001) explored the use of bright-light therapy as an intervention for depression in older nursing home residents and found that 1/2 hour of exposure to 10,000 lux of bright light for 5 days produced clinically significant improvements in moderately to severely depressed subjects. Nurses can use Display 25-5 as a guide to educating older adults about health promotion interventions and alternative health care practices that can be used for depression.

DISPLAY 25-5
Health Education About Preventing or Alleviating Depression

Participation in exercise on a regular basis (e.g., ½ hour 3 to 5 times a week) may prevent or alleviate depression.

Nutritional Considerations

- Ensure adequate intake of (or use supplements of) the following nutrients: vitamins B and C, magnesium, potassium, and selenium.
- Include foods that are high in tryptophan (e.g., eggs, milk, fish, nuts, turkey, bananas, soybeans, pumpkin seeds).
- Include food sources of phenylalanine (e.g., meat, fish, poultry, soybeans, chocolate, watercress, sunflower seeds, black beans).
- Avoid intake of large amounts of caffeine and artificial sweeteners (e.g., aspartame).

St. John's wort, 300 mg three times daily, may be effective in reducing the symptoms of mild to moderate depression, but do not take this with antidepressants.

Additional Therapies That May be Effective for Reducing Symptoms

- Avoidance of nicotine
- Individual counseling and group therapies
- Bright-light therapy, ½ hour daily
- Aromatherapy (inhaled or applied to the skin): rose, basil, jasmine, bergamot, lavender, chamomile, clary sage
- Art, dance, music, drama, yoga, t'ai chi, qigong, massage, imagery, meditation, relaxation, stress management, spiritual healing
- Acupuncture, acupressure, reflexology

DISPLAY 25-6
Nursing Interventions for People Who Are Potentially Suicidal

Communicating With Someone Who Is Potentially Suicidal

- Be direct and honest; do not be afraid to ask direct questions, such as "Are you thinking of hurting yourself?"
- Express feelings of concern and confidence.
- Acknowledge the person's feelings of helplessness and hopelessness.
- Encourage the person to talk about the precipitating event, if there is one.
- Emphasize that suicide is only one of several options; then explore other options.
- Emphasize positive relationships; talk about the negative impact of suicide on survivors.
- Maintain a nonjudgmental attitude.
- Make a contract: ask the person to agree to do certain things for limited amounts of time and to call for help if he or she cannot keep the agreement.
- Discuss the problems openly with the family and caregivers.

Crisis Intervention

- Focus on the immediate precipitating event.
- Reduce the immediate danger by removing the implements, interfering with the plan, and providing constant supervision.
- Obtain psychiatric help; call a suicide hot line or activate emergency psychiatric services if necessary.

Preventing Suicide in Older Adults

Gerontological nurses do not usually deal with suicidal older adults in the course of their routine duties, but they may have to plan immediate interventions when they identify a patient at risk. The most important intervention is to seek out psychiatric resources and activate protective service agencies, rather than attempting to deal with potentially suicidal people without the help of specialized resources. All communities have some emergency psychiatric services, and nurses can either make referrals directly or discuss these resources with older adults and their caregivers. Some guidelines for working with people who are potentially suicidal are listed in Display 25-6.

EVALUATING EFFECTIVENESS OF NURSING INTERVENTIONS

Nursing care of depressed older adults is evaluated by documenting improved coping skills and diminished manifestations of depression. For example, the person may report diminished feelings of hopelessness and improved appetite and sleep. Another measure that would reflect improved quality of life would be that the older adult expresses interest in and participates in meaningful activities. Effectiveness of nursing interventions also could be evaluated by whether the older adult has begun taking antidepressant medications and participating in individual or group therapies.

Nursing care of older adults who are at high risk for self-harm would be evaluated by the prevention of harm. Another measure would be the degree to which the older adult develops coping skills to deal with the issues that underlie suicidal thoughts. Nursing care also could be evaluated by whether the older adult obtains mental health services to address underlying problems.

CHAPTER SUMMARY

Late-life depression occurs because of a combination of factors, including many psychosocial influences and biologic factors (e.g., age-related nervous system changes). Common risk factors that contribute to depression include physical illness, functional impairments, psychosocial factors, impaired cognitive function, and medication and chemical effects. Functional consequences of late-life depression include numerous physical manifestations (e.g., eating and sleep disturbances), emotional manifestations (e.g., sad affect, low self-esteem), and cognitive components (e.g., memory and attention deficits). Late-life depression has a significant negative effect on quality of life, and the most serious functional consequence is a high risk for suicide.

Nursing assessment must address the unique manifestations of depression in older adults and the differences between dementia and depression. Nurses also must assess the risk for suicide and cultural factors in the expression of depression. Applicable nursing diagnoses include Powerlessness, Hopelessness, Ineffective Individual Coping, and Risk for Suicide. Health promotion interventions are directed toward alleviating risk factors and improving psychosocial function. Nursing interventions include providing counseling and educating older adults about health promotion interventions and alternative health care practices. Nurses also provide health education about medical interventions, such as antidepressants and ECT. In addition, nurses have important responsibilities in facilitating referrals for mental health services, particularly when suicidal ideation is part of the depression.

■ CONCLUDING CASE STUDY AND NURSING CARE PLAN

➤ Mrs. D. is 81 years old and recently has been diagnosed as having vascular dementia. She lives with her husband, who has diabetes, macular degeneration, and severe arthritis. Mrs. D. had managed all household and financial responsibilities until about 1 year ago, when she began having trouble with her memory. Mrs. D. was evaluated at the geriatric assessment program where you work, and she was advised to stop driving and to arrange for some help with complex tasks, such as bill paying and grocery shopping. Two months after the initial evaluation, Mrs. D. returns for follow-up and informs you that she limits her driving to short, daytime trips in familiar areas. When asked about getting help with complex tasks, she states, "I just don't have any energy to make all those calls you suggested. Besides, I don't want anyone else looking at my finances or going to the store for me."

■ Nursing Assessment

A mental status assessment indicates that Mrs. D.'s level of cognitive impairment is unchanged since her initial evaluation. She has prominent deficits in calculation, short-term memory, abstract thinking, problem solving, and language skills. Your psychosocial assessment reveals that Mrs. D. has a very sad affect and low self-esteem, and she expresses feelings of hopelessness and helplessness. She admits to being overwhelmed with feelings of responsibility for herself and her husband, and she says she feels "paralyzed because there's no light at the end of the tunnel."

When you ask about her daily life, Mrs. D. says she spends most of her time at home because she hasn't had the energy to go out. She admits that she doesn't sleep well and that she has difficulty falling asleep at night. She naps for a couple of hours in the morning and in the afternoon because "I feel tired all the time and I can't go out and do things anyway." Her appetite is poor, and in the past 2 months, her weight has declined from 140 pounds to 126 pounds (her height is 5′6″). She complains of constipation and "heartburn."

When you ask about meaningful activities, she tells you she no longer goes to her weekly bowling club because it meets in the evening and she doesn't want to drive at night. She also has given up her church activities (Thursday discussion club and Sunday service) because she does not want to inconvenience anyone by having them drive her. She feels it's "demeaning to have to tell my friends that I need a ride." She used to enjoy reading, but she hasn't felt like going to the library, and she's not interested in any of the books she has at home.

■ Nursing Diagnosis

You use the nursing diagnosis of Ineffective Individual Coping, related to depression and declining cognitive abilities. Evidence comes from Mrs. D.'s sad affect, low self-esteem, loss of interest in activities, feelings of hopelessness and helplessness, and inability to address

DISPLAY 25-7 • NURSING CARE PLAN FOR MRS. D.

EXPECTED OUTCOME	NURSING INTRVENTIONS	NURSING EVALUATION
Mrs. D. will be able to identify her coping patterns.	• Ask Mrs. D. to describe her prior experiences in dealing with her husband's illness. • Help Mrs. D. to identify coping strategies that have been helpful in the past.	• Mrs. D. will recognize and acknowledge the coping strategies that have been helpful in the past.
Mrs. D. will learn about depression and be encouraged to obtain further evaluation of her depression.	• Talk with Mrs. D. about her signs and symptoms of depression, emphasizing the fact that depression is a treatable condition. • Discuss the relationship between depression and the inability to cope effectively with stressful situations. • Ask Mrs. D. if she is willing to see a geropsychiatrist or talk to her primary care practitioner for further evaluation and treatment. • Explain that antidepressant medications can be very effective when used in conjunction with counseling.	• Mrs. D. will follow through with an appointment with a geropsychiatrist or talk with her primary care practitioner.
Effective coping strategies for addressing Mrs. D.'s declining abilities will be identified.	• Discuss with Mrs. D. several options for ongoing support and counseling to assist her in coping with her declining abilities (e.g., the "Something for You" support group for people with memory loss; or individual counseling sessions with the social worker who is affiliated with the geriatric assessment program). • Emphasize the importance of developing short-term goals that can be addressed through problem solving (e.g., suggest that Mrs. D. begin to address her lack of meaningful activities by going to the library for reading material).	• Mrs. D. will attend one support group on a trial basis and talk with you about the experience at her next appointment in 1 month. • Mrs. D. will make an appointment for counseling with the social worker. • Mrs. D. will participate in one meaningful activity each week for the next month.

her problems effectively. Physical manifestations are her poor appetite, weight loss, sleep disturbances, and complaints about constipation and heartburn.

■ Nursing Care Plan

The nursing care plan you develop for Mrs. D. is shown in Display 25-7.

 CRITICAL THINKING EXERCISES

1. Address the following questions in relation to Mrs. D., the subject of the case study.
   • What risk factors are likely contributing to Mrs. D.'s depression?
   • What further assessment information would you obtain?

   • If you applied the Geriatric Depression Scale (Figure 25-2) to Mrs. D., what score do you think she would have?
   • What additional interventions would you suggest for Mrs. D.?
2. Think of an older adult in your personal life or professional practice who is or has been depressed. What are (were) the risk factors in that person's situation that might play (have played) a part in the depression?
3. Describe at least four cultural variations in the way depression might be expressed.
4. What assessment observations would you make and what questions would you ask to differentiate between dementia and depression in older adults?
5. Make up a case example of someone who is potentially suicidal and who would require all four

levels of suicide assessment. Describe how you would phrase the questions for each of the levels.

6. Describe a teaching plan for an 84-year-old woman for whom Paxil, 10 mg daily, has been prescribed.

EDUCATIONAL RESOURCES

Depression and Bipolar Support Alliance (DBSA)
730 North Franklin, Suite 501, Chicago, IL 60610-7224
(800) 826-3632
http://www.ndmda.org

National Center for Complementary and Alternative Medicine
NCCAM Clearinghouse,
P.O. Box 7923
Gaithersburg, MD 20898
(888) 644-6226
http://nccam.nih.gov/

National Institute of Mental Health DEPRESSION Awareness, Recognition, and Treatment Program (D/ART)
6001 Executive Boulevard, Rm. 8184, MSC 9663,
Bethesda, MD 20892-9663
(866) 615-6464
http://www.nimh.nih.gov

National Mental Health Association
2001 N. Beauregard Street, 12th Floor,
Alexandria, VA 22311
(800) 969-6642
http://www.nmha.org

National Senior Service Corps
1201 New York Avenue, NW,
Washington, DC 20525
(800) 424-8867
http://www.seniorcorps.org

U.S. Department of Health and Human Services Agency for Healthcare Research and Quality
AHRQ Publications Clearinghouse
P.O. Box 8547,
Silver Spring, MD 20907-8547
http://www.ahcpr.gov

REFERENCES

Agency for Healthcare Research and Quality. (2002, May 20). *U.S. Preventive Services Task Force now finds sufficient evidence to recommend screening adults for depression.* Retrieved from http://www.ahrq.gov/news/press/pr2002/deprespr.htm.

American Psychiatric Association. (1994). *Diagnostic and statistical manual of mental disorders (DSM-IV)* (4th ed.). Washington, DC: Author.

Andrews, M. M., & Boyle, J. S. (2003). *Transcultural concepts in nursing care* (4th ed.). Philadelphia: Lippincott Williams & Wilkins.

Bartels, S. J., Coakley, E., Oxman, T. E., Constantion, G., Oslin, D., Chen, H., et al. (2002). Suicidal and death ideation in older primary care patients with depression, anxiety, and at-risk alcohol use. *American Journal of Geriatric Psychiatry, 10,* 417–427.

Beck, A. T. (1967). *Depression: Clinical, experimental and theoretical aspects.* New York: Harper & Row.

Beck, A. T., Rush, A. J., Shaw, B., & Emery, G. (1979). *Cognitive therapy of depression.* New York: Guilford Press.

Blazer, D. G. (1993). *Depression in late life* (2nd ed.). St. Louis: C. V. Mosby.

Blazer, D. G. (2002a). *Depression in late life* (3rd ed.). New York: Springer.

Blazer, D.G. (2002b). The prevalence of depression symptoms. *Journal of Gerontology: Medical Sciences, 57A,* M150–M151.

Blazer, D. G. (2002c). Self-efficacy and depression in late life: A primary prevention proposal. *Aging & Mental Health, 6*(4), 315–324.

Blazer, D. G. (2003). Depression in late life: Review and commentary. *Journal of Gerontology: Medical Sciences, 58A,* 249–265.

Blazer, D. G., Hybels, C. F., & Pieper, C. F. (2001). The association of depression and mortality in elderly persons: A case for multiple independent pathways. *Journal of Gerontology: Medical Sciences, 56A,* M505–M509.

Blow, F. C., & Barry, K. L. (2000). Older patients with at-risk and problem drinking patterns: New developments in brief interventions. *Journal of Geriatric Psychiatry and Neurology, 13,* 115–123.

Brown, M. N., Lapane, K. L., & Luisi, A. F. (2002). The management of depression in older nursing home residents. *Journal of the American Geriatrics Society, 50,* 69–76.

Burvill, P. W. (1996). Suicide in the multiethnic elderly population of Australia, 1979–1990. In J. L. Pearson & Y. Conwell (Eds.), *Suicide and aging: International perspectives* (pp. 187–201). New York: Springer.

Bush, D. E., Ziegelstein, R. C., Tayback, M., Richter, D., Stevens, S., Zahalsky, H., et al. (2001). Even minimal symptoms of depression increase mortality risk after acute myocardial infarction. *American Journal of Cardiology, 88,* 337–341.

Carpenito, L. J. (2002). *Nursing diagnosis: Application to clinical practice* (9th ed.). Philadelphia: Lippincott Williams & Wilkins.

Conwell, Y., Pearson, J. L. (2002). Suicidal behaviors in older adults. *American Journal of Geriatric Psychiatry, 10*(4), 359–361.

Corin, E. (1996). From a cultural stance: Suicide and aging in a changing world. In J. L. Pearson and Y. Conwell (Eds.), *Suicide and aging: International perspectives* (pp. 205–224). New York: Springer.

Dalton, S. O., Johansen, C., Lellemjaer, L., Norgard, B., Sorensen, H. T., & Olsen, J. H. (2003). Use of selective serotonin reuptake inhibitors and risk of upper gastrointestinal tract bleeding. *Archives of Internal Medicine, 163,* 59–64.

Doraiswamy, P. M., Khan, Z. M., Donahue, R. M. J., & Richard, N. E. (2002). The spectrum of quality-of-life impairments in recurrent geriatric depression. *Journal of Gerontology: Medical Sciences, 57A,* M134–M127.

Fabacher, D. A., Raccio-Robak, N., McErlean, M. A., Milano, P. M., & Verdile, V. P. (2002). Validation of a brief screening tool to detect depression in elderly ED patients. *American Journal of Emergency Medicine, 20*(2), 99–102.

Flint, A. J. (2002). The complexity and challenge of non-major depression in late life. *American Journal of Geriatric Psychiatry, 10,* 229–232.

Gaster, B., & Holroyd, J. (2000). St. John's wort for depression. *Archives of Internal Medicine, 160,* 152–156.

Geddes, J. R., Carney, S. M., Davies, C., Furakawa, T. A., Kupfer, D. J., Frank, E., & Goodwin, G. M. (2003). Relapse prevention with antidepressant drug treatment in

depressive disorders: A systematic review. *Lancet,
361*(9358), 653–661.

Glick, I. D., Suppes, T., DeBarrista, C., Hu, R. J., & Marder,
S. (2001). Psychopharmacologic treatment strategies for
depression, bipolar disorder, and schizophrenia. *Annals of
Internal Medicine, 134,* 47–60.

Goldstein, M. Z. (2002). Depression and anxiety in older
women. *Primary Care; Clinics in Office Practice, 29*(1),
69–80.

Han, B. (2002). Depressive symptoms and self rated health
in community dwelling older adults. *Journal of the
American Geriatrics Society, 50,* 1549–1556.

Hybels, C. F., Blazer, D. G., & Pieper, C. F. (2001). Toward a
threshold for subthreshold depression: Analysis of correlates of depression by severity of symptoms using data
from an elderly community. *Gerontologist, 4,* 357–365.

Iowa Intervention Project. J. C. McCloskey & G. M. Bulechek
(Eds.) (2000). *Nursing interventions classification* (NIC)
(3rd ed.). St. Louis: Mosby.

Judd, L. L., & Akiskal, H. S. (2002). The clinical and public
health relevance of current research on subthreshold
depressive symptoms to elderly patients. *American Journal
of Geriatric Psychiatry, 10,* 233–238.

Kelly, K. G., & Zisselman, M. (2000). Update on electroconvulsive therapy (ECT) in older adults. *Journal of the American Geriatrics Society, 48,* 560–566.

Kiosses, D. N., Klimstra, S., Murphy, C., & Alesopoulos, G.S.
(2001). Executive dysfunction and disability in elderly
patients with major depression. *American Journal of
Geriatric Psychiatry, 9,* 269–274.

Kockler, M., & Heun, R. (2002). Gender differences of
depressive symptoms in depressed and nondepressed elderly persons. *International Journal of Geriatric Psychiatry,
17,* 65–72.

Kujala, I., Rosenvinge, B., & Bekkelund, S. I. (2002). Clinical
outcome and adverse effects of electroconvulsive therapy
in elderly psychiatric patients. *Journal of Psychiatry Neurology, 15,* 73–76.

Kurlowicz, L. (1999). The Geriatric Depression Scale (GDS).
Geriatric Nursing, 20, 212–213.

Kurlowicz, L. H., & NICHE faculty. (1997). Nursing standards of practice protocol: Depression in elderly patients.
Geriatric Nursing, 18, 192–199.

Landreville, P., Landry, J., Baillargeon, L., Guerette, A., &
Matteau, E. (2001). Older adults' acceptance of psycho-
logical and pharmacological treatments for depression.
Journal of Gerontology: Psychological Sciences, 56B,
P285–P291.

Lavretsky, H., & Kumar, A. (2002). Clinically significant
non-major depression. *American Journal of Geriatric Psychiatry, 10,* 239–255.

Lenze, E. J., Rogers, J. C., Martire, L. M., Mulsant, B. H.,
Rollman, B. L., Dew, M. A., et al. (2001). The association
of late life depression and anxiety with physical disability.
American Journal of Geriatric Psychiatry, 9, 113–135.

Lipson, J. G., Dibble, S. L., & Minarik, P. A. (1996). *Culture
& nursing care: A pocket guide.* San Francisco: UCSF
Nursing Press.

MacMahon, B., & Pugh, T. F. (1970). *Epidemiology: Principles and methods.* Boston: Little, Brown & Company.

Manly, D. T., Oakley, S. P., & Bloch, R. M. (2000). Electroconvulsive therapy in old-old patients. *American Journal
of Geriatric Psychiatry, 8,* 232–236.

Mann, J. J. (2002). A current perspective of suicide and
attempted suicide. *Annals of Internal Medicine, 136,*
302–311.

McCurren, C. (2002). Assessment for depression among
nursing home elders: Evaluation of the MDS mood
assessment. *Geriatric Nursing, 23*(2), 103–107.

McKenna, M. A. (2003). Transcultural nursing care of
older adults. In M. A. Andrews & J. S. Boyle. *Transcultural concepts in nursing care* (pp. 209–246). Philadelphia:
Lippincott Williams & Wilkins.

Mehta, K. M., Yaffe, K., & Covinsky, K. E. (2002). Cognitive
impairment, depressive symptoms, and functional decline
in older people. *Journal of the American Geriatrics Society,
50,* 1045–1050.

Meyers, B. S. (2002). Treatment and course of geriatric
depression: Questions raised by an evolving clinical science. *American Journal of Geriatric Psychiatry, 10,*
497–502.

Meyers, B. S., Klimstra, S. A., Gabriele, M., Hamilton,
M., Kakuman, T., Tirumalasetti, F., et al. (2001). Contin-
uation treatment of delusional depression in older adults.
American Journal of Geriatric Society, 9, 415–422.

Miller, M. D., Lenze, E. J., Dew, M. A., Whyte, E., Weber, E.,
Begley, A. E., et al. (2002). Effect of cerebrovascular risk
factors on depression treatment outcome in later life.
American Journal of Geriatric Psychiatry, 10, 592–598.

Minicuci, N., Maggi, S., Pavan, M., Enzi, G., & Crepaldi, G.
(2002). Prevalence rate and correlates of depressive symptoms in older individuals: The Vento study. *Journal of
Gerontology: Medical Sciences, 57A,* M155–M161.

Moretti, R., Torre, P., Antonello, R. M., Cazzato, G., & Bava,
A. (2002). Depression and Alzheimer's disease: Symptom
or comorbidity? *American Journal of Alzheimer's Disease
and Other Dementias, 17,* 338–344.

National Center for Health Statistics. (2002). *Health, United
States, 2001* (Table 47). Hyattsville, MD: U.S. Department
of Health and Human Services.

National Institute of Mental Health. (2001). *Depression
research at the National Institute of Mental Health.*
Retrieved from http://www.nimh.gov.publicat/depres-
fact.cfm.

Nygaard, I., Turvey, C., Burns, T. L., Crischilles, E., & Wallace,
R. (2003). Urinary incontinence and depression in middle-
aged United States women. *Obstetrics and Gynecology, 101,*
149–156.

Olin, J. T., Katz, I. R., Meyers, B. S., Schneider, L. S., &
Lebowitz, B. D. (2002a). Provisional diagnostic criteria
for depression of Alzheimer disease. *American Journal of
Geriatric Psychiatry, 10,* 129–141.

Olin, J. T., Schneider, L. S., Katz, I. R., Meyers, B. S., Alex-
opoulos, G. S., Breitner, J. C., et al. (2002b). Provisional
diagnostic criteria for depression of Alzheimer disease.
American Journal of Geriatric Psychiatry, 10, 125–128.

Oslin, D. W., Datto, C. J., Kallan. M. J., Katz, I. R., Edell, W.
S., TenHave, T., et al. (2002). Association between medical comorbidity and treatment outcomes in late life
depression. *Journal of the American Geriatrics Society, 50,*
823–828.

Oxman, T. E., Barrett, J. E., Sengupta, A., & Williams, J. W.
Jr. (2000). The relationship of aging and dysthymia in primary care. *American Journal of Geriatric Psychiatry, 8,*
318–326.

Oxman, T. E., & Sengupta, A. (2002). Treatment of minor
depression. *American Journal of Geriatric Psychiatry, 10,*
256–264.

Penninx, B. W. J. H., Rejeski, W. J., Pandya, J., Miller, M. E.,
Di Bari, M., Applegate, W. B., Pahor, M. (2002). Exercise
and depressive symptoms: A comparison of aerobic and
resistance exercise effects on emotional and physical

function in older persons with high and low depressive symptomatology. *Journal of Gerontology: Psychological Sciences, 57B,* P124–P132.

Piven, M. L. (2001). Detection of depression in the cognitively intact older adult protocol. *Journal of Gerontological Nursing, 27*(11), 8–14.

Piven, M. L., & Buckwalter, K. C. (2001). Depression. In M. L. Maas, K. C. Buckwalter, M. D. Hardy, T. Tripp-Reimer, M. G. Titler, & J. P. Specht (Eds.), *Nursing care of older adults: Diagnoses, outcomes, and interventions* (pp. 521–542). St. Louis: Mosby.

Reker, G. T. (1997). Personal meaning, optimism, and choice: Existential predictors of depression in community and institutional elderly. *Gerontologist, 37,* 709–716.

Remick, R. A. (2002). Diagnosis and management of depression in primary care: A clinical update and review. *Canadian Medical Association Journal, 167,* 1253–1260.

Robison, J., Gruman, C., Gaztambide, S., & Blank, K. (2002). Screening for depression in middle aged and older Puerto Rican primary care patients. *Journal of Gerontology: Medical Science, 57A,* M308–M314.

Roff, S. (2001). Suicide and the elderly. *Journal of Gerontological Social Work, 35*(2), 21–36.

Romanelli, J., Fauerbach, J. A., Bush, D. E., & Ziegelstein, R. C. (2002). The significance of depression in older patients after myocardial infarction. *Journal of the American Geriatric Society, 50,* 817–822.

Rozzini, R., Giovanni, B., Sabatini, T., & Trabucchi, M. (2002). Response to "The association of depression and mortality in elderly persons." *Journal of Gerontology: Medical Sciences, 578A,* M144.

Seligman, M. E. P. (1981). A learned helplessness point of view. In L. P. Rehm (Ed.), *Behavior therapy for depression.* (pp. 123–141). New York: Academic Press.

Simpson, S., Baldwin, R. C., Jackson, A., Burns, A., & Thomas, P. (2000). Is the clinical expression of late-life depression influenced by brain changes? MRI subcortical neuroanatomical correlates of depressive symptoms. *International Psychogeriatrics, 12,* 425–434.

Singh, N. A., Clements, K. M., & Singh, M. A. F. (2001). The efficacy of exercise as a long term antidepressant in elderly subjects: A randomized, controlled trial. *Journal of Gerontology: Medical Sciences, 56A,* M497–M504.

Snow, V., Lascher, S., & Mottur-Pilson, C. (2000). Pharmacologic treatment of acute major depression and dysthymia. *Annals of Internal Medicine, 132,* 738–742.

Stolley, J. M. (2001). Ineffective individual coping. In M. L. Maas, K. C. Buckwalter, M. D. Hardy, T. Tripp-Reimer, M. G. Titler, & J. P. Specht (Eds.), *Nursing care of older adults: Diagnoses, outcomes, and interventions* (pp. 766–781). St. Louis: Mosby.

Strawbridge, W. J., Deleger, S., Roberts, R. E., & Kaplan, G. A. (2002). Physical activity reduces the risk of subsequent depression for older adults. *American Journal of Epidemiology, 156,* 328–334.

Sumaya, I. C., Rienzi, B. M., Deegan, J. F., & Moss, D. E. (2001). Bright light treatment decreases depression in institutionalized older adults: A placebo controlled crossover study. *Journal of Gerontology: Medical Sciences, 56A,* M356–M360.

Sutcliffe, C., Cordingley, L., Burns, A., Mozley, C. G., Bagley, H., Challis, D., et al. (2000). A new version of the Geriatric Depression Scale for nursing and residential home populations: The Geriatric Depression Scale. *International Psychogeriatrics, 12*(2), 173–181.

Tateno, A., Kimura, M., & Robinson, R. G. (2002). Phenomenological characteristics of poststroke depression. *American Journal of Geriatric Psychiatry, 10,* 575–581.

Thobaben, M. (2002). Screening for depression: Ask clients two simple questions. *Home Health Care Management & Practice, 15*(1), 82–83.

Turvey, C. L., Conwell, Y., Jones, M. P., Phillips, C., Simonsick, E., & Pearson, J. L. (2002). Risk factors for late life suicide. *American Journal of Geriatric Psychiatry, 10,* 398–406.

Ugarriza, D. N. (2002). Elderly women's explanation of depression. *Journal of Gerontological Nursing, 28*(5), 22–29.

Uncapher, H., & Arean, P. A. (2000). Physicians are less willing to treat suicidal ideation in older patients. *Journal of the American Geriatrics Society, 48,* 188–192.

Unutzer, K., Patrick, D. L., Marmon, T., Simon, G. E., & Katon, W. J. (2002). Depressive symptoms and mortality in a prospective study of 2,558 older adults. *American Journal of Geriatric Psychiatry, 10,* 521–530.

Waern, M., Rubenowitz, E., Runeson, B., Skoog, I., Wilhelmson, K., & Allebeck, P. (2002). Burden of illness and suicide in elderly people: A case-control study. *British Medical Journal, 324*(7350), 1355.

Williams, J. W., Mulrow, C. D., Chiquettee, E., Noel, P. H., Aguilar, C., Cornell, J., et al. (2000). A systematic review of newer pharmacotherapies for depression in adults. *Annals of Internal Medicine, 132,* 743–756.

Xavier, F. M. F., Farraza, M. P. T., Argimon, I., Trentini, C. M., Poyares, D., Bertollucci, P. H., et al. (2002). The DSM-IV "minor depression" disorder in the oldest-old: Prevalence rate, sleep patterns, memory function and quality of life in elderly people of Italian descent in Southern Brazil. *International Journal of Geriatric Psychiatry, 17,* 107–116.

Younger, S., Clark, D., Ochmig-Lindroth, R., & Stein, R. (1990). Availability of knowledgeable informants for a psychological autopsy of suicides committed by elderly people. *Journal of the American Geriatrics Society, 38,* 1169–1175.

Elder Abuse and Neglect

Because elder abuse is the most complex and serious negative functional consequence that affects vulnerable older adults, these situations challenge gerontological nurses to apply their highest level of nursing skills. In this chapter, elder abuse is viewed as a serious impairment of overall function and is discussed from the perspective of the functional consequences theory.

OVERVIEW

Elder abuse is defined as the maltreatment of older people. This maltreatment can be intentional or unintentional, and it can result from the actions or inactions of other people, usually caregivers. Self-neglect is a type of elder abuse that occurs when older people fail to provide themselves with adequate food, shelter, medical care, and other life essentials. Certain members of any population are vulnerable to abuse and neglect by virtue of being physically or psychosocially impaired or subjugated. In colonial times, tensions between adult children and their parents over property sometimes produced hostility when parents became enfeebled and would not relinquish control. Moreover, the witch-burnings of the 16th and 17th centuries targeted old women in particular, possibly because of the burdens they placed on family resources and their access to property desired by younger relatives (Stearns, 1986). In industrialized societies today, vulnerable groups are protected and cared for through legislative mandates and social programs. For many decades, children and people with mental retardation have been protected in the United States and many other countries. In recent decades, two additional groups have been recognized as being in need of protection: victims of domestic violence, and abused or neglected older people. Although the problem of abused or neglected older adults is not new, elder abuse as a social problem has a short history in the United States.

Awareness of elder abuse as a social problem began in the 1950s and 1960s as the writings of Geneva Mathiasen and Gertrude Hall introduced the concept of protecting vulnerable adults. Centers like the Benjamin Rose Institute in Cleveland, Ohio, developed the concept in the early 1970s through initial demonstration projects, usually specifically related to self-neglect. Awareness of physical abuse, however, did not surface until the late 1970s, and awareness of other types of elder abuse (e.g., domestic violence against elders) arose during the 1980s. The late 1980s also witnessed the growing criminalization of elder abuse, a movement that peaked during the late 1990s. During this phase, consumer fraud, including scams and con games, was subsumed under elder abuse. In the new millennium, elder abuse is so broadly conceived that addressing it requires the widest range of professional disciplines, systems, and settings. It almost has become a concept with limitless boundaries and certainly is one that lacks a universally accepted definition.

Elder Abuse as a Social Problem

Recognition by public officials of the problem of domestic elder abuse can be traced to 1977, when congressional hearings on child abuse suggested that the entire scope of family violence be considered. In 1978, the term "battered parent" was first used by Suzanne Steinmetz at a congressional hearing on domestic violence, and that same year the Department of Health and Human Services awarded two grants for elder abuse research. In 1979, the first congressional hearing dealing exclusively with elder abuse was held by the U.S. House Select Committee on Aging. During the 1980s, further hearings were held, several bills were introduced in Congress, and

attention was called to the need for federal legislation to address the issue of elder abuse. Although federal legislation was not passed at that time, much public interest was stimulated, and state legislatures began to address the issue. By the mid-1990s, all states had passed some form of adult protective services or abuse-reporting laws. A major step was taken on the federal level in 1989 with the establishment of what is now called the National Center on Elder Abuse, which operates under the auspices of the National Association of State Units on Aging.

During the late 1980s, a decade after the first research on the subject, elder abuse emerged from the shadows of child and spousal abuse to receive public recognition as a major social problem on its own. Evidence of this can be seen in such newspaper and magazine headlines as "Old and Beaten" and "Woman Gets Four-Year Term for Torturing Her Father," as well as in discussion of the subject on popular television talk shows and news programs. Finally, elder abuse and neglect are topics of concern considered at every major aging-related conference and in public policy agendas. For example, federal government agencies have sponsored several national forums on elder abuse since 2000. Some of the most important involved the U.S. Departments of Justice and Health and Human Services, namely Our Aging Population: Promoting Empowerment, Preventing Victimization, and Implementing Coordinated Interventions and the National Policy Summit on Elder Abuse. These forums suggest increasing activity at the federal level regarding elder abuse, recognition that problem resolution requires both service and criminal justice approaches, and interest in interorganizational collaboration to make that happen. Both of these forums resulted in national action agendas with structures established to carry them forward.

Elder abuse has emerged as a major social problem and a significant aspect of family violence for several reasons. First, reports of elder abuse are increasing. This increase is attributable, at least in part, to the fact that the older people who are most likely to experience maltreatment and self-neglect, that is, women and people who are very old or frail and impaired, are the groups whose numbers are increasing at the fastest rate. In addition, adult children increasingly are called upon to care for their elderly parents. Some children, however, do not have the skills or resources to undertake this responsibility successfully. Abuse and neglect may be the unfortunate outcomes in such situations. Elder abuse also may be increasing because fewer adult children are available to share caregiving responsibilities as a result of population mobility and other factors. Therefore, the stress and burden of caregiving accelerates for those who are available. Finally, reports of elder abuse have increased because formal reporting systems are now in place and professionals and the public are more aware of abuse-reporting laws and adult protective services.

Second, because of the growing number of older people, increased attention is being directed toward all matters affecting this population, with special attention directed toward problems that affect the most vulnerable of the aged (e.g., abused elders). Problem recognition has been facilitated by the mushrooming of studies on elder abuse and the subsequent promulgation of experts to champion interest in the subject. A new generation of scholars, including Margaret Hudson and Mark Lachs, have joined pioneers like Suzanne Steinmetz and Karl Pillemer to keep attention focused on elder abuse through research and publications. In addition, congressional hearings and educational programs have stimulated public and professional interest in the issue. Finally, such organizations as the National Committee for the Prevention of Elder Abuse and the National Association of Adult Protective Services Administrators have promoted professional networking and perform key advocacy roles in directing public policy toward elder abuse.

Elder abuse was first formally brought to the attention of gerontological practitioners in 1975 through a letter to the editor of the *British Medical Journal,* referring to granny-battering (Burston, 1975). That same year, Robert Butler discussed the battered older person syndrome in his Pulitzer Prize-winning book *Why Survive? Being Old in America* (Butler, 1975). By the late 1970s, articles on the subject began appearing in the gerontological literature in both England and the United States. Research on elder abuse began in 1979 with a study at the Chronic Illness Center in Cleveland, Ohio. The study, which reviewed 404 cases handled by nurses, social workers, and other staff, revealed that nearly 10 % of the agency's elderly clients had suffered abuse or neglect during the previous year (Lau & Kosberg, 1979). This study also identified specific types of elder abuse, including physical and psychological abuse, misuse of property, and violation of rights.

Gerontological nurses have been in the forefront of research and publications on elder abuse. In the late 1970s, articles on the subject began appearing in nursing journals, such as *Nursing Research, Geriatric Nursing, Emergency Nursing, Journal of Gerontological Nursing,* and *Journal of Advanced Nursing.* In the mid-1980s, the first clinically oriented texts on elder abuse were coauthored by nurses (Fulmer & O'Malley, 1987; Quinn & Tomita, 1986). Since the mid-1990s, nursing has been represented in the field of elder

abuse through publications (e.g., Quinn, 1997) and the continuing research of Hudson (1994) aimed at defining elder abuse, Phillips (2000; Phillips, et al., 2000) on unraveling its dynamics, and Podnieks (1999) in understanding and treating elder abuse in Canada.

Elder Abuse Incidence and Causes

Elder abuse is neither a rare nor an isolated phenomenon in the United States and other industrialized countries. Rather, all indicators suggest that maltreatment of vulnerable older adults is widespread and occurs among all subgroups of the aged population. Although estimates of elder abuse range from 1 % to 6 %, it is widely agreed that it is difficult to be confident about the accuracy of these estimates because of significant underreporting of cases and differing definitions of elder abuse and neglect. Studies suggest that most maltreatment is repeated, is seldom reported to authorities, and represents more than one form of abuse. Moreover, although the problem can affect any older person, it is most likely to occur among those with certain characteristics. The typical abuse victim is a woman of advanced age who has few social contacts and lives alone or with the abuser. She usually has at least one physical or mental impairment that limits her activities of daily living (ADLs), and she usually depends on the abuser for care.

The National Elder Abuse Incidence Study is one of the most comprehensive examinations of elder abuse in the United States to date (National Center on Elder Abuse, 1998). It used a methodology that considered the number of new cases seen in 1996 by adult protective services staff and sentinels in community agencies having frequent contact with older adults in a representative sample of 20 counties in 15 states. Analysis of the results suggested that nationally, an estimated 551,011 older adults living in a domestic setting experienced elder abuse (including self-neglect) that year. Only one in five of those situations was reported to adult protective services. Two thirds involved a perpetrator, usually an adult child. Perpetrators were most likely to inflict (in descending order of occurrence): neglect, psychological abuse, exploitation, and physical abuse. The profile of the victim revealed a woman of advanced old age, unable or minimally able to care for herself, confused, and often depressed. Reporters of elder abuse situations were most commonly family members, hospital staff, and law enforcement personnel. Additional results from this national elder abuse incidence study are available at http://www.elderabusecenter.org.

Earlier studies identified different profiles of the typical abused elder by type of abuse. Victims of physical abuse, for example, are more likely to be younger and married, whereas victims of neglect are more likely to be older and single (Wolf et al., 1986). By comparison, victims of self-neglect are more likely to be older, living alone, and isolated from family, and to have dementia, mental illness, or substance abuse (Longres, 1995; O'Brien et al., 1999). There may be some association between type of abuse and the sex of the perpetrator, with men being more likely to exploit or physically abuse elders and women being more likely to physically neglect or psychologically abuse elders.

Research on the causes of elder abuse is still evolving, and much of what is known is derived from speculation or analogy with other abused populations. In the early 1980s, lengthy lists of likely explanations included causative factors such as ageism, retaliation, caregiver stress, caregiver unemployment, environmental conditions, increased life expectancy, resentment of dependence, lack of community resources, lack of financial resources, lack of close family ties, violence as a way of life, a history of personal and mental problems, and a history of alcohol and drug abuse. A summary of research on elder abuse dynamics suggests that, along with characteristics of victims and perpetrators, social context and cultural norms also must be considered in understanding elder abuse (Kosberg & Nahmiash, 1996). Financial difficulties, a legacy of violence, sharing a household, and intrafamily conflict may contribute to abuse occurrence. Likewise, cultural norms such as ageism, sexism, and stereotyping people with disabilities provide a climate that can foster elder abuse.

Recent studies of specific types of maltreatment indicate that elder abuse results from multiple, interrelated variables. Lachs and Pillemer (1995) summarized these variables according to characteristics associated with victims and those associated with perpetrators (Display 26-1). In summary, research on the causes of elder abuse is pointing in the following directions:

- Causation varies by form of abuse.
- The etiology of any form of abuse is a composite of several interrelated variables.
- The origins of elder abuse are found in both the victim and the perpetrator as well as in the relationship between the two.
- The etiology of elder abuse differs from that suggested for other abused populations in important ways (e.g., elder abuse is uniquely associated with ageism).

DISPLAY 26-1
Elder Abuse Profiles

Characteristics of the Perpetrator

- Substance abuse
- Psychiatric disorder
- History of violence
- Dependence on the victim
- Stress

Characteristics of the Victim

- Social isolation
- Chronic illness or functional limitation
- Cognitive impairment
- Shared living arrangement with the perpetrator

CULTURAL CONSIDERATIONS

Questions about cultural variations in elder abuse are under investigation, and several studies that address this issue are summarized in Culture Box 26-1. Collections of related research have been published in books and as special journal issues (Tatara, 1997a; 1999). Studies also have been showcased at the 1997 National Conference on Understanding and Combating Elder Abuse in Minority Populations. Moreover, major research initiatives are ongoing to identify differences in perceptions and attitudes toward elder abuse among older adults within racial and ethnic groups in the United States and, using translated survey instruments, among the elderly populations of other countries as well. Analysis of collected data is occurring at the University of California at Los Angeles.

Cultural variation extends beyond race and ethnicity, of course. Although research in this area is minimal, early explorations suggest differences among such other minority groups as older gays and lesbians. For instance, Cook-Daniels (1997) proposed that older gays and lesbians may be more vulnerable to elder abuse, especially self-neglect, because of social isolation stemming from living in a homophobic social environment. For many, this has resulted in a history of hiding, a value of independence, and a fear of encountering homophobia, particularly from senior service providers.

Strong family ties and respect for others that are inherent values in the Hispanic culture may minimize the incidence of elder abuse, but strong family ties and male/female roles may reduce the incidence of reporting it in the Hispanic community (Montoya, 1997).

- Korean-American elderly women were more likely to judge situations as abusive than either Caucasians or African Americans (Moon & Williams, 1993).
- A study of four ethnic groups in two urban areas found comparability among European Americans, African Americans, Puerto Ricans, and Japanese Americans in the importance placed on psychological abuse and neglect as forms of mistreatment (Anetzberger et al., 1996).
- Asian Indians consider ignoring and not visiting the worst things that family members can do to elderly members (Nagpaul, 1997).
- An investigation of two geographically distinct Plains Indian reservations revealed that elder abuse was more common in the reservation that had the higher unemployment and substance abuse rates and little potential income from the land (Krassen Maxwell & Maxwell, 1992).
- Financial abuse was the most prevalent form of mistreatment among African Americans in rural North Carolina (Griffin, 1994).
- Research that is currently being conducted under the auspices of the National Center on Elder Abuse indicates that Korean Americans hold the most divergent perspectives and attitudes about elder abuse among the six ethnic groups studied (Tatara, 1997b).
- In studies examining within-group differences among two Native American groups and five Caucasian American groups in North Carolina, differences were noted with regard to perceptions of the boundaries of elder abuse (Hudson et al., 1998; 2000).

RISK FACTORS THAT CONTRIBUTE TO ELDER ABUSE AND NEGLECT

Researchers are just beginning to identify specific risk factors for elder abuse. Perhaps the most accurate conclusion that can be drawn at this time is that several serious risk factors must be present for elder abuse to occur. Because these risk factors generally develop over a long period, it is not always possible to identify a specific point in time at which elder abuse begins. Moreover, risk factors often originate from several sources; they usually are present in the older adult, the caregiver or perpetrator, and the environment. Two characteristics, however, tend to be common to all elder abuse situations, regardless of the type of abuse: the invisibility of the problem and the vulnerability of the older person.

Invisibility

Elder abuse is unlike most problems affecting older adults in that one of its major risk factors is invisibility. The vast majority of elder abuse and neglect cases are not reported, even in states with good reporting and intervention models. Elder abuse has remained hidden for so long and continues to be as invisible as it is for several reasons. First, older people usually have less contact with the community than do other segments of the population, and their circumstances thus remain hidden for longer periods of time. By comparison, children are required to attend school and thus can be observed by teachers and counselors. Because retired older people are not required or expected to be anywhere, the potential exists for them to remain at home, unobserved, for some time.

The second reason for the invisibility of elder abuse involves the reticence of older people to admit to being abused or neglected. Self-reports are unusual. Sometimes this reflects the elder's desire to protect the abuser, who typically is a family member. Older people may also fear reprisal or believe that the alternatives, such as nursing home admission, may be worse than the present situation.

The last reason for the invisibility of elder abuse reflects society's negative feelings about aging. The myths and stereotypes associated with old age provide a negative image of the last stage of life. One consequence of this image has been a tendency to avoid older people and to ignore their circumstances. As a society, we maintain a strong denial of our own aging, but we hold an even stronger denial of the social problems associated with vulnerable old people. Another consequence of the negative image associated with old age has been the subjection of older adults to ridicule and even attack through such vehicles as messages on greeting cards and portrayals in the media.

Vulnerability

The one characteristic that abused or neglected older people have in common is their vulnerability. In sociologic terms, they might be described as needing protective services: they are functionally impaired to such a degree that they need formal support services. People who need protective services typically are unable to maintain minimal social standards of care; are unable to meet their own needs for food, shelter, or warmth; are unable to manage their own financial affairs; or represent a danger to themselves or others as a consequence of mental impairment. Moreover, people in need of protective services do not have relatives or others able and willing to provide adequate and appropriate assistance, and rarely seek services for themselves (Luppens & Lau, 1983; Byers & Lamanna, 1993; Anetzberger, in press). Examples of psychosocial impairments associated with vulnerability are depression, global cognitive impairment, and lifelong dependent or vulnerable personality.

Anetzberger (1990) has identified four sets of characteristics that can render individuals vulnerable to elder abuse: (1) personal characteristics, such as impairment and isolation; (2) situational characteristics, such as poverty and pathologic caregivers; (3) environmental factors, including deteriorated housing and crime-ridden neighborhoods; and (4) social factors, such as learned helplessness and growing up in a violent subculture. These characteristics tend to increase vulnerability to elder abuse, especially repeated or chronic maltreatment and self-neglect.

Psychosocial Factors

Common psychosocial factors that increase the vulnerability of older people include cognitive impairments, mental illness, and social and environmental influences. As indicated previously, many abused older adults become vulnerable as a result of impaired cognitive function. Impaired judgment, inability to make safe decisions, and loss of contact with reality are specific impairments that can lead to abuse and neglect. Cognitive impairment may be caused by an underlying dementia, delirium, or depression, or by a combination of pathologic processes. Therefore, anything that can cause cognitive impairments, such as dementia, physiologic disturbances, or adverse medication effects, must be considered a risk factor for impaired psychosocial function. When the older adult denies the cognitive impairment or refuses help or evaluation, the risk increases. Older people who live alone and are aware of their impairments may be afraid of acknowledging them because they fear that they have an untreatable problem that will require nursing home care. This fear may lead to social isolation, the overlooking of treatable or reversible causes of impairment, or a progressive but unnecessary decline in function.

Some attention has been focused on dementia as a risk factor for being physically abused. Pillemer and Suitor (1992), for example, identified predictors of both violent feelings and violence based on interviews with 236 family caregivers caring for people with dementia. Predictors of violent feelings included physical aggression and disruptive behaviors by the care recipient, along with a shared living situation. Predictors of violence included being a spouse and being very old. In a similar study of 184 patients with Alzheimer's disease and their primary caregivers, Paveza and colleagues (1992) found that important correlates to physical abuse included caregiver depression and a living arrangement in which the older person is residing with immediate family, without a spouse. A correlation also has been found

between self-neglect and dementia. For instance, Longres (1994) found that one third of self-neglecters in his statewide sample were impaired as a result of dementia. Similarly, half of all patients referred to a geriatric assessment center because of self-neglect suffered from dementia, compared with only 30 percent of patients referred for other reasons (Dyer et al., 2000).

Long-term mental illness predisposes an older adult to abuse or neglect, especially in combination with other factors, such as dementia or the loss of a significant social support. Families who describe an older adult as "always somewhat eccentric" may be masking their own denial of a long-term, progressive problem. Characteristics of depression that contribute to its role in self-neglect include social isolation, lack of interest in caring for oneself, and a negative outlook on life. Thus, any condition that is a risk factor for depression also must be considered a risk factor for elder abuse. Additional risk factors arise from social and environmental sources. The lack of a support system is one of the most common contributing factors to self-neglect, especially in old-old people who may have outlived most of the people who once provided support and tangible services. This is especially problematic for people who have been lifelong recluses or who have no children or extended family. More often than not, a combination of risk factors will be present in the older adult, the caregiver, and the environment.

Caregiver Factors

Caregiving itself is not the cause of elder abuse. Rather, it can provide a context for abuse occurrence when those assuming the caregiving role are incapable of doing so because of life stresses, pathologic characteristics, or lack of empathy for older people or people with disabilities. The volatility of caregiving can be heightened further when the caregiver sees the older adult's behaviors as being difficult or provocative (Anetzberger, 2000). Some psychosocial impairment usually can be identified in the caregiver who perpetrates abuse. Any of the psychosocial risk factors for abuse or neglect in older adults can also apply to their caregivers, particularly if the caregivers themselves are old. Caregivers who are physically abusive are more likely to have a psychopathologic condition than nonabusive caregivers. Psychosocial factors that can contribute to abusive and potentially abusive caregivers include a perception of social isolation, a recent decline in health, dependence and coresidence, an external locus of control, and poor interpersonal relations with the dependent elder (Anetzberger, 1987; Bendik, 1992; Wolf, 1997). It is not unusual to have a mutually neglectful or abusive situation when an older married couple has several of the psychosocial risk factors just identified and is, in addition, socially isolated. For example, a couple who both have dementia may unintentionally abuse each other and neglect themselves.

Figure 26-1 illustrates a screening tool that has been validated for use in identifying abuse indicators (Reis & Nahmiash, 1998).

> Mrs. B. is an 82-year-old divorced and widowed mother of four. She lives in a senior citizens' apartment located in the downtown area of a large city. The building is regularly serviced by subsidized transportation to grocery stores and shopping malls and has a nutrition center on the ground floor. Mrs. B.'s eldest son died in an accident 12 years ago. Her daughter lives 65 miles away, but visits once a week to do the grocery shopping and other errands. Two sons live within 4 miles of their mother's apartment. Mrs. B. lived in the home of one son and his wife until they argued 1 year ago. The other son lives alone in a small apartment and visits his mother two or three times weekly and frequently takes her to lunch or dinner. Mrs. B. has been hospitalized for major depression eight times since her eldest son's death. She also has been diagnosed as having hypertension, rheumatoid arthritis, and non–insulin-dependent diabetes.

Mrs. B. was referred to a home health agency for follow-up after her last hospital stay because her medication regimen, which she had followed for 6 years, had been changed while she was in the hospital. At the time of discharge, Mrs. B. was given a 30-day supply of medications set out in daily-dose medication containers for her. She was to take DiaBeta, 2.5 mg, once a day; Inderal, 40 mg, twice a day; Paxil, 20 mg, once a day; folic acid, 1 mg, once a day; and methotrexate, 2.5 mg, four tablets each Wednesday. Scheduled medication times were 8:00 AM and 8:00 PM. The home health nurse was to instruct Mrs. B. in her medication regimen, including what medications she was to take, how she was to take them, what each medication was expected to do, and possible side effects. The nurse was also to assess Mrs. B.'s ability to follow instructions and her adherence to the medication regimen.

Because Mrs. B.'s vision was impaired from diabetes, she had difficulty managing her complex medication regimen. The visiting nurse arranged for unit-dose packaging for Mrs. B.'s prescriptions and visited twice a day for 2 days to observe Mrs. B.'s ability to take her medications accurately. On the third morning, the nurse telephoned Mrs. B. at 8:15 AM and asked if Mrs. B. had any problems taking her pills. Mrs. B. happily reported that she had taken all the pills, including the four methotrexate, without any difficulty. The nurse then scheduled Mrs. B. to be

seen 3 times a week for ongoing assessment for several weeks.

THINKING POINTS

> What are the factors that contribute to the risk of Mrs. B. becoming abused or neglected?
> What are the factors that protect Mrs. B. from becoming abused or neglected?
> As the visiting nurse, what concerns would you have about Mrs. B. when you discharge her from home care, and how would you address these concerns?

FUNCTIONAL CONSEQUENCES ASSOCIATED WITH ELDER ABUSE AND NEGLECT

The existence of one or more of the risk factors predisposes an older person to become the knowing or unknowing victim of elder abuse. Elder abuse may be illustrated by the following cases, which have come to the attention of health and social service professionals in both rural and urban communities:

1. A middle-aged alcoholic man hit his aged father during an argument. In turn, both were beaten by their sons/grandsons, who wanted money for drugs.
2. An elderly woman never left home because she feared her memory lapses would prevent her from finding the way back. When she did venture out, she fell on the porch, and the local office on aging was called. Outreach workers found she had no food in the house and was malnourished.
3. An unemployed couple kept their impaired grandparents confined to the house, refusing them visitors, abandoning them for days without adequate food, and denying them help for fear of losing access to their Social Security checks.
4. A son visited his mother in a nursing home and sexually assaulted her when staff members were not present.
5. A depressed elderly woman refused to take a needed medication with the result that her legs became so swollen that she could not leave her chair.
6. A woman in her 80s—who was weak, incontinent, and had hypertension—was abandoned in an emergency room with a note reading "Totally dependent! Handle with care."

CAREGIVER AND CARE RECEIVER
INDICATORS OF ABUSE (IOA)
FOR DISCRIMINATING ABUSE AND NON-ABUSE CASES

Items which indicate abuse are listed below. After a 2 - to 3 - hour home assessment (or other intensive contact with the caregiver and/or care-receiver) please rate each of the following items on a scale of 0 to 4, as described below. Do not omit any items. Rate according to your *current opinion*.
Scale: Estimated extent of Problem.

0 = non-existent

1 = slight

2 = moderate

3 = probably/severe

4 = yes/severe

00 = non-applicable

000 = don't know

_____ 1.   CAREGIVER: Has behaviour problems

_____ 2.   CAREGIVER: Is financially dependent

_____ 3.   CAREGIVER: Has mental/emotional difficulties

_____ 4.   Care-Receiver: Been abused in past

_____ 5.   Care-Receiver: Has marital/family conflict

_____ 6.   CAREGIVER: Has alcohol/medication problem

_____ 7.   CAREGIVER: Has unrealistic expectations

_____ 8.   Care-Receiver: Lacks understanding of medical condition

_____ 9.   CAREGIVER: Lacks understanding of medical condition

_____10.   CAREGIVER: Caregiving reluctancy

_____11.   Care-Receiver: Is socially isolated

_____12.   CAREGIVER: Has marital/family conflict

_____13.   CAREGIVER: Has poor current relationship

_____14.   CAREGIVER: Caregiving inexperience

_____15.   Care-Receiver: Lacks social support

_____16.   Care-Receiver: Has behaviour problems

_____17.   CAREGIVER: Is a blamer

_____18.   Care-Receiver: Is financially dependent

_____19.   Care-Receiver: Has unrealistic expectations

_____20.   Care-Receiver: Has alcohol/medication problem

_____21.   Care-Receiver: Has poor current relationship

_____22.   Care-Receiver: Has suspicious falls/injuries

_____23.   Care-Receiver: Has mental/emotional difficulties

_____24.   CAREGIVER: Had poor past relationship

_____25.   Care-Receiver: Is a blamer

_____26.   CAREGIVER and Care-Receiver kinship

(score if caregiver is not spouse)

_____27.   Care-Receiver: Is emotionally dependent

_____28.   Care-Receiver: No regular doctor

_____29.   CAREGIVER: Age (if caregiver is younger than 58 years)

FIGURE 26-1 A screening tool that has been validated for use in identifying abuse indicators. (From Reis, M., & Nahmiash, D. [1998]. Validation of the indicators of abuse [IOA] screen. *Gerontologist*, 38, 471–480. Copyright © The Gerontological Society of America. Used by permission of the publisher.)

These situations reflect the variety of forms of elder abuse. Most researchers and practitioners agree on the following forms of elder abuse: (1) physical abuse, including hitting and shoving; (2) psychological abuse, including threats and name calling; (3) physical neglect, including denying adequate food or medication; (4) psychological neglect, including failure to provide proper supervision or social interaction; (5) exploitation, including forcing the elder to change a will or a deed; and (6) violation of rights, including denying privacy or visitors. In addition, state laws include sexual abuse, abandonment, and unreasonable confinement as types of elder abuse and neglect (Roby & Sullivan, 2000). Recent attention also is on undue influence (i.e., the substitution of one person's will for the true desires of another) as a form of elder abuse (Quinn, 2002).

Although rape and other sexual violence perpetrated against older people received some attention during the late 1970s, the focus at that time was on sexual assault by strangers. During the 1990s, sexual assault by family members and paid caregivers became a widely recognized aspect of elder abuse. For example, older women are sexually abused by husbands, sons, or male nursing assistants. Reports of sexual assault against older people are not common, but the resulting physical and emotional consequences can be severe and long lasting. Research on reported sexual abuse found the typical victim to be an older woman residing in a nursing facility. Her abuser tends to be a man who is either a facility staff member or another resident. Most cases are never prosecuted because of insufficient evidence or because victims are unable to participate in the prosecution (Teaster et al., 2000).

Abandonment occurs when dependent older people are deserted by the people who are responsible for their care. Although most states do not specifically address this form of elder abuse in protective services or abuse reporting laws, abandonment of older people at hospital emergency rooms is a form of abuse that is increasing. This increase is attributable, at least in part, to the increasing numbers of dependent older adults and to public policies that encourage care of dependent people at home by family or other informal providers, some of whom feel ill equipped to assume this role physically, emotionally, or financially.

Self-neglect and self-harm are forms of elder abuse that differ from other types in that they have no perpetrator other than the older person himself or herself. In cases of self-neglect, the older person fails to meet essential needs, usually because of such factors as serious functional impairments or the desire to die. In cases of self-abuse, the older person causes injury or pain to herself or himself, including body mutilations.

Although until recently the elder abuse literature usually did not address situations that were mutually abusive or neglectful, nurses working in home settings have long encountered situations in which two people, often a married couple, abuse each other or are both neglected. These situations may be rooted in a long-term, mutually abusive relationship but usually evolve because of gradual declines in the functional abilities of both people. They also may be associated with the poor coping skills of a spouse or caregiver who is faced with increasing demands and little or no outside help. These situations are now being recognized as aspects of domestic violence.

Since the late 1980s, domestic violence against older adults has been recognized as another aspect of elder abuse. In the early 1990s, the American Association of Retired Persons (AARP) brought together elder abuse and domestic violence experts for a forum entitled "Abused Elders or Older Battered Women?" During the 1990s, the federal government and organizations such as the AARP and the Older Women's League developed programs and resource guides to address domestic violence among older adults. Although attempts have been made to address this aspect of elder abuse through research, public testimony, professional conferences, and intervention programs, very few viable programs address domestic violence and elders. Those that do tend to focus on screening tools and protocols for abuse identification and referral, safety planning procedures, emergency shelter arrangements, and support groups for older victims (Anetzberger, 2001; Brandl & Raymond, 1997; Nerenberg, 1996; Wolf, 2001).

➤ When Mr. P.'s wife died, this frail man sought care in the home of a neighbor who offered both board and care in exchange for his monthly Social Security check. In reality, the neighbor provided neither, but locked Mr. P. in the basement and gave him little food. If he complained about the treatment or refused to sign over his income or property, the caregiver hit or kicked him. After 4 years, the situation was discovered and reported to the county protective services agency. Mr. P. later sat in the social worker's office and sadly commented, "So this is what it's like to be a protective case."

 THINKING POINTS

➤ What type(s) of abuse does this case represent?
➤ What are some of the psychosocial consequences that Mr. P. is likely to have experienced in the past 4 years?
➤ What are some factors that contribute to this situation going on for 4 years?

NURSING ASSESSMENT OF ABUSED OR NEGLECTED OLDER ADULTS

Elder abuse is not so much assessed as it is detected, so that gerontological nurses often must assume the role of detective. Because elder abuse by its very nature is a hidden problem, assessment begins with a suspicion about its existence. Information may be purposefully withheld, and it is rarely volunteered, except in situations in which the older person or caregiver is desperate for help. Clues to elder abuse might first be noted when an older person is seen in an emergency room or admitted to a hospital. Most often, a home visit is an essential component of the assessment process, and gaining admission to the home usually is the first assessment challenge. Many times, the situation deteriorates so gradually that it is hard to determine the onset of abuse. In borderline situations, people who suspect that elder abuse is occurring often choose to ignore the clues in hopes that the situation will resolve itself without intervention.

Unique Aspects of Elder Abuse Assessment

Assessment of elder abuse differs from usual nursing assessment in several respects. First, one of the purposes of assessment of elder abuse is to determine whether legal interventions are appropriate or necessary, in contrast to usual health care situations in which the purpose of assessment is to plan interventions for addressing health and medical needs. In situations in which abuse is suspected, the primary concern usually is a determination of the safety of the older person. This approach is similar to emergency room nursing, in which basic life-preserving needs are addressed immediately and other needs are considered later.

Second, health care workers dealing with elder abuse often are quite limited in their goals. They sometimes have to accept basic safety as the only goal, especially when the elder and caregiver insist on choices that are not in accordance with what the health care workers would recommend. An assessment of safe function is crucial, therefore, because legal interventions can be made only in high-risk situations. Because the determination of safety often is based on medical and nursing information, the role of the nurse is especially important. In home settings in particular, the nurse may be the only health care professional who directly assesses the situation, and the nursing assessment may be the major determinant of recommendations for legal intervention.

Third, cases of elder abuse usually involve some element of resistance from the older person or caregiver. Only in rare situations do abused elders or their caregivers seek out the assistance of health care professionals. Although it might be impossible to establish a trusting relationship, the nurse must try, at the very least, to establish an accepting relationship. The initial assessment, therefore, is aimed at identifying ways of gaining access and at least passive acceptance.

Fourth, in contrast to most health care situations, the nurse may be viewed as a threat rather than a help. Nurses are not accustomed to being viewed as the "bad guy" and often must identify a way to minimize the perceived threat, even before the initial contact. This can be accomplished by identifying someone who both acknowledges that a problem exists and is willing to facilitate the introduction of a nurse. Any of the following might be helpful in gaining access and acceptance: neighbors; relatives (especially family members who do not live in the problematic home setting); staff from senior centers, offices on aging, or health care or community agencies; physicians or any other health professionals; or church-based people (e.g., clergy).

Fifth, when legal interventions are being considered, the legal rights of the person and the caregivers must be addressed. Nurses and other workers involved in elder abuse cases usually are uncomfortable making decisions that involve the rights of other adults. When legal and ethical issues are addressed in institutional settings, the decisions are guided by medical information and institutional policies, and the role of the physician usually is the most important. In home settings, however, there are few clear guidelines and little or no physician input.

Physical Health

The nursing assessment of physical abuse and neglect focuses on the following: nutrition, hydration, bruises and injuries, degree of frailty, and presence of pathologic conditions. Nutrition and hydration are important not only in determining the existence of physical neglect but also in determining the seriousness and urgency of the situation. In community settings, a determination of nutrition and hydration status is sometimes the crucial factor as to whether emergency or involuntary measures must be taken, or whether time can be allowed for working with the person in the home setting. The guidelines discussed in Chapter 14, particularly in Table 14-1 (Causes and Consequences of Nutrient Deficiencies), can be applied to the detection of malnutrition and dehydration.

Skin turgor over the extremities is not necessarily a reliable indicator of hydration, especially for very old people or for people who have lost weight. Examination of the mucous membranes and an assessment of skin turgor over the sternum or abdomen provide more accurate clues to dehydration. The absence of thirst sensation does not necessarily mean that the person is adequately hydrated because older people may have a diminished thirst response. On the other hand, the presence of thirst sensation is a definite indicator of dehydration, a physiologic disturbance, or an adverse medication effect. If a urine sample can be obtained, a measurement of specific gravity will provide information about hydration. When a urinometer is not available, a visual examination of urine concentration will provide some clues to hydration.

When any indicators of malnutrition or dehydration are identified, the next step is to determine whether the hydration or nutritional status can be improved adequately without removing the person from the setting. The role of the nurse can be especially important in assessing not only the nutrition and hydration status but also the measures required to alleviate these risks immediately. Sometimes, the provision of water and food is the most important intervention in neglect situations. In addition, this intervention is inexpensive and readily available and can be quite effective in establishing a relationship with a hungry or thirsty person!

Assessment of indicators of physical harm is an important aspect of the detection of physical abuse or neglect. Nurses are likely to see any of the following indicators: leg ulcers; pressure ulcers; dependent edema; poor wound healing; burns from stoves, cigarettes, or hot water; and bruises, swelling, or injuries from falls, especially repeated falls. The presence of more than one of these indicators at the same time, or over a short period of time, should raise high levels of suspicion about physical neglect. The possibility of drug or alcohol abuse also should be considered when any of these indicators is identified, especially if the person is also depressed or socially isolated. To detect physical abuse, the nurse looks for any indication of injury caused by people who live with or visit a vulnerable older adult. Examples are marks from cuts, bites, burns, or punctures; bruises or injuries, especially of the face, head, or trunk; bruises on both upper arms, as would result from being grabbed or shaken harshly; or bruises that reflect the shape of objects, like belts or hairbrushes. If evidence of injuries from falls is present, the nurse must consider the possibility that the person was shoved or otherwise caused to fall by someone else.

Physical abuse may also be caused indirectly, as by a caregiver who gives the person excessive amounts of alcohol or drugs, especially psychoactive medications. Sometimes caregivers who abuse drugs or alcohol will give these substances to the people for whom they care, especially if the dependent person is not able or willing to refuse. Caregivers also may administer excessive amounts of psychoactive medications to keep a dependent person quiet and less troublesome. Using psychoactive medications only for the caregiver's benefit and to the detriment of the person receiving the medication constitutes physical or psychological abuse. Any of the following clues to substance abuse may be observed: ataxia, somnolence, clouded mentation, slurred speech, staggering gait, or extrapyramidal manifestations. If there is evidence that the caregiver of a passive and dependent older person is a substance abuser, the nurse should be particularly suspicious about the possibility that the caregiver is giving drugs or alcohol to the older person.

Other aspects of physical neglect include withholding therapeutic medications or interfering with the person's medical care. Caregivers may decide not to purchase prescriptions or provide nursing care, medical equipment, or comfort items because they do not want to spend the necessary money. A caregiver's decision not to purchase these things without the willing consent of the older adult may represent physical abuse. For example, a caregiver may be unwilling to spend money for nursing assistance, even though this care is necessary for the dependent older adult. If the older adult has not freely chosen to forego this available help, then this may be considered physical neglect. If the caregiver is likely to inherit the money that is being saved by the lack of paid help, this may represent financial exploitation as well.

Because physical neglect can arise from the caregiver's lack of knowledge, it is essential to assess the caregiver's understanding of the dependent person's needs. For example, caregivers may have good intentions when they use adult briefs for the control of incontinence, but they may not understand the potential for skin breakdown. Caregivers may administer excessive amounts of psychoactive medications because they do not understand the correct dosing schedule. This is especially common when medications are ordered on an as-needed basis and the caregiver has not been given clear guidelines for determining when the medication is needed, or what the most effective dosage is. In these situations, nursing assessment of the caregiver's knowledge is especially important because educational interventions or the provision of additional services may alleviate the abuse.

Assessment of the degree of frailty of the older adult is another consideration in determining actual or potential physical abuse or neglect. For example, an older adult who is slightly obese and fully ambulatory would not have the same degree of risk for fall-related injuries as one who weighs only 78 pounds and ambulates unsteadily with a walker. Similarly, if the 75-year-old wife of an alcoholic man can easily escape to safety when he becomes violent, and she chooses to remain in the situation, she would not necessarily be considered a protective case; however, if the woman is cognitively impaired, physically frail, or unable to move quickly and is the target of his violence when he is inebriated, the situation could be defined as elder abuse.

In the presence of certain medical conditions, someone may be determined to be neglected if necessary treatments are not or cannot be provided. For example, it is essential to determine whether daily insulin injections can be provided for a person who is an insulin-dependent diabetic. In determining whether an older adult can function safely in community settings, the nurse must consider the person's ability to follow medical regimens and the consequences of noncompliance. If a medication regimen is necessary for the control of medical conditions, such as congestive heart failure, the nurse and primary care provider must assess the person's ability to comply and the consequences of noncompliance. Assessment also addresses the question of whether the medical regimen could be modified so that compliance would be facilitated while still allowing the person to remain in an independent setting. In planning care for people in home settings, an ideal regimen may have to be modified to gain an increase in the level of compliance. For example, an older person who is hospitalized might be maintained on a complex medication regimen that requires some medications to be administered before meals and others after meals, and some to be administered 4 times a day and others 3 times a day. Although this might be the ideal way to ensure optimal medication effectiveness and minimal adverse reactions while the person is hospitalized, such a regimen may be so complicated for the older person or the caregivers to carry out in a home setting that it might not be followed at all. In such situations, a thorough nursing assessment of the total medication regimen can lead to interventions (e.g., simplification of medication regimen and patient education about the medications) that alleviate the neglect.

Activities of Daily Living

One of the purposes of assessment in elder abuse situations is to determine the necessity of legal interventions when an older adult is at risk. Therefore, a nursing assessment of the person's potential for safe performance of ADLs is extremely important. For community-living older adults, an assessment of the home environment and the person's level of function in that environment is best conducted by health care workers who can directly observe the person at home. The assessment is based not only on direct observations but also on information provided by caregivers who observe the person's daily function. Home health aides can be a valuable source of information, and they usually have a greater degree of objectivity than family members. In some circumstances, it may be appropriate to involve occupational or physical therapists in the home assessment. When a difference of opinion exists, or when the nurse is unable to make a clear determination of the safety of the situation, a team conference may be helpful in reaching some agreement. Team conferences ideally include all of the people who function in assessment or caregiving capacities and who have some degree of objectivity. In cases of suspected elder abuse, the assessment team may include many informal sources of help, such as family and neighbors, as well as formal sources of help, such as nurses and social workers.

Personal dress, hygiene, and grooming are among the most visible aspects of daily function. Even in social settings, these aspects of daily function are appraised by others. People often are viewed as neglected when they do not comply with socially defined standards of cleanliness, particularly when an unpleasant odor is noted. Although poor hygiene and grooming are important reflections of many underlying problems, these aspects of ADLs do not necessarily reflect the person's safe function. When families and health care or social service workers first work with a neglected older person who is obviously in need of much personal care, they often are tempted to begin by assisting the person with bathing and grooming. Although the workers may view this as the most socially acceptable way to begin, the older person may view this approach as very threatening.

Once the nurse has assessed whether the poor hygiene is hazardous to the person's health, the nurse should assess the consequences of imposing assistance with personal care on someone who may be unwilling to accept help or to acknowledge a hygiene problem. The nurse may determine that immediate efforts to deal with personal hygiene would be detrimental to the immediate goal of establishing a relationship and the long-term goal of assisting with other aspects of daily function. When this is the case, the nurse may have to reinforce the principle that "people don't die of dirt" with caregivers and other workers. Without ignoring the need for assistance

Functional Limitation	Risks to Safety
Any mental or physical impairment in combination with social isolation and lack of a support system	Nutrition and hydration
Mobility limitations or seriously impaired vision, especially in combination with poor judgment	Falls
Cognitive impairments in ambulatory people	Wandering, getting lost
Bed-bound status or seriously impaired ambulation	Pressure sores
Cognitive impairment, especially poor judgment	Inability to get help
Poor judgment, especially when living in an unsafe neighborhood	Basic safety and security

TABLE 26-1 • Risks to Safety Associated With Functional Limitations

incompetent or incapacitated. The crucial element of assessing risk for elder abuse, therefore, is a determination of risk (i.e., danger to the person) rather than a determination of whether the decision would be judged by others as good or appropriate. When the competence of an older adult to make safe decisions regarding self-care is in doubt, nurses may be legally bound to make reports or consider other legal interventions. There are no federal guidelines for determining the mental capacity of abused or neglected older adults, and the legal criteria differ from state to state. The ethical and legal considerations involved in various legal interventions are discussed briefly in this chapter and more extensively in Chapter 6.

Support Resources

Support resources include those people, such as caregivers and friends, who influence a person's physical and psychosocial function. Some or all of the support people may directly cause the abusive situation or may actively or passively contribute to it. Therefore, the support resources used by the dependent adult are assessed in terms of both helpful and detrimental effects. In addition, support resources not currently being used are identified as potential sources of help.

When the support resources currently being used are the caregivers who perpetrate the abuse, the nurse must assess the potential for working with the caregivers to alleviate the negative consequences. Although it is not always easy to work with abusive caregivers, it may be even more difficult to eliminate their influence over an older adult. During the assessment, therefore, the nurse must attempt to identify any strengths of the caregiver and any willingness to change the situation voluntarily. If the caregiver has good intentions but lacks the knowledge to provide adequate care, then educational interventions and role modeling may be effective. If the caregiver is extremely stressed, then respite, along with individual or group support and counseling, may be an effective intervention. In mutually abusive situations in which the designated caregiver also could be defined as abused or neglected, the nurse should attempt to identify any outside sources of support that have not been tapped. For example, in a mutually abusive situation involving a socially isolated married couple, the nurse might identify a relative or friend who is willing to assist with caregiving or decision-making responsibilities.

In situations of neglect, there usually are very few support services to assess, and the task of the nurse is to identify potential sources of help. In assessing potential support resources, the nurse also must identify the barriers that interfere with the use of these

with personal care, the nurse may need to emphasize the importance of addressing issues of nutrition, hydration, and safety first, and avoiding less important issues that could interfere with the acceptance of services.

Adequate nutrition, hydration, and an ability to obtain help in an emergency are the basic human needs that are most often called into question in cases of elder abuse. Other basic needs may also be compromised, usually in relation to specific functional impairments and environmental circumstances. For instance, for people who are bed-bound or who have very limited function, bowel and bladder elimination may be a basic need. For people with mobility limitations or serious vision impairments, safe ambulation and the ability to avoid falls are important considerations. Table 26-1 summarizes some of the specific functional and environmental conditions that present risks to basic needs.

Psychosocial Function

Assessment of psychosocial function is discussed at length in Chapter 10. In cases of elder abuse, the most important aspect of psychosocial function is assessment of the person's capacity for reasonable judgments about self-care. This is difficult because the determination of someone's ability to make appropriate judgments is based, at least in part, on subjective criteria and opinions. When judgment is impaired to the point that the person is at serious risk and does not acknowledge the risk, the person usually is considered resources. The assessment of barriers to the use of resources is discussed in Chapter 10 and is summarized in Display 10-8. It is especially important to identify these barriers because simple interventions, such as provision of information or assistance with transportation, may be effective in eliminating them. Cultural influences also must be assessed in relation to the use of support resources, as discussed in Chapter 9.

Environmental Influences

As with other aspects of elder abuse, the primary purposes of assessing the environment are to identify the factors that create risks and to determine which of these factors can be alleviated through interventions. With regard to the immediate living conditions, the nurse must assess whether minimal standards of safety and cleanliness are being maintained. When nurses assess home environments that are terribly cluttered, they must make some determination of both the meaning and the consequences of the clutter. A massive collection of clutter, like poor personal hygiene, reflects an underlying disorder and may or may not be a risk factor that needs to be addressed. Consequences of clutter range from socially unacceptable appearances to serious risks to health and safety. Therefore, the nurse must assess the person's ability to maneuver in the environment during daily activities as well as the person's safety in emergency situations, such as a fire. When nurses and other workers are initially exposed to massive amounts of clutter, their first impulse may be to think of a way to eliminate some of it. If this reaction is communicated to the resident of the cluttered home, however, it may become impossible to establish an accepting relationship, and the older adult may reject any further interventions. In assessing the home environment, therefore, nurses must be nonjudgmental, except in circumstances in which the risks are so great that immediate action must be taken.

The nurse also should assess the neighborhood environment for its impact on the safety of the person. This is especially important when the older person lives in an area of high crime or extreme isolation and is vulnerable by virtue of impaired judgment, physical frailty, or a combination of physical and psychosocial impairments. People who are only moderately forgetful may be safe in an apartment or a suburban neighborhood where neighbors watch out for them. In a high-crime neighborhood, however, forgetting to lock the doors or to take other precautions may place the person at increased risk for physical harm, financial exploitation, or other serious abuses. Likewise, in a rural environment, social isolation may increase the risks for vulnerable elderly people.

Finally, seasonal conditions can be a determinant of risk for elder abuse for those who live in climates characterized by extreme heat or cold. For example, a person who does not pay utility bills may not be in any danger as long as the weather is mild, but when the temperature turns cold, that person would be at risk for hypothermia. The same is true for people who occasionally wander outside without dressing appropriately. As long as the neighborhood is safe and the weather mild, they may be relatively safe; however, they may be at increased risk during the cold months, especially if they do not wear proper foot covering. If the person has any of the risk factors for hypothermia or heat-related illness discussed in Chapter 21, these additional risk factors also must be considered.

Threats to Life

The most immediate consideration in determining whether legal interventions are necessary is the assessment of threats to life. In home settings, it is often the nurse who assesses the urgency of the situation and whose opinion is used as the basis of legal interventions. Situations often are viewed as being of crisis proportions when they are first discovered, and the immediate reaction of the person who discovers the situation may be to remove a person from the environment. Many times, however, the person may not want to leave the home setting, or there may be no better setting in which the person can receive care immediately. In these situations, the nurse may be asked to assess the urgency and seriousness of the situation and to provide an opinion about whether or not legal interventions are justified. The nurse often is viewed as the person who can either convince the elder to accept help or convince the caregivers and social workers that the present situation is tolerable. Nurses are sometimes successful at convincing a person to accept help, especially if they assure the person that, with proper help, the situation can be improved.

In situations in which the caregiver is the abuser, the nurse and other team members must assess whether the caregiver presents a threat to the life of the dependent older person. If there is any evidence or history of physical violence on the part of the caregiver, and if the dependent elder does not have the ability to escape or otherwise defend himself or herself, a threat to life may exist. Threats to life also may exist if any of the following circumstances are present: (1) untreated wounds or infections; (2) inability to administer insulin correctly; (3) progressive gangrene or ulcerated conditions; (4) inability to adhere to therapeutic regimens; (5) consistent wandering in unsafe neighborhoods or in very cold weather; (6) misuse (usually unintentional) of certain medications, such as digitalis or insulin; or (7) excessive use of drugs or alcohol, either self-induced or caregiver-induced. In any of these circumstances, the nurse may be the health professional whose opinion is essential in determining the consequences of action or inaction.

When the nurse does not have firsthand knowledge of the abused or neglected older person before being notified of a crisis situation, the first question that should be asked, if only in the nurse's mind, is whether this is truly a crisis, or is merely a crisis in the eyes of the person who just discovered the situation. Situations that appear to be the most appalling may actually represent a gradual deterioration over several months or years. Therefore, the immediate assessment is aimed at determining whether there are currently any threats to the life of the abused elder, such as malnutrition, dehydration, or an untreated medical condition. Finally, suicide potential must be assessed, especially in self-neglected elders who also are depressed and expressing feelings of hopelessness. All of the principles of suicide assessment, discussed in Chapter 25, can be applied to the abused and neglected elder.

Cultural Aspects

Definitions and perceptions of elder abuse and neglect are influenced to a great extent by cultural norms. For example, Asian Indians may consider not visiting an older family member to be a form of psychological neglect, but Anglo-Americans may consider it a way of respecting privacy and autonomy. Cultural factors also have a strong influence on caregiver roles and responsibilities. Most families have culturally influenced expectations about which family members should provide care to dependent elders and about whether it is acceptable to enlist the aid of paid caregivers. In some families, there may be conflicts about these expectations, particularly between older and younger generations. Sometimes these conflicts may need to be identified and addressed before elder abuse or neglect can be resolved.

Nurses must identify cultural factors that influence the care that is provided—or not provided—to older adults. Culture Box 26-2 lists some of the assessment questions that should be considered in identifying cultural influences. In addition, cultural assessment information on the following topics also should be considered: communication and psychosocial assessment (see Chapters 9 and 10), nutrition (see Chapter 14), sources of health care and modes of treatment (see Chapter 5), dementia (see Chapter 24), and depression (see Chapter 25). Brownell (1997)

CULTURE BOX 26-2

Cultural Considerations in Assessing Elder Abuse and Neglect

- What are the family and cultural expectations concerning family caregivers? (For example, is it acceptable to employ paid caregivers, or are family members expected to provide all the care?)
- Do family members differ in their perceptions about caregiving responsibilities?
- What are the family and cultural perspectives on autonomy and independence?
- Do family members differ in their perspectives on autonomy and independence?
- How are decisions made about care of the older adult? (For example, is it a patriarchal or matriarchal family?)
- Who are the acceptable sources of social support and personal assistance?
- Who are the acceptable sources of health care (e.g., herbalists, spiritual healers, Native American practitioners)?
- What are the acceptable health care practices (e.g., herbs, homeopathy, acupuncture, faith healing, folk remedies)?
- Are there language barriers that influence the care that is provided or that limit the number of care providers?
- How does skin color affect assessment of bruises, pressure sores, and other skin changes?

---

describes the use of a Culturagram as a screening tool to promote culturally sensitive assessment and detection of family abuse among immigrant elders.

▶ Mrs. K. is 80 years old and had resided in a nursing facility for 1 year until she recently was discharged at her request but "against medical advice" with no prescriptions for her medications or medical referral for home care. She has complex health conditions, including osteoarthritis, coronary artery disease, congestive heart failure, chronic obstructive pulmonary disease (COPD), depression, and insulin-dependent diabetes. Although alert and oriented, Mrs. K. has major deficits in her ability to perform daily living tasks. She also depends on a walker for ambulation and has a history of falling, including a fall that resulted in a hip fracture and her admission to a nursing facility.

Mrs. K.'s support system is limited. Her son lives in another state but functions as power-of-attorney and provides some telephone reassurance. Her daughter is estranged from Mrs. K. and at their last meeting was verbally abusive to her. Mrs. K.'s older brother visits a few times weekly to help with meal preparation, grocery shopping, transportation, and medication pickups. More extensive assistance is impossible owing to his own health problems.

Shortly after returning home, Mrs. K.'s precarious health status rapidly deteriorated. She became severely short of breath, requiring continuous oxygen. She began to hallucinate in the evening, believing that she alone had the responsibility of feeding all of the children in the neighborhood. As her fears increased, so too did the calls to her brother. Eventually she made several calls every night, overwhelming and exhausting him.

 THINKING POINTS

➤ What form(s) of elder abuse is (are) represented?

➤ What are signs or indicators of abuse that you as a nurse would be able to identify?

➤ What factors contribute to Mrs. K.'s current risks?

➤ How will you proceed in conducting a nursing assessment of Mrs. K.?

➤ What barriers might you encounter in conducting the assessment? How will you overcome them?

NURSING DIAGNOSIS

Because elder abuse and neglect are so broad and complex, various nursing diagnoses are applicable, depending on the situation. A nursing diagnosis that would apply to many elder abuse situations in which family members are caregivers is Disabled Family Coping. This is defined as "the state in which a family demonstrates, or is at risk to demonstrate, destructive behavior in response to an inability to manage internal or external stressors due to inadequate resources (physical, psychological, cognitive)" (Carpenito, 2002, p. 280). Related factors include changes in family roles, unrealistic expectations about caregiving, and changes in the health status of the older adult. If the nursing assessment identifies several stressors primarily related to family caregiving, the nursing diagnosis of Caregiver Role Strain might be used. This is defined as "a state in which an individual is experiencing physical, emotional, social, and/or financial burden(s) in the process of caregiving to another" (Carpenito, 2002, p. 161). Related factors involving the caregiver include ineffective coping patterns, functional or cognitive impairments, and insufficient resources (e.g., respite, financial assets, assistance with care). Related factors involving the dependent older adult include increased dependence and the presence of difficult or unsafe behaviors (e.g., paranoia, wandering, incontinence).

The nursing diagnosis of Risk for Injury might be used for older adults who are in self-neglecting situations, especially if the person lives alone and is physically and psychosocially impaired. The nursing diagnosis of Decisional Conflict might apply to abused or neglected older adults who live in an environment

that places them at risk for harm because they are unable to make decisions about alternative environments. Related factors include fear, lack of information about alternatives, and impaired decision-making ability.

OUTCOMES

Care for older adults with the nursing diagnosis of Disabled Family Coping is directed toward identifying and addressing the contributing factors, such as multiple stressors associated with elder care. Outcome criteria are established according to the contributing factors. For example, if a change in the health status of the dependent older adult is a contributing factor, the outcome would be that the older adult functions at the highest possible level. Another outcome would be that resources for assisting with the care of the dependent person would be identified and used. If family caregivers are experiencing multiple stressors, a goal would be to alleviate some of the caregiving burden. This would be accomplished by identifying appropriate resources and facilitating referrals for care. A related outcome in many situations would be that barriers to accepting services are addressed and eliminated. This might be accomplished through counseling and case management services provided by a nurse or social worker.

If abused or neglected elders are at risk for harm and they or their caregivers resist voluntary interventions, then the "highest nursing-sensitive patient outcome priority is to ensure the safety of the mistreated elder while respecting the patient's autonomy" (Cowen, 2001, p. 106). Interventions often include legal interventions, such as reporting the situation to the appropriate public agency. Nurses may feel torn ethically between the right of the person to refuse treatment and the obligation to report abuse and neglect situations, as discussed later in this chapter. Usually, outcomes for these situations are achieved through coordinated efforts with adult protective services providers and concerned and cooperative family caregivers.

 ## NURSING INTERVENTIONS TO ADDRESS ELDER ABUSE

Elder abuse is a compilation of several or many nursing and social problems involving the older person, the caregivers, and the environment. Nurses identify the various underlying problems, then plan and implement appropriate interventions for each problem. A unique aspect of elder abuse, however, is the inherent complexity and difficulty of most situations. From a health care perspective, abused elders would be described as the intensive care patients of the community. Like intensive care patients in hospitals, abused elders demand the highest level of skill from a variety of professionals. In cases of elder abuse, however, the team members are not specialized health care professionals, but rather are community-based workers and people who provide informal support.

A second unique aspect of interventions for elder abuse is the fact that many abused elders have some impairment in their ability to make decisions. In some cases of abuse, the decision-making abilities of the caregivers also may be impaired; the caregiver may not be a competent decision maker or may not be acting in the best interest of the dependent elder. Most cases of elder abuse present a decision-making challenge to both professional and family caregivers. Nurses and other health care professionals generally are not prepared to deal with the underlying legal and ethical issues, or to assume the role of advocate for older adults. Even when they are prepared, most are uncomfortable either making or participating in decisions for other adults.

Interventions for elder abuse are implemented in community settings, over a long period of time, by a team of formal and informal care providers. Nurses working in home and community settings have the most direct opportunities for both the prevention of and interventions for elder abuse. A study of the most effective intervention strategies for abused older adults concluded that "the most accepted and successful strategies for the abused older adults are general nursing and medical strategies offered by health professions of the home care team" (Nahmiash & Reis, 2000, pp. 66–67). Nurses in institutional settings, however, have many opportunities for detecting elder abuse, working with caregivers, and facilitating referrals to appropriate community agencies. Because the role of the nurse in institutional settings is quite different from that of the nurse in community settings, each of these areas is discussed separately below.

Role of the Nurse in Institutional Settings

Nurses in acute and long-term care settings can intervene in cases of elder abuse through their work with caregivers and their participation in discharge planning. When elder abuse is rooted in the caregiver's lack of information about adequate caregiving measures, the nurse can teach the caregiver about the person's care before discharge. In addition, when nurses are concerned about a caregiver's abilities, they can initiate a referral to a home care or public nursing

agency for follow-up. In some cases, the nurse may ascertain that a situation requires skilled nursing care, which is usually covered by health insurance for at least a few visits. If the nurse has serious questions about a discharge plan that seems inadequate, a referral to a protective services agency may be made so that the situation can be monitored on a long-term basis.

Caregivers of dependent older adults who have been placed temporarily in institutional settings often seek advice from nurses about care management. They may be ambivalent about taking the person home or may be unsure or unrealistic about their own ability to provide appropriate care or to cope with the stress of the situation. In some cases, caregivers may indirectly be seeking permission not to provide care at home. In these situations, nurses often are in the best position to facilitate communication among all the decision makers, including the primary care provider, the older adult, and the various family members who are responsible for care. When nurses identify caregiver concerns, they can suggest individual counseling or support groups. One of the most effective ways to prevent elder abuse is to provide support and education for caregivers, and the best opportunities for this may arise when the dependent older adult is in a hospital or nursing home. Nurses can encourage caregivers to use a period of institutionalization to reevaluate their own abilities to provide care at home as well as their own need to accept additional support and assistance.

Role of the Nurse in Community Settings

Although home health aides are the health care workers most likely to observe clues to elder abuse in home settings, they often are ill prepared to detect or address elder abuse. Nurses in home care agencies, therefore, have a tremendous responsibility to work closely with home health aides, in both recognizing and intervening in situations of elder abuse. Home care nurses must educate home health aides about the detection of elder abuse and should be available if home health aides have questions or concerns about what they observe. If the home situation cannot be discussed openly during supervisory visits, the nurse may have to arrange a time for private discussion with the home health aide. In situations in which the older adult requires a significant degree of physical care or supervision, the services of a home health aide may be the most effective means of preventing elder abuse. Often, however, the retention of a home health aide in such difficult situations depends largely on the degree of support and guidance provided by a professional nurse.

When home health aides or home care nurses detect evidence of abuse, they must decide whether or not a referral to a protective services agency is warranted. Decisions about reporting actual or suspected abuse may present an ethical dilemma for the nurse, as discussed later in this chapter. If an abuse situation is rooted in caregiver stress, the caregiver may voluntarily agree to accept help if the nurse suggests counseling resources.

Nurses in home settings also have many opportunities for teaching caregivers about adequate care through verbal and written instruction. In addition to teaching caregivers directly about the provision of physical care and the management of difficult behaviors, nurses and home health aides also can serve as role models. Some caregivers may have great difficulty managing complex medication regimens; in such cases, the nurse can simplify these regimens through the use of charts and specially designed medication organizers. Nurses also can educate caregivers about basic care needs, such as nutrition, exercise, and elimination. For example, nurses may suggest innovative ways of meeting the nutritional requirements of an elderly person who does not eat adequately. Home care nurses have the advantage of observing many creative and effective techniques used by caregivers that have never been described in any nursing texts. Thus, experienced home care nurses are continually expanding their repertoire of techniques for physical care and behavioral management, and these techniques can then be passed on to other family caregivers.

Nurses in other community settings, such as clinics or senior centers, also have opportunities to intervene in elder abuse. In these settings, nurses often come in contact with spouses who have assumed a caregiving role and need advice about resources to assist with the care of the dependent spouse. Nurses also will encounter older people who neglect themselves and need support services at home. Older adults and their caregivers may not be aware of the many community-based services that are available, and the nurse may be the only person with whom they have any contact. Community-based resources, such as group meal programs, home-delivered meals, or adult day care centers, may be an effective way of preventing or alleviating some situations of elder abuse or neglect. Nurses can facilitate referrals for whatever services are appropriate. If nurses are not familiar with specific community services, they can educate the older adult or caregiver about the general kinds of services available and their advantages. Every geographic area of the United States has an area agency on aging, and nurses can suggest that older adults and caregivers use this agency as a source of information about specific

programs. Information about local agencies on aging also is available by contacting the Eldercare Locator at (800) 677-1116 or http://www.eldercare.gov.

Role of the Nurse in Multidisciplinary Teams

Because elder abuse situations usually are very complex, nursing interventions are implemented in conjunction with other nonnursing interventions, using a multidisciplinary team approach. When nurses assume the role of case manager, they may have to be quite creative in finding other team members with whom to work. In community settings, the nurse is usually the health care person who can identify the need for health services and facilitate appropriate referrals. In working with homebound people, nurses may need to identify essential resources for an initial medical evaluation or for ongoing monitoring. In many areas of the country, primary care providers are resuming the old-fashioned practice of making home visits. Nurses can determine whether such a home visit is warranted and then find an appropriate primary care provider to provide this service. In addition, with the growing demand for home health services, an increased number of diagnostic tests can be performed in the home (e.g., radiographs, blood tests, and electrocardiograms). In many situations, these diagnostic tests are essential for determining whether involuntary care measures are justified. For instance, if the older adult refuses to go out of the home for care, home-based diagnostic measures may provide the evidence needed to convince the person or the primary care provider that hospitalization is warranted. On the other hand, results of these diagnostic tests also may be used to convince caregivers, protective services workers, and involved professionals that hospitalization is unnecessary.

Nurses can also facilitate referrals for services that decrease the burden of caregiving responsibilities and improve an older adult's self-esteem and level of independence. For instance, speech, physical, and occupational therapy may be useful in improving the older person's ability to communicate, ambulate, and perform ADLs. Referrals for skilled nursing and other skilled care services usually are made at the time of discharge from an institution, but if the person has not received institutional care, these services may not have been suggested. The nurse making a home visit may be the first health professional to suggest these resources. Sometimes, when referrals are suggested as part of a discharge plan following a stay at a health care facility, either the older adult or the family may be reluctant to pursue those services at that time. Although an older adult or his or her family may have refused such services, he or she may be more receptive at another time to accepting help. If a person's condition has recently changed, the nurse may be able to obtain an order from the primary care provider for certain services that are covered under Medicare or managed care. Nurses in home care agencies who provide skilled care usually are happy to discuss health care services with anyone who calls for information, and these nurses can offer advice about the possibility of having services covered by health insurance. For example, a change in medications might qualify a person for skilled nursing care, and a fall might qualify a person for skilled physical therapy.

Nurses also can suggest medical equipment and assistive devices that would improve the person's function and relieve some of the caregiver's responsibilities. Some durable medical equipment is covered by health insurance, and medical supply companies usually are quite helpful in advising people about specific equipment. Caregivers may be unaware of disposable supplies and the many assistive devices that are available, and they may be responsive to suggestions from the nurse about obtaining and using these items. Any interventions that improve unsafe situations may prevent or alleviate elder abuse or neglect.

Finally, nurses sometimes assume responsibility for facilitating referrals to services aimed at reducing caregiver stress or dealing with caregiver problems. For example, participation in Alcoholics Anonymous may be an effective intervention in situations in which abuse is related to the caregiver's alcoholism. Mental health counseling or support groups may be helpful when abuse is related to caregiver stress. Respite services can be provided through in-home care, by companions or home health aides, or through the participation of the dependent older person in an adult day care program. Sometimes, even a limited amount of respite will be sufficient to prevent or alleviate elder abuse in situations in which the caregiver is stressed and overburdened.

Prevention and Treatment Interventions

The range of interventions that may be needed by abused elders and their caregivers or abusers is great. These interventions can be categorized according to basic function: (1) core, or essential, integrative services; (2) emergency services, which are appropriate during crises or just before or after abuse or neglect occurs; (3) support services, or services used for managing the problem and improving the situation; (4) rehabilitative services, or services that help to diminish the likelihood of abuse or neglect by addressing the problems of either the victim or the perpetrator; and (5) preventive services, which include programs directed toward changing society in ways that diminish the likelihood of maltreatment or self-neglect.

Figure 26-2 identifies some of the specific types of services, arranged by function, that may be needed in elder abuse situations. Probably no community has either a full array of needed services or enough of any particular service to deal adequately with the scope of the problem locally. In recent years, however, communities throughout the country have made notable progress in understanding and addressing elder abuse and neglect. Nurses have been identified as having primary responsibility for implementing the most successful prevention and treatment interventions directed toward both the caregivers and abused or neglected older persons. Not only are they highly qualified as health professionals to address the complex issues involved with elder abuse, but they also are recognized as among the most accepted professionals by older adults (Nahmiash & Reis, 2000).

➤ Mr. and Mrs. G. have been married for more than 50 years and have six children, four of whom live in their area. Because of Mrs. G.'s memory loss in recent years, Mr. G. has allowed home care workers into the house to help her with eating and to perform personal care. The workers report that Mr. G. yells at his wife when she forgets things. On more than one occasion, they witnessed him attempting to force feed her when she failed to eat an entire meal. After the couple has gone to their bedroom in the evening, the night workers have reported hearing screams, crying, and slapping sounds coming from behind the closed bedroom door. In the morning, Mrs. G. had bruises on her body and bumps on her head. When asked, Mr. G. denied hitting his wife. Mrs. G. cried when questioned, never providing an explanation for her injuries.

Mr. G. is reluctant to consider additional services, like adult day care, fearing that the couple's savings will evaporate. He had Mrs. G. change doctors several times in recent years because "they don't do anything to really help her." The children who live nearby have said that they do not want to get involved in their parents' situation. They describe years of their father physically and verbally abusing their mother and fear what might happen if any action is taken now.

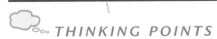 **THINKING POINTS**

➤ What interventions might be helpful in addressing the elder abuse evident in this situation?

➤ What is the role of the home care nurse in introducing and implementing these interventions?

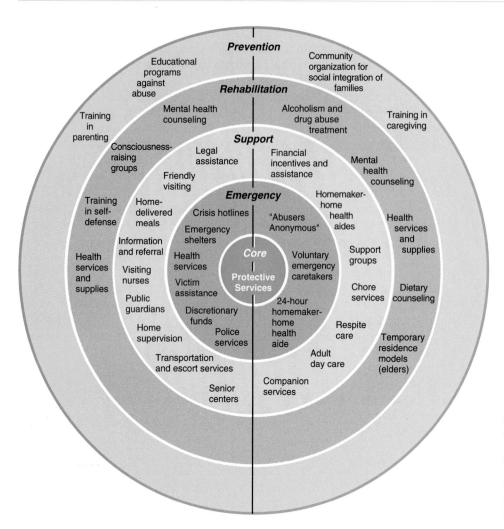

FIGURE 26-2 Types of services needed by abused older adults and their caregivers. (From Anetzberger, G. J. [1982]. *Report of the Elder Abuse Project: Recommendations for addressing the problem of elder abuse in Cuyahoga County.* Cleveland, OH: Federation for Community Planning. Used with permission.)

➤ What barriers might be encountered in acceptance of the interventions?

➤ As the home care nurse in this situation, how will you help to overcome these barriers?

LEGAL INTERVENTIONS

Adult Protective Services Law

Philosophically, adult protective services law provides protection for the person who is abused, for the person offering assistance, and for society from possible dangers posed by the person. Elder abuse reporting and adult protective services laws differ among the 50 states in terms of their provisions. In part, this reflects a lack of federal guidance or incentive in this area. Partly, too, it suggests the diversity of percep-

tions and arrangements for dealing with the complex problem of elder abuse that exists throughout the country.

Interest in state adult protective services law began in the mid-1960s and peaked during the early 1980s. Four major reasons account for this recent interest. First, growth in the elderly population has resulted in increased concern about all matters related to this population. As the proportion of those aged 65 years and older expanded (from 8.1% of the population in 1950 to 12.4% in 2000), so did public policies related to the needs of older people. In this regard, protective services law simply represents one policy promoting the welfare of older adults. In addition, it reflects increased public awareness that older people can be disproportionately impaired and disadvantaged and, therefore, disproportionately dependent on caregivers, who may or may not have the best interest of their charges at heart. Public outrage over nursing home abuse, in particular, has led to protective measures, like protective services law, encouraging safety and improved care for older people in dependent situations.

Second, as discussed earlier, adult protective services law grew out of an increased public awareness of the problem of elder abuse. With this increased awareness came the demand for state laws to address this area of family violence. Today, every state has some kind of adult protective services or elder abuse reporting law, and all were enacted or amended in the 1980s, except for three that were enacted between 1973 and 1977.

The third factor promoting interest in adult protective services law has been the belief that other laws are inadequate for protecting older people. Guardianship law often is regarded as restrictive and antiquated. Because the intent of the criminal code is to punish offenders rather than to assist victims, it fails to correct the conditions leading to or resulting from elder abuse. In addition, the criminal code typically does not address neglect and the many forms of exploitation experienced by older people. Finally, under many domestic violence laws, a battered person must seek relief by charging the perpetrator, who may be a relative, with abusive behavior. Usually, an older person is unwilling to do this, and so remains at risk. None of these protective laws, therefore, adequately meet the safety needs of older people.

The fourth reason for interest in adult protective services law concerns the passage of protective laws for other populations subject to maltreatment. Protective services laws for older adults have been enacted on the coattails of similar laws for abused children and spouses and have been modeled after the child abuse laws. In part, this is justified. If adults are impaired, then they are often in dependent situations, much as are small children. Even the most severely impaired adults, however, are not just children who have grown up or become dependent. They are categorically different under the law by virtue of the rights and responsibilities inherent in adult status. Therefore, statutes that do not recognize this fact—and some adult protective services laws do not—reflect a bias against older people and a stereotyping of people who are disabled.

Purpose and Structure

Laws protecting maltreated and self-neglected older people usually have four purposes: (1) to promote the identification and referral of abuse or neglect; (2) to convey public and centralized authority for addressing protective matters; (3) to establish a system of protective services to prevent, correct, or discontinue

abuse or neglect that is discovered; and (4) to permit, under certain circumstances, involuntary access to the suspected victim of abuse for the purpose of investigation and service delivery. Usually, local departments of welfare or social services receive reports of abuse, although in some states, departments of aging or prosecutors' offices receive them.

Reports generally are accepted for neglect, exploitation, and physical, sexual, and psychological abuse; in several states, they also are accepted for abandonment and cruel punishment. In most states, reporting suspected abuse is mandatory for health, social service, and safety professionals and paraprofessionals. People in these categories can be penalized for failure to report; the typical penalty is a charge of a misdemeanor, with or without financial penalty. In some states, however, imprisonment, civil liability for damages, or notification of the state licensing board may be the consequence of failure to report. Most state laws also protect the confidentiality of reports and the identity of all people involved in making them.

Response to a report on the part of the public authority responsible for implementation usually is prompt; sometimes, the law mandates a response within 24 to 72 hours of receipt of a report. In this context, response means investigation of the situation, which generally includes a home visit with the alleged victim and consultation with people knowledgeable about the situation. Service intervention for endangered older people often can include health care, support services, protective placement, emergency services, or financial management. Under most state laws, intervention must be accepted voluntarily by mentally capable older adults. Less than 10% of adult protective services clients receive interventions without their consent (Duke, 1997). Likewise, most laws emphasize the principles of self-determination, use of the least restrictive interventions, and due process in their implementation.

The intent of adult protective services law is to protect the vulnerable aged. That this intent has not always or everywhere been realized is a result of factors that limit the effective and appropriate implementation of these laws, such as the following:

- Only a handful of states have enacted elder abuse reporting or adult protective services law with any accompanying appropriations. Therefore, most public authorities have had to implement the laws using already-diminished state and federal dollars.
- Alleged perpetrators and people failing to report elder abuse or neglect rarely are prosecuted and,

given the vague wording of many statutes, may not be prosecutable (Tatara, 1995).

- The public authority is seldom accountable to anyone, including the court, with the result that it can and sometimes does assume unreasonable control over elderly clients.

Responsibilities of Nurses

Despite its limitations, adult protective services law reduces the endangerment of, and secures the help required by, thousands of abused and neglected older adults every year (Lachs et al., 1996). Although the primary role in law implementation is assumed by the protective services worker, nurses play an essential secondary role. This role includes five dimensions: reporting, assessment, consultation, court testimony, and acute and ongoing care. Only reporting, however, tends to be explicitly stated in law.

Reporting. As health care professionals, nurses are the category of mandatory reporters most frequently identified in adult abuse and protective services laws. Personnel in long-term care facilities and mental health professionals are the second and third most commonly cited in state law as mandatory reporters (Roby & Sullivan, 2000). This is appropriate because the various duties ordinarily assumed by nurses place them in a critical position for witnessing the consequences of abuse and neglect. In addition, a primary role of nurses is to foster collaboration between health care professionals as abuse reporters and adult protective services or law enforcement officials as abuse investigators or service providers.

Mandatory reporting laws do not require reporters to know whether abuse or neglect has occurred, but merely to report it if they suspect its occurrence. The responsibility for problem verification rests with the public agency charged with law implementation, not with the reporter or referral source. Suspecting elder abuse means detecting signs of violence, such as bruises, welts, or fractures. It also means recognizing conditions resulting from the deprivation of proper shelter, food, or medical care, such as frostbite, malnutrition, oversedation, or mental changes.

Most mandatory reporting laws provide immunity for people reporting elder abuse or neglect. On this basis, nurses can report suspected cases of maltreatment or self-neglect without fear of civil or criminal liability, so long as the report is made in good faith and without malicious purpose. A few laws specifically offer immunity in the workplace. Accordingly, nurses cannot be fired, transferred, or demoted for making a report.

The locus of responsibility for making the report, in all states, rests with the individual nurse. Even if the nurse is part of a large agency or hospital, he or she cannot delegate that responsibility to someone else, be it a supervisor or an attending physician. The nurse alone has the responsibility for reporting, and for the consequences—both legal and moral—of failing to do so.

This does not mean that it may not be advantageous to establish a protocol concerning such reporting. Many agencies and hospitals have done this. Protocols and detection teams do not erode individual responsibility in this matter, however. They simply clarify roles and enhance the credibility of the report. Excellent examples of elder abuse detection protocols are available, and they should be considered for use by nurses in all health care settings involving multiple professions and levels of authority. Display 26-2 illustrates a typical protocol for hospital- or agency-based nurses.

Assessment. Protective services workers often call on nurses to assess older people suffering from abuse or neglect. Sometimes, this request comes during an emergency, when the client's life is believed to be endangered. More commonly, however, nurses are asked to make routine assessments of new protective clients, or of existing clients who are exhibiting changes in health status. Nurses often are the preferred health care worker for conducting such assessments owing to their holistic approach to health assessment, their availability through public health departments or visiting nurse associations, their willingness to make home visits, and the relative ease with which older people usually accept nurses.

Because assessment was discussed earlier in this chapter, only one aspect requires further examination here. Established assessment instruments are often developed and used in institutional settings and home care agencies. Such an instrument can be used to:

- Summarize observations
- Facilitate the collection of vital information
- Organize the information in one document
- Ensure that important information is collected
- Provide a basis for referral or action
- Offer documentation for possible court action

Assessment instruments for various aspects of elder abuse and neglect are widely available (Cowen, 2001). Whatever instrument is adopted for this purpose, however, it should be able to assess and document the following:

- Background data (e.g., client's name and address)
- Signs of maltreatment or self-neglect according to type (e.g., bruises or welts in cases of suspected physical abuse)

DISPLAY 26-2
Sample Protocol for Nurses with Regard to Elder Abuse

Perform an Initial Assessment

- Gather data on the client's clinical presentation; observe the client and interview the client, caregivers, or both.
- Analyze data that raise a suspicion of abuse, neglect, or exploitation; consider objective findings and whether these fit the explanations; consider client–caregiver interactions.

If There Is Reason for Suspicion, Use an Assessment Guide

If There Is Continued Suspicion, Consult the Abuse Detection Team

- Report pertinent findings to the primary nurse.
- Summarize findings from the assessment guide on progress notes.
- Discuss the information with the assigned primary care provider and social worker as soon as possible.
- Determine the need to report abuse or neglect to authorities charged with investigation under law.

- Document additional facts, and whether a report was made, in the progress notes.

Meet with the Client and Caregivers to Inform Them of the Intent to Report

- Include representatives from at least two health care, social service, or other professional disciplines in the meeting.
- Document the interaction and the results of the meeting in the progress notes.

Follow-up Actions

- Provide a report to the appropriate abuse detection team member for handling and distribution.
- Identify any security measures that must be taken to protect the client.
- Implement appropriate interventions.

Source: Cleveland Metropolitan General/Highland View Hospital. (1987). *Statement of policy and procedure: Abuse/neglect cases, reporting of suspected elder abuse* (unpublished manuscript).

- Severity of signs (e.g., an immediate life threat)
- Indicators of maltreatment intentionality (e.g., a caregiver who will not allow the nurse to be alone with the client)
- Symptoms of acute or chronic illness or impairment (e.g., incontinence)
- Functional incapacity (e.g., an inability to dress or toilet without assistance)
- Aggravating social conditions (e.g., a client who lives alone and is socially isolated)
- Source of information (e.g., agency referral)
- Recommended action (e.g., referral of the case to home health care service providers)

Consultation. Nurses serve as an important resource for protective services workers when questions arise regarding the health status of clients. In such situations, telephone contact between the nurse and protective services worker usually provides the necessary information. Typical questions relate to medications, continence, nutrition and hydration, and disease signs. Consultation ordinarily is an informal arrangement, based on established networks among service providers in a given community. Sometimes, however, consultation is formally organized through clinical consultation teams associated with protective services coalitions. Nurses also are used by protective services agencies to train workers in health assessment, disease identification and detection,

recognition of endangerment, and other topics. Training usually is accomplished through in-service programs, although it is occasionally presented within the context of workshops or conferences.

Court Testimony. Nationally, very few cases involve involuntary intervention through adult protective services law. In those that do, court assistance usually is sought to gain access, either to conduct an investigation or to deliver services. Sometimes, a caregiver or other person may refuse to allow intervention on behalf of the abused or neglected elder. When legal intervention is indicated, the older person usually is mentally impaired and unable to make decisions that would alleviate or eliminate the endangerment. Legal intervention may also be required on the basis of life-threatening circumstances. Cases requiring legal intervention involve the presentation of evidence to a judge or referee to document that the older person is abused or neglected, that he or she requires protective services, and that no other means of receiving protective services exist, except through court action. Much of this evidence is provided through records kept by protective services workers. Additional evidence is secured through mental or physical health evaluation by psychologists or physicians. Occasionally, however, the nurse who assessed the situation or offered care might be called on to offer testimony and submit records.

Testimony provides two types of evidence: direct observation and opinion. Direct observation is an eyewitness account of the health status or function of the older person. Expert opinion represents conclusions drawn from specific observations related to the situation and based on the training and experience of the expert witness. To be effective, opinion must never be overstated or relate to areas outside the nurse's scope of practice or expertise. Medical records are useful as evidence because they are maintained in the regular course of client care by people who understand the facts being documented. Characteristics of good documentation include timeliness, legibility, thoroughness, and objectivity. In addition, corrections to medical records must be obvious and clear, removing any doubt about the destruction of relevant evidence.

Acute and Ongoing Care. As discussed earlier in the section on Nursing Interventions to Address Elder Abuse, nurses provide essential care and treatment for abused and neglected older people. They help correct conditions caused by maltreatment and self-neglect, and they prevent their recurrence through such activities as treating injuries, monitoring medications, educating caregivers, obtaining assistive devices, and facilitating service referrals. In this role, as in others, nurses work cooperatively with other professionals and with paraprofessionals, applying their training and experience in an attempt to help the victims of elder abuse.

Ethical Issues

Ethical issues in adult protective services are similar to ethical issues in medicine and other fields. Rather than having clear answers and absolute rights and wrongs, there are usually differing perspectives and different implications, depending on what course of action is taken. Law, community pressures, and personal concepts of professionalism lead to the erroneous assumption that a problem, such as maltreatment or self-neglect, can easily or simply be resolved. However, protective situations involving older people are rarely easily resolved.

One aspect of the dilemma surrounding ethical issues in adult protective services is the fact that all adults in American society have rights—including freedom from intrusion, the right to fair treatment, freedom from unnecessary restraint, and the right to self-determination—but these rights can be taken away through the use of legal measures. Professionals often are reluctant to initiate legal measures that take away the rights of other adults. For example, unless an older adult has been judged to be incompetent by a court of law, he or she has the right to be protected from intrusion, even by well-intentioned professionals. In adult protective services situations, this right is threatened, and services can be imposed on an older person who does not willingly agree to assistance.

Another aspect of the dilemma involves the characteristics of protective situations that sometimes make respecting personal rights so difficult. The following characteristics of protective situations sometimes make respecting personal rights difficult:

- In situations that are urgent or dangerous, it is hard to walk away, even when the older person asks to be left alone.
- Public pressure to do something, no matter what, places pressure on care providers who are trying to resolve the situation while respecting the rights of the older person.
- Contradictory societal values may pit individual rights against other values, such as paternalism and protectionism.
- The goals of nurses are directed toward helping others. This presents difficulties for nurses when others do not accept their help, especially when the lack of help has detrimental consequences.
- Serious decisions often have to be made without an adequate base of information. Older adults may be too impaired to provide accurate information, the situation may not allow time for a good assessment, or pertinent information may be withheld by the older person or the caregivers.
- The questionable mental status of many abused or neglected elders places decision-making responsibility in the hands of other people. One option in these situations is to seek guardianship or another form of surrogate decision making. Although this option may deprive the person of certain rights unnecessarily, not pursuing it might mean that basic human needs are not being met adequately, or at all.
- The intrusive nature of legal interventions, including protective services law, robs older adults of fundamental rights. Mandatory reporting provisions, for example, by their very nature, invade privacy. Likewise, the sharing of information among agencies involved in case planning infringes on confidentiality.

Ethical dilemmas about particular situations sometimes can be resolved by applying practice guidelines (Anetzberger et al., 1997) or a hierarchy of principles, such as the one in Display 26-3 (Anetzberger, 1999). The principles of adult protective services, which were developed from long-term experience

---

DISPLAY 26-3
Principles of Adult Protective Services

I. **Freedom over Safety.** The client has a right to choose to live at risk of harm, providing she or he is capable of making that choice, harms no one, and commits no crime.

II. **Self-Determination.** The client has a right to personal choices and decisions until such time that she or he delegates, or the court grants, the responsibility to someone else.

III. **Participation in Decision Making.** The client has a right to receive information to make informed decisions and to participate in all decision making affecting her or his circumstances to the extent that she or he is able.

IV. **Least Restrictive Alternative.** The client has a right to service alternatives that maximize choice and minimize lifestyle disruption.

V. **Primacy of the Adult.** The worker has a responsibility to serve the client, not the community people concerned about appearances, the landlord concerned about crime, or the family concerned about finances.

VI. **Confidentiality.** The client has a right to privacy and secrecy.

VII. **Benefit of Doubt.** If there is evidence that the client is making a reasoned choice, the worker has a responsibility to see that the benefit of doubt is in her or his favor.

VIII. **Do No Harm.** The worker has a responsibility to take no action that places the client at greater risk of harm.

IX. **Avoidance of Blame.** The worker has a responsibility to understand the origins of any maltreatment and to commit no action that would antagonize the perpetrator and so reduce the chances of terminating the maltreatment.

X. **Maintenance of the Family.** The worker has a responsibility to deal with the maltreatment as a family problem, if the perpetrator is a family member, and to try to find the necessary family services to resolve the problem.

Anetzberger, G. J. (1999). Ethical issues in personal safety. In T. F. Johnson (Ed.), *Handbook on ethical issues in aging* (pp. 187–219). Westport, CT: Greenwood Press.

---

with abused elders, are arranged from the most to the least important considerations with regard to interventions for abused or neglected elders.

Adult protective services are fraught with ethical dilemmas. Some of these dilemmas are related to the five basic roles—reporter, investigator, service provider, administrator, and planner—assumed by professionals. Each role has a particular sphere of responsibility in addressing elder abuse and neglect. The reporter detects the situation and describes it to someone authorized by law to deal with it. The investigator is the legal agent who assesses the situation and determines the need for protective services. The service provider offers interventions for correcting or discontinuing maltreatment or self-neglect. The administrator manages a protective services program. Finally, the planner develops policies and programs, as well as community education initiatives, aimed at preventing or treating the problem.

Professional workers in each of these roles face different ethical issues. Issues of the reporter role include questions about whether to make a report and the consequences of doing so. The role of the investigator involves confronting questions about privacy, openness, and confidentiality. The service provider deals with issues about the rights of the elder, the rights of the caregivers, and the degree of risk for the elder. Program planners and administrators face dilemmas about service priorities and the lack of

funds, staff, and other critical resources. Nurses most often deal with ethical issues in their roles as reporters, investigators, and service providers. Table 26-2 identifies some of the ethical problems, as well as related solutions, that nurses may encounter in their roles in adult protective services.

Additional Legal Interventions

Adult protective services law cannot address every situation of elder endangerment or abuse. In particular, it has limited application when considerable property needs protection, the maltreatment is significant and repeated, the older person's mental impairment is substantial and permanent, or the goal is to prevent maltreatment rather than to treat it. Under these conditions, other legal interventions should be considered in conjunction with, or as alternatives to, adult protective services (discussed in Chapter 6).

Determining the Need for Legal Intervention

Older people who are mentally impaired may require legal intervention. This is especially true when the impairment substantially reduces insight, judgment, memory, or cognition, all of which are essential for living in a complex and ordered society. Without these abilities, the following functional consequences may occur: bills may go unpaid, personal

TABLE 26-2 • Ethical Questions and Suggested Solutions Regarding Abused Elders

Ethical Question/Implications	Suggested Solution
When do I report elder abuse? (If I report too soon, I may needlessly invade someone's privacy. If I wait, the situation may worsen.)	Report elder abuse when you believe that, without intervention, the situation will deteriorate or endanger the elder.
What if my report places the elder in more danger, or labels someone inaccurately? What if it causes the elder to shy away from me and my agency?	Report elder abuse if you believe that the protective services system can reduce the risk better than the current interventions.
How do I decide if the elder or the caregiver receives priority? (If my priority is the elder, I may alienate his or her family members, who serve as the primary sources of care. If my priority is the family, then the care plan may be contrary to the elder's wishes and may not adequately respect his or her rights.)	With certain exceptions, the elder should receive priority. These exceptions are limited to circumstances in which the elder has been judged to be incompetent by a court of law or is endangering others by his or her behavior.
Is it more important to maintain standards of confidentiality than to comply with a reporting law?	State law takes precedence over professional standards.
Does the right of an elder to refuse services extend to total self-neglect and intentional suicide? How can I know that endangered elders clearly understand the consequences of their self-neglect? How can I accept abandoning the situation?	Ethical dilemmas such as these often can be resolved through the use of a hierarchy of values or principles, such as those summarized in Display 26-3.
Can emergency services be thrust upon an elder who would have refused them under ordinary circumstances? If the elder's life is endangered, then is it not my primary responsibility to use my nursing skills in life-saving ways, no matter what the elder chooses? Even if the elder might have refused services in the past, does that mean he or she absolutely would refuse them now?	If the elder is incapable of deciding whether to accept or reject emergency services, then these services should be provided, subject to the constraints of the protective services law. This offers the elder essential protection, but recognizes his or her right to refuse ongoing services when the emergency has subsided and he or she is capable of making decisions on his or her own behalf.

hygiene may be ignored, prescribed medications may be forgotten, the home environment may deteriorate, and unscrupulous people may abscond with property. Although nurses are not the primary people responsible for determining the appropriateness of legal interventions, they often are called on to assist in assessing a person's abilities. This is appropriate because nurses often are in the best position to assess the person's abilities to meet basic human needs.

A complete assessment and home evaluation usually requires the involvement of a multidisciplinary team. These teams have been established as special units in some hospitals. Other teams are components of agencies offering protective or case management services to older people and their families. In either instance, multidisciplinary teams include professionals who offer the perspectives of law, nursing, medicine, psychiatry, social work, and rehabilitation therapy. Additional disciplines are included if the situation requires. When legal interventions are being considered, the multidisciplinary team must conduct a complete assessment, including assessment of the person's ability to function safely in the home environment, the involvement of the family and significant others in meeting basic needs, and the ability of the older person to participate in developing a safe and realistic plan of action.

Whenever feasible, problems should be remedied using services rather than legal intervention. For example, an impairment may improve or a risk may be decreased through the use of resources, such as counseling, telephone reassurance, adult day care, home-delivered meals, caregiver support groups, or homemaker/home health aide services. Alternatively, residence in a protected setting may be necessary. Assisted-living settings and board and care settings offer full accommodations, including meals, as well as a range of services, such as social interaction and transportation, while ensuring the continuance of community living and personal freedom.

Assessment is emphasized here because knowledge of the nature of the older person's impairment, functional limitations, and personal or social resources is essential. Without this knowledge, it becomes impossible to determine appropriate interventions. Generally, legal intervention is indicated when assessment reveals all of the following conditions: (1) decisions must be made about the older person's health, living arrangements, money, or property; (2) the older person is unable to make sound decisions related to these matters because of impaired mental function; (3) there is a risk to the older person's health, safety, money, or property as a result; and (4) the risk would be reduced or eliminated if someone else made decisions on behalf of the older person in these matters.

Considerations in the Choice of Legal Interventions

Three features of legal interventions should be considered in selecting those most appropriate for addressing an older person's needs: voluntary versus involuntary nature of the action; temporary versus long-term intervention; and limited versus extensive loss of personal freedom (Bookin, 1992). Some legal interventions are voluntary and, therefore, require the consent of the older person before they are implemented. Money management, power of attorney, and various types of bank accounts, such as joint or direct deposit, are all interventions of this nature. Other legal interventions, such as guardianship or civil commitment, are either voluntary or involuntary, but they tend to be used on an involuntary basis when others in the community believe that the older person's safety or property is in jeopardy. Because these legal interventions involve a much more extensive loss of personal freedom than voluntary ones, they should be employed with extreme caution. A key consideration in the choice of legal interventions is determining the competency of the person to make decisions. This is discussed at length in Chapter 6.

Some legal interventions are temporary, or can be terminated whenever the older person elects. These characteristics apply to all voluntary measures but do not apply to most involuntary ones. Some measures, like guardianship, may be easier to initiate than to discontinue. Others, like civil commitment, may be accompanied by long-term stigma, even when the intervention is terminated. Finally, domestic violence law or the criminal code may be used to deal with abusers and should be included in the range of legal interventions available to abused older adults.

EVALUATING EFFECTIVENESS OF NURSING INTERVENTIONS

Nursing care of abused or neglected older adults is evaluated by the extent to which nursing goals are achieved. If a nursing goal is to alleviate the contributing factor of unnecessary dependence, the care is evaluated by whether the older adult is functioning at a higher level of independence. If a nursing goal is to address caregiver stress, the nursing care might be evaluated by the caregiver accepting help with the care, attending caregiver support groups, and expressing less stress about their caregiving responsibilities. When the nursing goal is to protect an incompetent older adult from harm, nursing care might be evalu-

ated by the extent to which the least restrictive legal interventions are implemented. In such cases, nursing care is evaluated in terms of protecting the older adult from harm while also protecting his or her rights.

CHAPTER SUMMARY

Elder abuse and neglect is one of the most complex issues involved in the nursing care of older adults because it usually involves multiple aspects of health care as well as legal and ethical considerations regarding the rights of the older person. Conclusions derived from studies indicate that elder abuse causation is extremely complex, with many variables associated with both the victim and the perpetrator. Factors that increase the risk for elder abuse include invisibility and vulnerability of the elder and numerous psychosocial factors affecting both older adults and their caregivers. Types of elder abuse include self-neglect, physical or psychological abuse or neglect by others, exploitation, sexual abuse, violation of rights, and abandonment.

Nursing assessment of elder abuse begins with a suspicion of abuse or neglect and involves the careful detection of clues. Assessment is accomplished best through the coordinated efforts of members of a multidisciplinary team. Nurses assess many aspects of physical and psychosocial function, with emphasis on safe function and identification of threats to life. Nursing diagnoses to address elder abuse and neglect include Disabled Family Coping, Caregiver Role Strain, and Risk for Injury. Nursing outcomes include the alleviation of contributing factors and the protection of vulnerable older adults.

Nurses assume many roles, particularly with regard to adult protective services laws. Responsibilities of nurses include reporting, assessing, consulting, court testimony, caregiver education, and direct nursing care. Nurses need to be familiar with the range of services and the legal interventions that might be used for abused or neglected older adults. Ethical considerations can be addressed by applying principles of adult protective services.

➤ Recall that Mrs. B. is 82 years old and lives in a senior citizens apartment. After 2 months of receiving skilled nursing visits, Mrs. B. was discharged from the home care agency because she was successfully managing her medications and other aspects of functioning adequately. Several months after she was discharged, the nurse in the Wellness Clinic at the senior citizens apartment noted a change in her mannerisms, accompanied by slurred speech and an unbalanced gait. Mrs. B. had bruises on her arms, knees, and forehead, but insisted that she had not fallen. After further investigation, the nurse found that her blood pressure was 210/104 mm Hg and that her blood glucose level was 410 mg/dL on the glucometer that the nurse kept in the clinic. A pill count revealed that Mrs. B. had not taken her medications for 2½ days. After a consultation with her primary care provider, Mrs. B. was admitted to the hospital. Tests revealed that she had suffered a stroke, resulting in left-sided weakness and short-term memory loss.

Mrs. B. left the hospital against medical advice and returned to her apartment, initially refusing visits from the home health nurse. She insisted that her children come and administer her medications and prepare her meals because she was unable to do this for herself. Mrs. B. reasoned that she had cared for her children when they were young, so they should come when she needed them. The children tried to assist Mrs. B. for 4 days but were unable to meet both her demands and those of their jobs and families. Mrs. B. reluctantly agreed to a visit from the home health nurse who had visited her before. She expected that she would see the nurse once and that the nurse would "make my children do right."

Mrs. B.'s children were present for the initial assessment. Mrs. B. was unable to stand or transfer to the commode without help. She could not take her pills correctly, even by using the chart and color-coded boxes. Mrs. B. flatly refused to consider admission to a nursing facility to receive therapy to regain her strength, and she would not consider living with her daughter or either son. The family told the nurse that they were exhausted and on the "verge of a breakdown" and could not continue to provide the care that Mrs. B. needed. The nurse explained to Mrs. B. that it was not safe for her to remain in her apartment without assistance. She suggested that she hire an aide until other arrangements could be made because her children were not obligated to lose their jobs or jeopardize their family relationships to care for her. Mrs. B. accused her children of being greedy and caring only about themselves. She said that children have a duty to care for their parents and that she wasn't going to "have strangers doing the things that decent children should be doing." She directed her concluding remarks at the nurse, stating, "What's more, I don't need you to come back either, because all you want to do is side with my children."

 THINKING POINTS

➤ What strategies would you use to establish a relationship with Mrs. B.?

➤ What additional assessment information would you want to obtain, and how would you obtain it?

➤ What would your next steps be in working with Mrs. B.?

➤ How would you work with the family?

➤ What other resources would you involve in planning and providing care for Mrs. B.?

➤ What criteria would you use for making a referral for adult protective services?

CRITICAL THINKING EXERCISES

1. Identify factors in each of the following categories that contribute to elder abuse and neglect in the United States:
   - Demographic statistics
   - Changes in families
   - Health care systems
   - Health status and other characteristics of older adults
   - Social awareness
2. What is different about the nursing assessment of abused or neglected elders compared with the nursing assessment of other older adults?
3. What do you believe about family caregiving responsibilities? How would you deal with a family whose values about caregiving differed significantly from yours?
4. What are your beliefs about the degree of risk a frail elder should be allowed to take?
5. Under what circumstances should an elder be denied the right to remain in his or her own home?

EDUCATIONAL RESOURCES

Clearinghouse on Abuse and Neglect of the Elderly (CANE)
University of Delaware, Newark, DE 19716
(302) 831-3525
http://www.elderabusecenter.org

National Center on Elder Abuse
1201 15th Street, NW, Suite 350, Washington, DC, 20005-2800
(202) 898-2586
http://www.elderabusecenter.org

National Clearinghouse on Family Violence, Health Canada
Address Locator: 1907D1
Jeanne Mance Building, Tunney's Pasture, Ottawa, ON K1A 1B4
(800) 267-1291
http://www.hc-sc.gc.ca/hppb/familyviolence/

National Committee for the Prevention of Elder Abuse
1101 Vermont Avenue, NW, Suite 1001, Washington, DC 20005
(202) 682-4140
http://www.preventelderabuse.org

National Eldercare Locator
(800) 677-1116
http://www.eldercare.gov

REFERENCES

Anetzberger, G. J. (1987). *The etiology of elder abuse by adult offspring.* Springfield, IL: Charles C Thomas.

Anetzberger, G. J. (1990). Abuse, neglect and self-neglect: Issues of vulnerability. In Z. Hanel, P. Ehrlich, & R. Hubbard (Eds.), *The vulnerable aged: People, services, and policies* (pp.140–148). New York: Springer.

Anetzberger, G. J. (1997). Elderly adult survivors of family violence: Implications for clinical practice. *Violence Against Women, 3*(5), 499–514.

Anetzberger, G. J. (1999). Ethical issues in personal safety. In T. F. Johnson (Ed.), *Handbook on ethical issues in aging* (pp.187–219). Westport, CT: Greenwood Press.

Anetzberger, G. J. (2000). Caregiving: Primary cause of elder abuse? *Generations, 24*(11), 46–51.

Anetzberger, G. J. (2001). Elder abuse identification and referral: The importance of screening tools and referral protocols. *Journal of Elder Abuse & Neglect, 13*(2), 3–22.

Anetzberger, G. J. (In press). Adult protective services. In D. J. Ekerdt (Ed.), *The Macmillan encyclopedia of aging.* New York: Macmillan Reference USA.

Anetzberger, G. J., Dayton, C., & McMonagle, P. (1997). A community dialogue series on ethics and elder abuse: Guidelines for decision-making. *Journal of Elder Abuse & Neglect, 9*(1), 33–50.

Anetzberger, G. J., Korbin, J. E., & Tomito, S. K. (1996). Defining elder mistreatment in four ethnic groups across two generations. *Journal of Cross-Cultural Gerontology, 11,* 187–211.

Bendik, M. (1992). Reaching the breaking point: Dangers of mistreatment in elder caregiving situations. *Journal of Elder Abuse & Neglect, 4*(3), 39–59.

Bookin, D. (Ed.). (1992). *Working with impaired elders in the community: A guide to the decisions-making process and legal interventions.* Cleveland, OH: Federation for Community Planning.

Brandl, B., & Raymond, J. (1997). Unrecognized elder abuse victims: Older abused women. *Journal of Case Management, 6*(2), 62–68.

Brownell, P. (1997). The application of the Culturagram in cross-cultural practice with elder abuse victims. *Journal of Elder Abuse & Neglect, 9*(2), 19–33.

Burston, G. R. (1975). Granny-battering. *British Medical Journal, 3,* 592.

Butler, R. N. (1975). *Why survive? Being old in America.* New York: Harper & Row.

Byers, B., & Lamanna, R. A. (1993). Adult protective services and elder self-endangering. In B. Byers & J. E. Hendricks (Eds.), *Adult protective services: Research and practice* (pp. 61–85). Springfield, IL: Charles C. Thomas.

Carpenito, L. J. (2002). *Nursing diagnosis: Application to clinical practice* (9th ed.). Philadelphia: Lippincott Williams & Wilkins.

Cook-Daniels, L. (1997). Lesbian, gay male, bisexual and transgendered elders: Elder abuse and neglect issues. *Journal of Elder Abuse & Neglect, 9*(2), 35–49.

Cowen, P. S. (2001). Elder mistreatment. In M. L. Maas, K. C. Buckwalter, M. D. Hardy, T. Tripp-Reimer, M. G. Titler, & J. P. Specht (Eds.), *Nursing care of older adults:*

Diagnoses, outcomes, and interventions (pp. 93–120). St. Louis: Mosby.

Duke, J. (1997). A national study of involuntary protective services to adult protective services clients. *Journal of Elder Abuse & Neglect, 9*(1), 51–68.

Dyer, C. B., Pavlik, V. N., Murphy, K. P. & Hyman, D. J. (2000). The high prevalence of depression and dementia in elder abuse or neglect. *Journal of the American Geriatric Society, 48,* 205–208.

Fulmer, T. T., & O'Malley, T. A. (1987). *Inadequate care of the elderly: A health care perspective on abuse and neglect.* New York: Springer.

Griffin, L. W. (1994). Elder maltreatment among rural African-Americans. *Journal of Elder Abuse & Neglect, 6*(1), 1–27.

Hudson, M. F. (1994). Elder abuse: Its meaning to middle-aged and older adults. Part II: Pilot results. *Journal of Elder Abuse & Neglect, 6*(1), 55–82.

Hudson, M. F., Armachain, W. D. Beasley, C. M., & Carlson, J. R. (1998). Elder abuse: Two Native American views. *Gerontologist, 38,* 538–548.

Hudson, M. F., Beasley, C., Benedict, R. H., Carlson, J. R., Craig, B. F., Herman, C., & Mason, S. C. (2000). Elder abuse: Some Caucasian-American views. *Journal of Elder Abuse & Neglect, 12*(1), 89–114.

Kosberg, J. L., & Nahmiash, D. (1996). Characteristics of victims and perpetrators and milieus of abuse and neglect. In A. Baumhover & S. C. Beall (Eds.), *Abuse, neglect, and exploitation of older persons: Strategies for assessment and interventions* (pp. 31–49). Baltimore: Health Professionals Press.

Krassen Maxwell, E., & Maxwell, R. J. (1992). Insults to the body civil: Mistreatment of the elderly in two Plains Indian tribes. *Journal of Cross-Cultural Gerontology, 7,* 3–23.

Lachs, M. S., & Pillemer, K. (1995). Current concepts: Abuse and neglect of elderly persons. *New England Journal of Medicine, 332,* 437–443.

Lachs, M. S., Williams, C., O'Brien, S., Hurst, L., & Horwitz, R. (1996). Older adults: An 11-year longitudinal study of adult protective service use. *Archives of Internal Medicine, 156,* 449–453.

Lau, E., & Kosberg, J. (1979). Abuse of the elderly by informal care providers. *Aging, 299/300,* 10–15.

Longres, J. F. (1994). Self-neglect and social control: A modest test of an issue. *Journal of Gerontological Social Work, 22*(3/4), 3–20.

Longres, J. F. (1995). Self-neglect among the elderly. *Journal of Elder Abuse & Neglect, 7*(1), 69–86.

Luppens, J., & Lau, E. (1983). The mentally and physically impaired elderly relative: Consequences for family care. In J. I. Kosberg (Ed.), *Abuse and maltreatment of the elderly: Causes and interventions* (pp. 204–219). Boston: John Wright-PSG.

Montoya, V. (1997). Understanding and combating elder abuse in Hispanic communities. *Journal of Elder Abuse & Neglect, 9*(2), 5–17.

Moon, A., & Williams, O. (1993). Perceptions of elder abuse and help-seeking patterns among African-American, Caucasian American, and Korean-American elderly women. *Gerontologist, 33,* 386–395.

Nagpaul, K. (1997). Elder abuse among Asian Indians: Traditional versus modern perspectives. *Journal of Elder Abuse & Neglect, 9*(2), 77–92.

Nahmiash, D., & Reis, M. (2000). Most successful intervention strategies for abused older adults. *Journal of Elder Abuse & Neglect, 12*(3/4), 53–70.

National Center on Elder Abuse. (1998, September). *The National elder abuse incidence study: Final report.* Washington, DC: Author.

Nerenberg, L (1996). *Older battered women: Integrating aging and domestic violence services.* Washington, DC: National Center on Elder Abuse.

O'Brien, J. G., Thibault, J. M., Turner, L. C, & Laird-Fick, H. S. (1999). *Self-neglect: Challenges for helping professionals* (pp. 1–19). New York: Haworth Press.

Paveza, G. J., Cohen, D., Eisdorfer, C., Freels, S., Semla, T., Ashford, J. W., et al. (1992). Severe family violence and Alzheimer's disease: Prevalence and risk factors. *Gerontologist, 32,* 493–497.

Phillips, L. (2000). Domestic violence and aging women. *Geriatric Nursing, 21*(4), 188–198.

Phillips, L. R., Torres de Ardon, E., & Briones, G. S. (2000). Abuse of female caregivers by care recipients: Another form of elder abuse. *Journal of Elder Abuse & Neglect, 12*(3/4), 123–143.

Pillemer, K. A., & Suitor, J. J. (1992). Violence and violent feelings: What causes them among family caregivers? *Journal of Gerontology: Social Sciences, 47,* S165–S172.

Podnieks, E. (1999). Support groups: A chance at human connection for abused older adults. In J. Pritchard (Eds.), *Elder abuse work: Best practice in Britain and Canada* (pp. 457–483). London: Jessica Kingsley Publishers.

Quinn, M. J. (1997). *Elder abuse and neglect: Causes, diagnosis, and intervention strategies* (2nd ed.) New York: Springer.

Quinn, M. J. (2002). Undue influence and elder abuse: Recognition and intervention strategies. *Geriatric Nursing, 23,* 11–15.

Quinn, M. J., & Tomita, S. K. (1986). *Elder abuse and neglect: Causes, diagnosis, and intervention strategies.* New York: Springer.

Reis, M., & Nahmiash, D. (1998). Validation of the indicators of abuse (IOA) screen. *Gerontologist, 38,* 471–480.

Roby, J. L., & Sullivan, R. (2000). Adult protective service laws: A comparison of state statutes from definition to case closure. *Journal of Elder Abuse & Neglect 12*(3/4), 17–51.

Stearns, P. J. (1986). Old age family conflict: The perspective of the past. In K. A. Pillemer & R. S. Wolf (Eds.), *Elder abuse: Conflict in the family* (pp. 2–24). Dover, MA: Auburn House.

Tatara, T. (1995). *An analysis of state laws addressing elder abuse, neglect, and exploitation.* Washington, DC: National Center on Elder Abuse.

Tatara, T. (Ed.). (1997a). Elder abuse in minority population. *Journal of Elder Abuse & Neglect, 9*(2).

Tatara, T., (1997b, November). *Attitudes toward elder mistreatment and reporting: A multicultural study.* Paper presented at the Annual Scientific Meeting of the Gerontological Society of America, Cincinnati, OH.

Tatara, T. (Ed.). (1999). *Understanding elder abuse in minority population.* Philadelphia: Brunner/Mazel.

Teaster, P. B., Roberta, K. A., Duke, J. O., & Kim, M. (2000). Sexual abuse of older adults: Preliminary findings of cases in Virginia. *Journal of Elder Abuse & Neglect, 12*(3/4), 1–16.

Wolf, R. S. (1997). Elder abuse and neglect: Causes and consequences. *Journal of Geriatric Psychiatry, 30*(1), 153–174.

Wolf, R. S. (2001). Support groups for older victims of domestic violence. *Journal of Women & Aging, 13*(4), 71–83.

Wolf, R., S., Godkin, M. A., & Pillemer, K. A. (1986). Maltreatment of the elderly: A comparative analysis. *Pride Institute Journal of Long-Term Home Health Care, 5*(4), 10–17.

Review of Physiologic Aspects of Function

This appendix serves as a guide to applying the functional consequences theory to the specific aspects of physiologic function covered in Part 4. The numbers in parentheses refer to the figures, tables, displays, and culture boxes that provide detailed information about age-related changes, risk factors, negative functional consequences, nursing assessment, and nursing interventions. In addition, this outline identifies positive functional consequences for each aspect of functioning.

I. Hearing

Age-Related Changes (Table 12-1)

- External ear: thicker hair, thinner skin, increased keratin
- Middle ear: less resilient tympanic membrane, calcified ossicles, stiffer muscles and ligaments
- Inner ear and auditory nervous system: fewer neurons and hair cells, diminished blood supply, degeneration of spiral ganglion and central processing systems

Risk Factors

- Prolonged exposure to noise (Figure 12-1)
- Genetic predisposition to otosclerosis
- Past or present use of ototoxic medications (Display 12-1)
- Systemic diseases (e.g., diabetes, Paget's disease)
- Auditory diseases (e.g., Meniere's disease)
- Background noise

Negative Functional Consequences (Figure 12-2; Table 12-1)

- Presbycusis (diminished ability to hear high-pitched sounds, especially in the presence of background noise)
- Predisposition to impacted cerumen
- Diminished sensory input, impaired social interaction

Nursing Assessment (Displays 12-2, 12-3, and 12-4)

- Screening tool: The Hearing Handicap Inventory for the Elderly (Figure 12-3)
- Past and present risk factors (e.g., use of ototoxic medications, noise exposure, family history of otosclerosis)
- Attitudes about hearing aids if impairment is present
- Impact of hearing impairment on communication and quality of life
- Behavioral cues to impaired hearing
- Otoscopic examination for impacted cerumen
- Tuning-fork tests for hearing

Nursing Interventions (Displays 12-5, 12-6, and 12-7)

- Teaching older adults about hearing
- Removing and preventing impacted cerumen
- Teaching older adults about the use and care of a hearing aid
- Communicating with hearing-impaired older adults
- Compensating for hearing deficits by using hearing devices and hearing aids (Figure 12-4)

Positive Functional Consequences

- Improved communication
- Improved social interactions
- Safer functional level

II. Vision

Age-Related Changes (Table 13-1)

- Corneal yellowing and opacity; changes in curvature
- Increase in lens size and density
- Decreased pupillary size; atrophy of ciliary muscle
- Fewer photoreceptor cells and a diminished blood supply in the retina

Risk Factors

- Environmental factors (e.g., glare, poor lighting)
- Pathologic conditions (e.g., diabetes, hypertension)
- Adverse medication effects

Negative Functional Consequences (Figure 13-3; Table 13-1)

- Presbyopia (diminished ability to focus on near objects)
- Need for 3 to 5 times more light than previously
- Increased sensitivity to glare
- Slowed response to changes in illumination
- Altered color perception
- Difficulty with night driving
- Increased risk for unsafe mobility
- Increased difficulty in performing activities of daily living (ADLs)

Nursing Assessment (Figures 13-2 and 13-4; Displays 13-1, 13-2, and 13-3)

- Past and present risk factors and diseases that affect vision
- Influence of vision changes on performance of ADLs
- Source of and attitudes about ophthalmologic evaluation
- Attitudes regarding use of low-vision aids
- Vision screening tests

Nursing Interventions (Displays 13-4, 13-5, 13-6, 13-7, 13-8, and 13-9)

- Teaching about prevention of eye disease
- Teaching about comfort measures for dry eyes
- Modifying the environment to improve safety and functioning (e.g., optimal illumination)
- Using low-vision aids for improving visual performance

Positive Functional Consequences

- Improved visual performance
- Increased safety
- Improved independence in performing ADLs
- Improved quality of life

III. Digestion and Nutrition

Age-Related Changes

- Diminished smell and taste sensation
- Less efficient chewing
- Loss of elasticity in intestinal wall
- Slower motility throughout gastrointestinal tract

- Need for fewer calories but same amount of nutrients

Risk Factors

- Inadequate oral care
- Conditions that may lead to nutritional deficiencies (Table 14-1)
- Any pathologic process or functional impairment that interferes with the ability to obtain, prepare, consume, or enjoy food
- Medication effects (Table 14-2)
- Psychosocial factors (e.g., depression)
- Cultural and socioeconomic factors (Culture Box 14-1)
- Environmental factors
- Behaviors based on myths and misunderstandings

Negative Functional Consequences (Figure 14-1)

- Difficulty with preparing meals
- Diminished food enjoyment
- Impaired digestion
- Decreased absorption of nutrients
- Tendency to develop constipation as a result of risk factors

Nursing Assessment (Figure 14-2; Displays 14-1, 14-2, and 14-3)

- Usual nutrient intake and eating pattern
- Risks that interfere with any aspect of eating
- Symptoms of gastrointestinal dysfunction
- Identifying risks that interfere with any aspect of obtaining, preparing, eating, and enjoying food
- Physical examination and laboratory data regarding nutritional status

Nursing Interventions (Figure 14-3; Displays 14-4, 14-5, 14-6, and 14-7)

- Teaching older adults about nutrition and digestion
- Applying the daily food guide to older adults
- Modifying the environment in institutional settings to improve nutrition
- Promoting oral and dental health
- Using referrals to community resources (e.g., home-delivered meals, group meal programs)

Positive Functional Consequences

- Optimal nutrition
- Prevention of constipation
- Improved overall functional level, including mental performance and psychosocial function
- Improved quality of life

IV. Urinary Function

Age-Related Changes

- Kidney: diminished blood flow, decreased number of nephrons, changes in tubules
- Urinary muscles: hypertrophy of bladder muscle, replacement of smooth muscle with connective tissue, relaxation of pelvic floor
- Neurologic control: degenerative changes in cerebral cortex

Risk Factors

- Behaviors based on myths and misunderstandings
- Functional impairments that affect control over socially appropriate urinary elimination
- Pathologic conditions (e.g., vaginitis, benign prostatic hypertrophy, urinary tract infections)
- Medication effects (Table 15-1)
- Dietary and lifestyle factors (e.g., obesity, intake of caffeinated beverages)
- Environmental factors (Display 15-1)

Negative Functional Consequences (Figure 15-1)

- Decreased glomerular filtration rate
- Decreased efficiency of homeostatic mechanisms
- Delayed excretion of water-soluble medications
- Diminished bladder capacity, urinary urgency, and frequency
- Decreased interval between the signal of the need to void and the actual emptying of the bladder
- Chronic residual urine and consequent predisposition to bacteriuria
- Urinary incontinence
- Diminished quality of life due to urinary incontinence

Nursing Assessment (Figure 15-2; Displays 15-2, 15-3, and 15-4)

- Normal voiding patterns
- Risk factors that increase the potential for incontinence
- Risk factors that influence renal function and the maintenance of homeostasis
- Symptoms of impaired urinary elimination
- Misunderstandings about urinary elimination; attitudes about incontinence
- Psychosocial consequences of incontinence
- Signs of impaired urinary elimination

Nursing Interventions (Table 15-2; Displays 15-5, 15-6, 15-7, 15-8, and 15-9)

- Teaching older adults about preventing urinary incontinence
- Pelvic muscle exercises for preventing and managing urinary incontinence
- Environmental modifications
- Teaching about medications
- Devices and procedures for urinary incontinence
- Continence products

Positive Functional Consequences

- Prevention or alleviation of incontinence
- Improved psychosocial function and quality of life

V. Cardiovascular Function

Age-Related Changes

- Arterial stiffening
- Hypertrophy of the left ventricular wall
- Thicker, less elastic, more dilated veins
- Increased peripheral resistance
- Altered baroreflex mechanisms

Risk Factors

- Inactivity, physical deconditioning
- Obesity
- Cigarette smoking
- Pathologic conditions (diabetes, hypertension, hypothyroidism)
- Dietary habits that contribute to hyperlipidemia
- Conditions that predispose the person to postural hypotension (Display 16-1)

Negative Functional Consequences (Figure 16-1)

- Increased blood pressure
- Diminished adaptive response to exercise
- Increased susceptibility to cardiac arrhythmias
- Increased susceptibility to orthostatic and postprandial hypotension
- Decreased cerebral blood flow
- Varicosities, increased susceptibility to venous stasis

Nursing Assessment (Figure 16-2; Table 16-1; Displays 16-2, 16-3, and 16-4)

- Heart rate, rhythm, and sounds
- Blood pressure, including hypertension and hypotension
- Risk for cardiovascular disease

Nursing Interventions (Displays 16-5, 16-6, 16-7, and 16-8)

- Health education about optimal cardiovascular function
- Nutrition and lifestyle interventions (e.g., diet, exercise)

- Teaching about medications for primary and secondary prevention of cardiovascular disease
- Medication, nutrition, and lifestyle interventions for hypertension (Culture Box 16-1)
- Medication, nutrition, and lifestyle interventions for hyperlipidemia
- Prevention and management of orthostatic and postprandial hypotension

Positive Functional Consequences

- Improved cardiovascular performance
- Prevention of cardiovascular disease
- Optimal oxygen perfusion of all body organs and tissues
- Diminished risk for falls due to prevention and management of hypotension
- Improved quality of life

VI. Respiratory Function

Age-Related Changes (Tables 17-1 and 17-2)

- Upper airway changes (e.g., calcification of cartilage)
- Increased anteroposterior chest diameter
- Chest wall stiffness, weakened muscles
- Enlarged alveoli; thinner alveolar walls
- Alterations in lung volumes and airflow (Table 17-1)
- Diminished compensatory response to hypoxia and hypercapnia

Risk Factors

- Tobacco smoking
- Environmental factors (e.g., dry air, pollutants)
- Occupational hazards (Display 17-1)

Negative Functional Consequences (Figure 17-1; Table 17-2)

- Mouth breathing, diminished cough reflex, decreased efficiency of gag reflex
- Increased use of accessory muscles, increase in the energy expended for respiratory function
- Diminished efficiency of gas exchange, decreased arterial PO_2 levels
- Decreased vital capacity, slight decrease in overall efficiency
- Increased susceptibility to lower respiratory infections

Nursing Assessment (Displays 17-2 and 17-3)

- Overall respiratory function
- Detection of lower respiratory infections
- Smoking patterns and attitudes regarding smoking

Nursing Interventions (Displays 17-4 and 17-5)

- Teaching about prevention of pneumonia and influenza
- Health education about cigarette smoking

Positive Functional Consequences

- Prevention of pneumonia and influenza
- Early detection and management of lower respiratory infections

VII. Mobility and Safety

Age-Related Changes

- Diminished muscle mass
- Degenerative changes in joints
- Changes in central nervous system
- Osteoporosis

Risk Factors for Impaired Musculoskeletal Function and Osteoporosis (Display 18-1)

- Inactivity
- Inadequate calcium intake
- Female gender, small bones, increased age, cigarette smoking, long-term use of certain medications

Risk Factors for Falls and Fractures (Display 18-2)

- Age-related changes in gait, sensory function, and central nervous system
- Pathologic conditions and functional impairments
- Medication effects and interactions
- Environmental factors (glare, throw rugs, physical restraints)

Negative Functional Consequences (Figure 18-1)

- Diminished muscle strength, endurance, and coordination
- Increased difficulty in performing ADLs
- Increased susceptibility to falls
- Increased susceptibility to fractures

Nursing Assessment of Overall Musculoskeletal Function (Display 18-3)

- Ability to walk and perform ADLs safely
- Risk factors for osteoporosis (e.g., intake of calcium and vitamin D, history of fractures)

Nursing Assessment of Falls and Fear of Falling

- Fall risk assessment tools (Figure 18-2)
- Safety of the environment (Display 18-4)

Nursing Interventions to Promote Healthy Musculoskeletal Function (Display 18-5)

- Teaching older adults about exercise
- Health promotion teaching about osteoporosis (e.g., early detection and treatment, lifestyle interventions, nutritional interventions, medications)

Multidisciplinary Interventions to Prevent Falls and Fall-Related Injuries (Figures 18-3 and 18-4; Display 18-6)

- Identifying people who are at risk for falls
- Educating staff, patient/resident, and families about preventing falls
- Implementing fall prevention programs (e.g., eliminating risk factors, using monitoring devices)
- Preventing fall-related injuries
- Addressing fear of falling

Positive Functional Consequences

- Prevention of falls
- Prevention of fractures
- Improved quality of life
- Decreased health care expenditures

VIII. Skin

Age-Related Changes (Table 19-1)

- Decreased rate of epidermal proliferation
- Thinner dermis, flattened dermal–epidermal junction
- Diminished moisture content
- Decreased dermal blood supply
- Decreased number of sweat and sebaceous glands
- Decreased number of melanocytes and Langerhans' cells
- Changes in patterns of hair distribution (Figure 19-1)

Risk Factors

- Exposure to ultraviolet rays (sunlight)
- Adverse medication effects
- Personal hygiene practices
- Factors that increase the risk for skin breakdown (Figure 19-2)

Negative Functional Consequences (Figure 19-3; Table 19-1)

- Dry skin, discomfort
- Irregular pigmentation
- Increased susceptibility to injury, mechanical stress, ultraviolet radiation effects
- Delayed wound healing, increased susceptibility to infection

- Decreased tactile sensitivity, increased susceptibility to burns
- Decreased sweating and shivering, increased susceptibility to hypothermia and hyperthermia
- Increased susceptibility to skin cancer
- Increased risk for skin breakdown

Nursing Assessment (Figures 19-4 and 19-5; Tables 19-2 and 19-3; Displays 19-1 and 19-2)

- Identifying abnormal skin conditions
- Personal care practices
- Skin lesions common in older adults
- Risk for development of pressure sores

Nursing Interventions (Display 19-3)

- Health promotion teaching about maintaining healthy skin
- Preventing skin wrinkles
- Preventing dry skin
- Detecting and treating harmful skin lesions
- Preventing and managing pressure ulcers

Positive Functional Consequences

- Improved comfort level
- Prevention of burns and injuries

IX. Sleep and Rest

Age-Related Changes (Figure 20-1; Table 20-1)

- Time in bed and total sleep time
- Sleep efficiency and number of arousals
- Alterations in sleep stages and circadian rhythm
- Decreased time spent in deep sleep and dream stages

Risk Factors

- Psychosocial factors (beliefs and attitudes, anxiety, depression, lack of daytime activity)
- Environmental factors (noise, lack of privacy, conflicting needs)
- Physiologic factors affecting sleep (Table 20-2)
- Lack of daytime activity or stimulation
- Sleep apnea and neuromuscular disorders
- Adverse medication effects (Table 20-3)

Negative Functional Consequences (Figure 20-2)

- Longer time needed to fall asleep
- Aroused more easily
- Diminished quality of sleep
- Same quantity of sleep during 24 hours
- More time spent in bed

Nursing Assessment (Display 20-1)

- Perception of quality and quantity of sleep
- Factors that affect sleep
- Sleep pattern and habits
- Actual sleep pattern (observed in institutional settings)
- Sleep assessment tools (Figure 20-3)

Nursing Interventions (Figure 20-4; Table 20-4; Displays 20-2, 20-3, and 20-4)

- Teaching about interventions to promote healthy sleep patterns
- Modifying the environment
- Individualizing care in institutional settings
- Relaxation and mental imagery techniques to promote sleep
- Teaching about medications that affect sleep

Positive Functional Consequences

- Diminished daytime drowsiness
- Improved quality of life and overall functional level

X. Thermoregulation

Age-Related Changes

- Diminished subcutaneous tissue
- Decreased efficiency of vasoconstriction
- Delayed and diminished shivering
- Decreased peripheral circulation
- Decreased efficiency of sweating
- Diminished ability to acclimatize to heat

Risk Factors (Table 21-1)

- Environmental and socioeconomic influences
- Behaviors based on myths and misunderstandings
- Chemical effects and adverse medication effects
- Physiologic disturbances (e.g., cardiovascular or endocrine disorders)

Negative Functional Consequences (Figure 21-1)

- Diminished ability to respond to hot or cold environments
- Increased susceptibility to hypothermia and heat-related illnesses
- Diminished febrile response to infection
- Altered perception of environmental temperatures
- Psychosocial consequences of altered thermoregulation

Nursing Assessment (Display 21-1)

- Baseline body temperature and normal diurnal fluctuation

- Risk for altered thermoregulation
- Manifestations of hypothermia or hyperthermia
- Altered febrile response to illness

Nursing Interventions (Display 21-2)

- Addressing risk factors
- Maintaining normal body temperature
- Education regarding prevention of hypothermia and heat-related illnesses

Positive Functional Consequences

- Prevention of hypothermia and heat-related illnesses
- Awareness of normal temperature, and improved ability to detect an altered febrile response

XI. Sexual Function

Age-Related Changes

- Changes in reproductive organs in women
- Changes in reproductive organs in men

Risk Factors

- Attitudes and stereotypes of older adults
- Attitudes and stereotypes of caregivers
- Social circumstances (e.g., lack of partner)
- Constraints in long-term care settings (e.g., lack of privacy)
- Adverse effects of medications, alcohol, and nicotine (Display 22-1)
- Functional impairments and pathologic conditions
- Factors that affect the level of sexual activity of older adults

Negative Functional Consequences (Figure 22-1)

- Effects on male and female reproductive abilities
- More prolonged and less intense response to sexual stimulation (Table 22-1)
- Menopause and andropause
- Effects of risk factors on sexual interest and activity

Nursing Assessment (Displays 22-2 and 22-3)

- Assessment of personal attitudes toward sexuality and aging
- Cultural aspects of sexual function (Culture Box 22-1)
- Interview atmosphere and communication techniques
- Interview questions specific for older men and women

- General principles for assessing sexual function in older adults

Nursing Interventions (Displays 22-4, 22-5, 22-6, and 22-7)
- Role of the nurse in providing education about sexual function
- Health education regarding sexual function in older adults
- Health education about issues specific to women's sexual health (hormonal therapy, menopausal symptoms)

- Health education about issues specific to men's sexual health (testosterone therapy, erectile dysfunction) (Table 22-2)
- Addressing sexual needs of nursing home residents

Positive Functional Consequences
- Improved and prolonged enjoyment of sexual activity
- Improved attitudes of staff toward expressions of sexuality by residents in long-term care facilities
- Improved quality of life

Index

The letter f following a page number indicates a figure; the letter t following a page number indicates a table or display.